Thoracic Outlet Syndrome

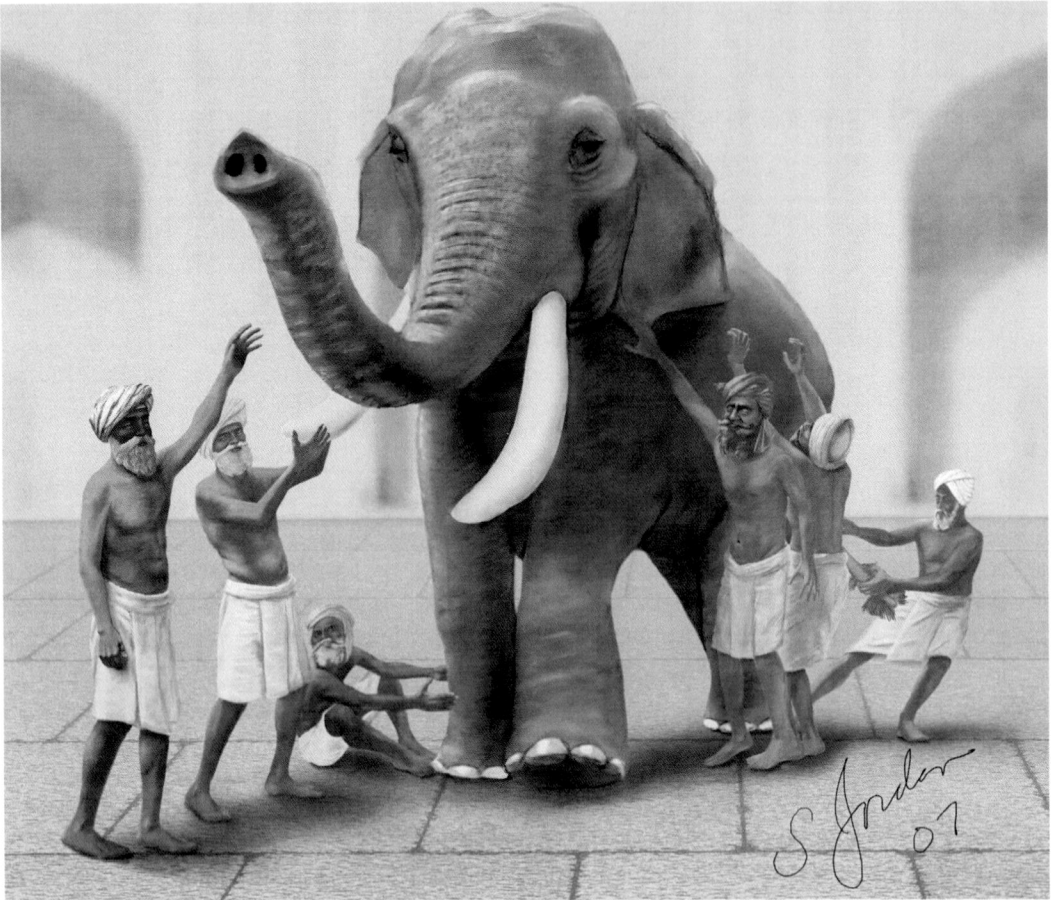

An old Hindi wise man told a story about six blind men meeting up with an elephant. Each blind man could feel only a part of the beast. One man felt a tusk and said that an elephant is similar to a spear. Another man touched a leg and said that an elephant is a big tree. Grabbing the trunk, one blind man claimed that the elephant is a big snake. With each blind man, the true nature of a whole elephant was misjudged because each one could only sense one part. The old Hindi wise man told us that truth is found by considering many different points of view.

In composing this book, we recognize that clinicians may view Thoracic Outlet Syndrome from many different perspectives. From the very beginning of this project, we hoped to incorporate as many of these different perspectives as we can, because it is our conviction that knowledge will arise out of a process of consensus while we try to reconcile the differences. In so doing, we honor the old Hindi wise man and the elephant.

Karl A. Illig • Robert W. Thompson
Julie Ann Freischlag • Dean M. Donahue
Sheldon E. Jordan • Peter I. Edgelow
Editors

Thoracic Outlet Syndrome

🐴 Springer

Editors
Karl A. Illig
Department of Surgery
Division of Vascular Surgery
University of South Florida
Tampa, Florida
USA

Robert W. Thompson
Department of Surgery
Section of Vascular Surgery
Washington University Center
for Thoracic Outlet Syndrome
Barnes-Jewish Hospital
St. Louis, Missouri
USA

Julie Ann Freischlag
Department of Surgery
John Hopkins Medical Institutions
Baltimore, Maryland
USA

Dean M. Donahue
Department of Thoracic Surgery
Massachusetts General Hospital
Boston, Massachusetts
USA

Sheldon E. Jordan
Department of Neurology
Neurological Associates
of West LA
Santa Monica
California
USA

Peter I. Edgelow
Graduate Program in Physical Therapy
UCSF/SFSU
Union City, California
USA

ISBN 978-1-4471-4365-9   ISBN 978-1-4471-4366-6   (eBook)
DOI 10.1007/978-1-4471-4366-6
Springer London Heidelberg New York Dordrecht

Library of Congress Control Number: 2013938870

Printed on acid-free paper

Springer is part of Springer Science+Business Media (www.springer.com)

Karl A. Illig: *Thanks to those who taught me that asking questions about what we do is fun, and to those who instilled within me a fairly unusual passion for the thoracic outlet and the patients who suffer from problems within it: Seymour Schwartz, Jim DeWeese, and Jim Adams, Harry Sax and Jim Peacock, Dave Feliciano, Dick Green, and Ken Ouriel. Thanks to several whose friendship has made an academic journey fun: Mike Singh, Joe Serletti, Walt Pegoli, Cinny Shortell, and Peter Knight. Thanks also to David Smith and Smitty, two new friends and colleagues who have provided amazing support and a wonderful and warm place to work. Finally, huge thanks to my co-editors and to all the authors of this volume; in addition to the knowledge I learned from each of you I count among you a mentor equally as valuable as any.*

Robert W. Thompson: *To the surgical mentors that have provided me with inspiration and instruction: Norm Thompson (dad), John Mannick, Ron Stoney, and Greg Sicard. To my colleagues in the care of patients with thoracic outlet syndrome, for being some of the most thoughtful, compassionate, and skilled physicians I have ever known; with special thanks to Richard Sanders, the Master. To my students, residents, and fellows, I am ever grateful that you keep me challenged and humbled in trying to pass on all of the pearls. To Della, Yvette, Robert, and Valerie, for your daily support and strength in our quest to help patients with thoracic outlet syndromes, and for your unflinching devotion to the mission. To my wonderful wife, Michelle, and the joy of our lives, Taylor Alexandra, who makes it all so worthwhile.*

Julie Ann Freischlag: *My experience with thoracic outlet syndrome began with Herb Machleder. Every Tuesday we would operate together when I was a vascular fellow at UCLA – his knowledge of the disease and his philosophy about the process of care for these patients was extraordinary – and I thank him to this day for the experience and mentorship. From my point of view this book is dedicated to all of our patients with this disease so that they receive better care and to our trainees who we hopefully will give the same teaching that Herb gave to me.*

Sheldon E. Jordan: *My experience with thoracic outlet syndrome began with Herb Machleder. He simply rose above the noise of controversy. In a clear, compassionate, and inquisitive fashion he approached the patients individually and as members of a population in need. He was remarkably unbiased, creative, and eclectic in his quest for better treatment of these patients. He is my hero.*

Dean M. Donahue: *I would like to dedicate this to the people who have taught me the most about TOS: my patients. I admire the courage you show dealing with this condition. I would like to thank my colleagues, who fortunately, are also my friends. You have inspired and encouraged me to reach for your lofty standards. I would like to acknowledge a very hard working office staff: Patricia Guerriero, Kathy Cocozella and Julie Garrity. You fight the TOS battle in the trenches every day. Mostly, I want to thank my entire family, especially my amazing wife Julie, and awesome children Trevor, Abby, Ally and Emily. This was only accomplished because of their love, understanding, and support.*

Peter I. Edgelow: *It has been an honor to assist in the birth of this text on Thoracic Outlet Syndrome. I owe much to Dr. Ronald Stoney, M.D., who introduced me to TOS by inviting me to observe surgery. What I learned led me to research the literature to explain the problem that Dr. Stoney first clarified. I also acknowledge the work of Dr. Herman Kabat, M.D., the originator of the Physical Therapy technique called Proprioceptive Neuromuscular Facilitation (PNF). His observation of weakness in the ulnar innervated thumb muscles and the reversal of this weakness following proprioceptive stimulation to the neck flexors filled in a gap in conservative treatment. Over the past 20 years, success with patients plus studies on the effects of trauma secondary to MVAs has provided an evidence base to support conservative care as clarified in the text. Lastly but by no means least, a grateful thanks to my wife Margaret for her editorial expertise and to our daughter Gillian who is the model for the DVD that demonstrates the exercises.*

Foreword

After a century of contributions to the Medical Literature, new ideas about neurovascular compression syndromes had apparently run aground. By the 1970s there was little of consequence in the contemporary literature, no ongoing investigative efforts, and except for a colorful monograph by artist Frank Netter, virtually no Medical School teaching of the subject. It was all too obvious that clinical understanding of "Thoracic Outlet Syndrome" was inadequate to meet the rising number of patients with these unique disorders.

Then, from the Basic Sciences, came a coherent view of the developmental anatomy of the Thoracic Outlet structures. Perhaps that was the spark that ignited the energy of a new generation of collaborative Neurologists, Physicians, Surgeons, and Radiologists to rethink the conceptual framework, integrate what was known, and create a new multidisciplinary forum for the generation of new knowledge. Clinical scholarship in this area flourished, guided by Peer Reviewed Research and Evidence Based Medicine. The result, from one perspective as a State Disability Examiner; "TOS disabled" Musicians were returning to their orchestras, Professional and Student Athletes to their teams. Workers returned to office, shop, and construction site. When viewed in the setting of just a few years past, these accomplishments cannot be overrated.

Thoracic Outlet Syndrome, the textbook, represents the first thorough compilation of what has come to be known of these disorders. And for this time in history, it has been put together in one elegant text.

It should be immediately apparent, when you review the roster of Editors, the list of 52 Authors from 27 cities and 20 University Medical Centers, that this is no Monograph, or idiosyncratic look at a subject, but the collective wisdom and experience of a diverse group of outstanding Clinicians and Clinical Scientists from the major medical and rehabilitative disciplines. From this perspective comes a comprehensive, cohesive, eminently literate account of the conceptual framework that encompasses the Thoracic Outlet disorders. The anatomic and physiologic fundamentals and the basis for the diagnostic and therapeutic algorithms are in detail.

The arrangement of the three sections (Neurogenic, Arterial, and Venous) and their major subdivisions of; Pathologic Anatomy/Physiology, Diagnosis, and Therapy, give the reader insight into the thoughtful pedagogic framework of the text. The management algorithms and therapeutic options cover a multitude of permutations, and practically every validated treatment variation.

All the "FAQs" are addressed: The myriad issues that accompany unexpected disability; Psychosocial, Vocational, Medico legal, even to Patient's assessments of their experiences, articulate and critical. One cannot help but sense the compassion, attention to detail, technical skill, and thoughtful rehabilitation that populates these pages. The clinician, from whatever discipline, comes away from this text with understanding, and fresh diagnostic and therapeutic confidence for dealing with what is now one of the most common disorders to encumber the modern workplace.

There has been an empty slot on the Reference Shelf, a hole in the Medical Curriculum, a space on the office desk, a 150 year lapse. The Editors and Authors of *Thoracic Outlet Syndrome* have filled that gap, with a textbook worthy of the task. Above all else, will be the improved care of a group of young men and women eager to be productive. It is hard to imagine there is a group among the healing sciences, from students to experienced clinicians and practitioners, who will not benefit from picking up and reading these pages.

CA, USA   Herbert I. Machleder, MD

Preface

Thoracic outlet syndrome (TOS) is a condition estimated to affect as many as 80 of every 1,000 patients in the United States. While estimates vary widely based in part on lack of consensus as to the definition of the syndrome, between 2,500 and 3,000 first rib resections are performed yearly in this country.

What is TOS? In reality, *it is at least three separate conditions*. Neurogenic TOS (NTOS), by far the most common (perhaps 95 % of cases), refers to the condition where the brachial plexus is compressed at the scalene triangle or retropectoral space, and is manifest as local and extremity pain and neurologic symptoms often exacerbated by lifting the arms overhead. Venous TOS (VTOS), accounting for about 4 % of cases, refers to the situation where the subclavian vein is compressed by the structures making up the costoclavicular junction, and presents as acute or chronic venous thrombosis or injury or occasionally intermittent positional obstruction. Finally, arterial TOS (ATOS), the rarest form of the condition, refers to the situation where arterial injury occurs as the result of abnormal bony or ligamentous structures at the outlet, and presents as occlusion of or embolization from an abnormal artery in this area. To further the confusion regarding terminology, VTOS and ATOS are sometimes lumped together as "vascular" TOS, and many patients with NTOS will have easily reproducible arterial abnormalities shown by history or physical exam.

TOS is perhaps the most common surgical condition that has not had a textbook specifically devoted to it. Several single-author monographs exist (and another is planned), notably Sanders' *Thoracic Outlet Syndrome: A Common Sequela of Neck Injuries* (Philadelphia: Lippincott, 1991) and Machleder's *Vascular Disorders of the Upper Extremity* (Hoboken: Wiley, 1999), but while seminal works these are both obviously directed at special cases of TOS and date from more than a decade ago. There are numerous reasons why a multidisciplinary, multi-author textbook is before you:

- TOS is a problem seen almost daily in most busy vascular surgery clinics and clinics of thoracic surgeons, neurosurgeons, and neurologist interested in this diagnosis.
- TOS is poorly understood by all but a handful of physicians.
- TOS is very poorly understood and hence very poorly diagnosed by the majority of primary care physicians, and almost unknown by the lay population.
- TOS is poorly treated by all but a handful of physicians and practitioners.

- Even by the "experts" – TOS is perhaps the most inconsistently treated and poorly assessed condition one can name:
  - There is little consensus as to pathophysiology.
  - There are no consistent diagnostic criteria to use.
  - There are no treatment algorithms consistently used by most clinicians.
  - There are no objective outcomes assessment tools, and thus trying to assess success or failure of treatment rests on very shaky ground.
  - As the condition is uncommon, almost no one has enough volume to truly assess what is helpful and what is not.

In short, and to summarize the problem in a few words, essentially no Level 1 evidence exists for anything we do in the treatment of this condition. It has been chilling for the editors to truly learn on what shaky ground we stand on when providing care for patients with TOS.

This textbook attempts to start the process of remedying this situation, by bringing together as many experts as possible who treat this disease and think and write about it critically. The book is divided into 13 parts. First is an overall summary of the problem, which includes reviews of terminology, embryology, and anatomy. Next, sections specifically addressing NTOS, VTOS, and ATOS each follow, each addressing specific anatomy and physiology, treatment pathways, and controversies and special questions we need to ask. Finally, a section most relevant to the condition as a whole is provided, which includes discussion of medicolegal and workman's compensation issues, psychological concerns, and "best practices" with regards to treating these patients – and essays, in their own words, by those affected by it. This book is designed as a clinical reference work. While it can certainly be read in its entirety (and should, by all who concentrate on this condition), it is designed to reside on a shelf in a busy surgical or neurologic clinic where individual chapters can be quickly referenced when a specific question arises in the course of daily practice. As such, we have tried to keep the chapters as short as possible, but in return some overlap and redundancy will be observed.

In summary, this condition can probably be best approached if we all "talk the same language," and this textbook is envisioned as a critical first step. The next task is probably to agree on unified diagnostic criteria and even treatment pathways so that we can begin to objectively assess what is the best possible care for these patients. Begun by the efforts of one of the authors (RT) using the Delphi process, we hope to accomplish this goal assisted by societal consensus statements, uniform registries, multi-institutional prospective randomized trials, and, ideally, "rare disease" funding.

TOS, while rare, is potentially a lifelong condition and is devastating to those affected. When coupled with the very poor state of knowledge and lack of interest by so many clinicians, the stage is set for suffering. We hope that the information that follows will help all to start to solve this problem.

Florida, USA	Karl A. Illig
Missouri, USA	Robert W. Thompson
Maryland, USA	Julie Ann Freischlag
Massachusetts, USA	Dean M. Donahue
California, USA	Sheldon E. Jordan
California, USA	Peter I. Edgelow

Terminology of Thoracic Outlet Syndrome and Related Problems

Dean Donahue, Peter Edgelow, Julie Freischlag, Karl Illig, Sheldon Jordan, Robert Thompson

As in any field of medicine or scientific endeavor, those who deal with Thoracic Outlet Syndrome (TOS) and related problems must understand and agree upon a unified terminology. TOS can be confusing, and the plethora of descriptions, eponyms, tests, maneuvers, and the like often make things worse. In several cases ("true" versus "disputed" TOS, for example), inappropriate terminology can even give the impression that the syndrome does not exist or that patients are imagining their complaints. Finally, accurate terminology allows professionals and patients alike to economically communicate with each other.

The following chapter sets forth a "vocabulary" of TOS, to be used in this textbook and, ideally, in the real world as well.

Thoracic Outlet Syndrome (TOS)

One of several conditions manifested by signs and symptoms attributable to compression or entrapment of vessels or nerves at the level of the thoracic outlet. The designation "syndrome" implies the presence of disability that is significant to the patient. It is critical to differentiate neurogenic (NTOS), venous (VTOS), and arterial (ATOS) as these are three separate syndromes, are treated in different ways, and have different natural histories and outcomes.

Note that the terms "**True TOS**" and "**Disputed TOS**" are no longer helpful, are of historical interest only, and should not be used. These terms arose in the era when diagnosis of NTOS was less precise and outcomes less assured, and suggest that controversy exists as to whether NTOS exists if motor dysfunction or wasting are not present, a proposition not supported by contemporary practice.

Aberrant Fibrous Bands

Fibrotic structures that course through or across the neurovascular structures at the scalene triangle, resulting in abnormal displacement or entrapment of these structures.

Adson Maneuver

A physical exam maneuver performed to evaluate for positional subclavian artery compression in the thoracic outlet. The patient is seated with their head rotated toward the asymptomatic side and extended. The arm is then extended and externally rotated during a single-breath hold while palpating the radial artery pulse at the wrist. The value of this test has been questioned because of a high frequency of positive results in asymptomatic individuals, and because it does not reliably demonstrate arterial wall changes characteristic of ATOS (i.e., subclavian artery aneurysms), and because it does not demonstrate or indicate brachial plexus nerve compression. In contrast, reproduction of upper extremity symptoms with arm elevation in the presence of a palpable radial pulse demonstrates that the symptoms are unrelated to arterial insufficiency, and more likely secondary to NTOS.

Anomalous First Rib

A true first rib (arising from T1) that exhibits an unusual shape or junction with the second rib.

Arterial TOS (ATOS)

Signs and symptoms attributed to "clinically significant" arterial compression within the thoracic outlet, such as subclavian artery occlusive lesions or aneurysms. ATOS is reserved for situations in which symptoms of arterial insufficiency or thromboembolism are dominant along with demonstrable structural pathology.

Axillary Artery Compression Syndrome

A form of ATOS characterized by arterial compression at the level of the humeral head or underneath the pectoralis minor muscle.

Axillosubclavian artery

The term encompassing the entire artery in the region of the thoracic outlet.

Brachial Plexus Neurolysis

A surgical technique used to mobilize the brachial plexus nerve roots from surrounding fibrous tissue, by operative dissection of scar tissue surrounding or interdigitating the nerves during thoracic outlet decompression. The term "neuroplasty" may also be used.

Brief Pain Inventory (BPI)

A well-validated and commonly used patient-reported survey form that incorporates scales for subjective pain as well as how the pain interferes with various functions. A whole-body diagram is used for mapping pain.

Cervical Rib

An anomalous extra rib arising from the C7 vertebra, which typically inserts onto the normal first rib, causing anterior displacement and/or compression of the brachial plexus and subclavian artery. Occurs in approximately 0.5 % of the general population and may be seen as either an incidental finding or in conjunction with one of the forms of TOS.

Cervicobrachial Syndrome

A constellation of neck and upper extremity signs and symptoms that may be attributable to musculoskeletal, neurologic, or vascular dysfunction of the neck, shoulder, or arm, not necessarily with a defined diagnosis. The designation "syndrome" implies the presence of disability that is significant to the patient. It is recognized that people may have minor signs and symptoms that may not be considered disabling, and that multiple pathophysiological conditions may coexist (e.g., NTOS may coexist with shoulder impingement). The term "cervicobrachial syndrome" may be used to describe patients with regional problems and with several potentially identifiable diagnoses, particularly at the time of initial presentation. Whenever possible, this term "cervicobrachial syndrome" should be followed by a full listing of indentified specific diagnoses.

Cervicobrachial Symptom Questionnaire (CBSQ)

A self-administered scale designed for evaluation of cervicobrachial syndrome. A total body diagram is included to test for widespread pain syndromes, and an oversized hand diagram is used to allow for precision in sensory maps. Questions have been added to screen for CRPS including allodynia, hyperalgesia, and for changes in color, temperature, and sweating.

Chemodenervation. Botulinum Toxin Chemodenervation

The use of intramuscular botulinum toxin injection to achieve synaptic block at cholinergic junctions, resulting in neuromuscular blockade with partial or complete paralysis of the targeted muscle(s). Effects are expected to last for several months. Conditions characterized by chronic excessive activation or spasm of muscles are often treated in this manner (see **Dystonia**). This approach has also been applied to NTOS.

Chiropractic

The health profession concerned with the diagnosis, treatment, and prevention of mechanical disorders of the musculoskeletal system, and the effects of these disorders on the functions of the nervous system and general health. There is an emphasis on manual treatments including spinal adjustment and other joint and soft-tissue manipulation.

Chronic Pain Syndrome

Pain that lasts beyond the usual expected duration for healing of an acute injury. Arbitrarily, time periods of 3 or 6 months have been used in the definition.

Complex Regional Pain Syndrome (CRPS)

A painful condition manifesting as regional pain (with or without other lesions described below) that appears to be disproportionate in time or intensity to the usual course of any known trauma or other lesion. Considered to be associated with local/regional overactivity of the sympathetic nerve system. A recent international symposium was held to achieve consensus as to additional signs and symptoms that are to be required for the diagnosis. This terminology replaces earlier terms in the present text, but it should be recognized that the previous terms Reflex Sympathetic Dystrophy (RSD) and/or Causalgia are often still used. The Budapest Criteria, used in this text, requires that symptoms must exist in three of four of the following categories: sensory symptoms (hyperesthesia or allodynia), vasomotor symptoms (skin color or temperature changes), symptoms related to sweating or edema, and symptoms from a category that includes motor (dystonia or weakness) or trophic (altered nail and hair growth and changes in skin texture).

Costochondritis

A condition produced by inflammation of the costal cartilage connecting the ribs to the sternum. This causes symptoms of anterior chest pain occasionally radiating to the back, upper abdomen, or arm. May mimic or overlap symptoms of NTOS attributable to brachial plexus compression at the subcoracoid (pectoralis minor) space, distinguishable by tenderness to palpation and exacerbation of neurogenic upper extremity symptoms.

Costoclavicular Space

The anatomic space between the first rib and clavicle, through which the subclavian vein passes.

Cumulative Trauma Disorder (CTD)

An older term not used in this text. See **work-related musculoskeletal disorder**.

Disabilities of the Arm, Shoulder, and Hand (DASH)

The DASH outcome measure is a 30-item, self-reported questionnaire designed and validated to measure physical function and symptoms in people with any of the several musculoskeletal disorders of the upper extremity.

"Disputed" TOS

A term historically referring to patients with signs and symptoms of NTOS but no objective hand muscle weakness or atrophy or electrophysiological abnormalities on nerve conduction testing. Because this term carries the implication that such patients with NTOS do not have a valid or treatable diagnosis, this term has been discarded in contemporary practice.

Double-Crush Syndrome; Multiple-Crush Syndrome

A condition in which peripheral nerve dysfunction may appear to be more evident or modified because of the cumulative effects of nerve compression at two or more points along its axonal course. Historically, discussions centered around the effects of compression on axonal transport mechanisms. More current discussions include reference to a variety of identified processes that produce sensitization of neural structures, working at a peripheral or central level of the neuraxis.

Dysesthesia

An unpleasant feeling of electrical sensation, pins and needles, or tingling.

Dystonia

A condition of postural disturbance, usually associated with pain, caused by abnormal activation or spasm of a muscle or muscle group. Electromyographic examination of affected muscles will demonstrate excessive activity of the recorded motor action potentials. The latter will differentiate postural disturbances or pain that may result from muscle shortening or contracture.

Elevated Arm Stress Test (EAST)

A timed, repetitive hand opening and closing activity with the hands held with the elbows flexed and shoulders abducted 90°. A positive test is scored (and time noted) if the patient experiences discomfort related to pain, sensory changes, or progressive weakness and fatigue that reproduces symptoms concordant with the patient's condition. Commonly performed for either 1 min (with an endpoint of symptom reproduction) or for 3 min (with an endpoint of inability to continue).

Effort Thrombosis of the Subclavian Vein (Paget-Schroetter Syndrome)

VTOS presenting with sudden, spontaneous, arm swelling and cyanotic discoloration, caused by thrombosis of the axillary-subclavian vein at the level of the first rib or costoclavicular space. Essentially an upper extremity deep vein thrombosis caused by mechanical compression injury to the subclavian vein at this location, often seemingly associated with a history of upper extremity "effort" caused by heavy lifting or overhead activity. The condition was originally described by Sir James Paget (1875) and Leopold von Schroetter (1884), and later summarized in a series of 320 cases by Sir E. S. R. Hughes in 1949.

Ergonomic

Pertaining to the biomechanics of work-related activities.

External Venolysis

Thorough surgical removal of the fibrous tissue sheath, distinct from the adventitia of the vein, which commonly surrounds the subclavian vein in patients with VTOS. In many cases, external venolysis is associated with re-expansion of the underlying vein, which may be otherwise normal in diameter and consistency to palpation.

Fibromyalgia

A clinical syndrome characterized by the presence of chronic widespread pain in combination with fatigue, non-restorative sleep, and cognitive change along with a variety of bodily complaints. The American College of Rheumatology has recently updated diagnostic criteria for this disorder.

Gilliat-Sumner Hand

Atrophy (wasting) of the hand muscles, along with electrophysiological abnormalities on nerve conduction studies, attributed to chronic compression of the brachial plexus nerve roots by a cervical rib or anomalous fibrous band at the level of the thoracic outlet. Originally described by Gilliat et al. in 1970.

Interventional Pain Management

Techniques having in common percutaneous or minimally invasive approaches for the control of acute or chronic pain.

Katz Diagram

A validated and commonly used instrument, first used for carpal tunnel syndrome, which can be used for a patient to map out areas of paresthesias or sensory loss in the hand and arm.

Maximal Medical Improvement (MMI)

The situation at a point in time after treatment where further substantial improvement in subjective complaints and functional status is not anticipated. Specifically used in adjucating worker's compensation claims to define when treatment for a given condition has come to a conclusion.

Myofascial Pain

Regional pain with the presence of palpably firm areas of muscle which are tender. When the firm areas of muscle are needled or firmly percussed there is an experience of pain which may extend to a more distant location (**"trigger points"**). Muscle twitches may also be seen during percussion or needling of the muscle area.

Neurogenic Pain; Neuropathic Pain

Pain initiated or caused by a primary lesion, dysfunction, or transitory perturbation in the peripheral or central nervous system.

Neurogenic TOS (NTOS)

The category of Thoracic Outlet Syndrome caused by compression and/or irritation of neural elements of the brachial plexus, either at the level of the supraclavicular scalene triangle and/or the infraclavicular subcoracoid (pectoralis minor) space.

Neurography

Imaging of nerves. Specifically used to describe functional imaging, typically using contrast-enhanced magnetic resonance techniques, to elucidate and localize areas of nerve dysfunction.

Occupational Therapy (OT)

The health profession that facilitates functional participation in the actions and activities that individuals want and need to do during daily life, particularly through the therapeutic use of everyday and work-related activities.

Pain Management

The medical discipline that uses interventional, pharmaceutical, psychological, and rehabilitative techniques for the control of acute or chronic pain.

Paresthesia(s)

The feeling of electrical sensation, tingling, or pins and needles which is indicative of nerve stimulation or dysfunction (see "**dysesthesia**").

Pectoralis Minor Block

An injection of local anesthetic and/or other agents into the pectoralis minor muscle in an attempt to diagnose, evaluate, or treat pathologic brachial plexus nerve compression in this area.

Pectoralis Minor Syndrome

A form of NTOS manifested by signs and symptoms attributable to compression or entrapment of the brachial plexus nerves at the level of the pectoralis minor tendon, as it passes from the chest wall to the coracoid process.

Pectoralis Minor Tenotomy

A surgical procedure used to treat pectoralis minor syndrome, in which the tendon of the pectoralis minor muscle is divided close to its insertion on the coracoid process.

Peripheral Neuropathy

Dysfunction of nerves outside of the spinal cord, i.e., peripheral nerves.

Persistent Neurogenic TOS

Disabling symptoms of NTOS that have not improved despite previous treatment, typically assessed at least 3 months after an operative procedure. Distinguished from "**recurrent neurogenic TOS**," in which symptoms are improved for a period of at least 3 months after an operative procedure but subsequently return at a later interval.

Phalen's Test

A physical exam maneuver in which the patient holds the wrists in complete and forced flexion (pushing the dorsal surfaces of both hands together) for 30–60 s. A positive result (symptoms in the median nerve distribution) is predictive of carpal tunnel syndrome.

Physical Medicine and Rehabilitation (PMR)

The discipline of medicine that focuses on the evaluation and treatment of musculoskeletal problems, including long-term rehabilitation for acute and/or chronic problems.

Physical Therapy (PT)

The health profession that focuses on treatment techniques to promote the ability to move, reduce pain, restore function, and prevent disability.

Quality-of-Life (QOL)

The concept of the benefit or quality of a person's life as a whole. Semiobjectively assessed by measuring functional health and general well being, most commonly by self-administered patient questionnaires, such as the SF-36 form.

Recurrent Neurogenic TOS

Return of symptoms attributable to NTOS after a period of remission, typically for at least 3 months, following a particular form of treatment.

Reflex Sympathetic Dystrophy (RSD)

An older term for the condition now classified as complex regional pain syndrome.

Repetitive Motion Disorder, Repetitive Trauma Disorder

Older terms for **work-related musculoskeletal disorder**.

Scalene Block

An injection of local anesthetic and/or other agents into the anterior scalene muscle in an attempt to diagnose, evaluate, or treat pathologic brachial plexus nerve root compression in this area. Typically performed with electromyographic monitoring and radiographic- or ultrasound-guided needle tip placement. Unless otherwise specified, may also include injection into the middle scalene, pectoralis minor, and/or subclavius muscles.

Scalenectomy

Surgical procedure in which the anterior and middle scalene muscles are excised as part of an operation for thoracic outlet decompression. Distinguished from "scalenotomy" which refers to a procedure in which the insertion of the scalene muscle(s) is divided from the first rib but the muscle is not excised.

Sensitization

A process related to the peripheral or central nervous system which results in regional or generalized pain that appears to be disproportionate in time or intensity to the usual course of any known trauma or other lesion. **Allodynia** is the experience of pain when a person is stimulated in a manner which is not usually experienced as painful (e.g., pain with light touch). **Hyperesthesia** is the experience of excessive pain when stimulated in a manner that would produce only minimal pain in a normal individual.

SF-36

A well validated and widely used self-administered or interview-assisted questionnaire that is used to measure and monitor functional health and general well being. Short forms are sometimes substituted for the original 36 item scale (i.e., SF-24, SF-12).

Spurling's Test

A physical exam maneuver involving ipsilateral rotation and extension of the neck and downward pressure on the head, which produces pain and paresthesias from the neck to the ipsilateral limb, associated with degenerative cervical spine disease.

Subclavius Muscle

The muscle originating on the undersurface of the clavicle and inserting on the first rib by terminating in the costoclavicular ligament. This muscle may contribute to subclavian vein compression in VTOS.

Subclavius Muscle Block

An injection of local anesthetic and/or other agents into the subclavius muscle in an attempt to diagnose, otherwise evaluate, or treat pathologic compression of the brachial plexus nerve roots in this area.

Sympathectomy

Surgical procedure involving removal of a part of the cervical sympathetic chain, usually from the level of the stellate ganglion to the T3 sympathetic ganglion, used to treat sympathetic hyperactivity as a component of NTOS or CRPS. Aside from its use in these conditions, sympathectomy is most frequently performed for palmar and/or axillary hyperhydrosis.

Tenotomy

A term used to describe surgical division of a muscle or its tendon, distinguished from procedures involving resection of the muscle.

Thoracic Outlet

The general term for the anatomic region beginning at the base of the neck, behind the clavicle and overlying the first rib, and extending to the subcoracoid (beneath the insertion of the pectoralis minor) space. The principal nerves and blood vessels to the arm pass through the thoracic outlet. Several distinct spaces are considered to exist within the thoracic outlet, where compression of different structures may occur at different locations, including the scalene triangle, the costoclavicular space, and the subcoracoid space. Occasionally the term "**thoracic inlet**" is used to denote the venous portion of this area (constoclavicular junction), but this term is confusing and should be avoided.

Tinel's Sign

A physical exam maneuver used to detect an irritated peripheral nerve. Light tapping (percussing) over the nerve (such as over the carpal tunnel or the cubital canal) elicits a sensation of tingling or "pins and needles" in the distribution of the nerve if it is inflamed or irritated at that location.

Upper Limb Tension Test (ULTT)

A physical examination technique involving a series of sequential provocative maneuvers designed to place components of the brachial plexus on tension in an attempt to reproduce symptoms of NTOS. Sometimes referred to as the "straight-leg raising test" for the arm, it was first described by R. L. Elvey in 1979.

Vascular TOS

A general term for venous and/or arterial TOS.

Venous TOS (VTOS)

Intermittent positional obstruction or thrombotic occlusion of the axillo-subclavian vein at the level of the first rib. Thrombotic occlusion is also referred to as subclavian vein **effort thrombosis** or **Paget-Schroetter syndrome**.

Whiplash injury

Generally refers to an acute injury to the soft tissues of neck (as opposed to the bones) caused by sudden flexion and extension movements.

Winged Scapula

Any abnormal scapular position in relation to the chest wall. Medial or posterior winging of the scapula results from paralysis and/or atrophy of the serratus anterior muscle secondary to injury and/or dysfunction of the long thoracic nerve, and is characterized by an inability to keep the scapula close to the chest wall during arm elevation and abduction and subsequent weakness and inability to perform these movements. Lateral winging of the scapula results from weakness of the trapezius and/or rhomboid muscles.

Workers Compensation

The system that has been developed under government supervision to provide treatment to workers who have been injured on the job site or in the course of employment-related duties.

Workplace Injury

An injury that occurs while at work and in the course of employment-related duties.

Work-Related Musculoskeletal Disorders (WMSDs)

Any musculoskeletal disorder caused by chronic physical workplace stress. These disorders can be caused by activities which are frequent and repetitive or by activities that involve sustained awkward postures. This term unites syndromes such as repetitive motion injuries, repetitive strain or stress injuries, cumulative trauma disorders, occupational cervicobrachial disorders, occupational overuse syndromes, regional musculoskeletal disorders, etc.

Contents

Contributors

Kevin J. Adrian BS, JD St. Louis, MO, USA

Zarina S. Ali, MD Department of Neurosurgery,
University of Pennsylvania Hospital, Philadelphia, PA, USA

Stephen J. Annest, MD, FACS Department of Vascular Surgery,
Presbyterian St. Luke's Medical Center, Vascular Institute of the Rockies,
Denver, CO, USA

George J. Arnaoutakis, MD Department of Surgery,
Johns Hopkins Hospital, Baltimore, MD, USA

Ali Azizzadeh, MD, FACS Department of Cardiothoracic
and Vascular Surgery, University of Texas Medical School,
Memorial Hermann Heart and Vascular Institute, Houston, TX, USA

Matthew Becher, Pharm D Candidate Presbyterian St Luke's Medical
Center and Rocky Mountain Hospital for Children, Denver, CO, USA

Nicholas Bennett, Pharm D Candidate Presbyterian St Luke's Medical
Center and Rocky Mountain Hospital for Children, Denver, CO, USA

Francis J. Caputo, MD Division of Vascular and Endovascular Surgery,
Department of Surgery, Cooper University Hospital, Camden, NJ, USA

David C. Cassada, MD, FACS Division for Vascular Surgery,
Stroobants Heart Center, Centra Lynchburg General Hospital,
Lynchburg, VA, USA

David C. Chang, PhD, MPH, MBA Department of Surgery,
University of California, San Diego, CA, USA

Charles R. Crane, MD Department of Certified Pain Management,
American Board of Physical Medicine and Rehabilitation,
American Board of Electrodiagnostic Medicine, Dallas, TX, USA

Michael Darcy, MD Department of Radiology, Mallinckrodt Institute of
Radiology, Barnes Jewish Hospital, St. Louis, MO, USA

Dean M. Donahue, MD Department of Thoracic Surgery,
Massachusetts General Hospital, Boston, MA, USA

Adam J. Doyle, MD Department of Surgery,
University of Rochester Medical Center, Rochester, NY, USA

Matthew R. Driskill, MSPT Department of Outpatient Musculoskeletal,
The Rehabilitation Institute of St. Louis, St. Louis, MO, USA

Michelle M. Dugan, MSN, FNP-BC Department of Neurosurgery,
University of Rochester Medical Center, Rochester, NY, USA

Peter I. Edgelow, DPT Graduate Program in Physical Therapy,
UCSF/SFSU, Union City, CA, USA

Wladislaw Ellis, MD Private Practice, Neurology/Psychiatry,
Berkeley, CA, USA

Dana Emery, OT/L, BS Department of Occupational Therapy,
University of Rochester Medical Center, Rochester, NY, USA

Valerie B. Emery, RN, ANP Section of Vascular Surgery,
Center for Thoracic Outlet Syndrome, School of Medicine,
Washington University, Saint Louis, MO, USA

Anna B. Evans, Pharm D Candidate Presbyterian St Luke's Medical
Center and Rocky Mountain Hospital for Children, Denver, CO, USA

Dustin J. Fanciullo, MD, RPVI Private Practice, Vascular Surgery,
Rochester, NY, USA

Richard L. Feinberg, MD Department of Vascular Surgery,
John Hopkins University School of Medicine, Columbia, MD, USA

Beverly Field, PhD Department of Anesthesiology,
Washington University School of Medicine, St. Louis, MO, USA

Kathryn Fowler, MD Mallinckrodt Institute of Radiology,
Washington University School of Medicine,
St. Louis, MO, USA

Gary M. Franklin, MD, MPH Departments of Environmental
and Occupational Health Sciences, Neurology, and Health Services,
University of Washington, Seattle, WA, USA

Julie Ann Freischlag, MD Department of Surgery,
Johns Hopkins Medical Institutions, Baltimore, MD, USA

Hugh A. Gelabert, MD Division of Vascular Surgery,
UCLA David Geffen School of Medicine, Los Angeles, CA, USA

David L. Gillespie, MD Department of Surgery,
University of Rochester Medical Center, Rochester, NY, USA

Christopher Gilligan, BA, MPhil, MD, MBA
Department of Anesthesia, Critical Care and Pain Medicine,
Massachusetts General Hospital, Center for Pain Medicine,
Boston, MA, USA

Carolyn Glass, MD, MS Department of Vascular Surgery, Strong Memorial Hospital, Rochester, NY, USA

Richard M. Green, MD Department of Surgery, Lenox Hill Hospital, New York, NY, USA

Linda M. Harris, MD Department of Surgery, Kaleida Health, Buffalo, NY, USA

Nancy L. Harthun, MD, MS Department of Surgery, Johns Hopkins Bayview Medical Center, Baltimore, MD, USA

Gregory G. Heuer, MD, PhD Department of Neurosurgery, Children's Hospital of Philadelphia, Philadelphia, PA, USA

Karl A. Illig, MD Department of Surgery, Division of Vascular Surgery, University of South Florida, Tampa, FL, USA

Kaj H. Johansen, MD, PhD Department of Vascular Surgery, Swedish Heart and Vascular Institute, Seattle, WA, USA

Sheldon E. Jordan, MD, FAAN Department of Neurology, Neurological Associates of West Los Angeles, Santa Monica, CA, USA

David G. Kline, MD Department of Neurosurgery, LSUHSC Neurosurgery (retired), Lenoir, NC, USA

Purandath Lall, MD Department of Surgery, VA WNY Health Care System, Buffalo, NY, USA

Jason T. Lee, MD Department of Surgery, Stanford University Medical Center, Stanford, CA, USA

Ying Wei Lum, MD Division of Vascular Surgery, John Hopkins Hospital, Baltimore, MD, USA

Bennett I. Machanic, MD, FAAN Department of Internal Medicine and Neurology, Rose Medical Center, University of Colorado, School of Medicine, Denver, CO, USA

Herbert I. Machleder, MD Department of Surgery, University of California, Los Angeles (UCLA), Los Angeles, CA, USA

Andrew J. Meltzer, MD Division of Vascular and Endovascular Surgery, Weill Cornell Medical College, New York – Presbyterian, Weill Cornell Medical Center, New York, NY, USA

Stephan Moll, MD Department of Hematology, University of North Carolina School of Medicine, Chapel Hill, NC, USA

Vamsi Narra, MD FRCR Mallinckrodt Institute of Radiology, Washington University School of Medicine, St. Louis, MO, USA

Louis L. Nguyen, MD, MBA, MPH Department of Vascular
and Endovascular Surgery, Brigham and Women's Hospital,
Boston, MA, USA

Emil F. Pascarelli, MD Department of Medicine, College of Physicians
and Surgeons, Columbia University, Santa Monica, CA, USA

Amit N. Patel, MD Department of Cardiothoracic Surgery,
School of Medicine, The University of Utah, Salt Lake City, UT, USA

William H. Pearce, MD Department of Surgery,
Division of Vascular Surgery, Feinberg School of Medicine,
Northwestern University, Chicago, IL, USA

Gregory J. Pearl, MD Department of Vascular Surgery,
Baylor University Medical Center, Dallas, TX, USA

J. Mark Pool, MD Cardiac, Vascular and Thoracic Surgical Associates,
Texas Health Presbyterian Hospital of Dallas,
Dallas, TX, USA

Joshua Prager, MD, MS Departments of Anesthesiology and Internal
Medicine, UCLA, Los Angeles, CA, USA

Constantine A. Raptis, MD Mallinckrodt Institute of Radiology,
Washington University School of Medicine, St. Louis, MO, USA

Rahul Rastogi, MD Department of Anesthesiology,
Washington University School of Medicine, St. Louis, MO, USA

James P. Rathmell, MD Department of Anesthesia, Critical Care
and Pain Medicine, Massachusetts General Hospital, Center for Pain
Medicine, Boston, MA, USA

Thomas Reifsnyder, MD Department of Surgery,
Johns Hopkins Bayview Medical Center, Baltimore, MD, USA

Marta J. Rozanski, MD Department of Anesthesia,
Critical Care and Pain Medicine, Massachusetts General Hospital
Center for Pain Medicine, Boston, MA, USA

Richard J. Sanders, MD Department of Surgery,
HealthONE Presbyterian-St. Lukes Hospital, Denver, CO, USA

Darren B. Schneider, MD   Division of Vascular and Endovascular
Surgery, Weill Cornell Medical College, New York – Presbyterian,
Weill Cornell Medical Center, New York, NY, USA

Carlos A. Selmonosky, MD Department of Medicine,
Inova Fairfax Hospital, Falls Church, VA, USA

Mohammadali M. Shoja Neuroscience Research Center,
Tabriz University of Medical Sciences, Tabriz, Iran

Poblete Raul Silva, MD Equipo De Cirugia Vascular, Depto Cirugia, Hospital Militar de Santiago, Santiago, Chile

Michael J. Singh, MD, FACS, RPVI Department of Surgery, University of Rochester Medical Center, Rochester, NY, USA

Gabriel C. Tender, MD Department of Neurosurgery, Louisiana State University in New Orleans, New Orleans, LA, USA

Robert W. Thompson, MD Department of Surgery, Section of Vascular Surgery, Center for Thoracic Outlet Syndrome, Washington University, Barnes-Jewish Hospital, St. Louis, MO, USA

Charles Philip Toussaint, MD Department of Neurosurgery, University of South Carolina School of Medicine, Columbia, SC, USA

R. Shane Tubbs, PhD Section Pediatric Neurosurgery, Children's Hospital, Birmingham, AL, USA

Harold C. Urschel Jr. MD Department of Cardiovascular and Thoracic Surgery, University of Texas Southwestern Medical School, Dallas, TX, USA

Marc A. Weinberg, DC Active Health Center, North Palm Beach, FL, USA

Anna Weiss, MD Department of Surgery, University of California, San Diego, CA, USA

Scott Werden, MD Vanguard Specialty Imaging, Sunnyvale, CA, USA

Anna M. Wittenberg, MPH Department of Internal Medicine/ Cardiovascular Division, Barnes-Jewish Hospital, St. Louis, MO, USA

Eric L. Zager, MD Department of Neurosurgery, University of Pennsylvania Hospital, Philadelphia, PA, USA

Part I

Background and Basic Principles

A Brief History of the Thoracic Outlet Compression Syndromes

1

Herbert I. Machleder

Abstract

The History of the Thoracic Outlet Compression Syndromes has evolved over the past 150 years, from the first well documented case in 1861, to series of patients now treated in modern prospective randomized trials. This evolution has been driven by clinical and basic research contributions from major University Medical Centers and Clinics around the globe.

The three major manifestations; Arterial, Venous, and Neurogenic were drawn together in a dramatic, tragic, and eventually transcendent series of events, summarized in a single clinical case, by the great American Neurologist William S. Fields in 1986.

The complex developmental anatomy, of this key evolutionary departure of Primates from the rest of the Mammals, remained the conundrum that shrouded the thoracic outlet from clarity. The contributions of; Embryologists, Anatomists, Neurophysiologists and Neuropathologists, coupled with astute observations of generations of Clinicians, now clearly define this unique anatomic site, and its hazards.

In reviewing this historical sequence the reader encounters a fascinating account, of a disorder that affects a diverse population including; Musicians, Athletes, Industrial Workers, as well as those who toil at Data Entry. The history also well illustrates the twists and turns of scientific discovery and clinical application, that have always encumbered our efforts to study, understand, and effectively alleviate a disorder, that can range from a curious annoyance to major disability.

Prologue

It was sometime in winter of 1994 when a newspaper reporter came upon a tattered, homeless, and destitute man living in a crude cardboard shelter under a Houston bridge. How could this be; JR Richard once one of the highest paid and most talented "All-Star" pitchers of the Houston

H.I. Machleder, MD
Department of Surgery,
University of California, Los Angeles (UCLA),
10833 LeConte Blvd, Los Angeles,
CA 90095-6904, USA
e-mail: hmachled@ucla.edu

K.A. Illig et al. (eds.), *Thoracic Outlet Syndrome*,
DOI 10.1007/978-1-4471-4366-6_1, © Springer-Verlag London 2013

Astros? A giant of a man both in size (6′8) and accomplishment, brought low by an odd, poorly understood disorder [1]. It remained for another iconic figure to decipher the diagnosis, the Neurologist William Fields; referred to by his contemporaries as a physician who was a "Giant" in the field of Neurology (whose members are not noted for hyperbole), and whose contributions were "monumental" [2].

After examining Richard, and studying his case, Fields wrote, in his definitive style, "All shoulder girdle compression syndromes have one common feature, namely; compression of the brachial plexus, the subclavian artery, and subclavian vein, usually between the first rib and the clavicle. With elevation of the upper limb, there is a scissorlike approximation of the clavicle superiorly and the first rib inferiorly. Grouping the various conditions under the single heading of *thoracic outlet syndrome* should be considered in all neurologic and vascular complaints of the arm previously reported as scalenus anticus, hyperabduction, costoclavicuar, cervical rib, fractured clavicle, cervicobracial compression, pneumatic hammer, effort vein thrombosis, subcoracoid pectoralis minor, and first thoracic rib syndrome" [3].

As is often said in the vernacular, "…there you have it!" the essential history of Thoracic Outlet Compression Syndrome (TOS) in a paragraph. A group of seemingly inconsequential developmental and acquired abnormalities that can hide for a lifetime in obscurity, or, under certain conditions of occupational, recreational, or cumulative trauma, result in a syndrome of dramatic and unremitting disability.

Historical Evolution

The commonality of the often disparate abnormalities and complaints associated with TOS was not always so evident, but has been slowly worked out over years of experimental research and clinical observation (beginning more than a century before JR Richards' case). This trajectory was laid out in a paper presented at a Festschrift for Charles Rob held in San Francisco California in 1993, "Thoracic Outlet Syndromes: new concepts from a century of discovery" [4].

The history of TOS as a medical diagnosis begins in 1861 on a rainy spring day in London, when "Charlotte D," a 26 year-old servant woman, was admitted to St. Bartholomew's Hospital with a painful, dysesthetic and somewhat ischemic left arm. The diagnosis of "cervical rib" was made, and surgical excision was undertaken by Mr. Holmes Coot. The case was beautifully described less than 2 weeks later in the journal Lancet [5].

These earliest cases fascinated both physicians and surgeons, as they diagnosed and treated mostly young patients with painful pulsatile masses in their necks, often associated with a cool, painful, dysesthetic upper extremity. The presence of a cervical rib was diagnosed by physical examination, this being almost half a century before the discovery of X-rays. The technically challenging but by and large successful treatment, often dramatically so, drew the attention of clinics around the world. After Coote's successful case, anomalous cervical rib and its syndrome were increasingly diagnosed, particularly after 1900 when recognition was facilitated by the growing use of radiographic imaging. A number of subsequent surgical reports appeared in the literature, and cervical rib excision became an accepted therapeutic approach when the rib was associated with upper-extremity neurovascular symptoms.

Paradoxically, the symptom complex was becoming increasingly recognizable in the industrializing cities in England and Australia, but without a detectible bony abnormality. In 1912, T. Wingate Todd reported a landmark clinical and anatomical study of a large number of men woman and children. He concluded that "symptoms of cervical rib" may be caused by an *apparently normal first dorsal rib*, and may be cured by its removal. His studies showed that there was a progressive and gradual descent of the shoulder girdle in advancing years such that the first and second thoracic nerves are gradually displaced and must travel upward until they have crossed the uppermost rib and then angulate downward to enter the arm. As a consequence of this configuration, any elevation of the rib or depression of the shoulder must stretch these lower connections with the brachial plexus. He also noted the resting and carrying positions that relieve and exacerbate this stretching [6].

In 1920 Stopford and Telford reported a group of patients seen in Manchester complaining of loss of grip strength, fatigue of the hand with exercise, weakness of the intrinsic muscles, loss of sensation in the distribution of the lower trunk of the brachial plexus, and vasomotor instability with episodes of cyanosis and coolness. They noted that after removal of the impinging portion of the first rib there was rapid resolution of the vasomotor and sensory changes and slow resolution of atrophic and motor changes [7]. This is, fascinatingly, quite a modern description of neurogenic TOS as reported now almost a full century later.

The Scalenectomy Era

Although the general anatomic region of the compressive abnormality had became quite evident, there was changing opinion about the key offending structure. Consequently, the disorder did not yet have a commonly accepted name! There was also considerable variation in opinion regarding the best mode of treatment, or surgical decompression.

At the Mayo Clinic Adson, the Chief of the Neurosurgical Service, began to treat "cervical rib" patients by removing the anterior scalene muscle. He reasoned that the compression originated superiorly and compressed the neurovascular structures against the unyielding bony structure beneath, and thus that relief of the superior compression would solve the problem with limited morbidity [8]. The popularity of this operation grew, particularly as it was far safer than resection of a cervical rib. Naffziger, who was chief of Neurosurgery at the University of California and President of the American College of Surgeons, also considered the anterior scalene muscle to be the key to the neurovascular compressive abnormalities in patients with "Cervical Rib Syndrome," even in the absence of an actual cervical rib, and thus first used the term "Scalenus Syndrome." [9] The widespread interest in this subject is highlighted by Ochsner, Gage, and DeBakey publishing a description of the disorder in a landmark paper entitled "Scalenus anticus (Naffziger) syndrome," giving credit to Naffziger (although Ochsner's paper antedated Naffziger's by 3 years!) [10].

The concept of dividing the scalene muscle flourished, albeit with both dramatic cures and less enthusiastically documented failures. In this period of time, before the widespread recognition of carpal tunnel syndrome, cervical disc disease and neuroforaminal compression, and other similar problems, the widespread application of scalenotomy was certain to lead to failures, particularly when applied to patients with predominantly upper plexus or median nerve distribution symptoms.

The anatomic variations seen during surgery suggested that a careful look at the embryology of the area might provide some insight into the etiology and interrelation of the structural elements. Some of the most illuminating basic research was done in Paris and Berlin [11, 12]. Milliez and Poitevin working at the Museum of Man at the Sorbonne in Paris, demonstrated that the scalene muscle mass is differentiated into specific muscle groups by passage of the developing neurovascular bundle. The persistence of certain muscle inclusions in the brachial plexus as well as muscle groups that traverse various elements of the brachial plexus is related to the original mass of the scalene variously segmented by the passage of these developing structures as the limb bud develops. These investigators also emphasized that anomalies at the thoracic outlet rarely exist in isolation as there is interaction in development of the different elements. Cervical rib development, for example, is determined by the formation of the spinal nerve roots. The regression of the C5 through C7 ribs is occasioned by the rapid development of the enlarging roots of the brachial plexus in the region of the limb bud. In cases of a C7 rib, there is only a small neural contribution from the T1 nerve root. The inhibition of rib development at that level is lost or reduced, and the size of the cervical rib is then related to the extent of the contribution of this T1 root to the brachial plexus.

When muscle histochemistry and fiber type analysis became available, these newer methods of muscle investigation were applied to the anterior scalene. The neuropathologist Anthony Verity recognized that in the post-traumatic situation there would be a gradual recruitment of sustained contracting Type 1 fibers, corresponding to the clinical observation of increased muscle tone, tenderness, and consequent compression [13]. This clinical and ultrastructural evidence formed the basis for a number of non-surgical treatment protocols for symptomatic relief of the neurogenic disability, including targeted physical therapy and chemodenervation of the anterior scalene [14–16], although this is getting ahead of ourselves.

The Era of First Rib Resection

In 1962 O Theron Clagett delivered his Presidential address to the American Thoracic Society. Subsequently published in the Journal of Thoracic and Cardiovascular Surgery, it described the evolution of his understanding of the compressive process and his application of first rib resection to patients with TOS. The posterior thoracoplasty approach was a difficult operation (for both patient and surgeon) and there was consequently relatively limited further clinical application [17]. The paper was a milestone, however, in turning attention away from the scalene muscle and back to the first Thoracic rib.

Renewed interest in first rib resection then followed a report in 1966 by David Roos, who reported a series of 15 patients treated by removal of the first thoracic rib from a transaxillary approach. The dramatic superiority of this technique was readily appreciated and became widely accepted [18]. Improved recognition of other problems that can be confused with TOS combined with a more effective operative approach to thoracic outlet compression led to demonstrably superior results in the treatment of patients with upper extremity neurogenic and neurovascular symptoms. Roos's superb ability in communicating the critical elements in the clinical workup as well as the operative details proved to be one of the keys to widespread acceptance of this approach, and the transaxillary procedure became

the standard operation for removal of the first thoracic rib by the early- to mid-1970s [19].

Unfortunately there remained a lack of familiarity with the complex developmental anomalies that occur in these patients leading to a definite incidence of poor surgical results soon followed by medical malpractice litigation. This turn of events was highlighted by Andrew Dale, a thoracic Surgeon from Nashville [20]. At the time of his paper's publication it was still the practice for journals to publish the full discussion that followed the paper's oral presentation, which was most interesting (and three full journal pages long!). The lively and instructive debate that followed his talk sounds surprisingly modern and illustrates the differences of opinion and lack of consensus that existed in the beginning of the 1980s, and he concluded the printed discussion with a quote from John Homans; "I enjoyed the discussion of my paper, but I wish I had not learned so much from it" (20, p. 1445).

The first good description of clinical anatomical observations was published by Roos in 1976, who described a constellation of abnormal bands and fibers that he had observed in the course of operative intervention [21]. Because of incomplete understanding of the embryology of the region at that time, Roos was able to identify the abnormalities only by number: Type I, Type II, etc. As research regarding the embryology and developmental anatomy of this area progressed, Makhoul was able to place all of the structural variations seen within a more comprehensive system [22]. As understanding of the various underlying anomalies developed it became apparent to many surgeons who had a focused interest in this entity, that simply removing the first rib was not the single best operation in all circumstances. Although removal of the rib would often lead to relief of symptoms, failure to identify and deal with other associated developmental abnormalities would often lead to recurrent (or residual) problems – first rib resection alone really only decompressed the soft tissue elements. Because of this the group at the University of California, Los Angeles (UCLA) have emphasized the fact that this operation, in general, should be considered *thoracic outlet decompression* [23]. Unfortunately for billing and coding reasons the term "first rib resection" had become firmly established by this point (and remains so), illustrating (in a negative sense) how evolving understanding can be encumbered by terminology!

The Concept of "Thoracic Outlet Compression Syndrome"

By the 1950s the term *"Thoracic Outlet Compression Syndrome"* began to appear in the medical literature. The *'Mayo Clinic Number'* of the 1946 Surgical Clinics of North America was devoted to a symposium on pain in the shoulder and arm. Eaton, the consultant in Neurology, described a group of disorders that he would 10 years later (in 1956) regularly refer to as the "thoracic outlet syndrome." He began his description in this way, "Almost always the patient seeks relief from pain and paresthesias of the upper extremity…" [24].

In 1958 Rob and Standeven reported ten cases of arterial occlusion as a complication of what they termed, "thoracic outlet compression syndrome", and thereby introduced the term to the surgical literature. They remarked at the often delayed diagnosis of thoracic outlet problems, suspecting that the subtle early manifestations of arterial compression were often masked by collateral formation. They further observed that, 'three cases have been recorded in the literature in which proximal spread of arterial thrombosis had reached the bifurcation of the innominate artery and caused hemiplegia.' It would be almost three decades later that J.R. Richard would suffer this identical consequence, on July 30, 1980, while pitching in the Houston Astrodome.

The arterial complications of TOS (ATOS) seemed to find particular occurrence in "throwing athletes." The variety of lesions, and the exceptional skill needed for both accurate identification and correction was well documented by Cormier, Yao, and Gelabert [25–27].

The Venous Abnormality

Although by 1980 compression of the axillosubclavian artery and brachial plexus in the thoracic outlet were well described, compression of the axillosubclavian vein (venous TOS; VTOS) was still an uncertain member of this syndrome. The phenomenon that had originally been described as the Paget-Schroetter Syndrome (based on the first two case reports) was later routinely referred to as *"spontaneous thrombosis of the axillosub-clavian vein"* or *"effort thrombosis."* The first designation was perhaps most accurate, reflecting as it did an acknowledged lack of understanding regarding the etiology. The second designation, however, was an imaginary construction, that was actually quite fanciful. In its original form it posited that an extreme Valsalva maneuver (the *"effort"*) would increase pressure in the innominate and jugular-subclavian venous system enough to invert and tear the retro-clavicular valve of the subclavian vein, in turn setting up a nidus for inflammation, fibrosis and thrombosis. The few reported pathologic examinations of resected specimens showed an area of fibrosis, chronic thrombus, and thickening which could be construed as possibly substantiating the hypothesis (today, of course, the term *"effort"* is used to refer to the fact that most patients with this problem are young, fit athletes) [28]. Finally, there was no recognition at this time that nonocclusive intermittent compression could also occur as part of this problem [29].

The more accurate explanation (chronic, extrinsic compression by the structures that make up the costoclavicular junction) was developed around the time that thrombolytic therapy began to be used, by means of which the thrombosed vein could be rapidly cleared of thrombus and the underlying structural abnormality then demonstrated by positional venography. The earliest attempts at treatment using this new paradigm were published in a series of case reports by Zimmerman [30], Taylor [31], and Perler [32] in the 1980s. The institution of a comprehensive approach to the Paget-Schroetter Syndrome was applied to a reasonable cohort of patients beginning in 1985 and reported by Kunkel in the Archives of Surgery in 1989 [33]. The key at this stage was the careful exclusion of any of the other possible causes of venous thrombosis (which had become legion as a consequence of using the brachial veins for all type of access). The management strategy for true effort thrombosis was further refined and results as applied to a large, meticulously controlled group of patients were reported in the Journal of Vascular Surgery by the UCLA group in 1993 at which time the staged, multidisciplinary approach of thrombolysis followed by thoracic outlet decompression had become widely accepted [34].

Where Are We Today?

At this point the three major components of the Thoracic Outlet Compression Syndrome are all clearly delineated, and treatment strategies relatively well tested and extensively documented. A major missing piece of the puzzle is, however, the lack of prospective randomized evidence for what we do, a problem that will hopefully be addressed in the next decade (see Chap. 41).

The "Holy Grail" of NTOS remains a search for a reliable and accurate objective test that clearly differentiates those who will improve with physical therapy or other nonsurgical options from those who require surgical decompression. A reliable electrophysiologic test would meet this need, but so far nerve testing has not proved to be of significant clinical benefit. Nerve conduction studies [35], F wave measurements [36], and Somatosensory Evoked Potentials [37–39] have all been extensively studied, but their predictive value remains unproven and they have occasionally proven to be a quagmire [40].

Epilogue

Although in their most obvious manifestations the congenital and acquired abnormalities of the thoracic outlet are considered discrete anomalies, they should more properly be viewed as part of a continuum of developmental variation (especially ATOS and NTOS). The particular spectrum of developmental variations seen may be significant as predisposing elements when complicated by either increased functional requirement or changes subsequent to trauma – in other words an environmental stress in the setting of an anatomic predisposition are usually both needed for TOS to exist.

Greater resilience of the arterial and venous systems seems to result in relatively innocuous symptoms until compression reaches levels of hemodynamic significance, or causes structural damage. It is evident that the threshold for neurogenic symptoms, from the brachial plexus, is lower than that for the vascular system.

Coincident with the range and continuum of developmental abnormalities, there is a range and continuum of compression of the normal structures traversing the thoracic outlet. Symptoms associated with the extremes of the compressive abnormalities are easy to distinguish, since they represent the "classic" cases: (1) Paget-Schroetter axillosubclavian vein occlusion [41]; (2) hand ischemia from thrombosis or embolization from the subclavian artery [42]; and (3) the "wasted hand" of cervical rib or band compression [43].

In addition to these "end-stage" conditions, it has been found important to recognize the full spectrum of symptoms that can arise from neurovascular compression at the thoracic outlet. The lesser degrees of compression will often be disabling, in settings of specific physical or occupational requirements.

References

1. Keith Knomes. "Resurrection: The J.R. Richard Story." IMDB 2005, Director; Greg Carter. Production; Bellinger-BotheaX films
2. Van Horn G, Grotta JC, William S, Fields MD. Texas medical center pioneer. Ann Neurol. 2004;56(2):314.
3. Fields WS, et al. Thoracic outlet syndrome: review and reference to stroke in a major league pitcher. AJR Am J Roentgenol. 1986;7:73–8.
4. Machleder HI. Thoracic outlet syndromes: new concepts from a century of discovery. Cardiovasc Surg. 1994;2(2): 137–45. LCCN-Sn93002438 ISSN 0967–2109.
5. Coote H. Exostosis of the left transverse process of the seventh cervical vertebrae, surrounded by blood vessels and nerves, successful removal. Lancet. 1861;i: 350–1.
6. Todd TW. The descent of the shoulder after birth. Its significance in the production of pressure symptoms on the lowest brachial trunk. Anat Anz. 1912;41:385–95.
7. Stopford JSB, Telford ED. Compression of the lower trunk of the brachial plexus by a first dorsal rib. Br J Surg. 1919;7:168–77.
8. Adson AW, Coffey JR. Cervical rib, a method of anterior approach for relief of symptoms by division of the scalenus anticus. Ann Surg. 1927;85:839–53.

9. Naffziger HC, Grant WT. Neuritis of the brachial plexus, mechanical in origin: the scalenus syndrome. Surg Gynecol Obstet. 1938;67:722–30.

10. Ochsner A, Gage M, DeBakey M. Scalenus anticus (Naffziger syndrome). Am J Surg. 1935;28:669–95.

11. Milliez PY *Contribution A L'Etude De L'Ontogenese Des Muscles Scalenes (Reconstruction D'Un Embryon De 2.5 cm)* June 28, 1991 Universite Paris 1 Pantheon-Sorbonne Musee De L'Homme, Museum D'Histoire Naturelle

12. Lang J. Tropographische Anatomie de Plexus brachialis und Thoracic Outlet Syndrom. Berlin: Walter de Gruyter; 1985.

13. Machleder HI, Moll F, Verity MA. The anterior scalene muscle in thoracic outlet compression syndrome. Histochemical and morphometric studies. Arch Surg. 1986;121:1141–4.

14. Pascarelli EF, Hsu YP. Understanding work-related upper extremity disorders. J Occup Rehabil. 2001;11(1):1–21.

15. Jordon SE, et al. Diagnosis of thoracic outlet syndrome using electrophysiologically guided anterior scalene blocks. Ann Vasc Surg. 1998;12:260–4.

16. Jordon SE, et al. Selective botulinum chemodenervation of the scalene muscles for treatment of neurogenic thoracic outlet syndrome. Ann Vasc Surg. 2000;14:365–9.

17. Clagett OT. Research and prosearch. J Thorac Cardiovasc Surg. 1962;44:153–66.

18. Roos DB. Transaxillary approach for first rib resection to relieve thoracic outlet syndrome. Ann Surg. 1966;163:354–8.

19. Roos DB. Experience with first rib resection for thoracic outlet syndrome. Ann Surg. 1971;173:429–33.

20. Dale WA. Thoracic outlet compression syndrome: Critique in 1982. Arch Surg. 1982;117:1437–45.

21. Roos DB. Congenital anomalies associated with thoracic outlet syndrome. Am J Surg. 1976;132:771–8.

22. Makhoul RG, et al. Developmental anomalies at the thoracic outlet: an analysis of 200 consecutive cases. J Vasc Surg. 1992;16:534–45.

23. Machleder HI. Transaxillary operative management of thoracic outlet syndrome. Current therapy in vascular surgery. 2nd ed. Philadelphia: B.C. Decker; 1991. ISBN 1-55664-262-8.

24. Eaton LM. Neurological causes of pain in the upper extremities; with particular reference to syndromes of protruded intervertebral disk in the cervical region and mechanical compression of the brachial plexus. Surg Clin North Am. 1946;4(6):810–32.

25. Cormier JM, et al. Arterial complications of the thoracic outlet syndrome: fifty-five operative cases. J Vasc Surg. 1989;9:778–87.

26. Durham JR, Yao JST, Pierce WH, et al. Arterial injuries in the thoracic outlet syndrome. J Vasc Surg. 1995;21:57–70.

27. Gelabert HA, et al. Diagnosis and management of arterial compression at the thoracic outlet. Ann Vasc Surg. 1997;11:359–66.

28. Adams JT, DeWeese JA. "Effort" thrombosis of the axillary and subclavian veins. J Trauma. 1971;11:923–30.

29. Adams JT, DeWeese JA, Mahoney EB, Rob CG. Intermittent subclavian vein obstruction without thrombosis. Surgery. 1968;68:147–65.

30. Zimmerman R, Morl H, et al. Urokinase therapy of subclavian-axillary vein thrombosis. Klin Wochenschr. 1981;59:851–6.

31. Taylor LM, Mcallister WR, et al. Thrombolytic therapy followed by first rib resection for spontaneous ("effort") subclavian vein thrombosis. Am J Surg. 1985;149:644–7.

32. Perler BA, Mitchel SE. Percutaneous transluminal angioplasty and transaxillary first rib resection: a multidisciplinary approach to the thoracic outlet compression syndrome. Am Surg. 1986;52:485–97.

33. Kunkel JM. Treatment of Paget-Schroetter syndrome. A staged, multidisciplinary approach. Arch Surg. 1989;124:1153–8.

34. Machleder HI. Evaluation of a new treatment strategy for Paget-Schroetter syndrome: spontaneous thrombosis of the axillary-subclavian vein. J Vasc Surg. 1993;17:305–17.

35. Daube JR. Nerve conduction studies in the thoracic outlet syndrome. Neurology. 1975;25:347–52.

36. Eisen A, et al. Application of F wave measurements in the differentiation of proximal and distal upper limb entrapments. Neurology. 1977;27:662–8.

37. Yiannikas C, Walsh JC. Somatosensory evoked responses in the diagnosis of thoracic outlet syndrome. J Neurol Neurosurg Psychiatry. 1983;46:234–40.

38. Machleder HI, Moll F, Nuwer M, Jordan S. Somatosensory evoked potentials in the assessment of thoracic outlet compression syndrome. J Vasc Surg. 1987;6:177–84.

39. Haghighi SS, et al. Sensory and motor evoked potential findings in patient with thoracic outlet syndrome. Electromyogr Clin Neurophysiol. 2005;45(3):149–54.

40. Relman AS. Editorial: responsibilities of authorship: where does the buck stop? N Engl J Med. 1984;310:1048–9.

41. Hughes ESR. Venous obstruction in the upper extremity (Paget-Schroetter's syndrome). Int Abstr Surg. 1949;88:89–127.

42. Machleder HI. Vascular disorders of the upper extremity. 3rd ed. Armonk: Wiley-Blackwell; 1999. ISBN 978-0-87993-409-5.

43. Gilliat RW, et al. Wasting of the hand associated with a cervical rib or band. J Neurol Neurosurg Psychiatry. 1970;33:615–24.

Embryology of the Thoracic Outlet

R. Shane Tubbs and Mohammadali M. Shoja

Abstract

The thoracic outlet is the area in the lower neck traversed by the brachial plexus and subclavian vessels between the thorax and axilla. This dynamic space is formed by the first thoracic vertebra, first rib, and manubrium of the sternum. The thoracic outlet changes in volume with the movement of the upper limbs, thorax, and neck, is occupied by scalene and prevertebral muscles and fibrous structures, and is limited by osseous structures – the clavicle, first rib, and cervical vertebrae and transverse processes. During upper limb abduction, patients with thoracic outlet syndrome (TOS) have been found to decrease the space of the outlet more compared to healthy individuals.

The thoracic outlet is the area in the lower neck traversed by the brachial plexus and subclavian vessels between the thorax and axilla. This dynamic space is formed by the first thoracic vertebra, first rib, and manubrium of the sternum (Fig. 2.1). The thoracic outlet changes in volume with the movement of the upper limbs, thorax, and neck, is occupied by scalene and prevertebral muscles and fibrous structures, and is limited by osseous structures – the clavicle, first rib, and cervical vertebrae and transverse processes. During upper limb abduction, patients with thoracic outlet syndrome (TOS) have been found to decrease the space of the outlet more compared to healthy individuals [1].

The embryogenesis of the thoracic outlet is a function of harmonious and timely growth of regional osseous, fibromuscular and neurovascular elements with the emerging upper limb bud. Any disturbance in the interaction or development of these elements affects spatial features of the outlet. From a morphological point of view, the thoracic outlet is a heterogeneous region with inter-individual variability and individuals with substantially distorted outlet contours or a crowded outlet are prone to develop TOS. In this chapter, the general aspects of the development of the thoracic outlet region are described followed by an overview of the embryology of common osseous and fibromuscular anomalies associated with TOS.

R.S. Tubbs, PhD (✉)
Section Pediatric Neurosurgery,
Children's Hospital, ACC 400 1600 7th Ave.
South, Birmingham, AL, 35233, USA
e-mail: shane.tubbs@chsys.org

M.M. Shoja
Neuroscience Research Center,
Tabriz University of Medical Sciences,
Tabriz, Iran

K.A. Illig et al. (eds.), *Thoracic Outlet Syndrome*,
DOI 10.1007/978-1-4471-4366-6_2, © Springer-Verlag London 2013

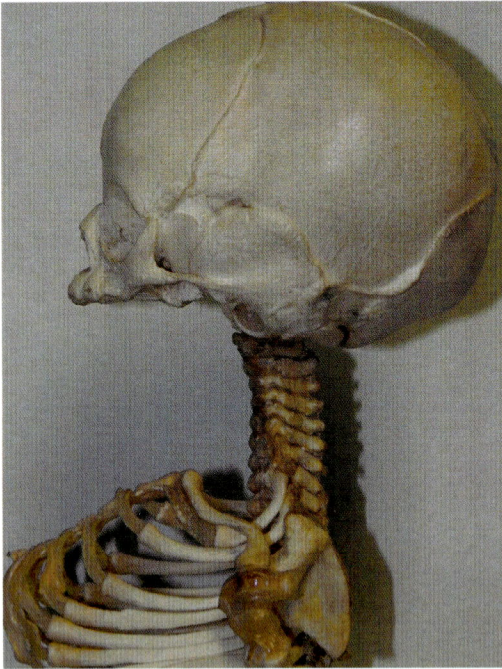

Fig. 2.1 Lateral view of the thoracic outlet from the skeleton of a 30 week old fetus. Notice the more horizontal nature of the manubrium as compared to the adult and the increased concavity of the first ribs

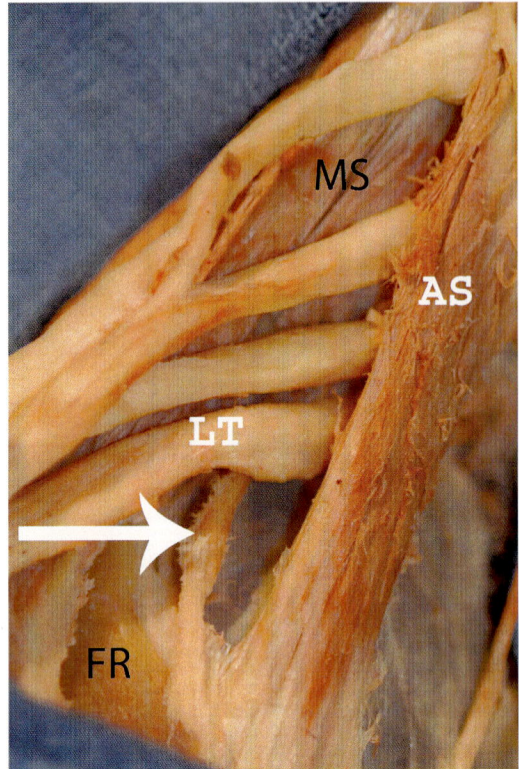

Fig. 2.2 Right neck from a cadaver found to harbor a cervical rib (*arrow*), which binds itself to the first rib (FR) via a fibrous band. Also note the middle (MS) and anterior scalene (AS) muscles and the lower trunk (LT) of the brachial plexus

Neurovascular Development

The subclavian vessels and brachial plexus traverse the thoracic outlet. The left subclavian artery arises from the left 7th intersegmental artery and from proximal to distal, the right subclavian artery arises from the fourth aortic arch, right dorsal aorta (between the 4th and the 7th intersegmental arteries), and the right 7th intersegmental artery. The subclavian veins form from the fusion of venous tributaries from the upper limb bud and the ventral rami that will form the brachial plexus begin budding from the neural tube by the end of the first month of gestation and grow toward their respective slerotomes and myotomes [2]. The slerotome of the upper thoracic region gives rise to the first thoracic vertebra. Normally, only the costal processes of the thoracic vertebrae give rise to ribs with the first rib joining the manubrium, which in turn is formed from the upper mesenchymal condensations that make up the sternebrae [2]. If the costal

elements of the seventh cervical vertebrae grow in a similar manner, an anomalous cervical rib forms.

Cervical Ribs

Anomalous elongation of the costal process of the seventh cervical vertebrae (cervical rib) (Fig. 2.2) has a wide range of frequency and has been reported to be present in 0.1–6.1 % of otherwise healthy individuals [3–5]. Although such variability can perhaps suggest that different ethnic groups could be more susceptible to thoracic outlet abnormalities, the validity of this assertion remains to be determined. During the development of the cervical vertebrae, cartilaginous costal elements are incorporated into the anterior and posterior tubercles and the intertubercular

Fig. 2.3 Schematic drawing of the right brachial plexus as it is deflected superiorly (especially the lower trunk formed by C8 and T1 ventral rami) by an anomalous cervical rib

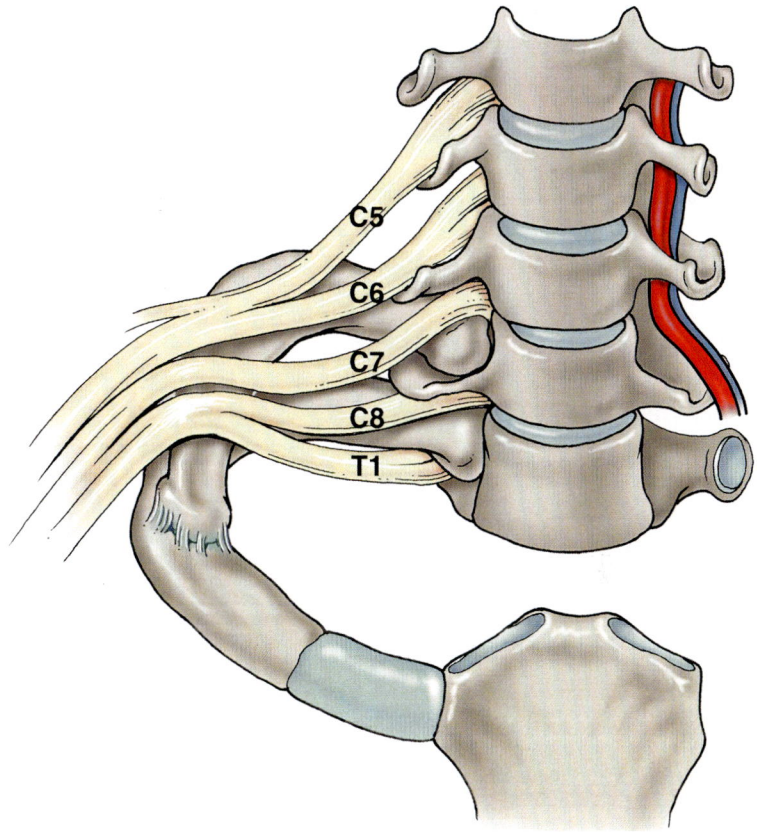

lamella of the transverse processes [6]. The anterior tubercle and intertubercular lamella of C7 are ill developed [7]. The endochondral ossification of the C7 costal element with the growth zone located at its medial margin acts as a precursor to a supernumerary rib [8]. A separate, ossified costal element of C7 has been seen in up to 63 % of stillborn human fetuses and as early as 14 weeks of gestation [9]. The dramatic reduction in the incidence of cervical ribs in adult humans implies an age-related process of absorption of the ossified costal element into the transverse processes of cervical vertebrae [3]. Cervical ribs may cause both neurogenic (Fig. 2.3) and vascular TOS [10]. The length of a supernumerary rib is also a determinant of the severity of compression. As cited in Makhoul and Machleder, Lang noted that cervical ribs greater than 5.6 cm pass beneath the subclavian artery and are more likely compress it [11]. Familial forms of TOS have been reported with apophysomegaly of the

C7 transverse process or formation of a cervical rib [12, 13]. An autosomal dominant inheritance has been suggested for such cases [14].

The mechanisms by which ossification of the C7 costal element and extent of growth and persistence of a cervical rib are directed have yet to be understood. Prenatal exposure to various toxic substances (e.g., valproic acid, retinoic acid, nitrous oxide, methanol) and disturbances in early organogenesis induce formation of cervical rib in some animals [15, 16]. An early attempt to understand the appearance of a cervical rib was made by Todd [17]. He attested that nerve and vessels at the thoracic outlet are the main limiting factors for the formation and size of cervical ribs. He distinguished several types of cervical ribs; some terminated behind the nerve trunk, some between the nerve and artery and others between the artery and vein, possibly indicating that the nerve, artery or vein, respectively, limits the growth of the cervical rib during embryogenesis.

Jones (as cited in Adson and Coffey [18]) suggested that with the outgrowing upper limb bud, the developing nerve trunks tend to course more or less obliquely. As the embryonic nerve trunk is proportionally larger than the ribs, the conflict between the obliquely oriented nerve and rib is in favor of the former, ultimately impeding the growth of the cervical rib.

Embryogenetics: Abnormalities in Hox gene expression affect the development of the thoracic outlet [19]. HOX genes are a cluster of homeobox-containing genes expressed along the anteroposterior axis of the developing skeleton which determine the segmental fate of the vertebral column [20, 21]. It has been postulated that formation of cervical ribs represent an error in HOX gene expression and thus the segmental identity of cervical and thoracic vertebrae [19, 22]. Alterations in homeotic transformation of the axial skeleton are often associated with fatal congenital malformations and are strongly selected against during development [23]. However, minor abnormalities such as formation of cervical ribs may escape this negative selection and persists through postnatal life.

Scalene Muscles

The scalene muscles occupy much of the thoracic outlet. Embryologically, the scalene muscles are derived from hypaxial mesoderm of hypomere of somital myotomes in much the same way as the intercostal muscles. While derivatives of the thoracic hypaxial mesoderm connect ribs, those of the lower cervical mesoderm extend from the transverse processes of cervical vertebrae to the upper ribs. Other local mesodermal components regress or transform into loose connective tissue or occasionally dense fibrous or ectopic/supernumerary muscular slips. Interestingly, in one series, single or multiple developmental anomalies were found in the thoracic outlet region in two thirds of surgical patients with TOS [11].

Developmental anomalies associated with TOS are classified into fibromuscular or osseous abnormalities [24, 25], and it is not uncommon to find a combination of both in a single patient [24].

Osseous abnormalities (e.g., cervical rib, abnormal first rib, or elongated C7 transverse process) are less common than fibromuscular anomalies, but are more likely to induce significant compressive symptoms or vascular TOS [26, 27]. Molecular aspects of these abnormalities (formation of dense fibrous or ectopic/supernumerary muscular strips) remain to be fully explored. It is known that precursor cells giving rise to hypaxial muscles undergo migration and myogenesis under the influence of various signals from dorsal ectoderm, lateral mesoderm and the developing limb buds [28, 29].

Congenital Anomalies of the Scalene Muscles: Congenital anomalies of the scalene muscles ranging from supernumerary muscle slips to muscle contraction and fibrosis account for a significant proportion of TOS. In one series, more than half of TOS patients without a cervical rib or other osseous abnormality had a scalene muscle anomaly crowding the interscalenic triangle [30]. Comments regarding the ontogeny of the scalene muscles are rarely found in the literature. Machelder [10] cited Millez and Poitevin who mentioned two relevant hypotheses: First, by the eighth week of gestation (2.5 cm embryo), a common scalene muscle mass develops and later separates into distinct muscle groups by traversing neurovascular bundles. As a consequence of segmentation defects, the scalenic mass may give rise to supernumerary muscle slips, e.g., scalenus minimus. Ectopic mesenchymal masses may transform into an anomalous muscle. The second hypothesis also states that supernumerary scalene muscles are remnants of the mesodermal mass, which normally regresses during embryogenesis.

More than ten fibromuscular anomalies of the thoracic outlet have been described in the literature. These anomalies may lead to compression of the brachial plexus anterior and/or posterior to the C5-T1 nerve trunks [26]. Anomalies posterior to the brachial plexus are more likely to cause symptomatic TOS [26]. Females have a predilection to combined anterior and posterior anomalies causing V-shaped impingement of the brachial plexus [26]. The most common anomaly is a ligamentous band that extends from the neck of the first rib to the inner surface of the first rib just behind the distal insertion of the anterior scalene onto the scalenic tubercle (called by some an "outlet band"). Ross found this anomaly in 146 (61 %) out of 241 operations for TOS [25]. The scalenus minimus and scalenus pleuralis muscles are well described and extend from C7 and/or rarely C6 transverse processes to the inner border of the first rib or the suprapleural fascia of Sibson, respectively [31]. The scalenus minimus is found in 15–88 % of thoracic outlets [32, 33]. This muscle passes between the subclavian artery anteriorly and the brachial plexus posteriorly, is occasionally replaced by a fibrous band or ligament, usually has attachment to Sibson's fascia, and can lead to irritation of the lower part of the brachial plexus [33, 34]. An anomalous distal insertion of the scalenus minimus onto the scalene

tubercle of the first rib causes elevation and compression of the subclavian artery [35]. It should be noted that many clinicians simply describe any muscle fibers that pass between the trunks of the brachial plexus as the scalenus minimus. Finally, a fibrotic band running from C7 to the first rib can be labeled as either a "middle scalene band" or simply as a non-ossified cervical rib.

In up to approximately 50 % of TOS patients without osseous anomalies, the distal insertion of the scalene medius is extended anteriorly behind the scalenus anterior. A common distal insertion of the anterior and middle scalene muscles, or overlapping distal insertions, referred to as intercostalization of the scalene muscle has been described [11]. Table 2.1 summarizes fibromuscular congenital anomalies associated with neurogenic TOS.

Table 2.1 Ross' classification of fibromuscular anomalies associated with neurogenic TOS

Involvement of upper and middle trunks of brachial plexus
A muscle strip that passes between C5 and C7, and connects the anterior and middle scalene muscles (interscalenic muscle)
An anomalous anterior scalene that is mixed with the middle scalene muscle superiorly and traverses between C5 anteriorly and C6-T1 posteriorly
An anterior scalene muscle with attachments to the epineurium of the upper trunk of brachial the plexus
A fused anterior-middle scalenic muscle mass through which the brachial plexus traverses
A vertical fibrous mass parallel to the vertebral column and anterior to the origin of the brachial plexus
Scalenus minimus muscle (see text)
A fibromuscular connection between the anterior and middle scalene muscles in the mid-portion of the inter-scalenic triangle
Involvement of lower trunk of brachial plexus
A fibrous band connecting the tip of an incomplete cervical rib to the mid-shaft of the first rib
A fibrous band connecting an elongated C7 transverse process to the upper surface of the first rib
A fibrous band connecting the neck of the first rib to the mid-shaft
An anomalous middle scalene muscle with an anterior extension of the distal insertion over the first rib
Scalenus minimus muscle (see text)
Scalenus pleuralis muscle (see text)
A fibromuscular band extending anteriorly from the lower portion of the middle scalene muscle beneath the lower trunk and subclavian vessels and attaching to the costal cartilage and sternum
A fibromuscular band extending anteriorly from the anterior scalene beneath the subclavian vein and attaching to the subclavius muscle and costoclavicular joint
A fibromuscular band along the posterior inner surface of the first rib
A fibromuscular band along the inner surface of the first rib from the rib neck to the sternum

Based on data from reference [36]
Note that other fibromuscular anomalies may exist that do not fit into the Ross classification, e.g., a fibrous band extending from the T1 vertebra to the inner surface of the first rib separating T1 from the C8 nerve root [32], a band from the C7 transverse process to the middle scalene separating the C8-T1 nerve root and subclavian artery from the C5–C7 nerve roots [32], a muscular slip from the anterior scalene attaching to the first rib between the subclavian artery and brachial plexus [26], etc.

References

1. Smedby O, Rostad H, Klaastad O, Lilleås F, Tillung T, Fosse E. Functional imaging of the thoracic outlet syndrome in an open MR scanner. Eur Radiol. 2000;10:597–600.

2. Larsen WJ, Sherman LS, Potter SS. Human embryology. 3rd ed. Philadelphia: Churchhill Livingstone; 2001.

3. Chernoff N, Rogers JM. Supernumerary ribs in developmental toxicity bioassays and in human populations: incidence and biological significance. J Toxicol Environ Health B Crit Rev. 2004;7:437–49.

4. Merks JH, Smets AM, Van Rijn RR, Kobes J, Caron HN, Maas M, Hennekam RC. Prevalence of rib anomalies in normal Caucasian children and childhood cancer patients. Eur J Med Genet. 2005;48:113–29.

5. Brewin J, Hill M, Ellis H. The prevalence of cervical ribs in a London population. Clin Anat. 2009;22:331–6.

6. Cave AJE. The morphology of the mammalian cervical pleurapophysis. J Zool. 1975;177:377–93.

7. O'Rahilly R, Müller F, Meyer DB. The human vertebral column at the end of the embryonic period proper. 2. The occipitocervical region. J Anat. 1983;136:181–95.

8. Meyer DB. The appearance of 'cervical ribs' during early human fetal development. Anat Rec. 1978; 190:481.

9. McNally E, Sandin B, Wilkins RA. The ossification of the costal element of the seventh cervical vertebra with particular reference to cervical ribs. J Anat. 1990; 170:125–9.

10. Machleder HI. Thoracic outlet syndrome. In: White RA, Hollier LH, editors. Vascular surgery: basic science and clinical correlations. 2nd ed. Malden: Blackwell Publishing; 2005. p. 146–61.

11. Makhoul RG, Machleder HI. Developmental anomalies at the thoracic outlet: an analysis of 200 consecutive cases. J Vasc Surg. 1992;16:534–42.

12. Weston WJ. Genetically determined cervical ribs; a family study. Br J Radiol. 1956;29:455–6.

13. Boles JM, Missoum A, Mocquard Y, Bastard J, Bellet M, Huu N, Goas JY. A familial case of thoracic outlet syndrome. Clinical, radiological study with treatment [French]. Sem Hop. 1981;57:1172–6.

14. Schapera J. Autosomal dominant inheritance of cervical ribs. Clin Genet. 1987;31:386–8.

15. Rengasamy P, Padmanabhan RR. Experimental studies on cervical and lumbar ribs in mouse embryos. Congenit Anom (Kyoto). 2004;44:156–71.

16. Steigenga MJ, Helmerhorst FM, de Koning J, Tijssen AM, Ruinard SA, Galis F. Evolutionary conserved structures as indicators of medical risks: increased incidence of cervical ribs after ovarian hyperstimulation in mice. J Anim Biol. 2006;56:63–8.

17. Todd TW. "Cervical Rib": Factors controlling its presence and its size. Its bearing on the morphology and development of the shoulder. J Anat Physiol. 1912; 46:244–88.

18. Adson AW, Coffey JR. Cervical rib: a method of anterior approach for relief of symptoms by division of the scalenus anticus. Ann Surg. 1927;85:839–57.

19. Galis F. Why do almost all mammals have seven cervical vertebrae? Developmental constraints, Hox genes, and cancer. J Exp Zool. 1999;285:19–26.

20. Burke AC, Nelson CE, Morgan BA, Tabin C. Hox genes and the evolution of vertebrate axial morphology. Development. 1995;121:333–46.

21. Ferrier DE, Holland PW. Ancient origin of the Hox gene cluster. Nat Rev Genet. 2001;2:33–8.

22. Horan GS, Kovàcs EN, Behringer RR, Featherstone MS. Mutations in paralogous Hox genes result in overlapping homeotic transformations of the axial skeleton: evidence for unique and redundant function. Dev Biol. 1995;169:359–72.

23. Galis F, Van Dooren TJ, Feuth JD, Metz JA, Witkam A, Ruinard S, Steigenga MJ, Wijnaendts LC. Extreme selection in humans against homeotic transformations of cervical vertebrae. Evolution. 2006;60:2643–54.

24. Roos DB. Pathophysiology of congenital anomalies in thoracic outlet syndrome. Acta Chir Belg. 1980; 79:353–61.

25. Roos DB. Congenital anomalies associated with thoracic outlet syndrome. Anatomy, symptoms, diagnosis, and treatment. Am J Surg. 1976;132:771–8.

26. Redenbach DM, Nelems B. A comparative study of structures comprising the thoracic outlet in 250 human cadavers and 72 surgical cases of thoracic outlet syndrome. Eur J Cardiothorac Surg. 1998;13:353–60.

27. Sanders RJ, Hammond SL. Management of cervical ribs and anomalous first ribs causing neurogenic thoracic outlet syndrome. J Vasc Surg. 2002;36:51–6.

28. Krüger M, Mennerich D, Fees S, Schäfer R, Mundlos S, Braun T. Sonic hedgehog is a survival factor for hypaxial muscles during mouse development. Development. 2001;128:743–52.

29. Ordahl CP, Williams BA, Denetclaw W. Determination and morphogenesis in myogenic progenitor cells: an experimental embryological approach. Curr Top Dev Biol. 2000;48:319–67.

30. Thomas GI, Jones TW, Stavney LS, Manhas DR. The middle scalene muscle and its contribution to the thoracic outlet syndrome. Am J Surg. 1983;145:589–92.

31. Bergman RA, Afifi AK, Miyauchi R. Illustrated encyclopedia of human anatomic variation: opus I: muscular system: alphabetical listing of muscles. http://www.anatomyatlases.org/AnatomicVariants/MuscularSystem/Text/S/04Scalenus.shtml. Accessed 15 Apr 2011.

32. Juvonen T, Satta J, Laitala P, Luukkonen K, Nissinen J. Anomalies at the thoracic outlet are frequent in the general population. Am J Surg. 1995;170:33–7.

33. Chen D, Fang Y, Li J, Gu Y. Anatomical study and clinical observation of thoracic outlet syndrome [Chinese]. Zhonghua Wai Ke Za Zhi. 1998;36:661–3.

34. Stott CF. A note on the scalenus minimus muscle. J Anat. 1928;62:359–61.

35. Boyd GI. Abnormality of subclavian artery associated with presence of the scalenus minimus. J Anat. 1934; 68:280–1.

36. Brantigan CO, Roos DB. Etiology of neurogenic thoracic outlet syndrome. Hand Clin. 2004;20:17–22.

Anatomy of the Thoracic Outlet and Related Structures

3

Richard J. Sanders

Abstract

Knowledge of anatomy is the key to understanding the thoracic outlet syndrome (TOS). By definition, TOS is hand and arm symptoms of pain, paresthesia, and weakness due to compression of the neurovascular bundle in the thoracic outlet area. While initially the scalene triangle was the focus of pathology in TOS, recent studies indicate that more than half of the patients thought to have TOS also have associated pectoralis minor compression, and in some patients this is the only diagnosis. Finally, it is important to recognize that the large majority of patients with anatomic abnormalities are asymptomatic unless neck trauma is also present – in other words, the mere presence of an abnormality does not mean it must be treated. Like many medical conditions, both an anatomic predisposition *plus* an environmental stressor are usually necessary for pathology to exist.

Introduction

Knowledge of anatomy is the key to understanding the thoracic outlet syndrome (TOS). By definition, TOS is hand and arm symptoms of pain, paresthesia, and weakness due to compression of the neurovascular bundle in the thoracic outlet area. While initially the scalene triangle was the focus of pathology in TOS, recent studies indicate that more than half of the patients thought to have TOS also have associated pectoralis minor compression, and in some patients this is the only diagnosis [1]. Finally, it is important to recognize that the large majority of patients with anatomic abnormalities are asymptomatic unless neck trauma is also present – in other words, the mere presence of an abnormality does not mean it must be treated. Like many medical conditions, both an anatomic predisposition *plus* an environmental stressor are usually necessary for pathology to exist.

R.J. Sanders, MD
Department of Surgery,
HealthONE Presbyterian-St. Lukes Hospital,
4545 E. 9th Ave #240, Denver, CO 80220, USA
e-mail: rsanders@ecentral.com

Anatomical Spaces

There are three anatomical spaces in the thoracic outlet area (Fig. 3.1a): The scalene triangle lying above the clavicle (Fig. 3.1b); the pectoralis minor

K.A. Illig et al. (eds.), *Thoracic Outlet Syndrome*,
DOI 10.1007/978-1-4471-4366-6_3, © Springer-Verlag London 2013

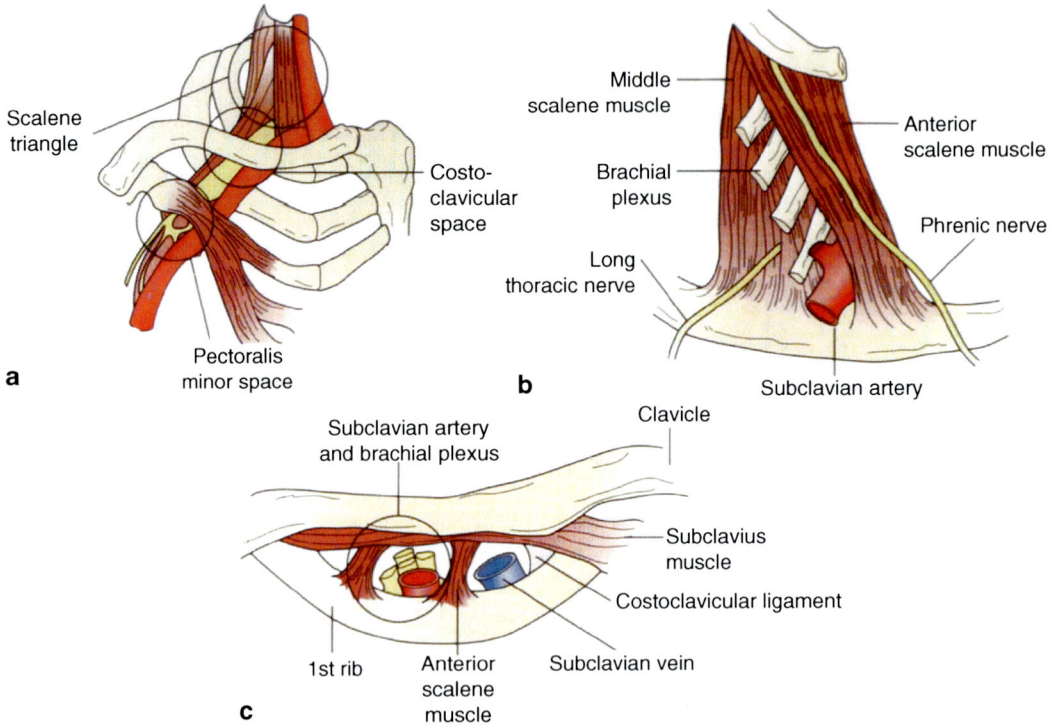

Fig. 3.1 Three spaces. (**a**) Anatomy showing the three spaces. (**b**) Scalene triangle with phrenic nerve passing from lateral to medial as it crosses anterior scalene muscle and long thoracic nerve exiting the middle scalene muscle. (**c**) Costoclavicular space (Reprinted from Sanders and Haug [2]. With permission from Lippincott Williams & Wilkins)

space, below the clavicle (Fig. 3.1c); and the costoclavicular space between clavicle and first rib. The neurovascular bundle, consisting of subclavian artery, vein, and brachial plexus, travels from the scalene triangle into the costoclavicular space and then through the pectoralis minor space. In this journey there is very little change in the vessels or the nerves (Fig. 3.2), and as a result the symptoms of nerve or vessel compression are about the same for each of the three spaces. The scalene triangle, unlike the other two spaces, contains only the subclavian artery and brachial plexus while the subclavian vein lies anterior to the triangle, anterior to the anterior scalene muscle.

Clinically, there is a small but significant difference in the symptoms of nerve compression in the scalene triangle versus the pectoralis minor space. Compression in the scalene triangle is usually associated with occipital headaches and significant neck pain due to trauma to the scalene muscles, while headaches and neck pain are absent or minimal when compression is in the other two spaces. When the arm is elevated, the neurovascular bundle rises against the pectoralis minor muscle which probably accounts for the onset of symptoms with the hyperextension maneuver (180° abduction) (Fig. 3.2) [3] and the elevated arm stress test (EAST or Roos test) [4].

The costoclavicular space is an area of potential compression in cases of clavicular fractures and subclavian vein obstruction, but it does not seem to be as important in neurogenic (NTOS) or arterial (ATOS) (Fig. 3.3).

Fig. 3.2 Thoracic outlet and pectoralis minor areas. Left arm is down, at the side. Note the subclavian and axillary artery and vein are essentially the same vessels one above and one below the clavicle. Right arm is elevated. This raises the axillary neurovascular bundle against the pectoralis minor muscle. This can constrict the axillary artery causing loss of the radial pulse and hand pallor and also pressure on the nerves of the brachial plexus causing paresthesia in the hand

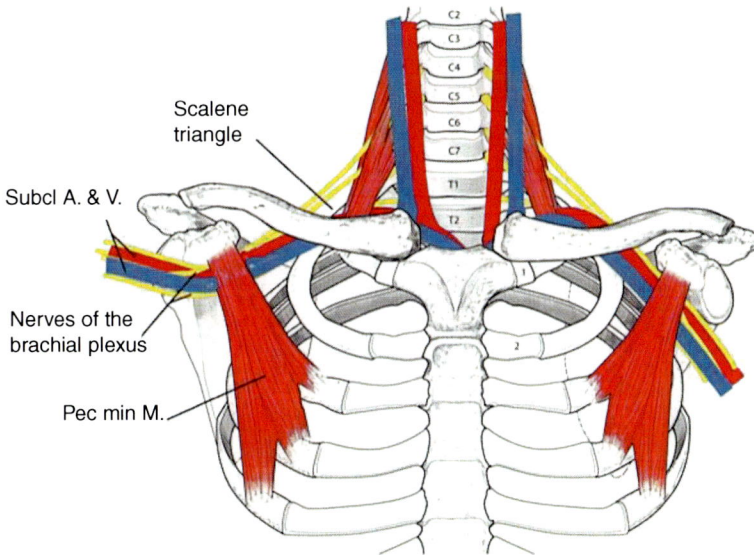

Fig. 3.3 Costoclavicular Space. Between the clavicle above and first rib below, all structures in the thoracic outlet area are seen. Note the subclavian vein is surrounded by costoclavicular ligament medially, subclavius muscle superiorly, anterior scalene muscle posteriorly, and first rib inferiorly. The subclavian vein is the structure most often compressed in this area and most often by costoclavicular ligament and/or subclavius muscle tendon

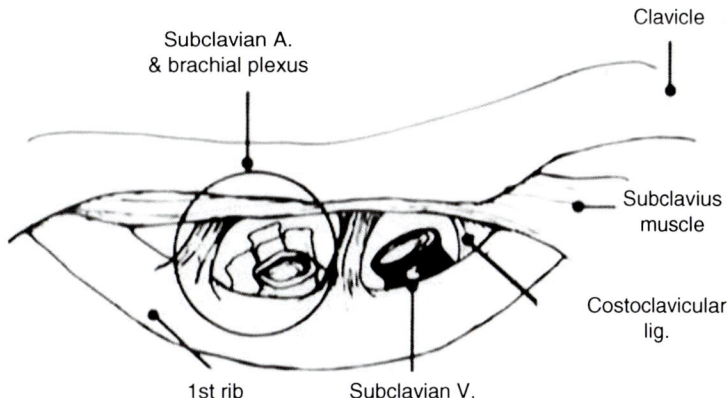

Cervical Ribs and Anomalous First Ribs

Cervical ribs arise from the transverse process of C7 and occur in about one in 140 people (0.7 %). They are more than twice as common in women than in men (70–30 %) [5]. Anomalous first ribs also have an incidence of 0.7 % and are equally as common in men as women [5]. The difference in gender distribution between the two types of ribs has yet to be explained.

In 1869 cervical ribs were classified into four groups [6]. From a clinical viewpoint, however, there are only two types: Complete or incomplete. About 30 % of cervical ribs are complete, and attach to the normal first rib either by a true joint or by fusion (Fig. 3.4). Incomplete cervical ribs are 0.5–3 cm long and invariably have a very tight, thick ligament extending from the tip of the cervical rib to the first rib (Fig. 3.5). Both complete and incomplete cervical ribs lie in the midst of the middle scalene muscle where their presence renders the scalene triangle tighter than triangles without cervical ribs.

Anomalous first ribs developed congenitally and are thinner, tend to lie more cephalad, and

Fig. 3.4 Complete cervical
rib with true joint to first rib
(Reprinted with permission
from Sanders [7], p. 1868.
With permission from
Elsevier)

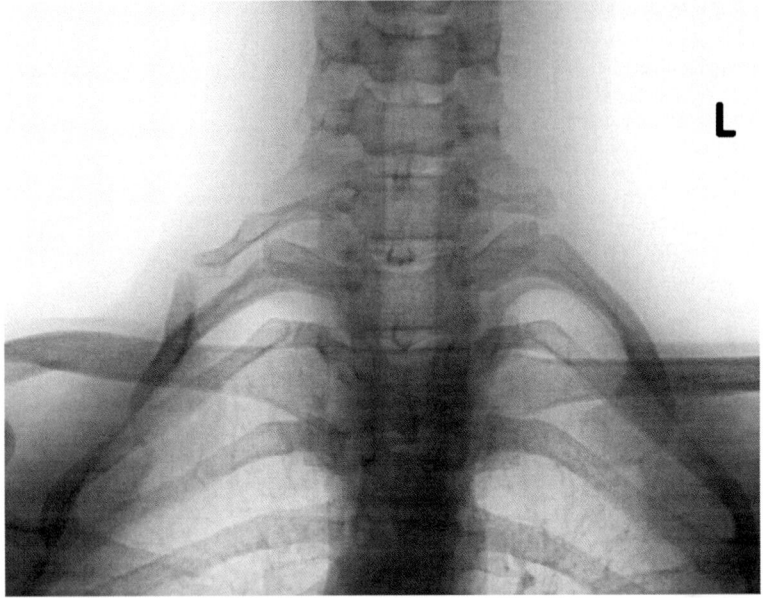

Fig. 3.4 Complete cervical rib with true joint to first rib (Reprinted with permission from Sanders [7], p. 1868. With permission from Elsevier)

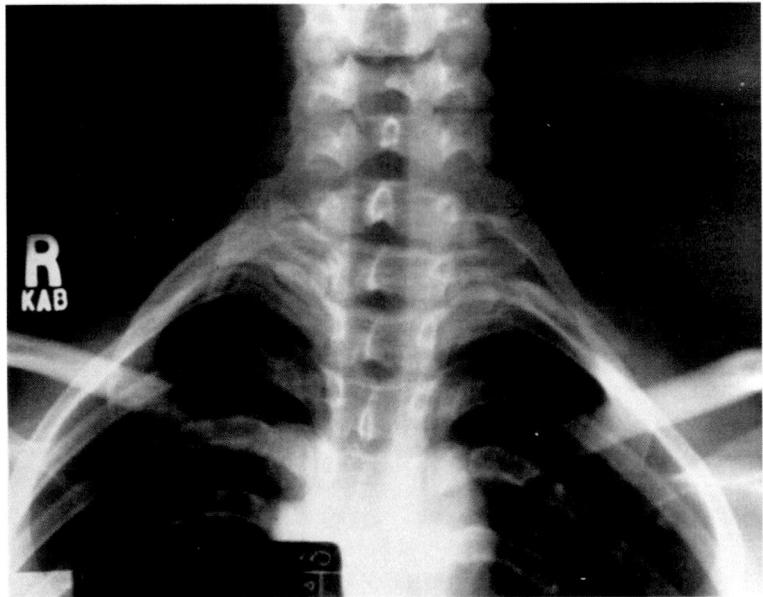

Fig. 3.5 Incomplete cervical ribs (Reprinted with permission from Sanders and Haug [2]. With permission from Lippincott Williams & Wilkins)

usually fuse to the second rib rather than the sternum as do normal first ribs. Seen on X-rays, anomalous first ribs are difficult to differentiate from cervical ribs. The best way to recognize them is to identify the T1 transverse process of the normal first rib on the contralateral side and see if the abnormal rib arises from the T1 or the C7 transverse process (Fig. 3.6).

From a clinical viewpoint both cervical and anomalous first ribs act in the same way, and differentiation between the two is primarily of academic interest only. Either can cause subclavian artery (ATOS) or brachial plexus (NTOS) compression. We have also seen one case of venous obstruction by an anomalous first rib causing VTOS.

Fig. 3.6 Anomalous right first rib. Note the normal second ribs bilaterally. Then note the normal left first rib and the anomalous right first rib both arising from transverse processes of T1 (Reprinted with permission from Sanders [7], p. 1869. With permission from Elsevier)

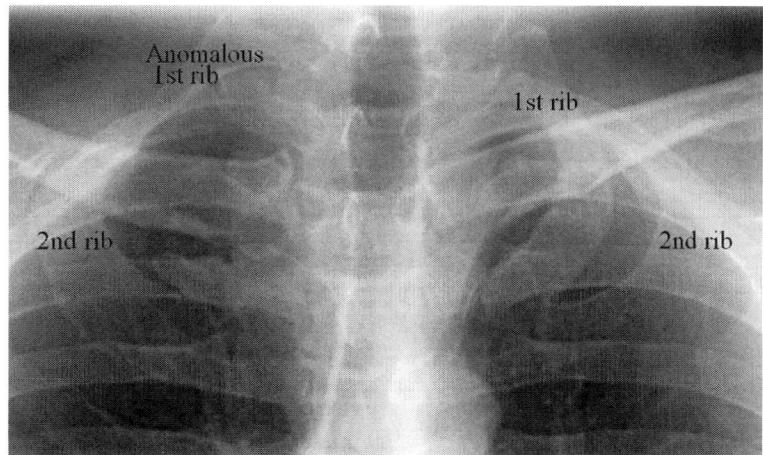

Cervical and anomalous first ribs are usually predisposing causes of NTOS. The majority of patients who posses them are asymptomatic. When symptoms of NTOS occur, it is usually following some type of hyperextension neck injury [8].

Ligaments and Bands

A variety of ligaments and bands attached to the first rib have been identified and classified [9]. These structures are present in 63 % of the normal population [10] and, as such, they are at best predisposing factors rather than causative factors of NTOS.

Nerves

In addition to the five nerve roots and their branches comprising the brachial plexus, other nerves also lie in the thoracic outlet area and are of extreme surgical importance. These include the phrenic, long thoracic, dorsal scapular, second intercostal brachial cutaneous, and supraclavicular nerves plus the cervical sympathetic chain.

Brachial Plexus (BP): The plexus arises from nerve roots C5 to C8 plus T1. The five nerve roots and the lower, middle, and upper trunks lie in the scalene triangle. The anterior and posterior divisions and cords form at the level of the costoclavicular space. By the time the BP reaches the pectoral space the cords and branches have formed (Fig. 3.7).

Phrenic nerve: The phrenic n. arises from branches of C3, C4, and C5. The C3 and C4 branches unite cephalad to the thoracic outlet area. As the combined two branches descend they cross the anterior scalene muscle (ASM) from lateral to medial (Fig. 3.1b). The C5 branch usually joins C3 and C4 near the spot where these two branches begin crossing the ASM, but the exact place where C5 joins them is quite variable. In some patients the C5 branch runs separately over ASM and may join the other two branches in the chest, and in a few patients (13 %) the C5 branch remains separate all the way to the diaphragm (when this occurs the C5 branch is called the accessory phrenic nerve) [12]. When performing supraclavicular scalenectomy it is important to identify the phrenic nerve (and any accessory phrenic nerves) before dissecting the ASM to recognize and avoid injuring them. The phrenic runs on the medial side of ASM in 84 % of necks but remains on the lateral side in 16 % [12].

Long thoracic nerve: The long thoracic nerve is formed by branches of C5, C6, and C7 with the C6 branch being the largest and most important. C5 and C6 branches arise cephalad to the scalene muscles and travel through the belly of middle scalene muscle (MSM) where they unite forming a single nerve. As the single nerve descends it exits the MSM, crosses the lateral edge of first rib (Fig. 3.1b), picks up the C7

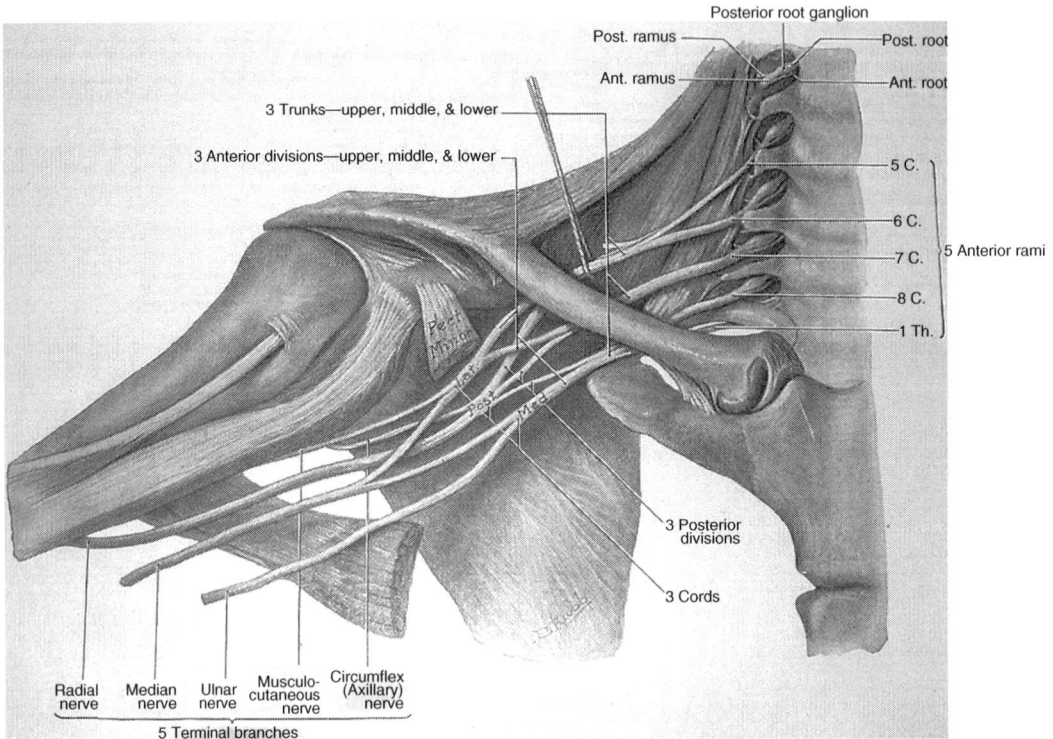

Posterior root ganglion
Post. ramus
Ant. ramus
Post. root
Ant. root
3 Trunks—upper, middle, & lower
3 Anterior divisions—upper, middle, & lower
5 C.
6 C.
7 C.
5 Anterior rami
8 C.
1 Th.
3 Posterior divisions
3 Cords
Radial nerve | Median nerve | Ulnar nerve | Musculo-cutaneous nerve | Circumflex (Axillary) nerve
5 Terminal branches

Fig. 3.7 Brachial plexus. Above the clavicle where the scalene triangle lies, the plexus is present as five nerve roots (C5 through T1) forming three trunks. Just below the clavicle in the costoclavicular space the trunks are starting to form divisions. Where the plexus travels through the pectoralis minor space the cords and branches appear (Reprinted from Grant [11]. With permission from Lippincott Williams & Wilkins)

branch, and eventually innervates the serratus anterior muscle. The C7 branch arises from the posterior aspect of C7, 2–4 cm below the top of ASM. It is a small branch which descends below the clavicle before it joins C5 and C6. However, in a minority of patients the C7 branch unites with the other two branches in the belly of MSM. When performing middle scale**notomy** or scale**nectomy** it is vital to dissect a few fibers at a time until the long thoracic branches are identified so they can be preserved.

Dorsal scapular nerve: The dorsal scapular nerve is the first branch arising from the C5 nerve root. It usually arises close to the C5 branch of the long thoracic nerve and the two branches descend a short distance together until the dorsal scapular nerve separates in the cephalic part of the MSM exiting through the lateral edge of that muscle and descending to innervate the rhomboid muscles and a portion of the levator scapulae muscle. Unlike the long thoracic nerve branches, the dorsal scapular nerve is only on the superior-lateral edge of MSM dissections; it is often not seen and easy to avoid.

Cervical sympathetic nerve chain: The cervical sympathetic nerve chain lies on the anterior surface of the cervical transverse processes, and is not seen when performing supraclavicular scalenectomy. However, when cautery is used to control bleeding from the MSM at the transverse process of scalene muscle origins, the electric current can reach the sympathetic nerve chain causing a Horner's syndrome. The Horner's may heal itself after a few months, but in some patients it is permanent. This can be avoided surgically by not dividing the scalenes on the transverse processes. It is best to stay at least a few mm away.

Fig. 3.8 Relationship of subclavian vein between clavicle and first rib. Subclavian vein can easily be compressed by costoclavicular ligament, subclavius tendon, or anterior scalene muscle (Reprinted with permission from Sanders and Haug [2], p. 236. With permission from Lippincott Williams & Wilkins)

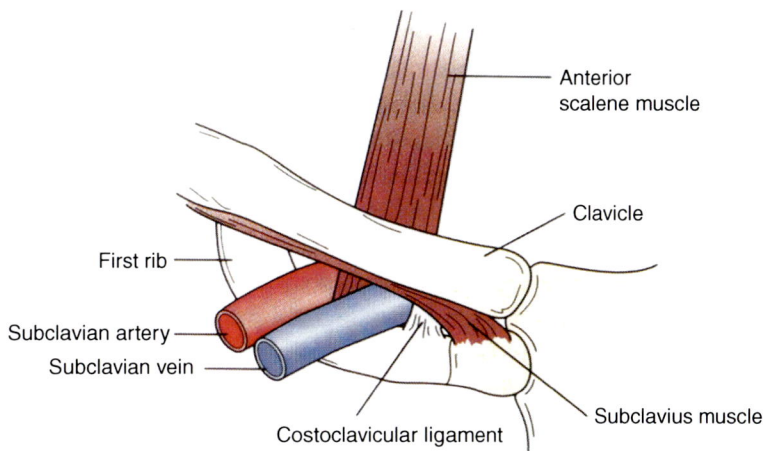

Subclavian and Axillary Vessels

The axillary artery and vein are continuations of subclavian vessels as they move laterally beneath the pectoralis minor muscle. Each vessel has a few small branches, but functionally the axillary artery and subclavian artery are regarded as a single large vessel traversing the thoracic outlet (the same is true of their accompanying veins). Only the subclavian artery lies in the scalene triangle while the subclavian vein lies anterior to the triangle, anterior to the ASM.

The subclavian vein is bounded by the subclavius tendon above, first rib below, ASM laterally, and costoclavicular ligament medially (Fig. 3.8). When the vein lies a little too medial, it lies against the costoclavicular ligament which sets up conditions for venous injury and subsequent thrombosis.

Prevenous phrenic nerve: In over 90 % of subjects the phrenic nerve descends into the chest *posterior* to the subclavian vein. In 5–7 % of patients, however, the phrenic lies superficial to the vein [13–15], and in this circumstance can partially obstruct the vein, a situation which has twice been reported [2, 16] (Fig. 3.9).

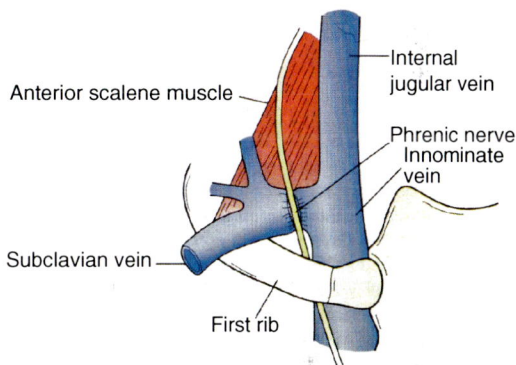

Scalene and Pectoralis Minor Muscles

The ASM and MSM originate at the transverse processes of the cervical spine and insert on the first rib. Hyperextension neck injuries stretch and

Fig. 3.9 Prevenous (anterior) phrenic nerve obstructing the subclavian vein (Reprinted with permission from Sanders and Haug [2], p. 237. With permission from Lippincott Williams & Wilkins)

tear some of the muscle fibers which then heal in part by forming scar tissue. The scarred muscle replaces the normal soft muscle which compresses the nerves of the brachial plexus causing the symptoms of NTOS.

The pectoralis minor muscle (PMM) originates on the anterior surfaces of ribs 3, 4, and 5 and inserts on the coracoid process of the scapula after passing over the top of the neurovascular bundle. When surgically dividing the PMM at the coracoid, removing 2 cm of the muscle will prevent the muscle end from reattaching to the top of the neurovascular bundle. Because the pectoral nerve to the pectoralis major muscle runs through PMM to reach the pectoralis major, care must be taken to avoid excising too much PMM to protect the pectoralis nerve.

Thoracic Duct

In the left neck the thoracic duct lies just posterior and inferior to the clavicle in the scalene fat pad. In addition, a fine network of tiny lymph channels run along the internal jugular vein. The lymph vessels are best avoided by being aware of the normal location of these structures. In supraclavicular TOS operations in the left neck, by avoiding dissection of the fat pad below the clavicle and by avoiding separating the fat pad from the internal jugular vein, lymph leaks are minimized. Following these guidelines will reduce lymphatic leaks, but will not totally eliminate them. In the right neck the only lymphatics are along the internal jugular vein, and lymph leaks in the right neck are rare.

Distribution of Pathology

The scalene triangle has traditionally been thought to be the space involved in over 95 % of patients with NTOS. Since recognizing the neurogenic pectoralis minor syndrome (nPMS) in 2004, more than 75 % of patients we have seen for NTOS seem to have nPMS; 70 % of them combined with NTOS (a double crush syndrome [17]) while the other 30 % have nPMS alone (unpublished data by author RJS).

References

1. Sanders RJ, Rao NM. The forgotten pectoralis minor syndrome: 100 operations for pectoralis minor syndrome alone or accompanied by neurogenic thoracic outlet syndrome. Ann Vasc Surg. 2010;24:701–8.
2. Sanders RJ, Haug CE. Thoracic outlet syndrome: a common sequela of neck injuries. Philadelphia: JB Lippincott; 1991. p. 237.
3. Wright IS. The neurovascular syndrome produced by hyperabduction of the arms. Am Heart J. 1945; 29:1–19.
4. Roos DB, Owens JC. Thoracic outlet syndrome. Arch Surg. 1966;93:71–4.
5. Haven H. Neurocirculatory scalenus anticus syndrome in the presence of developmental defects of the first rib. Yale J Biol Med. 1939;11:443–8.
6. Gruber W. Ueber die halsrippen des menschen mit vergleichend-anatomischen. Bemerkungen: St. Petersburg; 1869.
7. Sanders RJ. Thoracic outlet syndrome: general considerations. In: Cronenwett JL, Johnston KW, editors. Rutherford's vascular surgery. 7th ed. Philadelphia: Saunders; 2010. p. 1868.
8. Sanders RJ, Hammond SH. Management of cervical ribs and anomalous first ribs causing neurogenic thoracic outlet syndrome. J Vasc Surg. 2002;36:51–6.
9. Roos DB. New concepts of thoracic outlet syndrome that explain etiology, symptoms, diagnosis, and treatment. Vasc Surg. 1979;13:313–21.
10. Juvonen T, Satta J, Laitala P, Luukkonen K, Nissinen J. Anomalies at the thoracic outlet are frequent in the general population. Am J Surg. 1995;170:33–7.
11. Grant JCB. An atlas of anatomy. Baltimore: Williams & Wilkins Co.; 1947. 12.
12. Sanders RJ, Roos DB. The surgical anatomy of the scalene triangle. Contemp Surg. 1989;35:11–6.
13. Schroeder WE, Green FR. Phrenic nerve injuries; report of a case. Anatomical and experimental researches, and critical review of the literature. Am J Med Sci. 1902;123:196–220.
14. Hovelacque A, Monod O, Evrard H, Beuzart J. Etude anatomique du nerf phrenique pre-veineux. Ann Anat Pathol. 1936;13:518–22.
15. Hughes ESR. Venous obstruction in the upper extremity. Br J Surg. 1948;36:155–63.
16. Jackson NJ, Nanson EM. Intermittent subclavian vein obstruction. Br J Surg. 1961;49:303–6.
17. Upton ARM, McComas AJ. The double crush in nerve-entrapment syndromes. Lancet. 1973;2:359–62.

Clinical Incidence and Prevalence: Basic Data on the Current Scope of the Problem

Jason T. Lee, Sheldon E. Jordan, and Karl A. Illig

Abstract

The incidence and prevalence of TOS in the US is somewhat of an enigma, largely due to the absence of objective criteria for diagnosis and inconsistent reporting standards, but there are approximately 2,000 to 2,500 first rib resections performed in the US per year. This is a disease of younger individuals that has significant impact on the working cohort and can lead to significant disability and lost productivity if not recognized and treated. Surgery done for TOS in the United States is performed mostly for neurogenic reasons, and with excellent outcomes as a whole. Morbidity and mortality is minimal, and the majority of operations are being performed by vascular surgeons. The best outcomes are found in centers of higher volume and in teaching institutions. A better understanding of the incidence and prevalence of this condition will help the primary care physicians who initially hear about vague complaints and symptoms and must recognize these quickly enough to refer to the appropriate specialist for prompt therapy.

J.T. Lee, MD (✉)
Department of Surgery,
Stanford University Medical Center,
300 Pasteur Drive, Suite H3600,
Stanford, CA 94305, USA
e-mail: jtlee@stanford.edu

S.E. Jordan, MD, FAAN
Department of Neurology,
Neurological Associates of West Los Angeles,
2811 Wilshire Blvd, Suite 790,
Santa Monica, CA 90403, USA
e-mail: shellyj@aol.com

K.A. Illig, MD
Department of Surgery, Division of Vascular Surgery,
University of South Florida,
2 Tampa General Circle, STC 7016,
Tampa, FL 33606, USA
e-mail: killig@health.usf.edu

Thoracic outlet syndrome (TOS) continues to be a controversial diagnosis. Initially described in 1818, the term "TOS" was coined in 1956 by Peet et al. [1], and can grossly be categorized as vascular (arterial or venous) or neurogenic. While patients with vascular TOS present more objectively due to reproducible abnormalities, the lack of uniform imaging and diagnostic criteria for neurogenic TOS makes estimations of the overall incidence and prevalence of TOS particularly problematic, and in fact there has been significant controversy in some circles as to even the very existence of NTOS [2, 3].

Part of the diagnostic dilemma that impedes our understanding of the epidemiology of TOS is

K.A. Illig et al. (eds.), *Thoracic Outlet Syndrome*,
DOI 10.1007/978-1-4471-4366-6_4, © Springer-Verlag London 2013

historical, and stems from the strict diagnostic criteria of "true" NTOS outlined by Gilliatt et al. in 1970 [4]. Distinct anatomic and electrophysiologic findings include low compound muscle action potentials in the thenar and intrinsic muscles, abnormal sensory conduction of the ulnar nerve, prolonged F-wave latency of the ulnar nerve, and abnormal sensory conduction of the medial antebrachial cutaneous nerve. Because it is rare that patients evaluated meet these criteria for true NTOS (estimated at one case per million population), Wilbourn introduced the phrase "disputed" or nonspecific NTOS (NNTOS) [3]. Symptoms of patients with NNTOS will typically include arm discomfort, paresthesias of the inner surface of the hand and forearm, and weakness and atrophy of the thenar and intrinsic hand muscles of the affected side.

In a review of most series of surgery for neurogenic TOS, it is likely the majority of surgical patients include nonspecific NTOS, and when that is taken into account, most agree that neurogenic TOS is much more common than vascular TOS at a 20:1 ratio [5]. In terms of actual incidence in the United States population, estimates of cases of TOS range from 3 to 80 per 1,000 population [6]. Again, however, poor diagnostic criteria and lack of uniform definitions make this number an estimate, and given not all patients are surgical candidates or eventually get referred to surgery it makes the estimate potentially less accurate. One report found that patients with TOS are seen by an average of 4.7 physicians before appropriate conservative measures are instituted and by 6.7 physicians before surgery is performed [7].

Knowing that all forms of TOS are related to usage of the upper extremities, most consider the basic pathophysiology related to overuse injury, which further helps us understand and anticipate the population at risk. Patients with neurogenic varieties of TOS usually present in their 30s–50s and are more often women, with up to half of patients having a history of a hyperextension neck or shoulder injury such from an automobile accident or a fall to the floor [8]. Also very common is a work-related injury caused by repetitive movements or static posture. Occupations including secretarial work, manual labor, lifting of objects for delivery, truck drivers, and even surgeons are considered high-risk occupations for TOS. Predisposing anatomic factors to TOS include cervical ribs, anomalous first ribs, and congenitally narrowed scalene triangles. Cervical ribs are present in less than 1 % of the general population and are implicated as a predisposing factor in surgical TOS cases. Another common presentation is athletes with repetitive upper limb movements including swimmers, divers, water polo players, rowers, baseball pitchers, and football quarterbacks [9]. Athletes do not necessarily have a higher incidence, though, of TOS. Patients with anatomic risk factors will more often have vascular TOS, particularly venous TOS, in addition to neurogenic varieties of TOS, and often present in their 20s–30s. It is thought that arterial TOS, likely the most rare of all forms of TOS, is the most common cause of acute arterial thrombosis of the upper extremities in patients younger than 40 [10].

While most experts believe that obvious anatomic abnormalities coupled with TOS likely have a good outcome when the anatomy is corrected surgically, unfortunately the majority of patients do not have a cervical rib, abnormal band, or abnormal muscle slip. This leads to often conservative approaches when it comes to surgical intervention for TOS, particularly for NTOS that accounts for over 90 % of cases. To better understand the national perspective on surgery for TOS, we reviewed a decade's experience from United States administrative databases to get a snapshot of outcomes related to surgery for TOS [11].

ICD-9 procedure codes for rib resection and scalenectomy were linked back to specific diagnostic codes for either axillary/subclavian aneurysm or embolism (arterial TOS), subclavian DVT or thrombolysis procedure (venous TOS), and all others were considered operated upon for neurogenic etiologies. Over the past decade the number of cases performed for TOS in the United States remained relatively stable (Fig. 4.1). Of the 25,642 TOS operations coded in the National Inpatient Sample over 10 years, 96.7 % were done for neurogenic causes, 2.8 % for venous issues, and 0.5 % for arterial pathology. Most operations (<75 %) are performed in teaching hospitals, and the majority (>50 %) are done by

Fig. 4.1 The number of first rib resections performed in the United States from 1998 to 2007 (Reprinted from Lee et al. [11]. with permission from Elsevier)

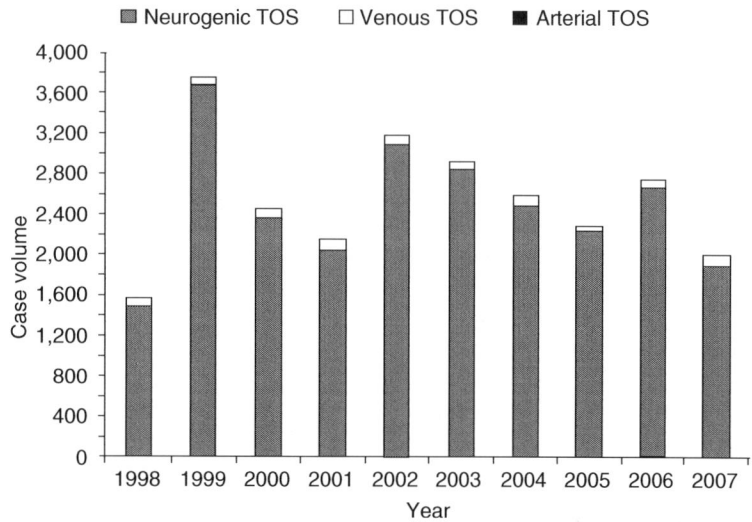

vascular surgeons. Neurogenic patients tend to be in their 30s–40s, compared to venous TOS patients in their 20s–30s, confirming what was postulated and observed in previous studies. Most importantly, high volume centers (>15 cases/year) outperformed low-volume centers in terms of lower complication rates, and has also been corroborated in teaching hospitals vs. non-teaching hospitals [12].

In summary, the incidence and prevalence of TOS in the United States is somewhat of an enigma. Poor diagnostic and radiographic confirmation challenge the accuracy of making a diagnosis of neurogenic TOS, and the relatively rarity of vascular forms of TOS compared to neurogenic type TOS further impairs accurate record keeping. It is clear though this is a disease of younger individuals that has significant impact on the working cohort and can lead to significant disability and lost productivity if not recognized and treated. Surgery done for TOS in the United States is performed mostly for neurogenic reasons, and with excellent outcomes as a whole. Morbidity and mortality is minimal, and the majority of operations are being performed by vascular surgeons. The best outcomes are found in centers of higher volume and in teaching institutions, which is not a surprise, given the nuances of both the diagnostic and treatment algorithms for surgical intervention. Future studies will need to focus on

better delineation and distinguishing forms of TOS to better recognize presentations and cohorts at higher risk for disability. Finally, a better understanding of the incidence and prevalence will help the primary care physicians who initially hear about vague complaints and symptoms and must recognize these quickly enough to refer to the appropriate specialist for prompt therapy.

Editorial Note: *Frequency of Undiagnosed Thoracic Outlet Syndrome in Medical Office Workers*

In our UCLA Vascular Surgery affiliated clinic, we prospectively evaluated subjects to determine the prevalence of NTOS in office workers not seeking medical attention. Twenty five office workers were examined with stress maneuvers, ultrasound examinations and application of a sensitive symptom survey instrument to detect mild levels of disability in everyday activities (CBSQ). Seven (28 %) complained of pain, fatigue and paresthesias with overhead activity on the CBSQ and had concordant symptoms with EAST consistent with a subclinical NTOS condition. Of the seven subclinical cases of NTOS, 5 (71 %) obliterated the radial pulse with 90° arm abduction and 4 (57 %) had ultrasound velocities of over 300 cm/s or showed an occlusion pattern for the subclavian artery during abduction. Five out of 18 (28 %) of the others without NTOS had loss of radial pulses with abduction and only 2 (11 %) had ultrasound velocities over 300 cm/s with abduction. Positional symptoms and signs are ubiquitous in subjects not seeking medical attention.

References

1. Peet RM, Henriksen JD, Anderson TP. Thoracic-outlet syndrome: evaluation of a therapeutic exercise program. Mayo Clin Proc. 1956;31:281–7.
2. Roos DB. The thoracic outlet syndrome is underrated. Arch Neurol. 1990;47:327–8.
3. Wilbourn A. The thoracic outlet syndrome is over-diagnosed. Arch Neurol. 1990;47:328–30.
4. Gilliatt RW, Le Quesne PM, Logue V, et al. Wasting of the hand associated with a cervical rib or band. J Neurol Neurosurg Psychiatry. 1970;33:615–24.
5. Lee JT, Laker S, Fredericson M. Thoracic outlet syndrome. PM R. 2010;2:64–70.
6. Huang JH, Zager EL. Thoracic outlet syndrome. Neurosurgery. 2004;55:897–902.
7. Landry GJ, Moneta GL, Taylor Jr LM, Edwards JM, Porter JM. Long-term functional outcome of neurogenic thoracic outlet syndrome in surgically and conservatively treated patients. J Vasc Surg. 2001;33:312–7.
8. Sanders RJ, Hammond SL, Rao NM. Thoracic outlet syndrome: a review. Neurologist. 2008;14:365–73.
9. Richardson AB. Thoracic outlet syndrome in aquatic athletes. Clin Sports Med. 1999;18:361–78.
10. Davidovic LB, Koncar IB, Pejkic SD, et al. Arterial complications of thoracic outlet syndrome. Am Surg. 2009;75:235–9.
11. Lee JT, Dua MM, Hernandez-Boussard TM, Illig KA. Surgery for TOS: a nationwide perspective. J Vasc Surg. 2011;53:100S–1S.
12. Chang DA, Lidor AO, Matsen SL, Freischlag JA. Reported in-hospital complications following rib resections for neurogenic TOS. Ann Vasc Surg. 2007;21:564–70.

Part II

Neurogenic TOS: General Principles

While exact proportion varies widely by practice, the majority of patients with problems at the thoracic outlet present with neurogenic compression – neurogenic thoracic outlet syndrome (NTOS). Proportional estimates in surgical populations range from 60 % (practitioners with an interest in venous TOS) to 98 % (the "classic" textbook description); neurologists may see only those with neurogenic symptoms. NTOS is felt to be caused by compression of the brachial plexus within the scalene triangle, as a result of narrowing of the space (bony deformity, muscular injury and fibrosis, or congenital predisposition) or inflammation of the plexus itself. Very closely related is the concept, only recognized in the past decade, that the nerves can also be compressed by the insertion of the pectoralis minor muscle, pectoralis minor syndrome (PMS). Whether a subgroup of NTOS or a separate entity that falls within the "double crush" concept is unknown, but as it is also commonly treated by NTOS physicians it is thoroughly dealt with here as well.

The classic patient with NTOS is found to have four general groups of symptoms and signs: Pain and numbness in the extremity, pain in the areas surrounding the base of the neck (including axilla, chest wall, breast, upper back, neck, and head), tenderness at the area of pathology (scalene triangle in classic NTOS and deltopectoral groove in PMS), and worsening of symptoms, especially in the hand and forearms, with maneuvers that either close off the triangle (arms overhead) or stretch the plexus (arms dangling; walking or driving with the arm unsupported). In addition, the majority, if thoroughly examined, report a history of trauma (some believe that trauma underlies all cases of NTOS, and if truly not described, that this trauma was minor enough to be forgotten). Many, many people are referred to TOS-focused practices with shoulder and hand symptoms, and the job of an interested practitioner is to rule out carpal tunnel syndrome, ulnar nerve entrapment, intrinsic shoulder problems, disk herniation, and many other problems. This is not at all an easy task, in part because of the lack of objective diagnostic criteria for this syndrome, and, at a deeper level, a lack of consensus as to what the syndrome is defined as. We have no gold standard, which significantly impairs our ability to identify lesions seen on imaging, as well.

The treatment of NTOS has evolved over the years, with surgical solutions ranging from scalenectomy alone to complete removal of most of the muscles and the entire rib with extensive neurolysis from the supraclavicular approach. Recently, significant interest has arisen in both diagnostic and therapeutic block techniques, which, if done correctly, seems to correlate well with surgical outcomes.

Essentially no prospective randomized data exist in this field. However, our knowledge is shaped by a respectfully large body of individual series, at times spanning more than three decades and describing more than 1,000 patients. Some complain that the patients never get any better, while others feel that their success rates with surgery are excellent. The latter group has somehow figured out how to identify those patients who

truly "have" NTOS – in other words, NTOS defined as those who improve with decompression done correctly. This suggests that there really is such a group – and our task, in the early twenty-first century, is to translate the "gut feelings" of those who see success into objective criteria that all can use.

The following section will explore this subject in detail, and present conventional and alternative points of view for each step in the treatment of these patients. Many surgical and nonsurgical options exist, and the benefits and failings of each will be discussed. Many, many patients see dramatic, life-changing benefit from proper treatment of this syndrome. How do we translate this into better patient care today, and how do we analyze such results to bring treatment of this syndrome to the same level as the rest of what we do?

NTOS for the Primary Care Team: When to Consider the Diagnosis?

Karl A. Illig and Dean M. Donahue

Abstract

Thoracic outlet syndrome (TOS) is a real but uncommon syndrome, and, as a result diagnosis is often delayed and referral to a specialist frequently comes later than the patient and physician would like. It is actually a spectrum of diseases, potentially involving the arteries, veins, or nerves (and these usually occur separately). By far the most common is *neurogenic* TOS (NTOS). This can be thought of as a chronic compressive brachial plexus problem – essentially a chronic compartment syndrome of the brachial plexus.

Considerable controversy and confusion exists regarding this problem. The entity is also associated with a high incidence of insurance claims, workman's compensation issues, and litigation. For these reasons and more, the current role of the primary care physician is probably identification that this problem potentially exists and referral to an interested and competent specialist.

In general, a putative diagnosis depends on three things: proper history, suggestive physical examination, and absence of obvious alternative diagnoses. An example of the first is a patient who complains of shoulder, neck, head, chest and arm problems with activity, elevation, or dangling, the second one with supraclavicular or infraclavicular tenderness, and the third absence of obvious cervical disk, rotator cuff, or carpal tunnel pathology. If these general findings are present, referral to a specialist is indicated.

K.A. Illig, MD (✉)
Department of Surgery, Division of Vascular Surgery,
University of South Florida, 2 Tampa General Circle,
STC 7016, Tampa, FL 33606, USA
e-mail: killig@health.usf.edu

D.M. Donahue, MD
Department of Thoracic Surgery, Massachusetts
General Hospital, Blake 1570, 55 Fruit Street,
Boston, MA 02114, USA
e-mail: donahue.dean@mgh.harvard.edu

Introduction

Thoracic outlet syndrome (TOS) is a real but uncommon syndrome, and, as a result, diagnosis is often delayed and referral to a specialist frequently comes later than the patient and physician would like. It is actually a spectrum of diseases, potentially involving the arteries, veins, or nerves (and these usually occur separately). By far the most common is *neurogenic* TOS (NTOS). This can be thought of as a chronic compressive brachial plexus problem – essentially a chronic compartment syndrome of the brachial plexus. Such compression can occur at the scalene triangle, pectoralis minor insertion site, or both.

Considerable controversy and confusion exists regarding this problem – for example, there has not been a multi-author textbook on this topic until now. The entity is also associated with a high incidence of insurance claims, workman's compensation issues, and litigation. For these reasons and more, the current role of the primary care physician is probably identification that this problem potentially exists and referral to an interested and competent specialist.

In general, a putative diagnosis depends on three things: proper history, suggestive physical examination, and absence of obvious alternative diagnoses. The classic example of the first is a patient who complains of shoulder, neck, head, chest and arm problems with activity, elevation, or dangling, the second one with supraclavicular or infraclavicular tenderness, and the third absence of obvious cervical disk, rotator cuff, or carpal tunnel pathology. If these general findings are present, referral to a specialist is indicated.

Epidemiology

NTOS is a rare entity, and as such the true incidence of NTOS is unknown – ominously, estimates vary from 1 to 80,000 per million! [1, 2]. Approximately 3,000 first rib resections are performed in the United States per year, an incidence of ten per million per year who undergo operation for any form of TOS. One of the difficulties in assessing the incidence of NTOS is the lack of reliable and reproducible sets of signs, diagnostic criteria, and objective laboratory tests, the latter factor being perhaps most important. NTOS is a candidate for the most poorly understood entity "commonly" seen in primary care and general surgical practices. A busy TOS surgeon serving a population of about 2,000,000 persons will see, for example, about five or ten patients per month (only half of whom will have obvious NTOS),

suggesting a true "new patient incidence" of about five per million persons per year. It is certainly an entity that most primary care providers should be familiar with.

Diagnosis

NTOS is a rare disease for which diagnostic criteria are subjective and medicolegal and workman's compensation issues significant, so most feel that the goal of the primary care physician should not be to make the definitive diagnosis (or provide definitive treatment) but rather to identify the group of patients who have a fairly high likelihood of having the syndrome. In other words, his or her level of suspicion should maximize sensitivity – all patients who might have TOS should be identified, even at the risk of some false positives. Specificity (everyone you think has TOS actually has it, but you miss some of those who have more subtle symptoms) and accuracy (you are always correct) are less important. Sending a patient to a specialist who is subsequently found to have something else is quite inexpensive and safe (and results in a happy patient), but denying early diagnosis and proper treatment to someone who ends up having NTOS is damaging to all. In other words, the primary care provider should cast a wide net and have a low index of suspicion. Many patients suffer symptoms for years without the diagnosis being considered, so increasing the level of suspicion for this entity will be of significant value.

The task of this chapter is thus to identify factors which should trigger an acceptable level of suspicion at the primary care level and lead to specialty referral. In general, there are three things which should trigger consideration of this diagnosis: An appropriate history, appropriate signs on physical examination, and absence of more common alternative diagnoses.

History

NTOS is essentially a compressive brachial plexopathy or "compartment syndrome" of the brachial plexus. Two reasonable hypotheses exist: first, the space surrounding the plexus is too small for the structures that pass through it, and, second, there is inflammation of the plexus (the plexus is "too big"). Such compression potentially occurs at two locations – the scalene triangle and the insertion of the pectoralis minor muscle on the coracoid process of the scapula (See Chap. 15).

Such compression causes temporary or permanent dysfunction of the nerves. Almost always, this injury is manifest as sensory changes; motor changes occur very late and, if present, indicate longstanding disease (see Chap. 10). Clinically, this is manifest as peripheral pain and numbness. Because local sensory nerves exit the plexus after the site of compression, it is very common to see upper arm, axillary, chest wall, trapezius, and occipital pain (such pain can also be the result of spasm and/or compensatory activation of neck muscles). Such a problem is often created by an event that stretches the plexus itself – a side-to-side whiplash injury, an injury that stretches the arm, or chronic workplace injury.

Exacerbating factors are critically important. Most commonly the symptoms described above are exacerbated by one of two things: Things that stretch the plexus (walking or driving with arms unsupported) or things that narrow the scalene triangle (arms overhead). The presence of either – most notably "it's worse when I put my arms over my head" – is a tipoff that NTOS may be present.

Physical Examination

Findings on examination very closely match what would be expected if this were a compressive problem at the brachial plexus or pectoralis minor insertion site – the area would be tender. Patients with NTOS almost invariably have point tenderness at one of two locations: the scalene triangle, low in the neck anterior to the sternocleidomastoid, or the pectoralis minor insertion site, just inferior to the mid- to medial portion of the clavicle. The typical patient with NTOS will be exquisitely tender to minor palpation, to the point that they violently withdraw. They may also have distal (hand and arm) neurologic symptoms reproduced by even minor palpation in these areas.

It should be noted that loss of pulses with arm abduction is quite common, and does not mean that NTOS (or any problem) exists. However, the subclavian artery runs through the scalene triangle along with the nerves, and thus arterial compression often occurs in patients with NTOS. Although many maneuvers are described, probably the only one of value at this point in the evaluation is the elevated arm stress test (EAST) which, in its simplest form, consists of having the patient perform repetitive hand opening and closing with arms overhead. Patients with NTOS will note (usually immediate) numbness, tingling, and pain on the affected side(s).

The presence of these symptoms and signs do not establish a diagnosis of NTOS, but do indicate that the diagnosis should be considered and further evaluation by an experienced specialist is warranted.

Exclusion of Other Problems

Finally, it is appropriate for the primary care provider to be able to exclude certain problems that may lead to symptoms suggestive of NTOS. The most common is cervical spine disease, which may include pathology of the intervertebral disc, facet or uncovertebral joints. Such a patient will likely not have supraclavicular tenderness, is more likely to have objective motor dysfunction, may have more acute pain, and is more likely to have pain with pressure applied to the vertex with the head extended (Spurling's test). In addition, putting the arm overhead typically relieves the pain of an acutely herniated disk, while it worsens symptoms due to NTOS. Occasionally carpal tunnel syndrome can be confused with NTOS. Such a patient, however, should not have any supraclavicular tenderness, should have minimal to no shoulder, neck, and chest symptoms, and should have tingling and reproduction of symptoms after tapping of the carpal tunnel (Tinel's sign). Rotator cuff pathology can also be confused with NTOS, but such a patient will have tenderness more laterally in the shoulder, absence of numbness and tingling distally, and absence of supraclavicular tenderness.

In general, while absence of supraclavicular or pectoralis minor insertion site tenderness does not necessarily exclude NTOS, any patient with significant tenderness at either of these locations should be considered to have NTOS and referred to an appropriate specialist.

What to Do Next

In general, recognition that NTOS might exist is enough to trigger a proper referral (and enough to gain the lifelong gratitude of your patient). One test is helpful to order before referral: Cervical spine radiographs. It is best to note "possible TOS;" this will alert the radiographer to pay special attention to the presence or absence of cervical ribs – if they are found (in the settings of appropriate symptoms), they significantly increase the chances of TOS in general being present.

What Not to Order

Nerve conduction studies and cross-sectional imaging (CT or MR) have not been shown to affect decision-making or outcomes in patients with NTOS. While the academic and research implications of both are fascinating, this is best left up to the TOS specialist, as protocols are complex, individualized, and primarily of research interest at this time.

Summary

The role of the primary care provider is to have this diagnosis in mind, and because this is a rare disease with substantial morbidity (and medicolegal

risk if not identified in a timely fashion), it is probably best to "cast a wide net" – maximize the sensitivity of one's diagnostic algorithm. As such, any of the following should immediately suggest that NTOS should be considered:

- Hand and arm numbness, tingling, and/or pain worsened by positioning the arms overhead or dangling,
- Hand and arm numbness, tingling, and/or pain with any degree of supraclavicular fossa or infraclavicular point tenderness, and
- Hand and arm numbness, tingling, and/or pain without another clear diagnosis.

These correspond to the three points above: something by history that suggests compression at the brachial plexus, something by exam that suggests inflammation and irritation at the scalene triangle or pectoralis minor insertion site, and absence of other things that are common and obvious. A cervical spine radiograph is the only pre-specialist objective test necessary.

NTOS is a real diagnosis, but one that is often made late – delayed by years in some cases. Outcomes, in turn, depend on the time from symptom onset to therapy (surgical and nonsurgical). If the primary care physician has a reasonable level of suspicion and can make the diagnosis early, he or she has significantly impacted the life of a patient. Do this and you are a hero.

References

1. Wilbourn AJ, Porter JM. Thoracic outlet syndromes. Spine. Spine State Art Rev. 1998;2(4):597–626.
2. Huang JH, Zager EL. Thoracic outlet syndrome. Neurosurgery. 2004;55:897–902 (discussion 902–3).

Anatomy and Pathophysiology of NTOS

6

Richard J. Sanders

Abstract

Neurogenic TOS is usually due to a combination of predisposing factors and a hyperextension neck injury. Predisposing factors include cervical rib variants and anomalous first ribs, a narrow scalene triangle, and various congenital bands and ligaments. The most common trauma is a whiplash injury, usually from a motor vehicle accident. The pathophysiology is felt to begin with trauma to the scalene muscles causing tearing of muscle fibers and hemorrhage with subsequent replacement of the blood with microscopic scar tissue throughout the scalene muscles. The now-tight muscles compress the nerve roots and trunks of the brachial plexus, subsequently causing the classic symptoms of extremity pain, paresthesias, and weakness. Further, the injured scalene muscles lead to neck pain and occipital headaches which are referred from the transverse process muscle origin.

Introduction

The usual etiology of neurogenic thoracic outlet syndrome (NTOS) is the combination of one or more predisposing anatomical variations or anomalies combined with a hyperextension neck injury. The eventual pathology created by this combination of factors is scarred scalene muscles which then compress the brachial plexus to produce symptoms.

R.J. Sanders, MD
Department of Surgery,
HealthONE Presbyterian-St. Lukes Hospital,
4545 E. 9th Ave #240, Denver, CO 80220, USA
e-mail: rsanders@ecentral.com

Predisposing Factors

Relatively minor trauma is a part of life, but some people are more likely than others to develop symptoms of NTOS, probably because they have variations of what is considered normal anatomy. Such a predisposition doesn't cause NTOS, but rather renders a person more likely to become symptomatic when a hyperextension neck injury occurs.

Scalene Muscle Variations Associated with NTOS

The *width of the scalene triangle* varies between 0.1 and 2.2 cm, averaging 1.1 cm [1]. In a cadaver study it was observed that 29 % of

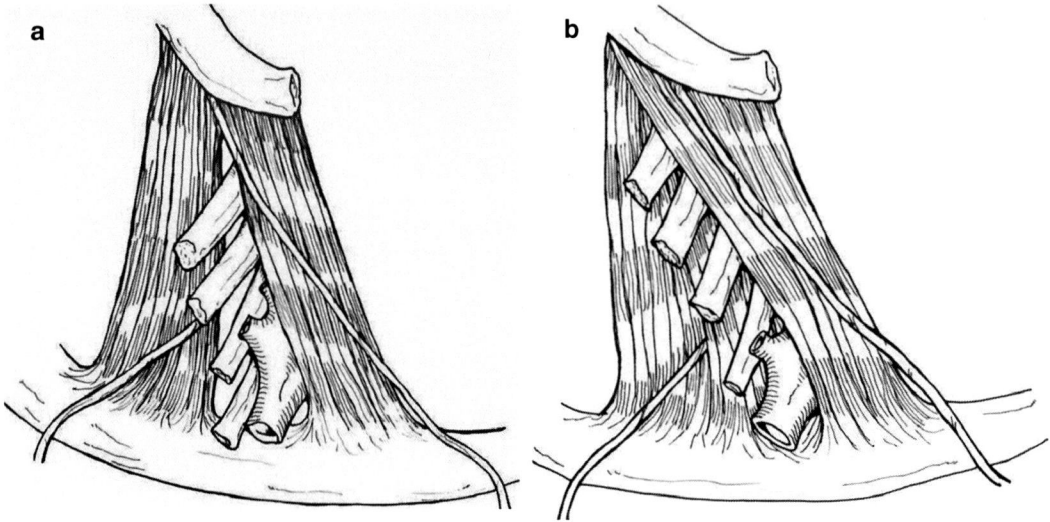

Fig. 6.1 Range of width of scalene triangle. (**a**) Usual width seen in cadavers. This is wider and nerves emerge a little lower than is seen in most NTOS patients. (**b**) Narrow tight triangle, the type seen in most NTOS patients. Nerves emerge higher and are in contact with muscle (Reprinted from Sanders and Roos [2]. With permission from Bobit Publishing)

scalene triangles were narrow compared to 39 % in NTOS patients (Fig. 6.1) [2]. In the same study, *interdigitating muscle fibers* between the anterior (ASM) and middle scalene muscles (MSM) were found to be much more common in patients undergoing operation for NTOS – present in 50 % of cases – than in control cadavers (23 %), a difference that was highly significant. [2]The *emergence of the C5 and C6 nerve roots* were found to be high in the apex of the scalene triangle in 80 % of patients operated on for NTOS as compared to only 40 % of cadaver controls, again highly significant. [2] Finally, *adherence of the ASM to the C5, C6, and C7 nerve roots* was found to be much more common in patients operated upon for NTOS as compared to cadaver controls, being present in 90 % vs. 29 %, 91 % vs. 40 %, and 62 % vs. 14 %, respectively, and *adherence of the MSM to C5 and C6* was found in 61 % of NTOS patients vs. 32 % of controls and 72 % of NTOS patients vs. 35 % of controls respectively. It should be noted that although this may reflect a causative factor, this high incidence of adherence could also be secondary to the original muscle trauma that caused the NTOS [2].

Scalene Muscle Variations That Do Not Correlate with NTOS

Congenital bands and ligaments have been classified into nine groups by Roos [3]. One or more of these are present in the majority of NTOS patients, but also in a high number of asymptomatic controls [4], and because most of the population has some such band it is unlikely that these represent significant predisposing factors for NTOS. In the cadaver study cited above, *splitting of ASM around C5 and C6* was actually more common in cadavers (45 %) than in patients operated upon for NTOS (23 %) [2]. Although this finding has been regarded by some as a predisposing factor, the data suggest the opposite. *Finally, the presence of a scalene minimus muscle* has been suggested as a predisposing factor for NTOS. Scalene minimus muscles, however, are found in as many as 71 % of (normal) cadavers [5].

Cervical and Anomalous First Ribs

Cervical ribs and anomalous first ribs occur in less than 1 % of the population, but the incidence of such anomalies in patients operated upon for

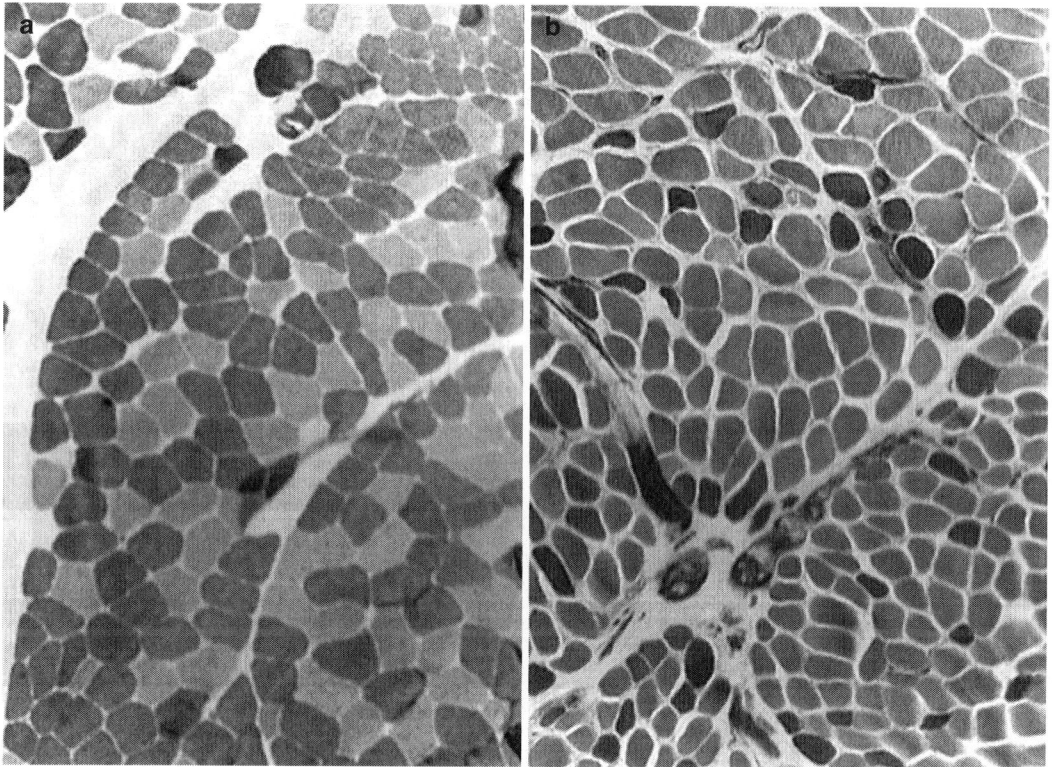

Fig. 6.2 (**a**) Control scalene muscle. Note equal distribution of type I and type II fibers. Also note minimal amount of connective tissue surrounding each muscle cell. (**b**) Scalene muscle of NTOS patient. Note predominance of type I fibers and decrease of type II fibers as well as type II atrophy and anisocytosis. Also note the large increase in connective tissue (or scar tissue) around individual muscle fibers (Reprinted from Sanders and Haug [7]. With permission from Lippincott Williams & Wilkins)

NTOS ranges from 4.5 to 57 % [6]. Most patients with cervical ribs are asymptomatic throughout their lifetimes. The onset of symptoms is preceded by neck trauma in 75 % of patients with incomplete cervical ribs, and in 50 % of patients with complete cervical ribs. In these patients the cervical or anomalous first rib remains a predisposition while neck trauma is still required for the syndrome to develop. However, the presence of an abnormal rib can be highly suggestive in patients who develop symptoms of NTOS without a clear history of neck trauma.

Pathology

Study of scalene muscles resected from NTOS patients has revealed two types of significant changes. First, the incidence of scar tissue (or connective tissue) is three times greater in NTOS patients than in controls (36 % vs. 14.5 %, $p = < 0.001$) (Fig. 6.2). Second, there is a significant reduction of type II fibers (from 47 % average to 22 %) and an increase in type I fibers (from 53 % average to 78 %). The type II fibers that remain, in addition, are atrophic and anisocytotic [8, 9].

Pathophysiology

Post-traumatic Onset

The large majority of NTOS patients give a history of some type of hyper-extension neck injury preceding the onset of symptoms. Whiplash injuries in motor vehicle accidents is the most common cause, but other causes include falls on ice, slippery floors, or downstairs, and athletic injuries. In these patients the usual sequence of symptom development is neck pain within the first 24 h followed within a few days by headaches and pain over the trapezius muscles. Anywhere from a few days to a several weeks later pain moves into the upper extremities and paresthesia develop in the fingers and hands. The major microscopic change seen, as noted above, is a significant increase in scar tissue spread diffusely throughout the scalene muscles.

Putting the history of an injury together with the pattern of symptom development and subsequent muscle pathology, a plausible explanation for the pathophysiology emerges. Following such an injury the initial neck pain is due to two things: cervical spine neck strain and acute tearing of the scalene muscle fibers. There is probably some intramuscular hemorrhage which causes muscle swelling and increased neck pain over the first few days. The symptoms of arm pain and paresthesia that develop in the first few days are probably due to swelling of the injured scalene muscles. If the muscle injury is mild enough so that there is minimal swelling, arm pain and paresthesias may not appear for a few weeks. These later arm and hand symptoms are then due to the healing process within the scalene muscles as intramuscular blood is absorbed and replaced by fibroblasts and collagen, resulting in scarring and overly tight muscles. Since the nerve roots are usually in contact with the scalene muscles, when the muscles become scarred they compress the nerve roots. It should be stressed that even though these muscles appear normal when viewed during surgery, the microscopic picture is not (Fig. 6.2). As discussed above, the predominance of type I and reduction of type II muscle fibers along with the significant fibrosis seen further confirms that there has been significant structural changes in the muscles.

In addition to the objective pathology described above, other lines of evidence further implicate the scalene muscles as the primary site of pathology in most cases. Scalene muscle block with local anesthetic can temporarily relieve symptoms and reverse physical findings within a few minute of injection, and correlates well with outcomes (See Chap. 20). Finally, most clinicians and investigators believe that surgically dividing or removing the scalene muscles is required for successful outcomes after thoracic outlet decompression for NTOS.

Repetitive Stress Injury (RSI)

People who perform repetitive activities (especially with the hands and arms in an awkward or fixed position) such as keyboard entry, assembly line work, sitting in one spot for several hours at a time, or work in an intrinsically awkward position (dentists or hygenists [10]) may also develop NTOS. In these patients multiple points of nerve compression are often seen, including problems at the carpal or cuboid tunnels and/or pectoralis minor insertion site. This observation collectively has been labeled "cumulative trauma syndrome," although the term has not entered widespread use. The underlying cause is felt to be due to the fact that resting muscles are lengthened by various abnormal positions, and activation of these lengthened muscles causes structural damage inside the muscle cells [11–13].

The Role of First Rib

What then is the role of the first rib, and why is first rib resection apparently as successful as scalenectomy in relieving symptoms? The answer may be that in performing first rib resection it is necessary to release the anterior and middle scalene muscles in order to remove the rib. Thus, scalenotomy is an essential part of every first rib resection, and patients improve primarily because anterior and middle scalenotomy was performed, not because the rib was removed. This view is supported by the fact that the results of anterior and middle scalenectomy without first rib resection have been as good as those of scalenectomy with first rib resection in carefully selected patients [14, 15].

Non-traumatic Onset

Finally, a minority of patients seem to spontaneously develop symptoms of NTOS even in the absence of a history of trauma. Although in many of these patients a history of neck trauma will be found with persistent history taking, there is still a small group, less than 15 % in our experience, in whom no history of trauma exists. In some of these patients a cervical rib or anomalous first rib may be the underlying cause, and in many the trauma may have been mild enough to escape the patient's notice (hence not recoverable by history taking). There remain in any practice a small number in whom the cause is obscure.

References

1. Daseler EH, Anson BJ. Surgical anatomy of the subclavian artery and its branches. Surg Gynecol Obstet. 1959;108:149–74.
2. Sanders RJ, Roos DB. The surgical anatomy of the scalene triangle. Contemp Surg. 1989;35:11–6.
3. Roos DB. New concepts of thoracic outlet syndrome that explain etiology, symptoms, diagnosis, and treatment. Vasc Surg. 1979;13:313–21.
4. Juvonen T, Satta J, Laitala P, Luukkonen K, Nissinen J. Anomalies at the thoracic outlet are frequent in the general population. Am J Surg. 1995;170:33–7.
5. Grant JCB. The musculature. In Morris's Human Anatomy, 10th ed. Philadelphia: The Blakeston Co; 1942. p. 419.
6. Sanders RJ, Hammond SH. Management of cervical ribs and anomalous first ribs causing neurogenic thoracic outlet syndrome. J Vasc Surg. 2002;36: 51–6.
7. Sanders RJ, Haug CE. Thoracic outlet syndrome: a common sequela of neck injuries. Philadelphia: Lipppincott; 1991. p. 60.
8. Sanders RJ, Jackson CGR, Banchero N, Pearce WH. Scalene muscle abnormalities in traumatic thoracic outlet syndrome. Am J Surg. 1990;159:231–6.
9. Machleder HI, Moll F, Verity A. The anterior scalene muscle in thoracic outlet compression syndrome: histochemical and morphometric studies. Arch Surg. 1986;121:1141–4.
10. Stockstill JW, Harn SD, Strickland D, Hruska R. Prevalence of upper extremity neuropathy in a clinical dentist population. J Am Dent Assoc. 1993;124: 67–72.
11. Faulkner JA, Brooks SV, Opiteck JA. Injury to skeletal muscle fibers during contractions: conditions and occurrence and prevention. Phys Ther. 1993;73: 911–21.
12. White SG, Sahrmann SA. A movement system balance approach to management of musculoskeletal pain. In: Grant R, editor. Physical therapy of the cervical and thoracic spine. New York: Churchill-Livingstone; 1994. p. 339–57.
13. Mackinnon SE, Novak CB. Clinical commentary: pathogenesis of cumulative trauma disorder. J Hand Surg Am. 1994;19:873–83.
14. Sanders RJ, Pearce WH. The treatment of thoracic outlet syndrome: a comparison of different operations. J Vasc Surg. 1989;10:626–34.
15. Cheng SWK, Reilly LM, Nelken NA, Ellis WV, Stoney RJ. Neurogenic thoracic outlet decompression: rationale for sparing the first rib. Cardiovasc Surg. 1995;3:617–23.

Clinical Presentation of Patients with NTOS

7

Sheldon E. Jordan

Abstract

The diagnosis of Neurogenic Thoracic Outlet Syndrome (NTOS) is often considered in patients presenting with neck, shoulder, and arm pain, sensory disturbance and weakness especially when these complaints are worsened when assuming certain postures or when performing activities such as reaching overhead. The label of NTOS should be considered when it explains a patient's suffering and disability; it is important for the clinician to differentiate ubiquitous complaints of innocuous positional numbness from those features of a condition that really are responsible for the patient's disability. The main goal of the clinician is to determine for whom NTOS targeted therapy would lead to both alleviation of suffering and improve functional impairment.

The task of making the diagnosis and finding patients who may benefit from NTOS targeted treatment starts with the discovery of certain positive features which suggest NTOS; the present chapter outlines this initial step in the diagnostic process. Conditions may mimic NTOS or may be comorbid with it having dramatic effects upon treatment outcomes; these conditions are discussed in Chap. 8.

Introduction

The diagnosis of Neurogenic Thoracic Outlet Syndrome (NTOS) is often considered in patients presenting with neck, shoulder, and arm pain, sensory disturbance and weakness especially when these complaints are worsened when assuming certain postures or when performing activities such as reaching overhead [1]. The label of NTOS should be considered when it explains a patient's suffering and disability; it is important for the clinician to differentiate ubiquitous complaints of innocuous positional numbness from those features of a condition that really are responsible for the patient's disability. The main goal of the clinician is to determine for whom NTOS targeted therapy would lead to both alleviation of suffering and improve functional impairment.

The task of making the diagnosis and finding patients who may benefit from NTOS targeted treatment starts with the discovery of certain positive

S.E. Jordan, MD, FAAN
Department of Neurology, Neurological Associates
of West Los Angeles, 2811 Wilshire Blvd., Suite 790,
Santa Monica, CA 90403, USA
e-mail: shellyj@aol.com

K.A. Illig et al. (eds.), *Thoracic Outlet Syndrome*,
DOI 10.1007/978-1-4471-4366-6_7, © Springer-Verlag London 2013

features which suggest NTOS; the present chapter outlines this initial step in the diagnostic process. Conditions may mimic NTOS or may be comorbid with it having dramatic effects upon treatment outcomes; these conditions are discussed in Chap. 8.

Positive Features that Suggest Possible NTOS

The diagnostic process starts with a search for features that may suggest NTOS in those patients who present with cervicobrachial pain after an acute injury or after a cumulative work related exposure [2–5]. Classically, the positive findings that suggest NTOS include a history of tingling, deadness, or weakness in the upper extremity which are exacerbated by maneuvers that compromise the thoracic outlet (arms overhead) or stretch the plexus (dangling). Similar findings may be elicited by bedside maneuvers that simulate a patient's experience. Pulse obliteration with arm abduction may be found to suggest combined neural and vascular compromise through the thoracic outlet. Actual muscle atrophy may occur on rare occasion. Sensitivity to palpation of the neural elements may be found in the supraclavicular fossa or over the pectoralis tendon insertion. These "classical" features are examined more closely in the following paragraphs.

History of Neurological Symptoms Affected by Position

Patients with NTOS typically have a history of tingling, pins and needles, deadness or electrical sensations, aching arm pain, and/or progressive and rapid fatigue of arm muscles when reaching overhead and in performing repetitive grasping and reaching movements. The absence of recurring positional sensory change, fatigue, or pain would make NTOS unlikely. The presence of a history of positional paresthesias with reaching overhead, although suggestive of NTOS, is nonspecific. In preparation for this chapter we surveyed 25 medical office workers that were not

patients and who were not seeing physicians for upper extremity complaints (unpublished data), and found that positional sensory change that mildly interfered with everyday activities was noted in 44 % of this group. A high prevalence among office workers of subclinical paresthesias separate from those due to carpal tunnel syndrome has been previously reported [6]. Positional sensory change and pain is also found in patients with carpal tunnel syndrome and can be used as basis for provocative testing [7–9]. Nocturnal numbness, which is often reported by NTOS patients, is also a common complaint in patients with carpal tunnel syndrome and ulnar compression neuropathy. Patients with NTOS may also report worsening of symptoms with dangling of the arm when walking.

Pulse Obliteration with Arm Hyperabduction and the Presence of Neurovascular Changes

Pulse obliteration may be observed with arm hyperabduction in patients with NTOS, although this finding alone is very common in normal individuals [10]. Nine subjects in our sample of 25 office workers had pulse obliteration at only 90° of arm abduction, and many more had obliteration with greater than 90° abduction. Cold hands, pallor, mottling, and mild cyanosis are frequently seen in otherwise normal women with mild forms of Raynaud's phenomenon.

Stress Maneuver Reproduction of Symptoms: EAST, Adson Maneuver, AER, Traction Test

Stress maneuvers have been described to reproduce those positional and effort related activities that may produce a sensory experience that is historically familiar to the patient.

Elevated Arm Stress Test (EAST)
Although a 3 min test was classically described by Roos, a 1 min stress test (1 min EAST) may be considered because many patients with NTOS

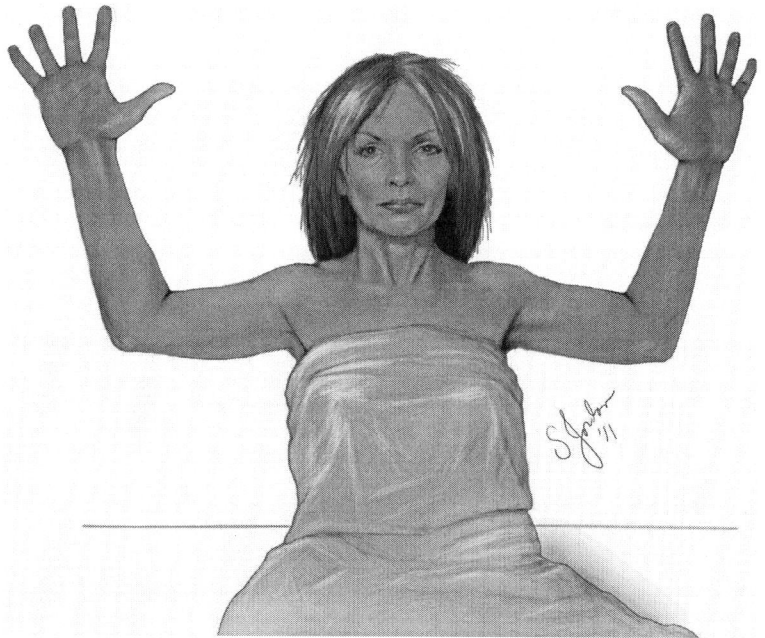

Fig. 7.1 Arm abduction and elbow flexion for the EAST test (Courtesy of Dr. Sheldon Jordan)

will have marked symptoms within a few seconds and patients with CRPS or fibromyalgia may experience many days of delayed onset muscular pain after a 3 min test (prolonged after-effects do not occur after a 1 min test in our experience testing 7,915 patients with this approach over the past 10 years in our UCLA Vascular Surgery affiliated clinic). The patient is asked to adduct the shoulder to 90°, flex the elbows at 90°, and face the hands forward while the hands are alternately opened and closed at a rate of one per second for a total of 60 s (see Fig. 7.1). At the end of this period, the patient is asked to rate the total amount of exercise induced discomfort including all components of aching pain, arm fatigue, and sensory changes including tingling, pins and needles, and deadness. The location of evoked symptoms and concordance with historical experiences are noted. Patients with carpal tunnel syndrome and sometimes ulnar neuropathy, CRPS, and fibromyalgia will all demonstrate increased symptoms with this test, so the location and quality of symptoms are critical to note in order to discriminate these patients from those with NTOS. In our 25 office worker sample, 12 (48 %) demonstrated a positive EAST. Similar results have been published [11].

The **Adson maneuver** (see Chap. 3) is performed by having the patient turn their head toward the pathologic side as the patient inhales with the arm extended; classically described to look for pulse changes, many use it to assess whether neurologic symptoms are exacerbated (see Fig. 7.2). The **arm abducted stress maneuver (AER)** and the **downward arm traction test** are other maneuvers that can be performed on patients with possible NTOS, the common goal in all being to reproduce distal symptoms by compromising the interscalene triangle and other components of the thoracic outlet. Unfortunately, while these tests are sensitive, low specificity limits their usefulness.

Supraclavicular Fossa and Infraclavicular Tenderness to Palpation

Another positive finding that is often considered to be suggestive of NTOS is that of tenderness to palpation at certain sites. Palpation over the scalene triangle will often produce extreme local pain as well as discomfort that radiates into the arm, chest, or axilla. A second area of compression, increasingly recognized, is the pectoralis minor muscle insertion site (see Chap. 15).

Fig. 7.2 Adson maneuver
(Courtesy of Dr. Sheldon
Jordan)

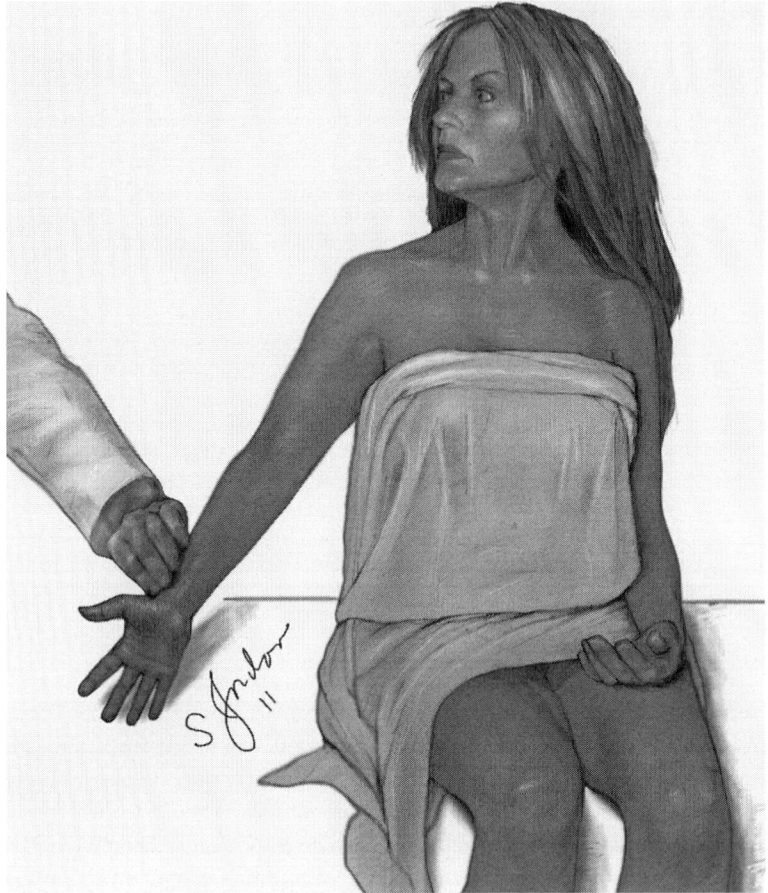

Patterns of Pain Radiation

Patients will very commonly complain of pain in areas radiating from the neck and proximal shoulder to the occiput and more generally to the head. Pain may radiate to the scapular region, down to the anterior chest, and to the axilla. Anterior chest pain, in particular, may confuse the clinician and lead to delays in diagnosis because a cardiogenic source of pain may be considered.

The Presence of Nerve "Irritability": The Tinel's Sign

Gentle tapping over a peripheral nerve may produce paresthesias that are perceived along the dermatomes of the targeted nerve. Although used commonly to assess the potential presence of carpal tunnel syndrome, its reliability, sensitivity,

and specificity has been extensively questioned even in these patients [12–16]. It is very difficult to achieve good inter-observer and intra-observer agreement because of the variability and targeting of effective striking force. In view of the variability of overlying soft tissues when using this test in patients with possible NTOS, particular over the interscalene triangle and the axilla, it is helpful to place a stationary finger over the course of the nerve with slight downwards pressure to ensure an accurate target for the striking finger. An alternative technique for eliciting paresthesia is to put 2 to 4 kilograms of pressure on the targeted nerve bundle (enough pressure to turn the fingernail beds white) and then to flick the palpating finger across the nerve. Using the tapping and flicking technique all of the patients in our clinical series of 110 patients, had inducible paresthesias down the arm when stimulation was applied to the plexus at the level of Erb's point or at the axilla. It is possible to elicit paresthesias at a proximal site of injury and at distal sites even when there is no separate identifiable distal injury [17]. Therefore, most of the patients in the clinical series with NTOS had a positive Tinel's sign over the plexus proximally and over the ulnar nerve at the elbow as well. Some of the patients also had a positive Tinel's sign over the median nerve at the wrist.

Weakness and Atrophy of Hand Muscles

Patients with NTOS may show atrophy of the intrinsic hand muscles involving both the thenar and hypothenar groups [18]. The latter is rare and was only present in 6 of 110 sequentially examined patients with possible NTOS in our clinic affiliated with the UCLA Vascular Surgery program. Objective weakness of the intrinsic muscles can be measured, although to ensure sensitivity calibrated finger ergometers are required [11]. As with any other form of muscle testing, the combination of motivation, painfulness of the effort, and examiner bias may interfere with testing accuracy. Patients with NTOS frequently have weakness of the adductor digiti minimi in the .25 to .5 kg range whereas normal individuals, including women typically demonstrate power at or above .5 kg for this muscle.

Utilization of Standardized Validated Questionnaires and Diagrams

As an adjunct to the formal history and physical examination and to monitor and quantify change, validated questionnaires and pain and sensory diagrams have been developed. The Disability of the Arm, Shoulder, and Hand (DASH) has been used in evaluating patients with cervicobrachial syndromes and demonstrates good sensitivity to effects of therapeutic interventions [19, 20]. It lacks, however, a sensory diagram that can be useful in focusing on sensory changes and it fails to test for conditions characterized by widespread pain or symptoms that may suggest CRPS. Besides detecting features consistent with NTOS, questionnaires must detect comorbid conditions that could drastically affect outcomes for NTOS-targeted therapy.

The CervicoBrachial Symptom Questionnaire (CBSQ) was developed to detect features typical of NTOS as well as to evaluate coexisting problems that significantly affect treatment (so-called "game changers"), incorporate a pain and sensory diagram (see Fig. 7.3), and be sensitive to the effects of therapy [21]. Because depression is often a comorbid and treatable condition, the Beck depression scale may be considered for an initial self administered battery as a patient presents for an initial visit. A CBSQ and Beck form can be filled out in 10–20 min and scoring is very fast (greater than 10 or 20 min for form completion becomes burdensome for patients who may have serious limitations in writing endurance). A family member is occasionally needed to be a scribe.

Additional Testing

Electromyography (EMG) will occasionally show increased polyphasic units or a drop out of units in the intrinsic hand muscles, although its sensitivity is low in patients with a clinical diagnosis of NTOS [22–25]. Evoked potential techniques have been described [24–30]; low sensitivity and specificity, muscle artifact contamination of the waveforms, and patient discomfort remain limiting factors. MRI scans will often show anatomical abnormalities that are consistent with NTOS; the frequent finding of anatomical changes in the thoracic outlet in autopsy studies of people dying without histories of NTOS, however, ensure a degree of non-specificity in image-based testing [31]. Furthermore, large prospective studies are still needed that would provide a correlation of cross sectional imaging "abnormalities" with clinical outcomes. The use of test injections of the scalenes for confirmation of the diagnosis and prediction of outcomes with targeted treatment is discussed in Chap. 20, "Scalene Test Blocks and Interventional Techniques in patients with NTOS."

Summary

Patients with possible NTOS present with neck and arm pain, sensory changes, and weakness which may be exacerbated by certain stress

Cervical Brachial Symptom Questionnaire

Mark where you feel pain with horizontal
or vertical lines. Mark sensory changes
with diagonal lines. If different pains or
sensory changes are caused by specific
items in the questionnaire, then indicate
by the question number.
Use next page if necessary

Name

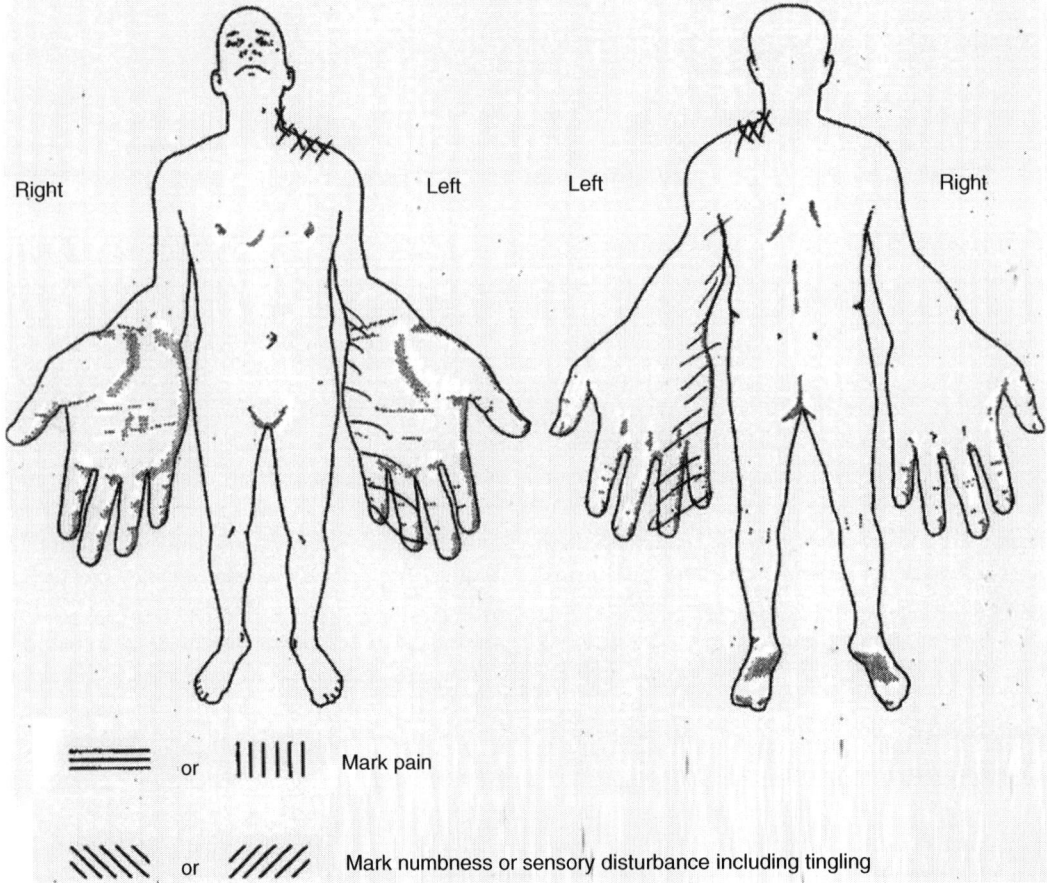

Right   Left   Left   Right

≡≡≡ or |||||| Mark pain

\\\\\ or ///// Mark numbness or sensory disturbance including tingling

Fig. 7.3 Pain and sensory diagram from CBSQ showing pattern of a typical TOS patient (Courtesy of Pain Physician, American Society of Interventional Pain Physicians)

maneuvers. As discussed in this chapter, the presence of these features in a patient's history and the reproduction of concordant experiences by bedside examination are two fundamental processes that start the diagnostic process.

The next step is to consider entities that simulate NTOS but are, in fact, separate entities. Often overlooked, however, is the need to recognize coexisting conditions that require treatment *in parallel with* NTOS-targeted treatment. Certain coexisting conditions have been associated with poor outcomes after NTOS-directed therapy and therefore require a change in the therapeutic approach; these are the "game-changers" that require a delay or denial of NTOS-targeted therapy. Chapter 8 addresses both the differential diagnosis and the critical "game-changers."

References

1. Machleder HI. Neurogenic thoracic outlet syndrome. In: Machleder HI, editor. Vascular disorders of the upper extremity. Armonk: Futura Publishing; 1998. p. 131–5.
2. Pascarelli EF. Dr. Pascarelli's complete guide to repetitive strain injury: what you need to know about RSI and carpal tunnel syndrome. Hoboken: Wiley; 2004.
3. Pecina M, Bojanic I. Overuse injuries of the musculoskeletal system. 2nd ed. Boca Raton: CRC Press; 2004.
4. Hadler NM. Occupational musculoskeletal disorders. Philadelphia: Lippincott Williams & Wilkins; 2005.
5. Nicholas JA, Hershman EB, Posner MA. The upper extremity in sports medicine. 2nd ed. St. Louis: Mosby; 1995.
6. Stevens JC, Witt JC, Smith BE, et al. The frequency of carpal tunnel syndrome in computer users at a medical facility. Neurology. 2001;56:1568–70.
7. Nord KM, Kapoor P, Fisher J, et al. False positive rate of thoracic outlet syndrome diagnostic maneuvers. Electromyogr Clin Neurophysiol. 2008;48:67–74.
8. Toomingas A, Hagberg M, Jorulf L, et al. Outcome of the abduction external rotation test among manual and office workers. Am J Ind Med. 1991;19:215–27.
9. Ahn DS. Hand elevation: a new test for carpal tunnel syndrome. Ann Plast Surg. 2001;46:120–4.
10. Rayan GM, Jensen G. Thoracic outlet syndrome: provocative examination maneuvers in a typical population. J Shoulder Elbow Surg. 1995;4:113–7.
11. Howard M, Lee C, Dellon AL. Documentation of brachial plexus compression (in the thoracic inlet) utilizing provocative neurosensory and muscular testing. J Reconstr Microsurg. 2003;19:303–12.
12. Lifchez SD, Means Jr KR, Dunn RE, et al. Intra- and inter-examiner variability in performing Tinel's test. J Hand Surg Am. 2010;35:212–6.
13. Bruske J, Bednarski M, Grzelec H, et al. The usefulness of the Phalen test and the Hoffmann-Tinel sign in the diagnosis of carpal tunnel syndrome. Acta Orthop Belg. 2002;68:141–5.
14. Salerno DF, Franzblau A, Werner RA, et al. Reliability of physical examination of the upper extremity among keyboard operators. Am J Ind Med. 2000;37: 423–30.
15. Kuhlman KA, Hennessey WJ. Sensitivity and specificity of carpal tunnel syndrome signs. Am J Phys Med Rehabil. 1997;76:451–7.
16. Heller L, Ring H, Costeff H, et al. Evaluation of Tinel's and Phalen's signs in diagnosis of the carpal tunnel syndrome. Eur Neurol. 1986;25:40–2.
17. Jabre JF. Distal "Tinel-like" percussion paresthesiae with proximal nerve lesions. Electromyogr Clin Neurophysiol. 1996;36:175–8.
18. Gilliatt RW, Le Quesne PM, Logue V. Wasting of the hand associated with a cervical rib or band. J Neurol Neurosurg Psychiatry. 1970;33:615–24.
19. Chang DC, Rotellini-Coltvet LA, Mukherjee D, et al. Surgical intervention for thoracic outlet syndrome improves patient's quality of life. J Vasc Surg. 2009;49:630–5.
20. Cordobes-Gual J, Lozano-Vilardell P, Torreguitart-Mirada N, et al. Prospective study of the functional recovery after surgery for thoracic outlet syndrome. Eur J Vasc Endovasc Surg. 2008;35:79–83.
21. Jordan SE, Ahn SS, Gelabert HA. Differentiation of thoracic outlet syndrome from treatment-resistant cervical brachial pain syndromes: development and utilization of a questionnaire, clinical examination and ultrasound evaluation. Pain Physician. 2007;10: 441–52.
22. Jordan SE, Machleder HI. Diagnosis of thoracic outlet syndrome using electrophysiologically guided anterior scalene blocks. Ann Vasc Surg. 1998;12:260–4.
23. Jordan S, Machleder HI. Electrodiagnostic evaluation of patients with painful syndromes affecting the upper extremities. In: Machleder HI, editor. Vascular disorders of the upper extremity. Armonk: Futura Publishing; 1998. p. 137–53.
24. Rousseff R, Tzvetanov P, Valkov I. Utility (or futility?) of electrodiagnosis in thoracic outlet syndrome. Electromyogr Clin Neurophysiol. 2005;45:131–3.
25. Gillard J, Perez-Cousin M, Hachulla E, et al. Diagnosing thoracic outlet syndrome: contribution of provocative tests, ultrasonography, electrophysiology, and helical computed tomography in 48 patients. Joint Bone Spine. 2001;68:416–24.
26. Machleder HI, Moll F, Nuwer M, Jordan S. Somatosensory evoked potentials in the assessment of thoracic outlet compression syndrome. J Vasc Surg. 1987;6:177–84.
27. Komanetsky RM, Novak CB, Mackinnon SE, et al. Somatosensory evoked potentials fail to diagnose thoracic outlet syndrome. J Hand Surg Am. 1996;21: 662–6.
28. Passero S, Paradiso C, Giannini F, et al. Diagnosis of thoracic outlet syndrome. Relative value of electrophysiological studies. Acta Neurol Scand. 1994;90: 179–85.
29. Yiannikas C, Walsh JC. Somatosensory evoked responses in the diagnosis of thoracic outlet syndrome. J Neurol Neurosurg Psychiatry. 1983;46:234–40.
30. Siivola J, Pokela R, Sulg I. Somatosensory evoked responses as a diagnostic aid in thoracic outlet syndrome. A postoperative study. Acta Chir Scand. 1983;149:147–50.
31. Juvonen T, Satta J, Laitala P, et al. Anomalies at the thoracic outlet are frequent in the general population. Am J Surg. 1995;170:33–7.

Differential Diagnosis in Patients with Possible NTOS

Sheldon E. Jordan

Abstract

Patients in whom the diagnosis of NTOS is being considered usually have neck and arm pain, sensory changes, and weakness that may be exacerbated by certain stress maneuvers. As discussed in Chap. 7, the presence of these features in a patient's history and the reproduction of concordant experiences by bedside examination are two fundamental processes that start the diagnostic process.

The diagnostic process then continues with a consideration of entities that simulate NTOS but are, in fact, separate entities. Equally important but often overlooked is the need to recognize certain conditions that commonly coexist with NTOS but are associated with a poor outcome to NTOS-directed therapy ("game changers") and, therefore, require a more dramatic change in the therapeutic approach.

Introduction

Patients in whom the diagnosis of NTOS is being considered usually have neck and arm pain, sensory changes, and weakness that may be exacerbated by certain stress maneuvers. As discussed in Chap. 7, the presence of these features in a patient's history and the reproduction of concordant experiences by bedside examination are two fundamental processes that start the diagnostic process.

S.E. Jordan, MD, FAAN
Department of Neurology,
Neurological Associates of West Los Angeles,
2811 Wilshire Blvd., Suite 790,
Santa Monica 90403, CA, USA
e-mail: shellyj@aol.com

The diagnostic process then continues with a consideration of entities that simulate NTOS but are, in fact, separate entities. Equally important but often overlooked is the need to recognize certain conditions that commonly coexist with NTOS but are associated with a poor outcome to NTOS-directed therapy ("game changers") and, therefore, require a more dramatic change in the therapeutic approach.

Coexisting, Confusing, and Complicating Factors

Conditions may coexist with NTOS that will require treatment in parallel with those that target NTOS itself. The presence of these coexisting conditions does not trump NTOS-directed

K.A. Illig et al. (eds.), *Thoracic Outlet Syndrome*,
DOI 10.1007/978-1-4471-4366-6_8, © Springer-Verlag London 2013

therapy, but rather directs the clinician to prioritize and coordinate treatment of each element so that the best outcomes are obtained.

There is a dearth of published studies that were designed to evaluate the frequency of coexisting conditions in those patients presenting with signs that might otherwise suggest NTOS, and we therefore reviewed our experience in preparation for this chapter.

Over the past 10 years, 7,915 patients visited our NTOS-directed neurology clinic affiliated with the UCLA Vascular Surgery service with a diagnosis of cervicobrachial syndrome and probable NTOS; 629 visits were new patient consultations. Each patient was seen an average of 13 times over this period. These patients had neck, shoulder, and/or arm pain as well as weakness, pain, and/or sensory changes with elevated arm stress testing.

One hundred and ten patients were prospectively and sequentially studied, as well, in order to determine how many ended up with NTOS as a major diagnosis that was substantially contributing to the patient's overall suffering and disability. Final diagnoses for the purposes of this analysis were determined by consideration of clinical signs and symptoms, response to test blockade [1–4], and evaluation of anatomic and electrophysiologic testing [5, 6] without consideration of response to NTOS-targeted therapy.

The majority of these patients were women (84 %). Forty-nine cases (45 %) were attributed to conditions at work (work-related musculoskeletal disorders; WRMD) while the remaining 61 (55 %) were caused by a variety of acute injuries including falls, lifting accidents, altercations, and auto accidents. Only one case was considered spontaneous. Bilateral complaints were common in this experience (58 %). Most importantly, NTOS rarely occurred as an isolated problem: only 11 out of 110 (10 %) patients were thought to have NTOS as a solitary diagnosis. Sixty one out of 110 (55 %) were found to have NTOS as a prominent factor in combination with other problems and in most of the remaining patients a component of the patient's overall clinical picture was compatible with NTOS but other conditions overshadowed this diagnosis (i.e., NTOS was a minor factor and other conditions were more important in contributing to the overall level of suffering and disability).

In 14 patients with NTOS as a *prominent* factor, thoracic outlet decompression was performed; 12 (86 %) had a good outcome as defined by reduction in rescue medications, fifty percent reduction in pain scale rating and improved activities of daily living. In nine patients who had thoracic outlet decompression in spite of having NTOS as a *minor* factor, none of them had a good outcome. It is apparent that having clinical features of NTOS alone is not sufficient in order to predict a good outcome to targeted surgery and the coexistence of other factors in a patient's cervicobrachial syndrome appears to play an important role in determination of outcomes when NTOS-targeted interventions are planned [2, 7–12].

In our experience, conditions that required independent or concurrent treatment included cervical spine disorders, cervical dystonia (CD), myofascial pain syndrome (MFPS), carpal tunnel syndrome (CTS), ulnar neuropathy (UN), headache, depression, and varied chronic musculoskeletal problems affecting the shoulder, elbow, and/or wrist.

Cervical Spine Disorders

Patients with cervical myeloradiculopathy may present with neck and shoulder pain and paresthesias and weakness in the upper limb. In contrast to patients with NTOS, numbness of fingers 4 and 5 are not commonly encountered in patients with cervical root compression because disc herniation and osteophytic spurs do not commonly occur at the C8 root level. Patients with cervical root syndromes also have more neck movement limitation and sensitivity to axial compression and extension as compared to patients with NTOS. Patients with cervical root irritation will often have a positive Spurling's sign (pain with downward forehead compression in a patient who is extending the neck, looking at the ceiling, with the head rotated toward the affected side). Pain radiation patterns can be quite similar to those due to NTOS but, by contrast, pain maximal in the supraclavicular fossa is less prominently noted. Although cervical disc abnormalities are common in otherwise normal individuals, a negative MRI of the cervical spine would likely exclude a compressive cervical radiculopathy in a patient presenting with a cervicobrachial syndrome (i.e., imaging has a very low false-negative rate in patients with cervical disk-related syndromes).

Patients with neck pain that radiates to the scapula may have pain generators innervated by facet nerves. These pain generators may coexist with NTOS in patients exposed to either occupational factors or to single accidents and may be a cause for persisting axial pain after technically successful NTOS surgery. Many such patients will have pain with palpation of the lateral masses of the neck in the area of facet joints. Selective blockade of facet innervation is required to confirm a diagnosis of a facet joint pain problem [13, 14].

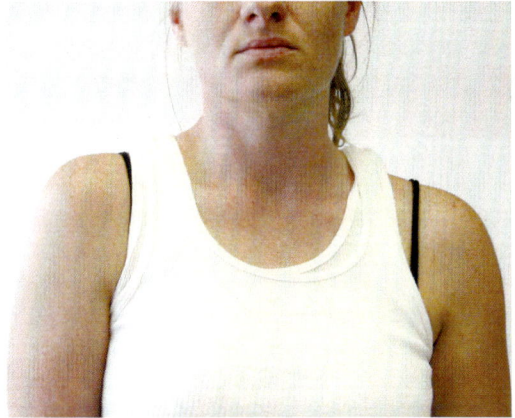

Fig. 8.1 Dystonic posture with shoulder elevation and protraction

Cervical Dystonia and Other Segmental Dystonias

Patients may present to a neurological clinic with spontaneous and prominent neck turning and tilting comprising a complete picture of cervical torsion dystonia (so-called torticollis); pain is a common complaint in these patients [15, 16]. In our experience, patients in the above category may have concomitant features of NTOS with hand numbness and positional worsening. The neck turning and the phasic and dystonic tremor-like movements as well as the characteristic ameliorating "trick gestures" that these patients exhibit are characteristic enough so that they are usually referred for neurological evaluation and botulinum chemodenervation early on in the illness; these patients do not often find their way to surgeons. When pain and positional numbness are predominant and dystonia less dramatic, however, these patients may be initially referred to non-neurological specialists such as orthopedic surgeons and thus ultimately find their way to a TOS surgeon.

There is an extensive literature describing patients with post traumatic and occupational dystonias [17–41]. As with spontaneous cases of torsion dystonia, patients with occupational dystonias may respond to botulinum chemodenervation of the affected muscles. When being evaluated by bedside examination, there may be a concern that postural change may result from shortening

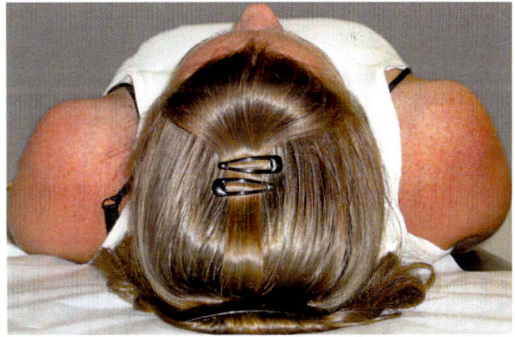

Fig. 8.2 Dystonic posture with shoulder elevation and protraction. Protraction can sometimes better seen with patient laying down

of muscles rather than active muscle contraction (see Figs. 8.1 and 8.2). Electromyography can easily distinguish passive muscle shortening from active contraction; the latter is associated with abundant spontaneous motor unit activity when the patient is trying to relax. It is critical to examine those muscles that are actually responsible for the patient's shoulder protraction, depression or elevation which may include the subclavius, pectoralis minor and other deep muscles. Combining ultrasound guidance with EMG is suggested in order to improve accurate muscle identification and to avoid a pneumothorax.

Myofascial Pain

The term "myofascial pain" refers to the presence of localized and regional pain associated with tender and palpably tight muscles. Needle insertion or tapping the tender muscle trigger point will produce pain that may radiate down the back or along the limb some distance from the targeted site. Many patients with muscle tenderness and tightness may not show active spontaneous motor unit activity by EMG which distinguishes this localized disturbance of muscle from patients with dystonia. The lack of active muscle contraction may be one reason why botulinum chemodenervation has not been uniformly effective in treating patients identified with myofascial pain [41–46]. NTOS patients will frequently demonstrate myofascial trigger points in the trapezii, levator scapulae, and rhomboid muscles.

Musculoskeletal Conditions of the Shoulder, Elbow and Hand

Many of the patients presenting with possible NTOS have coexisting identifiable musculoskeletal conditions that may have been treated with ergonomic adjustments, physical therapy, bracing, injections, or surgery, including elbow tendinitis, rotator cuff syndromes, frozen shoulder, or wrist tendinitis. Patients may be diagnosed with rotator cuff syndromes or tears of the labrum (SLAP lesions) only to develop prominent NTOS symptoms in spite of apparently technically adequate shoulder surgeries; this scenario was observed in 28 out of the 110 cervical brachial patients analyzed in our clinical series described above. Whether NTOS was the problem to start with or was created secondarily by such therapy is unknown.

Carpal Tunnel Syndrome

Carpal tunnel syndrome (CTS) refers to the condition where the median nerve is entrapped by the carpal tunnel at the wrist. The diagnosis of CTS is often based on the combination of clinical information along with electrodiagnostic testing, particularly when surgical release is anticipated [45]. The classic patient with CTS reports a history of paresthesias involving the

palmar aspect of the first three fingers and half of the ring finger (see Fig. 8.3). The Cervical Brachial Symptom Questionnaire (CBSQ) is useful to diagram symptoms; patients may show the classical pattern or fewer fingers may be involved (see Fig. 8.1). By contrast, patients with NTOS usually will diagram sensory disturbances involving the whole hand or involvement of fingers four and five with variable involvement of the ulnar forearm; there will be more proximal pain as well (Fig. 8.4). In addition, most (but not all) patients with CTS will have a positive Tinel's sign at the wrist over the median nerve while patients with NTOS almost uniformly have a positive Tinel's sign over the ulnar nerve at the cubital tunnel and over the plexus at the interscalene triangle or in the axilla. Both CTS and NTOS patients may have a history of worsening pain and paresthesias at night and with repetitive hand activities and with arm elevation. Ultimately, however, patients with CTS do not usually have the supraclavicular and proximal symptoms that are reported in patients with NTOS.

Nerve conduction studies across the wrist are often very helpful in distinguishing CTS from NTOS. Most patients with CTS will have slowed sensory or motor velocities for the median nerve at the wrist. If atrophy is present, patients with CTS will have weak and atrophic thenar muscles while those with severe NTOS will demonstrate more widespread atrophy involving the hypothenar muscles as well. The relative importance of NTOS or CTS in a patient with multifocal disease may be determined by analyzing the results of a scalene test block for TOS and the responses to wrist splinting or steroid injections for CTS.

Patients with Ulnar Neuropathy

Ulnar entrapment syndrome refers to symptoms created by compression of the ulnar nerve, the compression is localized to most often to the cubital tunnel at the elbow. According to the Washington State Department of Labor and Industries guidelines, patients with this diagnosis will have paresthesias involving the last two

Cervical Brachial Symptom Questionnaire

Name ————————————————————

————————————————————

Mark where you feel pain with hoizontal or vertical line.mark sensory changes with diagonal lines. If different pain or sensory changes are caused by specific items in the questionnaire,then indicate by the question number.
Use next page if necessary

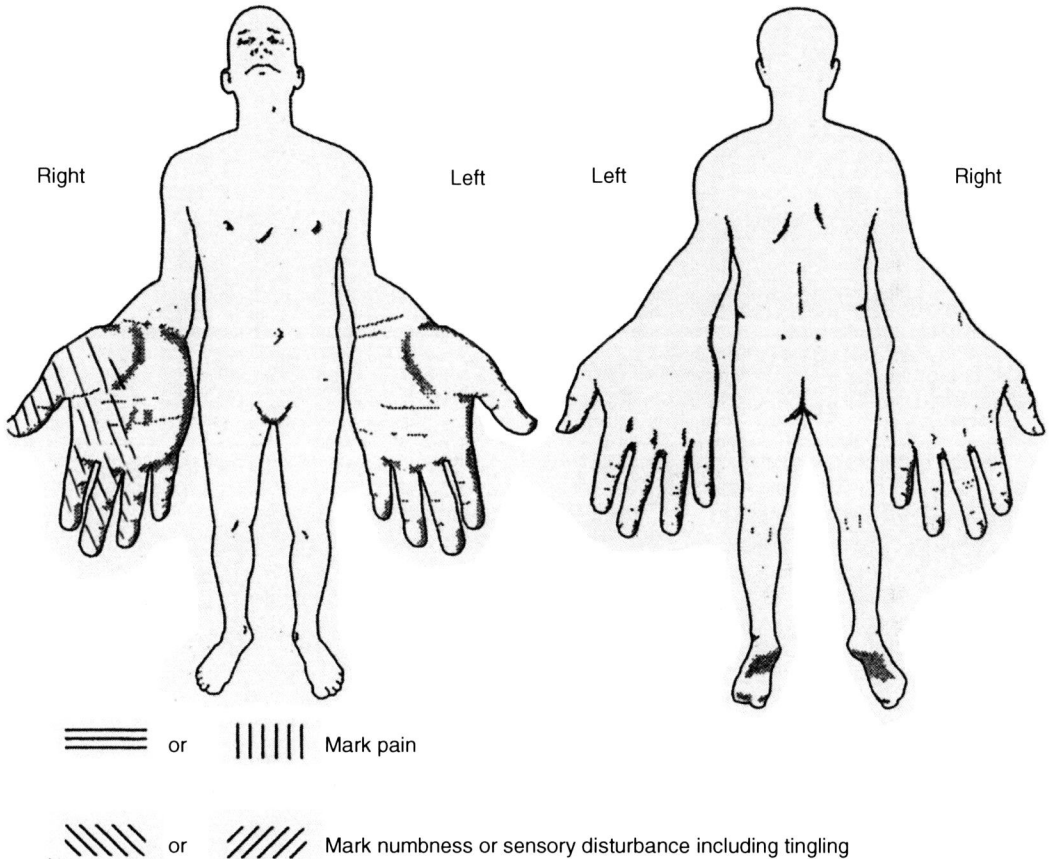

Right   Left   Left   Right

══════ or |||||| Mark pain

\\\\\\ or ////// Mark numbness or sensory disturbance including tingling

Fig. 8.3 CBSQ diagram for a patient with carpal tunnel syndrome (Courtesy of Pain Physician, American Society of Interventional Pain Physicians)

fingers usually associated with pain at the elbow and along the ulnar aspect of the forearm (see Fig. 8.5) [46]. Weakness may be demonstrated in the adductor pollicis muscle by asking a patient to grip a piece of paper between the finger tips of the index and thumb while the examiner tries to pull the paper away. Electrodiagnostic criteria have been suggested including the finding of motor conduction slowing specifically across the elbow. The technical difficulty in performing the electrophysiological test reliably has led to alternative proposals that utilize ultrasonic evaluation of the ulnar nerve. A Tinel's sign may be present at the elbow over the nerve and patients will often describe concordant paresthesias with elbow flexion after 1 min of positioning.

Cervical Brachial Symptom Questionnaire

Mark where you feel pain with hoizontal   Name _____
or vertical line.mark sensory changes   _____
with diagonal lines. If different pain or
sensory changes are caused by specific
items in the questionnaire,then indicate
by the question number.
Use next page if necessary

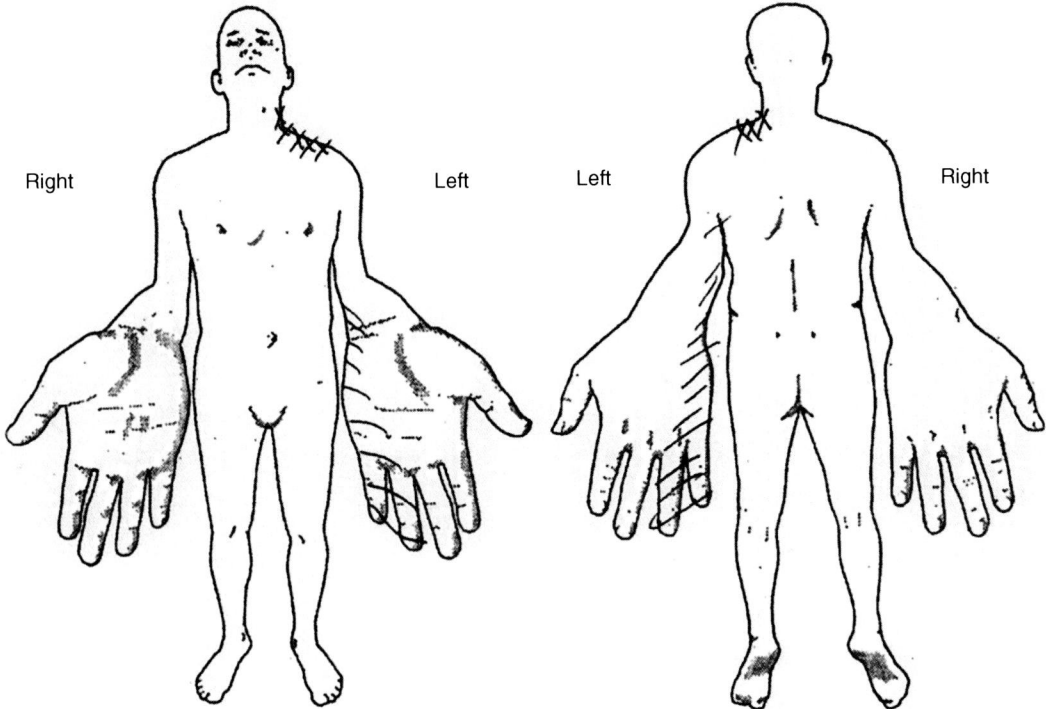

Fig. 8.4 CBSQ diagram for a patient with NTOS (Courtesy of Pain Physician, American Society of Interventional Pain Physicians)

Cervical Brachial Symptom Questionnaire

Mark where you feel pain with hoizontal or vertical line.mark sensory changes with diagonal lines. If different pain or sensory changes are caused by specific items in the questionnaire,then indicate by the question number.
Use next page if necessary

Name ─────────────────

Right   Left   Left   Right

≡≡≡ **or** ||||| Mark pain

\\\\\ **or** /////   Mark numbness or sensory disturbance including tingling

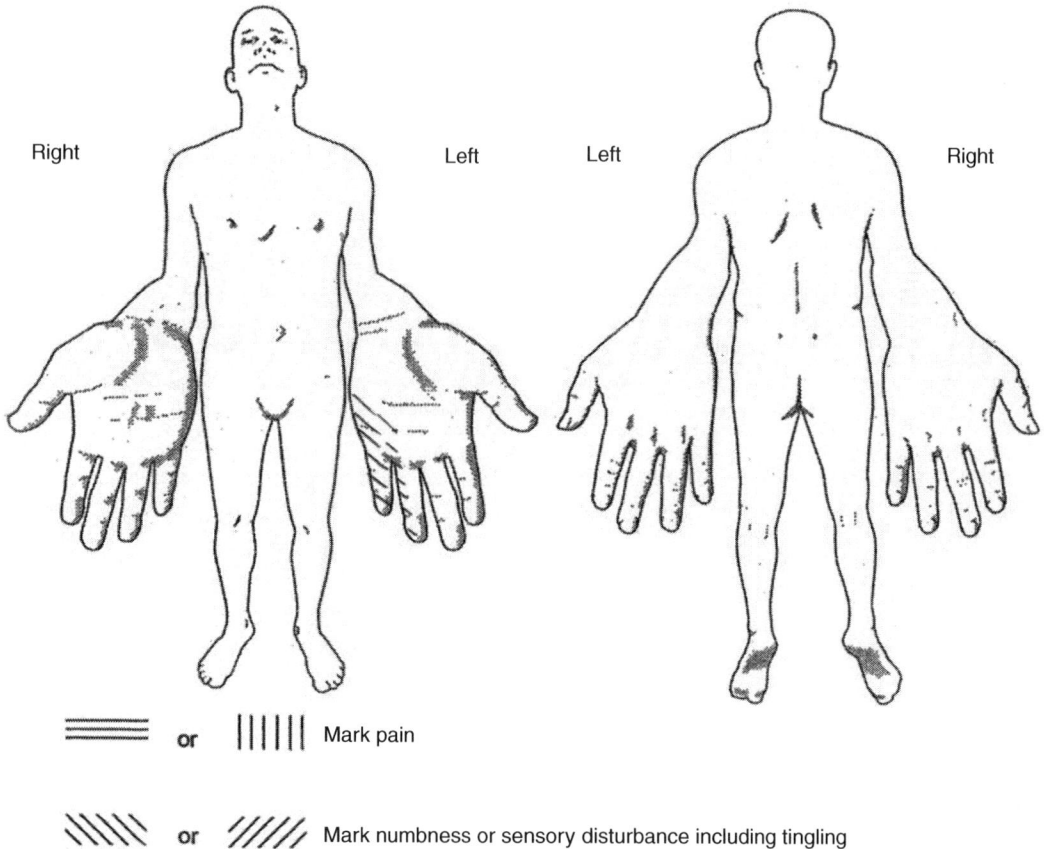

Fig. 8.5 CBSQ diagram for a patient with ulnar neuropathy (Courtesy of Pain Physician, American Society of Interventional Pain Physicians)

Chronic Headache

Many patients will continue to have disabling headaches after technically successful thoracic outlet decompression. The headaches may be caused by temporomandibular muscle dysfunction, frequent migraine, cervical facet arthritis, or occipital neuralgia. Referral to a neurologist or other physician specializing in the care of patients with these syndromes may be helpful.

Depression, Somatization and Iatrogenicity

Patients with chronic pain frequently express depressive symptoms; this condition adds to disability and will interfere with rehabilitation efforts. It is often proposed that stress and emotional upset will cause or worsen pain, a process often referred to as "somatization;" for this reason psychotropic medication, psychological counseling efforts, cognitive therapy, stress reduction techniques, and related interventions are often a part of multi-specialty pain management efforts.

Some observers have suggested that cumulative trauma disorders (including NTOS resulting from occupational factors) may result from an inability to cope with life stresses and may be partly iatrogenic in nature because of the doctor's role as an enabler [47, 48]. Such enabling may reinforce the sickness role when it leads to avoidance of unhappy work experiences and when it allows access to the rewards of entitlement programs (i.e., secondary gain). Physician and patient relationships after injury and physician participation in the process of litigation may contribute to this. In our 110 patient sample described above, 57 out of 72 patients (72 %) with NTOS were working and 26 (24 %) were being treated under the worker's compensation program; only two had pending litigation. In short, few of our NTOS patients were taking advantage of entitlement programs or expecting payouts from litigation.

The recent Australian experience with an "epidemic" of cervicobrachial occupational injuries which was mitigated by changes in physician willingness to diagnose these cases and the scaling back of entitlement programs is often cited as an example supporting the concept of iatrogenicity [49]. What is not often discussed in this context is the massive increase in alternative and complementary health care that occurred as clinical support from conventional medical circles waned, leading to an alternative explanation that a significant proportion of these patients simply migrated to alternative care when the conventional medical pathway became less available [49].

Conditions That Drastically Change Management: The "Game Changers"

There are certain conditions that command our attention because of the need to delay or avoid possible NTOS-targeted treatment, *as they predict a dismal outcome to conventional therapy*. In our 110-patient cohort, these "game changers" were not rare: 17 % had complex regional pain syndrome (CRPS), 15 % had opioid hyperalgesia, and 5 % fibromyalgia. While these conditions may coexist with or simulate NTOS, they predict unusually poor outcomes and thus it is imperative that they be recognized when present.

Complex Regional Pain Syndrome

CRPS may occur before or after thoracic outlet decompression in patients with any cervicobrachial syndrome. Both terminology and diagnosis may be confusing; diagnostic criteria have been recently updated by an international consortium (see Chap. 27) [50–53]. Patients with CRPS have widespread regional pain with markedly increased sensitivity to various somatosensory stimuli along with associated features such as dystonia, sweating, temperature change, swelling, discoloration, and late musculoskeletal changes including contracture and osteoporosis. It is important to recognize these patients early in the treatment process because surgical interventions and targeted injection therapy often fail. In our 110 patient series, only 34 % of individuals with CRPS had good outcomes after therapy versus 90 % of those without (p=0.0301).

Fibromyalgia

The term fibromyalgia refers to a chronic pain syndrome characterized by widespread achiness, pain and stiffness, soft tissue tenderness, general fatigue, and sleep disturbances. Original criteria were based on patients having chronic widespread pain and the presence of tenderness in at least 11 out of 18 specified sites on the body, but

Cervical Brachial Symptom Questionnaire

Mark where you feel pain with hoizontal
or vertical line.mark sensory changes
with diagonal lines. If different pain or
sensory changes are caused by specific
items in the questionnaire,then indicate
by the question number.
Use next page if necessary

Name ————————
       ————————

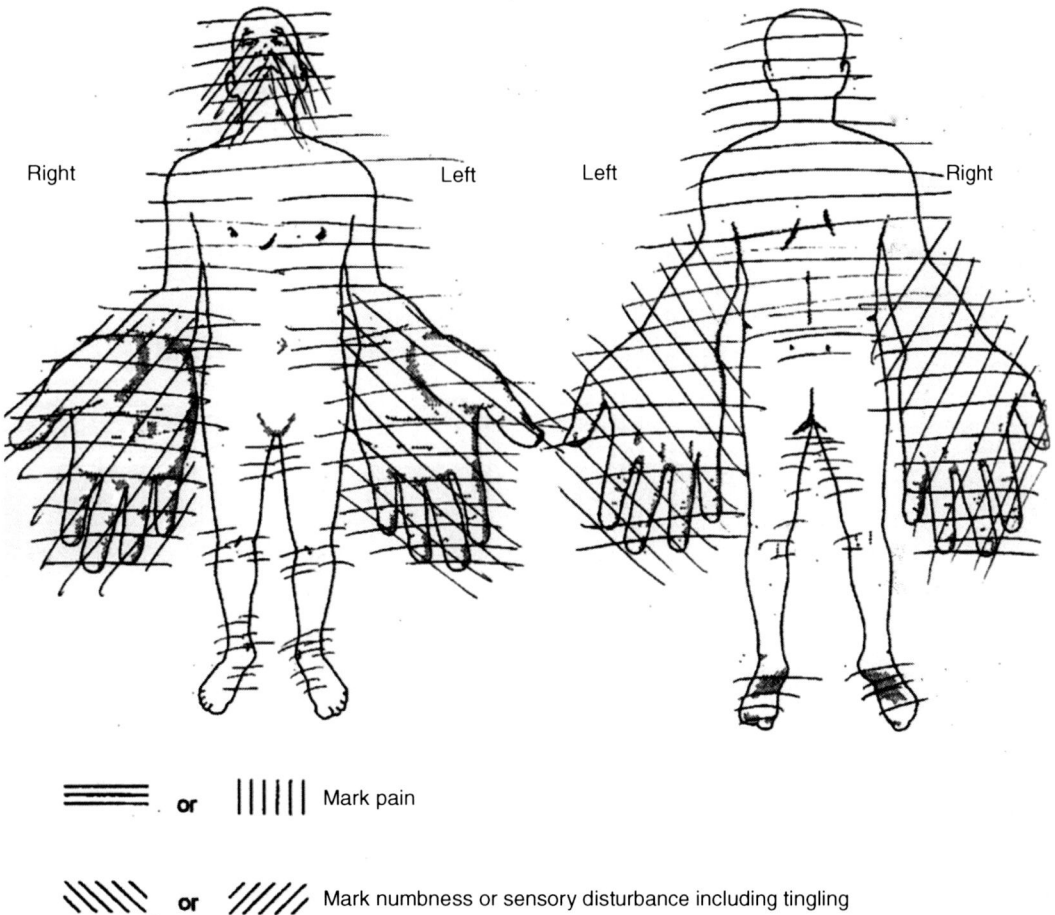

Right   Left   Left   Right

≡≡≡ or ||||||| Mark pain

\\\\\ or ///// Mark numbness or sensory disturbance including tingling

Fig. 8.6 CBSQ diagram for a patient with fibromyalgia (Courtesy of Pain Physician, American Society of Interventional Pain Physicians)

the American College of Rheumatology has recently updated and objectified diagnostic criteria [54]. These are, in part, based on scaled scores on the Widespread Pain Inventory (WPI) and Symptoms Severity Score (SSS). It should be noted that scales frequently used in for evaluation of patients with cervicobrachial syndromes such as the DASH do not address widespread pain. By contrast, the CBSQ concentrates on upper body complaints but allows the patient to map possible widespread pain on a figure of the body (see Fig. 8.6).

Fibromyalgia should be considered clinically when a patient has chronic pain in the upper and lower body, fatigue, non-refreshing sleep and a variety of functional complaints, often including functional bowel disease or pelvic organ dysfunction. These patients often endorse multiple system complaints on a review of systems intake form. They often have concomitant depression and may complain of problems with focus or memory. Multiple "allergies", food sensitivities and failed medical and surgical therapies may be present in the general history. Many of these patients, in our experience may conceal the diagnosis of fibromyalgia that was suggested by other physicians out of fear of rejection. By contrast, more "acceptable" labels may be openly discussed such a Lyme Disease, Chronic Epstein Barr infection, Lupus, vitamin deficiency, heavy metal toxicity, hypothyroidism, intestinal overgrowth, or whatever label the local "Urban Legend" expert health professional is selling.

Whether or not a particular physician is receptive to the idea of fibromyalgia as a distinct illness or that this label merely represents a "medicalization of misery", it is a reality that performing NTOS-targeted therapy for patients with chronic widespread pain and multi-organ complaints is unlikely to be successful. In our 110 patient sample, seven thoracic outlet decompressions were performed in the 16 patients with a diagnosis of fibromyalgia. The cases subjected to surgery had a poor outcome with minimal pain relief, no overall change in functional status, and no substantial change in the use of medications. Although surgery has been cited as an occasional trigger event for clinically recognizable fibromyalgia, most of these patients in our UCLA affiliated NTOS clinic had symptoms compatible with fibromyalgia and chronic widespread pain prior to TOS surgery.

The available literature generally describes poor outcomes for a variety of procedures and chronic excessive utilization of medical resources in patients with widespread pain and fibromyalgia [2, 53, 55–63]. Increased awareness of and better screening tools for this condition will ideally delay surgical plans and allow for suitable referral. If surgery is contemplated in these patients,

both doctor and patient should be aware of the potential for worsening of generalized symptoms and for the expectation of only modest functional gains in the long term with persisting poor quality of life assessments. An increased use of clinical resources will be expected in the post operative period.

Opioid Hyperalgesia

In patients with chronic use of opioids, tolerance and dependency may develop. In addition, some patients will have the appearance of worsened regional pain and overall pain sensitization associated with chronic exposure to high daily doses of opioids, so-called opioid hyperalgesia. Since these patients are highly tolerant, opioids no longer seem to produce effective analgesia. It seems obvious that such patients will have more difficulty than other patients in having adequate pain control in the post operative period after thoracic outlet decompression. In fact, outcomes after any NTOS-targeted therapy (including botulinum chemodenervation) are poor in patients with this condition. In our 110 patient sample, only 25 % of individuals with opioid hyperalgesia had successful outcomes after NTOS-targeted treatment as compared to 75 % of those without (p = 0.0004). Patients with opioid hyperalgesia again demonstrated a markedly increased utilization of medical services; these patients saw nearly twice as many physicians as compared to patients without opioid hyperalgesia (15 vs. 8 visits overall; p < 0.0002)

Summary

Patients with possible NTOS typically present with a multifactorial cervicobrachial syndrome. In order to achieve successful outcomes with NTOS-targeted therapy, a three step process should be considered. First of all, patients should demonstrate the presence of positive features typical of NTOS including numbness, fatigue, and pain exacerbated with overhead reaching in conjunction with evidence of pathology at the supraclavicular fossa and/or pectoralis minor insertion site. Secondly, other conditions (carpal tunnel syndrome or cervical disk disease) or coexisting conditions (depression or distal entrapment neuropathies) should be scrutinized and treated in parallel with NTOS. Third, it should be established that a patient does *not* show features of a condition that predicts failure of NTOS-targeted intervention (fibromyalgia, opioid hyperalgesia, or CRPS). Using this algorithm, a robust and repeatable diagnosis can be assured and patients who will have the highest likelihood of benefit from proper therapy can be identified.

References

1. Jordan SE, Ahn SS, Gelabert HA. Combining ultrasonography and electromyography for botulinum chemodenervation treatment of thoracic outlet syndrome: comparison with fluoroscopy and electromyography guidance. Pain Physician. 2007;10:541–6.
2. Jordan SE, Ahn SS, Gelabert HA. Differentiation of thoracic outlet syndrome from treatment-resistant cervical brachial pain syndromes: development and utilization of a questionnaire, clinical examination and ultrasound evaluation. Pain Physician. 2007;10:441–52.
3. Jordan SE, Ahn SS, Freischlag JA, et al. Selective botulinum chemodenervation of the scalene muscles for treatment of neurogenic thoracic outlet syndrome. Ann Vasc Surg. 2000;14:365–9.
4. Jordan SE, Machleder HI. Diagnosis of thoracic outlet syndrome using electrophysiologically guided anterior scalene blocks. Ann Vasc Surg. 1998;12:260–4.
5. Jordan S, Machleder HI. Electrodiagnostic evaluation of patients with painful syndromes affecting the upper extremities. In: Machleder HI, editor. Vascular disorders of the upper extremity. Armonk: Futura Publishing; 1998. p. 137–53.
6. Machleder HI, Moll F, Nuwer M, Jordan S. Somatosensory evoked potentials in the assessment of thoracic outlet compression syndrome. J Vasc Surg. 1987;6:177–84.
7. Axelrod DA, Proctor MC, Geisser ME, et al. Outcomes after surgery for thoracic outlet syndrome. J Vasc Surg. 2001;33:1220–5.
8. Franklin GM, Fulton-Kehoe D, Bradley C, et al. Outcome of surgery for thoracic outlet syndrome in Washington state workers' compensation. Neurology. 2000;54:1252–7.
9. Leffert RD. Thoracic outlet syndromes. Hand Clin. 1992;8:285–97.
10. Wood VE, Biondi J. Double-crush nerve compression in thoracic-outlet syndrome. J Bone Joint Surg Am. 1990;72:85–7.
11. Pascarelli E. Evaluation and treatment of repetitive motion disorders of the upper extremity in office workers and musicians. In: Machleder HI, editor. Vascular disorders of the upper extremity. Armonk: Futura Publising; 1998. p. 171–96.
12. Pascarelli EF, Hsu YP. Understanding work-related upper extremity disorders: clinical findings in 485 computer users, musicians, and others. J Occup Rehabil. 2001;11:1–21.
13. Falco FJ, Erhart S, Wargo BW, et al. Systematic review of diagnostic utility and therapeutic effectiveness of cervical facet joint interventions. Pain Physician. 2009;12:323–44.
14. Cohen SP, Bajwa ZH, Kraemer JJ, et al. Factors predicting success and failure for cervical facet radiofrequency denervation: a multi-center analysis. Reg Anesth Pain Med. 2007;32:495–503.
15. Chan J, Brin MF, Fahn S. Idiopathic cervical dystonia: clinical characteristics. Mov Disord. 1991;6:119–26.
16. Jankovic J, Leder S, Warner D, Schwartz K. Cervical dystonia: clinical findings and associated movement disorders. Neurology. 1991;41:1088–91.
17. Micheli F, Torres L, Diaz M, et al. Delayed onset limb dystonia following electric injury. Parkinsonism Relat Disord. 1998;4:39–42.
18. Carroll CG, Hawley JS, Ney JP. Post-traumatic shoulder dystonia in an active duty soldier. Mil Med. 2006;171:494–6.
19. Takemoto M, Ikenaga M, Tanaka C. Cervical dystonia induced by cervical spine surgery: a case report. Spine (Phila Pa 1976). 2006;31:E31–4.
20. Frei KP, Pathak M, Jenkins S, et al. Natural history of posttraumatic cervical dystonia. Mov Disord. 2004;19:1492–8.
21. O'Riordan S, Hutchinson M. Cervical dystonia following peripheral trauma–a case–control study. J Neurol. 2004;251:150–5.
22. Hollinger P, Burgunder J. Posttraumatic focal dystonia of the shoulder. Eur Neurol. 2000;44:153–5.
23. Wright RA, Ahlskog JE. Focal shoulder-elevation dystonia. Mov Disord. 2000;15:709–13.
24. Samii A, Pal PK, Schulzer M, et al. Post-traumatic cervical dystonia: a distinct entity? Can J Neurol Sci. 2000;27:55–9.
25. Thyagarajan D, Kompoliti K, Ford B. Post-traumatic shoulder 'dystonia': persistent abnormal postures of the shoulder after minor trauma. Neurology. 1998;51:1205–7.
26. Tarsy D. Comparison of acute- and delayed-onset posttraumatic cervical dystonia. Mov Disord. 1998;13:481–5.
27. Goldman S, Ahlskog JE. Posttraumatic cervical dystonia. Mayo Clin Proc. 1993;68:443–8.
28. Truong DD, Dubinsky R, Hermanowicz N, et al. Posttraumatic torticollis. Arch Neurol. 1991;48:221–3.
29. Tamagawa A, Uozumi T, Tsuji S. Occupational dystonia associated with production line work and PC work. Brain Nerve. 2007;59:553–9.

30. Altenmuller E, Jabusch HC. Focal dystonia in musicians: phenomenology, pathophysiology, triggering factors, and treatment. Med Probl Perform Art. 2010;25:3–9.

31. Abdo WF, Bloem BR, Eijk JJ, et al. Atypical dystonic shoulder movements following neuralgic amyotrophy. Mov Disord. 2009;24:293–6.

32. Baek W, Sheean G. Occupational dystonia affecting truncal muscles in a bricklayer. Mov Disord. 2007;22: 284–5.

33. Rodriguez AV, Kooh M, Guerra LA, et al. Musician's cramp: a case report and literature review. J Clin Rheumatol. 2005;11:274–6.

34. Schuele S, Jabusch HC, Lederman RJ, et al. Botulinum toxin injections in the treatment of musician's dystonia. Neurology. 2005;64:341–3.

35. Karp BI. Botulinum toxin treatment of occupational and focal hand dystonia. Mov Disord. 2004;19 Suppl 8:S116–9.

36. Defazio G, Berardelli A, Abbruzzese G, et al. Possible risk factors for primary adult onset dystonia: a case–control investigation by the Italian Movement Disorders Study Group. J Neurol Neurosurg Psychiatry. 1998;64:25–32.

37. Marsden CD, Sheehy MP. Writer's cramp. Trends Neurosci. 1990;13:148–53.

38. McDaniel KD, Cummings JL, Shain S. The "yips": a focal dystonia of golfers. Neurology. 1989;39:192–5.

39. Cohen LG, Hallett M. Hand cramps: clinical features and electromyographic patterns in a focal dystonia. Neurology. 1988;38:1005–12.

40. Qerama E, Fuglsang-Frederiksen A, Kasch H, et al. A double-blind, controlled study of botulinum toxin A in chronic myofascial pain. Neurology. 2006;67:241–5.

41. Gobel H, Heinze A, Reichel G, et al. Efficacy and safety of a single botulinum type A toxin complex treatment (Dysport) for the relief of upper back myofascial pain syndrome: results from a randomized double-blind placebo-controlled multicentre study. Pain. 2006;125:82–8.

42. Ojala T, Arokoski JP, Partanen J. The effect of small doses of botulinum toxin a on neck-shoulder myofascial pain syndrome: a double-blind, randomized, and controlled crossover trial. Clin J Pain. 2006;22:90–6.

43. Ferrante FM, Bearn L, Rothrock R, et al. Evidence against trigger point injection technique for the treatment of cervicothoracic myofascial pain with botulinum toxin type A. Anesthesiology. 2005;103:377–83.

44. Wheeler AH, Goolkasian P, Gretz SS. A randomized, double-blind, prospective pilot study of botulinum toxin injection for refractory, unilateral, cervicothoracic, paraspinal, myofascial pain syndrome. Spine (Phila Pa 1976). 1998;23:1662–6.

45. Keith MW, Masear V, Chung KC, et al. American Academy of Orthopaedic Surgeons Clinical Practice Guideline on diagnosis of carpal tunnel syndrome. J Bone Joint Surg Am. 2009;91:2478–9.

46. Ulnar Neuropathy at the Elbow (UNE) Diagnosis and treatment. http://www.lni.wa.gov/ClaimsIns/Files/OMD/UlnarNerve.pdf. Accessed 1 Jan 2010.

47. Hadler Nortin M. Occupational musculoskeletal disorders. Philadelphia: Lippincott Williams & Wilkins; 2005.

48. Yolande L. Constructing RSI: belief and desire. Sydney: UNSW Press; 2003.

49. Coulter ID, Willis MW. The rise and rise of complementary and alternative medicine: a sociological perspective. Med J Aust. 2004;180(11):587–9.

50. Harden RN. Objectification of the diagnostic criteria for CRPS. Pain Med. 2010;11:1212–5.

51. Harden RN, Bruehl S, Perez RS, et al. Validation of proposed diagnostic criteria (the "Budapest Criteria") for Complex Regional Pain Syndrome. Pain. 2010;150:268–74.

52. Harden RN, Bruehl S, Stanton-Hicks M, et al. Proposed new diagnostic criteria for complex regional pain syndrome. Pain Med. 2007;8:326–31.

53. Harden RN, Bruehl SP. Diagnosis of complex regional pain syndrome: signs, symptoms, and new empirically derived diagnostic criteria. Clin J Pain. 2006;22:415–9.

54. Wolfe F, Clauw DJ, Fitzcharles MA. Fibromyalgia criteria and severity scales for clinical and epidemiological studies: a modification of the ACR preliminary diagnostic criteria for fibromyalgia. J Rheumatol. 2011;38(6):1113–22. doi:10.3899/jrheum.100594.

55. Henry SL, Crawford JL, Puckett CL. Risk factors and complications in reduction mammaplasty: novel associations and preoperative assessment. Plast Reconstr Surg. 2009;124:1040–6.

56. Linder J, Ekholm KS, Jansen GB, et al. Long-term sick leavers with difficulty in resuming work: comparisons between psychiatric-somatic comorbidity and monodiagnosis. Int J Rehabil Res. 2009;32:20–35.

57. Pogatzki-Zahn EM, Englbrecht JS, Schug SA. Acute pain management in patients with fibromyalgia and other diffuse chronic pain syndromes. Curr Opin Anaesthesiol. 2009;22:627–33.

58. Linder J, Schuldt EK, Lundh G, et al. Long-term sick-leavers with fibromyalgia: comparing their multidisciplinarily assessed characteristics with those of others with chronic pain conditions and depression. J Multidiscip Healthc. 2009;2:23–37.

59. Burckhardt CS, Jones KD. Effects of chronic widespread pain on the health status and quality of life of women after breast cancer surgery. Health Qual Life Outcomes. 2005;3:30.

60. Muller A, Hartmann M, Eich W. Health care utilization in patients with fibromyalgia syndrome (FMS). Schmerz. 2000;14:77–83.

61. Velanovich V. The effect of chronic pain syndromes and psychoemotional disorders on symptomatic and quality-of-life outcomes of antireflux surgery. J Gastrointest Surg. 2003;7:53–8.

62. Straub TA. Endoscopic carpal tunnel release: a prospective analysis of factors associated with unsatisfactory results. Arthroscopy. 1999;15:269–74.

63. Wolfe F, Anderson J, Harkness D, et al. A prospective, longitudinal, multicenter study of service utilization and costs in fibromyalgia. Arthritis Rheum. 1997;40: 1560–70.

NTOS from the Physical Therapists' Point of View

Peter I. Edgelow

Abstract

The purpose of this chapter is to discuss the evaluation by a physical therapist of a patient who has been diagnosed as having neurogenic thoracic outlet syndrome (NTOS). Such an evaluation is designed to obtain the facts that will guide both the technique and vigor of treatment. The initial evaluation can be separated into three sections: First, subjective evaluation of the history of symptoms (with emphasis paid to characteristic pain patterns and their persistence), numeric assessment of current symptoms, and functional assessment (ideally using a standardized functional questionnaire). Second, an objective evaluation, including assessment of active movements and palpation, to determine both the sensitivity of the nervous system and to help differentiate various other problems from NTOS. Emphasis is placed on tests that are performed at every treatment session to assess the effect of the treatment. Finally, emphasis on evaluation of motor dysfunction (Kabat test), breathing, and neurodynamics of the brachial plexus are performed.

Introduction

Neurogenic thoracic outlet syndrome (NTOS) can present with signs and symptoms indicating the presence of neurological problems relating to the basic pathology as well as musculoskeletal consequences related to the chronicity of the condition. The purpose of the physical therapist's evaluation is threefold: First, examine the nervous system to determine its degree of sensitivity, second, to ascertain whether NTOS or another entity exists and, if both, to determine which predominates [1], and, third, obtain the data that will be needed to guide the technique(s) and vigor of treatment. The initial evaluation is separated into subjective and objective components.

Subjective Evaluation

The subjective evaluation includes a numeric rating of present symptoms, functional assessment using a standardized questionnaire, and history from onset to present time.

P.I. Edgelow, DPT
Graduate Program in Physical Therapy, UCSF/SFSU,
2429 Balmoral St, Union City, CA 94587, USA
e-mail: peteriedgelow@aol.com

K.A. Illig et al. (eds.), *Thoracic Outlet Syndrome*,
DOI 10.1007/978-1-4471-4366-6_9, © Springer-Verlag London 2013

Numeric assessment of present symptoms: The patient is asked to rate the intensity of pain at least and at worst on a 0–10 numeric pain rating scale (NPRS). The NPRS has high content validity; it directly measures the intensity of pain and has been shown to have correlations as high as r = .80 [2].

Functional assessment using a standardized functional questionnaire: The Disability Arm Shoulder Hand (DASH) questionnaire measures upper extremity function, and is ideal in this role. There are 30 questions, each with five possible answers ranging from 1 = normal to 5 = unable to do. Normal function is indicated by a score of 30 and maximum abnormal function, 120. The test-retest reliability is ICC = 0.96, and retesting after intervention can demonstrate change [3]. A problem encountered by this author is the difficulty of this and other standardized tests to pick up the subtle changes to be found over time in the NTOS population. The main value of the DASH assessment may be the fact that it provides a numeric value (albeit qualitative) that can be used as a measure of the severity of functional impairment between patients. A better answer to assessing change may be found in the Patient Specific Functional test [4].

History: The onset of symptoms in patients with NTOS is typically gradual. Characteristic symptomatic patterns emerge as these problems progress from acute to chronic. Symptoms can begin in the neck and spread to the arm and hand and other arm, or begin in the hand and progress to the arm, neck and other extremity. Pain, numbness, swelling, discoloration of the hand and temperature asymmetry in the hand can be specific to a peripheral nerve emanating from the brachial plexus, a cervical root or both. Symptoms can also include headache and, occasionally, low back and leg pain. As they progress, symptoms can be intermittent or constant and can vary in degree of severity from mild to severe. Rest or positional change or modification in performance of task eases mild symptoms, but not severe symptoms.

Objective Evaluation

Objective tests are divided into those tests that are done at the initial evaluation only, those tests that differentiate NTOS from other problems [1], and those tests that are repeated at every treatment to assess progress.

Testing at the Initial Evaluation

- **Postural observation/assessment:**
  - **Test:** Typical posture can include a forward head, together with scapular elevation and scapular protraction. There may be visible swelling in the supraclavicular fossa.
    - ○ **Goal:** Reduce forward head posture.
- **Active Movements:**
  - **Test:** All active movement tests must only be examined to the point of tension (the point at which the flexion withdrawal response, as defined below, is elicited) not to the point of pain or pain increase [5]. In the NTOS patient there are musculoskeletal dysfunctions as well as neurovascular dysfunctions. In examining the musculoskeletal consequences of the injury, movement is commonly evaluated to the point of pain or pain increase. If one evaluates the neurovascular consequences in the same way, there is a high probability that the examination itself will exacerbate the patient's condition. To avoid this increase in symptoms, movement tests should be examined to the point of tension only. If the examination is limited to this point of tension, then the possibility of a flare secondary to the evaluation will be minimized. In evaluating the nervous system to determine its sensitivity to movement one must instruct the patient to alert the examiner to the tension point in active range of motion. It is the relationship between the tension free range of motion (ROM) and the full ROM that measures the flexion withdrawal reflex that is initiated by the sensitized nervous system. The closer the tension point is to the end range of motion (EROM) the more likely that the restriction (tension) is musculoskeletal in origin. Typically in NTOS the tension point is found in the first 50 % of active ROM while the EROM may be close to normal.
- **Active movement and palpation tests: Measuring the sensitivity of the nervous system**

- **Test:** Active movements of the neck examined: neck flexion: neck extension, neck rotation right and neck rotation left. Note whether there is a pattern of cervical restriction vs. brachial plexus restriction. Cervical movements are commonly painful ipsilateral or sensitive in upper trapezius and intrascapular regions. NTOS is commonly sensitive in the contralateral neck movements more than the ipsilateral neck movements. i.e. Side bending of the neck towards the symptomatic arm eases the pain rather than increasing the pain with NTOS. Conversely, side bending the neck away from the symptomatic arm increases the pain, rather than eases the pain as in CR. (See Spurling's test).
  - ○ **Goal:** Increasing tension free ROM with reduction in pain, should be sufficient to allow increased function of the neck.
- **Test:** Active movements of upper extremities: Shoulder flexion with elbow extended tests shoulder ROM with a median nerve bias. Shoulder ROM with elbow flexed tests shoulder ROM with an ulnar bias and hand behind back tests shoulder ROM with a radial bias.
  - ○ **Goal**: Increasing tension free ROM with reduction in pain should be sufficient to allow increased function of the shoulder.
- **Test**: Tinel's tap test: at the carpal tunnel, Guyens canal, cubital tunnel and over the brachial plexus (Erb's point). The greater the number of positive Tinel's sites the greater the sensitivity of the nervous system.
  - ○ **Goal:** Decrease sensitivity of the nervous system, resulting in a negative tap test.
- **Test**: Palpation to assess tenderness: anterior scalene, subclavius and pectoralis minor.
  - ○ **Goal**: The more sites of tenderness, the more likely it is that the tender muscles are hyperactive. Therefore the goal is to reduce the hyperactivity of these dual functioning muscles. (Breathing, neck and shoulder girdle movements).
- **Test**: Sensation of numbness or paraesthesia more commonly C8/T1 in distribution.
  - ○ **Goal**: Normal sensitivity in C8-T1.

Tests Used to Differentiate NTOS from Other Problems (Most Commonly, at This Phase, Cervical Radiculitis)

- **Spurling's test.** A positive sign (incriminating a cervical disc problem) is pain or tingling referred to the ipsilateral arm. Referral to the contralateral arm suggests NTOS.
- Positioning the arm overhead eases the symptoms caused by cervical disk disease, while it aggravates the symptoms in NTOS. The elevated arm stress test (EAST) is a variant of this.
- Manual distraction of cervical spine eases symptoms caused by cervical disk disease, but aggravates those caused by NTOS.

Testing to Assess Changes Over Time

- **Test**: Hand temperature (conveniently measured with an infrared wine thermometer). Normal is symmetry between index and fifth digit and in high 80s low 90s. The hands may be cold with asymmetry between the index and little finger with the little finger commonly colder than the index finger [6]. The measurement error with the wine thermometer is estimated to be ±2°.
  - – **Goal**: Re-establish normal physiologic response to diaphragmatic breathing, walking, and repeated movements of the arms. The normal response is increasing hand temperature. In NTOS the response can be a decrease in temperature.
- **Test**: Patients with NTOS have a breathing pattern at rest that is upper chest, scalene, subclavius and pectoralis minor dominant rather than diaphragmatic.
  - – **Goal**: Calm the neurological system with parasympathetically sustained diaphragmatic breathing. Measure by increased tension free range of motion of the brachial plexus. Able to inhale 50 % without activating the scalenes [7, 8].
- **Test**: Even in NTOS, neurodynamic testing of sciatic plexus using straight leg raise (SLR) can be positive for abnormally restricted mobility and increased sensitivity. The extreme example is reproduction of hand symptoms with SLR.

Fig. 9.1 Right ULTT:
Starting position note that
the nervous system in its
resting position should be
relaxed and asymptomatic

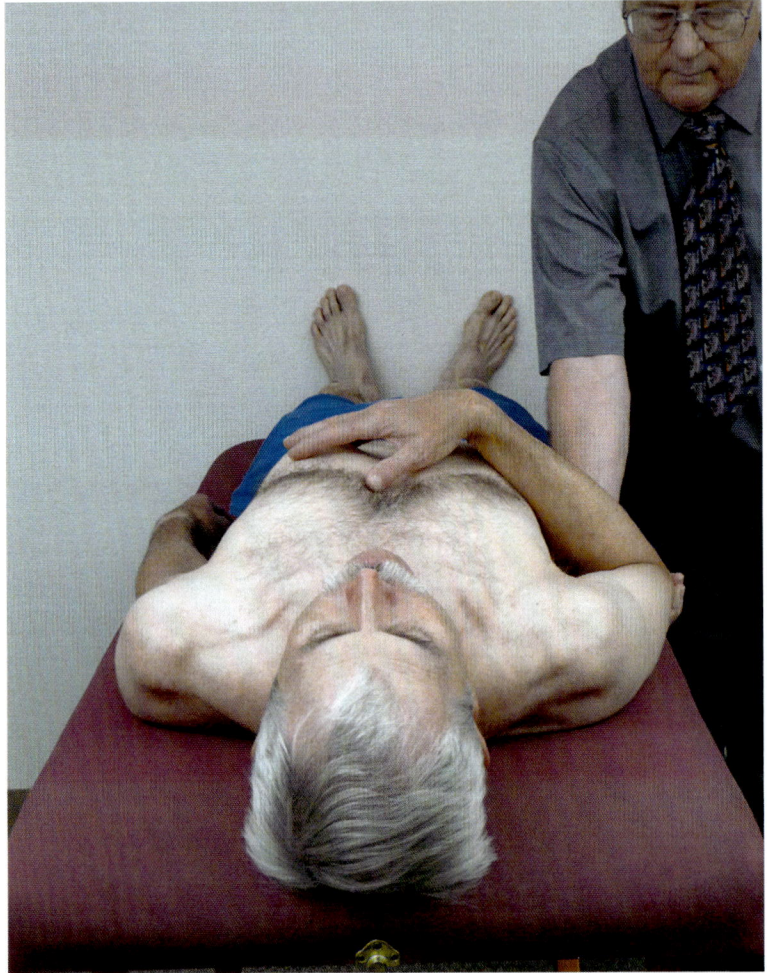

– **Goal**: Symmetrical (SLR) with pull in hamstrings and ROM 65° or greater.
- **Test**: Neurodynamic testing of upper limb tension test (ULTT) [8, 9]. I consider using the ULTT to assess the brachial plexus is as important as using the SLR to examine the sciatic plexus in symptoms of the lower extremity (Figs. 9.1, 9.2, 9.3 and 9.4). The ULTT limitation is not specific for a particular anatomical site but rather incriminates the nervous system as a whole in the symptom production [8, 9].
  – **Goal**: Use ULTT to assess increase in tension-free ROM of the brachial plexus which provides an objective measure of a decrease in neural sensitivity.
- **Test:** Cardiovascular assessment using a treadmill: Evaluate ability to walk without an increase in symptoms, record speed and time to a maximum of 20 min. Modify the speed and time and swing arms or support arms to avoid pain increase.
  – **Goal**: Swing arms, while walking at a speed of 3 mph, for 20 min, four times a day, without increase in symptoms.
- **Test**: Strength testing of the cervical spine, scapula, low back and thumb. Muscle weakness, if present, is mild and involves most commonly the thenar, hypothenar and interossei muscles innervated by the ulnar nerve. The traditional grip and pinch tests are within normal limits. To assess the relationship of the cervical spine stability and weakness of the thumb, examine with Kabat test (see Chap. 23). This test evaluates weakness of the intrinsic core stabilizers of the neck. It is also a sensitive measure of the dysfunction of the dynamics of

Fig. 9.2 Ending position before treatment Arm movements to take up the slack in the Brachial Plexus to initial point of tension. Assess symptoms at position of increase in tension. Record example as follows: Right ULTT: Symptoms of tension right IV and V digits at 40° of glenohumeral abduction and 180° of elbow extension without scapular depression without wrist and finger extension (This is a typical example of initial finding with NTOS)

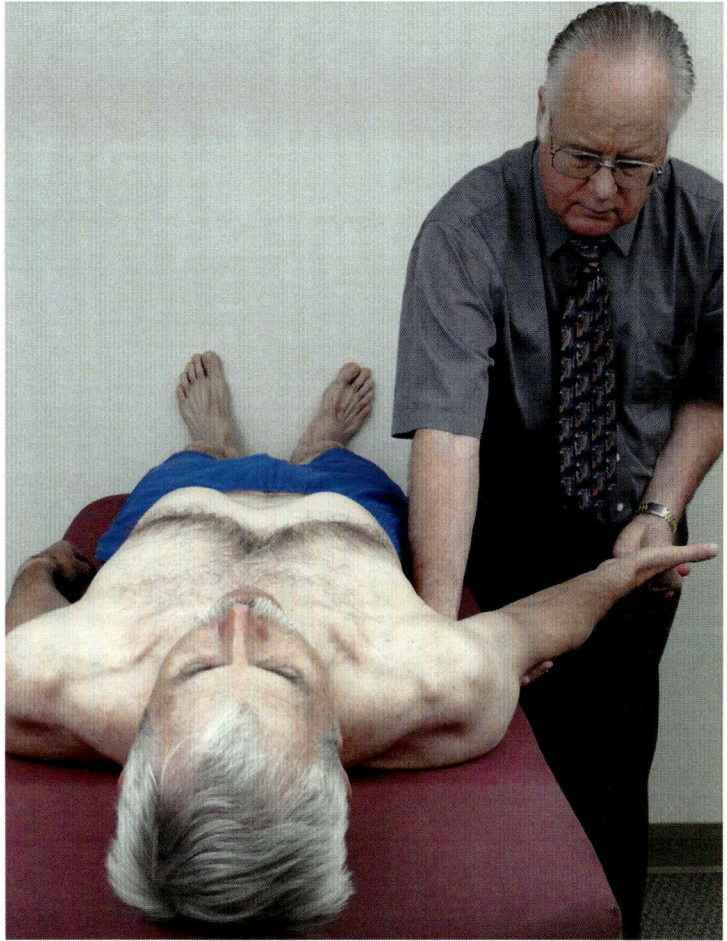

Fig. 9.3 End Range of Motion after a treatment technique such as diaphragmatic breathing. Sample of ULTT ending position demonstrating decrease in neural sensitivity. Assess symptoms at increase in tension position. Record as follows: Right ULTT, Symptoms of tension in IV and V digits at 90° of glenohumeral abduction and 180° of elbow extension without scapular depression and without wrist and finger extension. Typical example of NTOS as nervous system is decreasing in irritability. Commonly assessed by having the patient walk with a stride that does not increase pain and swinging the arms provided that also does not increase pain

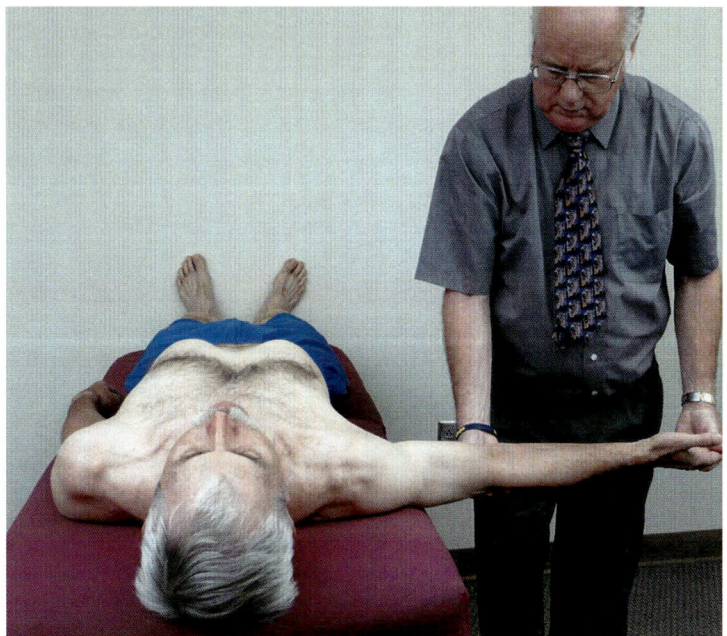

Fig. 9.4 Further increasing range of motion typical example with NTOS as nervous system is decreasing in irritability and now cannot find tension with full abduction of the arm unless take up more slack in the nervous system by hyperextending wrist and fingers. Record as follows: Right ULTT: Symptoms IV and V digits at 90° of glenohumeral abduction and 180° of elbow extension without scapular depression with wrist and finger extension

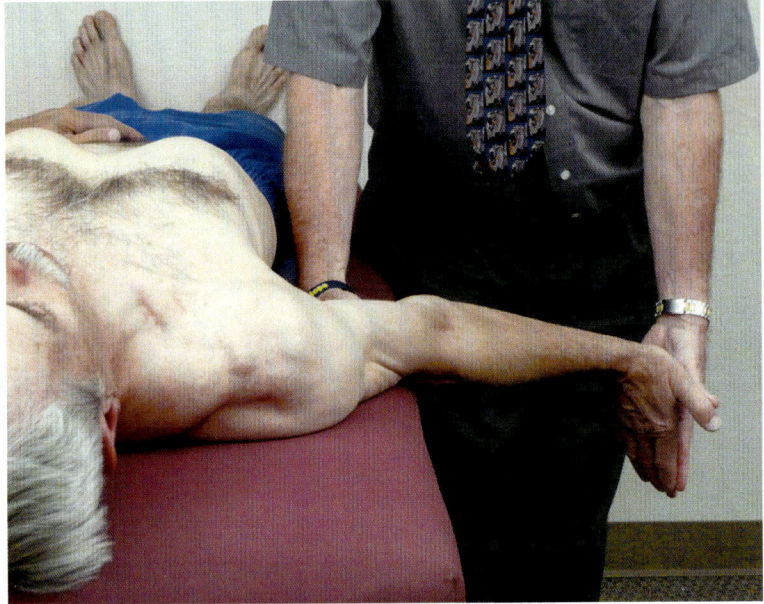

the neck and shoulder girdle stability. The physical therapist and the patient can use this test, plus the Thinker's Pose, to determine if an activity/exercise causes a unilateral weakness. These weaknesses and/or dysfunctions are associated with patient with a diagnosis of NTOS [10].

– **Goal**: To be strong in all postures and during all exercises when initially they were weak.

Herman Kabat, M.D., the originator of the physical therapy technique termed proprioceptive neuromuscular facilitation (PNF), recognized that in the evaluation of neuromotor control of the hand and its relationship to the cervical spine that following proprioceptive stimulation of the deep neck flexors the weakness in unilateral deep thumb flexor could be reversed with an immediate increase in strength of the weak thumb. The deep head of flexor pollicis brevis is tested isometrically in the shortened range of thumb adduction [11] (Fig. 9.5). For an accurate test care must be used to minimize activity from median innervated muscles such as opponens pollicis and the long flexor of the thumb and the fingers. If one thumb is weak, it is re-tested while the patient is doing the Thinker Pose (Fig. 9.6). The force is just enough to activate proprioceptors in the deep

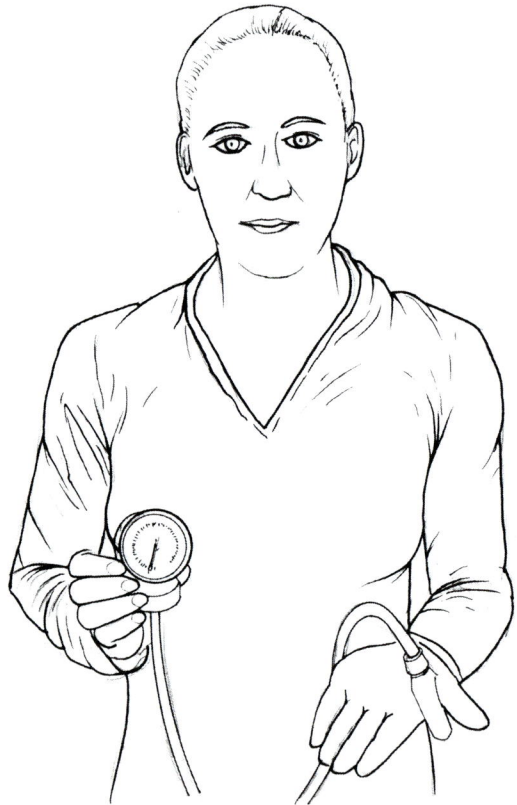

Fig. 9.5 Assessing strength of the ulnar innervated thumb muscles of the hand using an instrument as shown, the strength can be measured

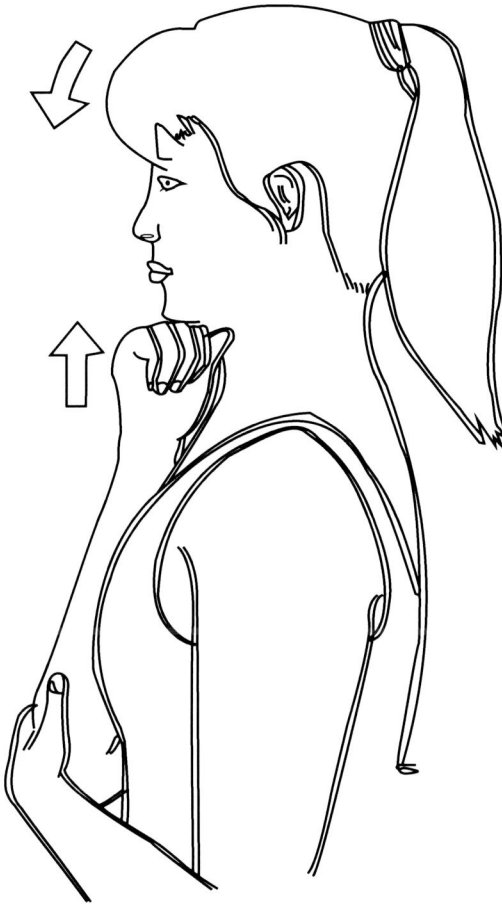

Fig. 9.6 "Thinker Pose"

neck flexors as the patient initiates movements of the trunk or upper extremities. The applied force should be thought of as a proprioceptive neuromuscular stimulus to the stabilizers of the neck rather than a strengthening stimulus, which could activate the scalenes as well as the deep neck flexors. If weakness is reversed, it is thought to be due to the isometric activation of the core stabilizers (deep neck flexors) with minimal or no activation of the scalenes, subclavius or pectoralis minor muscles. The hand weakness returns with stress to the neck in the form of minimal stress of gravity such as fully erect posture vs. relaxed forward head posture or flexed neck posture vs. relaxed resting posture. The patient who has a weak thumb that is strengthened by the "Thinker Pose" characteristically, has weakness in the stabilizers of the neck, lumbar spine and

stabilizers of the scapula. Test the patient at each treatment to assess whether they are functionally stable in neutral, fully erect and flexed postures. This would be accomplished when the thumb tests strong without input from the thinkers pose.

Comments

As in any medical condition, the purpose of the initial evaluation is to identify and characterize the problem at hand. It is a non-trivial point that the physical therapist's evaluation must not cause increased sensitivity of the nervous system, because the nervous systems' response to NTOS involves the whole nervous system generating an abnormal response to minimal movement/activity to begin with! The care provided by the physical therapist must provide a model for the patient the care they need to use to manage their problem. The ability to do a thorough evaluation without exacerbating the patient's symptoms will establish a foundation of confidence in the practitioner's skill and experience. In treatment, a change you can make during a visit may not be sustained but even so can provide the patient with the understanding that it is possible to reverse some of the symptoms and signs almost immediately. It may take repetition of dysfunctional symptoms to correct the neuromotor dysfunction, and it is possible to retrain such a normal neuromotor response with repetition also.

The more sensitive the nervous system is, the slower will be the progression of treatment. The usual goals of strengthening and stretching have to be monitored carefully and can be maladaptive if they increase the sensitivity of the nervous system. In patients with NTOS, the nervous system has been injured and the chronicity of the problem has resulted in the centralization of the pain.

Conclusion

The goals of the initial physical therapy evaluation are to examine the neurovascular system in order to develop a treatment plan and use the objective findings to assess progress.

References

1. Wainner R, Fritz J, Irrgang J, Boninger M, Delitto A, Allison S. Reliability and diagnostic accuracy of the clinical examination and patient self-report measures for cervical radiculopathy. Spine. 2003;28(1):52–62.

2. Jensen M, Karoly P, Braver S. The measurement of clinical pain intensity: a comparison of six methods. Pain. 1986;27:117–26.

3. Beaton D, Katz J, Fossel A, Wright J, Tarasuk V, Bombardier C. Measuring the whole or the parts? Validity, reliability, and responsiveness of the Disabilities of the Arm, Shoulder and Hand outcome measures in different regions of the upper extremity. J Hand Ther. 2001;14:128–46.

4. Stratford P, Gill C, Westeway M, Binkley J. Assessing disability and change on individual patients: a report of a patient specific measure. Physiother Can. 1995;47:258–63.

5. Coppieters M, Stappaerts K, Janssens K. Reliability of detecting "onset of pain" and "submaximal pain" during neural provocation of the upper quadrant. Physiother Res Int. 2002;7(3):146–56.

6. Ellis W, Cheng S. Intraoperative thermographic monitoring during neurogenic thoracic outlet decompressive surgery. Vasc Endovascular Surg. 2003;37(4):253–7.

7. McLaughlin L, Goldsmith CH, Coleman K. Breathing evaluation and retraining as an adjunct to manual therapy. Man Ther. 2011;16:51–2.

8. Shacklock M. Clinical neurodynamics: a new system of musculoskeletal treatment. 1st ed. Edinburgh: Elsevier; 2005.

9. Butler D. The sensitive nervous system. Unley: Noigroup Publications; 2000.

10. Jull G, Falla D, Treleaven J, Sterling M, O'Leary S. A therapeutic exercise approach for cervical disorders. 3rd ed. Churchill Livingston: Elsevier; 2005. Vol Chapter 32.

11. Kabat H. Low back and leg pain. St. Louis: Warren H. Green, Inc.; 1980.

The Gilliatt-Sumner Hand

Gabriel C. Tender and David G. Kline

Abstract

One form of NTOS results in the development of a clinical finding known as the Gilliatt-Sumner hand (GSH). The clinical features of GSH include weakness and atrophy of the thenar, hypothenar, and interossei intrinsic hand muscles. In addition, there is hypesthesia in the ulnar and medial antebrachial cutaneous distribution, but normal median nerve sensation. Electrical findings include decreased median and ulnar compound muscle action potentials (CMAP's) and ulnar and medial antebrachial cutaneous (MAC) sensory nerve action potentials (SNAP's). GSH has a frequent association with congenital anatomic variations which cause entrapment of the lower trunk of the brachial plexus. These variations include bony anomalies such as hypertrophic C7 transverse processes and cervical ribs, or soft tissue abnormalities like a cervical band, Sibson's fascia, or thickened medial border of the scalene muscle. In this subgroup of NTOS patients, a surgical decompression is indicated. Surgical results indicate that symptom progression is usually stopped, and often the pre-existing neurological deficits are reversed.

Historical Perspective

Neurogenic thoracic outlet syndrome (NTOS) is one of the most controversial entrapment neuropathies to diagnose and treat [1]. Historically, NTOS was divided into two categories: "true"

G.C. Tender, MD (✉)
Department of Neurosurgery, Louisiana State University in New Orleans, 2020 Gravier Street, Suite 744, New Orleans, LA 70112, USA
e-mail: gtende@lsuhsc.edu

D.G. Kline, MD
Department of Neurosurgery, LSUHSC Neurosurgery (retired), 7041 Globe Road, Lenoir, NC 28645, USA

and "disputed". The latter had poorly defined boundaries, whereas the term "true" NTOS was applied to patients who had a demonstrable, chronic C8, T1 and lower trunk brachial plexopathy, usually caused by congenital bony and soft tissue anomalies. In 1970, Gilliatt described the characteristic features of "true" NTOS: thenar, hypothenar, and interossei weakness and/or atrophy, plus ulnar and medial antebrachial cutaneous hypesthesia in the affected arm, but normal sensation in the median nerve distribution [2]. This constellation of clinical features, along with associated electrical findings, is now recognized as the Gilliatt-Sumner hand (GSH).

K.A. Illig et al. (eds.), *Thoracic Outlet Syndrome*,
DOI 10.1007/978-1-4471-4366-6_10, © Springer-Verlag London 2013

Given the infrequency of this syndrome, many symptoms are often misinterpreted as cervical radiculopathy, ulnar entrapment at elbow or wrist, or even advanced carpal tunnel syndrome. Electromyography helps in the differential diagnosis by showing normal ulnar conduction across the elbow, both median and ulnar decreased compound muscle action potentials (CMAP's) in hand intrinsics, and decreased ulnar and medial antebrachial cutaneous (MAC) sensory nerve action potentials (SNAP's), with normal median SNAP's [3, 4].

Anatomic Considerations in GSH

The surgical anatomy is described in detail in Chap. 6 of this book. Briefly, the spinal nerves and trunks of the brachial plexus are situated between the anterior and middle scalene muscles. The two scalene muscles and the first rib form the interscalenic triangle, the site of entrapment for most cases of TOS. The subclavian artery accompanies the lower trunk in the interscalenic triangle, in close proximity to the first rib, while the subclavian vein runs in front of the anterior scalene muscle.

Congenital anatomic variations can compromise the narrow passage of the nerve roots in the interscalenic triangle [1]. Bony anomalies include hypertrophic C7 transverse processes and cervical ribs [5]. More often, soft tissue abnormalities like a cervical band, Sibson's fascia, or thickened medial border of the scalene muscle are responsible for the entrapment.

We have used two approaches to decompress the lower brachial plexus involved by TOS: anterior supraclavicular and posterior subscapular. The anterior supraclavicular approach is better known to most neurosurgeons [6, 7] and is described in Chap. 29. The posterior subscapular approach is reserved for "complicated" cases: morbid obesity, large bony abnormalities (cervical ribs or very large C7 transverse processes), or cases with previous anterior neck operations [8, 9]. Skin incision is centered between the thoracic spinous processes and the medial edge of the scapula, in order to protect the spinal branch of

the accessory nerve and the ascending branch of the transverse cervical artery (Fig. 10.1, *upper left*). The major and minor rhomboids, and then the levator scapulae, and more superiorly a portion of the trapezius, are sectioned. The scapula is then retracted to an abducted and externally rotated position, by use of a chest retractor (Fig. 10.1, *upper right*). The first rib is exposed and is removed by rongeurs extraperiosteally, from the costotransverse articulation to the costo-clavicular ligament (Fig. 10.1, *lower left*). Removal of the posterior and middle scalene muscles exposes the lower spinal nerves and trunks of the brachial plexus, which are freed up by a complete 360° external neurolysis (Fig. 10.1, *lower right*). Care must be exercised to protect the long thoracic nerve as it originates from the posterior aspect of C6 as well as branches to it from C5 and C7, and sometimes C4 spinal nerves. Potential sites of compression by soft tissue, such as a fascial edge of middle scalene, Sibson's fascia, scalenus minimus, cervical rib or elongated C7 transverse process are removed. If necessary, the spinal nerves can be followed intraforaminally by removing part of the facet joint [8, 11].

If intraoperative nerve action potential (NAP) recordings are performed, the typical patient will have a markedly decreased or flat T1 to lower trunk NAP, moderately reduced C8 to LT NAP, and normal C7 to MT trace. Velocities are similarly affected, mostly in the T1 to LT traces, followed by C8 to LT traces and C7 to MT recordings [12, 13].

Potential complications of the posterior approach to the brachial plexus include intraoperative pleural rents, which can be recognized immediately and closed primarily, and scapular winging, which may be due to inadequate muscle layer closure.

Surgical Series

We reported a series of 33 patients with GSH who underwent surgical decompression of 34 limbs at LSUHSC [14]. All patients had weakness and atrophy of lumbricales, interossei, and thenar and hypothenar muscles. Three patients

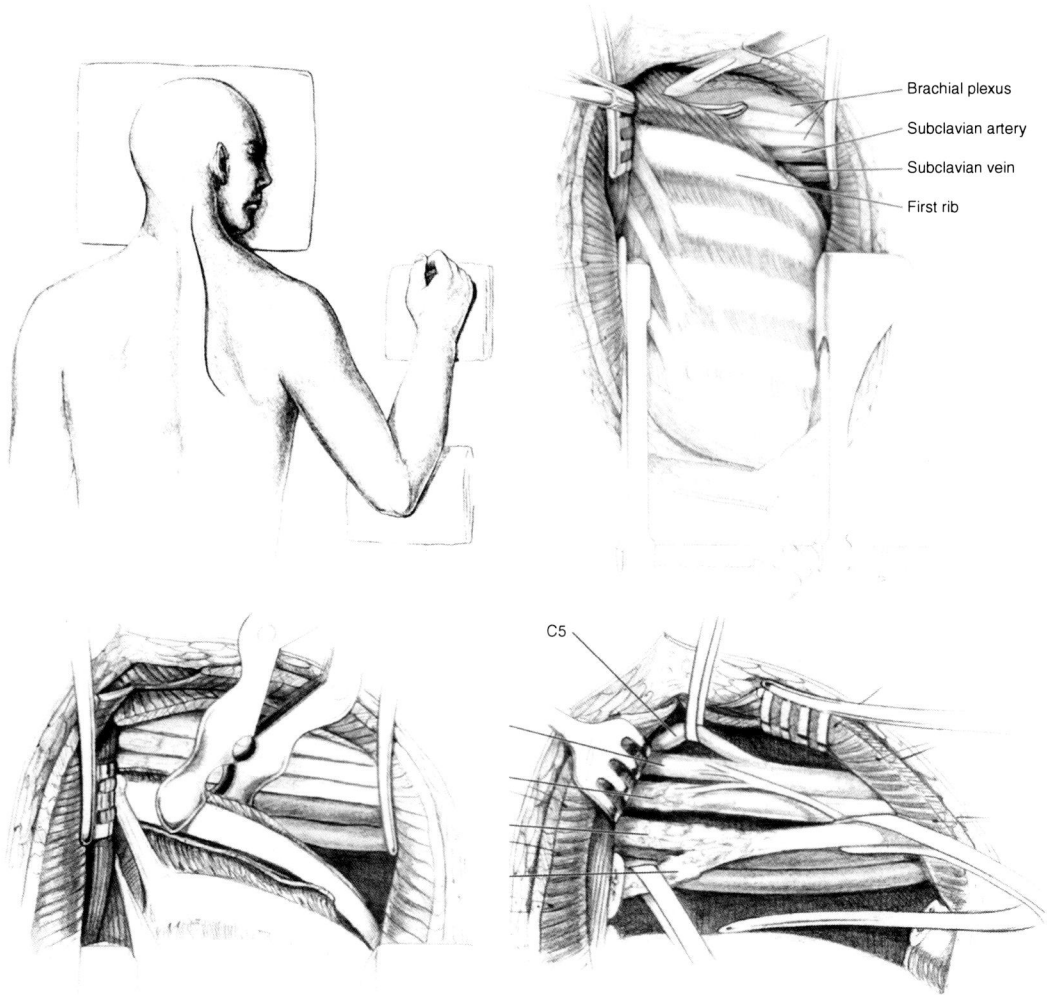

Fig. 10.1 Illustration depicting the posterior subscapular approach. *Upper left:* skin incision. The flexed elbow and arm are placed on a Mayo stand adjacent to the operating table. This can be lowered or elevated to change the position of the scapula. The skin incision is placed halfway between the scapular edge and the thoracic spinous processes. *Upper right:* scapular retraction. As the retractor is opened, the scapula is rotated laterally to expose the posterior aspect of the upper ribs. The posterior scalene muscle is detached from the superior surface of the first rib. *Lower left:* exposure of the inferior brachial plexus. The first rib is resected from the costotransverse articulation to the costoclavicular ligament. *Lower right:* the brachial plexus after neurolysis. The C8 and T1 spinal nerves appear thin and scarred. The long thoracic nerve originates from the posterior aspect of C6 and C7 spinal nerves at this level. The subclavian vessels are located anterior to the plexus (Reprinted from Kline et al. [10]. with permission from Elsevier)

also had weakness of finger extension, and four had flexor profundus weakness. Sensory examination usually paralleled motor function, but was less reliable. Pain was absent in about one third of the patients; when present, it was described as a dull, constant poorly localized ache radiating down the arm. Eleven of our patients had previous operations, none of which alleviated the TOS symptoms. We used the anterior supraclavicular approach in 19 limbs and the posterior subscapular approach in 15 limbs. The most common indications for a posterior approach were previous anterior neck operations and morbid obesity, since scar in the supraclavicular region, as well as working at an increased depth (i.e., in morbidly obese patients), make the exposure of the inferior plexal elements through an anterior approach extremely difficult.

Intraoperative NAPs are important in demonstrating the nerve pathology and localizing the level of injury. When compared to C5 to upper trunk, intraoperative NAPs showed a median reduction in velocity to 17 % for T1 to lower trunk (LT), and 30 % for C8 to LT. Similarly, the amplitude was reduced to 30 % for T1 to LT, and to 40 % for C8 to LT [14].

Results

Outcome was analyzed in terms of pain in the affected limb and motor function in the four muscle groups (thenar, hypothenar, lumbricales and interossei). Of the 21 patients who experienced pain preoperatively, six had complete resolution and 14 had partial improvement of the pain level postoperatively. Only one of the patients had significant residual pain at the 1 year follow-up visit.

Analysis of the pre and postoperative deficit showed significant improvement in 12 of 14 extremities with mild deficit preoperatively and partial improvement in 14 of 20 extremities with severe deficit. Disease progression was usually ameliorated by an adequate surgical decompression. None of the patients experienced new or worsening of preexisting deficits at 1 year follow up. Patients with mild deficit were more likely to recover than the ones with severe deficit, although return to normal motor function was seldom achieved.

Summary

In patients presenting with NTOS and the finding of a GSH, a surgical decompression is indicated. Analysis of our series of patients indicates that symptom progression is usually stopped, and often (over 50 % of patients) some deficit is reversed, if adequate decompression of the C8, T1 spinal nerves and lower trunk is achieved. Of importance, operative NAP recordings done on these patients indicate that conductive abnormalities

involve medial plexus elements, close to the spine, not lateral ones. Surgical decompression needs to involve the medial portion of the plexus, especially the C8 and T1 spinal nerves (sometimes incorrectly referred to as "nerve roots"). Electrical abnormalities included increased latencies and decreased amplitudes of NAP's recorded from T1 to lower trunk more than C8 to lower trunk more than C7 to middle trunk, respectively. Many of these patients recover some proportion of their motor function, although recovery is seldom complete. The pain syndrome, when present, is also improved by surgery in the majority of patients. Experience with not only the anterior but also the posterior exposure of the brachial plexus is helpful for optimal outcomes, especially in patients with prior operations, morbid obesity, or large bony abnormalities.

References

1. Cherington M, Wilbourn AJ. Neurovascular compression in the thoracic outlet syndrome. Ann Surg. 1999;230:829–30.
2. Gilliatt RW, Le Quesne PM, Logue V, Sumner AJ. Wasting of the hand associated with a cervical rib or band. J Neurol Neurosurg Psychiatry. 1970;33:615–24.
3. Glover JL, Worth RM, Bendick PJ, Hall PV, Markand OM. Evoked responses in the diagnosis of thoracic outlet syndrome. Surgery. 1981;89:86–93.
4. Le Forestier N, Moulonguet A, Maisonobe T, Leger JM, Bouche P. True neurogenic thoracic outlet syndrome: electrophysiological diagnosis in six cases. Muscle Nerve. 1998;21:1129–34.
5. Sanders RJ, Hammond SL. Management of cervical ribs and anomalous first ribs causing neurogenic thoracic outlet syndrome. J Vasc Surg. 2002;36:51–6.
6. Kline DG, Hackett ER, Happel LH. Surgery for lesions of the brachial plexus. Arch Neurol. 1986;43:170–81.
7. Tender GC, Kline DG. Anterior supraclavicular approach to the brachial plexus. Neurosurgery. 2006;58:ONS-360–4.
8. Dubuisson AS, Kline DG, Weinshel SS. Posterior subscapular approach to the brachial plexus. Report of 102 patients. J Neurosurg. 1993;79:319–30.
9. Tender GC, Kline DG. Posterior subscapular approach to the brachial plexus. Neurosurgery. 2005;57:377–81.
10. Kline DG, Hudson AR, Kim DH. Posterior subscapular approach to plexus. In: Kline DG, Hudson AR, Kim DH, editors. Atlas of peripheral nerve surgery. Philadelphia: W.B. Saunders Co.; 2001. p. 41–50.
11. Kline DG, Donner TR, Happel L, Smith B, Richter HP. Intraforaminal repair of plexus spinal nerves by a

posterior approach: an experimental study. J Neurosurg. 1992;76:459–70.

12. Robert EG, Happel LT, Kline DG. Intraoperative nerve action potential recordings: technical considerations, problems, and pitfalls. Neurosurgery. 2009;65: A97–104.

13. Tiel RL, Happel Jr LT, Kline DG. Nerve action potential recording method and equipment. Neurosurgery. 1996;39:103–8.

14. Tender GC, Thomas AJ, Thomas N, Kline DG. Gilliatt-Sumner hand revisited: a 25-year experience. Neurosurgery. 2004;55:883–90.

NTOS in the Pediatric Age Group

11

Hugh A. Gelabert

Abstract

NTOS in a child the consequences may be devastating form both a physical and emotional perspective. The rarity of the condition in children and adolescents frequently results in a delayed diagnosis, and children often present at a stage where the condition is severe and disabling. In this age group, injection of into the anterior scalene muscle also is a very specific test which may assist in establishing the diagnosis of NTOS. While most adults with NTOS will benefit from physical therapy, adolescents and children tend to have such acute and severe presentations that PT is seldom sufficient to achieve resolution. Controlling symptoms with chemodenervation using Botulinum toxin A may allow some patients to complete a school term before proceeding with surgical decompression. Surgical decompression of the thoracic outlet is the most effective means of alleviating severe, disabling symptoms in the pediatric population.

Introduction

NTOS typically presents with pain and paresthesia. It may also include muscle wasting, atrophy and weakness in the upper extremity. When these occur in a child the consequences may be devastating form both a physical and emotional perspective. The incidence of pediatric aged patients presenting with TOS is undefined but known to be low – accordingly most pediatricians are unfamiliar with the condition. The diagnosis is low on the differential of upper extremity pain. Because of the rarity of the condition in children and adolescents, the recognition of NTOS is frequently delayed. Presentations are often at a stage where the condition is acute, severe and disabling.

Additional diagnostic features are often required for those not familiar with TOS to recognize its presence. This is one reason for the observed relative increased frequency of vascular TOS (versus NTOS) and also the observed frequency of skeletal anomalies (cervical ribs, scoliosis) noted in younger patients [1]. It is also for this reason the incidence of cervical ribs and true neurogenic presentations with wasting of the musculature of the hand and arm is increased in this patient population [2, 3].

H.A. Gelabert, MD
Division of Vascular Surgery, UCLA David Geffen
School of Medicine, 200 UCLA Medical Plaza, Ste 526,
Los Angeles, CA 90095-6904, USA
e-mail: hgelabert@mednet.ucla.edu

K.A. Illig et al. (eds.), *Thoracic Outlet Syndrome*,
DOI 10.1007/978-1-4471-4366-6_11, © Springer-Verlag London 2013

Diagnostic Approach

The initial approach to pediatric aged patients begins with a careful review of symptoms and presentation, as well as a meticulous physical examination of the patient. As the incidence of skeletal anomalies and cervical ribs is increased in this patient population, chest and cervical spine radiographs are essential.

While MRI imaging of the cervical spine is done in all adult presentations, it benefit is limited in the pediatric population. Given the younger ages, the probability of degenerative spine disease is very low. An MRI of the cervical spine is done where history may suggest possible spine injury, or where examination indicates skeletal anomalies, pain or sensitivity with movement of the neck. More recently use of MRI for evaluation of the thoracic outlet, the brachial plexus, subclavian artery and subclavian vein has gained popularity [4]. The value of these studies is that they may provide evidence of compression at the thoracic outlet.

Electrophysiologic testing such as electromyography (EMG), nerve conduction testing have long been used to identify conditions which may mimic the presentation of TOS – specifically peripheral compression of the ulnar and median nerves [5]. These tests provide only indirect evidence of NTOS. More specific to the diagnosis is the somato-sensory evoked potential examination (SSEP) [6]. Recently the use of the median antebrachial cutaneous (MAC) sensory neural action potential (SNAP) testing has been reported as having high sensitivity and specificity for the diagnosis of NTOS [7].

Anterior Scalene Muscle Block

Injection of lidocaine into the anterior scalene muscle is a very specific test which may assist in establishing the diagnosis of NTOS [8]. The qualifying criterion of a successful or positive block is the reduction of symptoms of pain or paresthesia by at least 50 %. A positive block will serve to confirm the diagnosis of NTOS, and indicates that the symptoms of NTOS are related to spasm of the anterior scalene muscle. It is the only test which can directly relate the patient's symptoms to a specific anatomical entity. Thus it serves to illuminate the mechanism which is responsible for the patient's symptoms. If the symptoms respond to a Lidocaine based scalene muscle block, it suggests that the patient may be a candidate for chemodenervation with a longer lasting agent such as Botox. The block also serves to predict a favorable result from surgical decompression. Finally the block serves to distinguish symptoms related to TOS from any other co-morbid conditions such as fibromyalgia or polymyalgia rheumatica.

Treatment

Initial treatment of NTOS without atrophy of the intrinsic hand muscles will involve physical therapy, medication and neuromuscular blockade. While most adults with NTOS will benefit from physical therapy, adolescents and children tend to have such acute and severe presentations that PT is seldom sufficient to achieve resolution. In most instances of severe NTOS, PT will afford temporary relief, but further treatment is required.

Medications which are used for control of NTOS symptoms may be of limited use in children and adolescents. The severity of symptoms and the strength of the medications may render the patients unable to maintain normal daily activities. Students may not be able to attend school; athletes may not be able to play sports while on medication. The efficacy of medication in achieving complete remission of symptoms in severe presentations is limited.

The pharmacological approach to NTOS in pediatric aged patients is similar to that used in adults: anti-inflammatory and narcotic medications may be provided to relieve pain; muscle relaxants are provided to reduce muscle spasm; anti-depressants (such as amitriptyline) or medications such as pregabalin, gabapentin or topiramate can be used for relief of nerve irritation.

Chemodenervation of the anterior scalene muscle, the pectoralis minor, subclavius and upper trapezius muscles is very effective both as diagnostic and therapeutic intervention [9, 10]. This technique is discussed in greater detail in Chap. 20. The impact of a successful chemodenervation may be dramatic. When it works it may result in complete relief of symptoms with no side-effects. For the pediatric aged patients this allows them to continue with school without pain and paresthesia. For athletes while it allows control of symptoms, it does not allow return to athletic competition. In practice we have found use of long-lasting chemodenervation with Botox to be helpful in allowing patients to complete their school term before proceeding with surgical decompression.

Surgical Decompression

Surgical decompression of the thoracic outlet is the most effective means of alleviating severe, disabling symptoms in the pediatric population. It is a challenging effort, as the impact of complications or poor outcomes is magnified by the young age and dependency of the patients. Surgical approaches which have been reported include trans-axillary first rib resection, supra-clavicular anterior and middle scalene muscle resection, and supra-clavicular first rib resection.

Given the rarity of NTOS in pediatric aged patients it is not surprising that there is a dearth of literature dedicated to this problem. Most reports combine both vascular and neurogenic TOS presentations. Additionally most reports include only a handful of patients and thus account for a limited experience.

The earliest report found on Medline search of TOS in a child was by Nichamin in 1962 [11]. The youngest TOS patient reported in the medical literature was a 6-year-old boy who developed a subclavian artery aneurysm related to TOS compression [12]. Yang reported four cases of NTOS in the adolescent population [13]. Vercellio reported eight TOS patients ranging 8–16 years of age, including two that presented with neurogenic symptoms [14]. Follow-up ranged from 6 months to 3 years [14]. Six patients did well, with one recurrence out of the seven surgically treated patients. Swierczynska reported three

teenaged patients with NTOS [15]. The authors noted that neuro-rehabilitation did not result in complete recovery, whereas the combination of rehabilitation with surgical treatment led to measurable improvement as recorded by SSEP testing. Maru reported a series of 12 patients (average age 16 year) with TOS, finding acute ischemic symptoms as the initial presentation in 38 %, venous symptoms in 24 %, and neurogenic symptoms in 38 % [16]. They observed that vascular TOS presentations are much more common in adolescents and that the results of surgical are good in all subtypes of patients with TOS.

The largest series of pediatric and adolescent TOS reports are from UCLA [2, 3] and St Christopher's Hospital in Philadelphia [17]. These series both report combined vascular and NTOS cases. Rigberg reported a series of 18 patients, of whom 12 had NTOS [2]. In comparing the neurogenic and vascular TOS presentation he observes that NTOS predominantly affects female patients, whereas the vascular presentations were predominantly male athletes. The authors also note the impact and severity of the TOS presentations: 14 of their 18 patients were forced to take leave from school due to severity of their symptoms. While the preferred surgical approach was trans-axillary first rib resection, 42 % of neurogenic patients also required scalenectomy. There were no complications, and all patients improved and were able to resume scholastic activities.

Arthur reported a series of 25 patients (ages 12–18 years) who underwent surgical decompression for vascular and neurogenic TOS [16]. They noted that vascular TOS presentations accounted for the majority 14 (66 %), and NTOS was seen in 11 (44 %). They noted that 3 of the 11 (27 %) NTOS patients had cervical ribs. Their follow up was limited and they reported that of five long-term follow up patients, only two were considered asymptomatic. The symptom severity was such that only one patient required a secondary operation (scalenectomy) which resulted in significant improvement.

The UCLA series has been recently updated with a report of 33 teenaged patients presenting with TOS [3]. Of these 21 (64 %) had NTOS

Table 11.1 Adolescents and TOS

	Number	%	Males	%	Females	%
All	33		8	24	25	75
Neurogenic	21	64	2	9	19	91
Vascular	12	36	6	50	6	50

Adolescents (ages 13–19) presenting with TOS: neurogenic TOS and vascular TOS (*TOS* Thoracic outlet syndrome)

Table 11.2 Cervical ribs: Adolescents and TOS

	No. patients	Cervical ribs	%
Neurogenic	21	5	23

Number of cervical ribs in adolescent TOS

(Table 11.1). Females accounted for 19 (91 %) of the NTOS patients. All told, the 21 patients underwent 27 operations: 22 trans-axillary first rib resections (one patient required bilateral surgery) and five scalene muscle resections for recurrent symptoms. Thus recurrence requiring re-operation occurred in 21 % of the neurogenic patients. The incidence of cervical ribs amongst the patients with NTOS was 24 %, (Table 11.2) much higher than reported in large series of adult patients [18]. The follow up ranged from 90 days to 3 years, with 85 % remaining symptom-free when last contacted. Although still having residual symptoms, the remaining three patients were all improved, and able to resume school and participate in athletics.

Conclusions

NTOS in the pediatric aged patient is an unusual and difficult entity to diagnose, often resulting in a delayed presentation. Accordingly patients frequently present with severe pain, and are disabled from participating in sports or school. The diagnosis of NTOS in pediatric patients is based on the history and findings of neurovascular compression at the thoracic outlet. Diagnostic testing serves the purpose of excluding competing diagnosis and confirming the diagnosis of NTOS. Anterior scalene muscle block is the most specific test for NTOS, and is the only test which can relate the patient's symptoms to the functional anatomy. Initial treatment of NTOS relies on physical therapy and medication. Use of Botox for chemodenervation may serve to alleviate symptoms while preparing for surgical decompression. Surgical decompression via first rib resection is highly effective in well selected patients. Experience with pediatric patients indicates that the need for secondary resection of the anterior scalene muscle may be required in up to 30 %. Long term results in pediatric patients are very good with long lasting effective symptomatic relief.

References

1. Collins JD, Saxton EH, Miller TQ, Ahn SS, Gelabert H, Carnes A. Scheuermann's disease as a model displaying the mechanism of venous obstruction in thoracic outlet syndrome and migraine patients: MRI and MRA. J Natl Med Assoc. 2003;95(4):298–306.
2. Rigberg DA, Gelabert H. The management of thoracic outlet syndrome in teenaged patients. Ann Vasc Surg. 2009;23(3):335–40. Epub 6 Sep 2008.
3. Gelabert H. Thoracic outlet syndrome in the adolescent patient. In: Eskandari MK, Morasch MD, Pearce WH, Yao JST, editors. New findings in vascular surgery. Shelton: People's Publishing House; 2010. p. 409–23.
4. Charon JP, Milne W, Sheppard DG, Houston JG. Evaluation of MR angiographic technique in the assessment of thoracic outlet syndrome. Clin Radiol. 2004;59(7):588–95.
5. Tolson TD. "EMG" for thoracic outlet syndrome. Hand Clin. 2004;20:37–42, vi.
6. Machleder HI, Moll F, Nuwer M, Jordan S. Somatosensory evoked potentials in the assessment of thoracic outlet compression syndrome. J Vasc Surg. 1987;6:177–84.
7. Seror P. Medial antebrachial cutaneous nerve conduction study, a new tool to demonstrate mild lower brachial plexus lesions. A report of 16 cases. Clin Neurophysiol. 2004;115(10):2316–22.
8. Jordan SE, Machleder HI. Diagnosis of thoracic outlet syndrome using electrophysiologically guided anterior scalene blocks. Ann Vasc Surg. 1998;12(3):260–4.
9. Jordan SE, Ahn SS, Freischlag JA, Gelabert HA, Machleder HI. Selective botulinum chemodenervation of the scalene muscles for treatment of neurogenic thoracic outlet syndrome. Ann Vasc Surg. 2000;14(4):365–9.
10. Torriani M, Gupta R, Donahue DM. Botulinum toxin injection in neurogenic thoracic outlet syndrome: results and experience using a ultrasound-guided approach. Skeletal Radiol. 2010;39(10):973–80.
11. Nichamin SJ. Cervical ribs in a young child with neurovascular compression and electroencephalographic manifestations. J Mich State Med Soc. 1962;61:708–11.

12. DiFiore JW, Reid JR, Drummond-Webb J. Thoracic outlet syndrome in a child – transaxillary resection of anomalous first rib. J Pediatr Surg. 2002;37:1220–2.

13. Yang J, Letts M. Thoracic outlet syndrome in children. J Pediatr Orthop. 1996;16(4):514–7.

14. Vercellio G, Baraldini V, Gatti C, Coletti M, Cipolat L. Thoracic outlet syndrome in paediatrics: clinical presentation, surgical treatment, and outcomes in a series of eight children. J Pediatr Surg. 2003;38:58–61.

15. Swierczynska A, Klusek R, Kroczka S. Neurorehabilitation in children with thoracic outlet syndrome and its assessment. Przegl Lek. 2005;62:1308–13.

16. Maru S, Dosluoglu H, Dryjski M, Cherr G, Curl GR, Harris LM. Thoracic outlet syndrome in children and young adults. Eur J Vasc Endovasc Surg. 2009;38(5): 565–6.

17. Arthur LG, Teich S, Hogan M, Caniano DA, Smead W. Pediatric thoracic outlet syndrome: a disorder with serious vascular complications. J Pediatr Surg. 2008; 43(6):1089–94.

18. Makhoul RG, Machleder HI. Developmental anomalies at the thoracic outlet: an analysis of 200 consecutive cases. J Vasc Surg. 1992;16(4):534–42 (discussion 542–5).

NTOS in the Competitive Athlete

12

Gregory J. Pearl

Abstract

The symptoms of NTOS in athletes may be nuanced, and are often specific to their athletic activities. There are many conditions with overlapping symptoms affecting the upper extremities which must be excluded in high performing athletes. Because they repeatedly are required to perform exaggerated and at times violent movements of the upper extremities, NTOS in this highly competitive group may pose unique treatment challenges.

Introduction

The symptoms of neurogenic thoracic outlet syndrome (NTOS) include pain, numbness, and parsenthesias in the arm or hand sometimes associated with neck or shoulder pain. These symptoms vary in location and severity depending on position or level of intensity of activity with the extremity. Physical examination typically reveals tenderness and spasm over the scalene triangle and symptoms may be reproduced with direct palpitation over the plexus or with provocative maneuvers. Diagnostic imaging and electrophysiological testing may be unremarkable but hold value in exclusion of other conditions that may cause similar or overlapping symptoms. Temporary relief or improvement in symptoms with scalene or pectoralis minor block with local anesthetic may lend support to the diagnosis of NTOS and may also be predictive of the response to decompression [1].

These same general characteristics are present in the athlete experiencing symptoms secondary to NTOS; however, the clinical presentation in this highly functioning competitive group may be nuanced and deserves special consideration. High performance athletes with NTOS, particularly those at the collegiate and professional levels, present with symptoms specific to their athletic activities and may pose unique challenges for the treatment team not encountered in the "non-athlete".

Athletic Activities Predisposing to NTOS

The athletes predisposed to the development of neurogenic symptoms are those who participate in sports requiring strenuous repetitive overhead

G.J. Pearl, MD
Department of Vascular Surgery,
Baylor University Medical Center,
621 N. Hall Street, Suite 100, Dallas, TX 75226, USA
e-mail: gregp@baylorhealth.edu

K.A. Illig et al. (eds.), *Thoracic Outlet Syndrome*,
DOI 10.1007/978-1-4471-4366-6_12, © Springer-Verlag London 2013

hand, arm and/or shoulder activities (Table 12.1). These athletes engage in exaggerated and at times violent movements of the extremity causing repetitive stretch injury to the scalene muscles culminating in acute and chronic inflammation, spasm and ultimately fibrosis. These changes in the muscle lead to compression and irritation of the cervical nerve roots and brachial plexus causing neck pain, shoulder pain, and upper extremity pain, numbness and weakness.

In addition to these typical symptoms, the competitive athlete may also present with complaints elicited by certain provocative movements unique to their own specific sports related activities. The prototypical athlete who illustrates this point is the throwing athlete. The baseball pitcher with NTOS will complain of arm fatigue and loss of stamina with throwing, decrease in pitching velocity, and loss of grip strength and "feel" for the ball. Complaints of persistence of these symptoms with a sense of a "dead arm" that may last for several days following a throwing session are common, whereas in the non-athlete, symptoms typically abate more quickly. One well known major league starting baseball pitcher treated by the author reported that he had always been known for his ability to pitch into the late innings of the game. With the development of his neurogenic symptoms provoked by throwing, he was able to only pitch one or two innings before his arm because so fatigued he could not continue to throw and would be forced to leave the game. He had also experienced a 7–10 mph decline in the speed of his fastball concurrent with the fatigue, which is another common manifestation of NTOS in the throwing athlete.

A more subtle characteristic of NTOS seen in the baseball pitcher is the complaint of loss of "feel" for the ball. A baseball is covered in cowhide and stitched circumferentially with raised seams. The skilled throwing athlete puts movement on his pitches by varying the placement of his fingers in relation to the seams on the ball, as well as subtle variations in pressure applied to the ball by the fingertips and palmar surface on the throwing hand. The advanced pitcher with NTOS frequently complains of this elusive and insidious loss of perceptive feel for the baseball.

Misdiagnosed Conditions in Athletes with NTOS

An important characteristic seen in the athlete with NTOS is the common complaint of pain that may seem to be localized to the shoulder, biceps, elbow, and/or forearm. The localization of pain to a specific joint or muscle group in the athlete serves as a confounding factor, and may lead to misdiagnosis of a problem intrinsic to a particular joint or muscle group. Examples of misdiagnosis include a superior labral tear from anterior to posterior (SLAP lesion) in the shoulder, a bicep muscle strain, a medial collateral ligament strain, epicondylitis or cubital tunnel syndrome at the elbow, or pronator syndrome in the forearm. Incorrect diagnosis leads to a delay in the proper diagnosis of NTOS and the pursuit of appropriate and timely treatment (Table 12.2). The worst case is that in which the misdiagnosis culminates in an unnecessary operative procedure that does not address and correct the true underlying problem of NTOS and could ultimately

Table 12.1 Athletes predisposed to NTOS

| Baseball |
| Football |
| Softball |
| Tennis |
| Volleyball |
| Soccer |
| Golf |
| Track and Field |
| Swimmers |
| Gymnastics/Cheerleading |

Table 12.2 Diagnostic considerations in the athlete with NTOS

| Cervical strain |
| SLAP lesion (labral tear) |
| Biceps strain |
| Medial collateral ligament strain |
| Epicondylitis |
| Cubital tunnel syndrome |
| Pronator syndrome |
| Compartment syndrome |

jeopardize the career or at the very least, lead to a lost season for a professional or scholarship athlete [2]. A misdiagnosis and misdirected procedure that fails to alleviate the athlete's symptoms may lead to a sense of frustration or so much lost time that they may be released by their team, lose their scholarship, or be forced to give up their sport. In light of the frequency of confusing or overlapping symptoms in these high performing competitive athletes as it may affect the shoulder, biceps, elbow, forearm and hand, various imaging studies – typically deemed to be unnecessary in the general TOS population – may be necessary to help clarify the diagnosis. The vast majority of athletes referred to our practice for evaluation of NTOS have already undergone extensive imaging evaluation by the orthopedic and sports medicine team physicians which may include MRI of the shoulder, elbow or spine, MR arthrogram or even diagnostic arthroscopy.

Treatment and Results

Initial treatment of NTOS generally includes rest of the affected extremity, physical therapy to relax and stretch the scalene and pectoralis minor muscles and judicious use of muscle relaxants and anti-inflammatory agents. This will typically be continued for at least 4–6 weeks to gain maximum affect. Additional treatments that may be attempted, particularly in the athletic group, include corticosteroid injections into the symptomatic joint. However, in the setting of NTOS, the high performing competitive athlete rarely experiences satisfactory durable relief of their symptoms without surgical decompression. The lack of efficacy of conservative non-operative treatment may well be attributed to the forceful and repetitive nature of the activities inherent in this high performing group. By the time most athletes are referred to us for evaluation of TOS by the treating team physician or trainer, most felt they had already exhausted any hope of experiencing meaningful and satisfactory improvement with the non-operative program that would allow them to return to their expected high levels of functional performance. Additionally, the

athletes all had a sense of urgency to proceed with more definitive treatment arising from their frustration in failure to experience timely resolution or significant improvement of these symptoms that would allow them to return to competition.

In our practice at Baylor University Medical Center of Dallas in the past year, January 1, 2010 to December 31, 2010, 77 thoracic outlet decompressive procedures were performed in 75 patients. Of the 77 procedures, 73 were performed for NTOS. Forty-seven of the 75 patients treated over the past year with surgical decompression fell into the category of competitive athlete. Of the 47 athletes, 44 presented with and were treated for NTOS. Once a sound diagnosis of NTOS had been established and conservative management had been offered and failed, surgical options were carefully reviewed with the patient as well as expectations of outcome and the anticipated recovery process to return to full athletic activities. Our surgical treatment for NTOS in these competitive athletes is performed through a supraclavicular approach with a thorough anterior and middle scalenectomy, brachial plexus neurolysis and complete first rib resection [3]. We also recognize the potential importance of brachial plexus compression in the sub-pectoral space and the contribution to the neurogenic symptoms from compression at this site and when indicated, pectoralis minor tenotomy was performed concomitantly with the supraclavicular decompression. Following the operative procedure all patients were monitored overnight in the hospital with a small number spending a second night to ensure adequate analgesia with IV narcotics. Patients were seen for office follow-up 2–3 weeks following the surgery and then started into a post-operative rehab program with physical therapy and gradual resumption and progression to their athletic activities during the latter half of the program. The majority of the athletes returned to full activities by 10–12 weeks following surgical decompression.

Given the chronic nature of pre-existing nerve injury in some of these patients, the ability to predict and confidently assure the athlete that he or she will return to levels of physical ability that they had experienced prior to the development of

NTOS remains elusive [4]. There is currently very limited data regarding the predictability of outcomes in the treatment of NTOS in athletes. We have previously reported our outcomes and subsequent return to athletic activities and performance obtained via a mailed questionnaire to the patients [5]. This process proves to be quite cumbersome with less than satisfactory response from this group of young, busy and geographically mobile individuals. We are currently in the process of developing a tool to assess outcomes in this young, generally tech savvy group utilizing social media. Our hope is that this vehicle will facilitate a response rate that will allow us to more accurately and predictably assess the outcomes in this high performing, high achieving, and motivated group of individuals who have suffered disability and been unable to participate in their sport.

References

1. Jordan SE, Machleder HI. Diagnosis of thoracic outlet syndrome using electrophysiolocically guided anterior scalene blocks. Ann Vasc Surg. 1998;12:260–4.
2. Lowry to have circulatory problem fixed, ESPN.com; (2009, May 19). https://m.espn.go.com/mlb/story?storyId=4179864&wjb Accessed 2 May 2011.
3. Sanders RJ, Raymer S. The supraclavicular approach to scalenectomy and first rib resection: description of technique. J Vasc Surg. 1985;2:751–6.
4. Axelrod DA, Proctor MC, Geisser ME, Ross RS, Greenfield LJ. Outcome after surgery for thoracic outlet syndrome. J Vasc Surg. 2001;33:1220–5.
5. Thompson RW, Pearl GJ. Neurovascular injuries in the throwing shoulder. In: Denes JM, Ecahrache NS, Yocum LA, Altcherk DW, Andrews J, Wilk KE, editors. Sports medicine of baseball. Philadelphia: Lippincott Williams & Wilkins; 2011.

Cervical Ribs and NTOS

13

Dean M. Donahue

Abstract

Bone abnormalities of the C7 vertebrae include cervical ribs and elongated transverse processes, and represent space-occupying lesions within the confines of the thoracic outlet. These bone abnormalities, or the fibromuscular attachments between them and the underlying first thoracic rib, may cause irritation to the brachial plexus producing symptoms of NTOS. Conservative treatment may be the initial management, but is effective in a minority of patients. Surgical decompression of the thoracic outlet results in symptomatic improvement in most patients.

Embryology

In the developing human embryo, lateral costal processes form along each vertebrae of the entire spine. In the thorax these processes continue to grow to develop into ribs, but in the remainder of the spine they fuse with the vertebrae to become transverse processes. Abnormal development of these costal processes is most common at the seventh cervical vertebrae (C7) and likely is mediated by Hox genes [1]. This results in either a cervical rib or an elongated transverse process which extends beyond the transverse process of the first thoracic vertebrae (Fig. 13.1). While structural differences distinguish the two (see Chap. 81), it is unclear if there is a clinically significant difference between cervical ribs and an elongated transverse process of C7. Previous series of TOS patients frequently report their incidence of cervical ribs based on plain cervical spine or chest radiographs, raising the possibility of misidentification due to radiographic similarities (Fig. 13.2). Incomplete cervical ribs terminate without bone articulation with the underlying first thoracic rib or manubrium, and represent approximately two-thirds of cases. Complete ribs articulate with the underlying rib or manubrium, and have a higher incidence of developing symptoms spontaneously – without a history of trauma or repetitive strain. Complete ribs also appear to be the only cause of subclavian artery aneurysm associated with TOS.

D.M. Donahue, MD
Department of Thoracic Surgery,
Massachusetts General Hospital, Blake 1570,
55 Fruit Street, Boston, MA 02114, USA
e-mail: donahue.dean@mgh.harvard.edu

K.A. Illig et al. (eds.), *Thoracic Outlet Syndrome*,
DOI 10.1007/978-1-4471-4366-6_13, © Springer-Verlag London 2013

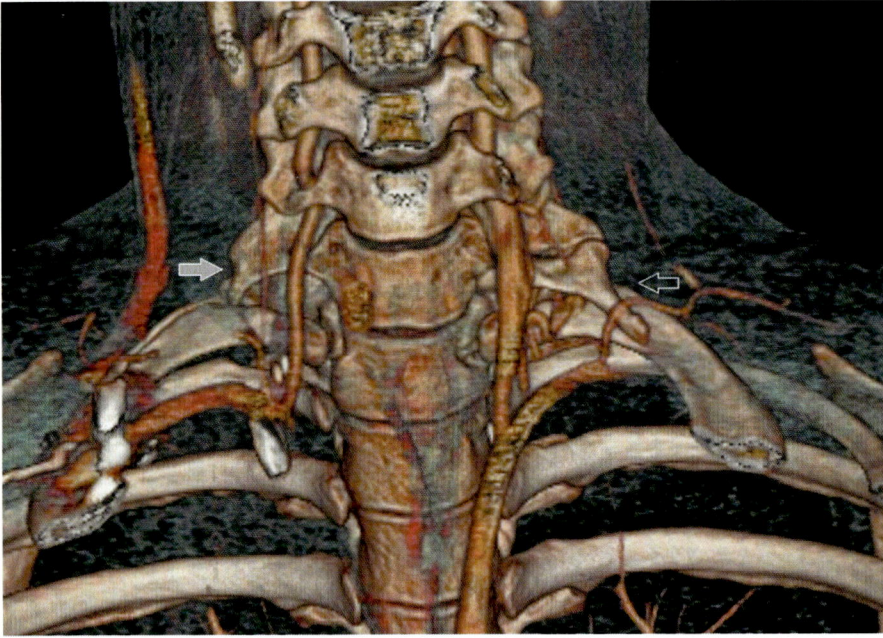

Fig. 13.1 CT scan with 3-dimensional reconstruction of a patient with symmetrical bilateral symptoms of TOS. An incomplete cervical rib (*open arrow*) with an articulation to the transverse process of the C7 vertebrae is seen on the *left*. An elongated transverse process of the C7 vertebrae extending beyond the transverse process of the first thoracic vertebrae is seen on the *right side* (*solid arrow*). At surgery, dense tissue bands were found attaching each bone abnormality to the first thoracic rib

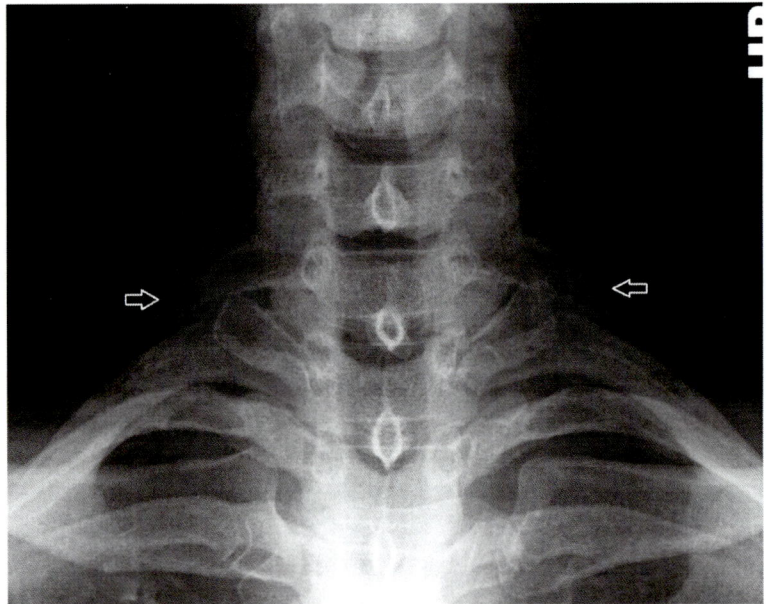

Fig. 13.2 Plain radiograph of the anterior cervical spine. This was initially interpreted as showing bilateral cervical ribs (*open arrows*), but a CT scan demonstrated that these bone projections originating from the C7 vertebrae were elongated transverse processes

Epidemiology, Pathophysiology, and Clinical Presentation

The exact incidence of bone abnormalities of the C7 vertebrae is not known. An analysis of 12 studies shows the prevalence of cervical ribs ranging from 0 to 3 %, with two showing the prevalence of an elongated C7 transverse process as 2.2–21 % [2]. A review of 1,352 digital chest radiographs over a 1 year period reported the incidence of cervical ribs as 1.09 % in females and 0.42 % in males, and the incidence of an elongated C7 transverse process was 3.43 % in females and 1.13 % in males [3]. The presence or absence of symptoms in these patients was not reported. It is believed that most cervical ribs are asymptomatic, and patients with bilateral cervical ribs may have only unilateral symptoms. Series of patients with TOS have reported the incidence of cervical ribs ranging from 4.5 to 8.5 % [4, 5]. Female patients outnumber males by a 4:1 ratio, with the age at presentation typically between 20 and 50 years-old. Symptoms can develop spontaneously, but approximately 80 % of patients report a prior history of trauma – the majority being motor vehicle accidents or repetitive strain injury.

The mechanism by which these bone abnormalities produce symptoms is assumed to be from direct irritation or impingement of the brachial plexus from the aberrant bone or from fibromuscular tissues originating from the bone abnormality at C7. These tissues are consistently found at surgery, as reported by Nelems and colleagues [6]. Because the lower trunk is closest to these abnormal structures, localized symptoms frequently involve the medial arm and hand. Tubbs and colleagues described the macroscopic and microscopic findings in two cadavers with cervical ribs found out of a series of 475 autopsies [7] (the pre-morbid presence of TOS symptoms in these cadavers was not known). The lower trunk of the brachial plexus in the two cervical rib cases showed fibrosis of the epineurium, perineurium and fascicles as well as hyalinized blood vessels and intraneural collagenous nodules. These findings were not present in age match control autopsies without cervical ribs.

Pain in the neck and arm is present in 80–95 % of patients presenting with NTOS and cervical ribs, with approximately half reporting pain in the upper chest, hand or occipital headaches. Paresthesias are reported by most patients, more commonly in the hand than the arm. Localization of pain and paresthesia to either a medial or lateral distribution is also more common in the hand compared to the upper arm or forearm. When localized, symptoms are reported in dermatomes innervated by the lower trunk of the brachial plexus in 70–90 % of cases.

Physical exam findings frequently included tenderness and a positive Tinel's sign at the scalene region. Subjective complaints of arm and hand weakness or decreased coordination are found in approximately 60 % of patients, but muscle weakness on exam is reproducibly demonstrated in approximately 10 %. Positional testing such as placing the arm at 90° of abduction with external rotation, or modified upper extremity tension testing reproduces symptoms in over 90 % of patients. The role of additional radiographic and electromyographic diagnostic techniques is covered elsewhere in the text. A full evaluation for other potential causes of symptoms suggestive of TOS should be performed in patients with cervical ribs.

Treatment

The initial treatment of patients with cervical ribs and symptoms of TOS is frequently physical therapy (PT), although some view the presence of an objective bony abnormality as an indication to proceed with operation without this step. Patients with cervical ribs that present with either acute vascular complications or evidence of atrophy of the intrinsic hand muscles typically are offered surgery as the initial treatment. PT addresses the strength and mobility abnormalities that create postural compromise of the thoracic outlet. This abnormal posture creates cervicothoracic spine and shoulder dysfunction resulting in retraction and depression of the clavicle during arm elevation.

In the author's experience, 25 % of patients with cervical ribs had greater than 50 % improvement in their symptoms of pain following treatment from an experienced therapist. The symptomatic improvement was significant enough that surgical treatment was declined, illustrating the fact that the presence of a bony abnormality per se, even in a symptomatic patient, is not necessarily an automatic indication for surgery (unpublished data).

Patients with cervical ribs who are refractory to conservative treatment benefit from surgical intervention after other potential causes have been investigated. There is no consensus regarding the surgical approach or the extent of resection. Options include resecting the cervical rib, the first thoracic rib or both, and no robust data exists supporting either option. It may be that a smaller cervical rib (<5 mm) needs only the soft tissue attachments resected along with the first thoracic rib, but resecting both ribs ensures adequate decompression of the thoracic outlet. The exposure can be obtained from either a transaxillary or supraclavicular approach, with the author favoring the latter along with resection of the anterior scalene muscle and neurolysis of the brachial plexus performed under magnification.

The largest series limited to patients with TOS and cervical ribs was published by Sanders and colleagues [4]. They reported the surgical results of 37 patients, and found "good to excellent" results in 72 %, "fair" in 17 and an 11 % failure rate. These patients had all failed to improve after 3–12 months of PT. The intraneural pathology of the brachial plexus reported by Tubbs may explain persistent symptoms some patients may experience in spite of decompression including neurolysis. While only speculation, it may be that decompression of symptomatic patients prevents ongoing nerve damage resulting from cervical ribs. As some patients with cervical ribs remain asymptomatic throughout their entire lives, there appears to be no role for surgery in incidentally found cervical ribs.

Summary

Cervical ribs or an elongated transverse process of the C7 vertebrae represent space-occupying lesions within the limited confines of the thoracic outlet. These bone abnormalities, or the fibromuscular attachments between them and the underlying first thoracic rib, may cause irritation to the brachial plexus producing symptoms of NTOS. These symptoms typically include pain in the neck and arm, with paresthesias of the hand. Conservative treatment may be the initial management, but is effective in a minority of patients. Surgical decompression of the thoracic outlet, with resection of the anomalous bone, the first thoracic rib or both, results in symptomatic improvement in most patients.

References

1. Galis F. Why do almost all mammals have seven cervical vertebrae? Developmental constraints, Hox genes, and cancer. J Exp Zool (Mol Dev Evol). 1999;285:19–26.
2. Tague RG. Sacralization is not associated with elongated cervical costal process and cervical rib. Clin Anat. 2011;24:209–17.
3. Brewin J, Hill M, Ellis H. The prevalence of cervical ribs in a London population. Clin Anat. 2009;22:331–6.
4. Sanders RJ, Hammond SL. Management of cervical ribs and anomalous first ribs causing neurogenic thoracic outlet syndrome. J Vasc Surg. 2002;36:51–6.
5. Makhoul RG, Machleder HI. Developmental anomalies at the thoracic outlet: an analysis of 200 consecutive cases. J Vasc Surg. 1992;16:534–45.
6. Reddenbach DM, Nelems B. A comparative study of structures comprising the thoracic outlet in 250 human cadavers and 72 surgical cases of thoracic outlet syndrome. Eur J Cardiothorac Surg. 1998;13(4):353–60.
7. Tubbs RS, Louis Jr RG, Wartmannn CT, et al. Histopathological basis for neurogenic thoracic outlet syndrome. J Neurosurg Spine. 2008;8:347–51.

NTOS and Repetitive Trauma Disorders

Emil F. Pascarelli

Abstract

The relationships between Neurogenic Thoracic Outlet Syndrome (NTOS) and the various forms of repetitive trauma disorders merit clarification. In many patients there is a link between NTOS and the various forms of repetitive trauma disorders. These disorders appear to, in part, stem from nerve involvement in the brachial plexus often related to poor posture. This in turn impairs peripheral muscle function when coupled with sustained overuse. Muscle regeneration is impaired due to a lack of activation of satellite cells located between muscle fibers and the basal lamina. Satellite cells create new muscle fibers under conditions of good circulation, intact nerve impulses and optimal hormonal factors. Our study and that of others show that about 70 % of persons with these trauma disorders have clinical evidence of NTOS. This association results in muscle damage particularly when associated with eccentric contraction of loaded stretched muscles. The degeneration-regeneration cycle of muscle is then impeded due to neurological circulatory abnormal factors decreasing the ability of satellite cells to repair damaged muscle. A logical continuum can be proposed under these circumstances linking NTOS with repetitive trauma in the peripheral nerves and muscles.

A Definition of Repetitive Trauma Disorders

The term Repetitive Trauma Disorders is used to describe work related soft tissue injuries, usually of the upper extremities. Other descriptive terms include Repetitive Strain Injury (RSI), Occupational Overuse Syndrome (OOS), Upper Extremity Musculoskeletal Disorder, Myofascial Pain Syndrome, and Cervical Brachial Pain Syndrome [1]. Carpal Tunnel Syndrome (CTS) is a peripheral median nerve entity that is rarely associated with repetitive trauma disorders, and should not be employed as a synonym for Repetitive Trauma Disorders.

E.F. Pascarelli, MD
Department of Medicine, College of Physicians and Surgeons, Columbia University, 3 Sea Colony Drive, Santa Monica, CA 90405, USA
e-mail: efp1@columbia.edu

K.A. Illig et al. (eds.), *Thoracic Outlet Syndrome*,
DOI 10.1007/978-1-4471-4366-6_14, © Springer-Verlag London 2013

NTOS, Posture and the Relationship to Repetitive Trauma Disorders

NTOS is a malady primarily due to compression, traction or obstruction of nerves by muscular, bony and ligamentous obstacles that lie between the spine, brachial plexus and the lower border of the armpit. The diagnosis of NTOS is primarily based on clinical observations, although imaging and electro-physiologic testing may also be necessary [2]. All too often, when a clinical examination is not done, the examiner's conclusion is that the patient's symptoms are psychosomatic. A diagnosis of psychosomatic illness, without a clinical examination, could prevent the patient from getting necessary physical therapy treatment.

NTOS appears to be clinically related to repetitive trauma disorders, particularly when associated with postural dysfunction. In our clinical study of 485 persons with repetitive trauma [3] we found that 80 % had postural dysfunction and 70 % had NTOS at the time of initial examination. During this study we found diminished hand temperature in 20 % of subjects. This finding may be related to stimulus from sympathetic nerve fibers that contribute to the brachial plexus from the sympathetic chain. This merits further investigation and may contribute to clinical diagnosis. Sharan and colleagues confirm these results in studies of several thousand Indian patients with repetitive trauma from computer work associated with NTOS [4, 5]. Dr. Sharan points out that during repetitive work of the upper extremities, the muscles of the proximal parts around the shoulders and neck are in static contraction while the peripheral muscles are in dynamic contraction, resulting in tightness in the proximal muscles and overuse distally. The proximal muscle activity often leads to NTOS – particularly when combined with both postural deficiency and anatomical anomalies.

The onset of postural dysfunction has been clearly illustrated by Sucher [6, 7]. His triptych illustration shows the gradual occurrence of neurovascular compression. As posture deteriorates, shoulder protraction begins with sternomastoid muscle shortening, drawing the head both anteriorly and inferiorly. This is followed by adaptive shortening of scalene and pectoralis minor muscles [6]. This postural dysfunction causes narrowing of the costoclavicular space with elevation of ribs one through five, leading to neurovascular compression. Postural deterioration is key in the relationships between NTOS and repetitive trauma, as it affects the ability of peripheral muscles not only to function properly because of damage from eccentric activity, but also to impede regeneration of the muscle itself. Because skeletal muscle fibers tend to resist stretching, a fully extended muscle, when forced to lengthen because of an external load which is greater than the force the muscle can generate, is eccentric activity.

Posture and Localization of Brachial Plexus Injury

This postural displacement also produces a distortion in the brachial plexus. Cervical spine radiographs often show loss of the normal lordotic curve of the neck [3]. Several studies have described which of the involved trunks of the brachial plexus relate to various symptoms [2, 8–10]. Superior trunk compromise causes pain radiating into the shoulder down the arm and along the central portion of the shoulder blade. There can also be swelling of the face and neck and occasional atypical migraine headaches. Medial cord injury causes pain in front of the neck radiating down the forearm and the fourth and fifth fingers. Lateral cord injury causes pain below the clavicle with tingling of the thumb, index, middle fingers and palm. Occasionally, chest wall pain can be erroneously thought to be a cardiac event. Posterior cord injury causes tingling or burning over the triceps muscle as well as the lateral epicondyle. Often there is tingling and burning in the forearm, thumb, index and middle fingers. Inferior trunk injury causes dull aching in the forearm and tingling or burning of the fourth and fifth fingers often accompanied by weakness of the thumb muscles and intrinsic hand muscles. Note that inferior trunk injury is the most common set of symptoms associated with NTOS.

These findings are also frequently present in patients with repetitive trauma disorder, buttressing the likelihood of a link between the two entities.

Muscle Degeneration and Regeneration

Why should NTOS lead to the often debilitating symptoms of repetitive trauma? The postural changes described in this chapter can be postulated as causing a continuing compromise of nerve and musculoskeletal function, which ultimately results in diminished muscle regeneration. Machleder [11] pointed to the loss of type II muscle fibers with a preponderance of Type I fibers persisting in injured patients. In order to understand what occurs with muscle injury we must look to the degeneration-regeneration cycle described by Mauro and others [12, 13]. The discovery of the muscle satellite cell has led to a plausible explanation for the genesis of repetitive trauma disorder [14]. Evaluation of muscle injury requires a close look at the degeneration-regeneration process and its relation to the nervous system.

The muscle fiber complex consists of three basic components; the multinucleated, skeletal muscle fiber, its surrounding basal lamina and a population of mononuclear satellite cells capable of regenerating new muscle. These are premitotic cells found between the muscle fiber and the basal lamina. At birth, immature muscle fibers are associated with large numbers of satellite cells, which diminish with aging. The way in which muscles are used can increase injury. There is evidence to suggest [15, 16] that eccentric muscle contraction causing repetitive trauma can damage peripheral muscle cells, which are then phagocitized and replaced with new fibers by activated satellite cells. However, optimal blood supply and adequate nerve stimulus are two of several factors necessary for muscle regeneration. New muscle creation is impeded by the development of NTOS associated with the injured brachial plexus [17, 18]. The various brachial plexus injury patterns result in neuropraxia, causing a compromise of actual muscle and nerve function that leads to diminished regenerative capacity of the peripheral muscle, which has been injured by eccentric muscle overuse [14].

We can infer that as a result of these proximal and peripheral interactions, a strong relationship exists between NTOS and Repetitive Trauma. Overloaded eccentric muscles sustain damage ordinarily repaired by the degeneration-restoration mechanism of the satellite cell. As a result, healing is impaired by the action of NTOS on muscles which, failing to heal, prolong chronicity.

References

1. Pascarelli EF. Evaluation and treatment of repetitive motion disorders. In: Machleder HI, editor. Vascular disorders of the upper extremity. 3rd ed. Mt. Kisco: Futura; 1998. p. 171–83.
2. Schwartzman RJ. Brachial plexus traction injuries. Front Hand Rehabil. 1991;7:547–56.
3. Pascarelli EF, Hsu YP. Understanding work related upper extremity disorders: clinical findings in 485 computer users, musicians and others. J Occup Rehabil. 2001;11(1):1–21.
4. Sharan D, Parijat P, Ajeesh PS. Risk factors, clinical features and outcome of treatment of work related musculoskeletal disorders in on site occupational health clinics in Indian information technology companies. In: Proceedings of WDPI 2010: the first scientific conference on work disability, prevention and integration at Angers, France, 23 Sept 2010.
5. Sharan D, Ajeesch PS, Jacob BN, Kumar R. Risk factors, clinical features and outcome of treatment of work related musculoskeletal disorders in on site clinics in Indian IT companies. In: Proceedings of the 17th world ergonomics congress. Beijing, China, Aug 2009.
6. Sucher BM. Thoracic outlet syndrome – a myofacial variant: Part 2. Treatment. J Am Osteopath Assoc. 1990;90:810–23.
7. Idem Part 3. Structural and postural considerations. J Am Osteopath Assoc. 1993;334–45.
8. Mackinnon SE, Novak CB. Evaluation of the patient with thoracic outlet syndrome. Semin Thorac Cardiovasc Surg. 1996;8:190–200.
9. Roos DB. New concepts of thoracic outlet syndrome that explain etiology, symptoms, diagnosis and treatment. Vasc Surg. 1979;13:313–21.
10. Machleder HI. Introduction to neurovascular compression syndromes in the thoracic outlet. In: Machleder HI, editor. Vascular disorders of the upper extremity. 3rd ed. Mt. Kisco: Futurama; 1998. p. 109–35.

11. Machleder HI, Moll F, Verity A. The anterior scalene muscle in thoracic outlet compression syndrome: histochemical and morphometric studies. Arch Surg. 1986;121:1141–4.
12. Mauro A. Satellite cell of skeletal muscle fibers. J Biophys Biochem Cytol. 1961;9:493–5.
13. Campion DR. The muscle satellite cell: a review. Int Rev Cytol. 1984;87:225–51.
14. Carlson BM. The satellite cell and skeletal muscle regeneration: the degeneration and regeneration cycle in repetitive motion disorders of the upper extremity. In: American Academy of Orthopedic Surgeons-Symposium Rosemont IL; 1995. p. 313–22
15. Seddon HJ. Three types of nerve injury. Brain. 1943;66:237–8.
16. Armstrong RB, Warren III GL, Lowe A. Mechanisms in the initiation of contraction-induced skeletal muscle injury. In: Gordon S, Blain S, Fine L, editors. Repetitive motion disorders of the upper extremity. Rosemont: American Academy of Orthopedic Surgeons Symposium; 1995. p. 339–48.
17. Fridén J, Sjöström M, Erblom B. Myofibrillar damage following intense eccentric exercise in man. Int J Sports Med. 1983;4:45–51.
18. Armstrong RB, Warren JA. Mechanisms of exercise induced muscle fiber injury. Sports Med. 1991;12:184–207.

Pectoralis Minor Syndrome

15

Richard J. Sanders

Abstract

Pectoralis minor syndrome (PMS) is a subset of neurogenic thoracic outlet syndrome (TOS) that can cause upper extremity symptoms of pain, paresthesia, and/or weakness due to compression of the neurovascular bundle by the pectoralis minor muscle (PM). The most distinguishing symptoms and signs of PMS include pain and/or tenderness in the subclavicular anterior chest wall and axilla. The clinical diagnosis of PMS can be confirmed by an improvement in symptoms and physical findings following a PM muscle block with local anesthetic. Treatment begins with PM stretching exercises. If this is insufficient, PM tenotomy (PMT) is a low risk operation, which can be performed as an outpatient. When PMS is the only diagnosis the success rate of PMT is 90 %, but when PMS is accompanied by nerve compression at the level of the scalene triangle the success rate of isolated PMT is only 35 %. PMS should also be considered in all patients with recurrent neurogenic TOS, as this condition has been found in a substantial proportion of such patients.

Introduction

Pectoralis minor syndrome (PMS) is a subset of neurogenic thoracic outlet syndrome (TOS) that can cause upper extremity symptoms of paresthesias, pain, and/or weakness due to compression of the neurovascular bundle by the pectoralis minor muscle (PM) [1]. PMS may exist as an isolated condition or in combination with brachial plexus compression at the level of the supraclavicular scalene triangle (PMS + ST). Rarely, PMS may occur with predominant compression of vascular structures [2].

Anatomy

The PM muscle arises from the anterior surfaces of ribs 2, 3, 4, and 5 and it inserts on the coracoid process of the scapula (see Chaps. 3 and 6). The space deep to the PM muscle contains the axillary artery (usually the most cephalad), the axillary vein (caudal to the artery), and the nerves of the brachial plexus, which are found around the

R.J. Sanders, MD
Department of Surgery, HealthONE Presbyterian-St.
Lukes Hospital, 4545 E. 9th Ave, #240,
Denver, CO 80220, USA
e-mail: rsanders@ecentral.com

K.A. Illig et al. (eds.), *Thoracic Outlet Syndrome*,
DOI 10.1007/978-1-4471-4366-6_15, © Springer-Verlag London 2013

Table 15.1 Etiology of isolated pectoralis minor syndrome

Etiology	# of patients	Percent (%)
Auto accidents or non-work causes of neck trauma	15	38
Falls on the floor, ice, etc.	3	8
Work accidents and repetitive stress injury (RSI)	7	18
Sports: weight lifting, swimming, baseball, tennis	7	18
Spontaneous (Idiopathic)	7	18
Total	39	100

Adapted from Sanders and Rao [1], p. 701–8. With permission from Elsevier

artery and between the artery and vein. The latassimus dorsi and subscapularis muscles lie deep to the neurovascular structures. Perhaps because the brachial plexus nerves are usually the most superficial structures, lying closest to the PM tendon, these nerves are most often involved in extrinsic compression.

Etiology

In a recently published study of patients with PMS, either in isolation or accompanied by neurogenic TOS localized to the supraclavicular scalene triangle, injuries of various types were present in 82 % of patients, whereas PMS developed spontaneously in 18 % (Table 15.1) [1]. The most common type of injury in isolated PMS was an automobile accident, similar to previous observations on the etiology of neurogenic TOS (NTOS). A significant difference between isolated PMS and PMS + NTOS was the relatively high incidence of injuries in athletes in PMS (18 %). This group of athletes included a few teenage girls, all of whom were initially thought to have NTOS related to the scalene triangle but were found to have only PMS.

Symptoms

The most common symptom in patients with isolated PMS was paresthesia, although this was absent in 12 %. When compared to a group of patients who had PMS + NTOS, there was no statistically significant difference in the incidence of pain in the upper extremity. However, a major difference between the two groups was that those with isolated PMS had significantly fewer symptoms in the head and neck (Table 15.2). In NTOS related to the scalene triangle, neck trauma results in a high incidence of occipital headache, neck pain, and supraclavicular pain due to injury to the scalene muscles. In isolated PMS, neck pain is usually absent or less intense. Another indication of the lesser degree of intensity of injury in isolated PMS is the number of patients in each group still working (85 % for patients with isolated PMS compared to 57 % for patients with PMS + NTOS) (Table 15.2).

Physical Examination

Physical examination includes evaluation for tenderness to palpation over the scalene, trapezius, deltoid and biceps muscles, as well as the rotator cuff, elbow and forearm, testing for reductions in sensation to very light touch in the fingers, and testing responses to provocative maneuvers of neck rotation, head tilt, the upper limb tension test (ULTT) of Elvey, and the elevated arm stress test (EAST) [3]. There are fewer positive findings on physical examination in patients with isolated PMS than in those with PMS + NTOS (Table 15.3). In a recent study, the only three positive findings present in almost all patients with isolated PMS were tenderness to palpation over the subcoracoid PM muscle tendon and a positive response to the ULTT and the EAST [1]. All other positive physical examination findings were significantly more frequent in patients with PMS + NTOS than in patients with isolated PMS (Table 15.3).

Table 15.2
Presenting symptoms in patients with pectoralis minor syndrome

	Isolated PMS 39 patients 52 operations	PMS + NTOS 37 patients 48 operations	
Symptoms	% of patients (#)	% of patients (#)	P value[a]
Pain			
Occipital headache	31 (16)	81 (39)	<0.001
Neck	50 (26)	96 (46)	<0.001
Supraclavicular area	44 (23)	79 (38)	0.004
Trapezius	87 (45)	96 (46)	0.163
Subcoracoid anterior chest	69 (36)	92 (44)	0.059
Axilla	52 (27/50)	78 (29/37)	0.024
Shoulder	69 (36)	90 (43)	<0.001
Arm	71 (37)	88 (42)	0.053
Arm/hand weakness	58 (30)	88 (42)	0.002
Paresthesia	88 (46)	98 (47)	0.114
All five fingers	54 (28)	48 (23)	0.699
Fourth and fifth fingers	29 (15)	42 (20)	0.670
First–third fingers	6 (3)	8 (4)	0.710
None	12 (6)	2 (1)	0.110
Still working	85 (33/39)	57 (21/37)	0.011

Adapted from Sanders and Rao [1], p. 701–8. With permission from Elsevier
PMS pectoralis minor syndrome, *PMS + NTOS* with symptoms of neurogenic TOS related to the scalene triangle
[a]Fisher's exact test

Table 15.3
Physical exam findings in patients with pectoralis minor syndrome

	Isolated PMS 39 patients 52 operations	PMS + NTOS 37 patients 48 operations	
Physical exam finding	% of patients (#)	% of patients (#)	P value[a]
Pectoralis minor tenderness	92 (48)	100 (48)	0.119
Trapezius tenderness	29 (56)	88 (42)	0.008
Axillary tenderness	71 (32/44)	95 (38/40)	0.008
90° AER (EAST)	82 (40/50)	98 (45/46)	0.008
ULTT of Elvey	79 (40)	92 (46)	0.008
Scalene triangle tenderness	48 (24)	86 (43)	<0.001
Biceps tenderness	54 (28)	88 (44)	<0.001
Neck rotation	40 (22/51)	80 (41)	<0.001
Head tilt	49 (24/51)	76 (39)	<0.001
Decreased sensation to touch	31 (16/51)	48 (23)	

Adapted from Sanders and Rao [1], p. 701–8. With permission from Elsevier
AER abduction and external rotation, *EAST* elevated arm stress test, *ULTT* upper limb tension test, *PMS* pectoralis minor syndrome, *PMS + NTOS* with symptoms of neurogenic TOS related to the scalene triangle
[a]Fisher's exact test

Relationship to Neurogenic TOS

Although PMS was first described in 1945 [4], only four publications about this condition appeared over the next 59 years [5–8]. It was rediscovered in 1998 by Dr. George Thomas of Seattle; although he did not publish his observations, PMS was described in a 2004 paper on recurrent neurogenic TOS [9]. Since 2005, every patient we have seen for possible neurogenic TOS has been specifically questioned for symptoms of pain in the anterior chest wall and axilla, the key symptoms of PMS. On physical examination we have routinely checked for tenderness to palpation over the subcoracoid PM muscle and in the axilla. The surprising finding was that 75 % of all patients had positive findings of PMS. After complete clinical evaluation, 30 % were diagnosed with isolated PMS, while 70 % had PMS+NTOS. The essential difference between the two conditions is that isolated PMS presents with pain or tenderness in the anterior chest wall and axilla, along with symptoms in the upper extremity and few or no symptoms in the head and neck. Patients with NTOS present with similar extremity symptoms, but also frequently have neck pain and occipital headaches which can often be the predominating symptoms. Patients who present with all of the typical symptoms of NTOS plus pain or tenderness in the chest and axilla are given both diagnoses (PMS+NTOS), as a form of "double-crush" syndrome [10].

Although many symptoms of the two conditions are similar, patients with isolated PMS often do not have as intense or as severe symptoms as do patients with PMS+NTOS or those with NTOS predominantly localized to the scalene triangle. Patients with isolated PMS are rarely incapacitated by their symptoms and it is seldom that they stop working. If there are neck symptoms, they are more frequently mild and not a major complaint, and it is seldom that these patients complain of severe headaches. In patients with isolated PMS, physical examination produces milder positive responses than in those with PMS+NTOS or those with NTOS predominantly localized to the scalene triangle.

Diagnostic Tests

Selective Muscle Blocks

PM muscle block is a helpful and fairly reliable diagnostic test. It is performed by injecting 4 ml of 1 % lidocaine, with a #22 1.5-in. needle, directly into the PM muscle. This can be done with ultrasound control to identify the muscle, but it has also been done fairly accurately without ultrasound control by spreading the lidocaine over a 2-cm wide area, centered at the point of maximal tenderness on the anterior chest wall. The point of injection is 3 cm below the clavicle and into the point of maximum tenderness. Care must be taken to introduce the needle at a 45° angle pointing cephalad, to avoid entering the pleural cavity. After injecting 0.2–0.3 ml, the needle is moved so that the lidocaine is spread medially and laterally into and around the PM muscle. The depth of the needle is also moved with each small injection. Moving the needle in this manner helps ensure that a good portion of the lidocaine reaches the PM muscle. Each time the needle is moved, the syringe is also aspirated before injecting to ensure that a blood vessel is not entered. If blood is aspirated, the needle is withdrawn a few millimeters, repositioned, and the injection is continued.

The accidental injection of some of the lidocaine into the pectoralis major muscle or surrounding tissues does not influence the results of the PM muscle injection. However, if the injection is too deep, resulting in paresthesias in the patient's hand, this reflects that the nerves of the brachial plexus have been anesthetized. When this occurs and the paresthesias haven't resolved within several minutes, the block is considered inconclusive and must be repeated on another day. Fortunately, with a little experience, this seldom occurs.

Just prior to the PM muscle injection, the patient is asked to relate all symptoms of pain and paresthesias that are present, to serve as a baseline to evaluate the results of the block. Once a technically good block has been achieved, as evidenced by loss of tenderness to palpation over the area of the PM muscle, the patient is asked if symptoms that were present at rest have subsequently diminished or disappeared and the physical examination is repeated. A good response to the PM muscle block is indicated by improvement in symptoms at rest, plus improvement on physical examination in responses to provocative maneuvers, sensation to very light touch, and the absence of residual tender points.

Electrodiagnostic Testing

Electrophysiological studies can also be helpful in confirming a diagnosis of PMS. A complete electromyography/nerve conduction velocity (EMG/NCV) test is of value to rule out other neurological conditions, but is usually normal in PMS. However, a recently-described variation of NCV testing was introduced, with measurement of the lowest branch of the brachial plexus, the medial antebrachial cutaneous (MAC) sensory nerve [11]. This has proven to be more sensitive than any other nerve measurement in patients with brachial plexus compression either above or below the clavicle. In a study of patients with unilateral NTOS undergoing surgical treatment, 40 of 41 patients had at least one abnormality on MAC NCV testing [12]. This testing procedure has not yet been evaluated in patients with isolated PMS.

Treatment

Conservative

PM muscle stretching is the main treatment for isolated PMS. This is performed by standing in a corner of a room or in an open doorway. With arms outstretched to support weight on either the two walls of a corner, or on the door jams of an open door, body weight is allowed to fall forward until the patient feels a stretch in the chest wall. The stretch is held for 15–20 s and then released. This procedure is repeated three to four times, resting 20–30 s between stretches, for three times a day. In general, patients who have been symptomatic for only a few months usually respond well to this approach within 1–2 months.

Associated Conditions

In addition to PM muscle stretching, if a patient also has symptoms of NTOS localized to the supraclavicular scalene triangle, appropriate therapy for NTOS is added to the physical therapy stretching program. Evaluation for other associated or differential conditions should also be performed, and if found, such conditions should be more thoroughly assessed and treated. These conditions typically include cervical spine disease, shoulder pathology, and carpal, radial, pronator, and cubital tunnel syndromes.

Surgery

If symptoms do not improve with 2–3 months of conservative therapy, and if all other diagnoses have been treated as extensively as possible, pectoralis minor tenotomy (PMT) is the treatment of choice. This is a minimal-risk surgical procedure that can be performed as an outpatient, either under local anesthesia with heavy sedation or under general anesthesia. Recovery time following PMT is often only a few days, although patients will typically continue to have soreness in the chest for a few weeks postoperatively.

Technique of PMT

The patient is positioned supine with the arm elevated to expose the axilla, and a towel is placed under the shoulder (Fig. 15.1). The position of the incision is important: it should be a 5–7 cm transverse incision beginning at the anterior axillary fold, and placed 1 cm above the bottom of the axillary hairline. In this way, by placing the incision in the anterior portion of the axilla, there is a better chance of avoiding injury to the second intercostal-brachial cutaneous nerve. If this nerve is seen it is gently retracted without significant stretching; if this is not possible, the nerve is divided to avoid hyperesthesia and pain in the underarm (it is considered better to leave an area of numbness under the arm from a divided nerve than to cause burning pain from an overstretched nerve). Other incisions that have been used for

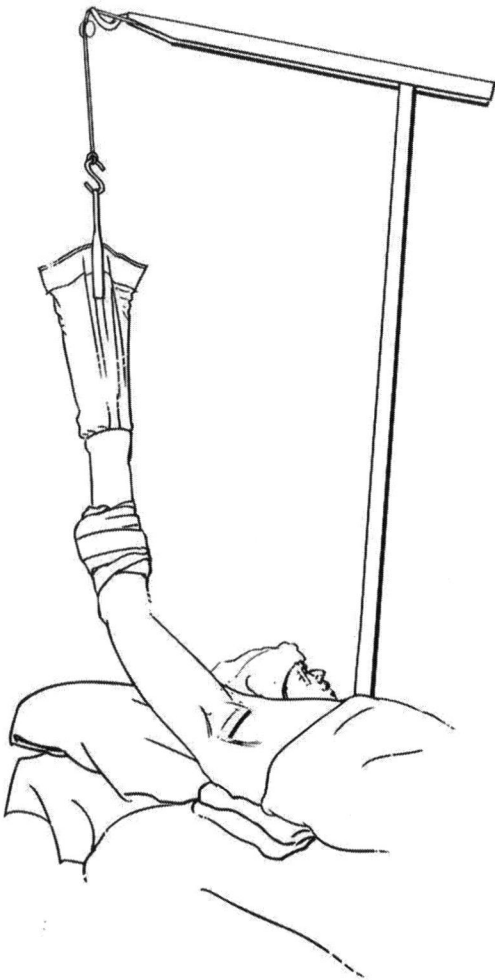

Fig. 15.1 Technique of transaxillary pectoralis minor tenotomy and partial myomectomy. The patient is positioned supine with a towel under operated shoulder. The arm is elevated with an orthopedic arm holder to expose the axilla. The transverse incision is 5–7 cm long, lying about 1 cm above the bottom of the hairline, and beginning at the anterior axillary fold. By placing the incision anteriorly, the chances of injuring the second intercostal-brachial cutaneous nerve are reduced, but not eliminated (Courtesy of Presbyterian-St. Lukes Hospital, Denver, Colorado by Wes Price)

PMT include the delto-pectoral groove on the anterior chest wall or an infraclavicular incision, with either providing equivalent exposure to that obtainable through the axilla.

Next, the subcutaneous tissue is divided and the pectoralis major muscle is exposed, and the coracoid process is identified by palpation and the PM muscle is visualized inserting into the coracoid process (Fig. 15.2). After isolating the PM muscle, it is divided at the coracoid with a cautery or harmonic scalpel. In some patients the PM muscle is difficult to identify because it is fused to the pectoralis major muscle. In these situations, the coracoid process is visualized and the fibers inserting on it are separated at that level, and the avascular plane is opened between the PM and pectoralis major muscles.

The divided end of the PM muscle is grasped with a clamp and elevated, and 2–3 cm of the muscle is excised to prevent the tendon from reattaching to the underlying neurovascular bundle postoperatively (Fig. 15.3). It is important not to excise too much of the PM muscle, to avoid injuring the pectoral nerve which runs through the PM to innervate the pectoralis major. Before closing, any thickened bands of clavipectoral fascia overlying the exposed axillary neurovascular bundle are also sharply divided (Fig. 15.4). The wound is closed without drainage using subcutaneous and subcuticular absorbable sutures.

Postoperative physical therapy is not necessary after isolated PMT, and patients can return to sedentary activities in a few days. However, it is recommended that patients refrain from using the arm for activities above the level of the shoulder for 2–3 months postoperatively. This is to permit the divided end of the PM muscle to adhere to the chest wall. It has been observed that in patients who resume vigorous activities with the arm too soon, pain and tenderness often develop over the chest wall, which can last a few months. When this occurs, one approach to treatment is by injecting the end of the PM muscle with a steroid solution and putting the arm at rest for several weeks. Even though the arm is placed at rest with this treatment, it is important that the patient continue to elevate the arm to 180° daily to avoid a frozen shoulder.

Results of Treatment

When PMS was the only diagnosis, 90 % of the patients had good improvement with surgical treatment (isolated PMT). However, when PMS

Fig. 15.2 Technique of transaxillary pectoralis minor tenotomy and partial myomectomy. After dividing the subcutaneous tissues, the edge of the pectoralis major muscle is identified first. The coracoid process is palpated although hard to visualize. The muscle descending from the coracoid is the pectoralis minor (PM) muscle. The neurovascular bundle lies immediately under the PM muscle but is usually covered by fat and is not visible. The PM muscle is freed on it lateral and medial sides (Courtesy of Presbyterian-St. Lukes Hospital, Denver, Colorado by Wes Price)

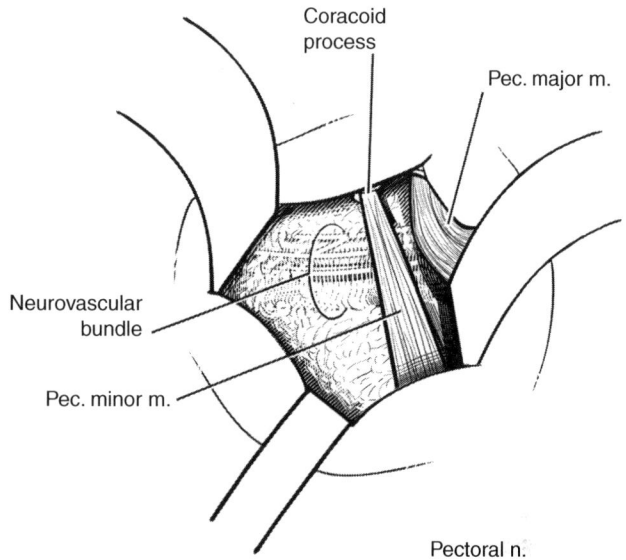

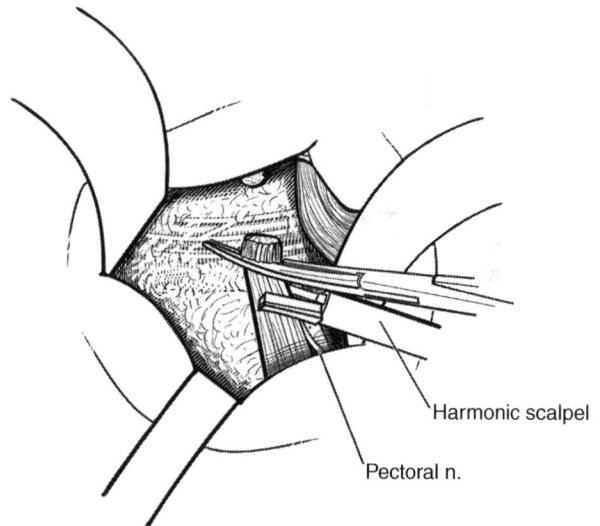

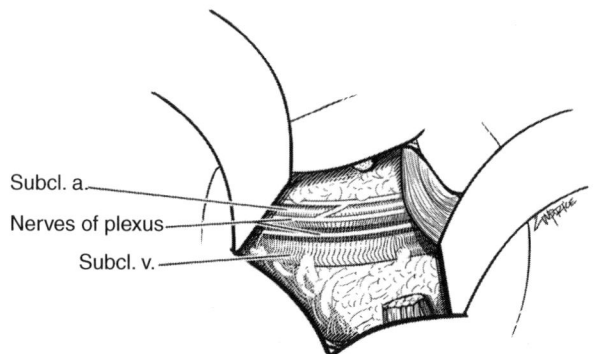

Fig. 15.3 Technique of transaxillary pectoralis minor tenotomy and partial myomectomy. The PM muscle is divided against the coracoid process with a harmonic scalpel or cautery. The end of the muscle is grasped with a long clamp, elevated, and 2–3 cm of muscle are excised to prevent postoperative attachment to the neurovascular bundle. Care is taken to look for and protect the pectoral nerve, which runs through the belly of the PM muscle to reach the pectoralis major. The nerve usually lies 3–5 cm from the coracoid process, so that limiting excision of the PM muscle to 2–3 cm is safe (Courtesy of Presbyterian-St. Lukes Hospital, Denver, Colorado by Wes Price)

Fig. 15.4 Technique of transaxillary pectoralis minor tenotomy and partial myomectomy. The completed operation shows the divided end of the PM muscle and the neurovascular bundle. There may be tight bands of clavipectoral fascia covering the bundle, which should be divided to prevent them from later compressing the nerves of the plexus (Courtesy of Presbyterian-St. Lukes Hospital, Denver, Colorado by Wes Price)

Table 15.4 Results of treatment with isolated pectoralis minor tenotomy

Diagnosis	# of operations	Outcomes at 1–3 years follow up, # of patients (%)		
		Excellent-good	Fair	Failure
Isolated PMS	52	47 (90 %)	1 (2 %)	4 (8 %)
PMS + NTOS	48	17 (35 %)	9 (19 %)	22 (46 %)

Adapted from Sanders and Rao [1], p. 701–8. With permission from Elsevier
PMS pectoralis minor syndrome, *PMS + NTOS* with symptoms of neurogenic TOS related to the scalene triangle

was associated with NTOS localized to the scalene triangle, only 35 % of patients had good improvement following surgery that had targeted the PMS alone (Table 15.4). The reason for offering isolated PMT to patients in both groups was that they had experienced very good improvement in symptoms following a selective PM muscle block. Indeed, the symptoms that continued were typically those of NTOS localized to the scalene triangle, and most of the patients who failed or had only fair improvement following isolated PMT went on to have more complete thoracic outlet decompression.

Pectoralis Minor Syndrome in Recurrent Neurogenic TOS

As noted in 2004, PMS can be the cause of recurrent or persistent symptoms in patients operated upon for NTOS [9]. For this reason, every patient with symptoms of recurrent NTOS should be carefully evaluated for PMS. If PMS is present and if the patient responds favorably to a selective PM muscle block, isolated PMT is recommended. In our experience with 65 operations in this setting, isolated PMT gave good symptom improvement in 69 %, fair improvement in 8 %, and no improvement in 23 % [13].

References

1. Sanders RJ, Rao NM. The forgotten pectoralis minor syndrome: 100 operations for pectoralis minor syndrome alone or accompanied by neurogenic thoracic outlet syndrome. Ann Vasc Surg. 2010;24:701–4.
2. Sanders RJ, Rao NM. Pectoralis minor obstruction of the axillary vein: report of six patients. J Vasc Surg. 2007;45:1206–11.
3. Sanders RJ, Hammond SL. Diagnosis of thoracic outlet syndrome. J Vasc Surg. 2007;46:601–4.
4. Wright IS. The neurovascular syndrome produced by hyperabduction of the arms: the immediate changes produced in 150 normal controls, and the effects on same persons of prolonged hyperabduction of the arms, as in sleeping, and in certain occupations. Am Heart J. 1945;29:1–19.
5. Lord Jr JW, Stone PW. Pectoralis minor tenotomy and anterior scalenotomy with special reference to the hyperabduction syndrome and "effort thrombosis" of the subclavian vein. Circulation. 1956;13: 537–42.
6. d'Huart. A propos de six case de syndrome du scalene anterieur traites par scalenotomie et section du petit pectoral. Ann Chir 1964; 18:205–9.
7. McIntyre DI. Subcoracoid neurovascular entrapment. Clin Orthop Relat Res. 1975;108:27–30.
8. Stallworth JM, Quinn GJ, Aiken AF. Is first rib resection necessary for relief of thoracic outlet syndrome? Ann Surg. 1977;185:581–92.
9. Ambrad-Chalela E, Thomas GI, Johansen KH. Recurrent neurogenic thoracic outlet syndrome. Am J Surg. 2004;187:505–10.
10. Upton ARM, McComas AJ. The double crush in nerve-entrapment syndromes. Lancet. 1973;2:359–62.
11. Seror O. Medial antebrachial cutaneous nerve conduction study, a new tool to demonstrate mild lower brachial plexus lesions: a report of 16 cases. Clin Neurophysiol. 2004;115:2316–22.
12. Machanic BI, Sanders RJ. Medial antebrachial cutaneous nerve measurements to diagnose neurogenic thoracic outlet syndrome. Ann Vasc Surg. 2008;22: 248–54.
13. Sanders RJ. Recurrent neurogenic thoracic outlet syndrome stressing the importance of pectoralis minor syndrome. Vasc Endovascular Surg. 2011;45: 33–8.

Double Crush Syndrome

16

Charles Philip Toussaint, Zarina S. Ali,
Gregory G. Heuer, and Eric L. Zager

Abstract

Upton and McComas formalized the hypothesis of the "double crush" syndrome (DCS) in 1973 (Upton and McComas Lancet 2:359–362, 1973) to describe the coexistence of multiple compressive lesions along the course of a peripheral nerve, postulating that entrapment of the peripheral nerve at one site renders the nerve susceptible to proximal and/or distal compression. By definition, augmented axonal injury occurs, representing more than just the combined independent effects of each lesion. This mechanism of neuronal injury is implicated in a variety of multi-focal neuropathies, including cervical radiculopathy and carpal tunnel syndrome (CTS), thoracic outlet syndrome and CTS, and cubital tunnel syndrome and Guyon's canal syndrome. The DCS hypothesis, however, is not universally accepted as an underlying mechanism of multi-focal neuropathies, and a critical review of this entity allows for a better understanding of the controversial theory.

Introduction

Upton and McComas formalized the hypothesis of the "double crush" syndrome (DCS) in 1973 [1] to describe the coexistence of multiple compressive lesions along the course of a peripheral nerve, postulating that entrapment of the peripheral nerve at one site renders the nerve susceptible to proximal and/or distal compression (Fig. 16.1). By definition, augmented axonal injury occurs, representing more than just the combined independent effects of each lesion. This mechanism of neuronal injury is implicated in a variety of multi-focal neuropathies, including cervical radiculopathy and carpal tunnel syndrome (CTS), thoracic outlet syndrome and CTS,

C.P. Toussaint, MD
Department of Neurosurgery,
University of South Carolina School of Medicine,
Columbia, SC 29203, USA

Z.S. Ali, MD • E.L. Zager, MD (✉)
Department of Neurosurgery,
University of Pennsylvania Hospital,
3400 Spruce St. Silverstein Pavilion 3rd Floor,
Philadelphia, PA 19104, USA
e-mail: eric.zager@uphs.upenn.edu

G.G. Heuer, MD, PhD
Department of Neurosurgery,
Children's Hospital of Philadelphia,
Philadelphia, PA 19104, USA

Fig. 16.1 Upton and McComas' diagram of the double-crush hypothesis. Anterograde axonal transport is represented in various states, including: (**a**)normal, (**b**) severe distal injury causing axon death with degeneration, (**c**) mild proximal compression causing only impaired axoplasmic flow, (**d**) mild distal lesion causing only limited impairment of axoplasmic flow, (**e**) combined mild proximal and distal lesions with aggregated axoplasmic flow impairment causing axon death and degeneration (Adapted from Upton and McComas [1]. With permission from Elsevier)

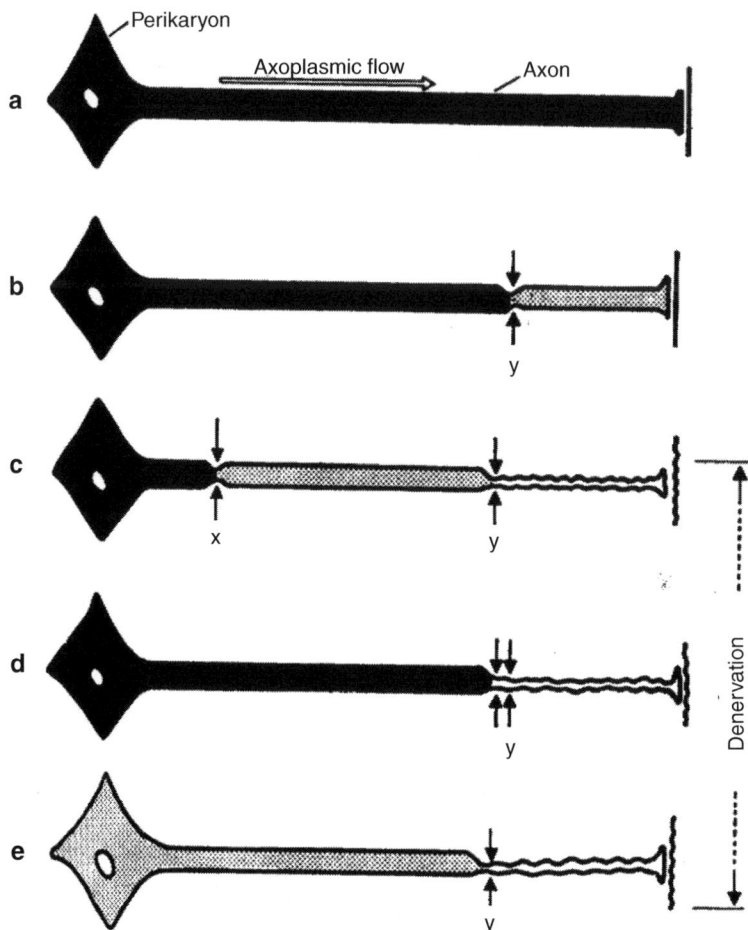

and cubital tunnel syndrome and Guyon's canal syndrome. The DCS hypothesis, however, is not universally accepted as an underlying mechanism of multi-focal neuropathies.

Etiology

An entrapment neuropathy is defined as a pressure-induced injury to a segment of a peripheral nerve secondary to anatomic or pathologic structures. Some patients have a predilection for entrapment neuropathies related to congenital narrowing of the nerve's osseous tunnel or thickening of an overlying retinaculum. Inflammation or edema of adjacent structures, such as tendons, may reduce the size of the passageway for the nerve, and mechanical forces on the nerve can

result in nerve compression. DCS involves *two or more sites of compression and/or entrapment* that interfere with normal neuronal function.

Animal studies have supported the concept that the loss of nerve function from two sites of compression is greater than the sum of the individual lesions [2].

Entrapment of a peripheral nerve can reduce its elasticity and ability to stretch through tethering and extra/intraneural fibrosis. This, in turn, predisposes the nerve to stretch injury, both proximally and distally [3]. Intrinsic neuropathy further renders the peripheral nerve susceptible to injury. Metabolic disorders such as diabetes mellitus, myxedema, uremia and pyridoxine deficiency can render the nerve less resilient to compression. Diabetes mellitus (DM) is the most frequently encountered metabolic neuropathy, and studies have shown an increased incidence of multiple nerve entrapments in patients with diabetic polyneuropathy [4]. Baba et al. have reported a 16 % incidence of ulnar nerve entrapment and carpal tunnel syndrome in patients with DM [5]. In contrast, motor neuron disease, such as amyotrophic lateral sclerosis, does not appear to make a peripheral nerve more susceptible to entrapment [6]. Ischemia also plays a role in nerve impairment from compression. Venous flow can be hindered with pressure as low as 20 mmHg, resulting in increased endoneural pressure and edema, which thereby restrict axonal flow [7].

Upton and McComas based their model of DCS on the dysfunction of axonal transport due to nerve compression or entrapment resulting in impaired distal "axoplasmic flow" and degeneration [1]. Anterograde flow of proteins and neurotransmitters from the cell body to the axon is imperative for proper nerve function. Compression along the course of a nerve can compromise this system. With 30 mmHg of pressure, axonal transport is impaired and at 50 mmHg, complete axonal block is seen [8]. With impaired axonal anterograde flow, the distal axon suffers and is likely more susceptible to injury. Retrograde flow within the axon is also important for proper nerve function, and it has also been suggested that impairment of retrograde flow makes the proximal nerve more susceptible to compression [9].

The mechanism of DCS relies on the presence of an anatomic continuity of nerve fibers between multiple lesion sites. However, sensory neurons are uniquely oriented such that their cell bodies lie in ganglia near the dorsal root in the spine. Anterograde axonal transport in sensory neurons occurs bidirectionally from the cell body into the peripheral nerve via postganglionic fibers, as well as into the nerve root via preganglionic fibers through separate microtubule systems. Given this, and other anatomic and pathophysiologic restrictions, Wilbourn and Gilliatt [10] and Morgan and Wilbourn [11] propose that the DCS hypothesis has limited application as a mechanism to explain multi-focal neuropathies, particularly those involving cervical radiculopathies.

A more comprehensive model is offered by Novak and Mackinnon, which suggests that certain postures or positions increase tension and pressure at sites where nerves are entrapped, causing vascular compromise and adaptive muscle shortening. These factors, in turn, result in neural edema, inflammation, fibrosis, decreased neural mobility and secondary compression [12].

Thoracic Outlet Syndrome and Double Crush Syndrome

Neurogenic thoracic outlet syndrome (NTOS) refers to the syndrome caused by compression of the brachial plexus along its path from the neck into the axilla and is the most common cause of brachial plexopathy. Criteria for diagnosis of NTOS are inconsistent and there are few objective criteria available to help. Patients with NTOS often present with vague or nonspecific symptoms of the forearm and hand that may overlap with carpal tunnel syndrome or cubital tunnel syndrome [13]. Wood and Biondi have reported a 44 % incidence of double crush syndrome in patients with NTOS, with the secondary site of compression being the carpal tunnel [14]. Other sites of secondary compression include the ulnar nerve at the cubital tunnel, the median nerve at the pronator teres, and the radial nerve at the radial tunnel. Narakas et al. reported a 10 % incidence of cubital tunnel syndrome in patients with NTOS [15]. Others feel that the co-incidence of CTS and NTOS approaches zero [16].

Clinically, the identification of such coexisting conditions can be difficult. Provocative tests, such as Tinel's sign, may be less reliable in DCS than in single entrapment neuropathies [17]. CTS may present with proximally referred symptoms that may be mistaken for a more proximal entrapment. Often, the presence of DCS is identified after the patient presents with persistent symptoms following decompression at a particular entrapment site. For example, Putters et al. reported a case of bilateral radial tunnel syndrome following surgery for bilateral thoracic outlet syndrome [18].

For the surgical treatment of NTOS and DCS, Yao and Osterman advocate treating the (almost always simpler) distal site of entrapment first, since this may allow the patient to improve to a point that he or she may not need the proximal decompression at the thoracic outlet [3]. Not surprisingly, Lascar et al. demonstrated worse outcomes following cubital tunnel surgery in patients with NTOS, as compared to patients with isolated cubital tunnel syndrome [19]. Similarly, Osterman demonstrated higher failure rates in carpal tunnel decompression in patients with DCS, as well as poorer post-operative functioning and return to work rates [20].

Conclusion

The "double crush" hypothesis is popular amongst clinicians due to the prevalence of multi-focal neuropathies, including NTOS and distal entrapment syndromes. However, the original hypothesis remains controversial; alternative models that incorporate the vascular compromise and associated adaptive muscular changes may offer a more comprehensive mechanism. While the diagnosis of NTOS alone is difficult to make, objectively identifying a coexistent distal entrapment further complicates matters. This potential diagnosis must be kept in mind, and thorough evaluation for "double crush" may be necessary since DCS may be implicated when one experiences less than satisfactory results following the surgical treatment of carpal tunnel or cubital tunnel syndrome.

References

1. Upton AR, McComas AJ. The double crush in nerve entrapment syndromes. Lancet. 1973;2(7825):359–62.
2. Nemoto K, Matsumoto N, Tazaki K, Horiuchi Y, Uchinishi K, Mori Y. An experimental study on the "double crush" hypothesis. J Hand Surg. 1987;12(4):552–9.
3. Yao J, Osterman A. Double crush syndrome. In: Slutsky DJ, Hentz V, editors. Peripheral nerve surgery. Philadelphia: Churchill Livingstone/Elsevier; 2006. p. 277–83.
4. Dellon AL, Mackinnon SE, Seiler WA. Susceptibility of the diabetic nerve to chronic compression. Ann Plast Surg. 1988;20(2):117–9.
5. Baba M, Ozaki I, Watahiki Y, Kudo M, Takebe K, Matsunaga M. Focal conduction delay at the carpal tunnel and the cubital fossa in diabetic polyneuropathy. Electromyogr Clin Neurophysiol. 1987;27(2):119–23.
6. Chaudhry V, Clawson LL. Entrapment of motor nerves in motor neuron disease: does double crush occur? J Neurol Neurosurg Psychiatry. 1997;62(1):71–6.
7. Rydevik B, Lundborg G, Bagge U. Effects of graded compression on intraneural blood blow. An in vivo study on rabbit tibial nerve. J Hand Surg. 1981;6(1):3–12.
8. Gelberman RH, Szabo RM, Williamson RV, Hargens AR, Yaru NC, Minteer-Convery MA. Tissue pressure threshold for peripheral nerve viability. Clin Orthop Relat Res. 1983;178:285–91.
9. Lundborg G, Myers R, Powell H. Nerve compression injury and increased endoneurial fluid pressure: a "miniature compartment syndrome". J Neurol Neurosurg Psychiatry. 1983;46(12):1119–24.
10. Wilbourn AJ, Gilliatt RW. Double-crush syndrome: a critical analysis. Neurology. 1997;49(1):21–9.
11. Morgan G, Wilbourn AJ. Cervical radiculopathy and coexisting distal entrapment neuropathies: double-crush syndromes? Neurology. 1998;50(1):78–83.
12. Novak CB, Mackinnon SE. Multiple nerve entrapment syndromes in office workers. Occup Med. 1999;14(1):39–59.
13. Simpson RL, Fern SA. Multiple compression neuropathies and the double-crush syndrome. Orthop Clin North Am. 1996;27(2):381–8.
14. Wood VE, Biondi J. Double-crush nerve compression in thoracic-outlet syndrome. J Bone Joint Surg Am. 1990;72(1):85–7.
15. Narakas A, Bonnard C, Egloff DV. The cervicothoracic outlet compression syndrome. Analysis of surgical treatment. Annales de chirurgie de la main: organe officiel des societes de chirurgie de la main. 1986;5(3):195–207.
16. Carroll RE, Hurst LC. The relationship of thoracic outlet syndrome and carpal tunnel syndrome. Clin Orthop Relat Res. 1982;164:149–53.
17. Lo SF, Chou LW, Meng NH, et al. Clinical characteristics and electrodiagnostic features in patients with carpal tunnel syndrome, double crush syndrome, and cervical radiculopathy. Rheumatol Int. 2012;32(5):1257–63.
18. Putters JL, Kaulesar Sukul DM, Johannes EJ. Bilateral thoracic outlet syndrome with bilateral radial tunnel syndrome: a double-crush phenomenon. Case report. Arch Orthop Trauma Surg. 1992;111(4):242–3.
19. Lascar T, Laulan J. Cubital tunnel syndrome: a retrospective review of 53 anterior subcutaneous transpositions. J Hand Surg. 2000;25(5):453–6.
20. Osterman AL. The double crush syndrome. Orthop Clin North Am. 1988;19(1):147–55.

Ergonomic and Postural Issues in NTOS

17

Marc A. Weinberg

Abstract

Ergonomics is the science of matching living conditions and job demands to the human body to optimize both health and productivity. Improper ergonomics can increase musculoskeletal disorders accounting for a large number of disabilities and loss of work days. The use of computers and related technologies by both adults and children can result in an adaptive change in posture. These abnormal postures and work-related factors may also pose a risk for the development of Neurogenic Thoracic Outlet Syndrome (NTOS). Good clinical outcomes can occur by combining work style behavior and ergonomic intervention with more traditional therapies.

Epidemiology of Ergonomic Abnormalities

Ergonomics, the science of matching living conditions and job demands to the human body, has two major goals: optimizing both health and productivity [1, 2]. Whether engaged in work, home or recreationally related activities, proper ergonomic design is necessary to help correct postural anomalies and to prevent injuries. These disorders are time dependent and may develop into long-term disabilities [2]. Improper ergonomics can increase work-related musculoskeletal disorders, and account for a large number of disabilities and loss of work days. It is one of the most expensive health problems in modern industrial societies, as 34 % of all injuries and illnesses resulting in absences from work in the United States in 2002 were related to musculoskeletal disorders [3].

It has been found that abnormal postures and work-related factors may pose a risk for the development of Neurogenic Thoracic Outlet Syndrome (NTOS) [4–7]. Specifically, a connection has been made between the stress of repetitive work and NTOS. Abnormal posture plays a major role in the cascade of physical events that are a prelude to certain upper extremity disorders [7] (see Table 17.1).

It is apparent that computers and related technologies are resulting in an adaptive change in our posture. The daily use of computers in the home and workplace has added to these ergonomic problems [8]. From an evolutionary standpoint, the adaptations to our working postures

M.A. Weinberg, DC
Active Health Center, 421 Northlake Blvd. Suite F,
North Palm Beach, FL 33408, USA
e-mail: drmarc@weinbergchiro.com

K.A. Illig et al. (eds.), *Thoracic Outlet Syndrome*,
DOI 10.1007/978-1-4471-4366-6_17, © Springer-Verlag London 2013

Table 17.1 The cascade of physical changes that can occur due to faulty posture and repetitive use syndrome

Postural misalignment and derangement including loss of the normal cervical lordotic curve, rigidity of the thoracic spine, protracted shoulders and head thrust forward position
Shortened scalene and pectoralis minor muscles
Space between the clavicles and the first rib becomes restricted
First ribs lift and diminish the costoclavicular space
Traction and scarring of the nerve bundles
Improper gliding of nerves through narrow canals or tendinous arches, compression from adjacent muscles, edema, synovial thickening, tendinitis, and angioedema secondary to chemical factors such as histamine release
Nerve entrapment and lack of nerve gliding in the neck
Development of secondary conditions such as thoracic outlet syndrome, medial or lateral epicondylitis, cubital tunnel syndrome, radial tunnel syndrome, carpal tunnel syndrome and deQuervain's tenosynovitis
Loss of peripheral pulses
Dual site ulnar nerve injury ("double crush syndrome")
Friction, compression and inflamation of nerves causing impaired nerve stimului
Impairment along the whole length of the nerve from possible longitudinal force on the nerve
Mechanical traction and mechanical damage of the nerves
Sympathetic nervous system overactivity
Diminished hand temperature
Complex regional pain syndrome (CRPS)
Shortening of forearm musculature causing impaired muscle regeneration
Myofascial pain syndrome

Adapted from Pascarelli and Hsu [7]. With permission from Springer Science+Business Media

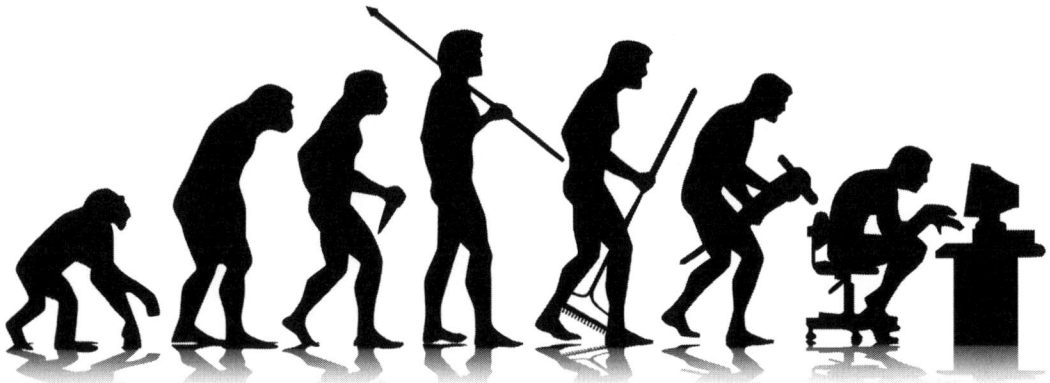

Fig. 17.1 A comical depiction of the "devolution" of the human posture

are being forced to occur over a relatively short period of time instead of the usual course of many thousands of years [9]. We live in a world of constantly advancing technology that may be causing a "devolution of human postural alignments" [10] (See Fig. 17.1). Our society is working harder, longer and in amounts that defies historical precedent and common sense. These physical and emotional demands are creating an epidemic of faulty ergonomic postural injuries [7, 11–13].

Ergonomic Effects on Children

Although there has been a surge of attention on ergonomics in the workplace, it is imperative that ergonomic discussion becomes commonplace in the home and, more importantly, with our children. The most important time of spinal and postural development is childhood and adolescence [14]. Children are switching from dynamic childhood activities, such as running, playing outside and participating in sports, to the more static activities of playing video games and "text chatting" [15–17]. This has become so prevalent that we now have common clinical complaints named for the actions that are causing the problems: Text Message Injuries (TMI's), "gamers' thumb" and "stylus finger" which are caused by repetitive use of mobile and gaming devices [17].

It has been found that postural defects from playing video games are many, but have specifically included protruding scapulae, increased lumbar lordosis and thoracic kyphosis. Children are spending only 4 h/week performing sports activities compared to 14 h/week watching TV and playing computer games. Children who did not participate in sports activities had a significantly higher probability of poor posture [15, 18].

An additional effect on posture in children and teens is the increase in educational demands placed on students today [19]. It has been shown that there is a correlation between the incidence of thoracic and low back pain in school children and adolescents and the use of heavy backpacks [20]. Forward head posture and subsequent TOS can also increase with the use of backpacks in school [21]. It has been suggested that a backpack weighing 15 % or more of body weight can have an adverse effect on cervical and shoulder posture in children in their early teens [21].

Pathophysiology of Abnormal Ergonomics

Faulty ergonomic postures have major influences on our bodies including increasing pressure on nerves in areas that are prone to entrapment, adaptive muscle shortening which subsequently compresses nerves, and hypertrophy of over-used muscles creating muscular imbalance [22]. Patients with a hyper-kyphotic thoracic curve

cause their neck to be in a forward posture position and that leads to a cascade of muscular changes, particularly protracted scapulae, anterior rotated shoulders and decreased clavicular mobility [23, 24]. These postures will all contribute to the development of NTOS by narrowing the spaces through which the neurovascular structures pass [24].

Additionally, altered posture will change breathing patterns over time. The resulting shallow breathing pattern results in hypertrophic development of the scalene muscles. This narrows the costoclavicular space as the muscles attempt to repetitively elevate the upper ribs during breathing [24]. A forward head posture may result in the loss of up to 30 % of vital lung capacity by blocking of the action of the scalene muscles as they elevate the first rib during inhalation [25].

Treatment Options

Clinical outcomes improve when work style behavior and ergonomic intervention are combined with more traditional therapies [26, 27]. Even with chronic cases, upper extremity symptomatology can be alleviated when therapy is combined with behavioral modification at home, work, school and sleep [22].

The first step for conservative management of NTOS is to physically assess the areas where the activities are being performed. This involves evaluating the workplace or home to ensure that there is proper body alignment and posture. Exercises, which may be taught by a Chiropractic Physician, Physical or Occupational Therapist who understand the biomechanics of TOS, can help strengthen muscles that improve posture and increase overall conditioning. This treatment assists in maintaining proper muscular balance and will help correct sitting and standing postures thereby decreasing pressure on the nerves and blood vessels [28, 29]. Simple modifications such as reducing mouse use, lowering the height of the keyboard, decreasing the number of hours at the keyboard, resting the arms on the desk surface, and providing a large forearm support

Table 17.2 Proper ergonomic sitting postures

Working postures

1. Head and neck are upright with trunk facing forward
2. Trunk is perpendicular to the floor with shoulders and upper arms in-line with the torso
3. Elbows are close to the body
4. Forearms, wrists, and hands are straight and in-line
5. Feet rest flat on the floor with thighs parallel to the floor and the lower legs perpendicular to floor

Seating

6. Use a backrest which provides support for the lower back
7. Ensure that there is a properly fitted seat
8. Armrests, if used, support both forearms while performing computer tasks and they do not interfere with movement

Keyboard/input device

9. Keyboard/input device platform(s) is stable and large enough to hold a keyboard and an input device (mouse or trackball) is located right next to the keyboard
10. Wrists and hands do not rest on sharp or hard edges

Monitor

11. Monitor screen is directly in front and is at or below eye level
12. Monitor distance allows reading of the screen without leaning of head, neck or trunk forward/backward

Work area

13. Thighs have sufficient clearance space between the top of the thighs and the computer table/keyboard platform
14. Legs and feet have sufficient clearance space under the work surface

Accessories

15. Document holder, if provided, is stable and large enough to hold documents and is the same height and distance as the monitor screen
16. Wrist/palm rest, if provided, is padded and free of sharp or square edges that push on the wrists and keeps forearms, wrists, and hands straight and in-line
17. Telephone can be used with head upright and shoulders relaxed

Reprinted from Department of Labor, Occupational Safety and Health Administration Website. OSHA Ergonomic Solutions: Computer Workstations eTool – Evaluation Checklist. http://www.osha.gov/SLTC/etools/computerworkstations/checklist.html. Accessed 5 May 2011

have all shown beneficial results [8, 13, 30, 31]. Encouraging specific seated postures may also reduce the risk of musculoskeletal symptoms and disorders [30, 31] (see Table 17.2 and Fig. 17.2).

Summary

The increasing incidence of TOS due to time spent on computers, video games, and mobile devices will be an important facet of future ergonomic studies. One of the most important aspects of conservative and ergonomic management of NTOS caused by postural involvement is early awareness and detection of the postural changes developing within the body, allowing intervention before the onset of significant symptomatology [32]. Being such a symptom-based society, early prevention and correction of abnormal postural development can only occur by increasing education and awareness of proper ergonomic postures and activities in the workplace, schools and in the home.

Fig. 17.2 Proper ergonomic position and support [Reprinted from Department of Labor, Occupational Safety and Health Administration. http://www.osha.gov/Publications/videoDisplay/videoDisplay.html. Working Safely with Video Display Terminals. OSHA 3092, 1997 (Revised)]

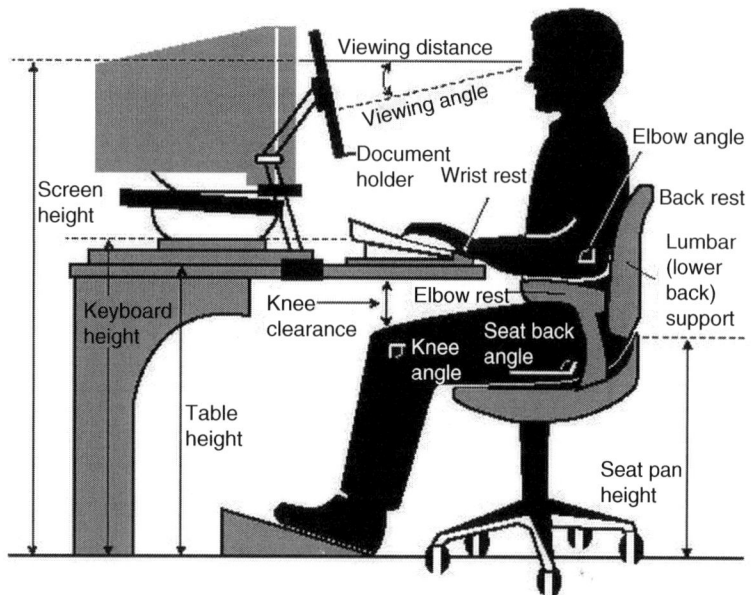

References

1. What is ergonomics. International ergonomics. http://www.iea.cc/01_what/What%20is%20Ergonomics.html. Accessed 6 May 2011.
2. Ergonomics. Lawrence Berkely National Laboratory. http://www.lbl.gov/ehs/ergo/index.shtml. Accessed 6 May 2011.
3. Wang PC, Rempel DM, Hurwitz EL, Harrison RJ, Janowitz I, Ritz BR. Self-reported pain and physical signs for musculoskeletal disorders in the upper body region among Los Angeles garment workers. Work. 2009;34(1):79–87.
4. Bernard BP, ed. Musculoskeletal disorders and workplace factors – a critical review of epidemiologic evidence for work-related musculoskeletal disorders of the neck, upper extremity, and low back. NIOSH; 1997. p. 3–25 (Publication no. 97-141).
5. Medical Treatment Guidelines. Washington State Department of Labor and Industries (effective 1 Oct 2010). http://www.lni.wa.gov/ClaimsIns/Files/OMD/MedTreat/ThoracicOutletNeurogenic.pdf. Accessed 6 May 2011.
6. Department of Labor, Occupational Safety and Health Administration. 29 CFR Part 1910, Ergonomics Program; Proposed Rule. Federal register/vol. 64, no. 225/Tuesday, November 14, 2000/Proposed Rules; 68432.
7. Pascarelli EF, Hsu YP. Understanding work-related upper extremity disorders: clinical findings in 485 computer users, musicians, and others. J Occup Rehabil. 2001;11(1):1–21.
8. Tornqvist EW, Hagberg M, Hagman M, Risberg EH, Toomingas A. The influence of working conditions and individual factors on the incidence of neck and upper limb symptoms among professional computer users. Int Arch Occup Environ Health. 2009;82(6):689–702.
9. Frequently asked questions about evolution. Public Broadcasting Station web site. http://www.pbs.org/wgbh/evolution/library/faq/cat06.html. Accessed 6 May 2011.
10. Mercer L. Posture therapy. Livestrong. http://www.livestrong.com/article/183967-posture-therapy/. Accessed 6 May 2011.
11. The Real Reasons You're Working So Hard … and what you can do about it. Bloomberg Businessweek. http://www.businessweek.com/magazine/content/05_40/b3953601.htm. Published 3 Oct 2005. Accessed 6 May 2011.
12. Gerr F, Marcus M, Ensor C, et al. A prospective study of computer users: I. Study design and incidence of musculoskeletal symptoms and disorders. Am J Ind Med. 2002;41(4):221–35.
13. Gerr F, Marcus M, Monteilh C. Epidemiology of musculoskeletal disorders among computer users:

lesson learned from the role of posture and keyboard use. J Electromyogr Kinesiol. 2004;14(1):25–31.

14. Lafond D, Descarreaux M, Normand MC, Harrison DE. Postural development in school children: a cross-sectional study. Chiropr Osteopat. 2007;15:1.

15. Kratenová J, Zejglicová K, Malý M, Filipová V. Prevalence and risk factors of poor posture in school children in the Czech Republic. J Sch Health. 2007;77(3):131–7.

16. Too much texting can be a pain in the neck, Researchers begin to study the physiological effects of text messaging on college students. Temple University web site. http://news.temple.edu/news/too-much-texting-can-be-pain-neck. 19 Nov 2009. Accessed 6 May 2011.

17. Blackberry use can damage thumb. BBC NEWS. http://news.bbc.co.uk/go/pr/fr/-/2/hi/health/4222365.stm. 31 Jan 2005. Accessed 6 May 2011.

18. Salminen JJ, Oksanen A, Mäki P, Pentti J, Kujala UM. Leisure time physical activity in the young. Correlation with low-back pain, spinal mobility and trunk muscle strength in 15-year-old school children. Int J Sports Med. 1993;14(7):406–10.

19. 'Race to Nowhere': are students working harder and hurting themselves in the process? Local parents and experts weigh in. The Daily Herald web site. http://www.dailyherald.com/article/20110301/news/703019902. Updated 3 Mar 2011. Accessed 6 May 2011.

20. Korovessis P, Koureas G, Papazisis Z. Correlation between backpack weight and way of carrying, sagittal and frontal spinal curvatures, athletic activity, and dorsal and low back pain in schoolchildren and adolescents. J Spinal Disord Tech. 2004;17(1):33–40.

21. Chansirinukor W, Wilson D, Grimmer K, Dansie B. Effects of backpacks on students: measurement of cervical and shoulder posture. Aust J Physiother. 2001;47(2):110–6.

22. Novak CB, Mackinnon SE. Repetitive use and static postures: a source of nerve compression and pain. J Hand Ther. 1997;10(2):151–9.

23. Warren H. Forward head/forward shoulders. Dynamic Chiropractic web site. http://www.dynamicchiropractic.com/mpacms/dc/article.php?id=36230(1999). Accessed Feb 2013.

24. Kisner C, Allen Colby L. Therapeutic exercise: foundations and techniques. 5th ed. Columbus: The Ohio State University School of Allied Medical Professionals; 2007. p. 359–61.

25. Cailliet R, Gross L. Rejuvenation strategy. New York: Doubleday & Co; 1987.

26. Meijer EM, Sluiter JK, Frings-Dresen MH. Is work-style a mediating factor for pain in the upper extremity over time? J Occup Rehabil. 2008;18(3):262–6.

27. Fabrizio P. Ergonomic intervention in the treatment of a patient with upper extremity and neck pain. Phys Ther. 2009;89(4):351–60.

28. Nicholas RA, Feuerstein M, Suchday S. Workstyle and upper-extremity symptoms: a biobehavioral perspective. J Occup Environ Med. 2004;47(4):352–61.

29. Devereux J, Vlachonikolis I, Buckle P. Epidemiological study to investigate potential interaction between physical and psychosocial factors at work that may increase the risk of symptoms of musculoskeletal disorder of the neck and upper limb. Occup Environ Med. 2002;59(4):269–77.

30. Marcus M, Gerr F, Monteilh C, et al. A prospective study of computer users: II. Postural risk factors for musculoskeletal symptoms and disorders. Am J Ind Med. 2002;41(4):236–49.

31. Rempel DM, Krause N, Goldberg R, Benner D, Hudes M, Goldner GU. A randomised controlled trial evaluating the effects of two workstation interventions on upper body pain and incident musculoskeletal disorders among computer operators. Occup Environ Med. 2006;63(5):300–6.

32. Beer S, Schlegel C, Hasegawa A. Conservative therapy in thoracic outlet syndrome. Literature review and pathogenetic considerations. Schweiz Med Wochenschr. 1997;127(15):617–22.

Radiographic Imaging in Diagnosis and Assessment of NTOS

Scott Werden

Abstract

The clinical diagnosis of NTOS remains controversial and challenging. Fortunately, modern medical imaging, particularly MRI, provides excellent evaluation of the brachial plexus, the surrounding soft tissues and bones, and the dynamic changes that occur in the thoracic outlet on movement of the upper extremity. This chapter details the imaging anatomy of the thoracic outlet, including the component anatomic tunnels that comprise the thoracic outlet, the brachial plexus, and the dynamic changes of the thoracic outlet seen on movement of the upper extremity. Imaging findings of NTOS, as defined by pathologic entrapment of the brachial plexus, are demonstrated and defined, including soft tissue anomalies, bony anomalies, and pathologic dynamic changes that cause narrowing of the anatomic tunnels of the thoracic outlet and resultant entrapment of the brachial plexus. A simple and straightforward algorithm for reviewing an imaging study of a patient with TOS is provided. The reader will understand the important anatomic landmarks and tunnels of the thoracic outlet, the soft tissue or bony anomalies and pathologic changes that occur in the thoracic outlet, and the difference between normal and abnormal changes that occur on movement of the upper extremity, along with the resulting entrapment of the brachial plexus.

Introduction

Neurogenic thoracic outlet syndrome (NTOS) is by far the most frequent type of TOS, making up 95–98 % of cases of thoracic outlet syndrome

S. Werden, MD
Vanguard Specialty Imaging,
1345 Lillian Ave., Sunnyvale, CA 94087-3523, USA
e-mail: mobileme4@me.com

[1–5]. NTOS has been and remains a considerable source of discussion and debate to the present day [6–9], and is frequently difficult to diagnose and treat. Provocative clinical tests for NTOS demonstrate limited accuracy and specificity [10–14]. Most of these tests depend upon evidence of arterial compression, which is a poor proxy for compression of the brachial plexus, given the complex anatomy and dynamic changes of the thoracic outlet [15]. Fortunately, current medical imaging has emerged as a valuable tool

K.A. Illig et al. (eds.), *Thoracic Outlet Syndrome*,
DOI 10.1007/978-1-4471-4366-6_18, © Springer-Verlag London 2013

Fig. 18.1 Normal scalene triangle, axial plane: The anterior (*A*) and middle (*M*) scalene muscles form the anterior and posterior borders of the scalene triangle. The brachial plexus roots and trunks (*arrowheads*) are surrounded by ample white fat within the scalene triangle. The posterior aspect of each first rib is seen (*R*) (Courtesy of Scott Werden, MD)

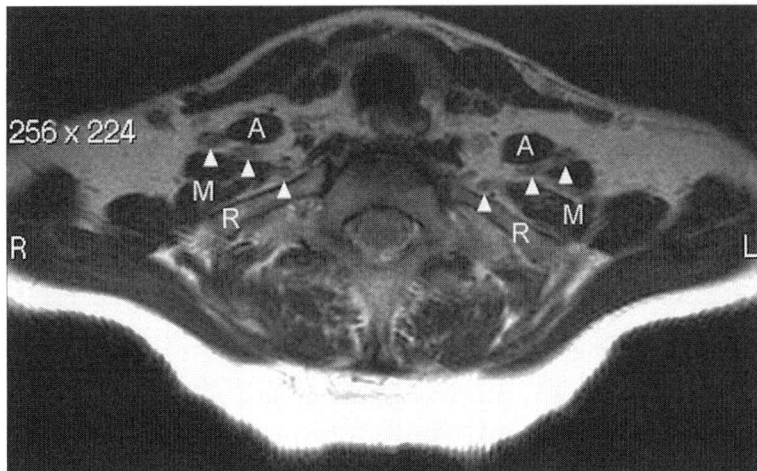

in understanding the anatomy and pathology underlying this syndrome. Imaging findings are most accurate and valuable when combined with an appropriate history and clinical examination, and should always be evaluated in conjunction with these clinical findings.

Imaging Anatomy

The thoracic outlet is the anatomic space at the junction of the neck, superior mediastinum, ipsilateral hemithorax, and ipsilateral upper extremity. Within the thoracic outlet, the great vessels and brachial plexus pass through a series of parallel and contiguous tunnels to converge in the upper extremity [12, 16, 17]. These tunnels have been classically defined as the scalene (or interscalene) triangle, the costoclavicular interval, the retropectoralis space and the prescalene space. NTOS results from impingement on the brachial plexus. The simplest way to evaluate a cross-sectional imaging study for the presence of NTOS is to follow the course of the brachial plexus from its constituent nerve roots through its terminal branches. This process will outline the borders of each anatomic tunnel, demonstrate those key structures that may cause impingement on the brachial plexus, and clarify the dynamic changes that occur on movement of the upper extremity. For this purpose, MRI will be used for all illustrations.

The anatomy of the thoracic outlet and the brachial plexus has been extensively studied by CT [15, 18–20], ultrasound [21, 22], and MRI [23–28]. As the nerve roots exit their respective neural foramina, they enter the scalene triangle (Figs. 18.1 and 18.2). The scalene triangle is bounded anteriorly by the anterior scalene muscle, posteriorly by the middle scalene muscle, and inferiorly by the first rib. The insertions of the anterior and middle scalene muscles on the first rib and the resultant gap between them is widely variable [14, 29–31].

The brachial plexus exits the scalene triangle and enters the costoclavicular interval (Fig. 18.3). The costoclavicular interval is bounded superiorly by the clavicle and subclavius muscle, and inferiorly by the first rib and serratus anterior muscle. The brachial plexus exits the costoclavicular interval and enters the retropectoralis space (Fig. 18.4). The retropectoralis space is obliquely oriented. Its anterior border is the pectoralis minor muscle, which originates from the third through fifth ribs medially and inferiorly, and inserts laterally and superiorly on the coracoid process. The coracoid process forms the superior border. Inferiorly and medially, the chest wall forms the posterior border of this space, while superiorly and laterally, the subscapularis muscle forms the posterior border. The brachial plexus passes through the superior half of the retropectoralis space to enter the axilla.

Fig. 18.2 Normal scalene triangle, sagittal plane: The anterior (*AS*) and middle (*MS*) scalene muscles and the first rib (*R*) form the borders of the scalene triangle (*Line 2*). The subclavian artery (*A*) and brachial plexus roots (*arrowheads*) are surrounded by ample white fat within the scalene triangle. The clavicle (*C*) and anterior scalene muscle form the borders of the prescalene space (*Line 1*), which transmits the subclavian vein (*V*) (Courtesy of Scott Werden, MD)

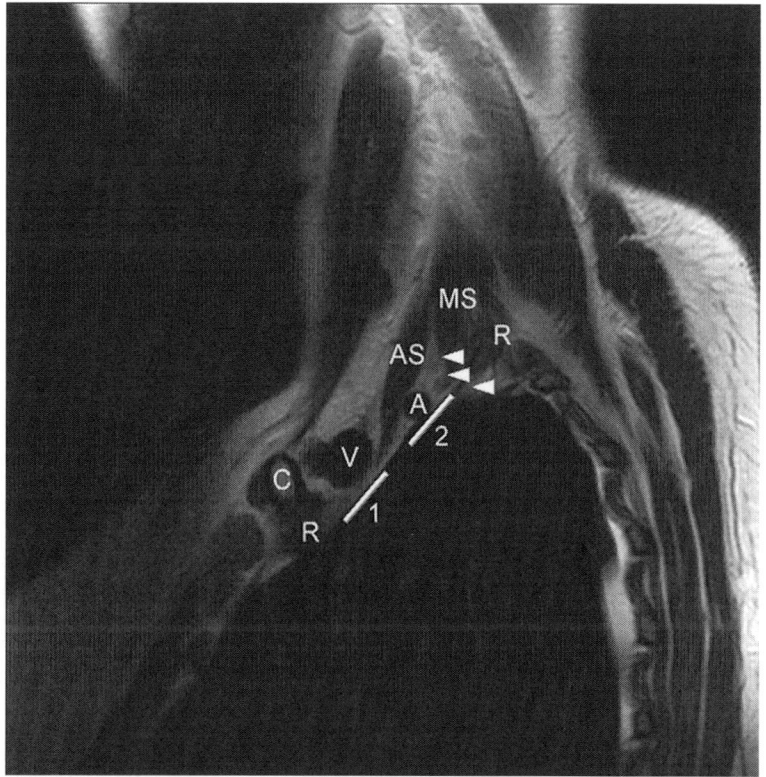

Fig. 18.3 Normal costo-clavicular interval, sagittal plane: The clavicle (*C*) and subclavius muscle (*S*) form the superior border of the costoclavicular interval, while the first rib (*R*) and serratus anterior muscle (*SA*) form the inferior border. The divisions of the brachial plexus (*arrowhead*), subclavian artery (*A*) and subclavian vein (*V*) are surrounded by ample white fat (Courtesy of Scott Werden, MD)

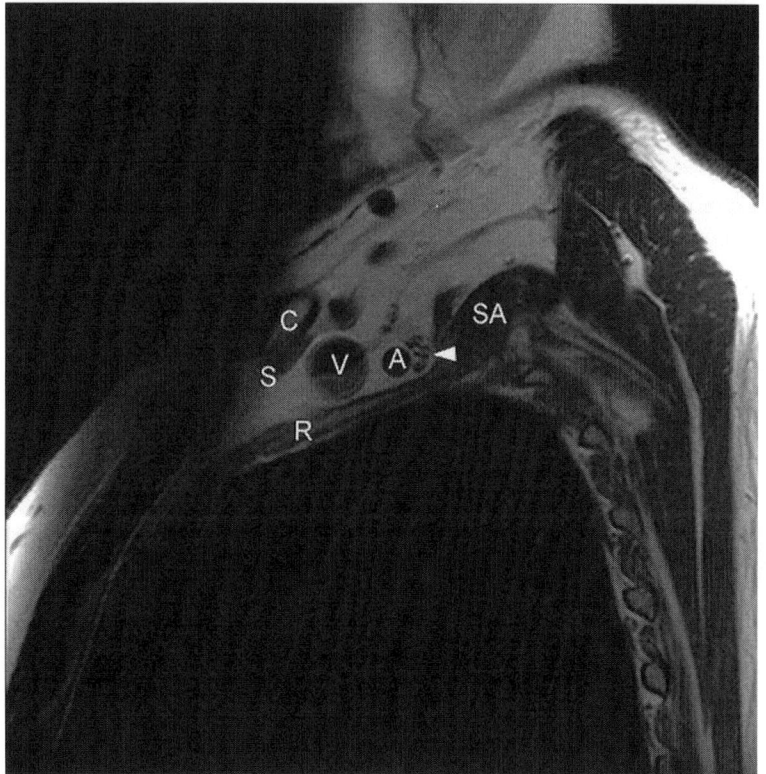

Fig. 18.4 Normal retropectoralis space, sagittal plane: The pectoralis minor muscle (*PM*) forms the anterior border, the subscapularis muscle (*SS*) forms the posterior border, and the coracoid process (*CP*) forms the superior border. Note that the origin of the pectoralis minor muscle is medial and inferior to this section. The lateral cord (*LC*), posterior cord (*PC*), and medial cord (*MC*) of the brachial plexus, the axillary artery (*A*) and the axillary vein (*V*) pass through the superior half of this space, and are surrounded by ample white fat (Courtesy of Scott Werden, MD)

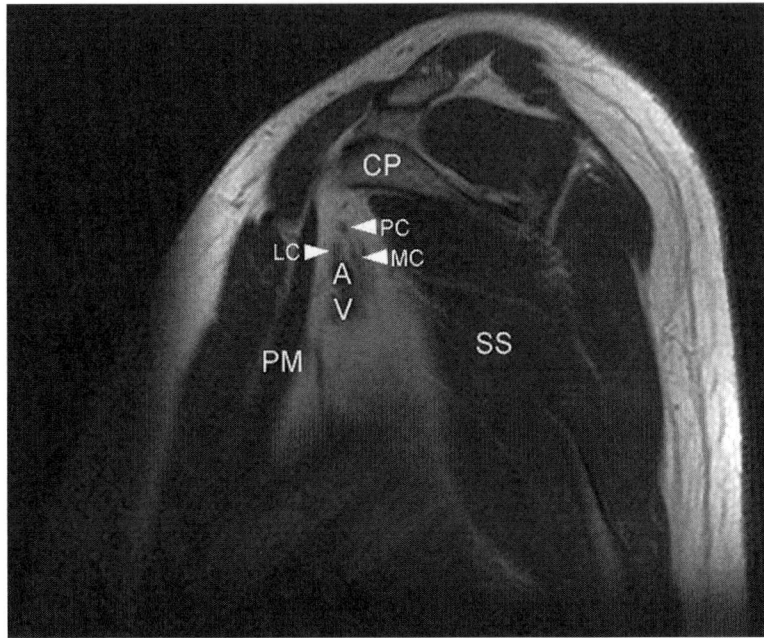

The prescalene space is bounded anteriorly by the clavicle and tendon of the subclavius muscle, and posteriorly by the insertion of the anterior scalene muscle (Fig. 18.2). The prescalene space parallels the scalene triangle, and transmits the subclavian vein, which then enters the costo-clavicular interval.

The composition and branching pattern of the brachial plexus is quite complex, but for imaging purposes it can be broken down into the following key components. The ventral rami of spinal nerve roots C5 through T1 exit their respective neural foramina, and form the superior, middle and inferior trunks within the scalene triangle. Each trunk divides into anterior and posterior divisions near the lateral margin of the first rib. These divisions form the lateral, posterior and medial cords in the retropectoralis space. The cords give rise to the terminal branches lateral to the coracoid process, in the axilla (Figs. 18.1–18.4) [32, 33].

rib. Additionally, there is ventilatory motion of the first rib. While discussion of the motion of these structures is beyond the scope of this chapter, a few key points are worth noting regarding normal dynamic changes of the thoracic outlet:

1. In the scalene triangle, the angle between the first rib and the horizontal plane constitutes the predominant dynamic element (Fig. 18.5).
2. In the costoclavicular interval, the first rib acts as a relatively fixed 'hard floor', while motion of the clavicle constitutes the predominant dynamic element (Fig. 18.6).
3. In the retropectoralis space, there is complex motion of the pectoralis minor and the scapula, including the coracoid process and subscapularis muscle, relative to the chest wall (Fig. 18.7).
4. In the prescalene space, the anterior scalene muscle is relatively fixed, while motion of the clavicle constitutes the predominant dynamic element (Fig. 18.5).

Dynamic Changes

The shoulder joint has the greatest range of motion of any joint in the body, involving complex movement of the scapula, clavicle, and first

Anatomic Variants and Pathology

Pathologic abnormalities of the thoracic outlet may be categorized as static or dynamic. Static abnormalities create impingement on the brachial

Fig. 18.5 Normal scalene triangle, sagittal plane, with hyperabduction-external rotation: The first rib (*R*) angle relative to the horizontal plane decreases slightly on abduction, but the scalene triangle dimensions do not significantly change, and there is no effacement of fat surrounding the brachial plexus and subclavian artery (*A*) in the scalene triangle (*solid line*) (Courtesy of Scott Werden, MD)

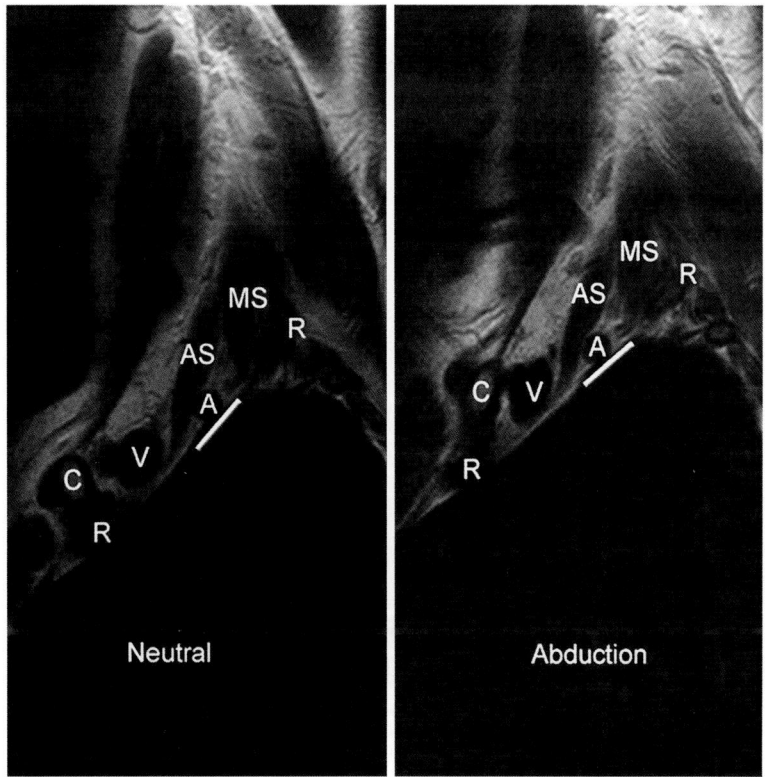

Fig. 18.6 Normal costo-clavicular interval, sagittal plane, with hyperabduction-external rotation: The first rib (*R*) angle relative to the horizontal plane decreases slightly on abduction, but the clavicle (*C*) moves considerably in a posterior direction, decreasing the dimensions of the costoclavicular interval. Note that despite this maneuver, there is no effacement of fat around the brachial plexus (*arrowheads*), subclavian artery (*A*), and subclavian vein (*V*), and there is no change in the shape or caliber of the arterial or venous flow voids (Courtesy of Scott Werden, MD)

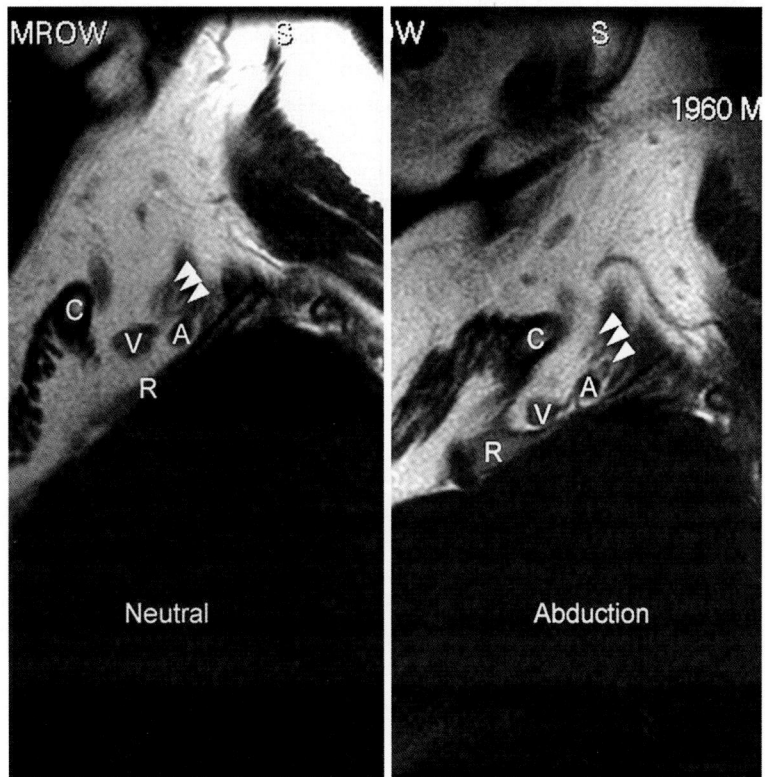

Fig. 18.7 Normal retropectoralis space, sagittal plane,
with hyperabduction-external
rotation: The pectoralis
minor muscle (*PM*) moves
posteriorly, but the scapula,
coracoid process (*CP*) and
subscapularis muscle (*SS*)
move as well, with minor
narrowing of this space. Note
there is no effacement of fat
around the lateral cord (*LC*),
posterior cord (*PC*), and
medial cord (*MC*) of the
brachial plexus, the axillary
artery (*A*) or the axillary vein
(*V*). Note that the neurovascular bundle moves cephalad,
closer to the coracoid
process, but without loss of
the fat plane inferior to the
coracoid process (Courtesy
of Scott Werden, MD)

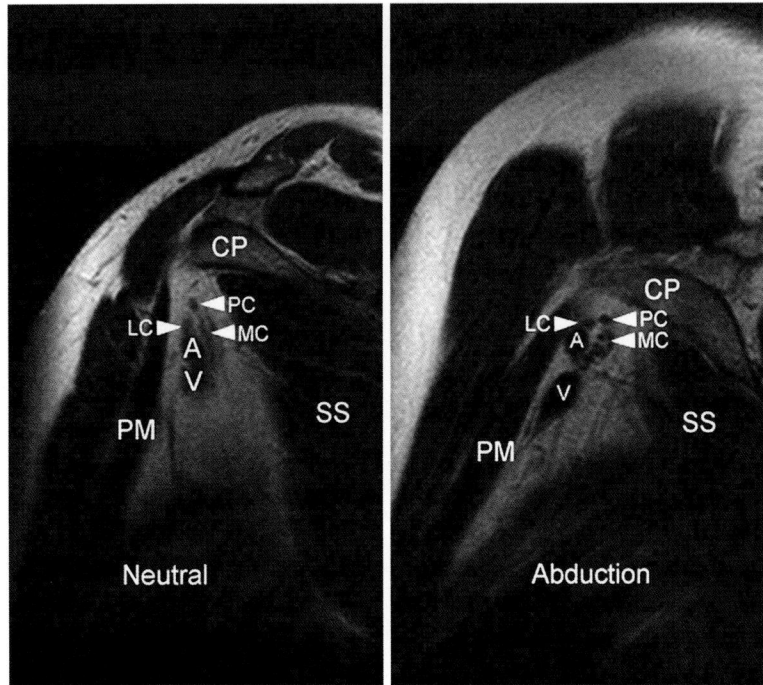

plexus independent of dynamic changes of the
upper extremity. Dynamic abnormalities create
impingement on the brachial plexus via movement of the upper extremity. Static and dynamic
abnormalities may combine to create impingement on the brachial plexus when neither abnormality is sufficient to cause impingement on its
own, or may compound impingement when each
abnormality is independently causing impingement. The following description of pathologic
entities should be considered a 'checklist' of possible causes of NTOS as one follows the course
of the brachial plexus from central to peripheral.

Static Pathology

Bony Abnormalities

Bony abnormalities were the first anatomic
abnormalities noted in patients with TOS, as
early as 1821 [34]. The first successful surgery
for thoracic outlet syndrome successfully
removed an elongated C7 transverse process in
1861 [35]. The association of TOS with bony
elements was reinforced with the development of
radiography in the late nineteenth century. Several

bony abnormalities have been shown to cause
TOS:

1. Cervical rib [35–37]
2. Anomalous first rib, including first rib exostosis or pseudarthrosis [38–41]
3. Elongated C7 transverse process (due to associated fibrous bands) [42–44]
4. First rib fracture or hypertrophic callous [39,
   41, 45, 46]
5. First rib neoplasm [47–49]
6. Anomalous clavicle [50–52]
7. Clavicular fracture [19, 41, 53, 54] or dislocation [55]
8. Clavicular neoplasm, hematoma, osteomyelitis or other pathology [41, 56]

Although neurogenic TOS is far more frequent than arterial TOS, patients with arterial
TOS are much more likely to have bony abnormalities than are patients with neurogenic TOS.
Bony abnormalities are particularly likely in the
presence of post-stenotic dilation or an arterial
aneurysm [41, 57].

Fibromuscular Abnormalities

Early TOS cases associated with bony abnormalities were of the arterial type. In the early 1900s,

Fig. 18.8 NTOS patient, scalene triangle, sagittal plane: The anterior scalene muscle (*AS*) and middle scalene muscle (*MS*) have markedly broadened insertions on the first rib (*R*), causing marked narrowing of the scalene triangle (*line*) and near-complete effacement of fat around the brachial plexus roots and subclavian artery (*A*). Compare to normal scalene triangle (Fig. 18.2) (Courtesy of Scott Werden, MD)

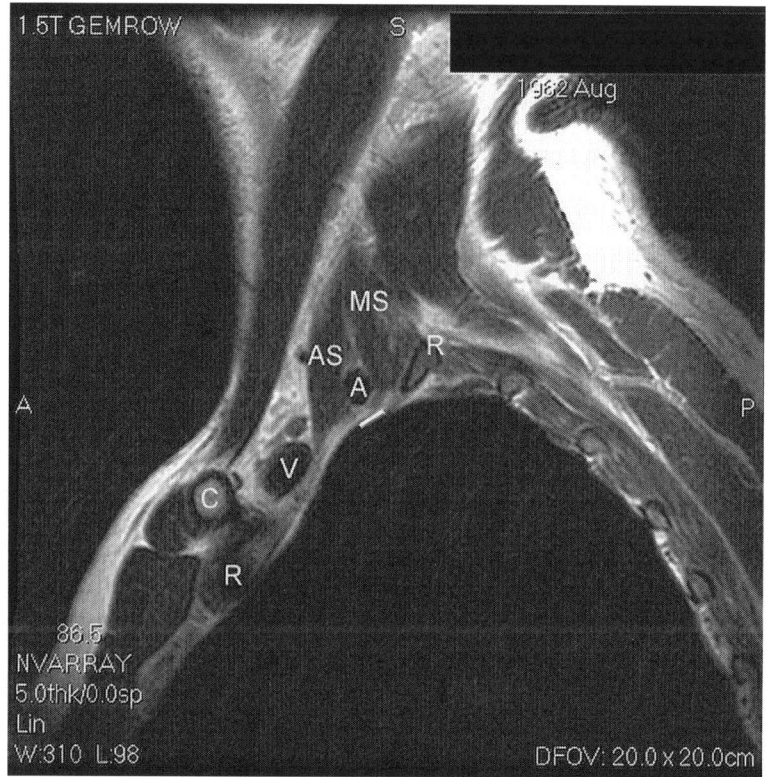

NTOS was described, first in the presence of bony abnormalities, and then in the absence of bony abnormalities [58–61]. Fibromuscular abnormalities of the thoracic outlet were described and proposed as the causative element for this syndrome. These fibromuscular abnormalities may be developmental or acquired.

Developmental anomalies of the scalene muscles, supernumerary muscles, and anomalous fibrous bands occur frequently in the thoracic outlet. Riolan first described the scalene minimus muscle in the early seventeenth century. Other anomalies have been described in detail since at least 1911 [14, 58]. The anterior scalene muscle was first implicated in NTOS in the 1920s, including the "Scalenus anticus syndrome" [37, 62, 63]. Roos further defined 13 types of fibromuscular abnormalities found at surgery [44, 64, 65]. The presence of an anatomic anomaly has been associated with better surgical outcome [66].

Acquired abnormalities include overuse and repetitive stress syndromes, trauma, and surgery. Neoplasms of the lung apex and supraclavicular fossa may occupy space or directly involve the brachial plexus.

A simplified approach to these complex anomalies is suggested, categorized by defined space:

1. Scalene triangle
   (a) Developmental anomalies
       (i) Abnormal scalene origins
       (ii) Abnormal scalene insertions (Figs. 18.8 and 18.9)
       (iii) Abnormal connections between anterior and middle scalene muscles
       (iv) Supernumerary muscles, including scalene minimus (Fig. 18.10) [14, 29–31, 36, 58, 67–71], accessory middle scalene muscle [72], anomalous trapezius muscle [73], and others [74–77]
       (v) Fibrous bands, including those arising from cervical ribs or C7 transverse processes and those inserting on the endothoracic fascia overlying the parietal pleura at the lung apex (Fig. 18.9) [44, 67, 68]

Fig. 18.9 NTOS patient, scalene triangle, sagittal plane: The anterior scalene muscle (*AS*) has a second, anomalous insertion (*arrowhead 1*) on the first rib (*R*), posterior to the subclavian artery (*A*). A small fibrous band (*arrowhead 2*) passes between the roots of the brachial plexus to insert on the first rib adjacent to this anomalous insertion. The scalene triangle is markedly narrowed. Compare to normal scalene triangle (Fig. 18.2) (Courtesy of Scott Werden, MD)

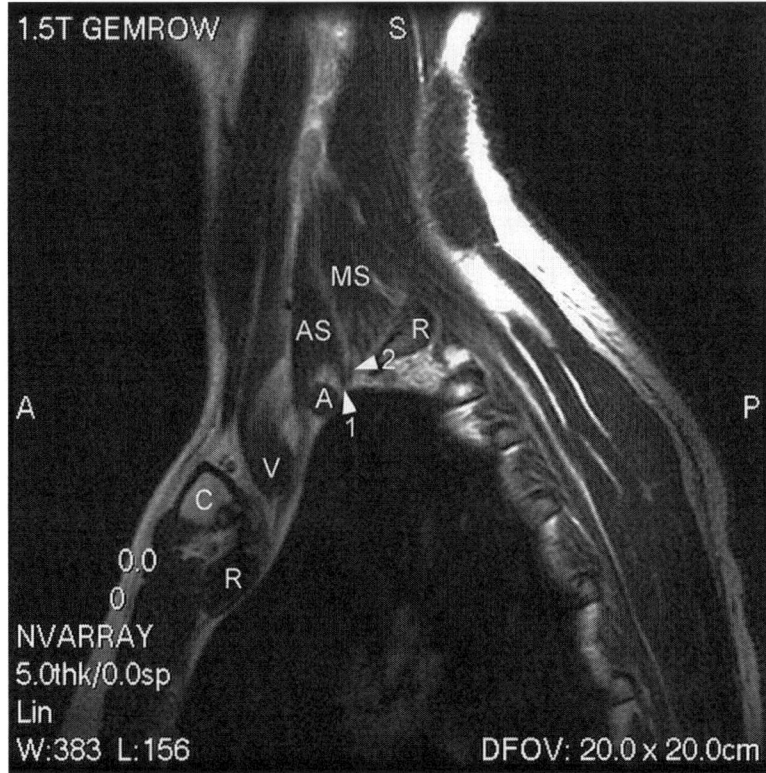

Fig. 18.10 NTOS patient, costoclavicular interval, sagittal plane: A scalene minimus muscle (*arrow*) is present, causing narrowing of the scalene triangle and effacement of fat around the C7 and C8 nerve roots (*arrowheads*). Anterior scalene muscle (*AS*), middle scalene muscle (*MS*), subclavian artery (*A*) and vein (*V*), and first rib (*R*) noted (Courtesy of Scott Werden, MD)

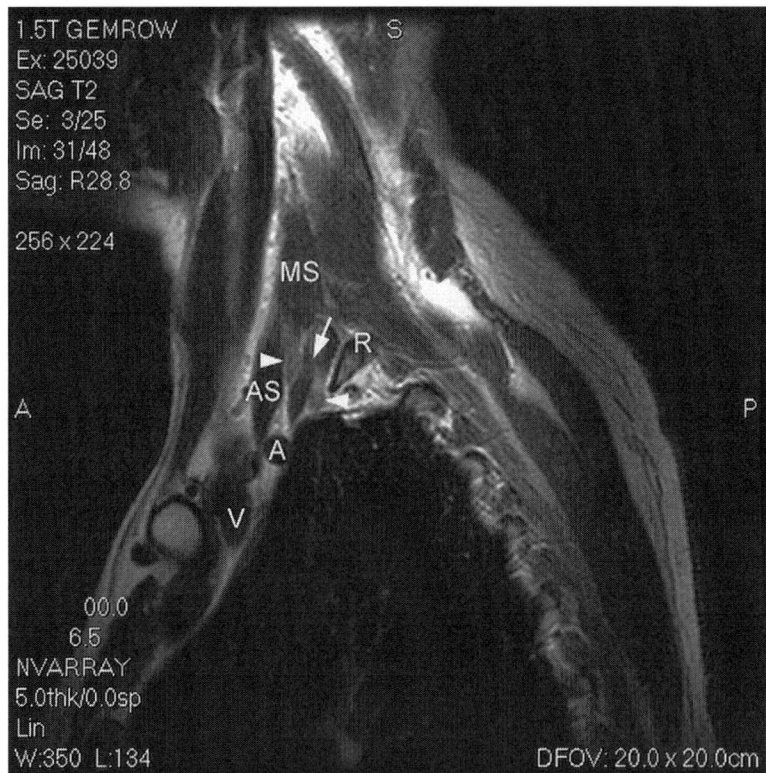

(b) Acquired abnormalities
   (i) Hypertrophy [44, 63, 78], including athletes [79–82]
   (ii) Post-traumatic changes [83, 84]
   (iii) Post-surgical changes
2. Costoclavicular interval
   (a) Developmental anomalies of the subclavius muscle (including the subclavius posticus [85, 86] or other subclavius anomalies [51]) or serratus anterior muscle
   (b) Acquired abnormalities, including hypertrophy of the subclavius muscle [81, 87, 88] or serratus anterior muscle [46]
3. Retropectoralis space
   (a) Developmental anomalies of the pectoralis minor, such as the pectoralis minimus [89]
   (b) Acquired abnormalities, including hypertrophy of the pectoralis minor, seen in weightlifters and overhead athletes [79–82]
4. Axilla
   (a) Developmental anomalies, including an anomaly of the latissimus dorsi, the axillary arch of Langer [90]
   (b) Acquired abnormalities, including muscular hypertrophy, aneurysm of the posterior humeral circumflex artery, and axillary artery dissection [78, 91–93]

Brachial Plexus Abnormalities

There are variations of the brachial plexus which may predispose the plexus to compression, even in the absence of fibromuscular or bony anomalies or dynamic compression [71, 94–96]:
1. Abnormal branching pattern of the brachial plexus
   • The pre-fixed brachial plexus receives an additional contribution from the C4 nerve root.
   • The post-fixed brachial plexus receives an additional contribution from the T2 nerve root.
2. Abnormal course of the brachial plexus
   • Components of the brachial plexus may pass anterior to the anterior scalene muscle or directly through the anterior scalene muscle.

Dynamic Pathology

CT and MRI studies have clarified the dynamic changes that occur in the anatomic tunnels of the thoracic outlet on motion of the ipsilateral upper extremity [11, 15, 25, 41, 45, 81, 86, 88, 97–103]. On hyperabduction-external rotation, imaging demonstrates:
1. No significant narrowing of the scalene triangle.
2. Significant narrowing of the costoclavicular interval in NTOS patients.
3. Narrowing of the retropectoralis space, but less in NTOS patients than in normal subjects.
4. Frequent significant narrowing of the prescalene space in both NTOS patients and normal subjects.

In the scalene triangle, the angle of inclination of the first rib decreases on hyperabduction-external rotation in both normal subjects and NTOS patients, although it decreases to a greater degree in NTOS patients (Fig. 18.5). However, there is no significant narrowing of the scalene triangle in either population.

The costoclavicular interval narrows significantly on hyperabduction-external rotation in both normal subjects (Fig. 18.6) and in NTOS patients (Fig. 18.11). This narrowing is significantly greater in NTOS patients. While there is no specific measurement threshold that defines NTOS, the close proximity of bone and brachial plexus or the effacement of fat planes surrounding the brachial plexus is considered diagnostic of nerve impingement (Fig. 18.11) [11, 88, 100].

In the retropectoralis space, the space between the pectoralis minor and the subscapularis narrows on hyperabduction-external rotation, and the neurovascular bundle shifts superiorly, towards the coracoid process (Fig. 18.7). A fat plane separates the neurovascular bundle from the inferior surface of the coracoid process and from the surrounding muscles. Brachial plexus impingement in NTOS patients has been hypothesized on the basis of two proposed mechanisms.

The first mechanism suggests that narrowing of the anteroposterior width of the retropectoralis space causes impingement. However, while narrowing occurs (Fig. 18.7), it is less severe in NTOS patients than in normal subjects [11, 88]. Additionally, the neurovascular bundle shifts to the wider cephalad portion of the retropectoralis space, where the coracoid process limits posterior motion of the pectoralis minor.

Fig. 18.11 NTOS patient, costoclavicular interval, sagittal plane, with hyperabduction-external rotation: Note marked thickening and loss of definition of the brachial plexus (*arrowheads*) as it passes through the costoclavicular interval with the arms in neutral position. On abduction, there is marked compression of the brachial plexus between the clavicle (*C*) and first rib (*R*), with complete effacement of perineural fat. Note also the decreased caliber of the subclavian artery (*A*) and subclavian vein (*V*), which were confirmed on *MR* angiography Courtesy of Scott Werden, MD

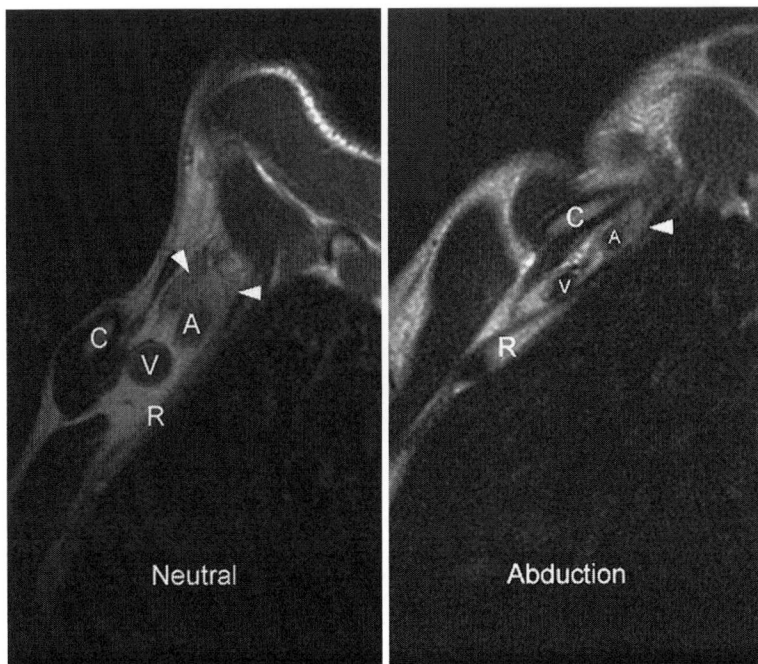

The second mechanism suggests that the brachial plexus becomes taut beneath the coracoid process. In 1922, Todd reported the results of an experiment he performed by sleeping with his own arm hyperabducted for 8 years, which resulted in trophic changes of his hand. In 1945, Wright studied 150 controls and five patients who reported neurovascular symptoms related to sleeping with their arm hyperabducted. Wright hypothesized that the neurovascular bundle came under tension as it traversed the coracoid process on hyperabduction. However, imaging fails to demonstrate such a mechanism [11, 25, 88, 100] (Fig. 18.7).

Narrowing of the prescalene space with compression of the subclavian vein on hyperabduction-external rotation is frequent in both normal subjects and TOS patients, but does not equate with venous TOS [20, 25, 88, 100].

Imaging Algorithm-MRI or CT

MRI or CT should be performed with the patient's arms in the neutral position, and then with the arms in hyperabduction-external rotation. The volume of imaging should extend from the cervical spine medially to the axilla laterally. Sagittal and axial MRI images are usually sufficient.

The primary goal of any imaging test intended to diagnose NTOS is to assess for impingement on the brachial plexus or its components. The first step is to evaluate the course of the brachial plexus, as outlined in the Imaging Anatomy section, looking for abnormalities of each of the anatomic tunnels in turn, and for impingement on the brachial plexus caused by those entities listed in the Pathology section. Evaluation of the brachial plexus should include any intrinsic lesion of the brachial plexus. The next step is to evaluate the hyperabduction-external rotation images, as described in the Dynamic Pathology section. Evaluation of the cervical spine to rule out central canal or neural foraminal stenosis, and of the lung apices and supraclavicular fossa soft tissues to rule out a soft tissue mass involving the brachial plexus should be performed.

Finally, MR angiography should be considered, as there is frequently an element of vascular compression in patients with brachial plexus compression. Vascular compression can be evaluated with nearly the same search pattern, including the prescalene space, after which the great vessels and brachial plexus converge to enter the upper extremity.

Imaging Modality Selection

Selection of the appropriate imaging modality in a patient with TOS depends on the type of TOS and the clinical question in a particular patient. Commonly used modalities include radiographs, CT, ultrasound, and MRI.

Radiographs

1. Advantages
   - Widely available
   - Inexpensive
   - Low ionizing radiation dose
   - Widely understood by physicians
2. Disadvantages
   - 2-dimensional only
   - Extremely limited soft tissue evaluation

CT Scan [39, 45, 48, 52, 97, 99, 101, 103–106]

1. Advantages
   - Excellent bony detail in three dimensions
   - CT angiograms provide excellent vascular detail
   - Fair soft tissue contrast
   - Cross-sectional imaging allows excellent evaluation of anatomic relationships
   - Faster examination than MRI
   - Widely available
2. Disadvantages
   - Poor demonstration of soft tissue abnormalities associated with TOS [19, 46]
   - Higher dose of ionizing radiation than other modalities
   - Angiograms require iodinated contrast material, with attendant nephrotoxicity and allergic contrast reaction risk
   - Artifacts caused by bones and by contrast in the accompanying arteries, especially on the side of injection

- Direct imaging is performed only in the axial plane

Ultrasound [99, 107, 108]

1. Advantages
   - No ionizing radiation
   - Allows real-time and dynamic evaluation of blood flow in arteries and veins
   - Allows assessment in any arm position
   - Allows assessment in any patient position-supine, sitting, decubitus or standing
   - Allows assessment in any anatomical plane
2. Disadvantages
   - Acoustic window is limited
     - Bone or lung creates sonographic 'blind spots'
       Cannot directly see the costoclavicular interval, although blood flow can be evaluated proximal and distal to the interval
   - Highly operator-dependent
     - Few sonographers understand the complex anatomy or expected dynamic changes
   - Limited soft tissue differentiation
     - High-frequency transducers required for evaluation of smaller structures may be limited in larger patients or patients with a short neck [117]

MRI [11, 19, 23, 24, 56, 81, 86, 88, 100, 109–114]

1. Advantages
   - Superior soft tissue contrast, characterization and differentiation
     - Allows differentiation of nerves [109, 110, 112, 115, 116], muscle, fat, lung, fluid
     - Can selectively emphasize or de-emphasize specific soft tissues, such as fat, fluid, nerves or blood vessels
   - No ionizing radiation
   - Direct imaging in any plane
2. Disadvantages
   - Lengthier examination than radiographs, CT, and ultrasound
     - The patient must keep their arms in a potentially painful position for a longer period of time

- Often more expensive than other examinations
- Not as widely available as other tests
  - More technically demanding examination for technologists and radiologists
- More complex and difficult to understand for non-radiologists

In the author's practice, MRI has become the imaging modality of choice in patients with NTOS. While bony abnormalities are easily detected on radiography or CT, they are more frequently associated with arterial TOS than with neurogenic TOS. Soft tissue abnormalities are more frequently associated with neurogenic TOS, are frequently invisible on radiography and CT, and are well-seen on MRI.

As a final note, imaging findings should always be interpreted in the setting of appropriate clinical findings, as is true with any imaging test. Developmental anomalies or acquired abnormalities are not always sufficient to cause TOS, but the combination of clinical diagnosis of TOS and demonstration of anatomic anomalies or pathologic changes is a powerful confirmatory tool in these patients.

References

1. Sanders RJ, Hammond SL, Rao NM. Thoracic outlet syndrome: a review. Neurologist. 2008;14(6):365–73.
2. Brantigan CO, Roos DB. Diagnosing thoracic outlet syndrome. Hand Clin. 2004;20(1):27–36.
3. Atasoy E. Thoracic outlet compression syndrome. Orthop Clin North Am. 1996;27(2):265–303.
4. Atasoy E. History of thoracic outlet syndrome. Hand Clin. 2004;20(1):15–6, v.
5. Fugate M, Rotellini-Coltvet L, Freischlag J. Current management of thoracic outlet syndrome. Curr Treat Options Cardiovasc Med. 2009;11(2):176–83.
6. Wilbourn AJ. The thoracic outlet syndrome is overdiagnosed. Arch Neurol. 1990;47(3):328–30.
7. Roos DB. The thoracic outlet syndrome is underrated. Arch Neurol. 1990;47(3):327–8.
8. Wilbourn AJ. Thoracic outlet syndrome is overdiagnosed. Muscle Nerve. 1999;22(1):130–6, discussion 136–7.
9. Roos DB. Thoracic outlet syndrome is underdiagnosed. Muscle Nerve. 1999;22(1):126–9, discussion 137–8.
10. Plewa MC, Delinger M. The false-positive rate of thoracic outlet syndrome shoulder maneuvers in healthy subjects. Acad Emerg Med. 1998;5(4):337–42 (Official journal of the Society for Academic Emergency).
11. Demirbag D, Unlu E, Ozdemir F, et al. The relationship between magnetic resonance imaging findings and postural maneuver and physical examination tests in patients with thoracic outlet syndrome: results of a double-blind, controlled study. Arch Phys Med Rehabil. 2007;88(7):844–51.
12. Rayan GM. Thoracic outlet syndrome. J Shoulder Elbow Surg. 1998;7(4):440–51.
13. Rayan G, Jensen C. Thoracic outlet syndrome: provocative examination maneuvers in a typical population. J Shoulder Elbow Surg. 1995;4:113–7.
14. Telford ED, Mottershead S. Pressure at the cervicobrachial junction. J Bone Joint Surg Br. 1948;30-B(2):249.
15. Remy-Jardin M, Doyen J, Remy J, Artaud D, Fribourg M, Duhamel A. Functional anatomy of the thoracic outlet: evaluation with spiral CT. Radiology. 1997;205(3):843–51.
16. Ranney D. Thoracic outlet: an anatomical redefinition that makes clinical sense. Clin Anat. 1996;9(1):50–2.
17. Atasoy E. Thoracic outlet syndrome: anatomy. Hand Clin. 2004;20(1):7–14, v.
18. Chiles C, Davis KW, Williams DW. Navigating the thoracic inlet. Radiographics. 1999;19(5):1161–76 (A review publication of the Radiological Society of North America, Inc.).
19. Rapoport S, Blair DN, McCarthy SM, Desser TS, Hammers LW, Sostman HD. Brachial plexus: correlation of MR imaging with CT and pathologic findings. Radiology. 1988;167(1):161–5.
20. Matsumura JS, Rilling WS, Pearce WH, Nemcek AA, Vogelzang RL, Yao JS. Helical computed tomography of the normal thoracic outlet. J Vasc Surg. 1997;26(5):776–83.
21. Perlas A, Chan VWS, Simons M. Brachial plexus examination and localization using ultrasound and electrical stimulation: a volunteer study. Anesthesiology. 2003;99(2):429–35.
22. Sheppard DG, Iyer RB, Fenstermacher MJ. Brachial plexus: demonstration at US. Radiology. 1998;208(2):402–6.
23. van Es HW, Bollen TL, van Heesewijk HPM. MRI of the brachial plexus: a pictorial review. Eur J Radiol. 2010;74(2):391–402.
24. Van Es HW. MRI of the brachial plexus. Eur Radiol. 2001;11(2):325–36.
25. Demondion X, Boutry N, Drizenko A, Paul C, Francke JP, Cotten A. Thoracic outlet: anatomic correlation with MR imaging. AJR Am J Roentgenol. 2000;175(2):417–22.
26. Sherrier RH, Sostman HD. Magnetic resonance imaging of the brachial plexus. J Thorac Imaging. 1993;8(1):27–33.
27. Blair DN, Rapoport S, Sostman HD, Blair OC. Normal brachial plexus: MR imaging. Radiology. 1987;165(3):763–7.
28. Kellman GM, Kneeland JB, Middleton WD, et al. MR imaging of the supraclavicular region: normal anatomy. AJR Am J Roentgenol. 1987;148(1):77–82.

29. Juvonen T, Satta J, Laitala P, Luukkonen K, Nissinen J. Anomalies at the thoracic outlet are frequent in the general population. Am J Surg. 1995;170(1):33–7.
30. Kirgis HD, Reed AF. Significant anatomic relations in the syndrome of the scalene muscles. Ann Surg. 1948;127(6):1182–201.
31. Gage M, Parnell H. Scalenusanticus syndrome. Am J Surg. 1947;73(2):252–68.
32. Leinberry CF, Wehbé MA. Brachial plexus anatomy. Hand Clin. 2004;20(1):1–5.
33. Bowen BC, Pattany PM, Saraf-Lavi E, Maravilla KR. The brachial plexus: normal anatomy, pathology, and MR imaging. Neuroimaging Clin N Am. 2004;14(1):59–85, vii–viii.
34. Cooper A, Travers B. On exostosis. 3rd ed. 1821. p. 167–224.
35. Coote H. Exostosis of the left transverse process of the seventh cervical vertebra, surrounded by blood vessels and nerves-successful removal. Lancet. 1861;1:360–1.
36. Todd TW. "Cervical Rib": factors controlling its presence and its size. Its bearing on the morphology and development of the shoulder. J Anat Physiol. 1912;46(Pt 3):244–88.
37. Adson AW, Coffey JR. Cervical rib: a method of anterior approach for relief of symptoms by division of the scalenus anticus. Ann Surg. 1927;85(6):839.
38. Dow DR. The anatomy of rudimentary first thoracic ribs with special reference to the arrangement of the brachial plexus. J Anat. 1925;59(Pt 2):166.
39. Sabapathy SR, Venkatramani H, Bhardwaj P. Pseudarthrosis of cervical rib: an unusual cause of thoracic outlet syndrome. J Hand Surg Am. 2010;35(12):2018–21.
40. Sanders RJ, Hammond SL. Management of cervical ribs and anomalous first ribs causing neurogenic thoracic outlet syndrome. J Vasc Surg. 2002;36(1):51–6.
41. Criado E, Berguer R, Greenfield L. The spectrum of arterial compression at the thoracic outlet. J Vasc Surg. 2010;52(2):406–11.
42. Gilliatt R, Le Quesne P, Logue V, Sumner AJ. Wasting of the hand associated with a cervical rib or band. Br Med J. 1970;33(5):615–24.
43. Roos DB. Experience with first rib resection for thoracic outlet syndrome. Ann Surg. 1971;173(3):429–42.
44. Roos D. Congenital anomalies associated with thoracic outlet syndrome: anatomy, symptoms, diagnosis, and treatment. Am J Surg. 1976;132(6):771–8.
45. Terabayashi N, Ohno T, Nishimoto Y, et al. Nonunion of a first rib fracture causing thoracic outlet syndrome in a basketball player: a case report. J Shoulder Elbow Surg. 2010;19(6):e20–3.
46. Panegyres P, Moore N, Gibson R. Thoracic outlet syndromes and magnetic resonance imaging. Brain. 1993;116(Pt 4):823–41.
47. O'Brien PJ, Ramasunder S, Cox MW. Venous thoracic outlet syndrome secondary to first rib osteochondroma in a pediatric patient. J Vasc Surg. 2011; 53(3):811–3.
48. Yeow KM, Hsieh HC. Thoracic outlet syndrome caused by first rib hemangioma. J Vasc Surg. 2001; 33(5):1118–21.
49. Haniuda M, Morimoto M, Nishimura H. A case of chondrosarcoma arising from the left first rib. Kyobu Geka. 1990;43(10):835–8 (The Japanese journal of thoracic surgery).
50. Nehme A, Tricoire J, Giordano G, Rouge D, Chiron P, Puget J. Coracoclavicular joints. Reflections upon incidence, pathophysiology and etiology of the different forms. Surg Radiol Anat. 2004;26(1):33–8.
51. Hama H, Matsusue Y, Ito H, Yamamuro T. Thoracic outlet syndrome associated with an anomalous coracoclavicular joint. A case report. J Bone Joint Surg Am. 1993;75(9):1368–9.
52. Khu KJ, Midha R. Clavicle pseudarthrosis: a rare cause of thoracic outlet syndrome. Can J Neurol Sci. 2010;37(6):863–5.
53. Bilbey JH, Lamond RG, Mattrey RF. MR imaging of disorders of the brachial plexus. J Magn Reson Imaging. 1994;4(1):13–8.
54. Kitsis CK, Marino AJ, Krikler SJ, Birch R. Late complications following clavicular fractures and their operative management. Injury. 2003;34(1):69–74.
55. Jain S, Monbaliu D, Thompson JF. Thoracic outlet syndrome caused by chronic retrosternal dislocation of the clavicle. Successful treatment by transaxillary resection of the first rib. J Bone Joint Surg Br. 2002; 84(1):116–8.
56. Kapickis M. Neurogenic thoracic outlet syndrome caused by subacute clavicle osteomyelitis. Acta Chir Latviensis. 2011;10(2):124–6.
57. Durham JR, Yao JS, Pearce WH, Nuber GM, McCarthy WJ. Arterial injuries in the thoracic outlet syndrome. J Vasc Surg. 1995;21(1):57–69, discussion 70.
58. Todd TW. The relations of the thoracic operculum considered in reference to the anatomy of cervical ribs of surgical importance. J Anat Physiol. 1911;45(Pt 3):293–304.
59. Stopford JSB, Telford ED. Compression of the lower trunk of the brachial plexus by a first dorsal rib. With a note on the surgical treatment. Br J Surg. 1919; 7(26):168–77.
60. Brickner W. Brachial plexus pressure by the normal first rib. Ann Surg. 1927;85(6):858–72.
61. Murphy T. Brachial neuritis caused by pressure of first rib. Aust Med J. 1910;15:582–5.
62. Ochsner A, Gage M. Scalenusanticus (Naffziger) syndrome. Am J Surg. 1935;28:669.
63. Swank RL, Simeone FA. The scalenus anticus syndrome: types, their characterization, diagnosis and treatment. Arch Neurol Psychiatry. 1944;51(5):432.
64. Roos D. New concepts of thoracic outlet syndrome that explain etiology, symptoms, diagnosis, and treatment. Vasc Endovascular Surg. 1979;13(5):313–21.
65. Roos DB. Pathophysiology of congenital anomalies in thoracic outlet syndrome. Acta Chir Belg. 1980;79(5):353–61.

66. Lindgren SH, Ribbe EB, Norgren LE. Two year follow-up of patients operated on for thoracic outlet syndrome. Effects on sick-leave incidence. Eur J Vasc Surg. 1989;3(5):411–5.

67. Law AA. Adventitious ligaments simulating cervical ribs. Ann Surg. 1920;72(4):497.

68. Gaughran GRL. Suprapleural membrane and suprapleural bands. Anat Rec. 1964;148(4):553–9.

69. Poitevin L. Proximal compressions of the upper limb neurovascular bundle. An anatomic research study. Hand Clin. 1988;4(4):575–84.

70. Makhoul RG, Machleder HI. Developmental anomalies at the thoracic outlet: an analysis of 200 consecutive cases. J Vasc Surg. 1992;16(4):534–42, discussion 542–5.

71. Harry W, Bennett J, Guha S. Scalene muscles and the brachial plexus: anatomical variations and their clinical significance. Clin Anat. 1997;10(4):250–2.

72. Paraskevas G, Ioannidis O, Papaziogas B, Natsis K, Spanidou S, Kitsoulis P. An accessory middle scalene muscle causing thoracic outlet syndrome. Folia Morphol (Warsz). 2007;66(3):194–7.

73. Hug U, Burg D, Meyer V. Cervical outlet syndrome due to an accessory part of the trapezius muscle in the posterior triangle of the neck. J Hand Surg Eur Vol. 2000;25(3):311–3.

74. O'Sullivan ST, Kay SP. An unusual variant of the levator claviculae muscle encountered in exploration of the brachial plexus. J Hand Surg Br. 1998;23(1):134–5.

75. Darwish H, Ibrahim A. Three muscles in the upper costovertebral region: description and clinical anatomy. Clin Anat. 2009;22(3):352–7. doi:10.1002/ca.20773.

76. Rajanigandha V, Ranade A, Pai M, Rai R, Prabhu L, Nayak S. The scalenus accessorius muscle. Int J Morph. 2008;26(2):385–8.

77. Goubran E, Carlos J, Ayad S. A bifurcated anterior scalene muscle: a case report. Clin Chiropr. 2010;13(2):153–5.

78. Cooke R. Thoracic outlet syndrome-aspects of diagnosis in the differential diagnosis of hand-arm vibration syndrome. Occup Med. 2003;53(5):331–6.

79. Lee J, Laker S, Fredericson M. Thoracic outlet syndrome. PM R. 2010;2(1):64–70.

80. Safran MR. Nerve injury about the shoulder in athletes, part 2: long thoracic nerve, spinal accessory nerve, burners/stingers, thoracic outlet syndrome. Am J Sports Med. 2004;32(4):1063–76.

81. Esposito MD, Arrington JA, Blackshear MN, Murtagh FR, Silbiger ML. Thoracic outlet syndrome in a throwing athlete diagnosed with MRI and MRA. J Magn Reson Imaging. 1997;7(3):598–9.

82. Rayan G. Lower trunk brachial plexus compression neuropathy due to cervical rib in young athletes. Am J Sports Med. 1988;16(1):77–9.

83. Machleder HI, Moll F, Verity MA. The anterior scalene muscle in thoracic outlet compression syndrome. Histochemical and morphometric studies. Arch Surg. 1986;121(10):1141–4.

84. Sanders RJ, Ratzin Jackson CG, Banchero N, Pearce WH. Scalene muscle abnormalities in traumatic thoracic outlet syndrome. Am J Surg. 1990;159(2): 231–6.

85. Ozçakar L, Güney MS, Ozda F, et al. A sledgehammer on the brachial plexus: thoracic outlet syndrome, subclavius posticus muscle, and traction in aggregate. Arch Phys Med Rehabil. 2010;91(4):656–8.

86. Akita K, Ibukuro K, Yamaguchi K, Heima S, Sato T. The subclavius posticus muscle: a factor in arterial, venous or brachial plexus compression. Surg Radiol Anat. 2000;22(2):111–5.

87. Thompson JF, Winterborn RJ, Bays S, White H, Kinsella DC, Watkinson AF. Venous thoracic outlet compression and the paget-schroetter syndrome: a review and recommendations for management. Cardiovasc Intervent Radiol. 2011;34(5):903–10.

88. Demondion X, Bacqueville E, Paul C, Duquesnoy B, Hachulla E, Cotten A. Thoracic outlet: assessment with MR imaging in asymptomatic and symptomatic populations. Radiology. 2003;227(2):461–8.

89. Turgut H, Anil A, Peker T, Barut C. Insertion abnormality of bilateral pectoralis minimus. Surg Radiol Anat. 2000;22(1):55–7.

90. Clarys J, Barbaix E, Vanrompaey H, Caboor D, Vanroy P. The muscular arch of the axilla revisited: its possible role in the thoracic outlet and shoulder instability syndromes. Man Ther. 1996;1(3):133–9.

91. Duwayri YM, Emery VB, Driskill MR, et al. Positional compression of the axillary artery causing upper extremity thrombosis and embolism in the elite overhead throwing athlete. J Vasc Surg. 2011;53(5):1329–40.

92. Ikezawa T, Iwatsuka Y, Asano M, Kimura A, Sasamoto A, Ono Y. Upper extremity ischemia in athletes: embolism from the injured posterior circumflex humeral artery. Int J Angiol. 2000;9(3):138–40.

93. Gelabert HA, Machleder HI. Diagnosis and management of arterial compression at the thoracic outlet. Ann Vasc Surg. 1997;11(4):359–66.

94. Uysal II, Seker M, Karabulut AK, Büyükmumcu M, Ziylan T. Brachial plexus variations in human fetuses. Neurosurgery. 2003;53(3):676–84, discussion 684.

95. Natsis K, Totlis T, Tsikaras P, Anastasopoulos N, Skandalakis P, Koebke J. Variations of the course of the upper trunk of the brachial plexus and their clinical significance for the thoracic outlet syndrome: a study on 93 cadavers. Am Surg. 2006;72(2):188–92.

96. Pellerin M, Kimball Z, Tubbs RS, et al. The prefixed and postfixed brachial plexus: a review with surgical implications. Surg Radiol Anat. 2010;32(3):251–60.

97. Lindgren K, Manninen H, Rytkönen H. Case of the month. Thoracic outlet syndrome-a functional disturbance of the thoracic upper aperture? Muscle Nerve. 1995. doi:10.1002/mus.880180508.

98. Remy-Jardin M, Remy J, Masson P, et al. CT angiography of thoracic outlet syndrome: evaluation of imaging protocols for the detection of arterial stenosis. J Comput Assist Tomogr. 2000;24(3):349.

99. Gillard J, Pérez-Cousin M, Hachulla E, et al. Diagnosing thoracic outlet syndrome: contribution of provocative tests, ultrasonography, electrophysiology, and helical computed tomography in 48 patients. Joint Bone Spine. 2001;68(5):416–24.

100. Demondion X, Herbinet P, van Sint Jan S, Boutry N, Chantelot C, Cotten A. Imaging assessment of thoracic outlet syndrome. Radiographics. 2006;26(6):1735–50 (A review publication of the Radiological Society of North America, Inc.).

101. Nord KM, Kapoor P, Fisher J, et al. False positive rate of thoracic outlet syndrome diagnostic maneuvers. Electromyogr Clin Neurophysiol. 2008;48(2):67–74.

102. Ozçakar L, Dönmez G, Yörübulut M, et al. Paget-schroetter syndrome forerunning the diagnosis of thoracic outlet syndrome and thrombophilia. Clin Appl Thromb Hemost. 2010;16(3):351–5.

103. Laban MM, Zierenberg AT, Yadavalli S, Zaidan S. Clavicle-induced narrowing of the thoracic outlet during shoulder abduction as imaged by computed tomographic angiography and enhanced by three-dimensional reformation. Am J Phys Med Rehabil. 2011;90(7):572–8.

104. Remy-Jardin M, Remy J, Masson P, et al. Helical CT angiography of thoracic outlet syndrome: functional anatomy. AJR Am J Roentgenol. 2000;174(6):1667–74.

105. Brantigan CO, Johnston RJ, Roos DB. Appendix: use of multidetector CT and three-dimensional reconstructions in thoracic outlet syndrome: a preliminary report. Hand Clin. 2004;20(1):123–6, viii.

106. Bilbey JH, Müller NL, Connell DG, Luoma AA, Nelems B. Thoracic outlet syndrome: evaluation with CT. Radiology. 1989;171(2):381–4.

107. Longley DG, Yedlicka JW, Molina EJ, Schwabacher S, Hunter DW, Letourneau JG. Thoracic outlet syndrome: evaluation of the subclavian vessels by color duplex sonography. AJR Am J Roentgenol. 1992;158(3):623–30.

108. Odderson IR, Chun ES, Kolokythas O, Zierler RE. Use of sonography in thoracic outlet syndrome due to a dystonic pectoralis minor. J Ultrasound Med. 2009;28(9):1235–8 (Official journal of the American Institute of Ultrasound in Medicine).

109. Vargas MI, Viallon M, Nguyen D, Beaulieu JY, Delavelle J, Becker M. New approaches in imaging of the brachial plexus. Eur J Radiol. 2010;74(2):403–10.

110. Chin C. Magnetic resonance neurography. In: Nerve and vascular injuries in sports medicine. New York: Springer; 2009. p. 27–39.

111. Filler A. MR Neurography and diffusion tensor imaging: origins, history and clinical impact of the first 50,000 cases with an assessment of efficacy and utility in a prospective 5,000 patient study group. Neurosurgery 2009;65(Suppl 4):A29.

112. Filler A, Maravilla K, Tsuruda J. MR neurography and muscle MR imaging for image diagnosis of disorders affecting the peripheral nerves and musculature. Neurol Clin. 2004;22(3):643–82.

113. van Es H. MR imaging of the brachial plexus. Utrecht: University Hospital; 1997.

114. Es HW, Witkamp TD, Feldberg MAM. MRI of the brachial plexus and its region: anatomy and pathology. Eur Radiol. 1995;5(2):145–51.

115. Filler A. MR neurography and brachial plexus neurolysis in the management of thoracic outlet syndromes. In: Yao J, Pearce W, editors. Advances in vascular surgery. 2002. p. 499–523.

116. Maravilla K, Bowen B. Imaging of the peripheral nervous system: evaluation of peripheral neuropathy and plexopathy. AJNR Am J Neuroradiol. 1998;19(6):1011–23.

117. Demondion X, Herbinet P, Boutry N, Fontaine C, Francke J-P, Cotten A. Sonographic mapping of the normal brachial plexus. American Journal of Neuroradiology 2003;24(7):1303–9.

Electrophysiological Assessment and Nerve Function in NTOS

19

Bennett I. Machanic

Abstract

Electro-diagnosis of NTOS has been challenging for several years, and conventional needle electrode and nerve conduction velocity techniques have proven disappointing. Currently, newer techniques using cervical root stimulation and measurements of medial antebrachial cutaneous nerve function appear to provide far improved clinical correlations for presence of NTOS, and should be included in any electro-diagnostic evaluation. Traditional approaches such as somatosensory evoked potentials, stimulation at Erb's point, and F-wave determinations have been discredited, and provide little substantive information.

Historical Perspective

Electrical recording of internal bodily physiological functions has long been employed in clinical medicine. The electrocardiogram records cardiac activity, the electroencephalogram records cerebral activity, and electromyography evaluates both muscle and nerve. For many decades, there has been hope that electro-diagnostic techniques could be applied reliably in the confirmation of neurogenic thoracic outlet syndrome (NTOS), similar to substantiating carpal tunnel syndrome or cervical radiculopathy. Unfortunately, due to disappointing lack of correlation when traditional electro-diagnostic approaches were employed,

B.I. Machanic, MD, FAAN
Department of Internal Medicine and Neurology,
Rose Medical Center, University of Colorado,
School of Medicine, 4545 East 9th Avenue,
Suite # 240, Denver, CO 80220, USA
e-mail: bmach5@aol.com

skepticism regarding the value of electromyography emerged. In 1999, Roos commented about the absence of "more sensitive techniques" to confirm NTOS [1]. However, in the past few years, technical advances have clarified physical examination findings, localized pathology, and even correlated with surgical outcomes. These procedures use both direct and indirect electrical measurements of the brachial plexus, and can confirm anatomical pathology over the lower brachial plexus.

Classically, a number of electrophysiological findings were thought to be useful in confirming brachial plexus pathology. Gilliatt studied patients with cervical ribs or bands and described a reduced ulnar sensory nerve action potential (SNAP) consistent with a lesion at or distal to the dorsal root ganglion of C-8. They also noted reduced thenar M-wave voltage indicating pathology localized in the brachial plexus [2, 3]. In 1979 Wulff and Gilliatt noted some afflicted patients demonstrating a prolonged latency of hypothenar F-wave response to ulnar nerve stimulation in the affected hand [4]. During the 1980s, multiple reports of abnormal ulnar nerve somatosensory evoked potentials (SSEP) in patients with thoracic outlet syndrome appeared in the literature [5, 6]. However, in 1988 Aminoff reported on 23 patients with suspected brachial plexopathies [7]. Five of the patients were labeled as having NTOS, and diagnosis was confirmed by diminution of ulnar sensory nerve action potentials, abnormal thenar muscle motor responses, and some needle electrode abnormalities in ulnar innervated muscles. However, ulnar F-wave responses and SSEP measurements failed to confirm the above findings. Ten patients with non-NTOS were also studied, and had normal electro-diagnostic studies. Of interest, the investigators were aware of "nerve root stimulation in evaluating conduction across the lower trunk and medial cord of the brachial plexus" but had no experience utilizing this technique. This paper did re-emphasize the prior failure of supraclavicular stimulation at Erb's point to confirm pathology in the brachial plexus, especially in regards to NTOS [8, 9].

Traditional Electrophysiologic Nerve Testing

During the 1980's, it was felt that the most useful and well established electro-diagnostic criteria to evaluate NTOS utilized needle electrode electromyography (EMG) and conventional nerve conduction studies [6]. Diagnosis of "true thoracic outlet syndrome" was based on needle electrode findings of chronic neurogenic changes in small hand muscles, and diminished amplitude of ulnar SNAP's, in the presence of otherwise normal nerve conduction velocities [10]. The value of ulnar nerve SSEP determinations was discredited by a Mayo Clinic study in 1988 [11]. Of the 20 patients clinically diagnosed with TOS, nerve conduction studies and needle electrode examinations were abnormal in 30 %, yet only 15 % of these patients possessed abnormal SSEPs. It was concluded that ulnar SSEP's would only be

abnormal if the EMG data was also abnormal and therefore was "probably not worthwhile."

Due to the fact that multiple patients with TOS failed to show EMG abnormalities, with traditional techniques, a number of papers described an entity called "disputed thoracic outlet syndrome" [12]. Concerns of the risks involved in surgery for TOS emphasized that there were "no reliable confirming or diagnostic tools" available pre-operatively [13]. Some reports also suggested a diagnostic confusion between NTOS and carpal tunnel syndrome [14], and comments stating that there were "no generally accepted electro diagnostic abnormalities" appeared in the literature in 1999 [1].

Cervical Root Stimulation (CRS)

As has been previously witnessed in the history of medical progress, little attention was initially paid to clarifying approaches to electro-diagnosis of TOSI. In 1975 a new technique was introduced by MacLean and Taylor [15]. They performed direct measurements of the brachial plexus by placing a needle electrode subcutaneously just laterally, next to the C-7 vertebral body, and were able to establish reliable measurements of conduction velocity across the lower brachial plexus. Subsequent studies of cadavers provided a profile of expected normal values and a refinement of early techniques [16]. The technique of CRS was described in 1983, and normal nerve conduction velocity values across the lower brachial plexus were documented [17, 18]. This approach seemed also of some potential benefit in evaluation of cervical radiculopathy [19]. Electrical stimulation at the root level provided an approach to directly measure through the vertebral foramen and across the brachial plexus. This contrasted with the failures of Erb's point stimulation techniques that were too distal and imprecise to document focal plexus pathology such as medial cord compression, and have now been discredited as having little value in diagnosis of NTOS [9]. Application of electrical currents through implanted needle electrodes instead of surface electrodes raised fears of damage to nerve and muscle. A safety study demonstrated that the maximal temperature elevation at the needle tip was 2.5 °C, and 2,000 consecutive patients experienced no adverse events [20].

Medial Antebrachial Cutaneous Nerve (MACN) Testing

Another valuable approach was described in 1993, when Nishida tested the MACN in "true thoracic outlet" syndrome, and recommended this technique as an adjunct in the early diagnosis of NTOS [21]. Asymmetrical low voltage MACN potential testing abnormalities seemed more frequent than low voltage ulnar SNAP's, in the symptomatic arm. Subsequently, Kothari described electro-diagnostic results of MACN studies in eight patients who possessed clinical symptoms and signs of NTOS [22]. The MACN voltage results were abnormal in all eight, and correlated with abnormal ulnar SNAP's in seven patients. It was suggested that the MACN sensory study be performed when other standard electrophysiological tests proved inconclusive. In 2004, Seror reported usage of MACN conduction studies in 16 patients with mild lower brachial plexus lesions. This further established the value of this approach in patients who otherwise possessed normal electro-diagnostic studies [23]. Only 4 out of 16 patients demonstrated any needle electrode abnormalities in C8-T1 innervated muscles, and none demonstrated abnormal median compound motor action potentials (CMAP) or low ulnar SNAP's. Accordingly, this study comments "MACN testing may be the only abnormal result of an electro-diagnostic examination … to characterize these mild lower brachial plexus lesions".

Anatomically, the MACN is the lowest branch of the brachial plexus, with sensory fibers traveling through the lower trunk and medial cord of the brachial plexus, and, specifically derived from the C8-T1 roots. Functionally, it provides sensation over a portion of the medial forearm. The MACN carries predominately T1 fibers, and may correlate with NTOS in a more sensitive fashion due to the presence of more stretching and angulations of the T1 fibers as compared to the C8 fibers [24]. An older observation amongst electromyographers, who studied NTOS, was the finding of occasional low voltage median CMAP's associated with normal ulnar CMAP's, which has been considered to represent T1 pathology, also [22].

From the data involving both direct brachial plexus measurements (CRS) and the studies detailing work with MACN evaluations, it appears that electro-diagnostic testing can be used quite reliably to document the presence of NTOS. Incorporating both these newer techniques with classical approaches, 41 patients diagnosed with NTOS were studied pre-operatively, and in a few cases, post-operatively [25]. All of these patients possessed both chronic and advanced clinical symptoms and signs. In 40 of these individuals, electro-diagnostic abnormalities were present. C8 nerve root stimulation showed slowing of conduction velocity over the lower brachial plexus in 54 % of tested individuals. MACN amplitudes were measured bilaterally with 61 % of patients showing a 50 % amplitude reduction, and 73 % with prolongation of SNAP latency on the involved side. Additional electro-diagnostic pathology in ten patients studied post-operatively demonstrated needle electrode abnormalities in C8-T1 muscles, decreased ulnar SNAP voltages, and even presence of carpal tunnel syndrome and cubital tunnel syndrome (unpublished data). Patients who experienced a successful surgical outcome, showed improved electrical results postoperatively. C8 nerve root stimulation showed improved conduction velocity in four tested patients, each with positive surgical outcomes. In seven patients with excellent outcomes, the MACN amplitude returned to normal, but in the two patients without surgical response, the amplitudes did not substantially alter.

Summary

It is now abundantly clear that electro-diagnostic testing for NTOS is of substantial value in not only confirming the diagnosis, but also of benefit in confirming or disconfirming surgical

Table 19.1 Electro-diagnostic technical approaches

Cervical root stimulation: Insert the needle perpendicular to the skin 1 cm slightly lateral and caudal to the C7 spinous process. The recording site should be over the hypothenar eminence, abductor digiti quinti. The evoked response form should be identical to that obtained when stimulating at the wrist or proximal to the elbow, and distance measurements can be taken from the neck to just below the axilla. Do not use Erb's point as a distance marker! Proximal conduction velocity in the literature across the plexus employing C8 stimulation techniques range from 63 to 74 m/s [18]. Steel calipers are more accurate than tape measures (Conservative values were used in the Machanic and Sanders study, 56 m/s or below to indicate pathology)

MACN testing: Place the recording disc electrodes 12 cm distal to the antecubital fossa, over the dermatomal distribution of the MACN. Stimulate over the medial forearm about 1–2 cm proximal to the antecubital fossa. Carefully increase stimulation voltage, as too high a voltage will cause a CMAP to obscure the SNAP response in some cases. Compare both sides. The most acceptable abnormality is a voltage asymmetry of 50 % or more. Latency prolongation is less reliable, but if asymmetrical, may be helpful. Best here to gain experience by testing normals and establishing lab values for both latency and voltage (In the Machanic and Sanders study, a latency beyond 2.4 ms and a voltage below 10 μV was felt to be abnormal, but the literature values do vary, and local standardization is recommended)

outcomes. The medical literature does support the usage of a variety of approaches that can provide clinical correlations. The following techniques have proven of value:

1. Needle electrode examination of cervical paraspinal and upper extremity muscles can evaluate and correlate cervical radiculopathy, brachial plexopathy, carpal tunnel syndrome, cubital tunnel syndrome, and myopathy. Specific to NTOS, neurogenic changes in C8-T1 innervated small muscles of the hand can be identified.

2. Conventional nerve conduction velocity studies can confirm presence of carpal tunnel syndrome, ulnar neuropathy, radial neuropathy, etc. Specific to NTOS, low amplitude ulnar SNAP, low amplitude median CMAP, and very rarely, low amplitude ulnar CMAP may be identified.

3. CRS studies are of proven benefit, but are technically challenging and not as consistently useful as MACN studies. It is important to note that abnormalities indicate pathophysiology, but anatomically do not rule out an alternative process such as metastasis, diabetes, vasculitis, Parsonage-Turner Syndrome, etc.

4. MACN studies are perhaps now the gold standard, and should always be performed on patients with suspected NTOS. However, they may be nonspecific, and like CRS studies can be abnormal in patients with brachial plexopathy of other etiologies.

The literature does suggest highest correlation and yields, if all of the above approaches are included in the electro-diagnostic evaluation. NOT RECOMMENDED due to limited value or redundancy in evaluation of NTOS: Erb's point stimulation and measurements, SSEP's of median and ulnar nerves, and F wave studies (See Table 19.1 for technical aspects for electro-diagnostic testing).

References

1. Roos DB. Thoracic outlet syndrome is under-diagnosed. Muscle Nerve. 1999;22:126–9.
2. Gilliatt RW, LeQuesne PM, Logue V, Sumner AJ. Wasting of the hand associated with a cervical rib or band. J Neurol Neurosurg Psychiatry. 1970;33:615–24.
3. Gilliatt RW, Williston RG, Dietz V, Williams IR. Peripheral nerve conduction in patients with a cervical rib or band. Ann Neurol. 1978;4:124–9.
4. Wulff CH, Gilliatt RW. F waves in patients with hand wasting caused by a cervical rib or band. Muscle Nerve. 1979;2:452–7.
5. Yiannikas C, Walsh JC. Somatosensory evoked potentials in the diagnosis of thoracic outlet syndrome. J Neurol Neurosurg Psychiatry. 1983;46:234–40.
6. Veilleux M, Stevens JC, Campbell JK. Value of somatosensory evoked potentials in the diagnosis of thoracic outlet syndrome. Muscle Nerve. 1986;9:655.
7. Aminoff MJ, Olney RK, Parry GJ, Raskin NJ. Relative utility of different electrophysiologic techniques in the evaluation of brachial plexopathies. Neurology. 1988;38:546–50.
8. Cherington M. Ulnar conduction velocity in thoracic outlet syndrome. N Engl J Med. 1976;294:1185.

9. Wilbourn AJ, Lederman RJ. Evidence for conduction delay in thoracic outlet syndrome is challenged. N Engl J Med. 1984;310:1052–3.

10. Smith T, Toyaberg W. Diagnosis of thoracic outlet syndrome. Arch Neurol. 1987;44:1161–3.

11. Veilleux M, Stevens JC, Campbell JK. Somatosensory evoked potentials: lack of value for diagnosis of thoracic outlet syndrome. Muscle Nerve. 1988;11:571–5.

12. Wilbourn AJ. Thoracic outlet syndrome: a plea for conservatism. Neurosurg Clin N Am. 1991;2:235–45.

13. Cherington M, Happer I, Machanic B, Parry L. Surgery for thoracic outlet syndrome may be hazardous to your health. Muscle Nerve. 1986;9:632–4.

14. Nord K, et al. Evaluation of thoracic outlet syndrome diagnostic maneuvers in carpal tunnel syndrome patients. Rev Neurol Dis. 2005;2:199–200.

15. MacLean IC, Taylor RS. Nerve root stimulation to evaluate brachial plexus conduction. Abstracts of communications of the fifth international congress of electromyography. Rochester, Mn. 1975. p. 47.

16. Livingstone EF, DeLisa JA, Halar EM. Electrodiagnostic values through the thoracic outlet using C8 root needle studies, F-waves, and cervical somatosensory evoked potentials. Arch Phys Med Rehabil. 1984;65:726–30.

17. Goodgold J, Eberstein A. Electrodiagnosis of neuromuscular diseases. Baltimore: Williams & Wilkins; 1983. p. 217.

18. Kimura J. Electrodiagnosis in diseases of nerve and muscle. Philadelphia: FA Davis; 1983. p. 119–22.

19. Berger AR, Busis NA, Logigian EL, Wierzbicka M, Shahani BJ. Cervical root stimulation in the diagnosis of radiculopathy. Neurology. 1987;37:329–32.

20. Pease WS, Fatehi MT, Johnson EW. Monopolar needle stimulation: safety considerations. Arch Phys Med Rehabil. 1989;70:412–4.

21. Nishida T, Price SJ, Minieta MM. Medial antecubital cutaneous nerve conduction in true thoracic outlet syndrome. Electromyogr Clin Neurophysiol. 1993;33:285–8.

22. Kothari MJ, MacIntosh K, Heistand M, Logigian EL. Medial antebrachial cutaneous sensory studies in the evaluation of neurogenic thoracic outlet syndrome. Muscle Nerve. 1998;21:647–9.

23. Seror P. Medial antebrachial cutaneous nerve conduction study, a new tool to demonstrate mild lower brachial plexus lesions. A report of 16 cases. Clin Neurophysiol. 2004;115:2316–22.

24. Levin KH, Wilbourn AJ, Maggiano HJ. Cervical rib and median sternotomy related brachial plexopathies. Neurology. 1998;63:1407–13.

25. Machanic BI, Sanders RJ. Medial antebrachial cutaneous nerve measurements to diagnose neurogenic thoracic outlet syndrome. Ann Vasc Surg. 2008;22:248–54.

Scalene Test Blocks and Interventional Techniques in Patients with TOS

20

Sheldon E. Jordan

Abstract

For targeted therapy such as TOS surgery to be effective, it must be determined that a particular patient has a disability actually caused by TOS and that this component overshadows any coexisting causes of disability. When the TOS component of a cervicobrachial syndrome is temporarily reversed with selective blockade it is expected that the longer term benefits of a targeted approach may be predicted. The present chapter will discuss the evolution and implementation of scalene test blocks in performing the role of predicting outcomes to TOS targeted therapy. For those patients who are not TOS surgical candidates other pain interventional techniques are discussed.

Introduction

For targeted therapy such as TOS surgery to be effective, it must be determined that a particular patient has a disability actually caused by TOS and that this component overshadows any coexisting causes of disability. When the TOS component of a cervicobrachial syndrome is temporarily reversed with selective blockade it is expected that the longer term benefits of a targeted approach may be predicted. The present chapter will discuss the evolution and implementation of scalene test blocks in performing the role of predicting outcomes to TOS targeted therapy.

S.E. Jordan, MD, FAAN
Department of Neurology,
Neurological Associates of West Los Angeles,
2811 Wilshire Blvd. Suite 790,
Santa Monica, CA 90403, USA
e-mail: shellyj@aol.com

For those patients who are not TOS surgical candidates other pain interventional techniques are discussed.

A scalene test block is designed to provide diagnostic information that would help a clinician decide on a therapy that targets NTOS specifically. As discussed in Chap. 8, many patients with features of NTOS may have coexisting conditions that overshadow NTOS in causing disability. A scalene test block is designed for the purposes of temporarily reversing the TOS component for a few hours in order to demonstrate a resulting substantial improvement in the performance of activities that would typically be limited by pain, rapid development of fatigue or numbness. In this manner, the patient and clinician is able to preview what may happen after targeted therapy is applied so that NTOS decompression surgery may be considered with a greater degree of confidence. The scalene test block is able to produce a temporary relief by virtue of producing temporary paralysis of the muscle due to anesthetic blockade at the level of the intramuscular nerve branches. Potential direct effects of muscle paralysis include relaxation of neurovascular compression between tightened muscles at the interscalene triangle as well as potential dropping of the top rib while upward tension is lost from the scalene muscle. Other direct effects may result from blockade of painful sensory input from the muscles. Indirect effects that may confound analysis include placebo effects and examiner biases which both need to be minimized. Occasionally weeks or months of therapeutic benefit may result from scalene test injections, although the procedure is designed primarily for diagnostic purposes.

Over the years, the test has evolved so that it has become highly predictive of good outcomes following thoracic outlet decompression. It is worthwhile to consider a historical view; as refinements have been added incrementally, the incremental benefits in test accuracy can attest to the needs for these refinements.

Evolution of the Scalene Test Block and Presently Utilized Protocols

TOS Test Blocks: Single Site Injection, Surface Landmarks

In an initial account, scalene test blockade was performed using surface landmarks only without imaging or electrophysiological guidance. There were no corrections for placebo effects or examiner bias. Inadvertent spread of anesthetic to unintended sites was occasionally observed [1].

TOS Test Blocks: Single Site Injection, EMG Guidance

Another early technique utilized electromyographic and stimulation guidance [2]. The anterior scalene was the sole anesthetic target with this approach. The high rate of false negatives

(50 %) was thought to be caused a failure to block more distal sites of potential compression. Furthermore, inadvertent injection of anesthetic outside of the targeted muscle due to accidental needle advancement could not be detected as the EMG signal is lost during actual fluid injection. Inaccurate placement of injectant was as least partially problematic because some patients would experience numbness of the thumb due to C6 blockade or develop a clinically evident sympathetic block.

TOS Test Blocks: Multiple Site Injection, Fluoroscopic and EMG Guidance

More accurate targeting was achieved when fluoroscopic guidance was added to EMG guidance [3, 4]. Although CT and MRI guidance were considered, these imaging modes were rapidly abandoned because of cost, the slow pace of patient flow and the intrinsic inability to track misplaced injectant flow as these modalities lack a real time mode. Radiation exposure was also problematic for CT guidance.

In the final 5 years of a protocol combining fluoroscopic guidance and EMG, 497 test block injections were performed in our UCLA Vascular Surgery affiliated clinic; there were two pneumothoraces and there were occasional inadvertent blocks of the C6 root or sympathetic blockade. There were insufficient safeguards to minimize and account for placebo effects and potential examiner biases.

TOS Test Blocks: Multiple Site Injection, Double Blinding, Randomized Comparative Intramuscular Nerve Blockade with Ultrasound and EMG Guidance and a Specific Instruction Set

The most recent iteration of the test block for NTOS has included controls for placebo effects and examiner bias. Live combined ultrasound guidance and EMG guidance is performed to ensure accurate injectant placement and confirm delivery of small volumes of injectant to the motor

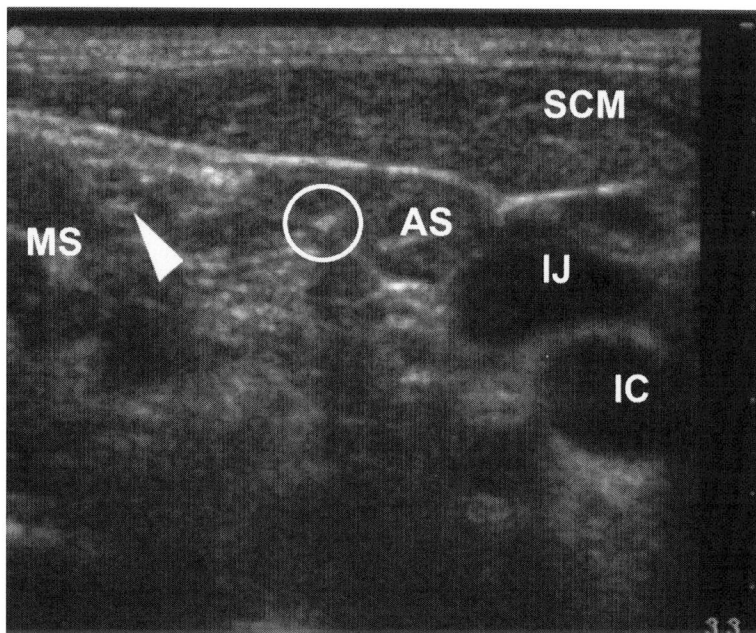

Fig. 20.1 Needle tip in anterior scalene muscle prior to injection (inside *circle*). The *arrow* points to C6 nerve root which may reached by leakage of injectant

innervation within the muscle targeted without spread across tissue planes. A full target set is included to be sure that more distal sites of TOS compression are not missed. Accuracy in predicting outcome to TOS targeted therapy is markedly improved compared to historical approaches.

A detailed description for the present scalene test protocol is as follows: patients are first instructed about the need and the nature of double blinding. They are told that either chloroprocaine (with a 1 h duration) or marcaine (with a 5 h duration) will be injected into the targeted muscles including the anterior scalene, subclavius, pectoralis minor. They are shown how to keep an hourly pain diary that measures pain, numbness and weakness at rest and with stress maneuvers (including the 1 min EAST) every hour while awake and the following morning. They are also asked to perform activities that characteristically cause discomfort. They are carefully coached to focus on either a 1 h or a 5 h response. The identity of injection is determined by coin flip by the surgical nurse and then documented in a form placed in a sealed envelope. Patient expectations are reviewed prior to the procedure to be sure that there is a full understanding of what is being measured.

During the procedure, the patient is awake and secured in a semi rotated supine position on a surgical table with the upper body elevated 30° and the shoulder is rotated off the table with a wedge. Combined electromyographic monitoring and live ultrasound is performed throughout. The muscles of interest are targeted in the mid belly region with 25 gauge Teflon coated hypodermic EMG and injection needle (see Fig. 20.1). EMG recording may confirm high frequency motor unit activity when the patient is at rest consistent with clinically observed dystonia. Motor thresholds are then determined by observing a twitch on the ultrasound at approximately 1 mA constant current stimulation at final needle positioning. The procedure targets the intramuscular nerve terminal branches. The patient is instructed to respond when the effects of stimulation are perceived, and the nurse records pain intensity and relative concordance with historical pain patterns. The recording nurse is blinded to the muscle being injected and there is no verbal identification of target identity. Control muscles, such as the trapezius and sternocleidomastoid, are similarly targeted but only injected with saline. The anterior scalene, subclavius and pectoralis minor are sequentially subjected to the above targeting maneuvers and then injected with 1 cc of anesthetic and 1 mg of dexamethasone. Live ultrasound is continued throughout to be sure that the injectant flows along the targeted muscle and not into the plexus.

The pain diaries are mailed or faxed to the examiner the following day and interpreted prior to revealing the identity of the injectant. A valid positive response consists of a greater than 50 % reduction in the pain scale scoring at rest and with stress maneuvers for a time period that is consistent with the identity of the injectant. Provocation testing during the procedure should reveal concordant pain responses from the scalene, subclavius or pectoralis muscles and not from control muscles.

Over the 5 years prior to writing this chapter, 879 combined ultrasound and EMG guided TOS test blocks were performed in our UCLA Vascular Surgery affiliated clinic. There were no instances of inadvertent anesthesia of the plexus or C6 root, sympathetic blockade, pneumothorax or hematomas. Of the 110 consecutive cases of cervicobrachial syndrome that were closely analyzed, 64 out of 67 with a positive block had a good outcome (defined as more than 50 % improvement in numerical pain scores and improvement in work and home activities and reduction in rescue medications for at least 3 months for chemodenervation and 1 year for surgery) to targeted therapy (botulinum chemodenervation or thoracic outlet decompression) yielding a true positive rate of 96 %. Further, 14 of 15 patients who had a positive block had a good outcome after surgery for a true positive rate of 93 %. By contrast, only 3 of the 11 with a negative test block had a good outcome, yielding a false negative rate of 27 %.

The 96 % true positive rate is better than that in our previously published series (86 %; Fisher exact p=0.0433) [4]. The false negative rates for the two series, 0 and 27 %, respectively, were not significantly different. The improvement in the true positive rate likely results from enhancements that were designed to minimize placebo effects. Using comparative blocks is a commonly used strategy to cut down on placebo effects [5, 6]; it is proposed that direct effects of an anesthetic block should last as long as the physiological effects of a local anesthetic. Unexpectedly long or short responses are proposed to represent placebo responses or other non specific effects. In a sequential and prospective comparison of protocols when 41 patients were given nonspecific instructions during the consent procedure only 12, or 29 %, had experienced responses that were commensurate with the specific anesthetic; many had improvements that lasted days or weeks. By contrast, 20 of 26 patients (77 %) who were treated with a specific instruction set had a commensurate response. In other words by using specific and controlled instructions as outlined above, the placebo and non-specific response rate was cut down from 71 to 23 % (Fisher Exact p=0.0002).

In the series of 110 patients analyzed sequentially above, there were seven poor outcomes to targeted therapy in patients who had a positive test block at other facilities that did not follow the above protocol. Double blinding was not practiced by these centers.

The EMG component of the present protocol confirms the presence of excessive motor unit activity and is a critical addition in two circumstances. First, it will confirm the ultrasound appearance of intramuscular needle tip penetration and help identify illusions of penetration due to needle tip invagination of the muscle surface. The second benefit is the ability to monitor an intramuscular location when the ultrasound image of the tip is obscured by the clavicle while trying to target the subclavius muscle (see Fig. 20.2). Live ultrasound is helpful in demonstrating patterns of injectant flow in real time; incomplete filling or leakage will lead to an immediate adjustment of needle tip positioning (see Figs. 20.3 and 20.4).

Ultrasound Guided Stellate Blocks

Sympathetic blockade targeting the Stellate ganglion and cervical sympathetic chain has been used for treating patient with complex regional pain syndrome (CRPS). Anterior cervical approaches utilizing surface landmarks or fluoroscopic imaging have been recently replaced with ultrasound guided targeting of the cervical sympathetic chain and ganglia using and anterolateral approach [7–9]. The lateral approach with ultrasound appears to minimize complications such as vascular laceration with

Fig. 20.2 Needle tip obscured by clavicular shadow (*C*). *Arrows* along line of needle shaft

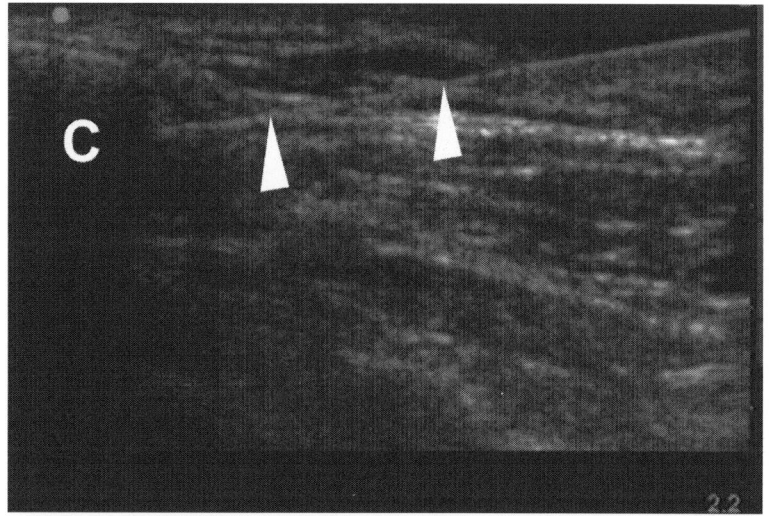

Fig. 20.3 Needle tip (inside *circle*) within pectoralis minor

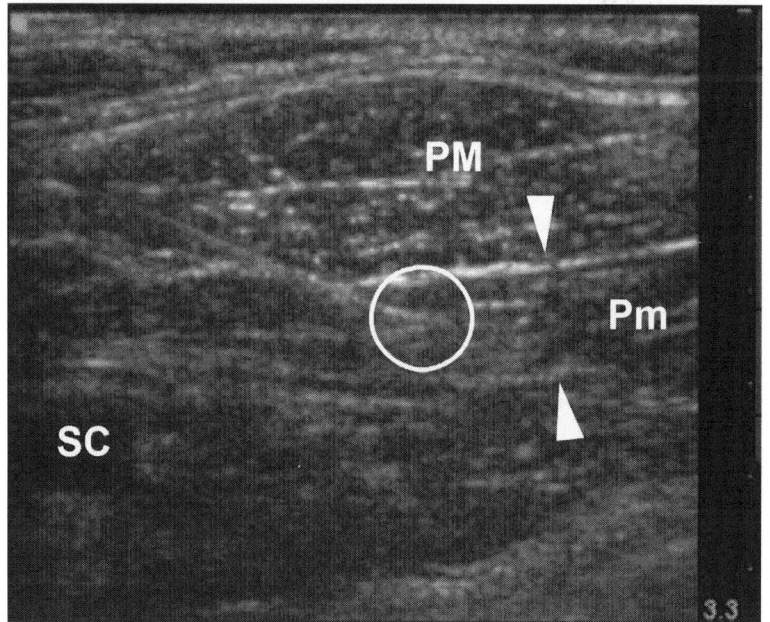

hematoma formation, inadvertent spinal injection, inadvertent esophageal injection, hoarseness, dysphagia, and pneumothorax. In our experience, 290 combined ultrasound and EMG guided stellate ganglion blocks have been performed. The technique is similar to published accounts except that EMG guidance is used with a Teflon insulated recording and injecting needle to be sure that the needle tip is not in the longus colli muscle, but just superficial to it. Live ultrasound confirms spread along the prevertebral fascial plane. Most of the patients developed a Horner's Syndrome for hours, but no complications have been seen. Most patients with CRPS have at least temporary relief of hand and arm symptoms and several degrees warming of the extremity by thermographic monitoring. Some patients may not have pain relief in the hands due to bypassing of the stellate ganglion and cervical sympathetic chain by hand sympathetic innervation directly from T2. A direct approach to the T2, T3 sympathetics may be performed percutaneously with fluoroscopic guidance for the latter patients.

Fig. 20.4 Needle tip (inside *circle*) within pectoralis minor showing filling of injectant throughout the muscle belly

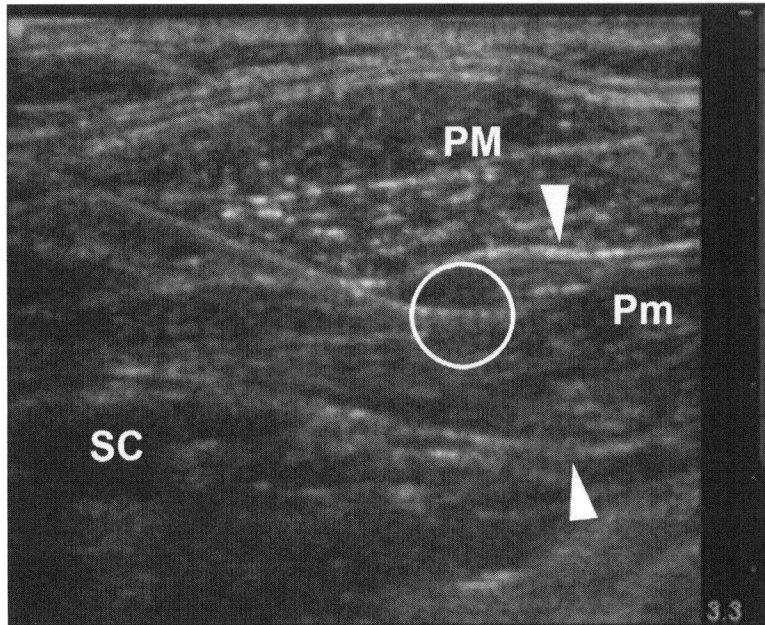

Ultrasound Guided Brachial Plexus Blocks

Ultrasound monitoring has improved techniques of brachial plexus blocks for peri-operative applications [10]. Ultrasound guided selective brachial plexus blocks may also be added to the therapeutic regimen for patients who have recurrent neuropathic pain after thoracic outlet decompression. As with other regional nerve injection techniques, pulsed radiofrequency and hyaluronidase injections may be added in attempts to create a longer duration of effect. In our experience, 84 ultrasound guided brachial plexus blocks have been performed. Most often the lower trunk was specifically targeted. Most patients achieved 1–3 months of relief. Complications have been rare: one patient with von Willebrand's disease had a hematoma that resolved without further intervention and one patient had a temporary paresthesias in the hand.

Suprascapular and Axillary Blocks

Ultrasound and fluoroscopically guided suprascapular blocks with pulsed radiofrequency have been described for chronic shoulder pain [11–13].

If a patient still has shoulder complaints which may not be amenable to surgery, then suprascapular blocks may be performed along with pulsed radiofrequency to help reduce the ongoing pain problem.

Facet Blocks

For patients with axial and periscapular pain, cervical facet-generated pain may be considered. Several authors have discussed the possibility of diagnosing facet generated pain by performing comparative blocks of the facet innervation. Prolonged benefit may be provided when patient with a positive test injection are subsequently treated with radiofrequency ablation of the facet nerves [14–18].

Botulinum Chemodenervation

There is an abundant literature describing the evaluation and treatment of spontaneous dystonias as well as dystonias associated with occupational exposures and trauma [19–43]. Although some authors have pointed out distinctions between the two groups, many similarities can be pointed out. Both classes of patients may have pain in the neck and shoulder muscles, and both classes may demonstrate excessive motor unit activity in the scalene muscles and may have radiating symptoms due to neural compression.

It was the latter revelation that suggested the initial trial of botulinum toxin type A (Botox, Allergan, Inc, Irvine, CA) for patients with TOS who may demonstrate excessive tension in the scalenes and other shoulder muscles. Furthermore, a muscle biopsy study from our group seemed to demonstrate that many patients with TOS may have histochemical evidence compatible with chronic ongoing excessive muscle activity in the scalene muscles [44]. As we had been routinely performing EMG guided scalene blocks at that time, it was further demonstrated that many of the TOS patients had electromyographic evidence of excessive motor unit activity. This excessive muscle activity appeared to be a potentially treatable with botulinum toxin injections.

Botulinum: Single Site Injections for TOS and Dystonia

As with the scalene test block experience, an historical account of incremental improvements in botulinum chemodenervation over the years can be used to point out important improvements that appear to be crucial in maximizing good outcomes when this approach is used for patients with TOS.

In the 1990's, our group started using botulinum chemodenervation targeting the anterior and middle scalene muscles as well as the painfully dystonic trapezius muscles using EMG and stimulation guidance [3]. All patients were confirmed to have NTOS by provocative and anesthetic scalene block testing, and all patients had EMG confirmation of excessive motor unit activity in the anterior and middle scalene muscles. Live mode fluoroscopy confirmed filling of contrast along muscle planes without leakage. There was, however, no ability to separately monitor the flow patterns of the subsequently injected toxin or for reconfirmation of needle positioning after the completion of injections, and this was thought to be responsible for the two out of 22 patients who had developed transient dysphagia. A good

outcome was defined as a 50 % or better relief of pain at rest and with targeted functional activities involving repetitive reaching and grasping; this lasted for only 3 months and occurred in only 64 % of these patients. The low response rate was believed to be due to injection of only a single site for the neurovascular complaints (anterior and middle scalene muscles) and only a single site for shoulder pain (trapezius).

Christo and colleagues presented a series of single site botulinum injection using CT guidance into the anterior scalene muscle in 27 patients with a clinical diagnosis of TOS [45]. No other injections were performed for shoulder pain or for shoulder protraction or elevation dystonia. There was a 15 % reduction in Visual Analogue Pain scores (VAS) at 3 months, but no functional outcomes were measured. Torriani also reported on a series of ultrasound guided injections with botulinum toxin in patients with TOS with VAS pain scale improvement in 69 % lasting an average of 31 days [46]. Again, no functional outcomes were measured. Most of the patients had injection of the scalene muscles, although a few had injection of either the pectoralis minor or subclavius. Finlayson reported on randomized placebo controlled double blinded EMG guided single site injection of the scalene muscles in patients with a clinical diagnosis of TOS. The primary outcome was pain measured by VAS. Secondary outcomes included the SF-36, the DASH and days lost from work. No beneficial effect of botulinum chemodenervation was found [47].

Botulinum: Multiple Site Injections for TOS and Treatment of Dystonia

Several experiences suggested that multiple targets should be included when considering botulinum injections. The emergence of MRI imaging of TOS with stress positioning demonstrated that patients may have proximal as well as distal sites of compression, for example, at the costoclavicular space. It became apparent that full decompression of the thoracic outlet may require chemodenervation of muscles distal to the scalenes. Furthermore, it was our experience that patients who already had scalenectomy could still achieve relief with botulinum injections of the subclavius and pectoralis minor muscles. A newly developed strategy was to target all muscles that may be relevant for TOS as well as to treat all of the dystonic muscles that were causing postural disturbances or contributed to regional pain. The published comparison of multisite and single site injection for TOS demonstrated superiority of good response rates for the multisite protocol at 91 and 68 %, respectively (Fisher one tailed p=0.0201) [48]. Compared to the earlier reported mean duration of 3 months, the present duration of effect is a mean of 5.4 months with a range of 1.5–12 months with the most recent protocol. Although botulinum toxin type A is thought to have a muscular relaxation effect only as long as 3 months and a potential action on release of inflammatory factors for a similarly short time period, it appears that patients may have clinical improvements that last longer than the direct effects of botulinum toxin.

Over the most recent 2 year period, botulinum chemodenervation was performed on 382 occasions in our UCLA Vascular Surgery affiliated clinic with no instances of pneumothorax, hematoma, infection, dysphagia, dysphonia, or any other evidence of unintended muscular paralysis.

Concerns have been raised about the possibility of developing neutralizing antibodies with subsequent secondary resistance to botulinum toxin when using large doses and multiple targets. Over the past 10 years we have performed a total of 1,794 botulinum chemodenervation procedures in 522 patients in our UCLA Vascular Surgery affiliated clinic using multiple target injections and Botox doses in the 150–200 MU range. There have been only two patients with secondary resistance, both of whom responded to botulinum toxin type B. Our experience compares favorably to the published rate of developing neutralizing antibodies of approximately 1 % for patients injected with similarly large doses and multiple site injections [49, 50].

In summary, for patients with NTOS, several interventional injection techniques may be considered at different stages of the patient treatment plan. Test injections may be used in the pre-operative stage to confirm a diagnosis of TOS and to predict outcomes for surgical decompression. In patients who are not surgical candidates, brachial plexus injections, sympathetic blocks and botulinum chemodenervation can be done safely and may be helpful in reducing pain and providing for a higher level of functioning.

References

1. Sanders RJ, Haug CE. Thoracic outlet syndrome: a common sequela of neck injuries. Philadelphia: Lippincott Williams & Wilkins; 1991.
2. Jordan SE, Machleder HI. Diagnosis of thoracic outlet syndrome using electrophysiologically guided anterior scalene blocks. Ann Vasc Surg. 1998;12:260–4.
3. Jordan SE, Ahn SS, Freischlag JA, et al. Selective botulinum chemodenervation of the scalene muscles for treatment of neurogenic thoracic outlet syndrome. Ann Vasc Surg. 2000;14:365–9.
4. Jordan SE, Ahn SS, Gelabert HA. Differentiation of thoracic outlet syndrome from treatment-resistant cervical brachial pain syndromes: development and utilization of a questionnaire, clinical examination and ultrasound evaluation. Pain Physician. 2007;10:441–52.
5. Manchikanti L, Manchukonda R, Pampati V, et al. Prevalence of facet joint pain in chronic low back pain in postsurgical patients by controlled comparative local anesthetic blocks. Arch Phys Med Rehabil. 2007;88:449–55.
6. Schwarzer AC, Aprill CN, Derby R, et al. Clinical features of patients with pain stemming from the lumbar zygapophysial joints. Is the lumbar facet syndrome a clinical entity? Spine (Phila Pa 1976). 1994;19:1132–7.
7. Usui Y, Kobayashi T, Kakinuma H, et al. An anatomical basis for blocking of the deep cervical plexus and cervical sympathetic tract using an ultrasound-guided technique. Anesth Analg. 2010;110:964–8.
8. Gofeld M, Bhatia A, Abbas S, et al. Development and validation of a new technique for ultrasound-guided stellate ganglion block. Reg Anesth Pain Med. 2009;34:475–9.
9. Narouze S, Vydyanathan A, Patel N. Ultrasound-guided stellate ganglion block successfully prevented esophageal puncture. Pain Physician. 2007;10:747–52.
10. Zencirci B. Comparision of nerve stimulator and ultrasonography as the techniques applied for brachial plexus anesthesia. Int Arch Med. 2011;4:4.
11. Perlas A, Lobo G, Lo N, et al. Ultrasound-guided supraclavicular block: outcome of 510 consecutive cases. Reg Anesth Pain Med. 2009;34:171–6.

12. Eyigor C, Eyigor S, Korkmaz OK, et al. Intra-articular corticosteroid injections versus pulsed radiofrequency in painful shoulder: a prospective, randomized, single-blinded study. Clin J Pain. 2010;26:386–92.

13. Gurbet A, Turker G, Bozkurt M, et al. Efficacy of pulsed mode radiofrequency lesioning of the suprascapular nerve in chronic shoulder pain secondary to rotator cuff rupture. Agri. 2005;17:48–52.

14. Falco FJ, Erhart S, Wargo BW, et al. Systematic review of diagnostic utility and therapeutic effectiveness of cervical facet joint interventions. Pain Physician. 2009;12:323–44.

15. Manchikanti L, Singh V. Diagnosis of facet joint pain and prediction of success and failure for cervical facet radiofrequency denervation. Reg Anesth Pain Med. 2009;34:81–2.

16. Husted DS, Orton D, Schofferman J, et al. Effectiveness of repeated radiofrequency neurotomy for cervical facet joint pain. J Spinal Disord Tech. 2008;21:406–8.

17. Boswell MV, Colson JD, Sehgal N, et al. A systematic review of therapeutic facet joint interventions in chronic spinal pain. Pain Physician. 2007;10:229–53.

18. Manchikanti L, Singh V, Vilims BD, et al. Medial branch neurotomy in management of chronic spinal pain: systematic review of the evidence. Pain Physician. 2002;5:405–18.

19. Chan J, Brin MF, Fahn S. Idiopathic cervical dystonia: clinical characteristics. Mov Disord. 1991;6:119–26.

20. Jankovic J, Leder S, Warner D, Schwartz K. Cervical dystonia: clinical findings and associated movement disorders. Neurology. 1991;41:1088–91.

21. Micheli F, Torres L, Diaz M, et al. Delayed onset limb dystonia following electric injury. Parkinsonism Relat Disord. 1998;4:39–42.

22. Carroll CG, Hawley JS, Ney JP. Post-traumatic shoulder dystonia in an active duty soldier. Mil Med. 2006;171:494–6.

23. Takemoto M, Ikenaga M, Tanaka C, et al. Cervical dystonia induced by cervical spine surgery: a case report. Spine (Phila Pa 1976). 2006;31:E31–4.

24. Frei KP, Pathak M, Jenkins S, et al. Natural history of posttraumatic cervical dystonia. Mov Disord. 2004;19: 1492–8.

25. O'Riordan S, Hutchinson M. Cervical dystonia following peripheral trauma – a case-control study. J Neurol. 2004;251:150–5.

26. Hollinger P, Burgunder J. Posttraumatic focal dystonia of the shoulder. Eur Neurol. 2000;44:153–5.

27. Wright RA, Ahlskog JE. Focal shoulder-elevation dystonia. Mov Disord. 2000;15:709–13.

28. Samii A, Pal PK, Schulzer M, et al. Post-traumatic cervical dystonia: a distinct entity? Can J Neurol Sci. 2000;27:55–9.

29. Thyagarajan D, Kompoliti K, Ford B. Post-traumatic shoulder 'dystonia': persistent abnormal postures of the shoulder after minor trauma. Neurology. 1998;51:1205–7.

30. Tarsy D. Comparison of acute- and delayed-onset posttraumatic cervical dystonia. Mov Disord. 1998;13: 481–5.

31. Goldman S, Ahlskog JE. Posttraumatic cervical dystonia. Mayo Clin Proc. 1993;68:443–8.

32. Truong DD, Dubinsky R, Hermanowicz N, et al. Posttraumatic torticollis. Arch Neurol. 1991;48: 221–3.

33. Tamagawa A, Uozumi T, Tsuji S. Occupational dystonia associated with production line work and PC work. Brain Nerve. 2007;59:553–9.

34. Altenmuller E, Jabusch HC. Focal dystonia in musicians: phenomenology, pathophysiology, triggering factors, and treatment. Med Probl Perform Art. 2010;25:3–9.

35. Abdo WF, Bloem BR, Eijk JJ, et al. Atypical dystonic shoulder movements following neuralgic amyotrophy. Mov Disord. 2009;24:293–6.

36. Baek W, Sheean G. Occupational dystonia affecting truncal muscles in a bricklayer. Mov Disord. 2007;22: 284–5.

37. Rodriguez AV, Kooh M, Guerra LA, et al. Musician's cramp: a case report and literature review. J Clin Rheumatol. 2005;11:274–6.

38. Schuele S, Jabusch HC, Lederman RJ, et al. Botulinum toxin injections in the treatment of musician's dystonia. Neurology. 2005;64:341–3.

39. Karp BI. Botulinum toxin treatment of occupational and focal hand dystonia. Mov Disord. 2004;19 Suppl 8:S116–9.

40. Defazio G, Berardelli A, Abbruzzese G, et al. Possible risk factors for primary adult onset dystonia: a case-control investigation by the italian movement disorders study group. J Neurol Neurosurg Psychiatry. 1998;64:25–32.

41. Marsden CD, Sheehy MP. Writer's cramp. Trends Neurosci. 1990;13:148–53.

42. McDaniel KD, Cummings JL, Shain S. The "yips": a focal dystonia of golfers. Neurology. 1989;39: 192–5.

43. Cohen LG, Hallett M. Hand cramps: clinical features and electromyographic patterns in a focal dystonia. Neurology. 1988;38:1005–12.

44. Machleder HI, Moll F, Verity MA. The anterior scalene muscle in thoracic outlet compression syndrome. Histochemical and morphometric studies. Arch Surg. 1986;121:1141–4.

45. Christo PJ, Christo DK, Carinci AJ, et al. Single CT-guided chemodenervation of the anterior scalene muscle with botulinum toxin for neurogenic thoracic outlet syndrome. Pain Med. 2010;11:504–11.

46. Torriani M, Gupta R, Donahue DM. Botulinum toxin injection in neurogenic thoracic outlet syndrome: results and experience using a ultrasound-guided approach. Skeletal Radiol. 2010;39:973–80.

47. Finlayson HC, O'Connor RJ, Brasher PM, Travlos A. Botulinum toxin injection for management of thoracic outlet syndrome: a double-blind, randomized, controlled trial. Pain. 2011;152:2023–8.

48. Jordan SE, Ahn SS, Gelabert HA. Combining ultrasonography and electromyography for botulinum chemodenervation treatment of thoracic outlet syndrome:

comparison with fluoroscopy and electromyography guidance. Pain Physician. 2007;10:541–6.

49. Naumann M, Carruthers A, Carruthers J, et al. Meta-analysis of neutralizing antibody conversion with onabotulinumtoxinA (BOTOX(R)) across multiple indications. Mov Disord. 2010;25:2211–8.

50. Brin MF, Comella CL, Jankovic J, et al. Long-term treatment with botulinum toxin type A in cervical dystonia has low immunogenicity by mouse protection assay. Mov Disord. 2008;23:1353–60.

Development of Consensus-Based Diagnostic Criteria for NTOS

21

Robert W. Thompson

Abstract

The diagnosis of neurogenic thoracic outlet syndrome (NTOS) depends upon clinical suspicion, pattern-recognition, and exclusion of more common conditions that have overlapping features. In most patients a diagnosis of NTOS can be made or excluded on the basis of the clinical history, description of symptoms, and physical examination, with the provisional diagnosis being supplemented by a limited number of diagnostic studies. In this chapter we describe ongoing efforts by the Consortium for Outcomes Research and Education on Thoracic Outlet Syndrome (CORE-TOS) to develop and validate diagnostic criteria for NTOS, based on an expert group consensus approach using Delphi methodology, and present a preliminary set of diagnostic criteria. Careful follow-up studies using standardized assessment instruments, particularly through consortium efforts to involve larger number of patients than available at any single center, will provide further insight into the most accurate diagnostic and prognostic criteria for NTOS.

Introduction

Thoracic outlet syndromes are rare conditions caused by compression of neurovascular structures within the anatomic space posterior to the clavicle, above the first rib, and extending to the subcoracoid space. Neurogenic thoracic outlet syndrome (NTOS) is the most frequent of these conditions, representing 85–95 % of all patients. NTOS is due to brachial plexus nerve compression caused by a combination of (1) congenital variations in anatomy, such as a cervical rib, anomalous scalene musculature, and/or aberrant fibrofascial bands, coupled with (2) a history of neck or upper extremity injury or repetitive trauma that has resulted in spasm, fibrosis and other pathological changes in the scalene and/or pectoralis minor muscles [1–5]. Acquired changes in posture, abnormalities in neck and shoulder muscle mechanics, and excessive perineural fibrosis also contribute to brachial plexus nerve compression

R.W. Thompson, MD
Department of Surgery/Section of Vascular Surgery,
Center for Thoracic Outlet Syndrome,
Washington University, Barnes-Jewish Hospital,
660 S Euclid Avenue, Campus Box 8109/Suite 5101
Queeny Tower, St. Louis, MO 63110, USA
e-mail: thompson@wudosis.wustl.edu

K.A. Illig et al. (eds.), *Thoracic Outlet Syndrome*,
DOI 10.1007/978-1-4471-4366-6_21, © Springer-Verlag London 2013

Table 21.1 Differential diagnosis of NTOS

Carpal tunnel syndrome	Cubital canal syndrome	Rotator cuff tendinitis
Cervical spine strain	Cervical disc disease	Cervical arthritis
Fibromyositis	Brachial plexus injury	Acromioclavicular joint
Fibromyalgia	Vasculitis	Atheroembolism
Raynaud's syndrome	Scleroderma	CRPS/RSD
Cervical dystonia	Lymphedema	Psychogenic syndrome
Parsonage-turner syndrome	Nerve sheath neoplasm	Pancoast tumor
Catheter-induced thrombosis	Primary thrombosis	Arterial embolism

[6–9]. In some cases NTOS may be combined with cervical spine radiculopathy or additional peripheral nerve compression disorders (e.g., carpal tunnel, cubital canal, and/or radial canal syndromes), to produce what has been termed the "double-crush" phenomenon [10–13]. NTOS may also be part of a regional pain syndrome with multiple simultaneous sources of pain generation (e.g., shoulder dysfunction, fibromyalgia), or it may co-exist with complex regional pain syndrome (CRPS), with or without a sympathetic-mediated component [14–17].

In the presence of a congenital cervical rib, some patients with NTOS present with weakness, overt electrophysiological abnormalities and thenar or hypothenar muscle atrophy ("Gilliatt-Sumner hand") [18, 19]. Although this clinical presentation has been termed "true" NTOS, these findings may simply represent an advanced form of NTOS with longstanding and possibly irretrievable nerve injury. In contrast, most patients with NTOS exhibit varying degrees of sensory symptoms with no hand muscle weakness or atrophy, and normal or non-specific findings on conventional electrophysiological testing and/or imaging studies. These individuals are identified primarily through comprehensive clinical diagnosis and the exclusion of other conditions. Because there remain no validated objective tests by which to definitively establish the diagnosis of brachial plexus compression in such patients, these individuals are often considered to have "non-specific" or "disputed" NTOS. Such modifying terms for NTOS have not been found to be particularly helpful, either in understanding the condition or in clinical evaluation and management, and have been largely discarded by most investigators.

NTOS is clinically important because when unrecognized and/or inadequately treated, it can cause chronic pain syndromes and/or long-term restrictions in use of the upper extremities, and because it produces substantial disability in relatively young, active, and otherwise healthy individuals in the prime of working life. Accurate diagnosis of NTOS remains a significant challenge in clinical practice, yet properly identified patients can respond quite well to treatment. The various methods used in the diagnosis and treatment of NTOS are more specifically discussed in Chap. 7, "Clinical Presentation of Patients with NTOS."

Differential Diagnosis

Because the symptoms, diagnosis and management of NTOS often overlap with other upper extremity neurological and musculoskeletal disorders, this condition is associated with a particularly broad differential diagnosis (Table 21.1). Indeed, many unresolved issues surrounding NTOS revolve around defining the most accurate clinical criteria to differentiate this condition from other cervical-brachial syndromes and the optimal means to select patients for different forms of treatment. The diagnosis of NTOS depends upon clinical suspicion and pattern-recognition based on the history, description of symptoms, and targeted physical examination, along with the exclusion of more common conditions that have overlapping features. In most patients a provisional diagnosis of NTOS can be made or excluded on this basis. There has been a longstanding effort to establish testing procedures that can improve diagnostic accuracy and/or better predict outcomes of treatment, including various forms of soft tissue imaging [20–25], advances in electrophysiologic testing [26–29], the application of selective scalene and pectoralis muscle blocks, and ongoing refinement of clinical criteria [30, 31]. Although such tests and studies may be of value, both in excluding other conditions and in supporting the suspected diagnosis, with the exception of scalene/pectoralis muscle blocks, no single test is entirely specific for NTOS.

Initial Development of Consensus-Based Diagnostic Criteria

Comparisons of outcome for the treatment of NTOS are limited by the diverse diagnostic criteria used in various publications and a corresponding lack of uniformity in the patient populations represented. To help address this issue, the Consortium for Outcomes Research and Education on Thoracic Outlet Syndrome (CORE-TOS) was formed several years ago as a multidisciplinary effort to facilitate comparative-effectiveness research. One of the first tasks undertaken by the CORE-TOS group was to begin establishing a consensus-driven set of defined diagnostic criteria for NTOS. This was addressed utilizing a Delphi process approach, a group-consensus strategy that has been widely utilized in other specialties of medicine [32–35].

The Delphi method refers to a step-wise process by which an expert group reaches consensus on a given set of criteria for predicting a particular outcome. The main characteristics of the process are as follows: (1) A panel or group of experts is selected for their experience or opinions regarding the topic under study; (2) A facilitator is selected that facilitates, and receives the results of each survey in the initial and all subsequent steps, and processes the information received in each iteration and filters out irrelevant content; (3) An initial step intended to identify a set of features to be considered as potentially relevant to the topic under study; (4) A second step in which each member rates each of the selected features with regard to its frequency in individuals with the condition under study (diagnostic sensitivity) and

its frequency in individuals without the condition under study (reverse diagnostic specificity), with the ratings of each member of the group submitted to the facilitator along with any appropriate comments and criticisms explaining the rating, then having these ratings and comments collated by the facilitator in an anonymous manner and redistributed to members for further consideration; (5) A third step in which each member is asked to re-evaluate their previous ratings for each feature in light of the results submitted by other group members and the group as a whole, as well as the anonymous comments submitted by other group members, with each member encouraged to make modifications in their ratings, which are then resubmitted to the facilitator and collated in an anonymous manner and common and conflicting viewpoints continue to be elucidated; and (6) Repeat of steps 4 and 5 at least once more and perhaps more often, as needed, in order to reach a consensus where possible and to identify features for which clear consensus cannot be reached. The step-wise process inherent in the Delphi approach allows each group member to modify their responses based on the additional information received during each iteration of rating and commentary by the group. Maintaining the anonymity of ratings and responses helps to limit potential domination of the process by a few individuals, allows each group member equal opportunity to articulate opinion, promotes free expression of opinion and open critique, and encourages members to identify errors and correct their earlier judgments. These are some of the ways that the Delphi method helps overcome common problems in group dynamics and consensus building, separating it from other methodologies.

A panel of 12 experienced clinicians with expertise in the care of patients with NTOS participated in the survey process, initially developing a broad list of 223 clinical features considered to be potentially important in establishing a diagnosis of NTOS. This included features principally related to (a) clinical history, (b) description of symptoms, (c) physical examination findings, and (d) tests and studies. The data elements also included clinical features associated with poor

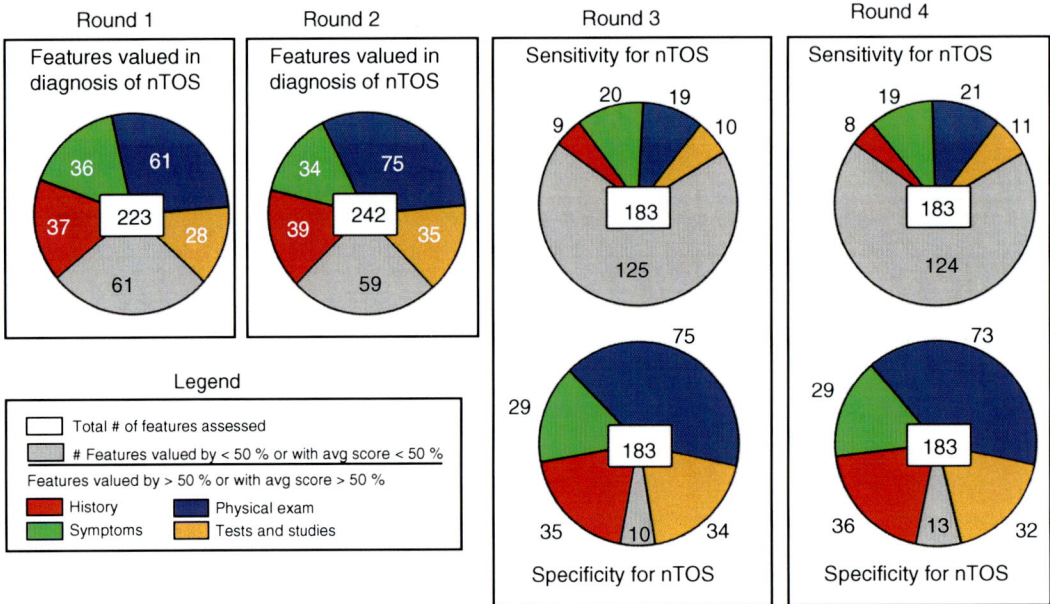

Fig. 21.1 Delphi process for diagnostic criteria of NTOS. The results of the first four rounds of the Delphi process are shown. Rounds 1 and 2 were qualitative surveys to identify features considered of value in diagnosis; rounds 3 and 4 were quantitative surveys to estimate sensitivity and specificity of features in diagnosis

clinical outcomes of treatment in patients with NTOS in previous studies, particularly signs and symptoms of depression, fibromyalgia, complex regional pain syndrome, peripheral nerve compression syndromes, and coexisting musculoskeletal disorders [30, 31].

In the first round of the Delphi survey, 162 of the initial 223 features were considered to be of potential diagnostic value by >50 % of the evaluators (Fig. 21.1). These features were then modified and/or consolidated during the feedback/discussion phase and additional features were added for more specificity. In a second round of survey evaluation the consensus panel evaluated 242 features, of which 183 were considered to be of potential value by >50 % of evaluators. In a third survey round, panel members were asked to score each of the identified features with respect to: (1) the "proportion of patients with a cervical-brachial syndrome attributed to NTOS that would be expected to exhibit that feature" (diagnostic sensitivity), and (2) the "proportion of patients with a cervical-brachial syndrome not attributed to NTOS that would be expected to exhibit that feature" (reverse diagnostic

specificity). Following analysis of the results and an additional feedback/discussion phase, the list of diagnostic features was consolidated to 62 that appeared to exhibit the greatest estimated diagnostic sensitivity, specificity, and accuracy (Table 21.2) [36].

Second-Stage Consensus-Based Diagnostic Criteria

While the initial consolidated list of diagnostic features provided some insight into the items upon which the expert panel reached greatest consensus, the main limitation of this stage was the absence of information about the relative "weights" that would be placed on different items in arriving at a clinical diagnosis. To define more valid consensus-based diagnostic criteria for NTOS, the expert panel next re-evaluated the series of items derived from the previous work with respect to the relative importance of each item in making a clinical diagnosis of NTOS, seeking to assess which items carried the greatest analytical strength as consensus-derived criteria. This approach was modeled after the survey

Table 21.2 Initial consensus-based diagnostic criteria for NTOS

Type and description of feature	+NTOS %	−NTOS %
Clinical history		
Symptoms not explained by other condition	100	1
Symptoms worsened by work	90	60
History of neck/arm injury (all types)	80	50
Repetitive strain injury	78	25
Age 15–35 years	70	60
Symptoms worse/minimally improved with conservative Rx	58	37
Substantial improvement with conservative Rx for TOS	15	5
History of cervical rib	10	1
Performance music or sports, arm overhead/weights	10	5
History of peripheral nerve surgery (median, ulnar)	8	6
History of previous treatment or surgery for TOS	5	3
History of clavicle or first rib fracture	4	2
Symptoms		
Paresthesias in digits 4 and 5	90	12
Complaint of hand/digit numbness	90	25
Symptom exacerbation with daily activities or work	90	60
Symptom exacerbation with arm use especially overhead	88	35
Pain interferes with sleep	85	37
Paresthesias radiate in ulnar distribution	83	20
Pain in neck, upper back, shoulder, and/or arm	83	70
Complaint of weakness in arm or hand	72	25
Paresthesias radiate from supraclavicular space	70	5
Headache occipital	60	20
Pain in hand/digits especially with arm use	50	23
Complaint of hand/digit swelling or coldness	50	22
Paresthesias in hand and/or all digits	43	15
Complaint of neck swelling	20	10
Physical examination		
Tenderness/pain on palpation scalene triangle	95	5
Upper limb tension test reproduces symptoms	95	20
Tenderness/pain on palpation >1 areas	90	30
Hand/digit paresthesias on passive arm elevation	90	10
Head tilt/neck rotation reproduces symptoms contra only	83	22
Palpable muscle spasm scalene triangle	80	5
Hand/digit paresthesias on palpation scalene triangle	80	5
Tinel's supraclavicular	80	15
Head tilt/neck rotation reproduces Sx ipsilateral only	80	30
Postural abnormalities (e.g., slumped head-forward)	68	20
Tenderness/pain on palpation pectoralis minor	60	10
3-Min EAST unable to complete or moderate symptoms	60	17
1-Min EAST unable to complete	55	5
Radial pulse ablated or diminished on arm elevation	55	17
Palpable muscle spasm pectoralis and/or trapezius	50	20
Pale hand upon arm elevation	50	10
Diminished sensation in hand/digits esp. digits 4/5	49	12
Hand/digit paresthesias on palpation pec minor	45	7

(continued)

Table 21.2 (continued)

Type and description of feature	+NTOS %	−NTOS %
Weakness of handgrip, intrinsic muscles or digit 5	44	18
Pain-limited ROM neck, shoulder, or arm	33	33
Tenderness/pain SCM, ant chest, rhomboid, or trap	29	21
Visible arm swelling, cyanosis, distended subcut veins	9	4
Hyperalgesia/allodynia neck	8	5
Palpable supraclavicular mass	5	2
Digital ischemia, ulceration, emboli, or Raynaud's	4	2
Thenar or hypothenar atrophy	4	5
Radial, brachial, or axillary pulse not *palpable* at rest	2	1
Indwelling subclavian vein access, past or present	1	3
Tests and studies		
Cervical imaging: Normal C-spine	80	50
Scalene muscle block moderate or dramatic improvement	79	3
Vascular lab: Diminished arterial pressures arm elevation	72	21
Venogram: Subclavian vein stenosis and/or thrombosis	34	15
Cervical imaging: Cervical rib or wide C7 affected side	13	1
Abnormal EMG/NC studies: Brachial plexus	8	5
Arteriogram: Subclavian artery aneurysm and/or stenosis	5	1
Vascular lab: Axillary-subclavian vein thrombosis	5	0

Using a Delphi process, each of 118 potential diagnostic features of NTOS were rated by an expert panel with regard to diagnostic sensitivity (+NTOS, the estimated percent of patients with NTOS that would exhibit the feature listed) and specificity (−NTOS, the estimated percent of patients without NTOS that would exhibit the feature listed). Data shown indicate the mean ratings for the entire 12-member panel of evaluators, for the 62 features exhibiting the highest rankings. Unpublished data from the Consortium for Outcomes Research and Education on Thoracic Outlet Syndrome (CORE-TOS)

construction and statistical analysis of Delphi-based survey results that has been used by Graham and Wright, in developing criteria for the diagnosis of carpal tunnel syndrome [32, 37, 38].

Survey Construction

For this purposes of this last survey, the diagnosis of neurogenic TOS was considered to represent symptoms caused by brachial plexus compression at the level of the scalene triangle and/or the subcoracoid (pectoralis minor) space. The diagnosis was also considered to represent a clinically significant condition that would warrant treatment, but without specifying the treatment that might be recommended. In addition, efforts were made to focus primarily on those items most important in establishing the diagnosis, rather than items that might be used principally in evaluating the severity of symptoms, degree of disability, prognosis, type of treatment to be

recommended, or the likelihood of response to treatment. Finally, the items considered were primarily those that would be potentially important (or not important) in reaching a diagnosis based on clinical features (patient characteristics, history, previous treatment, symptoms and physical examination), rather than the results of any specific tests or studies, but did include items referring to previous or current diagnoses, treatments, and test results. Additional items were included to indicate potential tests and studies to be performed beyond the clinical evaluation, in order to identify those considered important (or not important) in reaching a more definitive diagnosis of neurogenic TOS.

The survey instrument consisted of 194 items, with 118 related to clinical diagnosis (23 history, 40 symptoms, 55 examination), 60 related to previous tests, diagnoses, and treatments (30, 12, and 18, respectively), and 16 describing potential tests/studies to be performed. Panel members were asked to rate the importance of each item

Item 1361   History: Symptoms began after automobile collision

(−) NTOS ————————————————————————————————— (+) NTOS
−5   −4   −3   −2   −1   0   1   2   3   4   5
Extremely important   Completely unimportant   Extremely important

Clarification: The type of injury, diagnostic tests, or any treatment provided is not otherwise specified. The interval between injury and the onset of the current symptoms is not otherwise specified

Item 2153   History: Age 15–35 years

(−) NTOS ————————————————————————————————— (+) NTOS
−5   −4   −3   −2   −1   0   1   2   3   4   5
Extremely important   Completely unimportant   Extremely important

Item 1362   Symptoms: Headache frontal

(−) NTOS ————————————————————————————————— (+) NTOS
−5   −4   −3   −2   −1   0   1   2   3   4   5
Extremely important   Completely unimportant   Extremely important

Item 2736   Symptoms: Paresthesias radiating from supraclavicular space

(−) NTOS ————————————————————————————————— (+) NTOS
−5   −4   −3   −2   −1   0   1   2   3   4   5
Extremely important   Completely unimportant   Extremely important

Clarification: Distribution of paresthesias not otherwise specified

Item 2100   Symptoms: Pain in neck, upper back, shoulder, and/or upper arm

(−) NTOS ————————————————————————————————— (+) NTOS
−5   −4   −3   −2   −1   0   1   2   3   4   5
Extremely important   Completely unimportant   Extremely important

Item 3510   Previous tests: Arterial pressure waveforms = Diminished with arm elevation

(−) NTOS ————————————————————————————————— (+) NTOS
−5   −4   −3   −2   −1   0   1   2   3   4   5
Extremely important   Completely unimportant   Extremely important

Clarification: Refers to the side of the current symptoms. The previous test was considered to have been technically successful. The magnitude or proportion of symptoms attributed to this previous test result and any treatment recommendations based on this test result are not otherwise specified

Item 2297   Previous tests: EMG/NCS = Mild carpal tunnel syndrome

(−) NTOS ————————————————————————————————— (+) NTOS
−5   −4   −3   −2   −1   0   1   2   3   4   5
Extremely important   Completely unimportant   Extremely important

Clarification: Refers to the side of the current symptoms. Decreased nerve conduction velocity and/or amplitude, median nerve at the wrist. The magnitude or proportion of symptoms attributed to this previous test result and any treatment recommendations based on this test result are not otherwise specified

Item 2547   Previous Rx: Physical Rx for neck/shoulder, symptoms not improved

(−) NTOS ————————————————————————————————— (+) NTOS
−5   −4   −3   −2   −1   0   1   2   3   4   5
Extremely important   Completely unimportant   Extremely important

Clarification: Refers to the side of the current symptoms. Previous treatment was directed toward a neck and/or shoulder disorder, but the type of previous treatment is not otherwise specified. The previous treatment was considered to have addressed the abnormality for which the therapy was performed. The interval between the previous treatment and the current evaluation is not otherwise specified

Item 2056   Examination: Local tenderness/pain on palpation over scalene triangle

(−) NTOS ————————————————————————————————— (+) NTOS
−5   −4   −3   −2   −1   0   1   2   3   4   5
Extremely important   Completely unimportant   Extremely important

Item 2056   Examination: Spurling's test positive

(−) NTOS ————————————————————————————————— (+) NTOS
−5   −4   −3   −2   −1   0   1   2   3   4   5
Extremely important   Completely unimportant   Extremely important

Clarification: Refers to the side of the current symptoms. Spurling's test is performed by having the patient extend the neck and rotate the head toward the side of their pain. The test is positive if pain is exacerbated by this position. Spurling's test is often performed in evaluation of cervical spine disease

Item 1867   Examination: Positive 3-Min EAST

(−) NTOS ————————————————————————————————— (+) NTOS
−5   −4   −3   −2   −1   0   1   2   3   4   5
Extremely important   Completely unimportant   Extremely important

Clarification: EAST = Elevated arm stress test. Performed by having the patient place both arms in the elevated "surrender" position, then repetitively open and close the fists. A positive test is when the patient has reproduction of their characteristic upper extremity symptoms and has to discontinue the exam within the specified time period. A negative test is when the patient is able to complete the test for the specified time period. The 3-min EAST is often performed in evaluation of thoracic outlet syndrome

Item 1560   Examination: Hand or digit paresthesias on passive arm elevation

(−) NTOS ————————————————————————————————— (+) NTOS
−5   −4   −3   −2   −1   0   1   2   3   4   5
Extremely important   Completely unimportant   Extremely important

Clarification: Distribution of paresthesias is not otherwise specified

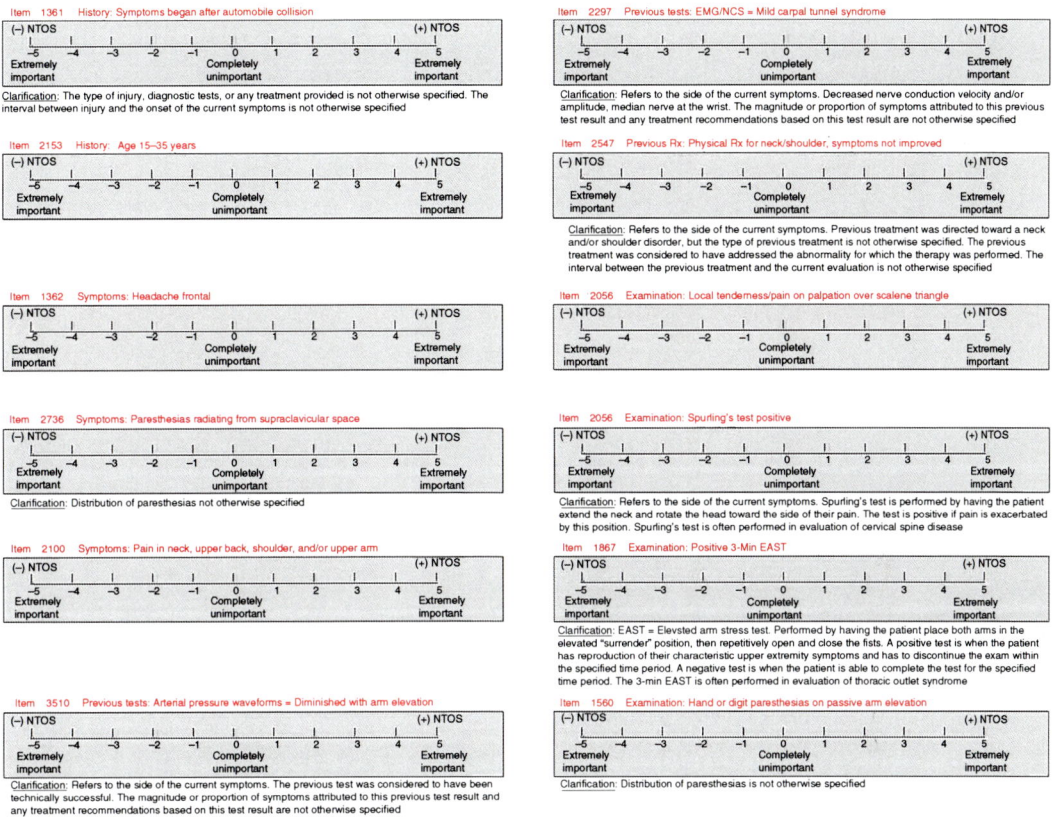

Fig. 21.2 Consensus survey of diagnostic criteria for NTOS. After identification of 178 features considered of potential value in the diagnosis of NTOS, a survey questionnaire was submitted to a 12-member expert consensus panel. Each panel member scored the diagnostic importance of each feature using an 11-point visual analog scale, ranging from −5 to +5. Several examples of the questions used in the survey instrument are shown (there were 23 items related to clinical history, 40 items related to symptoms, 12 items related to previous diagnoses, 18 items related to previous treatments, 30 items related to previous tests, and 55 items related to physical examination)

in reaching (positive) or excluding (negative) a clinical diagnosis of NTOS, using an 11-point horizontal visual analog scale (VAS), which ranged from a negative "extremely important" (−5.0), to neutral "completely unimportant" (0.0), to a positive "extremely important" (+5.0). The instructions reiterated that panel members should imagine how important a given item might be in helping reach a diagnosis of NTOS during a typical clinical evaluation in the office. It was indicated that items rated as extremely important should be those that one would require to be present in order to exclude or make a diagnosis of NTOS, whereas items rated as completely unimportant should be those that make

no difference in one's assessment of a patient for this diagnosis. Items that might help support or exclude a diagnosis of NTOS, but not considered essential, were expected to be rated at some relative level of intermediate importance. It was emphasized that although a given item might be frequently observed in patients with NTOS, that item may or may not be important in actually making a diagnosis. Similarly, a given item may indicate a certain magnitude of symptoms, extent of disability, or likelihood of responsiveness to treatment, but may or may not be important in reaching a clinical diagnosis. Several examples of the survey questions are illustrated in Fig. 21.2.

Table 21.3 Diagnostic criteria for NTOS, items of greatest diagnostic importance, subcategories related to clinical diagnosis

Rank	Item description	Mean ± SD	Variance
1	Local tenderness/pain on palpation scalene triangle	4.5 ± 0.7	0.47
2	Hand/digit paresthesias on palpation scalene triangle	4.2 ± 0.8	0.72
3	Known presence of a cervical rib	4.1 ± 1.0	1.04
4	Symptom exacerbation with overhead arm use	4.1 ± 0.8	0.59
5	Thenar or hypothenar atrophy	4.0 ± 1.5	2.15
6	Positive Tinel's supraclavicular	4.0 ± 1.0	1.01
7	Weakness of handgrip, intrinsic muscles or digit 5	3.8 ± 1.3	1.60
8	Diminished sensation in digits 4 and 5	3.8 ± 1.3	1.63
9	Paresthesias in digits 4 and 5	3.8 ± 1.0	0.99
10	Repetitive strain activities	3.7 ± 0.8	0.70
11	Paresthesias radiating from supraclavicular space	3.6 ± 1.6	2.46
12	Positive 1-min EAST	3.6 ± 1.6	2.60
13	Paresthesias radiating in ulnar distribution	3.5 ± 1.3	1.74
14	Symptoms exacerbated by driving	3.5 ± 0.9	0.74
15	Paresthesias radiating through arm to hand	3.4 ± 1.1	1.15
16	Hand and/or digit paresthesias on palpation pec minor	3.4 ± 1.6	2.53
17	Hand or digit paresthesias on passive arm elevation	3.4 ± 1.7	3.00
18	Complaint of weakness in hand, clumsiness	3.3 ± 1.2	1.52
19	Palpable muscle spasm scalene triangle	3.3 ± 1.4	1.84
20	Previous ipsilateral clavicle or first rib fracture	3.3 ± 1.4	1.98
21	Complaint of weakness in arm or hand	3.2 ± 1.1	1.28
22	Symptoms began after injury at work/change in activity	3.2 ± 1.1	1.28
23	Positive upper limb tension test	3.2 ± 1.6	2.68
24	Symptoms are exacerbated by work-related activities	3.2 ± 1.2	1.42
25	Occupation or recreation, overhead sports	3.1 ± 1.3	1.78
26	Complaint of hand and/or digit numbness	3.1 ± 2.2	4.69
27	Local tenderness/pain on palpation pectoralis minor	3.0 ± 1.4	1.87
118	Negative 3-min EAST	−3.2 ± 2.0	3.81

The importance of each feature related to Clinical Diagnosis of NTOS (n = 118) was scored using an 11-point visual analog scale (VAS), ranging from −5 to +5. Items were ranked by the mean score for the entire 12-member expert panel, with the data shown including the standard deviation and variance. There was a high degree of consistency in scoring by the overall panel (Cronbach's alpha = 0.901), indicating a high degree of consensus. Unpublished data from the Consortium for Outcomes Research and Education on Thoracic Outlet Syndrome (CORE-TOS)

Results and Analysis

There was excellent overall group consensus for the 118 items related to "Clinical Diagnosis", with an overall value for Cronbach's alpha, a measure of internal test consistency, of 0.901. There were 27 items (23 %) considered of great diagnostic importance (mean score > +3.00 or < −3.00), 32 items (27 %) considered of intermediate importance, and 57 items (48 %) considered unlikely to be important (mean score between −2.00 and +2.00). There were 71 items (60 %) with a group variance greater than 2.0, and the correlations for individual panelists and the group ranged from 0.553 to 0.886. The items considered of greatest diagnostic importance are summarized in Table 21.3 and those considered of no diagnostic importance are listed in Table 21.4.

For the 60 items related to "Previous Tests, Diagnoses, and Treatments", there was relatively low overall group consensus with a Cronbach's alpha of only 0.629. There were 13 items (22 %) considered of great diagnostic importance, 9 items (15 %) considered of intermediate importance,

Table 21.4 Diagnostic criteria for NTOS, items of no diagnostic importance, subcategories related to clinical diagnosis

Rank	Item description	Mean ± SD	Variance
76	2-point fingertip discrimination diminished (>5 mm)	0.9 ± 1.6	2.53
77	Symptoms began after chiropractic manipulation, neck	0.9 ± 2.1	4.22
78	Hyperalgesia/allodynia anterolateral neck	0.8 ± 1.8	3.21
79	Radial, brachial, or axillary pulses not palpable at rest	0.8 ± 2.7	7.54
80	Palpable muscle spasm pectoralis major and/or trapezius	0.6 ± 2.7	7.05
81	Phalen's sign negative	0.6 ± 1.6	2.45
82	Axial compression/traction test negative	0.6 ± 2.0	3.96
83	Digital ischemia, ulceration, or emboli	0.5 ± 3.9	15.10
84	Arm swelling, cyanosis, or distended subcutaneous veins	0.5 ± 3.1	9.34
85	Pain in upper back or neck, midline	0.3 ± 2.0	4.07
86	Normal hand color upon arm elevation	0.3 ± 1.0	1.01
87	Upper extremity deep tendon reflexes normal	0.3 ± 0.6	0.37
88	Local tenderness/pain on palpation over rhomboid muscles	0.2 ± 1.9	3.72
89	Obesity	0.2 ± 0.4	0.17
90	Hyperalgesia/allodynia entire upper extremity	0.0 ± 2.5	6.24
91	2-point fingertip discrimination normal	0.0 ± 0.3	0.12
92	Radiating pain in extensor forearm, not proximal to elbow	−0.3 ± 2.4	5.73
93	Diminished sensation in digits 1, 2 and 3	−0.3 ± 2.9	8.19
94	Symptoms present for < 6 weeks	−0.3 ± 1.7	2.87
95	Positive Tinel's test ulnar nerve at elbow	−0.4 ± 2.1	4.28
96	Headache frontal	−0.5 ± 1.6	2.57
97	Indwelling subclavian vein access, past or present	−0.5 ± 2.0	3.98
98	Relief of symptoms by shaking hand	−0.6 ± 1.9	3.69
99	Normal ROM neck, shoulder, and arm	−0.7 ± 1.8	3.34
100	Head tilt/neck rotation reproduces ipsilateral symptoms	−0.7 ± 2.4	5.54
101	Normal arterial pulses in all arm positions	−0.8 ± 1.0	0.96
102	Paresthesias radiating proximally from hand	−0.8 ± 2.5	6.38
103	Age > 50 years	−0.9 ± 1.1	1.20
104	Upper extremity deep tendon reflexes abnormal	−0.9 ± 1.9	3.74
105	Positive Tinel's test median nerve at wrist	−0.9 ± 2.2	4.73

The importance of each feature related to Clinical Diagnosis of NTOS (n = 118) was scored using an 11-point visual analog scale (VAS), ranging from −5 to +5. Items were ranked by the mean score for the entire 12-member expert panel, with the data shown including the standard deviation and variance. There was a high degree of consistency in scoring by the overall panel (Cronbach's alpha = 0.901), indicating a high degree of consensus. Unpublished data from the Consortium for Outcomes Research and Education on Thoracic Outlet Syndrome (CORE-TOS)

and 38 items (63 %) considered unlikely to be important. There were 41 items (68 %) with a group variance greater than 2.0, and the correlations for individual panelists and the group ranged from 0.412 to 0.888. The items considered of greatest diagnostic importance are summarized in Table 21.5.

For 16 items related to "Tests to be Performed", there were four items (25 %) considered of great diagnostic importance: "Anterior Scalene/ Pectoralis Minor Anesthetic Muscle Block"

(mean score +3.34), "Assess Response to Physical Therapy for NTOS" (mean score +3.28), "Cervical Spine Radiographs" (mean score +3.24), and "Chest X-Ray" (mean score +3.03). All 12 other items, including "Upper Extremity Arterial Doppler Studies" (mean score +1.70), were considered unlikely to be important. In this subset of items there were 15 (94 %) with a group variance greater than 2.0, indicating a wide spectrum of opinion.

Table 21.5 Diagnostic criteria for NTOS, items of greatest diagnostic importance, subcategories related to previous tests, diagnoses, and treatments

Rank	Item description	Mean ± SD	Variance
1	Anterior scalene muscle block = significant improvement	4.2 ± 1.5	2.12
2	Cervical radiographs = cervical rib or wide C7 process	4.1 ± 1.2	1.36
3	Combined ASM/PM muscle block = significant improvement	4.0 ± 1.5	2.24
4	Pectoralis minor muscle block = significant improvement	3.9 ± 1.6	2.39
5	Contralateral surgery for NTOS, symptoms improved	3.7 ± 1.5	2.12
6	Physical Rx for NTOS, symptoms improved	3.6 ± 1.4	2.02
7	EMG/NCS including MAC = abnormal MAC	3.4 ± 1.8	3.11
8	Ipsilateral surgery for NTOS, symptoms improved	3.4 ± 1.9	3.49
9	EMG/NCS: Abnormal for brachial plexus	3.3 ± 1.6	2.73
10	Ipsilateral pectoralis minor tenotomy, symptoms improved	3.2 ± 1.5	2.25
11	Upper extremity arteriogram = subclavian artery aneurysm	3.0 ± 3.2	10.12
59	Ipsilateral surgery for NTOS, symptoms not improved	−3.1 ± 1.3	1.75
60	Combined ASM/PM muscle block = no improvement	−3.2 ± 1.5	2.37

The importance of each feature related to Previous Tests, Diagnoses, and Treatments with regard to the diagnosis of NTOS (n = 60) was scored using an 11-point visual analog scale (VAS), ranging from −5 to +5. Items were ranked by the mean score for the entire 12-member expert panel, with the data shown including the standard deviation and variance. There was a relatively low degree of consistency in scoring by the overall panel (Cronbach's alpha = 0.629), indicating a lack of consensus. Unpublished data from the Consortium for Outcomes Research and Education on Thoracic Outlet Syndrome (CORE-TOS)

From the results of this last survey, the 28 items related to "Clinical Diagnosis" that were rated of greatest diagnostic importance were examined to identify potential quantitative and qualitative similarities. These items were then grouped and consolidated to establish terms that would reflect overlapping information from the similarly grouped items. These consolidated items indicated a series of 18 new items that, taken together, would be expected to capture the most important features needed to establish a clinical diagnosis of NTOS. These items are summarized as "provisional CORE-TOS criteria for the diagnosis of NTOS" in Table 21.6.

Future Directions

Given the provisional set of diagnostic criteria for NTOS developed through the Delphi process, the next steps in this effort are focused on re-testing these criteria in a different form of the survey process that employs a series of case scenarios. These case scenarios are developed in a manner that varies the presence or absence of each of the individual criteria, with expert evaluators providing numerical scores for the likelihood of the diagnosis of NTOS on a VAS for each case scenario. Statistical analysis of the results from this survey will be used to establish a logistic regression model for predicting the clinical diagnosis of NTOS. This statistical model will then be validated and tested further in case scenarios and in real patient populations. This effort will be supplemented by use of additional instruments used to evaluate the extent of symptoms and disability from NTOS, such as the DASH (Disabilities of the Arm, Shoulder, or Hand) [39–41], CBSQ (Cervical-Brachial Symptom Questionnaire) [30], BPI (Brief Pain Inventory) [42–44], and SF-12 (Medical Outcomes Study Short Form-12) [45], as well as other outcomes assessed following treatment, including return-to-work [46].

Acknowledgments The following individuals have participated in the CORE-TOS clinical research effort toward development of consensus-based diagnostic criteria for NTOS: David C. Cassada, MD, (Vascular Surgery) University of Tennessee, Knoxville, TN; Dean M. Donahue, MD, (Thoracic Surgery) Harvard Medical School and Massachusetts General Hospital, Boston, MA; Peter I. Edgelow, DPT, (Physical Therapy) Hayward Physical Therapy, San Francisco, CA; Julie A. Freischlag, MD, (Vascular Surgery) Johns Hopkins University and Johns Hopkins Hospital, Baltimore, MD; Hugh A.

Table 21.6 Provisional CORE-TOS criteria for the clinical diagnosis of NTOS

Unilateral or bilateral upper extremity symptoms that:

(1) Extend beyond the distribution of a single cervical nerve root or peripheral nerve

(2) Have been present for at least 12 weeks

(3) Have not been satisfactorily explained by another condition, and

(4) Meet at least one criteria in at least four of the following five categories:

Principal symptoms

　1A Pain in the neck, upper back, shoulder, arm and/or hand

　1B Numbness, paresthesias, and/or weakness in the arm, hand, or digits

Symptom characteristics

　2A Pain/paresthesias/weakness exacerbated with elevated arm positions

　2B Pain/paresthesias/weakness exacerbated with prolonged or repetitive arm/hand use, or by prolonged work on a keyboard or other repetitive strain

　2C Pain/paresthesias radiate down the arm from the supraclavicular or infraclavicular space

Clinical history

　3A symptoms began after occupational, recreational, or accidental injury of the head, neck or upper extremity, including repetitive upper extremity strain or overuse activity

　3B Previous clavicle or first rib fracture, or known cervical rib(s)

　3C Previous cervical spine or peripheral nerve surgery without sustained improvement

　3D Previous conservative or surgical treatment for TOS

Physical examination

　4A Local tenderness on palpation over scalene triangle or subcoracoid space

　4B Arm/hand/digit paresthesias on palpation over scalene triangle or subcoracoid space

　4C Weak handgrip, intrinsic muscles or digit 5, or thenar/hypothenar atrophy

Provocative maneuvers

　5A Positive upper limb tension test (ULTT)

　5B Positive 1- or 3-min elevated arm stress test (EAST)

Gelabert, MD, (Vascular Surgery) David Geffen School of Medicine at University of California-Los Angeles, Los Angeles, CA; Karl A. Illig, MD, (Vascular Surgery) University of South Florida, Tampa, FL; Kaj H. Johansen, MD, PhD, (Vascular Surgery) The Polyclinic Vascular Surgery Cherry Hill; Seattle, WA; Sheldon E. Jordan, MD, (Neurology) University of California-Los Angeles, Los Angeles, CA; Gregory J. Pearl, MD, (Vascular Surgery) Baylor University Medical Center and Baylor-Hamilton Heart and Vascular Hospital, Dallas, TX; Richard J. Sanders, MD, (Vascular Surgery) Rose Medical Center; Denver, CO; Carlos A. Selmonosky, MD, (Thoracic and Cardiovascular Surgery) Inova Fairfax Hospital, Falls Church, VA; and Robert W. Thompson, MD, (Vascular Surgery) Washington University School of Medicine and Barnes-Jewish Hospital, St. Louis, MO.

References

1. Sanders RJ. Thoracic outlet syndrome: a common sequelae of neck injuries. Philadelphia: J. B. Lippincott Company; 1991.

2. Mackinnon SE, Novak CB. Thoracic outlet syndrome. Curr Probl Surg. 2002;39(11):1070–145.

3. Thompson RW, Bartoli MA. Neurogenic thoracic outlet syndrome. In: Rutherford RB, editor. Vascular surgery. 6th ed. Philadelphia: Elsevier Saunders; 2005. p. 1347–65.

4. Sanders RJ, Hammond SL, Rao NM. Diagnosis of thoracic outlet syndrome. J Vasc Surg. 2007;46(3): 601–4.

5. Pascarelli EF, Hsu YP. Understanding work-related upper extremity disorders: clinical findings in 485 computer users, musicians, and others. J Occup Rehabil. 2001;11(1):1–21.

6. Novak CB. Thoracic outlet syndrome. Clin Plast Surg. 2003;30(2):175–88.

7. Lord JWJ, Stone PW. Pectoralis minor tenotomy and anterior scalenotomy with special reference to the hyperabduction syndrome and effort thrombosis of the subclavian vein. Circulation. 1956;13:537–42.

8. McIntyre DI. Subcoracoid neurovascular entrapment. Clin Orthop Relat Res. 1975;108:27–30.

9. Ambrad-Chalela E, Thomas GI, Johansen KH. Recurrent neurogenic thoracic outlet syndrome. Am J Surg. 2004;187(4):505–10.

10. Upton AR, McComas AJ. The double crush in nerve entrapment syndromes. Lancet. 1973;2:359–62.

11. Osterman AL. The double crush syndrome. Orthop Clin North Am. 1988;19:147–55.

12. Dellon AL, Mackinnon SE. Chronic nerve compression model for the double crush hypothesis. Ann Plast Surg. 1991;26:259–64.

13. Schenardi C. Whiplash injury. TOS and double crush syndrome. Forensic medical aspects. Acta Neurochir Suppl. 2005;92:25–7.

14. Goldenberg DL, Breekhardt C, Crofford L. Management of fibromyalgia syndrome. JAMA. 2004; 292:2388–95.

15. Wurtman RJ. Fibromyalgia and the complex regional pain syndrome: similarities in pathophysiology and treatment. Metab Clin Exp. 2010;59 Suppl 1:S37–40.

16. Schwartzmam RJ, Alexander GM, Grothusen J. Pathophysiology of complex regional pain syndrome. Expert Rev Neurother. 2006;6:669–81.

17. Albazaz R, Wong YT, Horner-Vanniasnkam S. Complex regional pain syndrome: a review. Ann Vasc Surg. 2008;22:297–306.

18. Gilliatt RW, Le Quesne PM, Logue V, Sumner AJ. Wasting of the hand associated with a cervical rib or band. J Neurol Neurosurg Psychiatry. 1970;33:615–24.

19. Tender GC, Thomas AJ, Thomas N, Kline DG. Gilliatt-sumner hand revisited: a 25-year experience. Neurosurgery. 2004;55:883–90.

20. Collins JD, Disher AC, Miller TQ. The anatomy of the brachial plexus as displayed by magnetic resonance imaging: technique and application. J Natl Med Assoc. 1995;87:489–98.

21. Saxton EH, Miller TQ, Collins JD. Migraine complicated by brachial plexopathy as displayed by MRI and MRA: aberrant subclavian artery and cervical ribs. J Natl Med Assoc. 1999;91:333–41.

22. van Es HW. MRI of the brachial plexus. Eur Radiol. 2001;11:325–36.

23. Demondion X, Bacqueville E, Paul C, Duquesnoy B, Hachulla E, Cotten A. Thoracic outlet: assessment with MR imaging in asymptomatic and symptomatic populations. Radiology. 2003;227:461–8.

24. Demondion X, Herbinet P, Van Sint Jan S, Boutry N, Chantelot C, Cotten A. Imaging assessment of thoracic outlet syndrome. Radiographics. 2006;26:1735–50.

25. Demirbag D, Unlu E, Ozdemir F, Genchellac H, Temizoz O, Ozdemir H, Demir MK. The relationship between magnetic resonance imaging findings and postural maneuver and physical examination tests in patients with thoracic outlet syndrome: results of a double-blind, controlled study. Arch Phys Med Rehabil. 2007;88(7):844–51.

26. Rubin M, Lange DJ. Sensory nerve abnormalities in brachial plexopathy. Eur Neurol. 1992;32:245–7.

27. Nishida T, Price SJ, Minieka MM. Medial antebrachial cutaneous nerve conduction in true neurogenic thoracic outlet syndrome. Electromyogr Clin Neurophysiol. 1993;33:285–8.

28. Cruz-Martinez A, Arpa J. Electrophysiological assessment in neurogenic thoracic outlet syndrome. Electromyogr Clin Neurophysiol. 2001;41:253–6.

29. Machanic BI, Sanders RJ. Medial antebrachial cutaneous nerve measurements to diagnose neurogenic thoracic outlet syndrome. Ann Vasc Surg. 2008;22(2):248–54.

30. Jordan SE, Ahn SS, Gelabert HA. Differentiation of thoracic outlet syndrome from treatment-resistant cervical brachial pain syndromes: development and utilization of a questionnaire, clinical examination and ultrasound evaluation. Pain Physician. 2007;10(3): 441–52.

31. Axelrod DA, Proctor MC, Geisser ME, Roth RS, Greenfield LJ. Outcomes after surgery for thoracic outlet syndrome. J Vasc Surg. 2001;33(6):1220–5.

32. Graham B, Regehr G, Wright JG. Delphi as a method to establish consensus for diagnostic criteria. J Clin Epidemiol. 2003;56(12):1150–6.

33. Holey EA, Feeley JL, Dixon J, Whittaker VJ. An exploration of the use of simple statistics to measure consensus and stability in delphi studies. BMC Med Res Methodol. 2007;7:52.

34. Kellum JA, Mehta RL, Levin A, Molitoris BA, Warnock DG, Shah SV, Joannidis M, Ronco C, Acute Kidney Injury Network. Development of a clinical research agenda for acute kidney injury using an international, interdisciplinary, three-step modified delphi process. Clin J Am Soc Nephrol. 2008;3:887–94.

35. Dahmen R, van der Wilden GJ, Lankhorst GJ, Boers M. Delphi process yielded consensus on terminology and research agenda for therapeutic footwear for neuropathic foot. J Clin Epidemiol. 2008;61:819–26.

36. Emery VB, Rastogi R, Driskill MR, Thompson RW. Diagnosis of neurogenic thoracic outlet syndrome. In: Eskandari MK, Morasch MD, Pearce WH, Yao JST, editors. Vascular surgery: therapeutic strategies. Shelton: People's Medical Publishing House-USA; 2010. p. 129–48.

37. Graham B, Dvali L, Regehr G, Wright JG. Variations in diagnostic criteria for carpal tunnel syndrome among ontario specialists. Am J Ind Med. 2006;49(1): 8–13.

38. Graham B, Regehr G, Naglie G, Wright JG. Development and validation of diagnostic criteria for carpal tunnel syndrome. J Hand Surg Am. 2006;31(6):919–24.

39. Hudak PL, Amadio PC, Bombardier C. Development of an upper extremity outcome measure: the DASH (disabilities of the arm, shoulder and hand). The Upper Extremity Collaborative Group (UECG). Am J Ind Med. 1996;29(6):602–8.

40. Kirkley A, Griffin S, Dainty K. Scoring systems for the functional assessment of the shoulder. Arthroscopy. 2003;19(10):1109–20.

41. Cordobes-Gual J, Lozano-Vilardell P, Torreguitart-Mirada N, Lara-Hernandez R, Riera-Vazquez R, Julia-Montoya J. Prospective study of the functional recovery after surgery for thoracic outlet syndrome. Eur J Vasc Endovasc Surg. 2008;35:79–83.

42. Keller S, Bann CM, Dodd SL, Schein J, Mendoza TR, Cleeland CS. Validity of the brief pain inventory for use in documenting the outcomes of patients with noncancer pain. Clin J Pain. 2004;20(5):309–18.

43. Zelman DC, Gore M, Dukes E, Tai KS, Brandenburg N. Validation of a modified version of the brief pain inventory for painful diabetic peripheral neuropathy. J Pain Symptom Manage. 2005;29(4):401–10.

44. Mendoza TR, Mayne T, Rublee D, Cleeland C. Reliability and validity of a modified brief pain inventory short form in patients with osteoarthritis. Eur J Pain. 2006;10(4):353–61.

45. Ware Jr J, Kosinski M, Keller SD. A 12-item short-form health survey: construction of scales and preliminary tests of reliability and validity. Med Care. 1996;34(3): 220–33.

46. Chang DC, Rotellini-Coltvet L, Mukherjee D, DeLeon R, Freischlag JA. Surgical intervention for thoracic outlet syndrome improves patients' quality of life. J Vasc Surg. 2009;49:630–5.

Pathways of Care and Treatment Options for Patients with NTOS

22

Valerie B. Emery and Robert W. Thompson

Abstract

Thoracic outlet syndrome (TOS) is a rare and complex group of disorders that may cause severe and disabling symptoms, and caring for patients with these conditions provides many challenges to health care providers. An organized, systematic, approach to the diagnosis and treatment of TOS provides an opportunity for specialists to deliver patient-centered care and to achieve optimal results with treatment. This specialized type of care is best delivered through the efforts of a multi-disciplinary team that consists of various specialists, including vascular surgery, thoracic surgery, neurology/neurosurgery, orthopedics, radiology, anesthesiology, pain management, physical therapy, and occupational therapy. This chapter will focus on the care path for managing patients with a diagnosis of neurogenic TOS (NTOS), as based on our experience at Washington University/Barnes-Jewish Hospital in St. Louis. Evaluation and care of patients with venous and arterial forms of TOS are covered elsewhere in this textbook.

V.B. Emery, RN, ANP (✉)
Section of Vascular Surgery,
Center for Thoracic Outlet Syndrome,
School of Medicine, Washington University,
666 South Eucld 5101 Queeny Towers,
Campus Box 8109, Saint Louis,
MO 63376, USA
e-mail: emeryv@wudosis.wustl.edu

R.W. Thompson, MD
Department of Surgery, Section of Vascular Surgery,
Center for Thoracic Outlet Syndrome,
Washington University, Barnes-Jewish
Hospital, 660 S Euclid Avenue, Campus
Box 8109/Suite 5101 Queeny Tower,
St. Louis, MO 63110, USA
e-mail: thompson@wudosis.wustl.edu

Initial Presentation

Patients presenting for evaluation of NTOS are referred from a variety of sources, including primary care physicians, neurologists/neurosurgeons, pain management physicians, orthopedic surgeons, sports medicine physicians, emergency room physicians, physical therapists, occupational therapists, and chiropractors. Another important route for presentation is patient self-referral, prompted by word-of-mouth, local news stories, and a rapidly increasing amount of information available on the internet.

The day of the initial office visit is carefully planned in order to provide a thorough review of

K.A. Illig et al. (eds.), *Thoracic Outlet Syndrome*,
DOI 10.1007/978-1-4471-4366-6_22, © Springer-Verlag London 2013

previous medical records and imaging studies, a detailed history, a comprehensive physical examination, and a determination regarding the likelihood of a clinical diagnosis of NTOS. The history will include pertinent information regarding the onset, duration, and type of symptoms experienced, the distribution of symptoms, any aggravating activities or other factors, and a description of any previous injury that preceded the onset of symptoms. The level of disability produced by the symptoms, particularly any interference with work-related activities, is carefully assessed.

The physical examination includes evaluation of the range of motion of the neck and upper extremity, any tenderness and/or reproduction of symptoms upon digital palpation over the supraclavicular (scalene triangle) and/or subcoracoid (pectoralis minor tendon) spaces, and screening for postural and/or movement abnormalities. Evidence for degenerative cervical spine disease is sought by localized tenderness, range-of-motion of the neck, and physical maneuvers (e.g., Spurling's sign). The cubital and carpal tunnel spaces are also palpated for tenderness and reproduction of paresthesias that might reflect ulnar and/or median nerve compression syndromes, respectively. The radial pulse is evaluated by palpation at rest as well as in the arm-elevated position to assess for positional ablation of the pulse (e.g., the Adson maneuver), taking care to maneuver the arm slowly in order to avoid vasospasm that might lead to inaccurate findings. It is also helpful to clarify if the patient's symptoms are aggravated by different degrees of arm elevation, and how this may or may not coincide with a decrease in the strength of the pulse; positional aggravation of arm/hand symptoms when the radial pulse is palpable serves to verify that the symptoms are not ischemic in nature but more likely due to nerve compression. Finally, provocative maneuvers specifically designed to assess the presence or absence of positional brachial plexus compression are an important part of the physical examination for NTOS, including the Upper Limb Tension Test (ULTT) and the 3-min Elevated Arm Stress Test (EAST).

The diagnosis of NTOS is ultimately established by a series of positive history and physical

Table 22.1 Etiology, differential diagnosis, and testing for neurogenic TOS

Etiologic factors contributing to NTOS
Anatomic variations and anomalies (cervical rib, scalene minimus muscle, fibrofascial bands)
Scalene/pectoralis muscle trauma
Bony trauma (clavicle fracture, first rib fracture)
Repetitive motion injury
Postural abnormalities and motion disturbances
Stereotypical findings in NTOS
History of whiplash-type neck trauma, fall on the arm or head, or repetitive motion injury
Symptoms of pain, numbness and tingling from neck to hand, typically all fingers
Symptoms vary day-to-day, consistently exacerbated by arm elevation
Supraclavicular/subcoracoid tenderness to palpation
Reproduction of symptoms upon supraclavicular/subcoracoid palpation
Positive upper limb tension test (ULTT)
Positive 3-min elevated arm stress test (EAST)
Principal differential diagnoses
Degenerative cervical spine disease (disc herniation, arthropathy, radiculopathy)
Primary shoulder joint pathology (rotator cuff tear, arthropathy, tendonitis)
Distal entrapment neuropathy (carpal tunnel syndrome, cubital canal syndrome)
Complex regional pain syndrome (CRPS)
Diagnostic testing in NTOS
Chest X-ray
Cervical spine imaging (CT, MRI)
Shoulder imaging (MRI)
EMG/NC studies
Cervical sympathetic block (stellate ganglion)
Scalene/pectoralis minor muscle block

exam findings coupled with the exclusion of other conditions that might produce similar symptoms (Table 22.1) [1–3]. The patient who presents with a history and physical examination findings that are not consistent with NTOS is referred to other specialists for further evaluation, in order to determine an alternative etiology for the symptoms. Additional diagnostic testing should be considered including cervical spine and shoulder imaging, as well as upper extremity electromyography and nerve conduction (EMG/NC) studies. In the absence of NTOS, the results of these diagnostic tests may indicate the need

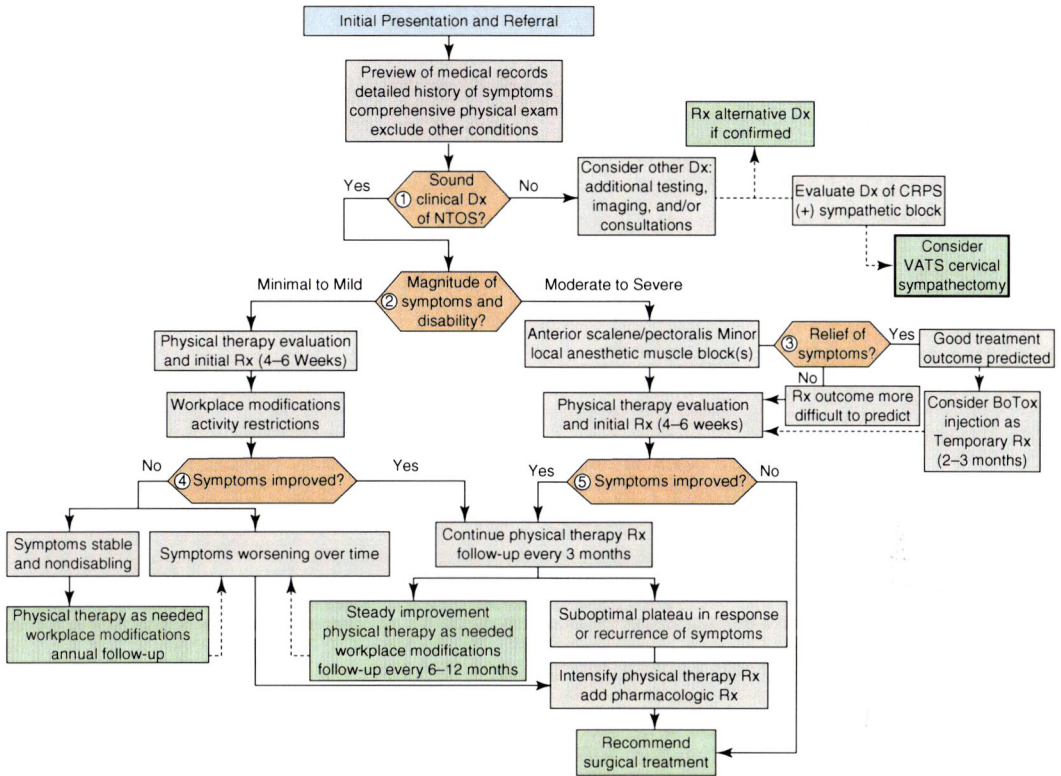

Fig. 22.1 Care-path for neurogenic TOS-I. Algorithm for the evaluation and management of patients presenting with NTOS, as developed at Washington University/Barnes-Jewish Hospital

for referral to an appropriate specialist in neurology, neurosurgery, orthopedics, and/or hand surgery (Fig. 22.1, *Box 1*).

Once a clinical diagnosis of NTOS has been established, the magnitude of symptoms and level of disability are assessed to guide further treatment (Fig. 22.1, *Box 2*). Patients with mild-to-minimal symptoms and disability are directed to conservative management for NTOS based primarily on physical therapy and occupational therapy, with the hope that some will achieve substantial improvement or at least a stabilization of symptoms (Fig. 22.1, *Box 4*). Patients with moderate-to-severe symptoms and disability, particularly when interfering with daily activities or work, longstanding in duration, and/or worsening over time, should undergo further diagnostic testing to provide support for the clinical diagnosis and to indicate the possible responsiveness to treatment.

Anterior Scalene/Pectoralis Minor Muscle Blocks

In the hands of a skilled and experienced interventionist, use of ultrasound- or fluoroscopically-guided anesthetic blocks of the anterior scalene and/or pectoralis minor muscles is an important component of the care path (Fig. 22.1, *Box 3*) [4, 5]. (See Chap. 27). Depending upon the constellation of symptoms and physical exam findings, a combined anterior scalene muscle and pectoralis minor muscle anesthetic block may be performed, to ensure that the response is not masked by persistent brachial plexus compression at one or the other location. It may also be appropriate to perform sequential, staged, anesthetic blocks, in which the patient will first undergo an isolated block of either the anterior scalene muscle or pectoralis minor muscle, followed at another time by a combined block or an isolated block of the site not previously tested. This is especially helpful in patients considered to have symptoms generated by brachial plexus compression at a single location, such as those with predominantly subcoracoid symptoms, for whom treatment isolated to the pectoralis minor might be considered. As discussed in Chap. 20, "Scalene Test Blocks and Interventional Techniques in patients with TOS," ideally the patient should be blinded as to the substance injected, but this is not always practical. The physician and staff directing the evaluation for NTOS should re-examine the patient as soon as possible following the procedure, in order to determine the extent and duration of the response. A positive response to an anterior scalene/pectoralis minor muscle block is achieved when the patient experiences a temporary improvement or relief of neurogenic symptoms with and without provocative maneuvers; this strongly supports the clinical diagnosis of NTOS and indicates a high likelihood that the patient will respond well to treatment, whether through conservative measures or surgery. In making this determination it is also important to consider that false-positive scalene/pectoralis minor muscle blocks may occasionally occur, due to placebo effects and/or examiner biases, such that appropriate effort should be made to minimize such effects.

Although anterior scalene/pectoralis minor blocks performed with local anesthetic are expected to be relatively short-acting (hours), in the event of a positive block it may also be reasonable to offer a similar procedure with injection of botulinum toxin to achieve a more durable result [6]. The effects of botulinum toxin on scalene muscle spasm are expected to last only 2–3 months, but in some cases the reduction in nerve irritation may extend to 5–6 months when accompanied by secondary scalene muscle atrophy. Because these effects remain temporary and do not serve as definitive treatment of the underlying condition, many physicians and patients prefer a potentially more durable approach in the form of surgical therapy.

The anterior scalene/pectoralis minor muscle block is considered negative if the patient experiences no relief of symptoms immediately after the procedure. While a negative block may be due to technical limitations (incomplete interruption of muscle spasm by the amount or location of anesthetic injected), it is important to note that this may also occur when spasm in the anterior scalene and/or pectoralis minor muscles is not a prominent cause of symptoms: in the presence of a fixed brachial plexus compression by bony or soft tissue anomalies, when there is extensive scalene/pectoralis muscle fibrosis that precludes responsiveness to the anesthetic, when middle scalene or subclavius muscle spasm make significant contributions to nerve irritation, or when there has been longstanding neural injury that may not be readily alleviated. Thus, a negative response cannot be used to exclude the diagnosis of NTOS, but serves to lower the likelihood that the patient will have a substantial response to treatment.

Complex Regional Pain Syndrome (CRPS)

Some patients seeking evaluation for NTOS present with symptoms of complex regional pain syndrome (CRPS, previously known as reflex sympathetic dystrophy), a sympathetic-mediated pain syndrome associated with extreme hypersensitivity to touch (allodynia) and vascular alterations in the hand (digital vasoconstriction and edema). CRPS may occur as an isolated condition that mimics some aspects of NTOS, or it may occur in conjunction with NTOS as a result of severe or longstanding brachial plexus compression (see Chap. 39). In these situations it has been our experience that a cervical sympathetic (stellate ganglion) block can be useful in augmenting the clinical diagnosis of CRPS and in separating the contribution of CRPS from any concomitant symptoms attributable to NTOS. Surgical cervical sympathectomy may be an appropriate consideration for CRPS in some patients, and we have used a positive response to stellate ganglion block to guide decision-making regarding the use of sympathectomy at the same time as thoracic outlet decompression in patients undergoing surgery for NTOS [7]. Patients presenting with isolated CRPS may also be treated with serial stellate ganglion blocks and/or surgical sympathectomy; when performed as an isolated procedure, cervical sympathectomy can be most effectively performed by video-assisted thoracoscopic surgery (VATS).

Physical Therapy and Occupational Therapy Evaluation and Treatment

Comprehensive evaluation by a physical therapist and/or occupational therapist that is experienced in the management of patients with NTOS is an essential part of the care path, regardless of the magnitude of symptoms or disability (Fig. 22.1, *Boxes 4 and 5*) [2, 8, 9]. Patients with mild-to-minimal symptoms should undergo an initial evaluation followed by a 6–8 week course of physical therapy treatment directed at relaxing and stretching the scalene and pectoralis minor muscles, improving shoulder girdle mechanics, and correcting postural changes. Occupational therapy can provide important additions to treatment, such as changes in workplace ergonomics, defined modifications and restrictions in upper extremity activity, and guided progression in workplace activity once an initial improvement in symptom control has been achieved. Patients with mild symptoms who improve with physical and occupational therapy should continue a home exercise program with office follow-up as needed. Physical and occupational therapy treatment should be repeated if symptoms return and/or progress in severity. These patients should also be considered for possible re-evaluation with more aggressive measures, including diagnostic blocks and surgical decompression.

Patients presenting with moderate-to-severe symptoms should be promptly evaluated by the physical and/or occupational therapist to evaluate the appropriateness and efficacy of any previous therapy that the patient may have undergone, and to outline an appropriate treatment plan for the presenting situation. An initial course of physical and occupational therapy treatment is undertaken, under the oversight and supervision by the specialist therapist. Patients who have had extensive therapy that is considered to have been appropriate for NTOS, and those in whom symptoms are aggravated by physical therapy such that effective

treatment will not be possible, are referred back to the initial treating physician for consideration of surgical treatment. Whenever feasible, the initial course of therapy should continue for 6–8 weeks, with oversight by the specialist therapist if treatment is to be implemented by another therapist closer to the place of residence, including frequent communication between therapists and physicians as needed. If symptoms appear to be improving during this time, physical and occupational therapy treatment will be continued as long as progress is observed at regular follow-up evaluations, typically every 6–8 weeks. Muscle relaxants, anti-inflammatory agents, and analgesics are also appropriate for patients with moderate to severe symptoms, particularly to assist with the effectiveness of conservative management.

Surgical Treatment

Thoracic outlet decompression is appropriate for patients who have a sound clinical diagnosis of NTOS and have failed to improve with physical therapy, particularly for those who have had a positive response to an anterior scalene and/or pectoralis minor muscle block [2, 10]. Surgical options preferred in our institution include pectoralis minor tenotomy; supraclavicular decompression with scalenectomy, brachial plexus neurolysis and first rib resection; or a combined procedure that includes both supraclavicular decompression and pectoralis minor tenotomy. In other institutions, transaxillary first rib resection is the preferred approach to thoracic outlet decompression for NTOS, with or without concomitant pectoralis minor tenotomy. It is notable that in the past 5 years there has been an increasing recognition of the role of brachial plexus compression at the level of the subcoracoid space in NTOS, along with an appreciation that initial treatment with an isolated pectoralis minor tenotomy may provide substantial symptom relief and greater ability to participate in physical therapy; thus, we currently favor the use of pectoralis minor tenotomy as the initial surgical treatment in patients in whom this site is the predominant location of neural compression [11]. In contrast,

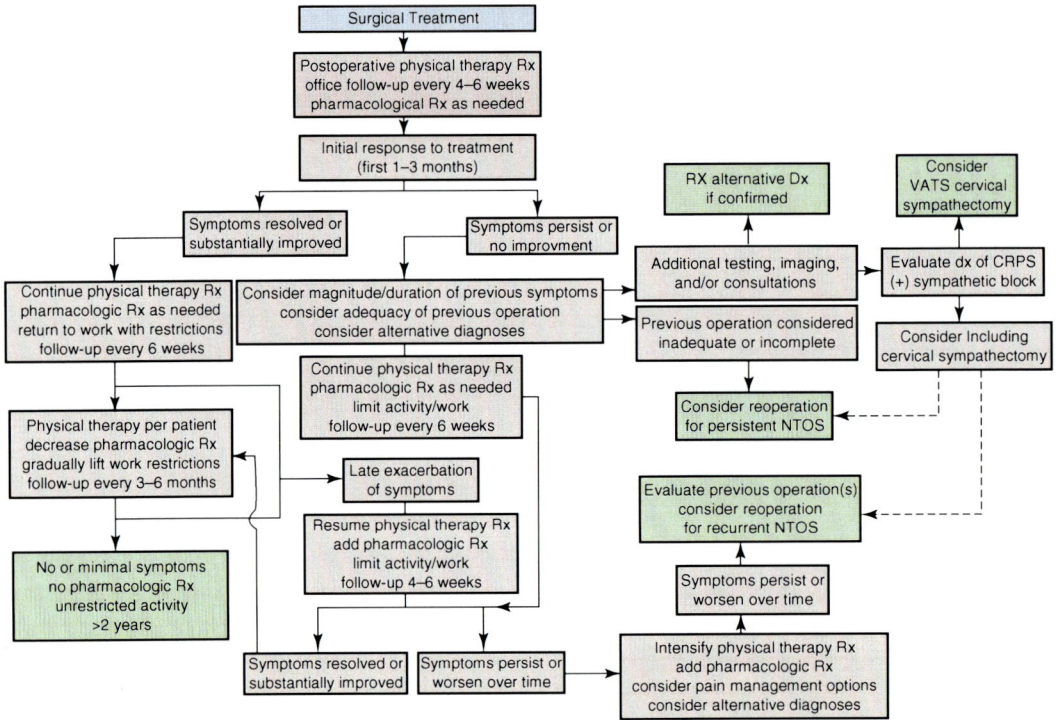

Fig. 22.2 Care-path for neurogenic TOS-II. Algorithm for the evaluation and management of patients that have undergone surgery for NTOS, as developed at Washington University/Barnes-Jewish Hospital

to achieve the most satisfactory results we recommend complete supraclavicular decompression, with or without concomitant pectoralis minor tenotomy, in patients who have evidence for substantial brachial plexus compression at the level of the scalene triangle.

Patients undergoing supraclavicular decompression for NTOS typically require a 3–5-day hospital stay. During the operative procedure, a small-caliber multihole catheter is inserted and placed in the surgical field alongside the brachial plexus, for continuous postoperative infusion of local anesthetic (0.5 % bupivacaine), to assist with post-operative pain management. A closed-suction drain is also placed in the surgical field to provide drainage of surgical fluids away from the area of the brachial plexus. During the first 24–48 h, the primary goal of care is to achieve good control of postoperative pain and anesthesia-related nausea. Once pain has been under adequate control utilizing continuous local anesthetic infusion and opioid narcotics administered

by intravenous patient-controlled analgesia (PCA), oral pain medications and muscle relaxants are started, the PCA is weaned, and the local anesthetic infusion device is discontinued (postoperative day 3). The patient is seen by an in-patient physical therapist beginning the day after surgery and provided with a series of range-of-motion exercises. Patients are discharged once the patient is tolerating a regular diet and pain and muscle spasm are sufficiently controlled with oral medications. Following hospital discharge the patient will undergo close monitoring and follow-up by the operating surgeon and treatment team, including the specialist physical therapist that was previously involved in the patient's care. Patients are seen on a regular follow-up schedule and are cared for on an indefinite basis, in recognition of the chronic nature of NTOS and the potential for later development of recurrent symptoms. Figure 22.2 outlines our current care path for the long-term management of patients having undergone surgical treatment for NTOS.

As noted above, isolated pectoralis minor tenotomy is an excellent treatment option in a select group of patients who present with symptoms of NTOS. Pectoralis minor tenotomy is a short (30 min) procedure that can be safely performed in the outpatient setting, with the patient being discharged home after recovery. We continue to prefer use of brief general anesthesia for pectoralis minor tenotomy; although intravenous sedation and local anesthesia is a feasible alternative, we have found it difficult to perform this procedure with a satisfactory level of patient comfort with this approach. Medications typically prescribed upon discharge home include a muscle relaxant and an opioid analgesic, limited up to 1 week from the operative procedure. Postoperative activity with the affected arm is minimally restricted until office follow-up and physical therapy re-evaluation within the first 2 weeks after surgery, at which time the patient is allowed to gradually increase activity. Physical therapy follow-up is continued on a long-term basis, along with ongoing management by the treating surgeon.

Follow-Up Care

Long-term management of the patient with NTOS requires on-going coordination of care from the thoracic outlet center team (Fig. 22.2). With proper selection for surgical treatment it is expected that approximately 80–90 % of patients will experience a substantial improvement in symptoms of NTOS within the first 3 months after operation. Patients who experience progressive and sustained improvement in symptoms following either conservative care or surgical treatment will need to maintain a home exercise program and physical therapy intervention as needed, and intermittent follow-up is provided on an indefinite basis. Patient that have not obtained improvement in symptoms following surgical treatment are considered to have persistent NTOS. In this event the diagnosis is reconsidered and additional evaluation for alternative conditions is carried out. The adequacy of the previous operation is also re-evaluated to determine if

additional surgical options should be considered early in the follow-up period.

Even in patients who have achieved substantial and sustained improvement in symptoms following treatment, there will be a small proportion that will develop recurrent symptoms over time [12, 13]. This typically occurs within 1–2 years after primary surgical treatment and is often associated with a secondary injury, which likely re-initiates wound-healing responses in the surgical field leading to additional scar tissue formation in the area of the brachial plexus. Recurrent symptoms may also occur following an inappropriate return to workplace activities that involve overhead or heavy use of the affected upper extremity or extensive repetitive motion, situations in which job retraining would have been better advised. Treatment options for recurrent NTOS include intensified physical therapy and pharmacologic management, trigger point injections for areas of focal muscle spasm, and injection of botulinum toxin to selected muscles. Reoperation is considered if the diagnosis of recurrent NTOS is sound and it is not possible to achieve adequate symptom control with conservative measures. In this event, operative re-exploration through a supraclavicular exposure is preferred, with brachial plexus neurolysis to remove fibrous scar tissue and achieve maximal mobility of the nerve roots. Any inadequacies of the initial operation are also corrected, such as removal of a first rib remnant or incompletely resected scalene muscle, along with consideration for pectoralis minor tenotomy if appropriate.

Patients with persistent symptoms of NTOS despite the use of maximum medical and surgical treatment may need chronic pain management with muscle relaxants, non-narcotic and/or narcotic analgesics, additional neurotropic medications, psychosocial support, and maintenance physical therapy. In some cases, additional interventional pain management techniques may also be appropriate and helpful (e.g., placement of a spinal cord stimulator). In addition to the other approaches described, patients that remain relatively stable but experience a temporary "flare" or exacerbation of chronic symptoms may benefit from a short-course of treatment

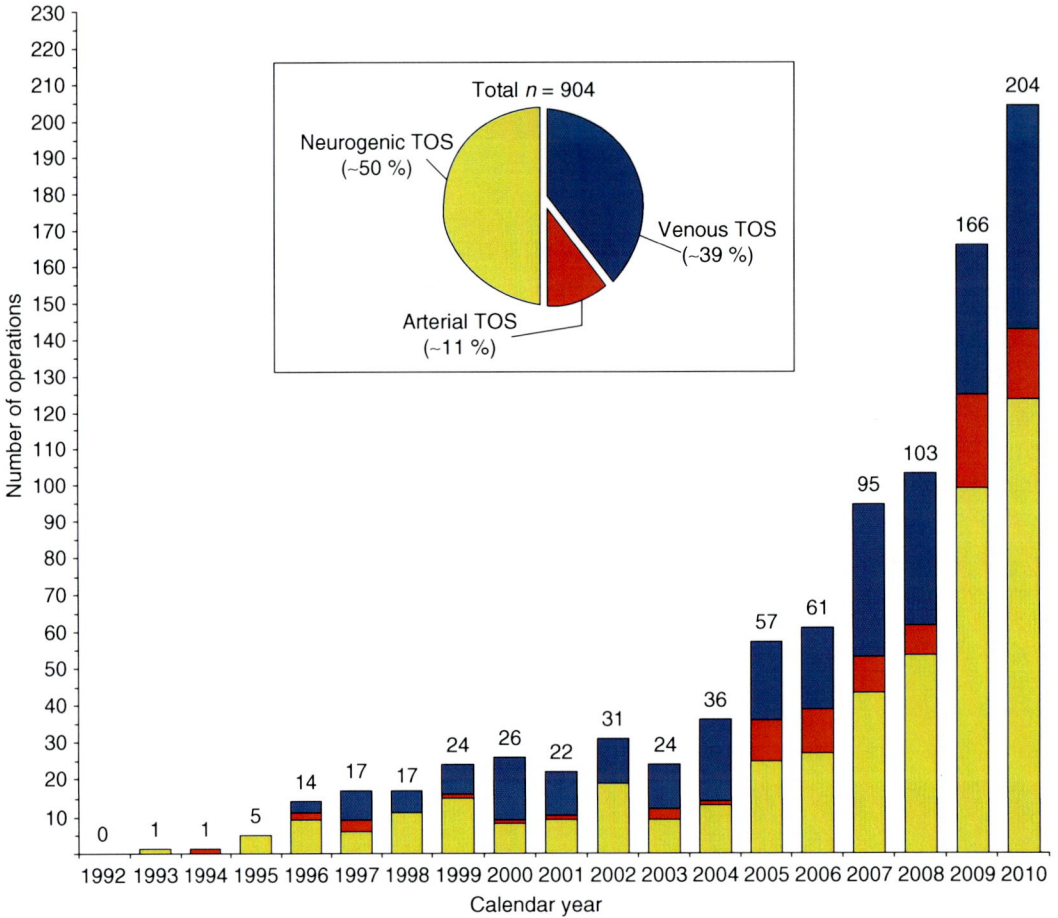

Fig. 22.3 Surgical treatment for TOS. Bar graph illustrating the number of operations for all forms of TOS performed at Washington University/Barnes-Jewish Hospital, 1992–2010

with glucocorticosteroids (e.g., methylprednisolone). Thus, patients with chronic symptoms may continue to experience periods of acute exacerbations that require on-going management and intervention, interspersed with periods of symptom stability and increased function.

The "Center" Approach to NTOS

Our experience indicates that patients with NTOS achieve excellent clinical and functional outcomes when their care is provided through a specialized center that utilizes a well-organized, multidisciplinary, and comprehensive approach to the diagnosis and management of all forms of

TOS. Several years ago we sought to accomplish this in our area by establishing the Center for Thoracic Outlet Syndrome at Washington University School of Medicine and Barnes-Jewish Hospital, located at a large tertiary-care academic medical center in a medium-size midwestern city. While the first patient with TOS that we treated was in 1993, over the next 15 years there was a gradual increase in the number of patients seen, coinciding with increasing local/regional recognition of our interests in TOS, good clinical outcomes, patient satisfaction, and word-of-mouth referrals (Fig. 22.3). A "Center" approach to TOS was more formally initiated in 2008–2009, with the additional of a dedicated nurse practitioner and medical assistant, a re-focusing of clinical practice to be almost entirely directed toward TOS, the inclusion of strong affiliations with specific physical and occupational therapists, pain management physicians, radiologists, and others with relevant expertise, and development of an informational website for patients, physicians, and practitioners (www.tos.wustl.edu). Being located within a large academic medical center has also allowed easy access to world-class consultants in orthopedics, sport medicine, neurology/neurosurgery and other areas, as well as superb facilities for radiologic and surgical procedures and inpatient care. These steps have allowed our group to evolve into a highly specialized center of excellence for the care of patients with all forms of TOS, in which we currently evaluate 7–8 new patients and perform 5–6 surgical procedures each week, and maintain a robust schedule of long-term follow-up for nearly 1,000 patients. While approximately 60 % of our patients are from the 6-county greater St. Louis metropolitan area, 20 % come from elsewhere in the adjacent states of Missouri and Illinois and another 20 % come from elsewhere in the U.S. Important components of our approach have been to provide care under the overall direction of a single individual with a clinical practice focused entirely on TOS and by taking a highly individualized approach to each patient while maintaining a broad view of the potential overlapping and coexisting diagnoses, to avoid taking a standardized "protocol-driven" approach for all patients. With this ongoing experience the members of our multidisciplinary team also meet on a monthly basis to provide interdisciplinary updates relevant to TOS, to review plans of care for specific patients, to discuss recent advances and controversies in the field, and to plan new educational and research initiatives. Through these efforts we believe we have been able to provide an organized, efficient, thorough and patient-centered approach to care of those presenting with neurogenic and other forms of TOS, and to help develop successful care-paths and management algorithms that are focused on achieving excellent results for an otherwise extremely challenging population of patients.

References

1. Sanders RJ, Hammond SL, Rao NM. Diagnosis of thoracic outlet syndrome. J Vasc Surg. 2007;46(3): 601–4.
2. Thompson RW, Driskill M. Thoracic outlet syndrome: neurogenic. In: Cronenwett JL, Johnston KW, editors. Rutherford's vascular surgery. 7th ed. Philadelphia: Elsevier; 2010. p. 1878–98.
3. Emery VB, Rastogi R, Driskill MR, Thompson RW. Diagnosis of neurogenic thoracic outlet syndrome. In: Eskandari MK, Morasch MD, Pearce WH, Yao JST, editors. Vascular surgery: therapeutic strategies. Shelton: People's Medical Publishing House-USA; 2010. p. 129–48.
4. Jordan SE, Machleder HI. Diagnosis of thoracic outlet syndrome using electrophysiologically guided anterior scalene blocks. Ann Vasc Surg. 1998;12(3): 260–4.
5. Jordan SE, Ahn SS, Gelabert HA. Differentiation of thoracic outlet syndrome from treatment-resistant cervical brachial pain syndromes: development and utilization of a questionnaire, clinical examination and ultrasound evaluation. Pain Physician. 2007;10(3): 441–52.
6. Jordan SE, Ahn SS, Freischlag JA, Gelabert HA, Machleder HI. Selective botulinum chemodenervation of the scalene muscles for treatment of neurogenic thoracic outlet syndrome. Ann Vasc Surg. 2000; 14(4):365–9.
7. Thompson RW. Treatment of thoracic outlet syndromes and cervical sympathectomy. In: Lumley JSP, Hoballah JJ, editors. Springer surgery atlas series: vascular surgery. London: Springer; 2009. p. 103–18.
8. Novak CB. Conservative management of thoracic outlet syndrome. Semin Thorac Cardiovasc Surg. 1996; 8(2):201–7.
9. Edgelow P. Neurovascular consequences of cumulative trauma disorders affecting the thoracic outlet: a patient centered treatment approach. In: Donatelli R, editor. Physical therapy of the shoulder. New York: Churchill Livingston; 2004. p. 205–38.
10. Thompson RW, Petrinec D, Toursarkissian B. Surgical treatment of thoracic outlet compression syndromes. II. Supraclavicular exploration and vascular reconstruction. Ann Vasc Surg. 1997;11(4):442–51.
11. Sanders RJ. Pectoralis minor syndrome. In: Eskandari MK, Morasch MD, Pearce WH, Yao JST, editors. Vascular surgery: therapeutic strategies. Shelton: People's Medical Publishing House-USA; 2010. p. 149–60.
12. Ambrad-Chalela E, Thomas GI, Johansen KH. Recurrent neurogenic thoracic outlet syndrome. Am J Surg. 2004;187(4):505–10.
13. Altobelli GG, Kudo T, Haas BT, Chandra FA, Moy JL, Ahn SS. Thoracic outlet syndrome: pattern of clinical success after operative decompression. J Vasc Surg. 2005;42(1):122–8.

Peter I. Edgelow

Abstract

Many, if not most patients with neurogenic thoracic outlet syndrome (NTOS) benefit from physical therapy, either as sole treatment or as an adjunct to surgery. Over the past few decades we have developed a protocol based on our perspective of the etiology and management of a variety of types of cumulative trauma disorders (including NTOS) which brings together the knowledge, experience and clinical findings to focus on the interactions of the structure and function of the human body and how it adapts to repetitive trauma whether that trauma is caused by accidents, life activities, or disease. The residual impairments and functional disabilities that result have factors in common that can be identified and corrected. Discussion of findings regarding evaluation and intervention effectiveness will be intertwined with specific clinical ideas for managing patients with these conditions. A model addressing the behavioral, biomechanical, cardiopulmonary and neurological aspects of chronic pain and repetitive strain injuries will broaden the traditional role of the orthopedic or neurological physical therapist. Further, this model will help to shift the traditional role of the physical therapist from a "hands on provider" to an educator/coach whose role is to empower the patient to take responsibility for improving quality of life.

Introduction

Many, if not most patients with neurogenic thoracic outlet syndrome (NTOS) benefit from physical therapy, either as sole treatment or as an adjunct to surgery. Over the past few decades we have developed a protocol based on our perspective of the etiology and management of a variety of types of cumulative trauma disorders (including NTOS). It brings together the knowledge, experience and clinical findings to focus on the interactions of the structure and function of the human body and how it adapts to repetitive trauma whether that trauma is caused by accidents, life activities, or disease.

P.I. Edgelow, DPT
Graduate Program in Physical Therapy, UCSF/SFSU,
2429 Balmoral St, Union City, CA 94587, USA
e-mail: peteriedgelow@aol.com

K.A. Illig et al. (eds.), *Thoracic Outlet Syndrome*,
DOI 10.1007/978-1-4471-4366-6_23, © Springer-Verlag London 2013

The Problem Seen as Loss of Motor Control

Over the past 20 years clinical observations and research suggest that following trauma to the cervical spine and/or thoracic outlet there is a motor control imbalance involving spinal and shoulder girdle muscular stability. There is also a breathing control problem due to accentuating the accessory breathing muscles more than the diaphragm [1–8]. Muscles that function primarily as stabilizers become hypoactive and muscles that function primarily as movers become hyperactive. This imbalance results in a problem of weakness or inhibition in the deep flexors of one of the ulnar innervated thumb flexors in addition to hypoactivity of the deep neck flexors, lower fibers of trapezius, serratus anterior and the abdominal corset. In tandem with this hypoactivity of the stabilizers [9–12], there is hyperactivity of the movers of the neck and ribs 1 through 5, including the anterior, middle and posterior scalenes, subclavius, pectoralis minor, upper trapezius, and levator scapulae. Histological analysis of scalene muscles removed during thoracic outlet decompression for NTOS demonstrates excess scar tissue within the muscles which results in a loss of flexibility, shortening of the muscle, and resultant narrowing of the muscular boundaries of the thoracic outlet [13].

The Problem Seen as Breathing Dysfunction

Epidemiologic evidence supports a link between breathing difficulties and back pain [14]. Since trunk muscles perform both postural and breathing functions, it is theorized that disruption in one function can negatively impact the other. Altered breathing mechanics can change respiratory chemistry and therefore pH, causing smooth muscle constriction, altered electrolyte balance, and decreased tissue oxygenation. These changes can profoundly impact any body system. Increased excitability in the muscular and nervous systems may be most relevant to a physical therapist. Respiratory function can be tested via capnography which measures CO_2 and end tidal CO_2 ($ETCO_2$), which closely

reflects arterial CO_2 in people with normal cardiopulmonary function. A case series of 29 outpatients with neck or back pain who had plateaued with manual therapy and exercise were found to have low $ETCO_2$ [15]. Breathing retraining improved $ETCO_2$, pain, and function in all patients, with 93 % achieving at least a clinically important change in either pain or function.

Many patients present with an accessory sternal breathing pattern in relaxed inhalation when they should be using the diaphragm. This could be a function of patterns of stress driven by sympathetic arousal or inhibition of a deep breath due to movement of the brachial plexus during breathing. The plexus behaves like cords that can be pulled or slid from both proximal and distal ends depending on the arm and spinal movements. Ultrasonography demonstrates that the plexus may also be made to bowstring in a cephalad direction over the first rib as the rib elevates under the plexus during inhalation [16–18].

The Problem Seen as Centralized Nociceptive Pain

Nociceptor inputs can trigger a prolonged but reversible increase in the excitability and synaptic efficacy of neurons in central nociceptive pathways. This central sensitization manifests as pain, hypersensitivity, pressure hyperalgesia, and enhanced temporal summation [19, 20]. The clinical result of such heightened mechano-sensitivity is the production of symptoms such as pain and paraesthesias with mechanical stresses in the nerves induced by normal body movements.

Conservative Treatment Protocol

A conservative protocol has been developed to correct the breathing dysfunction and core motor control dysfunction and calm the hyperesthesia of the brachial plexus. This protocol (the Edgelow Neuro Vascular Entrapment Syndrome Treatment; ENVEST) has been tested over the past 20 years in over 2,600 patients with severe neck and arm pain originating from the thoracic outlet.

Philosophy

The patient is a partner in the therapeutic process. The treatment protocol involves training the patient to become skilled in a series of exercises designed to reverse the neurovascular and musculoskeletal consequences of their injury. The patient is trained to recognize patterns of breathing dysfunction and through training be able to reset the inhalation to diaphragmatic and use exhalation to relax the hyperactive scalene, subclavius and pectoralis minor muscles.

Indications

The ENVEST program is indicated when a patient presents with neck and arm pain secondary to specific trauma or highly repetitive hand function that is performed in both an intellectually challenging activity with either self- or peer-directed pressure to perform [21]. These latter cases can include musicians, professional athletes and computer workers [22].

ENVEST Protocol

Following evaluation (see Chap. 9) the treatment protocol begins with learning to activate the stabilizers of the neck as well as diaphragmatic breathing to relax the scalene muscles. A useful mnemonic is ABC: **Activate** the stabilizer muscles of the neck and low back, perform **Breathing** training with emphasis on diaphragmatic inhale and abdominally assisted exhale, and end with **Cardiovascular** conditioning.

ACTIVATE the core stabilizers utilizing the THINKERS Pose (Fig. 23.1) and use biofeedback with a blood pressure cuff (Fig. 23.2) to activate the deep neck flexors without activating the scalenes.
1. Stabilize the neck, scapular and spinal stabilizers using the THINKER POSE.
2. Use pressure feedback to retrain the deep neck flexors.
3. Place the pressure device behind the neck. Set the pressure to 20 mmHg. NOD yes and raise the needle 2 mmHg while exhaling with pursed lips and inhale while relaxed at rest.

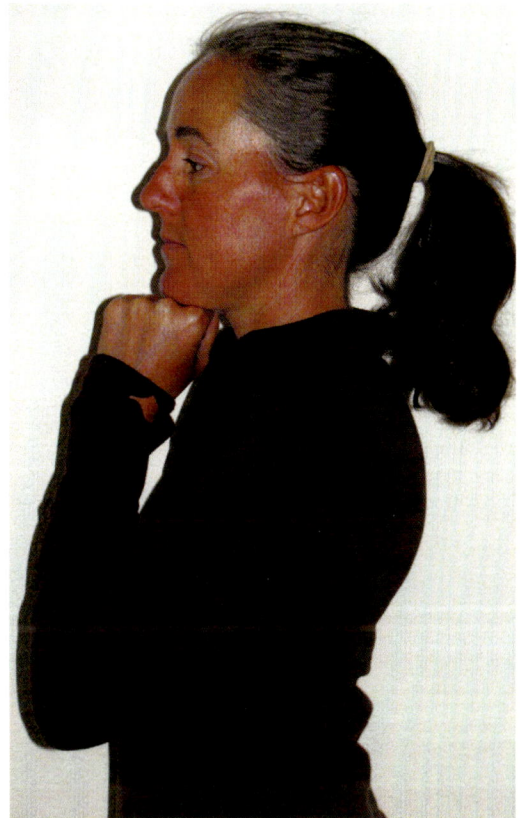

Fig. 23.1 The thinkers pose method of performing an isometric contraction of the deep neck flexors as a way of testing the identified weakness of one thumb adductor pollicis or flexor pollicis brevis (deep head). The force of the isometric contraction is minimized so as to avoid co-contraction of the scalenes. The thumb is again tested for strength during the isometric contraction. A strengthening response indicates weakness/hypoactivity of the deep neck flexors (Courtesy of Peter Edgelow)

4. Fix the pressure meter to a belt under a kitchen chair or clipped to a piece of dowel bridging two chairs so you can see it without holding it.
5. Do this four ways: (a). 1 nod per exhale, (b). Multiple nods per exhale, (c). 1 nod per exhale and hold 5 s, (d). 1 nod per exhale and hold 10 s. Once you can raise the needle 2 mmHg with good control in each of the four methods explained above, progress to doing the same with 4, 6, 8, and finally 10 mmHg.
6. Assess the strength of the thumb by using a device such as in Fig. 23.3. If there is asymmetry between thumbs the weaker thumb should become stronger following application of the

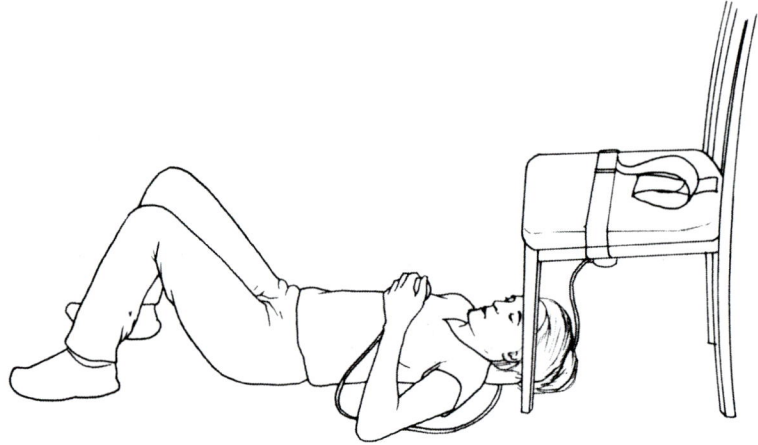

Fig. 23.2 Training position for using a blood pressure cuff to supply biofeedback for retraining the deep neck flexors. Modified from the work of G. Jull (Courtesy of Peter Edgelow)

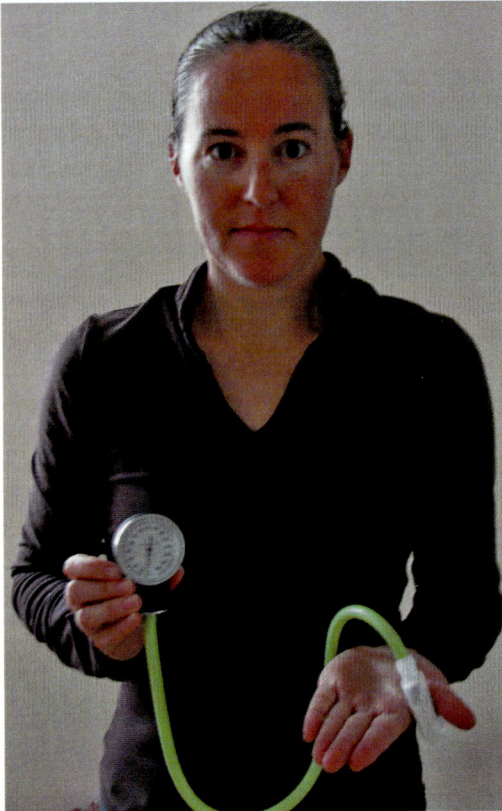

Fig. 23.3 The Thumbometer™ is constructed using a half ounce eye drop like bottle connected by a piece of Theratubing to the sphygmomanometer from a standard manual blood pressure cuff (Courtesy of Peter Edgelow)

thinkers pose. The activation exercises should not result in a weakening affect.

BREATHING training with emphasis on diaphragmatic inhalation and abdominally assisted exhalation.

1. Diaphragmatic breathing exercise: Part One (Fig. 23.4):

   (a) Instruct the patients to lie on their back on the floor without a pillow with knees bent. (Note: if they have to use a pillow because of neck pain then they should do so. Over time, the goal will be to slowly reduce the thickness of the pillow until they can perform the exercise without a pillow.) Support the involved extremity in the position of maximal comfort. The position of comfort will be found by placing the brachial plexus in its most tension-free anatomic position. Usually a wedge pillow to support the shoulder, with the elbow flexed to 90° will relieve tension in the neck and be most comfortable.

   (b) Patients should inhale through the nose and fill the lower lungs with air. This causes the abdomen to rise like a balloon filling up with air.

   (c) Patients then breathe out (exhale) through pursed lips, as if playing the flute. Exhaling should be accomplished by tightening the abdominal muscles, which has the effect of lowering the rib cage.

   (d) Patients are instructed to continue this rhythm of breathing, in through the nose and out through the mouth, making sure that the only motion that occurs is in the stomach. This is diaphragmatic breathing.

The patients then adds the following gentle and relaxed movements of the spine while keeping their neck and legs relaxed:

Fig. 23.4 Diaphragmatic
breathing exercise – Part one
(Courtesy of Peter Edgelow)

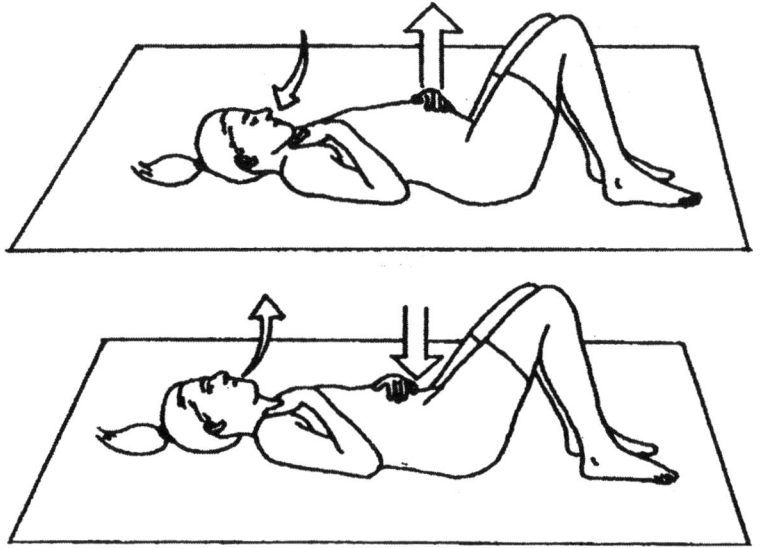

Fig. 23.5 Diaphragmatic
breathing exercise – Part
two. A rubber ball at the end
of a wooden dowel is used to
assist in depressing the first
rib as the patient flattens the
spine in conjunction with
exhalation (Courtesy of
Peter Edgelow)

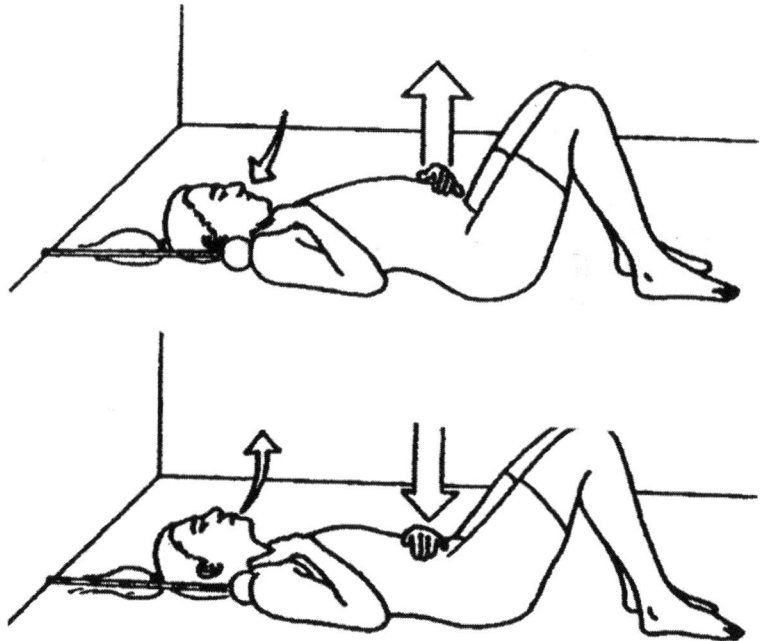

(e) Patients are instructed to slowly arch the low back as they inhale, shortening the spine and causing the chin to nod down while the neck is relaxed.

(f) Patients next slowly flatten the low back as they tighten the abdominal muscles and exhale, lengthening the spine and causing the chin to nod back up.

This gentle motion of the head and neck should occur without active contraction of the scalenes. The neck muscles should remain relaxed.

2. How to Perform the Diaphragmatic Breathing Exercise: Part Two (Fig. 23.5):

Patients are instructed to breathe as described in Part one, but they must add the rib mobilize ("ball on a stick").

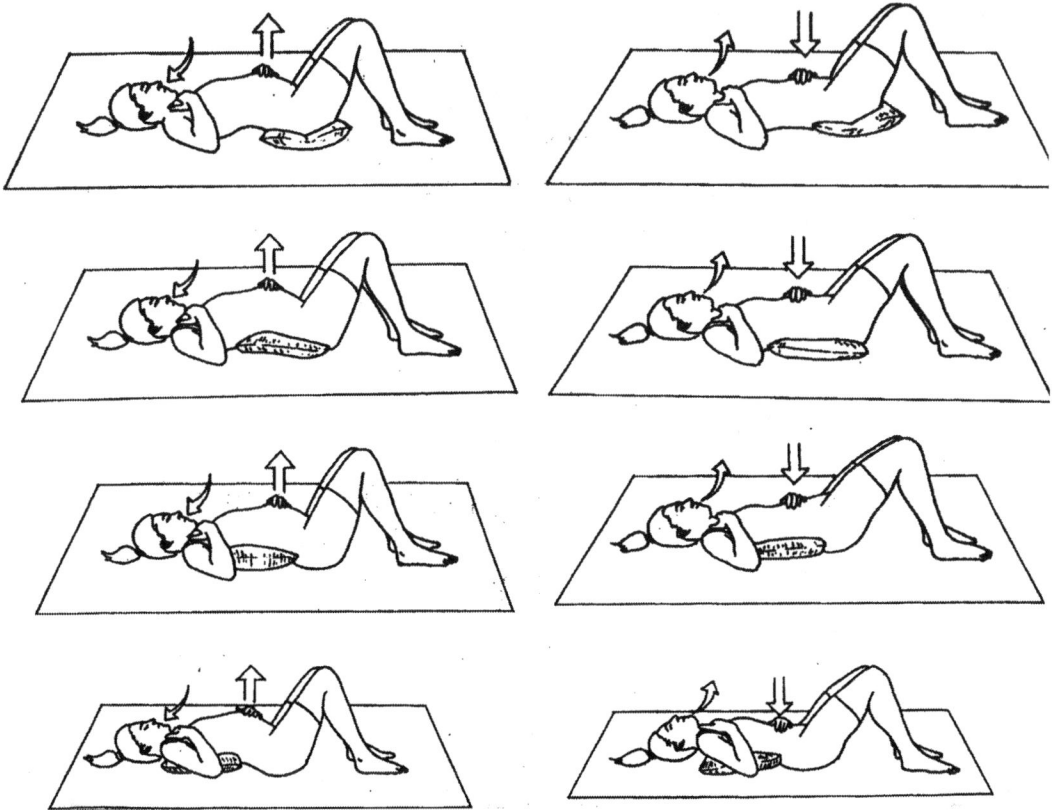

Fig. 23.6 Diaphragmatic breathing exercise – Part three. An air bag is partially inflated and used as a fulcrum to gently increase spinal extension. The air bag used in this exercise is made by Sealed Air Corp. and is called a Rapid Fill™ packaging bag. Dimensions are 14 by 18 in. (Courtesy of Peter Edgelow)

(a) Patients place the ball against the base of the neck, where the neck and shoulders meet. The end of the stick should be resting against the wall behind the patient and the ball should be resting on the floor.

(b) The ball assists with the depression of the first rib. As patients inhale, they move away from the ball; as they exhale, they move into the ball. Therefore as they exhale with contraction of the abdominal corset this pulls the ribs down as the contact with the ball against the posterior aspect of the first rib pushes the rib down.

3. How to Perform the Diaphragmatic Breathing Exercise: Part Three (Fig. 23.6):

(a) Patients are instructed to breathe as described in Part One while resting the pelvis on an air bag.

(b) Patients progress with the exercise, as they are able to tolerate it while breathing with the air bag positioned beneath the pelvis, the low back, the mid back, and the upper back.

This process is used to both increase spinal extension and help the patient perform an inhalation without scalene involvement and an exhalation resulting in relaxation of the accessory breathing muscles.

CARDIOVASCULAR conditioning. This consists primarily of aerobic walking three to four times a day provided there is no increase in pain. The patient is assessed on a treadmill. What speed and for how long with or without arm swing can they walk without increase in pain? Most patients cannot swing the arms without an increase in pain. Sometimes the hand will become colder. Slow progression over time resulting in increased speed to 3 mph and time to 20 min and being able to swing both arms without increased symptoms is the goal.

Treatment Progression

The initial **activate** phase of treatment is progressed by assessing scapular stability. The protocol by Watson is an excellent reference [1]. The pressure feedback is used to specifically retrain and strengthen the abdominal mechanism. Ethafoam rollers and the ball on a stick and the gymnastic ball are used to increase spinal and rib cage mobility. The gymnastic ball is used to improve balance, posture and breathing in sitting. Once the nervous system has calmed down and there is marked decrease in symptoms the next goal is to increase function. When a patient is inhibited from doing more because of fear of flaring the problem I have them read a book called Explain Pain [19]. Walking is progressed using a Feldenkrais: Walking Awareness Through Movement series of CD's [23]. For more detail one can obtain a DVD and/or refer to previously published material [24].

References

1. Watson L, Pizzari T, Balster S. Thoracic outlet syndrome part 2: conservative management of thoracic outlet syndrome. Man Ther. 2010;15(4):305–14.
2. Jull G, Kristjansson E, Dall'Alba P. Impairment in the cervical flexors: a comparison of whiplash and insidious onset neck pain patients. Man Ther. 2004;9(2): 89–94.
3. Jull G, Falla D, Treleaven J, Sterling M, O'Leary S. A therapeutic exercise approach for cervical disorders. 3rd ed. Edinburgh: Elsevier Churchill Livingston; 2005, Chapter 32.
4. Falla D, Jull G, Dall'Alba P, Rainoldi A, Merletti R. Electromyographic analysis of the deep neck flexors in performance of craniocervical flexion. Phys Ther. 2003;83:899–906.
5. Falla D, Bilenkij G, Jull G. Patients with chronic neck pain demonstrated altered patterns of muscle activation during performance of a functional upper limb task. Spine. 2004;29(13):1436–40.
6. Falla D. Unravelling the complexity of muscle impairment in chronic neck pain. Man Ther. 2004;9:125–33.

7. Woodhouse A, Vasseljen O. Altered motor control patterns in whiplash and chronic neck pain. BMC musculoskeletal disorders. http://www.biomedcentral.com/1471-2474/9/90 (2008). Accessed 25 May 2011.
8. Caldwell CSS, Van Dillen L. Use of a movement system impairment diagnosis for physical therapy in the management of a patient with shoulder pain. J Orthop Sports Phys Ther. 2007;37(9):551–63.
9. Janda V. Postural and phasic muscles in the pathogenesis of low back pain. Paper presented at: XIth Congress of the ISRD; Dublin, Ireland. 1969.
10. Janda V. Muscle weakness and inhibition (pseudoparesis) in back pain syndromes. In: Grieve G, editor. Modern manual therapy of the vertebral column. New York: Churchill Livingston; 1986. p. 197–201.
11. Comerford M, Mottram SL. Movement and stability dysfunction – contemporary developments. Man Ther. 2001;6(1):15–26.
12. Comerford M, Mottram SL. Functional stability retraining: principals and strategies for managing mechanical dysfunction. Man Ther. 2001;6(1):3–14.
13. Sanders R. Thoracic outlet syndrome: a common sequela of neck injuries. Philadelphia: J.B. Lippincott Co; 1991.
14. Smith MRA, Hodges P. Disorders of breathing and continence have a stronger association with back pain than obesity and physical activity. Aust J Physiother. 2006;52:11–6.
15. McLaughlin LGC, Goldsmith CH, Coleman K. Breathing evaluation and retraining as an adjunct to manual therapy. Man Ther. 2011;16:51–2.
16. Shacklock M. Clinical neurodynamics: a new system of musculoskeletal treatment. 1st ed. Oxford: Elsevier; 2005.
17. Fried R. The hyperventilation syndrome: research and clinical treatment. Baltimore: John Hopkins University Press; 1987.
18. Wilhelm F, Gervirtz R, Roth W. Respiratory dysregulation in anxiety, functional cardiac, and pain disorders assessment, phenomenology and treatment. Behav Modif. 2001;25(4):513–45.
19. Butler DS, Moseley GL. Explain pain. Adelaide, South Australia, Australia: Noigroup Publications, www.noigroup.com; 2003.
20. Woolf C. Central sensitization: implications for the diagnosis and treatment of pain. Pain. 2011;152(3 Suppl): S2–15.
21. Byl N, Wilson F, Merzenich M, et al. Sensory dysfunction associated with repetitive strain injuries of tendonitis and focal hand dystonia: a comparative study. J Orthop Sports Phys Ther. 1996;23(4):234–44.
22. Byl N, Nagarajan S, Newton N, McKenzie A. Effect of sensory discrimination training on structure and function in a musician with focal hand dystonia. Phys Ther Case Rep. 2000;3(3):94–113.
23. Reese M. Walking. Awareness through movement 5 CD set. 1-800-765-1907. 2004.
24. Edgelow P. Neurovascular consequences of cumulative trauma disorders affecting the thoracic outlet: a patient centered treatment approach. In: Donatelli R, editor. Physical therapy of the shoulder. 4th ed. New York: Churchill Livingston; 2004. p. 205–38.

Occupational Therapy Treatment for NTOS

24

Dana Emery

Abstract

When treating patients with neurogenic thoracic outlet syndrome (NTOS), the focus of occupational therapy (OT) is to decrease the impact of symptoms on daily activities, teach proper body mechanics and/or compensatory positioning, and prevent symptoms from further impacting the patient's life. OT can be used as the primary treatment for NTOS or as a part of the postoperative recovery process in patients who have undergone thoracic outlet decompression. A key to the alleviation of symptoms and an increase in recovery speed is teaching surgical and non-surgical patients to maintain appropriate posture while performing everyday activities. Providing the patient with information and skills needed regarding the positions that will close off the outlet and potentially increase symptoms and pain will aid the patient in independence in symptom management. Specific maneuvers include the avoidance of compression at the shoulder, side-lying sleep position, and the avoidance of prolonged or repetitive overhead arm use.

Introduction

When treating patients with neurogenic thoracic outlet syndrome (NTOS), the focus of occupational therapy (OT) is to decrease the impact of symptoms on daily activities, teach body proper mechanics and/or compensatory positioning, and prevent symptoms from further impacting the patient's life [1].

D. Emery, OT/L, BS
Department of Occupational Therapy,
University of Rochester Medical Center,
601 Elmwood Ave, Rochester, NY 14642, USA
e-mail: dana_emery@urmc.rochester.edu

Treatment Setting

An occupational therapist's practice in a multidisciplinary clinic setting can be crucial to patient outcomes. This approach involves the collaborative efforts of the physician, nurse practitioner, and occupational therapist to guide the appropriate level of intervention for each patient.

The occupational therapist participates in assessment of patients by performing examinations that provide important information for OT treatment planning. These tests include an assessment of function in daily activities, grip and pinch testing [2–4], sensory screening [5–7], and an evaluation of a patient's tolerance to peripheral nerve glides [8–12]. This assessment, in

K.A. Illig et al. (eds.), *Thoracic Outlet Syndrome*,
DOI 10.1007/978-1-4471-4366-6_24, © Springer-Verlag London 2013

conjunction with the standard provocative testing for TOS [13, 14], will assist the team in understanding the area of compression, severity of symptoms or rule out TOS all together.

In a specialized outpatient OT clinic, the therapist is able to be more detailed in their assessment of patients. This setting may identify patients with symptoms of TOS that have not yet seen a vascular surgeon; they may have been referred from a primary care physician or other discipline due to pain or dysfunction in daily activities, or job performance [15].

Primary Therapy for NTOS

For selected patients who do not require immediate surgery, the team may opt for a trial of OT before committing to a surgical approach. The goal of this phase of treatment is to "cure" the problem or, if this cannot be done, to mitigate symptoms and give the patient skills to cope with a chronic illness.

A thorough assessment of the patient will include a cervical screen [16–19], assessment of posture [12, 20], manual muscle testing, range of motion, grip and pinch assessments [3], pain assessment, sensory testing [6, 7], the relationship of vascular changes to upper extremity positioning [14], assessment of activities of daily living (ADL) and instrumental activities of daily living (IADL), which are tasks or activities that a patient does to maintain independence in the home or community, and determination of the patient's goals regarding treatment (Table 24.1). Following assessment, the occupational therapist establishes a frequency and expected duration of treatment, usually 1–2 times per week for 2–3 months. These visits are at longer intervals toward the end of the protocol to encourage independence in the exercise program and management of symptoms. If symptom management is not obtained in the designated time frame, or the patient's symptoms worsen at any point, the patient is referred back to the vascular surgeon [15, 21, 22].

The main focus of the OT approach to treatment is education. The patient is provided with written material to explain the anatomy of TOS, the structures involved, and how body position can exacerbate symptoms. For example, instruction may be given to correct slouching shoulders that may be worsening symptoms.

According to the protocol established by the OT department at the University of Rochester Medical Center, a critical early step is to address strengthening of scapular musculature, specifically the scapular retractors and depressors (Table 24.2). It is frequently noted that patients with TOS will exhibit protracted or forward-slouching shoulders. By strengthening the scapular retractors and depressors the shoulder becomes balanced and appropriate positioning of the shoulder is achieved. Because it is thought that restoring the ability of a nerve to glide will reduce pain, nerve glides are given within the home exercise program (Fig. 24.1), along with the scapular musculature strengthening. Walsh [23] describes nerve gliding as placing tension on the nerve at one point while releasing it at another with gliding occurring within the nerve itself or between the nerve and its interfacing tissue. The patient is instructed to stop before feeling pain while performing the nerve glide to avoid exacerbation of symptoms. With each visit the nerve glide is repeated and tolerance is documented to determine progress in elimination of paresthesias.

As the scapular muscle strength improves, allowing the patient to pull the shoulders back, the focus may be shifted to pelvic posturing in order to foster better overall body mechanics. It is frequently observed that correcting pelvic tilt will improve upper body posture. To maintain the correct shoulder position, the presence of posterior pelvic tilt (due to weak core musculature) must be eliminated.

Concurrent with the strengthening and nerve glide exercises is an ongoing assessment of the patients ADL and IADL tasks. The focus at this point is on improving positioning while completing these tasks, including how objects in the patient's environment and other environmental factors may be modified to improve task performance. An intake form is used (Table 24.1) to determine problem areas. These areas are simulated in the clinic with the occupational therapist present to modify position to avoid shoulder flexion above 90°, abduction above 90° or sustained overhead position. The same is done for

Table 24.1 A sample intake form

PLEASE RATE THE LEVEL OF DIFFICULTY FOR THE FOLLOWING TASKS

ACTIVITY	RATING	NEVER DO
BATHING	NO PROBLEM 1 2 3 4 CAN'T DO	
DRESSING	NO PROBLEM 1 2 3 4 CAN'T DO	
GROOMING	NO PROBLEM 1 2 3 4 CAN'T DO	
COOKING	NO PROBLEM 1 2 3 4 CAN'T DO	
HOUSEWORK	NO PROBLEM 1 2 3 4 CAN'T DO	
WRITING	NO PROBLEM 1 2 3 4 CAN'T DO	
RECREATIONAL ACTIVITY	NO PROBLEM 1 2 3 4 CAN'T DO	
LIGHT DUTY	NO PROBLEM 1 2 3 4 CAN'T DO	
NORMAL ACTIVITY	NO PROBLEM 1 2 3 4 CAN'T DO	

PLEASE RATE THE AVERAGE DISCOMFORT OR PAIN YOU HAVE HAD IN THE LAST

WEEK DURING THE FOLLOWING ACTIVITIES:

WHILE AT REST:	DURING BATHING/DRESSING/GROOMING
0 1 2 3 4 5 6 7 8 9 10 NO PAIN = 0 WORST POSSIBLE PAIN= 10	0 1 2 3 4 5 6 7 8 9 10 NO PAIN = 0 WORST POSSIBLE PAIN= 10
WHILE WORKING/IN SCHOOL	WHILE DOING LEISURE ACTIVITIES
0 1 2 3 4 5 6 7 8 9 10 NO PAIN = 0 WORST POSSIBLE PAIN= 10	0 1 2 3 4 5 6 7 8 9 10 NO PAIN = 0 WORST POSSIBLE PAIN= 10

Table 24.2 Muscles that control the scapua

Scapular protraction	*Scapular retractors*
Serratus anterior	Rhomboids
Pec minor	Trapezius
Pec major	Latissimus dorsi
Scapular depression	*Scapular elevation*
Pec minor	Levator scapulae
Trapezius (lower fibers)	Trapezius
Subclavius	
Lattisimus dorsi	
Scapular upward rotation	*Scapular downward rotation*
Trapezius	Pec minor
Serratus anterior	Pec major
	Subscapularis
	Latissimus dorsi

the patient's job tasks. Patients are instructed in proper sleep position, on their back, to allow passive opening of the thoracic outlet (Fig. 24.2).

The specific knowledge of the OT in task analysis is used here to educate and empower the patient to apply the lessons to their daily life. Without the patient's efforts to apply OT strategies to daily life, therapy will be ineffective.

Post Operative Treatment

For patients who need surgical intervention, the focus of OT in the acute phase is pain management. The patient is seen post operative day (POD) one for the initial assessment.

UNIVERSITY *of*
ROCHESTER
MEDICAL CENTER

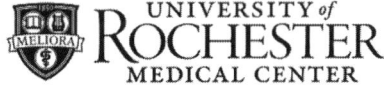

OCCUPATIONAL THERAPY

THORACIC OUTLET SYNDROME
POST OP HOME EXERCISE PROGRAM

- **POD #1-3 NERVE GLIDES/SCAPULAR STRENGTH**
  - ATTEMPT 10 REPETITIONS EVERY HOUR YOU ARE AWAKE
  - STOP JUST BEFORE YOU HAVE AN INCREASE IN SYMPTOMS
  - MAKE NOTE OF THE POSITION NUMBER YOU ENDED ON, TRY TO IMPROVE EACH SET OF 10 REPS
  - SQUEEZE SHOULDER BLADES TOGETHER 5 REPETITIONS
  - PRESS SHOULDER BLADES TOWARD FLOOR 5 REPETITIONS
- **POD #4-2 WEEKS POST OP NERVE GLIDES**
  - 10 REPETITIONS 3-4 TIMES PER DAY
  - STOP JUST BEFORE YOU HAVE AN INCREASE IN SYMPTOMS
  - NOTE THE POSITION NUMBER YOU ENDED ON TRYING TO IMPROVE WITH EACH SET YOU DO
  - SQUEEZE SHOULDER BLADES TOGETHER 10 REPETITIONS 1X/DAY
  - PRESS SHOULDER BLADES TOWARD FLOOR 10 REPETITIONS 1X/DAY
- **AFTER 2 WEEKS POST OP NERVE GLIDES**
  - 5 REPETITIONS 3-4 TIMES PER DAY
  - STOP JUST BEFORE YOU HAVE AN INCREASE IN SYMPTOMS
  - NOTING THE POSITION NUMBER AND TRYING TO IMPROVE WITH EACH SET
  - SQUEEZE SHOULDER BLADES TOGETHER 10 REPETITIONS 2-3X/DAY
  - PRESS SHOULDER BLADES TOWARD FLOOR 10 REPETITIONS 2-3X/DAY

Preoperative: **Postoperative:**

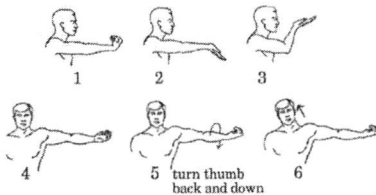

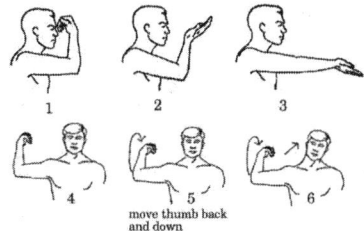

Hold _____ seconds
Repeat _____ times
Do _____ sessions per day

Hold _____ seconds
Repeat _____ times
Do _____ sessions per day

Fig. 24.1 Nerve glide handout used at the University of Rochester

Fig. 24.2 Proper positioning when supine

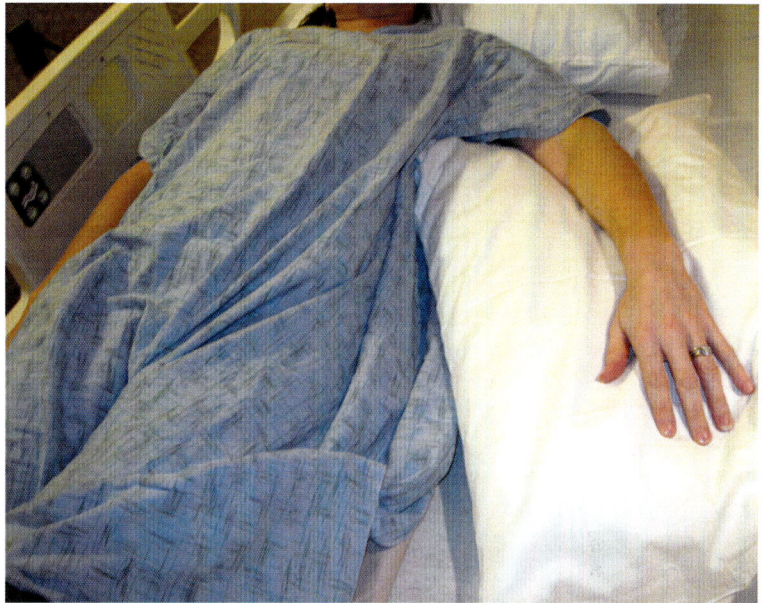

It is helpful for a family member or friend to be present at the time of the initial post operative visit as the patient may not be unable to remember instructions due to the lingering effects of the analgesic agents. The patient is given a post operative exercise program that starts as soon as they can participate and goes through week two post-op when they will be seen for their initial assessment as an outpatient in the Occupational Therapy Department.

The exercise program consists of nerve glides (Fig. 24.1), typically of the ulnar nerve, gentle active range of motion [12, 24] and scapular musculature exercises [12, 20] several times per hour to assist in edema control. Scapular exercises may not be tolerated POD#1, but the patient should attempt them daily. The frequency of nerve glides and range of motion in the exercise program are slowly decreases the as the patient approaches the 2-week mark and is using the extremity for normal activities.

The patient is also instructed in appropriate position to maintain and open the thoracic outlet during the acute stage [12]. It is important to educate the nursing staff, as well as the patient, to avoid shoulder flexion (raising arm in front of the body in the sagittal plane) positioning or range of motion above 90° or any position that "jam" the humeral head into the shoulder girdle, i.e. propping on multiple pillows while sitting in an arm chair (Fig. 24.3). The most effective way to position the arm while in supine is flat on the bed with one pillow arm at approximately 45° of shoulder abduction (moving arm away from the body in the coronal plane) (Fig. 24.2). Educational handouts are given at this time.

Aside from the positioning recommendations, the patient is restricted to no lifting over five pounds for the week after surgery. This is to avoid exacerbation of symptoms related to the surgical procedure. Patients are encouraged to move freely to complete their ADL tasks. The patient is also taught scar massage to begin POD#1 around the incision site. After the first week post-op, the patient is to begin scar massage on the incision line.

Occupational therapists should remind the patient that the first 48 h are the most uncomfortable and that following the exercise program will improve the pain due to the reduction of post-op edema and stiffness. It is also important to note, arterial and venous TOS patients recover much quicker and have less post-op pain than neurogenic TOS patients.

Fig. 24.3 Proper positioning when sitting

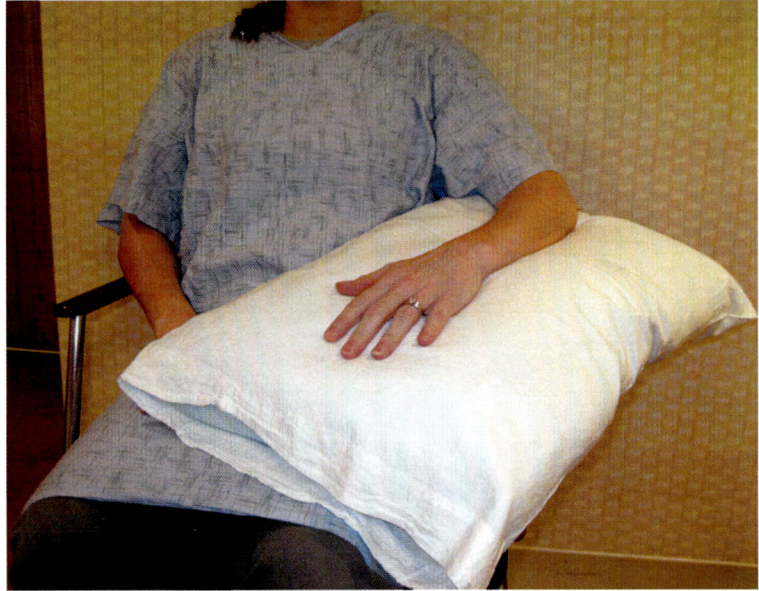

Follow up Outpatient OT

At the 2 week mark, the patient then begins out-patient OT for an individualized OT program which uses the same protocol referred to in the Surgical Prevention section of this chapter as a guide. As the patient works his or her way through the protocol, the frequency of visits is spaced far-ther out to wean OT treatment and allow the patient to attempt to manage the symptoms on their own.

Summary

The key to prevention of symptoms is teaching sur-gical and non surgical patients to maintain appro-priate posture while performing everyday activities. Providing the patient with information and skills needed regarding the positions that will close off the outlet [12, 15, 21, 22], potentially increase symptoms and pain will aid the patient in indepen-dence in symptom management. This includes avoiding slouching shoulders, side lying sleep position and avoidance of prolonged or repetitive overhead arm use. If the symptoms increase or return the patient is encouraged to contact the ther-apist or surgeon to reassess the problem.

References

1. Definition of occupational therapy practice for the AOTA Model Practice Act. 2011. www.aota.org/Practitioners/Advocacy/State/Resources/PracticeAct/36437.aspz. Adopted by Representative Assembly 5 Dec 2004. Accessed 31 May 2011.
2. Mathiowetz V. Reliability and validity of grip and pinch strength measurements. Crit Rev Phys Med Rehabil Med. 1991;2:201–12.
3. Mathiowetz V, Kashman N, Volland G, et al. Grip and pinch strength: normative data for adults. Arch Phys Med Rehabil. 1985;66:69–74.
4. Mathiowetz V, Weber K, Volland G, et al. Reliability and validity of grip and pinch strenght evaluations. Hand Surg. 1984;9A:222–6.
5. Jerosch-Herold C. Assessment of sensibility after nerve injury and repair: a systematic review of evi-dence for validity, reliability and responsiveness of tests. J Hand Surg. 2005;30:252–64.
6. Weinstein S. Fifty years of somatosensory research: from the Semmes-Weinstein monofilaments to the Weinsten Enhanced Sensory Tests. J Hand Ther. 1993;6:11–22.
7. Tomancik L. Directions for using Semmes-Weinstein monofilaments. San Jose: North Coast Medical; 1987.
8. Kleinrensink GJ, Stoeckart R, Mulder PG, et al. Upper limb tension tests as tools in the dagnosis of nerve and plexus lesions: anatomical and biomechanical aspects. Clin Biomech. 2000;16:717–8.
9. Millesi H, Zoch G, Rath T. Mechanical properties of peripheral nerves. Clin Orthop. 1995;314:76–83.
10. Wilgis EF, Murphy R. The significance of longitudi-nal excursion in peripheral nerves. Hand Clin. 1986; 2:761–6.

11. McLellan DL, Swash M. Longitudinal sliding of the median nerve during movements of the upper limb. J Neurol Neurosurg Psychiatry. 1976;39:566–70.

12. Novak CB. Conservative management of thoracic outlet syndrome. Semin Thorac Cardiovasc Surg. 1996;8:201.

13. Physical Therapy Corner. 2011. Thoracic outlet syndrome. http://www.nismat.org/ptcor/thoracic_outlet. Accessed 31 May 2011.

14. Rayan GM, Jensen C. Thoracic outlet syndrome: provacative examination maneuvers in a typical population. J Shoulder Elbow Surg. 1995;4:113–7.

15. Pascarelli EF, Hsu YP. Understanding work-related upper extremity disorters: clinical findings in 485 computers users, musicians and others. J Occup Rehabil. 2001;11:1–21.

16. Mackinnon SD, Dellon AL. Experimental study of chronic nerve compression clinical implications. Hand Clin. 1986;2:639–50.

17. Pechan J, Julius I. The pressure measurement in the ulnar nerve: a contribution to the pathophysiology of the cubital tunnel syndrome. J Biomech. 1975;8:75–9.

18. Sandmark H, Nisell R. Validity of five common manual neck pain provoking tests. Scand J Rehab Med. 1995;27:131–6.

19. Viikari-Juntara E, Porras M, Laasonen EM. Valididy of clinical tests in the diagnosis of root compression in cervical disc disease. Spine. 1989;14:253–7.

20. Watson LA, Pizzai T, Balster S. Thoracic outlet syndrome part 2: conservative management of thoracic outlet. Man Ther. 2010;15:305–14.

21. Sallstrom J, Schmidt H. Cervicobrachial disorders in certain occupations, with special reference to compression in the thoracic outlet. Am J Ind Med. 1984;6:45–52.

22. Wright IS. The neurovascular syndrome produced by hyperabduction of the arms. Am Heart J. 1945;29:1.

23. Walsh M. Rational and indications for the use of nerve mobilization and nerve gliding as a treatment approach. In: Hunter JS, Mackin EJ, Callahan AD, editors. Hunter, Mackin, Callahan's rehabilitation of the hand and upper extremity. 5th ed. Philadelphia: Mosby, Inc.; 2002. p. 771.

24. Tschakovsky ME, Sheriff DD. Immediate exercise hyperemia: contributions of the muscle pump vs. rapid vasodilation. J Appl Physiol. 2004;97:739–47.

Chiropractic Treatment of NTOS

25

Marc A. Weinberg

Abstract

Chiropractic as defined by the World Federation of Chiropractic is "a health profession concerned with the diagnosis, treatment and prevention of mechanical disorders of the musculoskeletal system, and the effects of these disorders on the functions of the nervous system and general health. There is an emphasis on manual treatments including spinal adjustment and other joint and soft-tissue manipulation." In patients with Neurogenic Thoracic Outlet Syndrome [NTOS] there may be mechanical compression of neural structures within the brachial plexus at one of several anatomical sites, several of which may be targeted by the techniques used in Chiropractic.

Introduction

Chiropractic as defined by the World Federation of Chiropractic is "a health profession concerned with the diagnosis, treatment and prevention of mechanical disorders of the musculoskeletal system, and the effects of these disorders on the functions of the nervous system and general health. There is an emphasis on manual treatments including spinal adjustment and other joint and soft-tissue manipulation" [1]. In patients with Neurogenic Thoracic Outlet Syndrome [NTOS] there may be mechanical compression of neural structures within the brachial plexus at one of six anatomical sites. The three most common areas of compression are between the scalene muscles; in the costoclavicular space; or behind the pectoralis minor tendon [2, 3]. These areas may be targeted by the techniques used in Chiropractic.

The Chiropractic Approach to NTOS

Chiropractors consider the importance of interconnectivity so that input upon the nervous system at one location may provoke a physiological response elsewhere within the nervous system [4–18]. Consequently, symptoms may manifest in seemingly unrelated tissues and organs [4, 6, 7, 9–20]. Additionally, it is thought that the proper function of the biomechanics of the cervical spine, thoracic spine and pectoral girdle are not independent of each other, but are each an integral component of

M.A. Weinberg, DC
Active Health Center,
421 Northlake Blvd., Suite F,
North Palm Beach, FL 33408, USA
e-mail: drmarc@weinbergchiro.com

Table 25.1 Generic types of chiropractic manipulative and adjustive techniques

A. Manual, articular manipulative, and adjustive procedures

1. Specific contact thrust procedures
   (a) High velocity thrust
   (b) High velocity thrust with recoil
   (c) Low velocity thrust
2. Nonspecific contact thrust procedures
3. Manual force, mechanically assisted procedures
   (a) Drop-tables and terminal point adjustive thrust
   (b) Flexion-distraction table adjustment
   (c) Pelvic block adjusting
4. Mechanical force, manually assisted procedures
   (a) Fixed stylus, compression wave adjustment
   (b) Moving stylus instrument adjustment

B. Manual, nonarticular manipulative, and adjustive procedures

1. Manual reflex and muscle relaxation procedures
   (a) Muscle energy techniques
   (b) Neurologic reflex techniques
   (c) Myofascial ischemic compression procedures
   (d) Miscellaneous soft tissue techniques
2. Miscellaneous procedures
   (a) Neural retraining techniques
   (b) Conceptual approaches

Reprinted from Mootz et al. [27]

a complex mechanical system [19, 21–23]. This holistic approach of re-establishing proper function to each joint and its physical communication with other related structures [24, 25], as well as giving focus to the neurologic innervation by removing nerve impingements, is the basis and cornerstone of the chiropractic approach to the management of many conditions including Neurogenic Thoracic Outlet Syndrome [NTOS] [1]. Most chiropractic techniques attempt to positively influence a patient's health by correcting biomechanical dysfunction through a chiropractic manipulation known as an adjustment [26]. The "dynamic thrust" style of adjusting is the most common method utilized; however many other methods are frequently used (See Table 25.1). Many chiropractic adjusting techniques can be administered with very little force while others can be slightly more aggressive (See Fig. 25.1) [26]. In the treatment of NTOS, the chiropractor will attempt to decrease nerve impingement by re-establishing normal function of the spine and upper extremity joints and musculature through chiropractic adjustments.

Assessment and Treatment

A chiropractor will complete a standard evaluation procedure which will include a history, physical and regional evaluation of the thoracic outlet and shoulder girdle, as well as a specialized assessment of the mechanical status of the patient [27]. Current research supports that NTOS can develop as a cascade of neuromuscular events secondarily to faulty posture, ergonomics, trauma and other factors [28]. It is important for the clinician to accurately diagnose the patient and rule out any unusual causes for the compression such as a space-occupying lesion, a vascular incident or some other relevant pathology [8]. Other specific causes to consider include anomalies such as a cervical rib, a fractured clavicle or an adaptive shortening of fascia [29]. Treatment of posturally related NTOS must address re-establishing normal mechanics of the cervical and thoracic spines, as well as the pectoral girdle [30]. The pectoral girdle evaluation is inclusive of the scapulothoracic, glenohumeral, acromioclavicular and sternoclavicular mechanisms [31] and even the integration of breathing mechanisms [32].

Although, more extensive research needs to be completed on the role of the proper function of the sterno-clavicular and acromioclavicular joint and its relation to TOS, chiropractors may be concerned with the finding of subluxaton or fixation in this patient population. In clinical experience, upper extremity symptomotology, (i.e. hand swelling, color changes, muscle weakness, paresthesias, etc.) related to TOS can be provocated when these joints are moved into certain positions and reduced after a low amplitude chiropractic adjustment (mobilization) is administered with the proper line of force.

Evaluation of strength, tone and balance of the cervical and related musculature is also important as imbalance can lead to a thickening and fibrosis of some of the muscles that make up the

Fig. 25.1 A low amplitude adjustment of an inferiorly subluxated (fixated) proximal clavicle is being performed on a 17-year-old TOS patient using the activator instrument

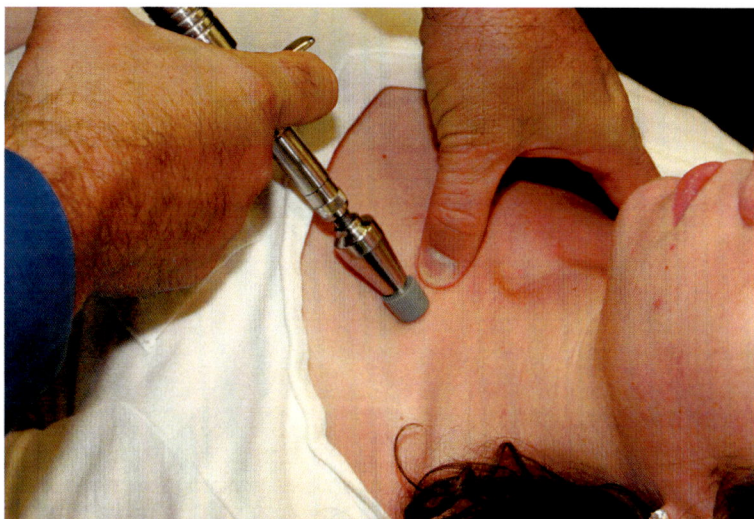

thoracic outlet and lead to further constriction [3]. Chiropractic Care has been effective for re-establishing proper bio-mechanical function to these structures [22, 33].

The Chronicity Factor

Long standing postural factors can cause numerous structural changes, which over time can lead to a "vicious cycle" of scalene and small pectoral muscle shortening. Additionally, some muscles are lengthened and are placed in a mechanically compromised position leading to muscular weakness, while others hypertrophy as they compensate for the faulty bio-mechanics [3]. The plethora of physical changes and symptoms that accompany TOS when developed over long periods of time may become chronically entrenched; therefore simultaneous treatment by both a chiropractor and a manual therapist is a good combination that may offer improved outcomes [30].

More research needs to be completed on the role that neck musculature weakness and imbalance plays in the development and perpetuation of TOS. There have been studies performed on the validity, repeatability and reliability of available technology for measuring neck strength and balance in the clinician's office [34, 35]. In practical use, it is helpful for a clinician to have an objective and repeatable method of assessing neck musculature strength. The Multi-Cervical Unit is a technology that fulfills that role and can also act as an objective way to assess, strengthen and balance the musculature of the neck [36–38]. Determining which muscles are weak and being able to isolate the rehabilitation of these individual muscle groups without exacerbation of the condition may be a key component to a positive long term prognosis of a TOS patient.

Thoracic Outlet Syndrome and the Breathing Mechanism

The breathing mechanism is an important component in the development of TOS. The scalenes and sternocleidomastoid are not normally used substantially in normal breathing [39]. Chiropractors will look for faulty and excessive movement patterns when assessing breathing dynamics (See Fig. 25.2) [32].

As a computer driven society, our faulty sitting ergonomics are continually forcing us into slumped seated postures. These postures lead to rounded shoulder and forward head posture and a shallow breathing pattern causing accessory muscle use and hypertrophy around the pectoral girdle. Neurovascular compression can occur from muscle hypertrophy in the scalenes [29, 40].

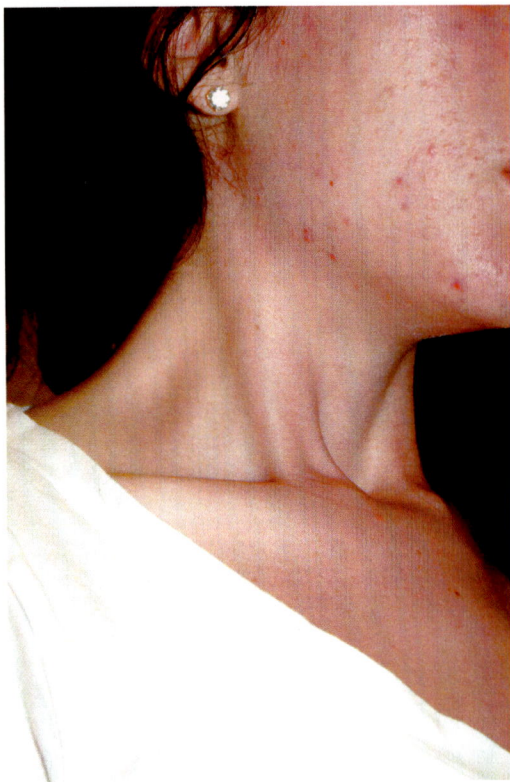

Fig. 25.2 Accessory muscle activation can be visualized on this TOS patient during normal inspiration

Therefore, a necessary part of TOS treatment is patient education on posture and proper abdominal breathing techniques to avoid the overuse syndrome of accessory breathing.

The Manual Challenge

In practice, the challenge that is faced when any manual therapy is performed on a patient with a compressive syndrome (i.e. Thoracic Outlet Syndrome, Carpal Tunnel Syndrome, Piriformis Syndrome, etc.) is being able to facilitate the body to decompress the offending structures without irritating the sensitive neurologic structures being compromised. Whether it is physical therapy, chiropractic treatment, massage or some other manual therapy, the apparent conundrum is that if the practitioner works too aggressively, irritation to the underlining neurology and thus an increase in the patient's pain can ensue. The

psychological factor that comes into play is that the patient assumes "the treatment is not working". The increased frustration level quickly leads the patient to consider more invasive treatment, with an expected quicker resolution. The actuality is that the treatment application may have been too aggressively initiated and therefore was never given an effective trial.

It is very important to introduce procedures, exercises or other aspects of treatment in a controlled conservative step-wise fashion. For example, a simple exercise performed improperly can quickly exacerbate a TOS patient, which will decrease the likelihood that they will continue with conservative care.

It is important for the practitioner to understand this psychology of the patient. By managing the patient's and their own expectations of a quick reduction of symptoms, it will assist in decreasing the frustration levels and ultimately increase the chance of a positive outcome with conservative management.

Chiropractic and Its Future Role in NTOS

It has been argued that there may be many benefits to the patients that seek conservative care for the management of NTOS [2, 3, 29, 30]. Some studies suggested that a multifaceted approach is better than a single approach [30]. The diagnosis of TOS appears to not only be one with a wide range of pathogenesis, but may also be inclusive of a variety of compressive entities. As more research is done, and there are more benchmarks to diagnose and assess the positive outcomes of treatment, Chiropractic will continue to grow and be a key component to the conservative treatment of NTOS.

References

1. World Chiropractic Federation Website. http://www.wfc.org/website/ (2011). Accessed 1 May 2011.
2. Medical Treatment Guidelines. Work-related neurogenic thoracic outlet syndrome: diagnosis and treatment. Washington State Department of Labor and Industries; Effective Oct 1, 2010.

3. Vanti C, Natalini L, Romeo A, Tosarelli D, Pillastrini P. Conservative treatment of thoracic outlet syndrome. A review of the literature. Eura Medicophys. 2007; 43(1):55–70.

4. Welch A, Boone R. Sympathetic and parasympathetic responses to specific diversified adjustments to chiropractic vertebral subluxations of the cervical and thoracic spine. J Chiropr Med. 2008;7(3):86–93.

5. Magee D, Zachazewski JE, Quillen WS. Scientific foundations and principles of practice in musculoskeletal rehabilitation. St. Louis: Saunders Elsevier; 2007. p. 187.

6. Ruskin AP. Sphenopalatine (nasal) ganglion: remote effects including "psychosomatic" symptoms, rage reaction, pain, and spasm. Arch Phys Med Rehabil. 1979;60(8):353–9.

7. Gunn CC. "Prespondylosis" and some pain syndromes following denervation supersensitivity. Spine (Phila Pa 1976). 1980;5(2):185–92.

8. Dahlin LB, Lundborg G. The neurone and its response to peripheral nerve compression. J Hand Surg Br. 1990;15(1):5–10.

9. Moore MK. Upper crossed syndrome and its relationship to cervicogenic headache. J Manipulative Physiol Ther. 2004;27(6):414–20.

10. Budgell BS. Reflex effects of subluxation: the autonomic nervous system. J Manipulative Physiol Ther. 2000;23(2):104–6.

11. Driscoll MD, Hall MJ. Effects of spinal manipulative therapy on autonomic activity and the cardiovascular system: a case study using the electrocardiogram and arterial tonometry [abstract]. J Manipulative Physiol Ther. 2000;23(8):545–50.

12. Igarashii Y, Budgell B. Case study response of arrhythmia to spinal manipulation: monitoring by ECG with analysis of heart-rate variability. Chiropr J Aust. 2000;30(3):92–5.

13. Carrick FR. Changes in brain function after manipulation of the cervical spine. J Manipulative Physiol Ther. 1997;8:529–45.

14. Tran T, Kirby J. The effect of upper thoracic adjustment upon the normal physiology of the heart. J Am Chiropr Assoc. 1977;11s:58–62.

15. Briggs L, Boone WR. Effects of a chiropractic adjustment on changes in pupillary diameter: a model for evaluating somatovisceral response. J Manipulative Physiol Ther. 1988;11(3):181–9.

16. Harris W, Wagnon RJ. The effects of chiropractic adjustments on distal skin temperature. J Manipulative Physiol Ther. 1987;10(2):57–60.

17. Eingorn AM, Muhs GJ. Rationale for assessing the effects of manipulative therapy on autonomic tone by analysis of heart rate variability. J Manipulative Physiol Ther. 1999;22(3):161–5.

18. Sato A, Swenson RS. Sympathetic nervous response to mechanical stress of the spinal column in rats. J Manipulative Physiol Ther. 1984;7(3):141–7.

19. Tyldeslye B, Grieve JI. Muscles, nerves and movement. In: Human occupation. Osney Mead: Blackwell Publishing Company; 2002. p. 80–6.

20. Palmgren PJ, Sandström PJ, Lundqvist FJ, Heikkilä H. Improvement after chiropractic care in cervicocephalic kinesthetic sensibility and subjective pain intensity in patients with nontraumatic chronic neck pain. J Manipulative Physiol Ther. 2006;29(2): 100–6.

21. Chila A, Fitzgerald M, American osteopathic association. Foundations of osteopathic medicine. Philadelphia: Lippincott Williams & Wilkins; 2010. p. 648–50.

22. Kuzmich D. The levator scapulae: making the con-NECK-tion. J Man Manipulative Ther. 1994;2(2): 42–54.

23. Innes K. What if – considerations, both practical and clinical for the cervicothoracic area. Dynamic Chiro. 1992;10(16), http://www.dynamicchiropractic.com/mpacms/dc/article.php?id=43394. Accessed Feb 2013.

24. Cleland JA, Childs JD, McRae M, Palmer JA, Stowell T. Immediate effects of thoracic manipulation in patients with neck pain: a randomized clinical trial. Man Ther. 2005;10(2):127–35.

25. Sucher BM, Heath DM. Thoracic outlet syndrome – a myofascial variant: part 3. Structural and postural considerations. J Am Osteopath Assoc. 1993;93(3):334. 340–345.

26. American Chiropractic Association. Spinal manipulation policy statement; Updated 2003.

27. Cherkin DC, Mootz RD. Chiropractic in the United States: training, practice, and research. Agency for health care policy and research. AHCPR publication no. 98-N002, Dec 1997.

28. Pascarelli EF, Hsu YP. Understanding work-related upper extremity disorders: clinical findings in 485 computer users, musicians, and others. J Occup Rehabil. 2001;11(1):1–21.

29. Kisner C, Allen Colby L. Therapeutic exercise: foundations and techniques. 5th ed. Columbus: The Ohio State University School of Allied Medical Professionals; 2007.

30. Cohen N. Non-operative care of a patient with thoracic outlet syndrome and cervical radiculopathy: a case report. J Am Chiropr Assoc. 2005;42(5): 9–13.

31. Woodward TW, Best TM. The painful shoulder: part I. Clinical evaluation. Am Fam Physician. 2000;61(10): 3079–88.

32. Murphy DR. Scalene trigger points: the great imitators. Dynamic Chiro. 1991;9(24), http://www.dynamicchiropractic.com/mpacms/dc/article.php?id=44643. Accessed Feb 2013.

33. Krauss J, Creighton D, Ely J, Podlewska-Ely J. The immediate effects of upper thoracic translatoric spinal manipulation on cervical pain and range of motion: a randomized clinical trial. J Man Manip Ther. 2008; 16(2):93–9.

34. Burnett AF, Naumann FL, Price RS, Sanders RH. A comparison of training methods to increase neck muscle strength. Work. 2005;25(3):205–10.

35. Burnett AF, Naumann FL, Burton EJ. Flight-training effect on the cervical muscle isometric strength of

trainee pilots. Aviat Space Environ Med. 2004;75(7): 611–5.

36. Pearson I, Reichert A, De Serres SJ, Dumas JP, Côté JN. Maximal voluntary isometric neck strength deficits in adults with whiplash-associated disorders and association with pain and fear of movement. J Orthop Sports Phys Ther. 2009;39(3):179–87.

37. Chiu TT, Sing KL. Evaluation of cervical range of motion and isometric neck muscle strength: reliability and validity. Clin Rehabil. 2002;16(8):851–8.

38. Chiu TT, Lam TH, Hedley AJ. Maximal isometric muscle strength of the cervical spine in healthy volunteers. Clin Rehabil. 2002;16(7):772–9.

39. Braun SR. Respiratory rate and pattern. In: Walker HK, Hall WD, Hurst JW, editors. Clinical methods: the history, physical, and laboratory examinations. 3rd ed. Boston: Butterworths; 1990 (Chapter 43).

40. Kera T, Maruyama H. The effect of posture on respiratory activity of the abdominal muscles. J Physiol Anthropol Appl Human Sci. 2005;24(4):259–65.

Complementary and Alternative Medicine and NTOS

26

Wladislaw Ellis and Karl A. Illig

Abstract

Symptom control is often difficult to achieve in individuals with NTOS, and conventional therapy can be inadequate. A wide variety of alternatives thus present themselves, as they do in other neuropathic pain syndromes. This chapter summarizes 20 years of experience with a wide variety of modalities, focusing on the relevance and effectiveness of new pharmaceutical and behavioural approaches mainly directed at pain control.

Given that physical therapy, opiates, muscle relaxants, anti-epileptics, NSAIDs, and operative interventions do not consistently give acceptable results in patients with NTOS and that symptoms can return even after the best post-operative result, alternative therapies continue to be relevant. These are modalities for which rigorous proof of mechanism or effectiveness is controversial or lacking, but may, nonetheless, be of benefit in patients with NTOS. Specifics vary, but their very existence underlines the inadequacy of much of our understanding and treatment of neuropathic pain, of which NTOS is an example. Finally, whether prescribed or not, patients may choose to treat themselves with such and even the most empiric clinician needs to have a sense of what issues are thus created.

Essentially by definition, proof of efficacy for many "alternative" therapies is lacking and as a result, the following descriptions are largely anecdotal. They are based, however, on 20 years of clinical observations in over 1,500 patients with diagnosis of NTOS. Controlled studies and further discussions of mechanisms are described in the appropriate citations. Modalities are presented roughly in order of effectiveness and possible mechanisms of action in NTOS are noted. The focus is on interventions that reduce or eliminate pain, the driving complaint in NTOS (to our knowledge, no "alternative therapy," used in this context, is thought to be marketed as a treatment for NTOS).

Careful physical therapy (e.g. Edgelow's protocol) emphasizing increased self awareness and gentle, appropriate movement is indispensible and is discussed at length in Chap. 23, Physical Therapy for NTOS [1–3]. The importance of proper technique is underscored by the frequent

W. Ellis, MD (✉)
Private Practice, Neurology/Psychiatry,
1220 Oxford St, Berkeley, CA 94709, USA
e-mail: wladislawellis@gmail.com

K.A. Illig, MD
Department of Surgery, Division of Vascular Surgery,
University of South Florida,
2 Tampa General Circle, STC 7016,
Tampa, FL 33606, USA
e-mail: killig@health.usf.edu

K.A. Illig et al. (eds.), *Thoracic Outlet Syndrome*,
DOI 10.1007/978-1-4471-4366-6_26, © Springer-Verlag London 2013

and significant injuries from inappropriate physical therapy or manipulations. Specific protocols such as Feldenkrais and Alexander work, developed initially to treat and prevent chronic re-injuries in athletes, are very useful for the same purpose in NTOS and are felt to work by sensitizing the patients to actions that potentially create damage and by hastening recovery from existing injury [4]. Proponents feel that the specific protocols need to be followed avidly for decent results.

Heparin, the most negatively charged molecule in the human, actively entrains, sequesters and degrades cytokines, chemokines, MMPs, growth factors, and related products untouched by NSAIDs and steroids, all of which in theory decrease and block neural inflammation [3–7]. Because of its anti-inflammatory and anti-proliferative effects, when injected peri-neurally in small amounts it can offer dramatic relief of pain [8]. Results are largely activity dependant and the propensity for easy re-injury continues in these patients. Duration of relief is variable and ranges from 10 to 14 days to many months probably reflecting the degree of neuro-fibrotic involvement as well as injection technique and other unknown factors.

Erythropoietin, as well as stimulating the production of red blood cells, is a neuroprotectant and seemingly normalizes function in both neurons and Schwann cells by inducing terminal differentiation with a consequent reduction in neurogenic inflammation [9–11]. Erythropoietin presumably acts in NTOS by inhibiting apoptotic pathways and normalizing hyperexcitable neurons. It provides excellent, lasting, pain relief starting 3–7 days after peri-neural injection of very small amounts [12]. Thromboembolic side effects are potentially limiting with caution demanding more extensive trials, despite the excellent results to date.

Nalbuphine, a kappa receptor agonist, works better than methadone or morphine in controlling pain, although nausea is a common side effect [13]. With the increasing amount of opiate tolerance in many patients, the fact that it acts on a different receptor makes it valuable. The main drawback is that it must be injected subcutaneously once or twice a day.

Expert, knowledgeable acupuncture can often relieve symptoms for up to a week [14]. Great controversy regarding the various proposed mechanisms of action exists and objective evidence is lacking, but it has been proposed that micro-injury at the site of needle insertion followed by locally intense stimulation seems to activate viscero-somatic and autonomic reflexes as well as extensive neural activity up to and including at the cerebral cortex [15–17]. Alternative explanations include systemic endorphin release and placebo effects. The traditional explanation of anatomical "meridians" and the elicitation of "Qi" (although used clinically by some) do not correspond to modern understanding of anatomy and physiology and is discounted by most.

Hypnosis with an experienced hypnotist and a patient able to be deeply hypnotized (critical) can be very helpful in multiple ways: changing activity patterns, pain and inflammation control, and by teaching autohypnosis for symptom flares [18, 19]. The precise mechanism(s) of action are clearly psychogenic but still remain largely unknown despite evidence of obvious (MRI, EEG) cerebral activation and the often dramatic ability to influence and change sensory and autonomic functioning. Debate continues as to whether hypnosis is truly a qualitatively different state of consciousness or merely a form of relaxation.

Nitroglycerine applied topically by patch to focus delivery, can reduce symptoms dramatically [20]. This is probably a result of local nitric oxide production leading to an increased anti-inflammatory effect: nitroglycerine is more effective than local anesthetic patches, supporting this mechanism of action. The major drawback is headache, of course, due to cerebral vasodilatation.

Octreotide, a neuropeptide inhibitor, is felt to alleviate the often ongoing neurogenic inflammation but, again, needs to be delivered locally by injection and has a short half-life [21]. For these reasons it is most useful in acute symptom flare-ups.

We have shown that pulsed high intensity magnetic stimulation can ameliorate pain in NTOS patients, but this has not been widely accepted by others [22, 23]. One explanation of this effect is that very quickly pulsed, Tesla-strength fields induce depolarization of affected peripheral nerves and muscles which relieves spasm and increases local circulation. Similar trials are currently being pursued at the NIH.

There is some literature on potential therapeutic effects of monochromatic infra-red (0.8–1.1 μm) laser light. Theories abound, and the consensus seems to be that the infra-red light normalizes aberrant mitochondrial ATP formation. How this translates into benefit, however, is unknown [24]. Anecdotally this can work very well, albeit in a minority of patients.

Much the same can be said for transcutaneous nerve stimulation (TNS), with some patients continuing to use it for years [25]. The transcutaneous electrical activation of local neural networks is thought to mimic the effects of acupuncture (see above) as well as activate descending spinal inhibitory signals. This is, of course, a widely used technique and it continues to be surprising that its precise mechanism of action is not better known (similar to acupuncture).

Vagal nerve stimulation may have a place in treating in treating pain and autonomic dysfunctions in failed thoracic outlet decompressions and is probably safer and more effective, in this context, than spinal cord stimulation [26]. It has not been studied widely for this condition.

Topical sphenopalatine ganglion blocks are felt to normalize autonomic dysfunction and can be very helpful in the same population (failure after surgical decompression) or when attempting to interrupt an on-going symptom flare [27]. Finding practitioners who are able to perform this is difficult.

Intraosseous blockade (usually in the ischium – but any accessible marrow bone will work) for chronic pain was explored in a few centers in the former Soviet Union, and might still be available in Moscow [28]. Our own experience with a visiting Soviet orthopedist was quite positive in a small group of patients.

Histone mimics, capsaicin, conotoxins, botulinum, cannabinoids, agents modulating inositol-3phosphate' and, not least, colchicine, all show promise using a wide variety of mechanisms [29, 30]. None of these has been studied widely.

Lastly, as every practitioner knows, the emotional state of the patient can affect treatment for better or worse. Appropriate and preemptive effective psychoactive pharmaceuticals and/or expert psychotherapy obviously have their place (see Chap. 57).

When dealing with chronic pain and related issues in this class of patients any of the options discussed above can be considered and all are ripe for further research and better definition of action and effectiveness. Recognizing and better understanding the neuro-inflammatory nature of why symptoms exist, increase, spread and change will be a significant step in our ability to modulate and reverse them. Achieving phenotypic changes for the better in localized pathology with transcription factors is possible and is being sought by a number of groups. We are hopeful.

Editorial Note: Complimentary and Alternative Medicine for TOS

There is no such thing as "conventional" and "alternative" (or "Eastern" or "Western," or "patriarchical" or "matriarchical" or any other artificial division) medicine – there is only medical treatment that can be shown to work in a rigorous, repeatable fashion, and that which cannot. While the definition is stable, therapies within each are not – phrenology, for example, was once accepted as a scientifically valid diagnostic tool, while many drugs we use today (leech saliva, for example) were first used in anecdotal fashion despite the criticism and scorn of mainstream science. The same standard should be applied to any therapy we wish to use on a human – does it work, and do the benefits exceed the risks – and we must strive to understand a mechanism of action that makes sense within the context of science and physiology. Keep in mind, however, that anything we now label as "alternative" may someday be part of our accepted armamentarium (and things we do today, in fact, may someday be shown not to work!).

This chapter presents "alternative" techniques for treatment of patients with NTOS (largely with chronic pain) in a rational and valid style (note that most of the references are from what most would describe as solid peer-reviewed sources). It is interesting that few patients with this problem seem to have latched upon things which clearly have no effect; the modalities presented here are all associated with reasonable mechanisms of action and bear study. Dr. Ellis and his colleagues have an extensive experience and the issues suggested in this chapter bear study by all.

References

1. Craig A. How do you feel? Interoception: the sense of the physiological condition of the body. Nat Rev Neurosci. 2002;3:655–65.
2. Edgelow P. Neurovascular consequences of cumulative trauma disorders affecting the thoracic outlet: a patient-centered approach. In: Donatelli R, editor. Physical therapy of the shoulder. 4th ed. St. Louis: Churchill-Livingston-Elsevier; 2004. p. 205–38.
3. Butler D. The sensitive nervous system. Adelaide: Noigroup Publications; 2000. p. 398–424.
4. Lundblad I, Elert J, Gerdle B. Randomized controlled trial of physiotherapy and Feldenkrais interventions in female workers with neck-shoulder complaints. J Occup Rehabil. 1999;9(3):179–94.
5. Engelberg H. Heparin and the prevention of atherosclerosis. Basic research and clinical application. New York: Wiley-Liss; 1990.
6. Glantz M, et al. Treatment of radiation-induced nervous system injury with heparin and warfarin. Neurology. 1994;40:2020–7.
7. Tyrrell D, et al. Heparin in inflammation: potential therapeutic applications beyond anticoagulation. Adv Pharmacol. 1999;46:151–208.
8. Ellis W. Heparin alleviates pain in nerve entrapments. Am J Pain Manag. 2003;13(2):54–9.
9. Brines M, Cerami A. Emerging biological roles for erythropoietin in the nervous system. Nat Rev Neurosci. 2005;6:484–94.
10. Campana W, Myers R. Exogenous erythropoietin protects against dorsal root ganglion apoptosis and pain following nerve root crush. Eur J Neurosci. 2003;18: 1497–506.
11. Bianchi R, et al. Erythropoietin both protects from and reverses experimental diabetic neuropathy. Proc Natl Acad Sci. 2004;101(3):823–8.
12. Ellis W. Erythropoietin as a novel analgesic for neuropathic pain. In: Abstracts of the 12th World Congress on Pain; control #08-A-1245-IASP. Glasgow 8/17-22; 2008.
13. Schmidt W, et al. Nalbuphine. Drug Alcohol Depend. 1985;14(3–4):339–62.
14. Napadow V. Hypothalamus and amygdala response to acupuncture stimuli in carpal tunnel syndrome. Pain. 2007;130(3):254–66.
15. Kendall D. Dao of Chinese medicine: understanding an ancient healing art. London/Hong Kong/New York: Oxford University Press; 2002.
16. Cheng R, Pomeranz B. A combined treatment with D-amino acids and electroacupuncture produces a greater analgesia than either treatment alone; naloxone reverses these effects. Pain. 1980;8: 231–6.
17. Chapman C, et al. Naloxone fails to reverse pain thresholds elevated by acupuncture: acupuncture analgesia reconsidered. Pain. 1983;16:13–31.
18. Moore L. Hypnotically-induced vasodilation in the treatment of repetitive strain injuries. Am J Clin Hypn. 1996;39(2):97–104.
19. Erickson M. The nature of hypnosis and suggestion. New York: Irvington Publishers; 1980.
20. Berrazueta J, et al. Successful treatment of shoulder pain due to supraspinatus tendinitis with transdermal nitroglycerine. A double blind study. Pain. 1996;66:63–7.
21. Ellis W. Octreotide, a small peptide, alleviates burning pain and hyperesthesia: a preliminary study. Pain Clinic. 1990;3(4):239–42.
22. Ellis W. Magnetic neuromuscular stimulation in humans. Automedica. 1989;11:15–8.
23. Zhadin M. Review of Russian literature on biological action of DC and low-frequency AC magnetic fields. Bioelectromagnetics. 2001;22:27–45.
24. Branco K, Naeser M. Carpal tunnel syndrome: clinical outcome after low-level laser acupuncture, microamps transcutaneous electrical nerve stimulation, and other alternative therapies– an open protocol study. J Altern Complement Med. 1999;5(1):5–26.
25. Mannheimer C, Carlson C. The analgesic effect of transcutaneous electrical nerve stimulation (TNS) in patients with rheumatoid arthritis. A comparative study of different pulse pattern. Pain. 1979;6: 329–34.
26. George M, et al. Vagus nerve stimulation therapy – a research update. Neurology. 2002;59:S56–61.
27. Ferrante F, et al. Sphenopalatine ganglion block for the treatment of myofascial pain of the head, neck, and shoulders. Reg Anesth Pain Med. 1998;23(1): 30–6.
28. Sokov E. Intramuscular and intraosseous blockade in the complex therapy of neurological signs in pelvic osteochondritis. J Neuropathol Psych named for SSKorsakov. 1988;88(4):57–61.
29. Li Z, et al. Inhibition of LPS-induced tumor necrosis factor-alpha production by colchicine and othe microtubule disrupting drugs. Immunobiology. 1996; 195(4–5):624–39.
30. Nicodeme E, et al. Suppression of inflammation by a synthetic histone mimic. Nature. 2010;468:1119–23.

Complex Regional Pain Syndrome and NTOS

Dean M. Donahue

Abstract

Complex regional pain syndrome (CRPS) is a chronic pain condition with defined diagnostic criteria that occasionally develops following an injury. It may develop in NTOS patients following the initial traumatic event resulting in both nerve injury and compression within the thoracic outlet, or from intraoperative nerve injury during treatment of NTOS. Both are rare occurrences, but this chapter will explore the possible mechanisms involved in CRPS.

Introduction

Chronic pain is the most common complaint in patients with neurogenic thoracic outlet syndrome (NTOS). The mechanism producing this pain is presumed to be from chronic nerve compression within the thoracic outlet. This compression would explain the associated sensory symptoms of paresthesia and numbness, as well as motor complaints such as weakness. An alternative or contributing factor could be mechanical stimulation of pain fibers (nociceptors) within the muscles of the thoracic outlet – possibly created

D.M. Donahue, MD
Department of Thoracic Surgery,
Massachusetts General Hospital, Blake 1570,
55 Fruit Street, Boson, MA 02114, USA
e-mail: donahue.dean@mgh.harvard.edu

by muscle dysfunction from postural abnormalities or repetitive strain injury.

Complex regional pain syndrome (CRPS) is a specific chronic pain condition which develops following an injury. It has defined diagnostic criteria, and is found in only a small number of patients with chronic, severe pain. CRPS is uncommon, but not rare in NTOS patients. Some patients with NTOS may have clinical features seen in CRPS without having all of the diagnostic criteria necessary. Clinical signs seen in some NTOS patients such as skin discoloration or edema may overlap with those seen in CRPS. The critical difference being that CRPS symptoms are out of proportion to the identified nerve injury. Nerve injury in NTOS patients that could potentially lead to CRPS are the traumatic event in a patient with pre-existing or subsequent thoracic outlet compression. The second results from intraoperative nerve injury during thoracic outlet decompression.

K.A. Illig et al. (eds.), *Thoracic Outlet Syndrome*,
DOI 10.1007/978-1-4471-4366-6_27, © Springer-Verlag London 2013

Classification of Pain: Nociceptive vs. Neuropathic

In evaluating patients with pain, it is important to understand two classifications of pain: nociceptive and neuropathic. Nociceptive pain involves stimulation of nociceptors in the skin, deep tissues or viscera, and is the common mechanism for experiencing pain from a direct injury. The stimulation of these pain fibers may be thermal, chemical or mechanical. Neuropathic pain results from damage or disease affecting the central or peripheral neurons. Characteristics of neuropathic pain include ongoing pain independent of stimulus, associated partial or complete sensory loss and abnormal summation of pain (i.e. the delivery of a consistent stimuli becomes increasingly painful). Examples of neuropathic pain include phantom limb pain, post-stroke pain, postherpetic neuralgia and CRPS.

Historical Perspective and Current Classification

The evolution of CRPS can be traced back to S. Weir Mitchell, a neurologist during the American Civil War. He found that 10 % of solders with major extremity injuries – including the brachial plexus – developed burning pain, abnormal skin perfusion with temperature asymmetry, swelling and excessive sweating. He termed this "causalgia" from the Greek word for burning. He noted that the symptoms often spread beyond the territory of the initial injury, and occasionally spread to the "mirror" site on the contralateral extremity. This condition was termed reflex sympathetic dystrophy (RSD) by Evans in 1946, as it was mistakenly believed that control of the microcirculation was exclusively limited to the autonomic nervous system [1]. In 1994 the International Association for the Study of Pain (IASP) used the term CRPS, and defined two groups of patients depending on the presence of a known nerve injury (Table 27.1) [2]. In each group, CRPS begins following a trauma or immobilization and has continued disproportionate pain, allodynia or hyperalgesia. Edema, skin

Table 27.1 The International Association for the Study of Pain (IASP) diagnostic criteria for CRPS

1. Continuing pain, allodynia (perception of pain from a nonpainful stimulus), or hyperalgesia (an exaggerated sense of pain) disproportionate to the inciting event.
2. A history of edema, changes in skin blood flow, or abnormal sudomotor activity in the area of pain.
3. The absence of any condition that would otherwise account for the signs and symptoms.

CRPS Type I (RSD) develop without a known nerve injury. CRPS Type II (causalgia) is diagnosed after an initiating noxious event or a cause of immobilization
Based on data from Merskey and Bogduk [2]

discoloration or abnormal sweating occurs at some point in time. In CRPS type I, patients may have had local trauma, but they do not have a known nerve injury. CPRS type II patients have an identified nerve injury. Since this classification, many patients thought to have CRPS-I are found to have a nerve injury on closer evaluation [3]. Many clinicians no longer separate these two groups, as the clinical presentation, pathophysiology and response to treatment are similar.

Because the IASP criteria were thought to be insufficiently specific, an international consortium convened in Budapest in 2003 to update the criteria used to diagnose cases of CRPS [4]. It was proposed that the original IASP criteria remain in use for diagnosing CRPS for research purposes. In addition, a less demanding set of criteria was proposed for clinically probable cases [5]. The "Budapest criteria" allows for a clinical diagnosis of CRPS to be made when the patient complains of pain which is out of proportion to the inciting event. In addition, four categories are evaluated for symptoms and signs. At least one symptom must be present in three of these four categories that include sensory complaints such as hyperesthesia, vasomotor complaints that include temperature or skin color changes, sudomotor or edematous changes and motor or trophic changes. There also had to be abnormal findings at the time of the physical exam in at least two of these four categories. Both the IASP and Budapest criteria require the absence of any condition that would otherwise explain the signs and symptoms.

Epidemiology and Clinical Features of CRPS

CRPS is typified by pain along with associated signs. It is a clinical diagnosis characterized by continuing pain, plus other features including skin hypersensitivity and microcirculatory abnormalities resulting in skin discoloration and edema. Abnormal sweating, bone resorption, and trophic changes in the skin, nails, hair or muscle can also be seen. Motor changes are frequently seen including dystonia, tremor and weakness. This condition can develop following any local trauma or period of extremity immobilization. The severity of CRPS symptoms is a wide spectrum, and appears to be disportionate to the initial injury. The role that TOS plays in causing a nerve injury leading to CRPS – as diagnosed by IASP criteria – is not defined, and examples in the literature are scarce. However, as outlined in Chap. 7, up to 10 % of patients with presumed TOS may have clinical features of CRPS. The clinical challenge is determining if the inciting nerve injury is from chronic compression within the thoracic outlet versus injury at another level.

The incidence of CRPS is reported to be 26.2 cases per 100,000 people annually, with at least 50,000 new cases of CRPS each year in the United States [6, 7]. Orthopedic injuries such as fractures and sprains are the most common precipitating factors. CRPS is four times more common in women, and typically occurs in middle-age adults. It is becoming increasingly clear that genetic factors likely play a role, and may explain why some patients with relatively minor injuries – such as following a needle stick or scald – develop CRPS [8].

Pathophysiology of CRPS

The pathophysiology of CRPS is unknown, but current evidence suggests a multifactorial process. The current model for the development of CRPS begins with tissue trauma and local nerve injury. This injury could be quite minimal, but in certain genetically predisposed individuals the response may lead to the development of CRPS.

The injury response begins with local inflammation, but in individuals who express a "CRPS-phenotype", the inflammatory response progresses down an abnormal pathway.

The abnormal response to local inflammation results in sensitization of the peripheral nociceptors [9]. There is some evidence to suggest that the affected nerves in CRPS are the "small fibers" of the peripheral nervous system. These fibers are thinly myelinated A-delta fibers, unmyelinated C-fibers and post-ganglionic sympathetic axons. Small fibers comprise 80 % of peripheral axons including pain receptors (nociceptors). They are also involved in controlling the microcirculation and sweat glands. Analysis of skin biopsies show an approximately 30 % decrease in small fiber nociceptors in CRPS-affected sites compared to uninvolved control sites [10]. This decrease is not seen in patients with chronic extremity pain, swelling and disuse from other painful conditions such as severe osteoarthritis. Examination of limbs amputated in CRPS patients showed a decrease in the number of small fiber axons with no change in myelinated nerves [11]. It is unclear why a decrease in the number of nociceptor fibers is associated with an increase in pain, but surviving small fibers in the region have reduced activation thresholds.

The abnormal response to injury in CRPS patients also appears to affect the sympathetic nervous system (SNS). There is a reduction in sympathetic outflow which could ultimately lead to an increased expression of adrenergic receptors on local nociceptors [12]. The SNS response may explain the inconsistent clinical response to local sympathetic blockade or surgical sympathectomy, yet increased sensitivity to circulating catecholamines. This is further outlined in Chap. 31.

Skin abnormalities such as discoloration, edema, temperature alterations and abnormal sweating led many to conclude that RSD was mediated by the sympathetic nervous system. However, some skin vessels do not contain any sympathetic innervation, and somatic small fibers also innervate the microcirculation [13]. Degeneration of small fibers within the nervi vasorum results in opening dermal arteriovenous shunts in the extremities causing blood to bypass tissue capillary beds. Thus, while the skin appears flushed, the tissues in CRPS-affected extremities may be ischemic as demonstrated by phosphorus magnetic resonance spectroscopy [14]. Neurogenic edema may result from capillary leakage mediated by inappropriate release of vasogenic peptides from malfunctioning small fibers.

CRPS also appears to affect the central nervous system as well. There is evidence to support the concept of "central sensitization", whereby an injury to peripheral afferent nerves triggers activation somatosensory nociceptive networks within the central nervous system [15]. This mechanism could explain both referred pain and the spread of pain beyond the initial area, and may be the final common pathway in neuropathic pain conditions. There also may be reorganization of the somatosensory cortex through a process referred to as "brain plasticity". The size and location of the sensory cortex associated with the CRPS-effected body part has been seen to change throughout the course of a patient's disease [16].

Treatment Strategies

Some cases of CRPS are mild, and will improve over time. Cases involving children and teenagers will frequently recover. Prior to treatment, other causes of neuropathy (i.e. diabetes, vitamin deficiency, Lyme disease, etc.) should be excluded. Patients who fail to improve should be evaluated for ongoing nerve injury from compression, scarring or neuroma formation. When nerve compression is clearly identified, decompression can provide effective treatment of CRPS. This is found in a very small minority of CRPS patients, and caution needs to be exercised before proceeding with surgery, as some patients can have a marked worsening of their pain following surgical treatment. Surgical sympathectomy for treatment of CRPS appears to have little role, and this is outlined further in Chap. 31.

Initial treatment of CRPS should address each component of patient's symptoms. Pain management allows patients to participate in physical therapy, thereby avoiding the complications of limb disuse. Physical therapeutic modalities such as mirror therapy or graded motor imagery have shown promise [17, 18], and neurogenic edema is treated by increasing activity, limb elevation and compression wrap or garments if tolerated.

In the absence of clinical trials in CRPS, data from randomized trials of other neuralgias involving focal peripheral nerve injuries such as postherpetic neuralgia (PHN) can guide therapy. Meta-analysis of PHN trials supports the use of oral tricyclic antidepressants, strong opioids, gabapentin, tramadol and pregabalin [19]. A more detailed strategy for management of neuropathic pain is outlined in Chap. 35. In CRPS patients, bone resorption is thought to be a source of "deep" pain that some experience, and is treated with bisphosphonates or nasal calcitonin. Smoking cessation and daily aspirin are advised because of the concern for tissue ischemia from microcirculatory abnormalities. Spinal cord stimulators have been shown to be effective in some patients with CRPS, particularly in patients with localized nerve injuries, and their role in treating chronic pain are discussed in Chap. 55.

References

1. Evans JA. Reflex sympathetic dystrophy; report of 57 cases. Ann Intern Med. 1947;26:417–26.
2. Merskey H, Bogduk N. Classification of chronic pain: descriptions of chronic pain syndromes and definitions of pain terms. 2nd ed. Seattle: IASP Press; 1994.
3. Oaklander AL. Role of minimal distal nerve injury in complex regional pain syndrome-I. Pain Med. 2010;11:1251–6.
4. Harden RN, Bruehl S. Diagnostic criteria: the statistical derivation of the four criterion factors. In: Wilson PR, Stanton-Hicks M, Harden RN, editors. CRPS: current diagnosis and therapy. Seattle: IASP Press; 2005. p. 45–58.
5. Harden RN, Bruehl S, Stanton-Hicks M, et al. Proposed new diagnostic criteria for complex regional pain syndrome. Pain Med. 2007;8:326–31.
6. De Mos M, de Bruijn AG, Huygen FJ, et al. The incidence of complex regional pain syndrome: a population based study. Pain. 2007;129:12–20.
7. Bruehl S, Chung OY. How common is complex regional pain syndrome-type 1? Pain. 2007;129:1–2.
8. de Rooij AM, de Mos M, Sturkenboom MC, Marinus J, van den Maagdenberg AM, van Hilten JJ. Familial occurrence of complex regional pain syndrome. Eur J Pain. 2009;13:171–7.

9. Cheng JK, Ji RR. Intracellular signaling in primary sensory neurons and persistent pain. Neurochem Res. 2008;33:1970–8.

10. Oaklander AL, Rissmiller JG, Gelman LB, Zheng L, Chang Y, Gott R. Evidence of focal small-fiber axonal degeneration in complex regional pain syndrome-1 (reflex sympathetic dystrophy). Pain. 2006;120: 235–43.

11. Albrecht PJ, Hines S, Eisenberg E. Pathologic alterations of cutaneous innervation and vasculature in affected limbs from patients with complex regional pain syndrome. Pain. 2006;120:244–66.

12. Schürmann M, Gradl G, Zaspel J, Kayser M, Löhr P, Andress HJ. Peripheral sympathetic function as a predictor of complex regional pain syndrome type I (CRPS 1) in patients with radial fracture. Auton Neurosci. 2000;86:127–34.

13. Holzer P. Control of the cutaneous vascular system by afferent neurons. In: Morris JL, Gibbons IL, editors. Autonomic innervations of the skin. Amsterdam/Holland: Hardwood Academic Publishers; 1997. p. 213–67.

14. Heerschap A, den Hollander JA, Reynen H, et al. Metabolic changes in reflex sympathetic dystrophy: a 31P NMR spectroscopy study. Muscle Nerve. 1993;16:367–73.

15. Ji RR, Woolf CJ. Neuronal plasticity and signal transduction in nociceptive neurons: implications for the initiation and maintenance of pathological pain. Neurobiol Dis. 2001;8:1–10.

16. Maihöfner C, Handwerker HO, Neundörfer B, Birklein F. Cortical reorganization during recovery from complex regional pain syndrome. Neurology. 2004;63:693–701.

17. Cacchio A, DeBlasis E, Necozione S, et al. Mirror therapy for chronic complex regional pain syndrome type I and stroke. N Engl J Med. 2009;361:634–6.

18. Daly AE, Bialocerkowski AE. Does evidence support physiotherapy management of adult complex regional pain syndrome type one? a systemic review. Eur J Pain. 2009;13:339–53.

19. Hempenstall K, Nurmikko TJ, Johnson RW, et al. Analgesic therapy in postherpetic neuralgia: a quantitative systematic review. PLoS Med. 2005;2:628–44.

Part III

Neurogenic TOS: Surgical Techniques

There are several different ways to approach the thoracic outlet for surgical treatment of neurogenic TOS. While much of what we do is based on what we're comfortable with and/or how we are trained, there are rational reasons for doing different operations for different problems. A useful way to think about this issue is based on what part of the thoracic outlet anatomy is thought to be most critical in the given situation. In other words, do you need to expose and control the brachial plexus and the posterior part of the first rib, or the costoclavicular junction and the anterior part of the first rib? Similarly, is there a cervical rib "up high" that needs correcting, or symptoms of upper or lower brachial plexus compression?

When treating a patient with neurogenic thoracic outlet syndrome (NTOS), the most critical structures to consider are the scalene muscles and associated anomalous structures or bands, the *mid- to posterior part* of the first rib, and any fibrous scar tissue around the brachial plexus nerves. Many clinicians and investigators believe that the brachial plexus itself should be fully dissected for optimal safety and best long-term results. The transaxillary approach, described below by Dr. Freischlag, is considered by many to be the most cosmetic, while the supraclavicular approach, described by Dr. Illig, allows the most thorough scalenectomy and brachial plexus neurolysis along with first rib resection. Interestingly, results seem to be very similar between the two when performed by experienced personnel, but there not yet satisfactory studies by which to make an accurate comparison. As described in another chapter, compression of the brachial plexus by the pectoralis minor muscle is increasingly recognized as an important part of NTOS in many patients, and Dr. Thompson discusses his strategy for operative correction of this problem. Cervical sympathectomy should be part of the armamentarium of all TOS surgeons, and this is described by Dr. Donahue. Finally, although not commonly performed, Dr. Urschel describes the posterior approach to thoracic outlet decompression, a technique that may be especially useful in reoperative situations.

Together these authors bring over a century of cumulative experience in the operating room with these problems. Every TOS surgeon should be familiar with each of these techniques, but ultimately which approach is better for which patient is an individualized decision.

Surgical Techniques: Operative Decompression Using the Transaxillary Approach for NTOS

28

George J. Arnaoutakis and Thomas Reifsnyder

Abstract

Most feel that patients with neurogenic thoracic outlet syndrome (NTOS) who are refractory to conservative management should undergo operative decompression. The ideal approach for NTOS should be based on the patient's symptoms and anatomy, and the surgeon's operative experience. The transaxillary approach was first described by Roos in 1966, and many surgeons prefer this approach because of its relative ease, low risk, and documented ability to improve patients' quality of life. This chapter describes the technical aspects of transaxillary first rib resection with attention to factors that influence short- and long-term outcome when performed in patients with NTOS.

Introduction

Most feel that patients with neurogenic thoracic outlet syndrome (NTOS) who are refractory to conservative management should undergo operative decompression. The ideal approach for NTOS should be based on the patient's symptoms and anatomy, and the surgeon's operative experience. The transaxillary approach was first described by Roos in 1966 [1]. Many surgeons prefer this approach because of its relative ease, low risk, and documented ability to improve patients' quality of life [2, 3].

Up to 95 % of TOS patients have neurogenic complaints [4]. Symptoms of NTOS include paresthesias, pain, and impaired strength in the affected shoulder, arm, or hand, along with occipital headaches and neck discomfort. There is commonly an antecedent history of hyperextension neck injury or repetitive neck trauma. Patients frequently manifest tenderness on palpation of the shoulder, mastoid region, supraclavicular fossa, or over the anterior scalene muscle.

Preoperative physical therapy is recommended for most patients with a diagnosis of NTOS, in an attempt to relieve symptoms through improved posture and to achieve greater range of motion. While many patients will improve with physical

G.J. Arnaoutakis, MD
Department of Surgery,
Johns Hopkins Hospital,
600 N. Wolfe Street, Blalock 655,
Baltimore, MD 21287, USA
e-mail: gja10@jhmi.edu

T. Reifsnyder, MD (✉)
Department of Surgery,
Johns Hopkins Bayview Medical Center,
4940 Eastern Ave. 5fl. A-Bldg,
Baltimore, MD 21224, USA
e-mail: treifsn1@jhmi.edu

Fig. 28.1 A photograph depicting proper patient positioning for *right* transaxillary first rib resection and use of the Machleder arm support with generous padding to prevent compression nerve injury. A padded axillary roll is placed under the dependent (*left*) axilla, and the patient is stabilized in the *left* lateral decubitus with the aid of a bean bag. The *dashed line* indicates the preferred location of the skin incision

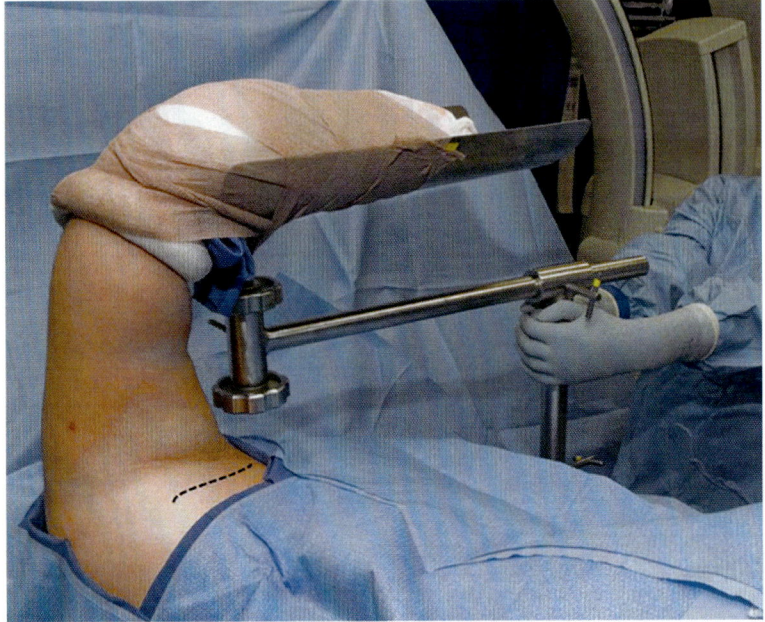

therapy and lifestyle alterations, patients with debilitating symptoms despite 8 weeks of physical therapy warrant surgical intervention.

Operative Technique

Prophylactic antibiotics (often a first generation cephalosporin) are administered immediately prior to the operation and prophylaxis for deep vein thrombosis should be instituted. Postoperative pain can be minimized by a preoperative intravenous dose of Ketorolac Tromethamine (Toradol).

Positioning

Induction of general anesthesia is performed. Short-acting neuromuscular blockade agents should be used for induction as normal nerve activity is desired for safer dissection around the brachial plexus. The patient is placed in the lateral decubitus position with the aid of a bean bag to facilitate positioning; care should be taken to pad the dependent axilla and maintain proper neck alignment. The sterile field includes the arm, axilla, and shoulder. An adjustable

Machleder arm support is affixed to the operating table with the vertical support bar attached at the level of the patient's chin. Extensive padding with sterile towels and cotton Sof-Rol (BSN Medical Inc., Rutherford College, NC) wrapped around the patient's arm prior to placement in the arm holder protects the median and ulnar nerves at the elbow joint. The arm is secured to the arm holder utilizing a Coban (3M Health Care, St. Paul, MN) self-adhesive wrap (Fig. 28.1). With proper positioning and arm retraction, visualization during the operation is excellent.

Exposure

After positioning the surgeon identifies the anterior border of the latissiumus dorsi muscle and the posterior border of the pectoralis major muscle. A transverse skin line incision is made between these two structures at the level of the inferior axillary hair line. The subcutaneous tissue is divided with electrocautery until thin areolar tissue just superficial to the chest wall is encountered. Self-retaining cerebellar or Weitlaner retractors are then inserted into the wound to maximize exposure. After encountering the chest wall—and if in the correct anatomic plane—gentle blunt dissection with the surgeon's fingers or a pair of Kitner peanut dissectors easily separates the soft tissues from it. This dissection proceeds in the cephalad direction and the second rib rapidly comes into view. The intercostobrachial nerve is located in the second intercostal space and is frequently difficult to avoid. Any injury causes numbness or dysesthesia of the medial aspect of the proximal arm, but this common complication generally resolves with time as long as the nerve is not divided. Raising the Machleder arm support at this point leads to optimal access to the first rib and thoracic outlet (Fig. 28.2). Deep wound retraction is provided by narrow Deaver or Wylie renal vein retractors. Fiber optic lighted Deaver retractors facilitate

visualization; the surgeon (and assistants) can also wear headlights. The first rib is identified cephalad and medial to the second rib; it is positively identified by noting the insertion of the anterior scalene muscle and direct visualization of the artery and vein. The first rib is generally encountered more cephalad than the non-expert would anticipate, and may initially be out of view medial to the second rib. A Kitner or peanut dissector is used to gently sweep away the loose fibrous tissue overlying the brachial plexus, subclavian artery and vein, and scalene muscles. There is occasionally a small branch of the subclavian artery that must be ligated and divided in order to widely expose the operative field.

The next step is to fully expose the rib. Depending on the patient's anatomy, it generally

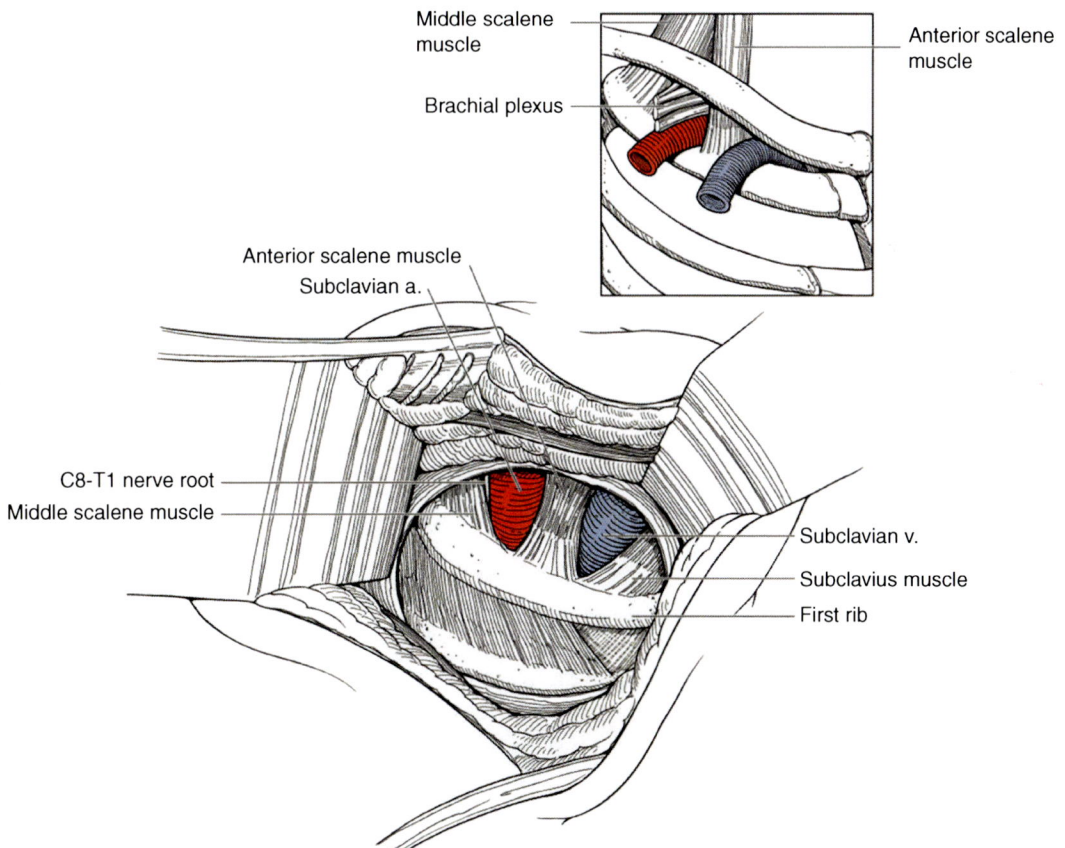

Fig. 28.2 Right-sided thoracic outlet anatomy from the surgeon's perspective as viewed through the operative field in a transaxillary approach. *Inset*, Normal anatomic field in a transaxillary approach. *Inset*, Normal anatomic

relationships of important thoracic *outlet* structures (Reprinted from Chaikof and Cambria [5]. With permission from Elsevier)

Fig. 28.3 A periosteal elevator is used to dissect along the superior surface of the first rib in order to divide intercostal muscle (Reprinted from Chaikof and Cambria [5]. With permission from Elsevier)

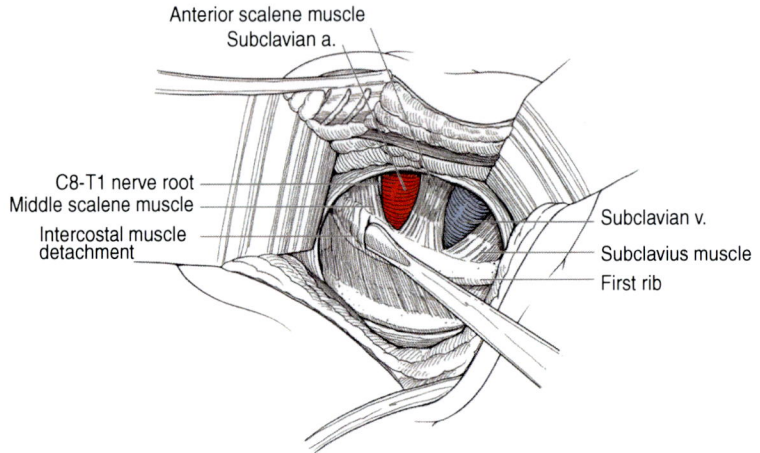

Anterior scalene muscle
Subclavian a.

C8-T1 nerve root
Middle scalene muscle
Intercostal muscle detachment

Subclavian v.
Subclavius muscle
First rib

is easiest to first clear the intercostal muscle attachments and periosteum laterally. A Cobb periosteal elevator works best, but any type of long elevator may be used (Fig. 28.3). The dissection proceeds in the anterior and posterior directions until all muscle attachments are separated from the rib and the inferior border is exposed. The elevator can then be used to elevate the first rib, separating it from the underlying parietal pleura. This mobilization should extend from a point posterior to the brachial plexus to a point anterior to the subclavian vein. Attention is then directed to the superior border of the first rib, where the periosteal elevator is used to bluntly divide the scalene medius fibers at their attachment to the rib. The long thoracic nerve courses along the lateral edge of the scalene medius muscle but is generally not visualized; sharp dissection should not be used for this step and dissection should be limited to the surface of the rib in order to protect the nerve.

During mobilization of the first rib, oozing of blood from dissected muscle can be controlled by temporarily packing the wound. Lowering the arm to collapse the wound will further assist with hemostasis. Periodic breaks are an important part of this operation to obtain hemostasis, temporarily relieve tension on the brachial plexus, and also to give the assistant a short break from a physically demanding operation.

The anterior scalene muscle should now clearly be identified as it attaches to the superior aspect of the first rib (Fig. 28.4). A right-angled clamp is passed behind the anterior scalene muscle near its insertion on the scalene tubercle. Gently lifting of the anterior scalene with the right-angled clamp protects the subclavian artery as it courses posterior to the muscle (Fig. 28.5). It is important to free several centimeters of the muscle prior to dividing it with Metzenbaum scissors (Fig. 28.6). This maneuver allows resection of a segment of the anterior scalene muscle, a move which has been shown to reduce recurrence rates when compared with simple division at its insertion point [6, 7]. Finally, the subclavius muscle will appear as a crescent-shaped ligamentous anterior attachment to the first rib adjacent to the subclavian vein. With care not to injure the subclavian vein, this can be sharply divided with scissors.

Rib Resection

After the rib is freely mobilized, a bone cutter is used to divide the first rib. Generally it is divided anteriorly and then posteriorly, although a patient's body habitus may render the reverse order easier (Fig. 28.7). Anteriorly the rib is divided adjacent to the subclavian vein and posteriorly as far back as possible, but complete visualization of the tips of the bone cutter should be the limiting factor to ensure that the nerve roots are not inadvertently injured. The rib is then

Fig. 28.4 An image of the gross anatomy from a close-up perspective of the right-sided thoracic outlet. The important relationships between the first rib, anterior scalene muscle, and subclavian vessels can be seen (Reprinted from Chaikof and Cambria [5]. With permission from Elsevier)

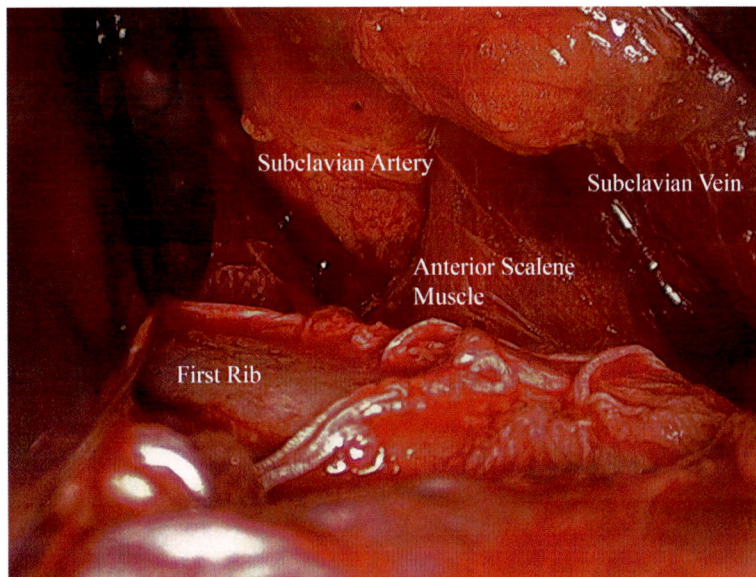

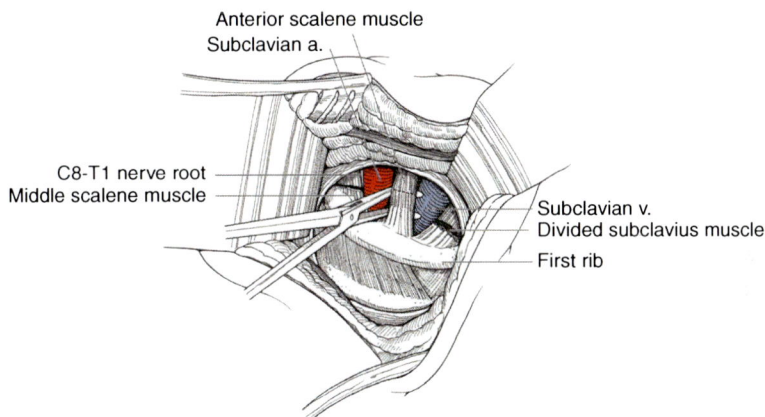

Fig. 28.5 A right-angled clamp is insinuated behind the anterior scalene muscle. Gentle elevation pulls the muscle away from the underlying subclavian artery thereby protecting the artery prior to dividing the muscle with scissors. The subclavius muscle is a crescent-shaped ligamentous attachment to the first rib adjacent to the subclavian vein. The subclavius muscle is sharply divided with scissors with care not to injure the subclavian vein (Reprinted from Chaikof and Cambria [5]. With permission from Elsevier)

removed, and typically the segment of bone resected is smaller than anticipated. A bone rongeur is used to excise residual rib and to smooth the cut ends until there is a near complete rib resection. A Roos retractor or similar instrument may be used to protect the nerves during use of the rongeur (Fig. 28.8).

It is important to ensure that no residual fibers from the anterior scalene muscle course beneath the subclavian artery and insert onto the thickened surface at the apex of the pleura (Sibson's fascia); any such fibers so identified should be divided.

Closure

The surgical field is inspected for bleeding. Temporarily packing the wound as described above reliably achieves hemostasis. The wound is then re-inspected, and any remaining bleeding is controlled

Fig. 28.6 The first rib is seen in the foreground of the operative photo taken during a *left* first rib resection. Metzenbaum scissors are used to sharply divide the anterior scalene muscle, with the *right* angled clamp elevating the muscle to protect the subclavian artery as it courses behind the muscle. The divided ends of the tendinous anterior scalene fibers can be seen (Reprinted from Chaikof and Cambria [5]. With permission from Elsevier)

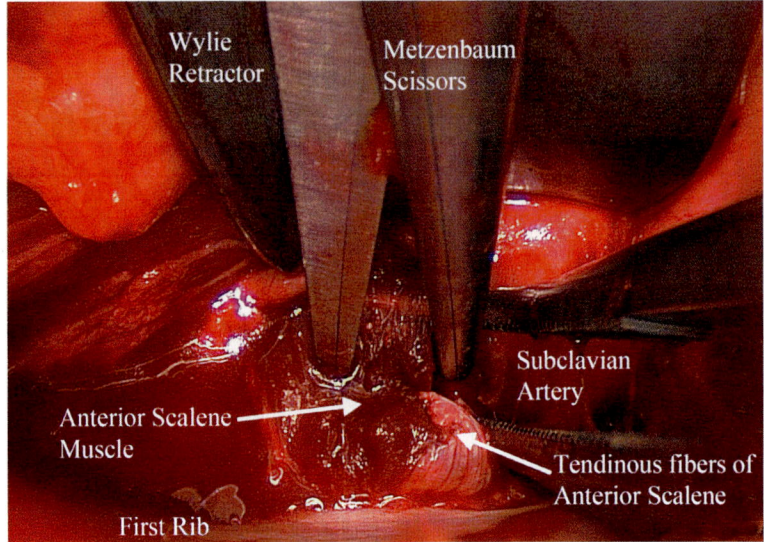

Fig. 28.7 A bone cutter is used to divide the first rib in its anterior and posterior direction. Once removed the rongeur is used to achieve smooth rib (Reprinted from Chaikof and Cambria [5]. With permission from Elsevier)

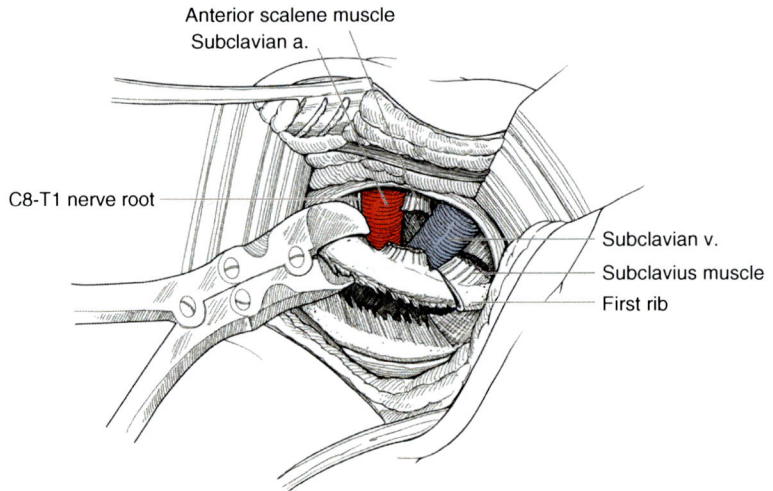

with judicious use of electrocautery. The wound is then filled with saline and several positive pressure ventilations are administered to assess for an air leak indicative of a postoperative pneumothorax; a small caliber (12 French) chest tube can be placed in the event of a significant air leak. If the irrigation drains into the pleural space but there is no air leak, the pleura has been breached but a chest tube may not be necessary. In this situation, a 12 or 14 French red rubber catheter is placed into the bed of the first rib and attached to gentle suction. The Machleder arm holder is lowered to providea tension free closure. The subcutaneous fascia is then closed around the tube on suction, but not tied. The anesthesia team then delivers a sustained Valsalva maneuver,

and the fascial suture is tied as the suction tube is rapidly removed. Closure is performed with absorbable 2–0 suture in the fascia and a 4–0 subcuticular skin closure.

Avoiding Injury to the Brachial Plexus

The brachial plexus is rarely injured during transaxillary first rib resection for TOS. However, because of the morbidity of neurologic injury, the surgeon should be vigilant on a few points. When a Machleder retractor is used to position the arm during the procedure, the arm should not be positioned at greater than 90° of abduction. The

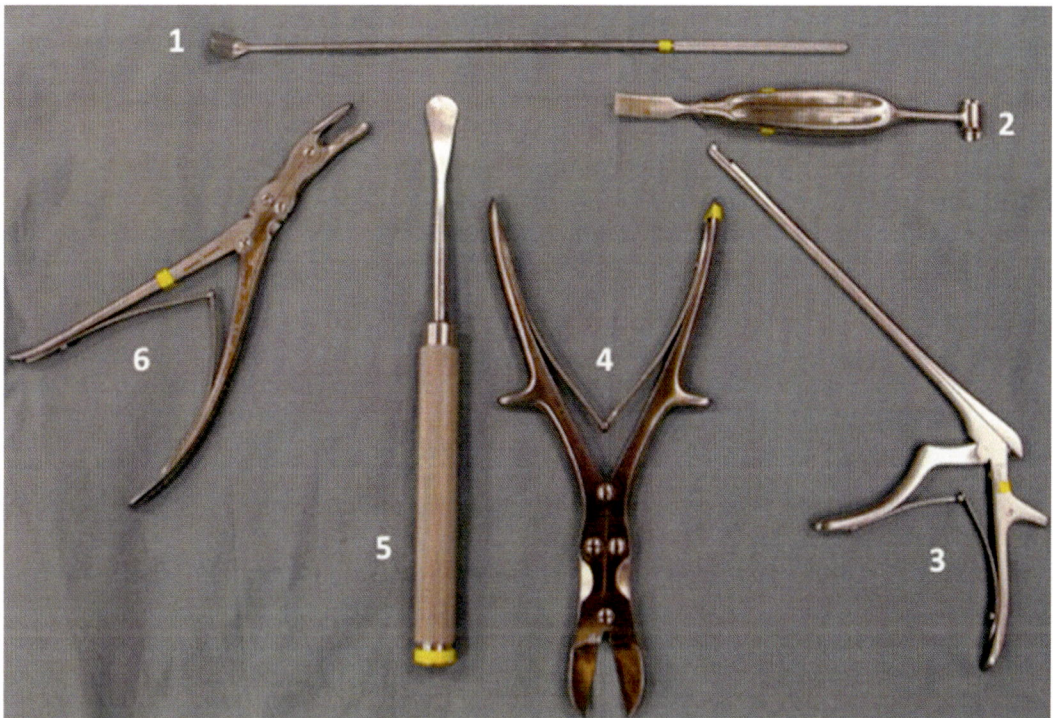

Fig. 28.8 From the top of the image in the clockwise direction, the instruments depicted are: *1* Roos retractor, *2* Alexander Periosteotome, *3* Kerrison Punch upbiting instrument, *4* Double action bone cutter, *5* Cobb periosteal elevator, and *6* Rongeur (Reprinted from Chaikof and Cambria [5]. With permission from Elsevier)

Machleder retractor should be adjusted periodically (every 20–25 min) to release tension on the brachial plexus. Because the operative field is narrowly confined, assistants holding retractors will have an impaired view. Therefore, the operating surgeon must constantly monitor the positioning of their retractors. Additionally, the brachial plexus is vulnerable to injury when dividing the rib or when using the rongeur to smooth the posterior rib stump. A good rule when using the bone cutters or rongeur is to check positioning at least twice before cutting once. Positioning a Roos retractor in front of the brachial plexus and gently displacing the nerve bundle offers protection when using the rongeur. Always keep the tips of any cutting instrument in view!

Postoperative Care

A chest radiograph is obtained in the recovery room. A small, clinically asymptomatic pneumothorax can be observed with a repeat chest radiograph performed the next morning. Patients are typically discharged from the hospital on postoperative day one if adequate oral analgesia has been achieved. Activity is restricted by the amount of post-operative pain. Occasionally, a short term sling may be used for patient comfort, but it is preferable to have the arm as mobile as tolerated.

Physical therapy should be prescribed after 2 weeks in all patients undergoing transaxillary first rib resection. Such therapy is critical to restore range of motion and strength, and may be required for 8–12 weeks.

Postoperative Complications

Vascular Injury

A national query identified injury to the subclavian vessels as the most common complication following transaxillary rib resection for neurogenic TOS, occurring in 1–2 % of cases

[8]. Patients experiencing a vascular injury have greater lengths of stay as well as increased hospital charges [2]. It is difficult to obtain proximal control of these vessels from the transaxillary approach, and therefore the surgeon should exercise extreme caution when dissecting near these vessels.

Nerve Injury

Major nerve injury has been traditionally regarded as the most common complication following surgery for TOS. However, large contemporary series disprove this belief, with rates of brachial plexus injury for patients undergoing transaxillary first rib resection being 0 % in many large series [2, 8]. Temporary or permanent numbness of the upper medial arm due to excessive traction or division of the intercostobrachial nerve occurs in up to 10 % of patients, but as discussed above these symptoms will usually improve over time.

Pneumothorax

Recognizable pneumothorax occurs in 2–10 % of patients [8]. Accordingly, an upright chest radiograph is routinely performed in the recovery room. Radiographically-detected pneumothoraces are frequently clinically insignificant, and patients require a chest tube only if symptomatic or the pneumothorax is enlarging. Adhering closely to the inferior surface of the first rib during blunt dissection will help protect against postoperative pneumothorax.

Recurrence

Symptoms of neurogenic TOS recur in 10–20 % of patients [7, 9] (discussed more thoroughly in Chap. 39, "Assessment and Treatment of Recurrent NTOS"). Two intraoperative factors are known to reduce recurrence rates: First, resecting a significant portion (2–3 cm) of the anterior scalene muscle (as opposed to simply dividing it at its insertion point) and, second, ensuring that the posterior edge of the first rib is resected sufficiently so as to leave as short a rib stump as technically feasible. Patients with spontaneous recurrence compared to those that are re-injured have worse outcomes when reoperation is performed. Most recurrences develop beyond 3 months but within 18 months of the initial operation [8], and therefore patients with neurogenic TOS should be followed for at least 2 years after first rib resection.

References

1. Roos DB. Transaxillary approach for first rib resection to relieve thoracic outlet syndrome. Ann Surg. 1966;163(3):354–8.
2. Chang DC, Lidor AO, Matsen SL, Freischlag JA. Reported in-hospital complications following rib resections for neurogenic thoracic outlet syndrome. Ann Vasc Surg. 2007;21(5):564–70.
3. Chang DC, Rotellini-Coltvet LA, Mukherjee D, De Leon R, Freischlag JA. Surgical intervention for thoracic outlet syndrome improves patient's quality of life. J Vasc Surg. 2009;49(3):630–5, discussion 5–7.
4. Sanders RJ, Hammond SL, Rao NM. Diagnosis of thoracic outlet syndrome. J Vasc Surg. 2007;46(3):601–4.
5. Chaikof E, Cambria R, editors. Atlas of vascular and endovascular surgery (in press)
6. Ambrad-Chalela E, Thomas GI, Johansen KH. Recurrent neurogenic thoracic outlet syndrome. Am J Surg. 2004;187(4):505–10.
7. Sanders RJ, Haug CE, Pearce WH. Recurrent thoracic outlet syndrome. J Vasc Surg. 1990;12(4):390–8, discussion 8–400.
8. Altobelli GG, Kudo T, Haas BT, Chandra FA, Moy JL, Ahn SS. Thoracic outlet syndrome: pattern of clinical success after operative decompression. J Vasc Surg. 2005;42(1):122–8.
9. Mingoli A, Feldhaus RJ, Farina C, Cavallari N, Sapienza P, di Marzo L, et al. Long-term outcome after transaxillary approach for thoracic outlet syndrome. Surgery. 1995;118(5):840–4.

Surgical Techniques: Operative Decompression Using the Supraclavicular Approach for NTOS

29

Karl A. Illig

Abstract

Supraclavicular exposure offers the benefits of complete scalenectomy, complete brachial plexus neurolysis, and excellent exposure for resection of the mid- and posterior first rib (and any other bony or soft tissue abnormalities), making it an excellent approach for the surgical treatment of patients with neurogenic thoracic outlet syndrome (TOS). Nonrandomized and noncontrolled data have not demonstrated any difference in outcomes when compared to transaxillary exposure in patients operated on for this problem, at least in the hands of experts using their preferred approach. In properly selected patients, an excellent-to-good outcome should be expected in approximately 80 % of patients using the supraclavicular approach for neurogenic TOS, and the recurrence rate may be lower than with other approaches. Temporary phrenic and/or long thoracic nerve dysfunction is not rare, occurring in between 5 and 10 % of patients, and pneumothorax is temporary and innocuous. With experience this exposure is an excellent solution in patients with neurogenic TOS, and has the flexibility to be readily applicable to the other forms of TOS.

Introduction

When treating a patient with neurogenic TOS, the most critical structures are the scalene muscles, the brachial plexus, and the middle to posterior part of the first rib. Many surgeons believe that to achieve the best results in thoracic outlet decompression, the scalene muscles should be entirely resected and fibrous scar tissue around the brachial plexus nerve roots should be fully excised. In addition, first rib resection is frequently advocated. For these reasons, many favor the supraclavicular approach for surgical treatment of neurogenic thoracic outlet syndrome. This approach has the following advantages:

- It provides the best exposure of the middle to posterior first rib, from the level of the anterior scalene tubercle to the transverse process of the spine.
- It allows complete removal of both the anterior and middle scalene muscles, which cannot be accomplished by other approaches.

K.A. Illig, MD
Department of Surgery, Division of Vascular Surgery, University of South Florida, 2 Tampa General Circle, STC 7016, Tampa, FL 33606, USA
e-mail: killig@health.usf.edu

K.A. Illig et al. (eds.), *Thoracic Outlet Syndrome*, DOI 10.1007/978-1-4471-4366-6_29, © Springer-Verlag London 2013

- It provides the best exposure of a cervical rib or other anomalous anatomical structures.
- It allows full exposure of the brachial plexus for complete neurolysis, which cannot be achieved by alternative approaches.
- The supine position provides easy access for inclusion of pectoralis minor tenotomy with the supraclavicular operation, even when performed on the contralateral side.
- This approach is the most versatile, allowing definitive treatment of all forms of TOS and unexpected abnormalities.
- May provides a greater degree of safety in surgical treatment given the better exposure than that achieved through alternative approaches.

The supraclavicular approach to thoracic outlet decompression was initially described by Sanders, and subsequently by Reilly and colleagues [1, 2]. Thompson and associates wrote what continues to be a useful description of this technique in 1997 [3]. Although the anatomy of the thoracic outlet has not changed, the following description reflects conceptual updates and advances in dealing with this challenging area, and presents results with another 15 years of experience.

Surgical Technique

No special preoperative preparation is needed. We ask all of our patients to wash their surgical site (in this case, the shoulder and supraclavicular region) with a surgical prep sponge the night before surgery. The base of the neck is a very well-perfused and clean area, and postoperative infection in this site is extremely rare. We also prescribe a scopolamine patch to be applied behind the ear the day before surgery, to help alleviate postoperative nausea related to the general anesthetic.

The operation is performed under general anesthesia with the patient in a semi-Fowler's position, placing the legs flat and the upper body elevated about 30°. A small inflatable pillow is placed across the shoulder blades, the head is turned to the opposite side, and the ipsilateral arm is tucked (alternatively, some prefer to leave

the arm out or to include it into the sterile field, so that the dynamics of the thoracic outlet can be assessed after decompression [3]). Such positioning provides excellent exposure to the supraclavicular region in a fashion that is comfortable for the surgeon and safe for the patient, and allows the surgeon to move between a position lateral to the shoulder or near the head, as the need for exposure dictates.

A transverse incision is made in the supraclavicular fossa one or two fingerbreadths above the clavicle, with the medial end at the lateral edge of the sternocleidomastoid muscle and extending almost to the anterior edge of the trapezius muscle (Fig. 29.1). The platysma layer is entered but the clavicular head of the sternocleidomastoid does not usually need to be divided. The surgeon then easily visualizes the supraclavicular scalene fat pad, with the omohyoid muscle traversing diagonally across the field. We retract the scalene fat pad upward using cautery to divide the inferior attachments, although some recommend moving this laterally or even inferiorly, and the omohyoid muscle is routinely divided.

As the fat pad is reflected laterally and upward, the anterior scalene muscle should come into view, with the phrenic nerve running vertically across its surface, and the brachial plexus nerve roots become apparent along the lateral edge of the anterior scalene. As has often been noted, the phrenic nerve is very easy to identify both because of its location and as it is the only peripheral nerve in the body that runs from lateral to medial as it descends. It usually (85 %) lies on top of the anterior scalene, but can occasionally be found within its fibers, relatively superficial and not associated with the muscle, or even lateral to or below it. Great caution should be used until the phrenic nerve is positively identified; such identification can be aided by noting that it arises from the brachial plexus high in the surgical field with the nerve and brachial plexus forming two sides of a small triangle. When in doubt, a handheld peripheral nerve stimulator can be used, to demonstrate abrupt contraction of the diaphragm when the phrenic nerve is directly stimulated. Following this the scalene fat pad is reflected

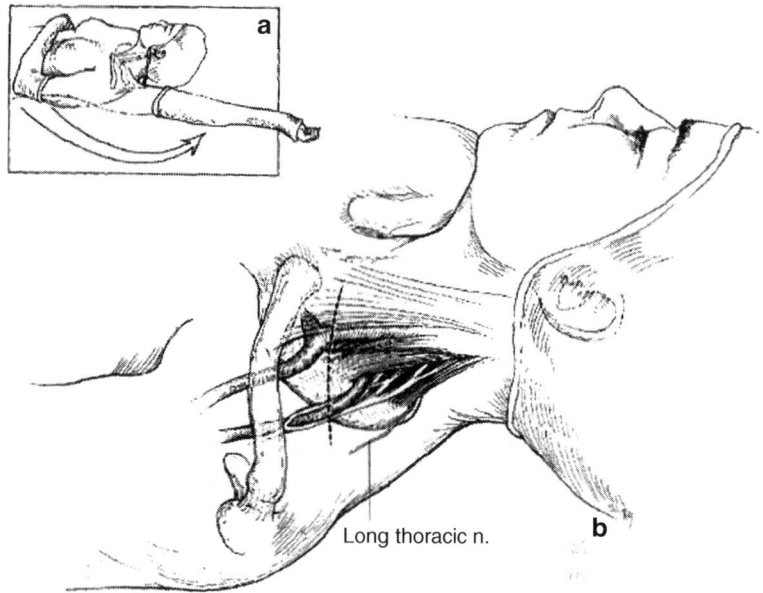

Fig. 29.1 Patient positioning and incision for supraclavicular exploration. (**a**) Many include the affected upper extremity in the sterile field, wrapped in a stockinette, to allow full range of motion during the course of the operation. (**b**) A skin crease incision is made 1–2 fingerbreadths above the clavicle, beginning over the clavicular head of the sternocleidomastoid, to allow full exposure of the structures associated with the scalene triangle (Reprinted from Thompson et al. [3]. With permission from Elsevier)

further, until the middle scalene muscle and the long thoracic nerve are also in view. A 3-arm self-retaining retractor is then put in place to maintain the exposure for the remainder of the procedure.

The anterior scalene muscle is next divided from its attachment to the first rib, with the phrenic nerve, subclavian artery and brachial plexus well protected (Fig. 29.2). It is probably best to perform this step with the scissors rather than the cautery, as this will help avoid any thermal injury to adjacent structures and any slight muscular bleeding from the muscle edge will stop spontaneously. The anterior scalene is then lifted and teased upward to expose the subclavian artery; gentle finger dissection is generally adequate to bring it off of its medial and posterior attachments, while sharp dissection is sometimes added to mobilize it medially off the brachial plexus. There are occasionally relatively large blood vessels that supply the muscle in this area; these can easily be clipped or divided between ligatures, as can the branches of the thyrocervical trunk. A characteristic finding at this point is that the muscle belly "disappears" underneath the previously described junction of the phrenic nerve and brachial plexus. We pass the anterior scalene muscle underneath to the medial side of

the phrenic nerve, allowing the muscle to then be traced further up to its origin on the transverse process of the cervical spine, where it is sharply divided while protecting the upper nerve roots of the brachial plexus. The entire anterior scalene muscle is thereby excised, usually providing a specimen 5–7 g in weight.

At this point, the anterior surface of the brachial plexus (and the subclavian artery) are quite apparent, with the phrenic nerve coursing over the empty space where the anterior scalene used to be (Fig. 29.3). The brachial plexus is now brought forward with gentle retraction to expose the middle scalene muscle. The main landmark to note at this point is the long thoracic nerve, which exits the antero-lateral border of the middle scalene muscle and courses inferolaterally (some classify the muscle posterior to the nerve as the posterior scalene, but no physical difference in fibers or actual separation is present). It is critical to identify this nerve, as otherwise blindly dividing the middle scalene will often result in injury. Once the nerve is identified, the muscle can be dissected free over the top of it, leaving muscle lateral and inferior to it. The long thoracic nerve arises from the brachial plexus in a matter analogous to the phrenic nerve medially, forming another small triangle at the top of the surgical

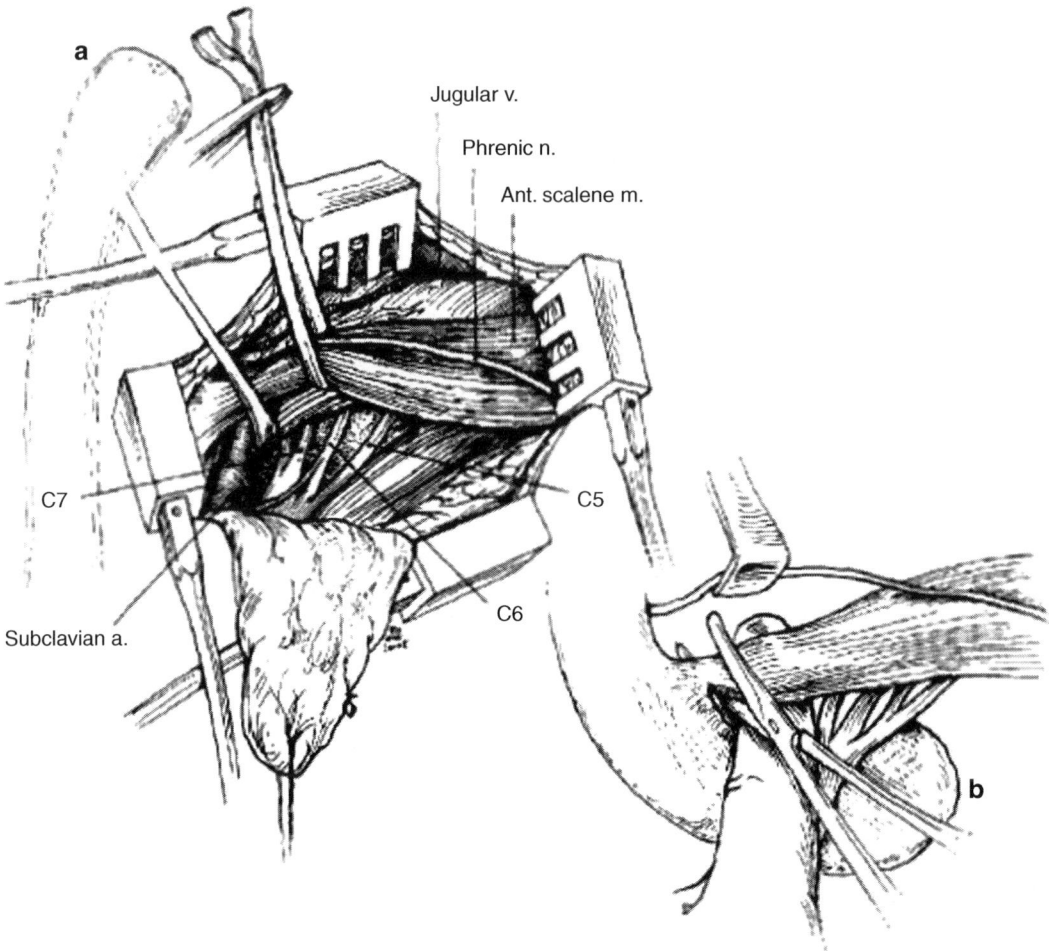

Fig. 29.2 Anterior scalenectomy. View is of the left side, from the side of the patient. (**a**) The anterior scalene muscle is circumferentially mobilized from the underlying subclavian artery and roots of the brachial plexus. The anterior scalene muscle is often firm and tendinous in this region, particularly posteriorly, and this space may be anatomically restricted. (**b**) The tendinous insertion of the muscle upon the first rib is sharply divided with scissors (or with the cautery if the phrenic nerve is well-separated from the insertion), with the surgeon's finger behind the insertion to protect the subclavian artery and brachial plexus (Reprinted from Thompson et al. [3]. With permission from Elsevier)

field. The middle scalene muscle is divided from the top of the lateral first rib, using scissors or cautery, until the first rib is cleanly exposed. The rib is often surprisingly deep in this location and the middle scalene can be 2 or 3 cm thick. If a cervical rib or fibrous band is present, it is typically exposed at this point, since it arises in the anatomical plane of the middle scalene muscle.

Two schools of thought exist regarding the need to remove the first rib. The majority of surgeons feel it should be removed in all cases, in order to ensure the greatest chance of a successful outcome with one operation. Other surgeons suggest that in "properly" selected patients, the results of surgical treatment without first rib resection seem to be just as good [4, 5]. If the first rib is to be removed, we complete the rib resection followed by brachial plexus neurolysis (see below); if preservation of the first rib is contemplated, brachial plexus neurolysis is completed first, followed by assessment and decision-making [3].

Once the first rib is identified, the cautery and a periosteal elevator are used to scrape the middle

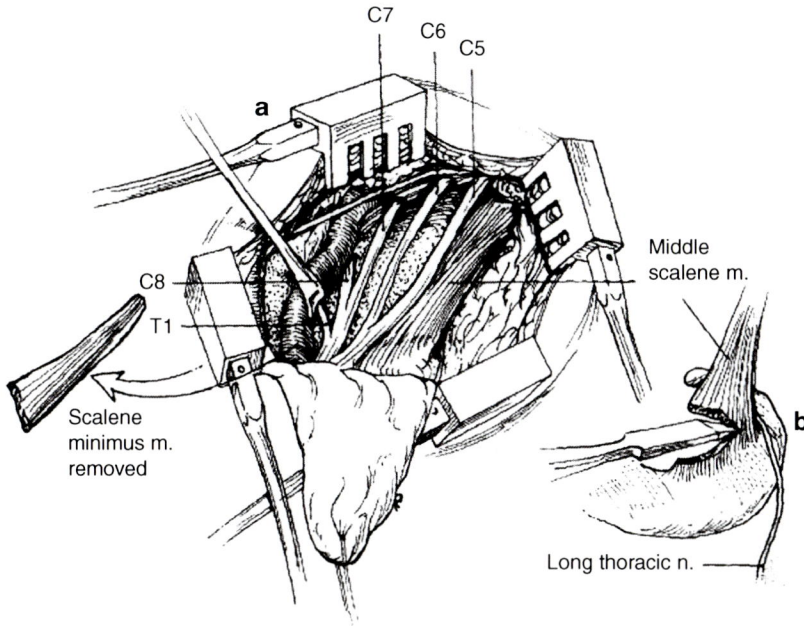

Fig. 29.3 Brachial plexus neurolysis and middle scale-nectomy. View is of the left side, from the side of the patient. (**a**) Complete dissection of the brachial plexus nerve roots from C5 to T1 is accomplished by resection of all inflammatory scar tissue and interdigitating muscle. The T1 nerve root should be seen exiting from beneath the neck of the first rib. (**b**) The long thoracic nerve is seen exiting from the middle scalene muscle, and this is used as a landmark to limit the lateral border of muscle resection. The middle scalene is detached from the first rib using a periosteal elevator or cautery, taking care to avoid injury to the nerve. All middle scalene muscle tissue lying anterior and medial to the course of the nerve is resected (Reprinted from Thompson et al. [3]. With permission from Elsevier)

scalene off its top surface (Fig. 29.3), both posteriorly (underneath the long thoracic nerve to the transverse process) and anteriorly (underneath the brachial plexus and subclavian artery). The middle scalene muscle is debulked as much as possible and passed from the field, a maneuver that yields a long segment of exposed posterior first rib. At this point, the rib is encircled using a right angle clamp, placing it under the medial and lateral borders (Fig. 29.4). Laterally, the exposure includes the intercostal muscles. With pressure upward on the right angle to minimize the chance of pleural entry, the medial, lateral and inferior attachments are divided by running the clamp back and forth as far posteriorly and anteriorly as possible; one can often safely undermine the rib edges extensively under the nerves and even the artery. Finally, small subclavian artery branches are divided and the subclavian artery is elevated to expose the middle to anterior portion of the first rib (although the costosternal junction itself cannot be

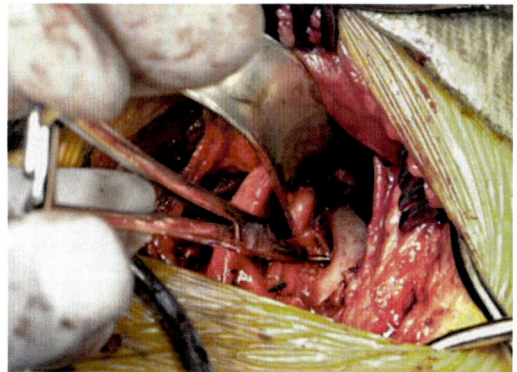

Fig. 29.4 Operative photograph of technique of clearing the first rib from the surrounding tissues. View is of the *left side*, from the side of the patient. A retractor is holding the brachial plexus medially, while a *right* angle clamp is being placed around and under the medial border of the posterior first rib

reached by means of a supraclavicular approach alone, the rib can be cleared and resected at least a centimeter anterior to the artery).

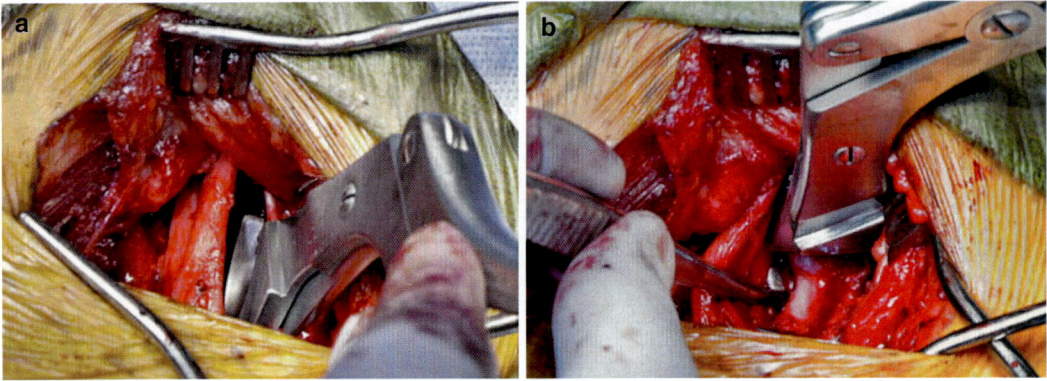

Fig. 29.5 Operative photographs of technique used to safely divide the first rib. View is of the left side, from the side of the patient. (**a**) A "guillotine-type" bone cutter is first inserted parallel to the rib and nerves, and the tip of the bottom blade placed under the rib. (**b**) With a forceps holding the brachial plexus medially, the rib cutter is then turned 90° and the bottom blade is observed to be free of the brachial plexus nerves. The rib cutter is then maneuvered as posteriorly as possible and the bone is cut. After anterior division and removal of the rib specimen, a bone rongeur is used to remove the remaining posterior rib to the level of the transverse process of the spine

At this point, a Stille-Gertz guillotine-type bone cutter is used to divide the posterior rib. It is safest to insert this instrument parallel to the rib, between the long thoracic nerve and plexus, and only move it perpendicular to surround the rib it when the lower blade can be positioned under the cleared lateral border of the posterior part of the rib. With retractor in place to make sure that the brachial plexus stays away from its blade, the rib is divided as far posteriorly as possible (Fig. 29.5). Finally, the rib is similarly divided about a centimeter anterior to the artery, just medial to the scalene tubercle, and passed away from the surgical field.

At this point the intact parietal pleura overlying the apex of the lung is at the base of the operative field, with the brachial plexus coursing across the middle of the field and the phrenic and long thoracic nerves running medially and laterally over the spaces formerly occupied by anterior and middle scalene muscles, respectively. A bone rongeur is used to remove the posterior part of the rib all the way back to its attachment with the transverse process of the spine. It is important that all periosteum and essentially all of the rib should be removed, and to persevere until the articular surface is seen. It is also critical to remember that the lowest part of the brachial plexus is the T1 nerve root; hence, one must be very careful in removing bone with a sharp instrument between two nerve roots (C7 above and T1 below). Finally, the rongeur is used to remove the anterior edge of the first rib, as far anteromedially as possible. It is not possible to go all the way to the level of the sternum from this approach, but one should ensure that the artery is well free of any part of the rib; this should go well into the point of anterior scalene insertion and ideally beyond the tubercle.

The final step at this point is to ensure that the brachial plexus itself is free of any investing muscle fibers and fibrous scar tissue. If there are muscle fibers that interdigitate between the nerve roots and trunks (e.g., a scalene "minimus" anomaly), they should be sharply debrided. Again, the difference in sensation between muscle and nerve is distinct enough so that nerve injury should be virtually impossible. The surgeon should persist until all five nerve roots are identified, mobilized, and well-cleared of scar tissue.

Over the past few years, we have routinely created a shallow tunnel using blunt fingertip dissection over the anterior surface of the brachial plexus as it courses underneath the clavicle toward the arm. We generally extend this tunnel to the level of the pectoralis minor muscle. In patients in whom a concomitant pectoralis minor tenotomy is to be performed, this maneuver can be useful in identifying the pectoralis minor muscle; however, we have not been able to accurately distinguish patients with or without pectoralis minor compression using this technique.

In an effort to prevent or limit the development of perineural scar tissue that might contribute to recurrent neurogenic TOS, we have used a hyaluronidate-based absorbable film (Seprafilm, Genzyme Biosurgery, Cambridge, MA) wrapped around the brachial plexus, as a temporary physical barrier between the nerves and adjacent tissues. Other surgeons utilize polylactide film (SurgiWrap, MAST Biosurgery, San Diego, CA) for the same purpose, with the advantage that this material can be secured in place with sutures and may resist absorption for 2–3 months rather than 2–3 weeks. Consideration has also been given to local injection or topical instillation of heparin or other substances, but to date no evidence exists showing the efficacy of any substance to address this problem.

We routinely place a closed-suction drain in all patients, typically using a #10 flat Jackson-Pratt or #19 fluted round Blake drain. If the pleural membrane has been entered, we put a few side holes in a red rubber catheter and place it within the pleural space, to be removed after wound closure to the level of the fascia (platysma layer), and have never had to place a chest tube after this maneuver (or after any supraclavicular exposure). Other surgeons intentionally open the pleura and place the closed-suction drain past the brachial plexus and extending into the chest cavity. The closed-suction drain exits via a separate stab wound placed posterolaterally in line with the incision for best cosmetic effect, and can be placed above or below the scalene fat pad. The scalene fat pad is placed back into its normal anatomic position and held in placed with several sutures, and the wound is closed in two layers.

Results

Sanders presented a very nice description of the evolution of operations for neurogenic TOS in 1996, and in so doing illustrated the results of various forms of decompression from his experience and from the published literature [6]. Although discussion is limited by the subjectivity of assessing success and varied definitions thereof, he reported "excellent, good, or fair" results in 87 % of patients undergoing supraclavicular scalenectomy with first rib resection in a series of 72 patients undergoing this operation over a 5-year period, when presumably, their technique was fully mature (interestingly, although not statistically significant, results are better than the concomitant group undergoing scalenectomy alone, a difference which persists even after later removal of the first rib in the latter group). It was also found that a work-related injury predicted a poorer outcome. Documented results are not any better than those in patients undergoing transaxillary exposure, although it must be stressed that such comparisons are uncontrolled, often historical, and, at this point, relatively dated.

The largest series of supraclavicular first rib resections was reported by Hempel in 1996 [7]. In their series of 637 patients undergoing 770 operations over a 28 year period, "good" or "excellent" results were achieved in 86 % of cases. Interestingly, they point out that results were much better in vascular TOS: all of those in this group had "excellent" results, while only 55 % of those with neurogenic TOS had "excellent" results (by extrapolation, "good" results or better were thereby seen in 75–80 % of patients operated on for neurogenic TOS).

Complications are probably more frequent after supraclavicular compared to transaxillary exposure, perhaps because the brachial plexus nerves and other structures are more thoroughly exposed during the course of complete scalenectomy. In a 2001 review, Sharp described a neurological complication rate of 38 % after supraclavicular exposure, but this resulted from three complications in only eight patients, all operated on for cervical ribs or vascular TOS [8]. True complication rates are also difficult to assess because most authors do not clearly differentiate those following transaxillary and supraclavicular exposures. Thompson estimates the rate of phrenic nerve dysfunction to be approximately 10 %, [9] and we have experienced at least three patients with long thoracic nerve dysfunction ("winged scapula") following 77 supraclavicular first rib resections over the past 5 years (4 %), although two of the three were transient. Brachial plexus injuries were found to occur in only 0.6 % of patients in a combined National Inpatient Sample inquiry combining transaxillary and supraclavicular operations [10]; this manuscript also provides a thorough literature review of this topic with brachial plexus injuries (very rare) broken down by exposure type. While less serious in the long term, pneumothorax requiring chest tube placement and thoracic duct injury requiring total parenteral nutrition or thoracic duct ligation can also occur, but are poorly documented in the literature. We have seen zero and two such complications over the past decade, respectively, and while Hempel describes pleural entry occurring in 20 % of cases, they also describe this as being innocuous [7].

Summary

In conclusion, supraclavicular exposure offers the theoretical benefit of complete scalenectomy and complete brachial plexus neurolysis, along with excellent exposure for first rib (and cervical rib) resection. Data, albeit nonrandomized, appear to show equivalent outcomes when compared with transaxillary exposure in patients operated on for neurogenic TOS (and perhaps slightly better for first rib resection as compared to scalenectomy alone). With proper selection for treatment, a good outcome should be expected in approximately 80 % of patients. Dysfunction of the phrenic and/or long thoracic nerves is not rare, occurring between 5 and 10 % of patients, but is almost always transient, and pneumothorax is temporary and innocuous. With ample experience

the supraclavicular exposure provides an excellent, versatile and safe approach in patients with neurogenic TOS.

References

1. Sanders RJ, Raymer S. The supraclavicular approach to scalenectomy and first rib resection: description of technique. J Vasc Surg. 1985;2:751–6.
2. Reilly LM, Stoney RJ. Supraclavicular approach for thoracic outlet decompression. J Vasc Surg. 1988;8:329–34.
3. Thompson RW, Petrinec D, Toursarkissian B. Surgical treatment of thoracic outlet compression syndromes. II. Supraclavicular exploration and vascular reconstruction. Ann Vasc Surg. 1997;11:442–51.
4. Sanders RJ, Pearce WH. The treatment of thoracic outlet syndrome: a comparison of different operations. J Vasc Surg. 1989;10:626–34.
5. Cheng SW, Reilly LM, Nelken NA, Ellis WV, Stoney RJ. Neurogenic thoracic outlet decompression: rationale for sparing the first rib. Cardiovasc Surg. 1995;3:617–23, discussion 624.
6. Sanders RJ. Results of the surgical treatment for thoracic outlet syndrome. Semin Thorac Cardiovasc Surg. 1996;8:221–8.
7. Hempel GK, Shutze WP, Anderson JF, Bukhari HI. 770 Consecutive supraclavicular first rib resections for thoracic outlet syndrome. Ann Vasc Surg. 1996;10:456–63.
8. Sharp WJ, Nowak LR, Zamani T, Kresowik TF, Hoballah JJ, Ballinger BA, et al. Long-term follow-up and patient satisfaction after surgery for thoracic outlet syndrome. Ann Vasc Surg. 2001;15:32–6.
9. Thompson RW, Driskill M. Thoracic outlet syndrome: neurogenic. In: Cronenwett JL, Johnston KW, editors. Rutherford's vascular surgery. 7th ed. Philadelphia: Elsevier; 2010. p. 1878–98.
10. Chang DC, Lidor AO, Matsen SL, Freischlag JA. Reported in-hospital complications following rib resections for neurogenic thoracic outlet syndrome. Ann Vasc Surg. 2007;21:564–70.

Robert W. Thompson

Abstract

Brachial plexus compression in neurogenic thoracic outlet syndrome (TOS) may occur either at the level of the supraclavicular scalene triangle and/or the infraclavicular subcoracoid space. As highlighted elsewhere by Sanders (Chap. 15), it has only recently been recognized that nerve compression at the level of the pectoralis minor muscle tendon can make a substantial contribution to symptoms in neurogenic TOS, and that in many cases nerve compression at this level may dominate over that occurring at the level of the scalene triangle. Untreated pectoralis minor compression of the brachial plexus may therefore represent an important factor in persistent or recurrent symptoms following operations for neurogenic TOS, and undoubtedly explains a proportion of surgical failures in previous clinical series. Moreover, it is now apparent that a significant number of patients may have a clinical diagnosis of neurogenic TOS represented by isolated brachial plexus compression at the level of the pectoralis minor muscle, for whom isolated pectoralis minor tenotomy may provide a minimally-invasive surgical option associated with rapid postoperative recovery and a high likelihood of clinical success. Recognition and treatment of this condition has therefore been an important step in our evolving understanding of neurogenic TOS.

Introduction

Brachial plexus compression in neurogenic thoracic outlet syndrome (TOS) may occur either at the level of the supraclavicular scalene triangle and/or the infraclavicular subcoracoid space. As highlighted elsewhere by Sanders (Chap. 15), it has only recently been recognized that nerve compression at the level of the pectoralis minor muscle tendon can make a substantial contribution to symptoms in neurogenic TOS, and that in

R.W. Thompson, MD
Department of Surgery,
Section of Vascular Surgery,
Center for Thoracic Outlet Syndrome,
Washington University, Barnes-Jewish Hospital,
660 S Euclid Avenue, Campus Box 8109/Suite 5101
Queeny Tower, St. Louis, MO 63110, USA
e-mail: thompson@wudosis.wustl.edu

K.A. Illig et al. (eds.), *Thoracic Outlet Syndrome*,
DOI 10.1007/978-1-4471-4366-6_30, © Springer-Verlag London 2013

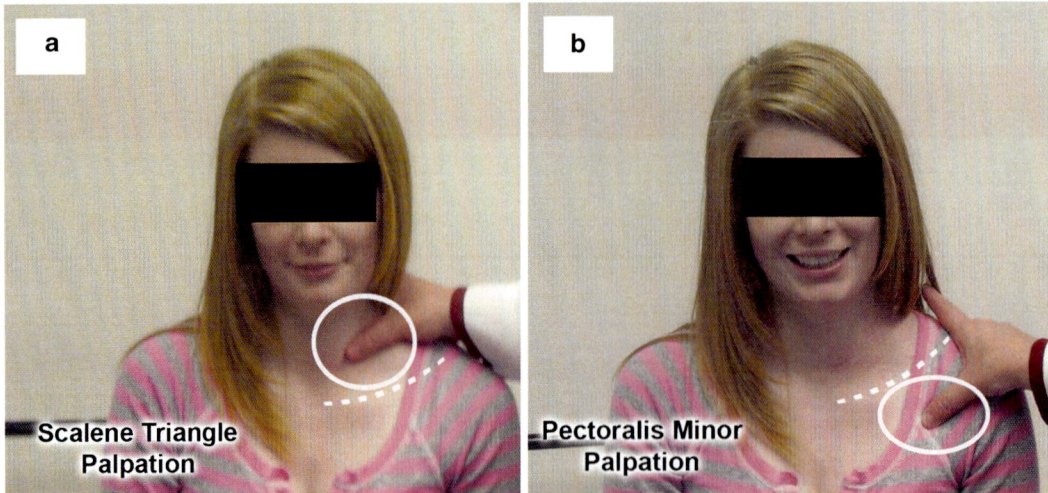

Fig. 30.1 Diagnosis of pectoralis minor compression in neurogenic TOS. Illustration of physical examination depicting localized tenderness and reproduction of upper extremity symptoms during palpation over the supraclavicular scalene triangle (**a**) and/or the infraclavicular subcoracoid (pectoralis minor) space (**b**). The position of the clavicle is shown by the *dashed line*

many cases nerve compression at this level may dominate over that occurring at the level of the scalene triangle [1, 2]. Untreated pectoralis minor compression of the brachial plexus may therefore represent an important factor in persistent or recurrent symptoms following operations for neurogenic TOS, and undoubtedly explains a proportion of surgical failures in previous clinical series [3]. Moreover, it is now apparent that a significant number of patients may have a clinical diagnosis of neurogenic TOS represented by isolated brachial plexus compression at the level of the pectoralis minor muscle, for whom isolated pectoralis minor tenotomy may provide a minimally-invasive surgical option associated with rapid postoperative recovery and a high likelihood of clinical success. Recognition and treatment of this condition has therefore been an important step in our evolving understanding of neurogenic TOS.

Diagnosis and Indications for Procedure

Pectoralis minor tenotomy is indicated for patients with disabling neurogenic TOS that have not had a satisfactory response to appropriately targeted physical therapy, in whom physical examination reveals significant tenderness and/or reproduction of upper extremity neurogenic symptoms upon palpation over the subcoracoid space. Symptoms suggesting pectoralis minor compression include infraclavicular, anterior chest wall, and/or axillary pain, but the nature of upper extremity symptoms and the response to upper extremity positional maneuvers is similar to that of patients with brachial plexus compression at the scalene triangle [2]. Physical examination is used to help distinguish whether there is brachial plexus nerve compression at the level of the pectoralis minor muscle in isolation, as the dominant source of symptoms, or in combination with compression at the level of the scalene triangle (Fig. 30.1). One valuable and specific examination maneuver is to demonstrate tenderness and/or reproduction of upper extremity symptoms during direct palpation over the subcoracoid space, which is resolved when the patient simultaneously contracts the pectoralis major muscle (Fig. 30.2).

In addition to physical examination, the response to radiographically-guided muscle blocks with local anesthetic can be particularly helpful to verify the presence of nerve compression exacerbated by pectoralis minor muscle

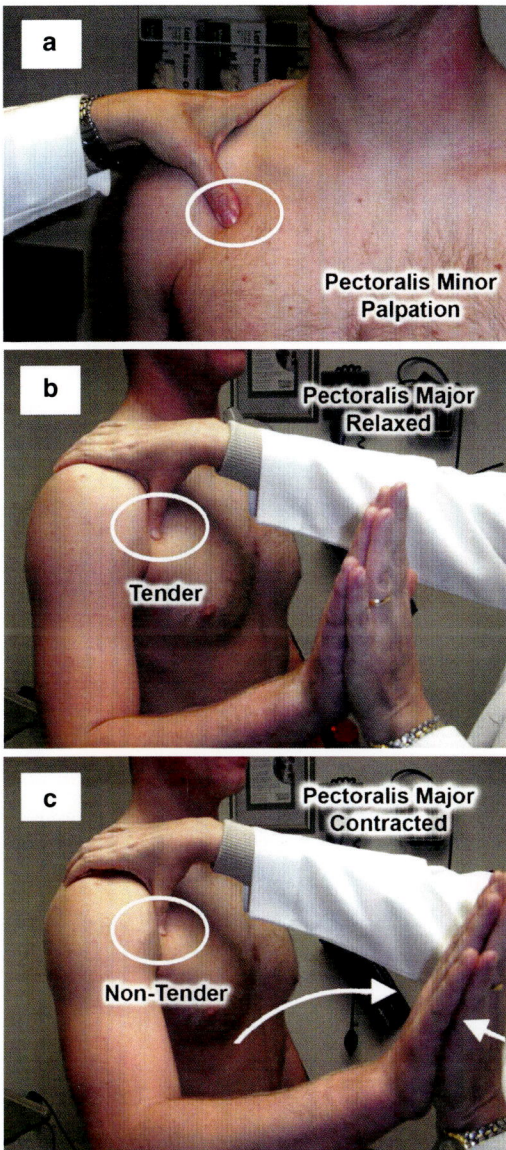

Fig. 30.2 Physical examination to distinguish pectoralis minor compression. Physical examination can often distinguish between pectoralis minor compression (neurogenic TOS) and more generalized pectoralis muscle tenderness. There is localized tenderness and reproduction of upper extremity symptoms during palpation over the infraclavicular subcoracoid (pectoralis minor) space (**a**). An important finding is the resolution of these findings when the patient simultaneously contracts the pectoralis major muscle, which prevents transmission of digital pressure to the underlying pectoralis minor tendon. In this maneuver, there is localized tenderness and reproduction of arm/hand symptoms during firm palpation over the subcoracoid space while the pectoralis major muscle is relaxed (**b**), but diminished symptoms during palpation with simultaneous flexion (contraction) of the pectoralis major muscle (**c**)

spasm [4]. Although we use combined anterior scalene and pectoralis minor muscle blocks in the evaluation of most patients with neurogenic TOS, an isolated pectoralis minor block is used when this is considered the dominant site of nerve compression and when isolated pectoralis minor tenotomy might be considered as an initial operative approach to treatment. Pectoralis minor muscle blocks can also be useful in patients with persistent or recurrent neurogenic TOS that have previously undergone transaxillary or supraclavicular decompression procedures, in whom pectoralis minor tenotomy may also be considered. A summary of the operations performed in our Center over the past 2 years demonstrates the increasing frequency with which pectoralis minor tenotomy is utilized for neurogenic TOS, with this procedure being included in approximately 80 % of all primary operations and as an isolated procedure in up to 30 % of patients (Fig. 30.3).

Surgical Techniques

Deltopectoral (Anterior) Approach

Under general anesthesia, the patient is positioned supine with the head of the bed elevated to 30° and the arms held comfortably at the side. The neck, upper chest and affected upper extremity are prepped into the field, with both sides prepped simultaneously for bilateral procedures. A short vertical incision is made in the deltopectoral groove, beginning approximately 1 in. below the coracoid process (Fig. 30.4a). The edges of the deltoid and pectoralis major muscles are gently spread apart from each other by blunt dissection (Fig. 30.4b), with the plane of dissection carried deeper medial to the cephalic vein (Fig. 30.4c). The lateral edge of the pectoralis major muscle is separated from its fascia and gently lifted in a medial direction with a small Deaver retractor. The plane underneath the pectoralis major muscle is separated by blunt fingertip dissection to further expose the underlying fascia over the pectoralis minor muscle, where the muscle can be easily identified by palpation (Fig. 30.4d). The fascia along the medial border of the pectoralis minor muscle is incised and the muscle is encircled using blunt fingertip dissection around its medial border. The fascia along the lateral border of the pectoralis muscle is then incised to ensure seperation of the pectoralis minor from the long head of the biceps muscle, which fuses with the pectoralis minor tendon

close to the coracoid process. The pectoralis minor tendon is then completely encircled near its insertion on the coracoid process, taking care to protect the underlying neurovascular bundle, and it is elevated with an umbilical tape or rubber tubing (Fig. 30.4e). The insertion of the pectora-

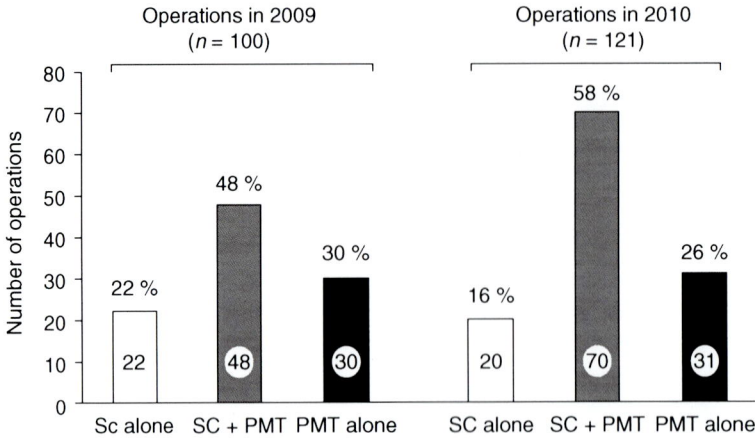

Fig. 30.3 Pectoralis minor tenotomy in the surgical treatment of neurogenic TOS. Bar graph illustrating the number of operations performed for neurogenic TOS at Washington University/Barnes-Jewish Hospital in St. Louis over a recent 2-year period. During 2009 and 2010, the proportion of operations that included pectoralis minor tenotomy (PMT) was 78 and 84 %, respectively, with approximately 30 % of patients undergoing isolated PMT. Supraclavicular (SC) thoracic outlet decompression consisted of complete anterior and middle scalenectomy, brachial plexus neurolysis and first rib resection, either alone or in combination with PMT

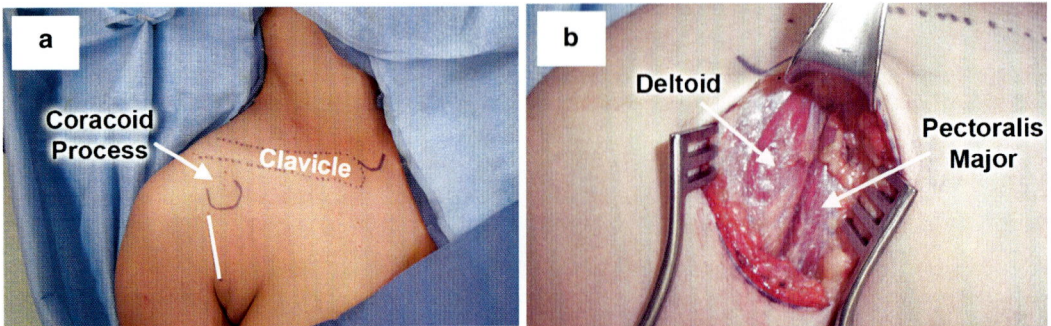

Fig. 30.4 Pectoralis minor tenotomy (deltopectoral approach). (**a**) Landmarks for pectoralis minor tenotomy include the clavicle and the coracoid process, which is easily palpable as a bony prominence inferior to the lateral aspect of the clavicle and medial to the shoulder. A short vertical incision is made in the deltopectoral groove (*white line*). (**b**) The edges of the deltoid and pectoralis major muscles are separated by blunt dissection. (**c**) The cephalic vein is identified as the deltoid and pectoralis major muscles are separated further, with the plane of dissection carried deeper medial to the vein along the lateral edge of pectoralis major. (**d**) The pectoralis major

muscle is lifted medially with a Deaver retractor to expose the underlying fascia over the pectoralis minor muscle. (**e**) The pectoralis minor muscle is encircled near its insertion on the coracoid process and elevated with an umbilical tape, prior to division with the electrocautery. (**f**) The edges of the divided pectoralis minor muscle have retracted to relieve compression of the underlying neurovascular structures (embedded in surrounding fat). The inferior edge of the muscle will be oversewn with a series of interrupted sutures for hemostasis and to facilitate its contraction underneath the pectoralis major muscle

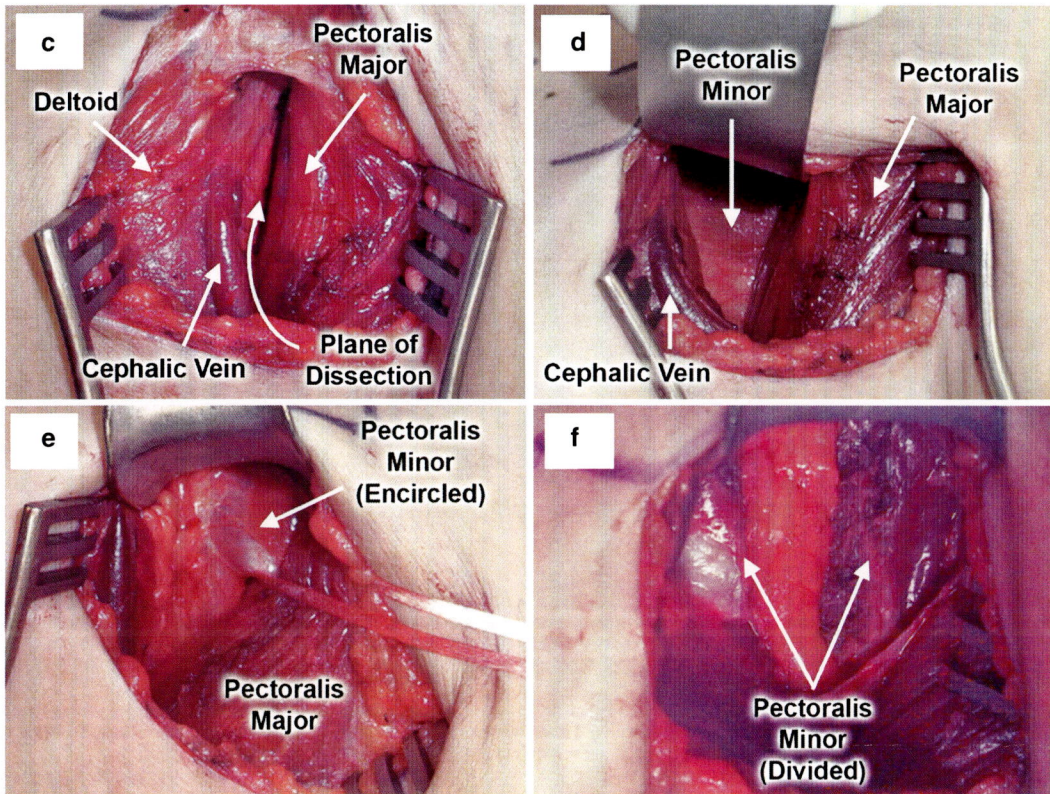

Fig. 30.4 (continued)

lis minor tendon on the coracoid process is exposed and isolated with a Richardson retractor, and the pectoralis minor muscle is injected with approximately 10 mL of 0.5 % bupivicaine. The muscle is then divided under direct vision with the electrocautery, within 2 cm of the coracoid process, with a finger placed behind the muscle to prevent thermal injury to the underlying neurovascular bundle. After the pectoralis minor muscle has been divided, the edges are seen to retract from each other to release any compression of the neurovascular bundle (Fig. 30.4f). The inferior edge of the divided muscle is oversewn with a series of interrupted figure-of-eight 2–0 silk sutures, to ensure hemostasis and to facilitate contraction of the muscle underneath the pectoralis major. The remaining clavipectoral fascia is also incised to the level of the clavicle, along with any other anomalous fascial bands that might be present overlying the brachial plexus, such as Langer's axillary arch [5]. No further dissection

of the brachial plexus nerves or the axillary vessels is performed. After infiltrating the edge of the pectoralis major muscle with a long-acting local anesthetic, the wound is irrigated and closed with several interrupted sutures in the deep subcutaneous layer followed by subcuticular closure of the skin, and dressed with a single steristrip.

Infraclavicular/Subclavicular (Anterior) Approach

Pectoralis minor tenotomy may be performed as a component of operations for venous or arterial TOS, in which an infraclavicular or paraclavicular approach is used, particularly to provide sufficient exposure for vascular reconstruction. In these situations the exposure obtained through a transverse infraclavicular incision is extended laterally far enough to directly expose the pectoralis minor muscle, and the muscle is divided near the coracoid process under direct vision with the electro-cautery. This permits easy exposure for vascular bypass graft reconstructions in which the periph-eral anastomosis is constructed at the level of the axillary vessels, and avoids any compression of the graft or anastomotic site which might otherwise occur from the overlying pectoralis minor muscle.

Transaxillary (Lateral) Approach

Utilizing either general or local anesthesia with heavy sedation, the patient is placed in a lateral position with the affected arm raised and held over the head. A transverse incision is made at the base of the axillary hairline and carried through the subcutaneous tissue to the chest wall. The second intercostal brachial cutaneous nerve is avoided by maintaining dissection along the anterior axillary fold. The edge of the pecto-ralis major muscle is identified and retracted anteromedially, and is used as a guide to expose the underlying pectoralis minor tendon at the level of the coracoid process. The pectoralis minor tendon is divided under direct vision with the electrocautery, and in some situations several centimeters of the muscle may also be excised.

Followup Care

Isolated pectoralis minor tenotomy, whether per-formed on one side or both, is conducted as an outpatient procedure, and the vast majority of patients are able to return home the same day. Muscle spasm, tightness and pain in the lateral pectoralis major muscle may occur over several days following operation, but has usually resolved within 1 week. Most patients are allowed full activity with the affected arm, and may return to work activities within several days (Fig. 30.5). We have not identified any specific limitations or restrictions in use of the upper extremity follow-ing pectoralis minor tenotomy, including in over-head throwing athletes. Furthermore, unlike patients that have undergone transaxillary first rib resection or supraclavicular scalenotomy, where muscle reattachment with recurrent symptoms is

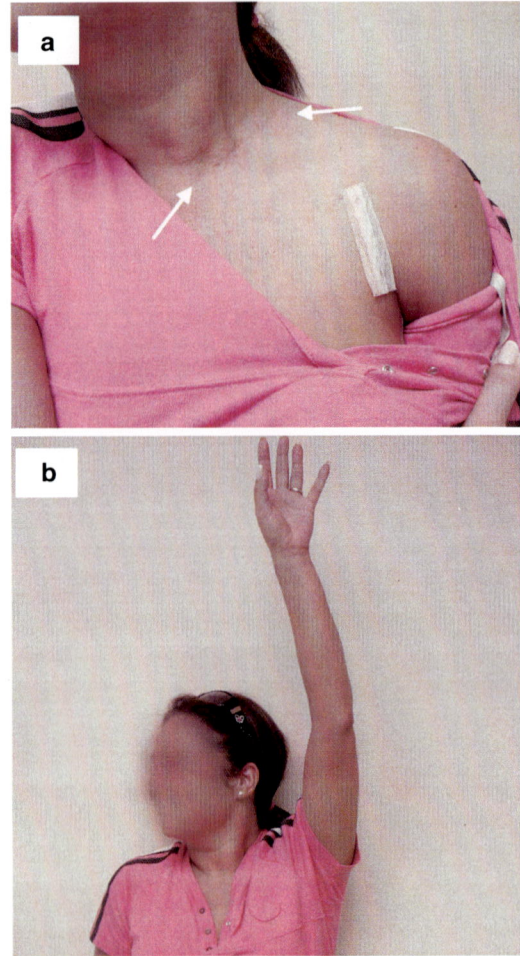

Fig. 30.5 Follow-up after pectoralis minor tenotomy. Photographs depicting a patient that had developed dis-abling symptoms of recurrent neurogenic TOS 9 months after supraclavicular thoracic outlet decompression, which were refractory to conservative measures. She was found to have no tenderness in the supraclavicular space, but had marked tenderness and reproduction of symptoms upon palpation over the subcoracoid area. Pectoralis minor tenotomy was performed as an isolated procedure through an anterior deltopectoral approach (**a**). The pectoralis minor tenotomy incision is covered by the steristrip dress-ing (the previous supraclavicular incision is indicated by the *arrows*). There was a complete resolution of symp-toms and a full range of motion demonstrated 2 weeks after operation (**b**)

a relatively frequent occurrence, during several years of follow-up we have not identified an instance in which there has been reattachment of the divided pectoralis minor or recurrent brachial plexus compression at this level.

References

1. Sanders RJ. Pectoralis minor syndrome. In: Eskandari MK, Morasch MD, Pearce WH, Yao JST, editors. Vascular surgery: therapeutic strategies. Shelton: People's Medical Publishing House-USA; 2010. p. 149–60.
2. Sanders RJ, Rao NM. The forgotten pectoralis minor syndrome: 100 operations for pectoralis minor syndrome alone or accompanied by neurogenic thoracic outlet syndrome. Ann Vasc Surg. 2010;24: 701–8.
3. Ambrad-Chalela E, Thomas GI, Johansen KH. Recurrent neurogenic thoracic outlet syndrome. Am J Surg. 2004;187(4):505–10.
4. Jordan SE, Ahn SS, Gelabert HA. Differentiation of thoracic outlet syndrome from treatment-resistant cervical brachial pain syndromes: development and utilization of a questionnaire, clinical examination and ultrasound evaluation. Pain Physician. 2007;10(3):441–52.
5. Ucerler H, Ikiz ZA, Pinan Y. Clinical importance of the muscular arch of the axilla (axillopectoral muscle, Langer's axillary arch). Acta Chir Belg. 2005; 105:326–8.

Dean M. Donahue

Abstract

Skin abnormalities, such as discoloration, edema, temperature alterations and abnormal sweating, have led many to conclude that Complex Regional Pain Syndrome (CRPS), previously known as Reflex Sympathetic Dystrophy (RSD), is mediated by the sympathetic nervous system. These previous clinical observations led to the concept that disrupting sympathetic innervation to an affected extremity, by chemical blockade or surgical disruption of the sympathetic chain, could improve symptoms. However, recent evidence has raised questions about the primary role of the sympathetic nervous system in CRPS/RSD, and clinical results from disruption of sympathetic innervation in patients with CRPS/RSD have remained inconsistent.

Introduction

Complex regional pain syndrome (CRPS) is a chronic pain condition that develops following a noxious event or period of limb immobilization. The clinical features include skin hypersensitivity, microcirculatory abnormalities resulting in skin discoloration and edema, and abnormal sweating. Resorption of bone as well as trophic changes in the skin, nails, hair or muscle may also be seen. A more detailed description of the clinical diagnostic criteria for this condition is outlined in Chap. 27. CRPS was previously known as reflex sympathetic dystrophy (RSD), because of the belief that the clinical findings were mediated by the autonomic nervous system [1]. In 1994, the International Association for the Study of Pain reclassified the term RSD as CRPS, and defined two groups of patients depending on the presence or absence of a known nerve injury [2]. More recently, alterations in the diagnostic criteria have been proposed, and many of these have been adopted into clinical practice [3]. Additional details regarding CRPS in the setting of thoracic outlet syndrome (TOS) are also outlined in Chaps. 13 and 92.

There has been speculation that the sympathetic nervous system plays a role in some patients with CRPS because physical findings suggest an increase in autonomic nerve activity. These findings, such as skin discoloration, edema, temperature alterations and abnormal sweating, have

D.M. Donahue, MD
Department of Thoracic Surgery,
Massachusetts General Hospital, Blake 1570,
55 Fruit Street, Boston, MA 02114, USA
e-mail: donahue.dean@mgh.harvard.edu

K.A. Illig et al. (eds.), *Thoracic Outlet Syndrome*,
DOI 10.1007/978-1-4471-4366-6_31, © Springer-Verlag London 2013

led to the idea that increased sympathetic outflow mediates these clinical features, and therefore may also augment pain in some patients. This concept, termed sympathetically-maintained pain, also led to speculation that if CRPS is mediated by excess sympathetic outflow, then symptoms could potentially be improved by disruption of the sympathetic nerves (sympathectomy).

Surgical Anatomy and the Evolution of Sympathectomy for CRPS

Sympathetic nerve fibers are contained within the sympathetic trunks. These are bilateral paraspinal structures composed of nerves and ganglia originating from white rami of the first thoracic (T1) to the second lumbar (L2) spinal nerves. The inferior cervical (stellate) ganglia lie between the transverse process of C7 and the neck of the first rib. In most cases, attempts to divide or ablate the sympathetic trunk are performed below the level of the stellate ganglia in order to avoid creating Horner's syndrome (ipsilateral papillary constriction, drooping of the eyelid, and hemifacial anhydrosis).

Under normal circumstances, increased sympathetic nervous system output to an extremity – the "fight or flight" response – results in cutaneous vasoconstriction, muscle bed vasodilation and sweating. These clinical features observed in RSD (now CRPS) first led clinicians to implicate the sympathetic nervous system in this condition. Treatment attempts to disrupt sympathetic innervation to an extremity, by performing surgical sympathectomy, date back more than 80 years [4]. In 1948, Shumaker reported the successful treatment of neuropathic pain by performing sympathectomy with either surgical division or alcohol injection; however, only short-term patient follow-up was reported [5]. Surgical sympathectomy has since been accomplished through either anterior, posterior or transaxillary approaches [6–8]. More recently, video assisted thoracoscopy (VATS) has been used for cervical sympathectomy in both thoracic outlet syndrome (TOS) with RSD, or more commonly, in primary hyperhidrosis [9, 10]. Each of these various surgical approaches provides ready access to the sympathetic nerve chain, at or just below the level of the first rib.

Because the initial clinical response to sympathectomy can be inconsistent, the use of temporary sympathetic blockade with local anesthetics has been performed as a diagnostic test. This is typically performed prior to proceeding with either surgical division of the sympathetic trunk or chemical nerve ablation with injection of phenol or alcohol. Interpretation of the results of these diagnostic injections may be difficult for several reasons. For example, the local anesthetic may spread to adjacent spinal nerves, thereby temporarily relieving pain through direct blockade of somatic afferents. Pain relief might also be achieved through the systemic absorption of the anesthetic. Finally, the response rates to temporary sympathetic blockade are often no higher than placebo [11]. Sympathetic blockade with oral adrenergic blocking agents, or by intravenous systemic infusion of phentolamine, have also provided inconsistent results in pain relief [12]. It has been proposed that sympathetic block with a combination of oral, intravenous and local injections may be the most reliable way to select appropriate candidates for permanent surgical or ablative sympathectomy; however, clinical results of this approach have not yet been published [13].

Other mechanisms have been proposed to evaluate the extent that the sympathetic nervous system might play in the pain experienced by individual patients. In those that have had a successful response to temporary sympathetic blockade with local injections, a subcutaneous injection of norepinephrine into the symptomatic extremity would be expected to result in increased pain, thereby adding further evidence in support of a sympathetically-maintained component of the chronic pain condition [14]. It is not yet known if this subgroup of patients would then more favorably respond to permanent sympathectomy with either chemical ablation or surgery.

Results of Sympathectomy in CRPS Patients

There are many retrospective, and some prospective, reports of both surgical and ablative sympathectomy in CRPS/RSD, but no strong evidence to suggest that it is superior to traditional pharmacotherapy treatment [15]. Most of these reports are limited by poorly defined diagnostic inclusion criteria for CRPS/RSD, small study sizes, and only short-term clinical follow-up. Placebo-controlled studies frequently report that the response rate to temporary sympathetic blockade is identical to that of placebo. A review of 37 reports, including 1,979 patients undergoing surgical sympathectomy for symptoms of neuropathic pain, found that 25 % of patients actually reported an increase in their symptoms [15]. Other complications in these patients have included compensatory hyperhidrosis (18.2 %), Horner's syndrome (6.2 %) and gustatory sweating (5 %). Though uncommon, significant cardiac rhythm disturbances have also been reported following thoracic sympathectomy [16]. To date there have been no randomized, blinded placebo-controlled trials evaluating the results and role of sympathectomy in CRPS/RSD, and the potential complications and varying success rates of these procedures remain a significant concern.

Cervical sympathectomy has been successfully performed during surgery for TOS in a group of patients who also demonstrated co-existing clinical signs to suggest autonomic dysfunction [17]. A total of 326 successful outcomes were described, but neither the diagnostic criteria for autonomic dysfunction, nor the total number of sympathectomies performed, were reported. First rib resection by either transaxillary, cervical or dorsal approaches provides adequate access to divide the cervical sympathetic trunk. However, any recommendation for use of these procedures remains confounded by the difficulties in patient selection and assessment of results that have been previously discussed.

The Role of the Sympathetic Nervous System in CRPS: Current Data

The clinical features of CRPS that implicate the sympathetic nervous system initially led to the idea that a direct link exists between sympathetic efferent nerves and sensory afferent fibers. These fibers travel together within a given peripheral nerve, and they share a close relationship within their respective areas of innervation [18]. However, recent studies by Campero using microneurography

have demonstrated no evidence that peripheral pain receptors (nociceptors) are activated by sympathetic fibers [19]. Additionally, physiological increases in sympathetic outflow to painful areas in patients with CRPS did not increase activity of local nociceptors.

Function of the sympathetic nervous system has been found to be both overactive and underactive in the symptomatic limbs of patients with CRPS. Signs of sympathetic deficit include increased extremity skin temperature and a loss of vasoconstrictor reflexes, occasionally referred to as "warm" CRPS. Sympathetic overactivity in these patients produces signs of coolness and increased sweating in the extremity [20]. It has been clinically observed that these changes develop over time in some CRPS patients, with the acute "warm" phase evolving into a chronic "cool" phase [21]. Regardless of skin temperature, sympathetic neurotransmittors (or their metabolites) measured in venous blood from the affected extremities of patients with CRPS are lower than those measured from the unaffected side, suggesting a local decrease in sympathetic neurotransmitter release [22–24]. This decrease in local sympathetic activity can be paradoxically accompanied by clinical signs of increased sympathetic function, such as vasoconstriction and hyperhidrosis. This discrepancy may reflect an increased sensitivity of peripheral adrenergic receptors to circulating catecholamines, rather than a direct effect through sympathetic fibers [25]. Given these findings, disruption of these sympathetic fibers may not address the underlying mechanism leading to the clinical features of autonomic dysfunction. This could explain the inconsistent and short-lived clinical results of sympathectomy in patients with CRPS.

There is further evidence suggesting that pathways other than the sympathetic nervous system have a role in mediating the clinical changes seen in the extremities of CRPS patients. There are also data suggesting that patients with chronic CRPS have abnormalities of the vascular endothelium-derived mediators, such as endothelin-1 and nitric oxide [26, 27]. Some skin vessels do not contain any sympathetic innervation, and somatic fibers have been found to innervate the microcirculation. Degeneration of non-sympathetic nerve fibers within the *nervi vasorum* results in opening dermal arteriovenous shunts in the extremities, causing blood to bypass tissue capillary beds [28]. Thus, while the skin appears flushed, the tissues in CRPS-affected extremities may be ischemic as demonstrated by phosphorus magnetic resonance spectroscopy [29]. Neurogenic edema may also result from capillary leakage mediated by the inappropriate release of vasogenic peptides from malfunctioning small fibers [30].

Thus, while there is some evidence to implicate a role for the sympathetic nervous system in some patients with chronic pain conditions, it does not seem to be the exclusive mediator of chronic pain and the degree of sympathetic involvement varies substantially between patients. While the occasional patient may show a temporary response to procedural interventions targeting the sympathetic system, the use of chemical or surgical sympathectomy in patients with CRPS must be approached cautiously.

References

1. Evans JA. Reflex sympathetic distrophy; report of 57 cases. Ann Int Med. 1947;26:417–26.
2. Merskey H, Bogduk N. Classification of chronic pain: descriptions of chronic pain syndromes and definitions of pain terms. 2nd ed. Seattle: IASP Press; 1994.
3. Harden RN, Bruehl S, Stanton-Hicks M, et al. Proposed new diagnostic criteria for complex regional pain syndrome. Pain Med. 2007;8:326–31.
4. Spurling RG. Causalgia of the upper extremity: treatment by dorsal sympathetic ganglionectomy. Arch Neurol Psychiatry. 1930;23:784.
5. Shumacker HB, Speigel IJ, Upjohn RH. Causalgia: the role of sympathetic interruption in treatment. Surg Gynecol Obstet. 1948;86:76–86.
6. Hempel GK, Rusher Jr AH, Wheeler CG, Hunt DG, Bukhari HI. Supraclavicular resection of the first rib for thoracic outlet syndrome. Am J Surg. 1981;141:213–5.
7. Smithwick RH. Modified dorsal sympathectomy for vascular spasm (Raynaud's disease) of the upper extremity. Ann Surg. 1936;104:339–46.
8. Atkins HJB. Sympathectomy by the axillary approach. Lancet. 1954;266:538–9.
9. Urschel Jr HC. Video-assisted sympathectomy and thoracic outlet syndrome. Chest Surg Clin N Am. 1993;3:299–306.
10. Cerfolio RJ, De Campos JR, Bryant AS, et al. The society of thoracic surgeons expert consensus for the surgical treatment of hyperhidrosis. Ann Thorac Surg. 2011;91:1642–8.
11. Price DD, Long S, Wilsey B, Rafii A. Analysis of peak magnitude and duration of analgesia produced by local anesthetics injected into sympathetic ganglia of complex regional pain syndrome patients. Clin J Pain. 1998;14:216–26.
12. Cohen SP, Kapoor SG, Rathmell JP. Intravenous infusion tests have limited utility for selecting long-term drug therapy in patients with chronic pain: a systematic review. Anesthesiology. 2009;111:416–31.
13. Raja SN, Campbell JN. Risk-benefit ratio for surgical sympathectomy: dilemmas in clinical decision making. J Pain. 2000;1:261–4.
14. Ali Z, Raja SN, Wesselmann U, et al. Intradermal injection of norepinephrine evokes pain in patients with sympathetically maintained pain. Pain. 2000;88:161–8.
15. Straube S, Derry S, Moore RA, McQuay HJ. Cervicothoracic or lumbar sympathectomy for neuropathic pain and complex regional pain syndrome. Cochrane Database Syst Rev 2010; (7):CD002918.
16. Lai CL, Chen WJ, Liu YB, et al. Bradycardia and permanent pacing after bilateral thoracoscopic T2-sympathectomy for primary hyperhidrosis. Pacing Clin Electrophysiol. 2001;24:524–5.
17. Urschel HC. Dorsal sympathectomy and management of thoracic outlet syndrome with VATS. Ann Thorac Surg. 1993;56:717–20.
18. Gibbs GF, Drummond PD, Finch PM, et al. Unravelling the pathophysiology of complex regional pain syndrome: focus on sympathetically maintained pain. Clin Exp Pharmacol Physiol. 2008;35:717–24.
19. Campero M, Bostock H, Baumann TK, et al. A search for activation of C nociceptors by sympathetic fibers in complex regional pain syndrome. Clin Neurophysiol. 2010;121:1072–9.
20. Wasner G, Schattschneider J, Heckmann K, et al. Vascular abnormalities in reflex sympathetic dystrophy (CRPS I): mechanisms and diagnostic value. Brain. 2001;124:587–99.
21. Birklein F, Riedl B, Sieweke N, et al. Neurological findings in complex regional pain syndromes: analysis of 145 cases. Acta Neurol Scand. 2000;101:262–9.
22. Drummond PD, Finch PM, Smythe GA. Reflex sympathetic dystrophy: the significance of differing plasma catecholamine concentrations in affected and unaffected limbs. Brain. 1991;114:2025–36.
23. Drummond PD, Finch PM, Edvinsson L, et al. Plasma neuropeptide Y in the symptomatic limb of patients with causalgic pain. Clin Auton Res. 1994;4:113–6.
24. Harden RN, Duc TA, Williams TR, et al. Norepinephrine and epinephrine levels in affected versus unaffected limbs in sympathetically maintained pain. Clin J Pain. 1994;10:324–30.
25. Jorum E, Orstavik K, Schmidt R, et al. Catecholamine induced excitation of nociceptors in sympathetically maintained pain. Pain. 2007;127:296–301.
26. Schattschneider J, Hartung K, Stengel M, et al. Endothelial dysfunction in cold type complex regional pain syndrome. Neurology. 2006;67:673–5.

27. Dayan L, Salman S, Norman D, et al. Exaggerated vasoconstriction in complex regional pain syndrome-1 is associated with impaired resistance artery endothelial function and local vascular reflexes. J Rheumatol. 2008;35:1339–45.

28. Albrecht PJ, Hines S, Eisenberg E, et al. Pathologic alterations of cutaneous innervation and vasculature in affected limbs from patients with complex regional pain syndrome. Pain. 2006;120:244–66.

29. Heerschap A, den Hollander JA, Reynen H, et al. Metabolic changes in reflex sympathetic dystrophy: a 31P NMR spectroscopy study. Muscle Nerve. 1993; 16:367–73.

30. Birklein F, Schmelz M. Neuropeptides, neurogenic inflammation and complex regional pain syndrome (CRPS). Neurosci Lett. 2008;437:199–202.

Surgical Techniques: Posterior Approach for Reoperative NTOS

32

Harold C. Urschel Jr.[†], Charles R. Crane, J. Mark Pool, and Amit N. Patel

Abstract

The treatment of recurrent neurogenic thoracic outlet syndrome (TOS) is an exceptional challenge. We believe that in patients with symptoms suggesting recurrent neurogenic TOS, the clinical diagnosis should be confirmed by objective nerve conduction velocity (NCV) testing, and that when NCVs are depressed in a patient whose symptoms are unrelieved by prolonged conservative therapy, a posterior reoperative procedure should be considered. Removal of any cervical or first rib remnants or regenerated fibrocartilage, along with neurolysis of C7, C8, and T1 nerve roots and the brachial plexus, is performed. Dorsal sympathectomy is typically included to minimize any contribution to symptoms that might be attributable to causalgia and sympathetic-maintained pain syndrome, and topical agents are employed to minimize formation of recurrent perineural scar tissue. In this chapter, we summarize results with this approach in a large number of patients.

[†]Deceased

H.C. Urschel Jr., MD (✉)
Department of Cardiovascular and Thoracic Surgery,
Baylor University Medical Center,
University of Texas Southwestern Medical School,
3600 Gaston Ave, Ste. 1201, Dallas, TX 75246, USA
e-mail: drurschel@me.com

C.R. Crane, MD
Department of Certified Pain Management,
American Board of Physical Medicine
and Rehabilitation, American Board
of Electrodiagnostic Medicine,
P.O. Box 550337, Dallas, TX 75355, USA

J.M. Pool, MD
Cardiac, Vascular and Thoracic Surgical Associates,
Texas Health Presbyterian Hospital of Dallas,
8230 Walnut Hill Lane, Suite 208,
Dallas, TX 75231, USA
e-mail: jmarkpool@gmail.com

A.N. Patel, MD
Department of Cardiothoracic Surgery,
School of Medicine, The University of Utah,
30 North, 1900 East, Suite 3C127,
Salt Lake City, UT 84132, USA
e-mail: dallaspatel@gmail.com

K.A. Illig et al. (eds.), *Thoracic Outlet Syndrome*,
DOI 10.1007/978-1-4471-4366-6_32, © Springer-Verlag London 2013

Introduction

The treatment of recurrent neurogenic thoracic outlet syndrome (TOS) is an exceptional challenge. We believe that in patients with symptoms suggesting recurrent neurogenic TOS, the clinical diagnosis should be confirmed by objective nerve conduction velocity (NCV) testing, and that when NCVs are depressed in a patient whose symptoms are unrelieved by prolonged conservative therapy, a posterior reoperative procedure should be considered. Removal of any cervical or first rib remnants or regenerated fibrocartilage, along with neurolysis of C7, C8, and T1 nerve roots and the brachial plexus, is performed. Dorsal sympathectomy is typically included to minimize any contribution to symptoms that might be attributable to causalgia and sympathetic-maintained pain syndrome, and topical agents are employed to minimize formation of recurrent perineural scar tissue. In this chapter, we summarize results with this approach in a large number of patients.

Electrophysiologic Testing

Objective nerve conduction velocity (NCV) testing is used to confirm the diagnosis of recurrent neurogenic TOS [1–4]. Over the past 50 years, ulnar NCV tests were performed on about 8,400 patients/year seen in consultation by the Department of Physical Medicine at Baylor University Medical Center for pain of the upper extremities. Over 700 were found to have varying degrees of neurovascular compression at the thoracic outlet, most of which could be treated conservatively.

Method for Measuring Conduction Velocities

Each patient was placed on the examination table with the arm fully extended at the elbow and in about 20° of abduction at the shoulder, to facilitate easy placement of the stimulation unit over the course of the ulnar nerve. Three needle electrodes were inserted serially into the hypothenar muscles or the first dorsal interosseous muscle,

with the ground electrode placed proximally, the reference electrode placed distally, and the recording electrode placed in between. In recording NCVs from the median nerve, the electrodes were placed in the thenar muscles in the same order described for the ulnar nerve.

The ulnar nerve was stimulated consecutively at four points: (1) At the proximal skin crease on the volar aspect of the wrist, about 2 cm proximal to the base of the metacarpal bones; (2) medially below the elbow, about 2.5 cm distal to the medial epicondyle of the humerus; (3) at a point over the medial aspect of the upper arm, midway between the axillary flexion line and the elbow flexion line; and (4) at Erb's point, located about 2.5 cm above the clavicle and slightly anterior to the edge of trapezus muscle, which is the nearest point to the lower trunk of the brachial plexus. For stimulation of the median nerve, the stimulation unit was placed closer to the lateral head of the sternocleidomastoid or slightly more superior.

Supramaximal stimulation was used at all points in order to obtain maximal response. The duration of the stimulus was 0.2 ms except for muscular individuals, where it was 0.5 ms. Time of stimulation, conduction delay and muscle response were recorded on the electrophysiologic testing device with time markers occurring each millisecond on the sweep. The conduction time, or latency of response to stimulation from the four points of stimulation to the recording electrode, were obtained from the digital recordings or calculated from the tracing on the screen. NCVs were calculated in m/s as the distance between two adjacent stimulation points (m) divided by the difference in latency (sec).

Clinical Diagnosis

The process of clinical differential diagnosis for recurrent neurogenic TOS is similar to that for patients that have previously undergone surgical treatment [5–9]. However, the indications for considering a reoperative procedure are more stringent than for a primary operation, in that longer periods of conservative therapy are usually involved.

In the group of our patients who were evaluated for recurrent neurogenic TOS, there was a substantial posterior stump of the first rib (>1 cm) remaining in 2,106 patients (all referred from outside physicians). Complete resection of the first rib at the initial procedure was observed in 199 patients, in whom recurrent symptoms were associated with excessive scar formation on the brachial plexus. We had performed the original surgical procedure on 98 of these 199 patients, for an overall reoperation rate of 2.5 % of 3,914 primary procedures. Even though some of our patients did not return to us for recurrent symptoms, this rate is much less than that reported in most other series. This may reflect our observation that few surgeons remove the rib completely at the time of the initial procedure, for fear of injuring the T1 or C8 nerve

roots, and that some surgeons also cover the end of the rib at the transverse process of the vertebra with the scalenus medius muscle.

Operative Technique

Posterior reoperations for recurrent thoracic outlet syndrome are performed through a muscle-splitting incision. Our preferred technique for such reoperations is the posterior, high thoracoplasty, muscle-splitting incision, with removal of any first rib stump, neurolysis of the C7, C8, and T1 nerve roots and the brachial plexus, and a dorsal sympathectomy (Fig. 32.1) [10].

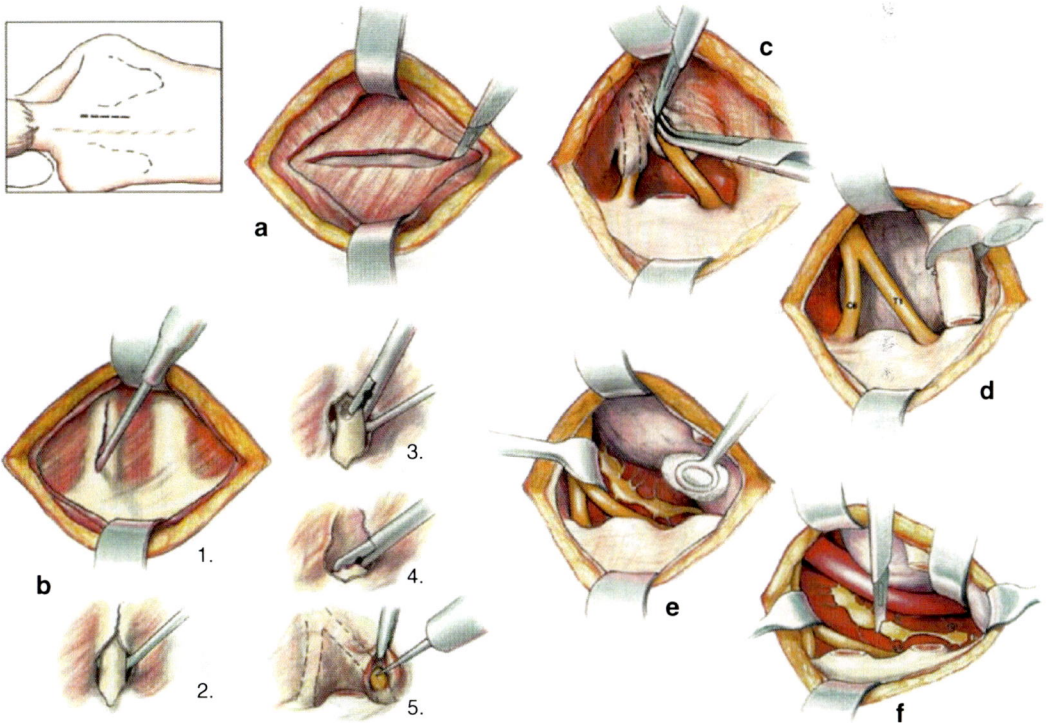

Fig. 32.1 Posterior approach for recurrent neurogenic TOS. Illustrations depicting surgical technique for posterior approach to thoracic outlet decompression, with removal of any first rib stump, neurolysis of the C7, C8, and T1 nerve roots and the brachial plexus, and a dorsal sympathectomy. The patient is placed in the lateral position and the incision is made between the scapula and the spine (*inset*). The incision is carried to the trapezius muscle and the trapezius and rhomboid muscles are split (**a**). After resecting the posterior superior serratus muscle, the first rib remnant is identified by retracting the sacrospinalis

muscle and incising the periosteum, exposed subperiosteally, and the head and neck of the remnant are excised using bone rongeurs (**b***1–5*). The C7, C8 and T1 nerve roots are identified and protected, and neurolysis is carried out to remove all of the surrounding scar tissue is removed as far forward as necessary (**c**). For dorsal sympathectomy, the head and neck of the second rib are dissected free and a short segment of the rib is resected (**d**), and the T2 and T3 ganglia, along with the intervening sympathetic chain, are exposed and resected (**e** and **f**)

The patient is placed in the lateral position with an axillary roll put under the "down" side. The upper arm is placed as for a thoracotomy. A 6-cm incision is made with its midpoint at the angle of the scapula, halfway between the scapula and the spinous processes (Fig. 32.1, inset). The incision is carried through the skin and subcutaneous tissue down to the trapezius muscle. The trapezius and rhomboid muscles are split (Fig. 32.1a).

The posterior superior serratus muscle is resected and the first rib stump is identified by retracting the sacrospinalis muscle medially (Fig. 32.1b). The electrocautery is used to expose the first rib remnant ("stump") and to open the periosteum. A periosteal elevator, or joker, is employed to remove the stump subperiosteally. The head and the neck of the rib usually have not been removed in the initial operation. The rib shears are used to divide the rib remnant, and the Urschel-Leksell reinforced and Urschel pituitary rongeurs are employed carefully to remove the head and neck of the rib. The T1 nerve root is identified grossly or with the help of a nerve stimulator.

Once the T1 nerve root is identified, neurolysis is carried out using a right-angle clamp, magnification, a knife, and special microscissors. A nerve stimulator may be helpful if extensive scarring is present. Neurolysis is extended to the C7 and C8 nerve roots and to the brachial plexus. All the scar tissue is removed as far forward as necessary, so that the nerve roots as well as the upper, middle, and lower trunks of the brachial plexus lie free. Care is taken not to injure the long thoracic nerve or any other brachial plexus branch. The subclavian artery and vein are decompressed through the same incision (Fig. 32.1c).

The second rib is dissected free and the cautery is used to open the periosteum linearly. A 2-cm segment of the rib is resected posteriorly, medial to the sacrospinalis muscle, in order to perform the dorsal sympathectomy (Fig. 32.1d). This exposure may also help identify the T1 nerve root. After the head and neck of the second rib are removed, the sympathetic chain is identified on the vertebra, or it may have been separated and found to lie on the pleura. The stellate

ganglion lies in an almost transverse rather than vertical position (Fig. 32.1e).

The T2 and T3 ganglia are dissected and clips are placed above the T2 and below the T3 ganglia. The gray (affegent) and white (efferent) rami communicans fibers to the T2 and T3 intercostal nerves are clipped and divided. The T2 and T3 sympathetic ganglia are removed along with the interposed sympathetic chain (Fig. 32.1f). The electrocautery is used to effect hemostasis and to char the area, 0.5 cm wide and 1.0 cm long, where the two ganglia and sympathetic chain had been removed. This is to discourage sprouting and regeneration of neural fibers from the sympathetic chain. After antibiotic solution is irrigated, methylprednisolone acetate and hyaluronic acid are also left on the areas of neurolysis to suppress scar tissue formation. The wound is closed in layers with interrupted nylon sutures in each of the muscle layers, absorbable sutures in the subcutaneous tissue, and metal clips in the skin. A large round Jackson-Pratt drain is placed in the area of neurolysis through a separate stab wound 2 cm below the inferior part of the incision, with care taken not to incorporate the drain while closing the muscle layers.

Results

The results of 2,305 procedures showed a moderately good early effect of a second operation for neurogenic TOS: 1,729 patients (75 %) had significant improvement, 369 (16 %) had fair improvement, and only 207 (9 %) did not improve (Table 32.1). Late results (5-year follow-up) in 528 extremities that underwent a second procedure revealed 396 (75 %) with good results and 132 (25 %) with fair to poor recovery; in addition, 48 patients (3.1 %) required a third surgical procedure.

The primary technical factors involved in recurrence seem to be related to incomplete extirpation of the first rib during the initial procedure. If a rib remnant is left (as performed by many surgeons outside of our group), osteocytes can grow from the end of the bone and produce

Table 32.1 Results of reoperations in 2,305 patients with recurrent neurogenic TOS

Outcome category	Symptom relief	Employment	Recreation limitation	No. of patients
Good	Complete	Full	None	1,729 (75 %)
Fair	Partial	Limitation	Moderate	369 (16 %)
Poor	None	No return	Severe	207 (9 %)

fibrocartilage and regenerated bone that can in turn compress the nerves. The risk of fibrosis may be higher in patients who produce keloids, in patients where postoperative hematomas are not drained, or in patients who undergo excessive early physical therapy after the first surgical procedure.

The transaxillary or supraclavicular route is usually preferred for the initial surgical procedure in patients with neurogenic TOS. Although the posterior approach may be used for primary operations, particularly in patients with large first ribs or cervical ribs, it is usually employed for reoperations. We prefer this approach because we believe that rib stumps or regenerated ribs can be more easily removed from a "virgin" posterior approach and because the nerve roots as well as the brachial plexus are easy to identify and access from the back. Reoperations for recurrent compression also usually incorporate a dorsal sympathectomy for causalgia-like symptoms, sympathetic maintained pain syndrome, or Raynaud's phenomenon, which can be readily accomplished through the posterior approach.

References

1. Krusen EM. Cervical pain syndromes. Arch Phys Med Rehabil. 1968;49(7):376–82.
2. Caldwell JW, Crane CR, Krusen EM. Nerve conduction studies: an aid in the diagnosis of the thoracic outlet syndrome. South Med J. 1971;64(2):210–2.
3. Greep JM, Lemmens HAJ, Roos DB, Urschel Jr HC. Pain in shoulder and arm: an integrated view. The Hague, the Netherlands: Martinus Nijhoff; 1979.
4. Urschel Jr HC, Razzuk MA, Wood RE, Perekh M, Paulson DL. Objective diagnosis (ulnar nerve conduction velocity) and current therapy of the thoracic outlet syndrome. Ann Thorac Surg. 1971;12(6):608–20.
5. Urschel Jr HC, Razzuk MA, Albers JE, Wood RE, Paulson DL. Reoperation for recurrent thoracic outlet syndrome. Ann Thorac Surg. 1976;21(1):19–25.
6. Urschel Jr HC, Razzuk MA. The failed operation for thoracic outlet syndrome: the difficultly of diagnosis and management. Ann Thorac Surg. 1986;42(5):523–8.
7. Urschel Jr HC. Reoperation for thoracic outlet syndrome. In: Grillo HC, Eschapasse H, editors. International trends in general thoracic surgery, vol. 2. St. Louis: CV Mosby; 1986.
8. Urschel Jr HC, Razzuk MA. Current management of thoracic outlet syndrome. N Eng J Med. 1972;286:21.
9. Urschel Jr HC, Razzuk MA. Neurovascular compression in the thoracic outlet: changing management over 50 years. Ann Surg. 1998;228(4):609–17.
10. Urschel Jr HC, Cooper J. Atlas of thoracic surgery. New York: Churchill Livingstone; 1995.

Part IV

Neurogenic TOS: Outcomes and Future Directions

NTOS: Postoperative Care

33

Stephen J. Annest, Richard J. Sanders,
Matthew Becher, Nicholas Bennett,
and Anna B. Evans

Abstract

Postoperative management for neurogenic thoracic outlet syndrome (TOS) begins with preoperative preparation of the patient. Obtaining informed consent includes reviewing with the patient the risks and complications of surgery, how soon symptoms will subside, and expectations for return to work and recreation. Postoperatively, a chest x-ray in the recovery room is obtained to detect pneumothorax, to look for apical fluid collection, and to view position of the hemidiaphragm. Medication for nausea, sleep, and pain should include anticipation of constipation from narcotics. Other postoperative considerations include deep vein thrombosis prophylaxis, diet, ambulation, and instructions for postoperative activity and physical therapy.

S.J. Annest, MD, FACS (✉)
Department of Vascular Surgery,
Presbyterian St. Luke's Medical Center,
Vascular Institute of the Rockies,
1601 East 19th Avenue, Suite 3950,
Denver, CO 80218, USA
e-mail: annest@vascularinstitute.com

R.J. Sanders, MD
Department of Surgery, HealthONE
Presbyterian-St. Lukes Hospital,
4545 E. 9th Ave, #240, Denver, CO 80220, USA
e-mail: rsanders@ecentral.com

M. Becher, PharmD • N. Bennett, PharmD Candidate
A.B. Evans, PharmD Candidate
Presbyterian St Luke's Medical Center and Rocky
Mountain Hospital for Children,
Denver, CO 80218, USA

Introduction

There are many variations of postoperative management. In this chapter we present a protocol the authors have used, and continue to update, for patients undergoing surgery for neurogenic TOS.

Preoperative Preparation

Prior to surgery, following an aviation check-list model, several topics are discussed with the patient: (1) Operative risks, benefits, and alternatives are reviewed. (2) Paresthesias usually improve within 24 h. (3) Incisional pain can persist in the neck, chest, and parascapular area, lasting 4–8 weeks after surgery. (4) Reduced range of motion of arm is expected for 3–4 weeks. (5) Good improvement in symptoms (50–60 %) takes 6–8 weeks, sometimes longer. Essentially, all patients can expect

K.A. Illig et al. (eds.), *Thoracic Outlet Syndrome*,
DOI 10.1007/978-1-4471-4366-6_33, © Springer-Verlag London 2013

some degree of residual symptoms; only rarely do patients note 100 % improvement. (6) The expected time off-work depends on the job performed before surgery: (a) with sedentary jobs, return may be possible in 1–2 weeks; (b) with jobs requiring keyboard use, absence from work may be necessary for 3–4 weeks, and when the patient returns, he/she initially works reduced hours, thereafter increasing time at work as symptoms allow; (c) for the patient whose work involves heavy labor, several weeks may be required before returning, and that patient might not ever be able to tolerate the rigors of the job, with some facing the possibility of a career change and job retraining. (6) The time required before resuming recreational activities depends on the severity of residual symptoms and the degree of recovery. (7) An appointment is made with physical therapy to explain the postoperative therapy routine. The commonly used drugs for pain management are listed by categories in the Table 33.1, along with dosages and routes of administration.

Day of Surgery

Operating Room

Prophylactic antibiotic (first generation cephalosporin unless patient allergy exists) is administered just prior to the incision. In the operating room, even after obtaining complete hemostasis, including the use of bone wax on the ends of the resected rib, blood and serum drains from the surfaces of the operative field. Therefore, suction drainage is always placed (our preferences are a 19-French round channel drain for transaxillary procedures and a 10-French round channel drain for supraclavicular procedures). If the pleura has been entered, it is not repaired. To avoid postoperative pneumothorax, the anesthesiologist expands the lung and maintains positive end expiratory pressure (PEEP) during wound closure. Even if the pleura is opened, a separate chest tube is not necessary. A small-caliber multi-hole local anesthetic infusion catheter is placed either in the subplatysmal space if a supraclavicular route is used or in the subcutaneous layer in transaxillary incisions, with the tip 1–2 cm beneath the incision

line for continuous infusion of local anesthetic. This catheter distributes local anesthetic and can be clamped if the patient experiences numbness or weakness, as the medication bathes the brachial plexus postoperatively. Injecting local anesthetic into the subcutaneous tissue at closure also helps to reduces incisional pain.

Post-anesthesia Care Unit (PACU)

A portable sitting anteroposterior (AP) chest x-ray is taken in deep inspiration. This film, available within minutes, allows the surgeon to assess diaphragmatic function, completeness of rib resection, the presence of intra-pleural air or fluid, and the presence of any fluid at the apex of the chest. As the patient awakens, evaluation of motor and sensory function is performed providing reassurance should subsequent weakness and/or numbness develop due to the local anesthetic infusion. Postoperative pain control in the PACU may be aided by use of a transcutaneous nerve stimulator (TNS unit) and by judicious use of intravenous narcotics and non-steroidal anti-inflammatory drugs. Patient-controlled analgesia (PCA) allows the patient to self-manage pain after waking from anesthesia. If the PCA is set up in the PACU, it becomes available immediately upon arrival to the surgical floor, lessening the chance of an unchecked increase in postoperative pain. A mild-moderate decrease in the hematocrit is often seen after surgery, in spite of seemingly insignificant intra-operative blood loss. A determination of the presence of bleeding that might be significant enough to require re-exploration is made by evaluating volume and nature of drain fluid, vital signs, and chest x-ray appearance.

Surgical Floor

Nausea

A scopolamine patch is placed pre-operatively on the patient's styloid process behind one ear and/or an intravenous anti-emetic (dexamethazone) is given.

Table 33.1 Potential pharmacological options for pain management following surgical intervention for neurogenic TOS

Type of medication	Primary uses and dose ranges	Routes
Narcotics		
Morphine	Breakthrough pain; acute/chronic pain	PO, IV, PR
	PO: 10–30 mg Q 3 h; IV/IM: 2.5–15 Q 2 h	
Comments	Start low, titrate to analgesia	
Hydromorphone	Breakthrough pain; acute/chronic Pain	PO, IV, PR, IM
	PO: 2.5–10 mg Q 3 h; IV/IM: 1–2 mg Q 4–6 h	
Comments	Start low, titrate to analgesia	
Oxycodone	Breakthrough pain; acute/chronic Pain	PO
	PO: 5 mg Q 6 h	
Comments	Start low, titrate to analgesia	
Fentanyl	Chronic pain	PO, IV, IM, TD
	Transdermal: 25mcg Q 72 h	
Comments	Transdermal formulation outlasts naloxone significantly	
Extended-release	Chronic pain	PO
Oxycodone	10 mg Q 12 h	
Methadone	Chronic pain	PO, IV, IM, SQ
	2.5–10 mg q 8–12 h	
Comments	High risk of accumulation/overdose in titration period	
Skeletal muscle relaxants		
Cyclobenzaprine	Chronic pain; adjunct	PO
	10–40 mg	
Carisoprodol	Chronic pain; adjunct	PO
	350 mg TID	
Baclofen	Chronic pain; adjunct	Oral/intrathecal
	5–10 mg TID	
Methocarbamol	Chronic pain; adjunct	Oral/injection
	1,500 mg QID	
Tricyclic antidepressants		
Amitriptyline	Chronic pain; adjunct	PO
	10–150 mg	
Comments	Start low, titrate to analgesia	
Nortriptyline	Chronic pain; adjunct	PO
	10–150 mg	
Comments	Start low, titrate to analgesia	
Gabapentin	Chronic pain; adjunct	PO
	300–1,800 mg/day	
Comments	Give in divided doses	
Pregabalin	Chronic pain; adjunct	PO
	50–300 mg/day	
Comments	Give in divided doses	
Non-steroidal anti-inflammatory drugs (NSAIDs)		
Ibuprofen	Acute/chronic pain; adjunct	PO, IV
	300–800 mg	
Comments	Given 3–4x daily	
Ketorolac	Acute/chronic pain; adjunct	IV
	10 mg every 4–6 h	
Comments	Max: 40 mg/day for 5 days	
Celecoxib	Acute/chronic pain; adjunct	PO
	200 mg daily</f	

Hygiene

The patient may shower after the drain is removed. Prior to that time sponge baths are allowed. This may require nurse or family assistance.

Activity

Assisted walking and bathroom privileges begin the evening of surgery. Each subsequent hospital day the patient is encouraged to increase activity, frequently walking in the hallway throughout the day.

Physical Therapy

Beginning on the first postoperative day, the patient is shown neck and shoulder stretches, instructed in diaphragmatic breathing exercises, and asked to begin limited wall-climbing or passive shoulder abduction, and forward flexion to stretch the shoulder and avoid development of a frozen shoulder. Postural correction maneuvers are started with clear instructions to stop any movement that induces "nerve pain" (e.g., paresthesias, burning, cold sensations, or shooting pain down the arm). The patient is requested to perform exercises throughout the day as tolerated, always stopping immediately upon experiencing the onset of increased pain other than incisional pain and muscle soreness.

Diet

In the absence of postoperative nausea, the patient may eat a select diet on the evening of surgery. During the first 24 h, intravenous maintenance fluids are provided as needed and as long as the PCA is in use.

Nurse Monitoring

An oxygen saturation monitor with alarm is utilized as long as the patient is receiving intrave-nous pain medication. Nasal oxygen is administered to maintain adequate oxygenation. Intravenous naloxone is ordered if necessary to counteract narcotic overdose.

Incentive Spirometry

Instruction is given on the use of the incentive spirometer and the patient is encouraged to perform deep diaphragmatic breathing exercises hourly while awake.

Anti-embolism Protection

Sequential compression devices (SCD) are worn constantly while in the hospital, removing them only when walking or in the lavatory. Prophylactic doses of low molecular weight heparin are administered in the sub-cutaneous abdominal wall daily, beginning 24 h postoperatively and continued until discharge, unless contraindicated.

Pain Management

Ice is placed on the incision and on the supra-clavicular fossa for 0.5 h every 2 h if the patient achieves comfort from its use. The patient is offered a heating pad if perceived to be beneficial. Transcutaneous local anesthetic patches may be placed under the arm, on the chest wall, and at the supraclavicular fossa, though not directly covering any incision. Deep heat rub is placed at bed-side to be applied by nursing staff or family a few times daily if desired. The PCA with narcotics is utilized during the first several postoperative hours, transitioning to oral pain medications as soon as improvement in pain level allows, usually during the evening of the first postoperative day.

Supportive Medication

This list includes judicious use of one or more muscle relaxants and anti-inflammatory drugs (along with an oral proton pump inhibitor for gastric protection), and sedatives for sleep if the degree of narcotic sedation allows.

Anti-constipation Medications

Use of postoperative narcotics frequently leads to constipation and obstipation, contributing substantially to patient discomfort. Therefore, daily bowel movements should be recorded. The patient and nursing staff join in assuring that a bowel movement occurs before discharge home and that a bowel program which results in bowel regularity continues after discharge. If the standard regiment fails, we have administered up to 3 quarts of polyethylene glycol-electrolyte solution (e.g., Go-LYTELY, Braintree Laboratories, Inc, Braintree, MA) while the patient is still in-hospital.

Drain Management

Output from the closed-suction drain is recorded every 8 h. To prevent air entry into the chest cavity, the nurse clamps the drain tubing before emptying. The drain can be removed when drainage is serous and minimal in amount. If drainage is chylous, the drain is left in place until lymph drainage stops.

Local Anesthetic Infusion Catheter

This small catheter placed at the time of surgery can be removed when the reservoir is empty or at discharge.

Discharge

Pain

Prescriptions are given for oral pain medications at the same dose as used in the hospital, with the plan to taper the level of narcotic used over the next few weeks in close communication with the patient.

Activity

The patient is advised against driving while taking narcotic pain medications. Walking is encouraged for up to an hour each day. The patient is expected to continue the same exercises that were performed while in the hospital. Activity is curtailed if "nerve pain" occurs.

Physical Therapy

Formal physical therapy sessions are scheduled to begin 1–2 weeks following hospital discharge.

Follow-Up

The patient is instructed to call the surgeon with any concerns. Office follow-up may occur anywhere from 1 week to 1 month after discharge. Often, immediate postoperative discomfort, which must simply be tolerated, will substantially resolve by 1 month after the operation.

Return to Work

The ability to safely and effectively return to one's job depends on the specific type of work and the extent of any residual symptoms. This is discussed with the patient both preoperatively and again in the first few weeks after discharge. For out of town patients, if the patient is doing well, a phone call discussion may suffice to determine the appropriate timing for return to work. When possible, we encourage returning to work part-time at least for the first several days.

Post-discharge Problems

Sensory Nerve Dysfunction

In the presence of intact motor nerve function of the upper extremity, dysfunction of sensory nerves of the brachial plexus, as manifested by paresthesias, can be expected to eventually resolve. Initial therapy is simply reassurance. However, cutaneous sensory nerves sometimes present a different problem. The second inter-costal-brachial cutaneous and supraclavicular sensory nerves are often temporarily irritated and can present with burning pain, hyperes-thesia, or dysesthesia. These symptoms often improve with time or by gently rubbing the pain-ful area (for example with a hairbrush) repeat-edly throughout the day over several weeks. If these symptoms persist after 3–4 months, we consider injection with a depot steroid and local anesthetic. If the injection gives only tem-porary relief, permanent relief can be obtained by neurectomy, going through the old incision under local anesthesia and excising the injured nerve. It is important to carefully localize the offending nerve prior to surgical exploration, as these small nerves can be difficult to find at operation.

Motor Nerve Dysfunction

Motor nerve injury can occur from cutting, trau-matizing, or stretching a nerve. If transected, the nerve should be repaired if it is recognized at the time of operation. Trauma and stretch injuries can only be monitored, but electrodiagnostic studies do not demonstrate injury for the first 4–6 weeks postoperatively. Physical and occupa-tional therapy, as directed by a physiatrist, is the mainstay of treatment.

Muscle Soreness

Patients can experience discomfort and muscle tightness occurring in muscles that have not been cut or dissected, including the sternocleidomas-toid, trapezius and rhomboid muscles. When present, physical therapy modalities, heat, and gentle stretching are utilized to relax and physi-ologically stretch painful, contracted muscles. Occasionally, injection of local anesthetic can assist in muscular relaxation.

Chest Wall Pain

Following pectoralis minor tenotomy, chest wall pain is treated with ice therapy, anti-inflammatory agents, transdermal analgesics, and progressive range-of-motion exercises, halting if and when they become uncomfortable. If persistent after 2–3 months, steroid and local anesthetic injec-tions may also be administered.

Chronic Regional Pain Syndrome (CRPS)

Rarely, a patient may manifests symptoms of coldness, hypersensitivity to touch, and burning pain. This suggests the presence of chronic regional pain syndrome (CRPS; previously termed "reflex sympathetic dystrophy" or RSD). This condition can be diagnosed and treated with a stellate ganglion cervical sympathetic block with local anesthetic, followed by initial treat-ment with physical therapy.

Delayed Recovery

Failure of the patient to steadily progress and improve following well-performed brachial plexus decompressive surgery raises the ques-tion of other pain generators. Diagnostic studies and appropriate consultations are initiated to find a solution.

Postoperative Pain Management in Thoracic Outlet Syndrome

Matthew Becher, Nicholas Bennett, and Anna B. Evans

Pain in neurogenic TOS precedes surgical inter-vention and is a consequence of surgery, resulting from inflammation due to tissue trauma inflicted during the surgical dissection and during nerve decompression [1]. Opioids have been the main-stay for treating moderate-to-severe postopera-tive pain; however, a multimodal approach for pain management is now preferred.

Narcotics

Opioids can have an important role immediately following surgery and to control chronic pain associated with neurogenic TOS. The variety of routes of administration and rapid onset of action make opioids a popular choice. Opioids act in the central nervous system (CNS) via the mu (OP3) opioid receptor to alter pain perception [1, 2]. Immediate-acting opioids are favorable in the inpatient setting and for breakthrough pain associated with chronic therapy. However, their effects decline relatively quickly. Sustained-release, longer-acting agents may keep a patient more comfortable, both in-hospital and after discharge. Opiates have many side effects: respiratory rate depression, sedation, hypotension, nausea, and obstipation are frequently seen during therapy [2]. Naloxone reverses the undesired effects of opiates. The opiate and its formulation should be taken into account; some opiates can outlast the effect of naloxone (particularly with extended-release and transdermal preparations). If a patient is to be on opioids chronically, a medication regimen to prevent constipation should be concomitantly instituted.

Muscle Relaxants

Muscle relaxants produce analgesia via CNS depression and alteration of pain perception [3]. Animal studies support mechanisms by which analgesia may also be produced through effects on serotonin receptors by cyclobenzaprine and on nociceptors by baclofen [4, 5]. Given the pathophysiology of neurogenic TOS and the mechanism of action of these agents, muscle relaxants may be used adjunctively with opioids for the treatment of chronic pain associated with TOS. In the absence of spasticity issues, these agents have little to no benefit post-operatively. Caution should be advised when combining these medications with other CNS depressants, such as opioids. Of all muscle relaxants, carisoprodol has the most addictive potential and may be best used for only 2–3 weeks at a time [6].

Anti-depressants

While not FDA-approved for the treatment of pain, tricyclic antidepressants (TCAs) are widely used in the management of pain for patients, with or without concomitant diagnosis of depression [3]. It is thought that the analgesic activity of TCAs is due to the re-uptake inhibition of norepinephrine and serotonin, and possibly potentiation of endogenous opioids. The inability of other serotonin inhibitors to produce marked analgesia indicates that the mechanism of TCA-produced analgesia is not completely understood. TCAs can be beneficial as adjunctive treatment to other therapies, not only augmenting pain relief, but also by treating concurrent depressive symptoms resulting from chronic pain. Due to their sedating effects, TCAs may also benefit patients by aiding sleep. The practitioner should inform patients that associated side effects often diminish with time, but that significant pain relief may require several weeks of therapy. While other classes of antidepressants have been used in the treatment of pain, the analgesia they produce is inferior to that of TCAs.

Nonsteroidal Anti-inflammatory Drugs (NSAIDs)

NSAIDs have been shown to be effective in a wide variety of postoperative pain states, including after thoracotomy [1]. These agents can be used preemptively prior to noxious stimuli, alone for mild to moderate pain, or in combination with opioid analgesics or local anesthetics to treat severe postoperative pain. The benefits of combining NSAIDS with morphine in the immediate postoperative period include not only improved pain control, but possible reduction of narcotic consumption, thereby offering the possibility of reduced postoperative nausea and vomiting, sedation and pruritus. The most commonly reported adverse effects associated with NSAIDS include surgical bleeding, gastrointestinal bleeding, oliguria, and renal failure. Factors that increase the risk for gastrointestinal ulcers and bleeding with NSAID use should be reviewed prior to initiating NSAID therapy. Cyclooxygenase-2 (COX-2) inhibitors may also be considered for postoperative pain management after TOS surgery. They are as effective as ketorolac in reducing pain and inflammation; however, are less likely to cause gastrointestinal ulceration or to promote bleeding.

Anticonvulsants

The symptoms of neurogenic TOS are associated with nerve irritation, resulting in pain, numbness, burning, prickling, itching, tingling, and weakness in the arm and hand. Following surgical intervention, tissue injury is known to cause a heightened response from the spinal cord, hyperalgesia, central sensitization and surgically-induced neuropathic pain [1]. Both gabapentin and pregabalin are indicated for the management of chronic neuropathic pain and may be considered in the multimodal approach for treating acute postoperative pain. In a recently published review [7], Dauri et al. concluded that both gabapentin and pregabalin are effective in reducing pain intensity and opioid consumption; however, the optimal dose, duration, and surgical population have yet to be established. Both gabapentin and pregabalin are well tolerated, with somnolence and dizziness being the most frequently reported side effects. Evidence supports tapering these agents to reduce the risk of adverse effects after chronic use.

References

1. Bhavani-Shankar KO. Management of postoperative pain. In: Basow DS, editor. UpToDate. Waltham: UpToDate; 2011.
2. Micromedex® Healthcare Series (electronic version). Thomson Micromedex, Greenwood Village, USA. http://0-www.thomsonhc.com.library.uchsc.edu:80 (cited: 15 Mar 2011).
3. Gold Standard, Inc. Morphine. Clinical pharmacology [database online]. Available at: http://www.clinicalpharmacology.com. Accessed 11 Mar 2011.
4. Bajwa Z. Overview of the treatment of chronic pain. In: Basow DS, editor. UpToDate. Waltham: UpToDate; 2011.
5. Gold Standard, Inc. Cyclobenzaprine. Clinical pharmacology [database online]. Available at: http://www.clinicalpharmacology.com. Accessed 15 Mar 2011.
6. Gold Standard, Inc. Baclofen. Clinical pharmacology [database online]. Available at: http://www.clinicalpharmacology.com. Accessed 10 Mar 2011.
7. Gold Standard, Inc. Carisprodol. Clinical pharmacology [database online]. Available at: http://www.clinicalpharmacology.com. Accessed: 15 Mar 2011.

Passive and Active Rehabilitation After First Rib Resection

34

Peter I. Edgelow

Abstract

It is clear to all that patients with neurogenic thoracic outlet syndrome (NTOS) require rehabilitation following first rib resection. The post-surgical treatment protocol described below has been designed using published research evidence together with 22 years of clinical experience treating pre- and post-surgical patients with (NTOS). Breathing training is performed before and after surgery. Pre-surgical breathing training is focused on relaxing the accessory breathing muscles by emphasizing the diaphragm. This helps to unload the hyperactive accessory breathing muscles. Post-operative training emphasizes diaphragmatic breathing to reduce the mechanical load on the surgical site but also emphasizes periodic full inhalation to maximize lymphatic flow and mobilize the brachial plexus in an attempt to reduce excessive scar formation around the surgical site. Manual cutaneous and subcutaneous mobilization of the scar, once it is healed enough to tolerate gentle stretching, is addressed, as are range of motion exercises to emphasize restoration of both neural and musculoskeletal movements. Retraining of the core stabilizers is helpful, as is cardiac re-conditioning with walking training. Finally, periods of rest are encouraged to minimize the opportunity of over-exercise and the symptom flares that this can cause.

Introduction

Patients with neurogenic thoracic outlet syndrome (NTOS) have symptoms that can benefit from appropriate physical therapy treatment. When a patient has an operation to remove the first rib and scalene muscles, however performed, it is both painful (leading to immobility) and intrinsically produces alterations in function. For both these reasons, rehabilitative physical therapy is critical in the treatment of such patients, both pre-operatively and post-operatively.

The major focus in active and passive rehabilitation after first rib resection is threefold: first, to restore maximum pulmonary status; second, to restore and maintain flexibility of the brachial plexus during the healing process; and third, to gradually help restore the ability to practice activities of daily living (ADL) during the

P.I. Edgelow, DPT
Graduate Program in Physical Therapy, UCSF/SFSU,
2429 Balmoral St, Union City, CA 94587, USA
e-mail: peteriedgelow@aol.com

K.A. Illig et al. (eds.), *Thoracic Outlet Syndrome*,
DOI 10.1007/978-1-4471-4366-6_34, © Springer-Verlag London 2013

recovery process. The psychosocial benefits of working closely and continuously with a therapist, who expresses care and concern for the patient during the long healing process, as well, is likely very beneficial. It is ideal if the patient has some experience with TOS-directed physical therapy (for example, diaphragmatic breathing) prior to surgery so they will have learned the exercises that they will need to continue after surgery. Finally, demonstration of a commitment to self-management pre-operatively probably predicts the patient's willingness to follow through with the exercises that can maximize the potentially successful surgical outcome.

Does physical therapy have any objectively - demonstrable benefits? Imaging studies (ultrasound) demonstrate that the amount of movement of the neck and shoulder girdle can change the space around the brachial plexus by more than 100 % [1–3]. It can also be demonstrated that the brachial plexus can move distally with movements of the arm and proximally with movements of the neck. In addition the plexus can also be made to bowstring in a cephalad direction over the first rib as the first rib elevates under the plexus with inhalation. [1] All of these movements can be beneficially altered by proper training. In addition, one can hypothesize that this degree of movement within the TO can act as a lymphatic pump. The lymphatic flow from the lower body, trunk, left arm and head drains through the left thoracic duct on its way back to the heart; whereas the lymphatic drainage to the right thoracic duct only includes lymph from the right arm and head. Therefore in a case of thoracic outlet decompressive surgery there is an increased lymphatic load on left TOD as compared to right TOD. The valves in the lymph vessels prevent backflow. It is likely, since the thoracic duct and the right lymphatic duct drain into the chest, the negative intrathoracic pressure during inhalation/exhalation aids lymphatic and venous circulation.

Breathing: Theory, Goals and Method

Many therapists believe that the most important factor upon which treatment rests is the pattern of breathing. Skilled breathing is required to restore maximum post operative pulmonary status. A goal is to return forced vital capacity to normal limits (3000+ cc). The specific goals of breathing training are to reduce stress at the surgical site (diaphragmatic inhalation), to mobilize the brachial plexus to assist in producing adequate elasticity as it heals, and to lower ribs two through five.

Breathing training should be started as soon as the patient can tolerate it following surgery. Patients should be trained to start with relaxed diaphragmatic breathing (50 % inhalation) to reduce stress on the surgical site. The patient should then practice periods of diaphragmatic breathing plus intercostal breathing (75 % inhalation) to mobilize the rib cage and, finally, end with accessory sternal breathing (inhale 100 %) to encourage movement of the brachial plexus, maximize lymphatic decongestion and maximize expansion of the upper lobes of the lungs. Caution must be used to ensure that the inhalation does not cause an increase in or production of symptoms. This is of importance in the case of bilateral disease where staged intervention is considered. While sternal breathing is appropriate for the post-operative side, a 100 % breath can be contraindicated for the not-yet operated upon side.

Healing

A worthy goal of therapy is to minimize scar tissue formation, both externally and within the body (i.e., surrounding the brachial plexus). The patient should be trained to mobilize the surgical site to minimize scar formation and limit any tethering of the neural elements.

The scar can be mobilized manually, once it has healed enough to tolerate gentle movement with the fingertips. The tension free motion of the upper limb can be measured before and after scar mobilization and a significant increase in mobility should be achievable (Figs. 34.1, 34.2, 34.3, 34.4 and 34.5)

Within the body, scarring around the brachial plexus can be mobilized using breathing exercises. This can be done with the neck in varying degrees of rotation and lateral bending

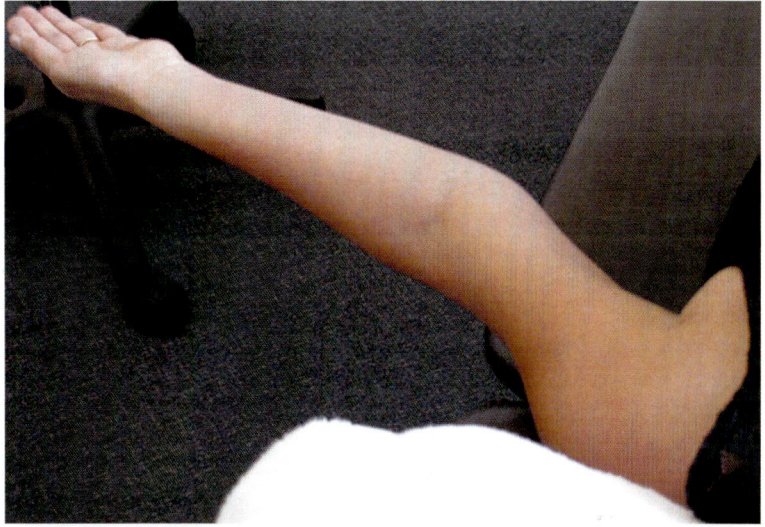

Fig. 34.1 Left ULTT: ending position. Brachial Plexus tension point pre-treatment. Assess symptoms at starting position. With the wrist in neutral flexion/extension and the fingers extended the arm on the surgical side is abducted until the patient feels an increase in tension, either at the surgical site or in the arm

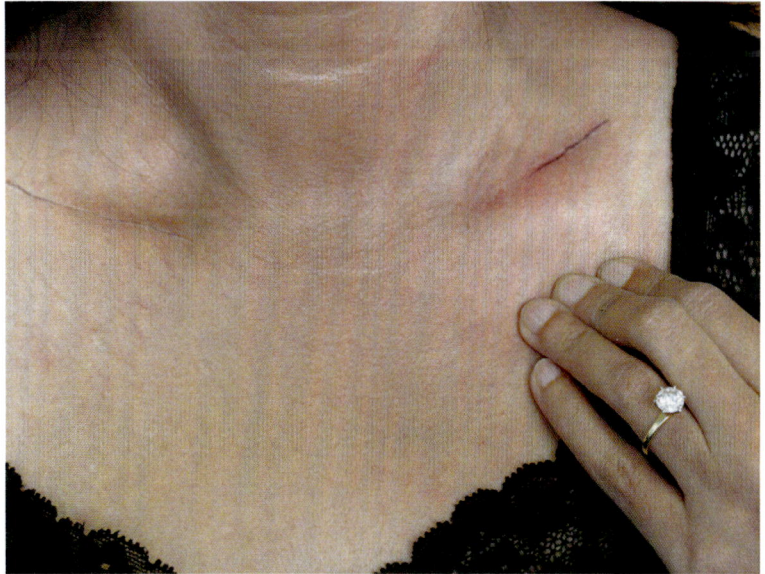

Fig. 34.2 Left scar self mobilization caudally. A treatment to mobilize the scar is performed manually

and during various positions of the arm. Such positions are designed to change the resting length of the nerve roots of the brachial plexus. Finally, the scar can be mobilized by movements of the shoulder girdle (elevation and protraction), as well.

Increasing the range of motion (ROM) of the musculoskeletal and neural systems is also critical. In order to assess ROM and decide whether limitations are due to neural irritability or musculoskeletal restriction, all joints in the upper extremity should be moved to the point of tension. If tension-free range ROM can be improved

by breathing modification or by slackening the nervous system distal to the site of maximum irritation by positioning, neural irritation is the source of limitation. If treatment involving gentle mobilization of the surgical scar results in an increase in tension-free ROM, the restriction is due to fascia and/or scar tissue rather than musculoskeletal limitation. If the initial ROM was as in Fig. 34.1 and shrugging the scapula results in an increase, like Fig. 34.5, then this restriction is neural [1, 4]. If the restriction is like Fig. 34.1 and scar mobilization or breathing does not increase ROM, then the shoulder should be examined

Fig. 34.3 Left scar self mobilization cephalad. A treatment to mobilize the scar is performed manually

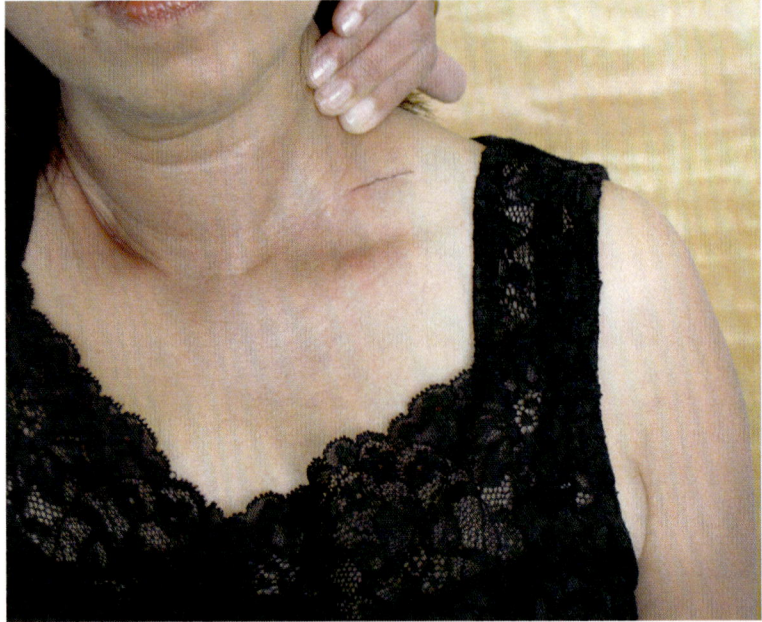

Fig. 34.4 Left scar self mobilization caudally and cephalad. A treatment to mobilize the scar is performed manually

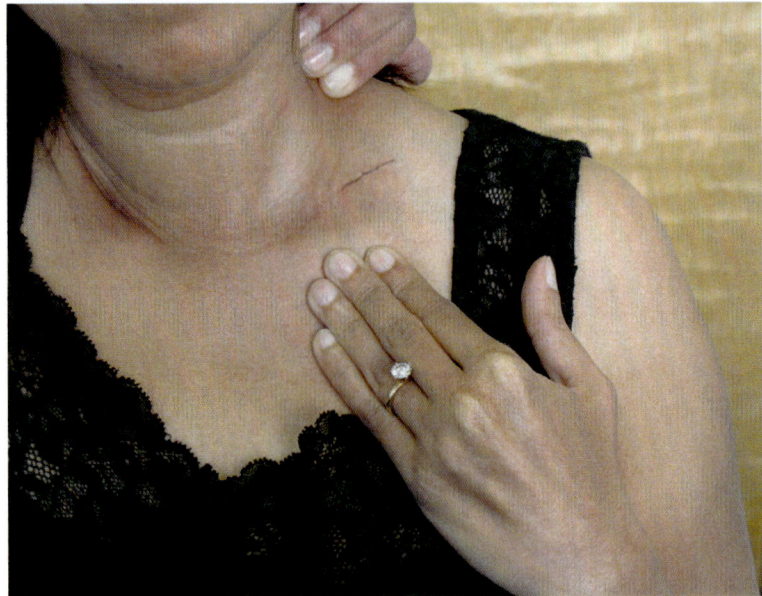

further by assessing whether there is capsular restriction in the glenohumeral joint.

The patient should be trained to perform ROM movements of the joints of the extremity beginning distally and working proximally with the goal of regaining full ROM in all joints while avoiding irritation of the nerves at the surgical site. For example, begin with the wrist and fingers, combining full flexion and extension, followed by forearm supination and pronation. The elbow should be moved in flexion, and extension. If there is tension that limits full ROM, the patient can be trained to activate the shoulder/scapular elevators ("shruggers") to

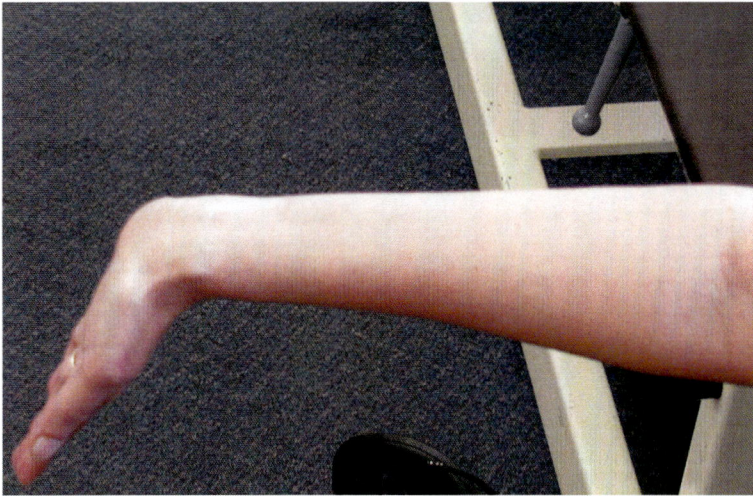

Fig. 34.5 Left ULTT: ending position. Brachial Plexus tension point post-treatment. Assess symptoms at ending position. Immediately post-treatment the arm is again, measured by abduction. The ROM was increased (wrist and finger extension), thereby demonstrating the efficacy of the technique. The patient is instructed to perform the same self-assessment, pre-treatment and post-treatment to prove the efficacy of the maneuver

slacken the brachial plexus. Lastly, have the patient move the shoulder joint and scapula in all directions. This is best performed by lying on one's side (the non-surgical shoulder) for scapular movements and supine for glenohumeral motion.

Ratio of Activity and Rest

It is important to develop a carefully graded exercise routine that builds on success and does not result in over exercise and the resulting symptom flare that can occur. Breathing exercises should be done four times a day for as many minutes as can be handled without an increase or production of pain (which generally will be from 5 to 20 min). A general rule is to increase "up time" and functional activities by no more than 10–20 % from any previous day. Pressure feedback (see Chap. 23) can be used to retrain the abdominal mechanism to stabilize the lumbar spine, lower the rib cage and monitor symptom production, as well as, to retrain the deep neck flexors that stabilize the cervical spine and hence unload the surgical site [5–7].

The scapular muscles (serratus anterior, lower trapezius, and rhomboids) [2, 8] can be retrained if they are weak. Finally, walking should be done initially for short time periods only, followed by gradually increasing time and distance as symptoms allow. While walking, note whether or not the arms can swing without pain. In the early post-operative period it may be helpful to periodically support the arms with hooking the thumb to a belt or support the arms with a fanny pack or a sling.

Conclusion

It is important for the therapist and patient to remember that the need for surgery was because the NTOS, even if responsive to a conservative physical therapy program, was not responsive enough to restore the level of function that is desired. In more chronic patients, there is sensitivity in the nervous system that can take several months to calm down following surgery. It is not desirable to have to deal with flares that are due to this sensitivity and the patient should be guided by the therapist in monitoring activity and rest, so as to minimize these flares [9].

References

1. Shacklock M. Clinical neurodynamics: a new system of musculoskeletal treatment. 1st ed. New York: Elsevier; 2005.
2. Watson L, Pizzari T, Balster S. Thoracic outlet syndrome part 2: conservative management of thoracic outlet syndrome. Man Ther. 2010;15(4):305–14.
3. McLaughlin LGC, Coleman K. Breathing evaluation and retraining as an adjunct to manual therapy. Man Ther. 2011;16:51–2.
4. Butler DS. The sensitive nervous system. Adelaide: Noigroup Publications; 2000.
5. Falla D. Unravelling the complexity of muscle impairment in chronic neck pain. Man Ther. 2004;9:125–33.
6. Falla D, Bilenkij G, Jull G. Patients with chronic neck pain demonstrated altered patterns of muscle activation during performance of a functional upper limb task. Spine. 2004;29(13):1436–40.
7. Jull G, Kristjansson E, Dall'Alba P. Impairment in the cervical flexors: a comparison of whiplash and insidious onset neck pain patients. Man Ther. 2004; 9(2):89–94.
8. Helgadottir H, Kristjansson E, Mottram S, Karduna AR, Jonsson Jr H. Altered scapular orientation during arm elevation in patients with insidious onset neck pain and whiplash – associated disorder. J Orthop Sports Phys Ther. 2010;40(12):784–90.
9. Butler DS, Moseley GL. Explain pain. Adelaide: Noigroup Publications, www.noigroup.com (2003).

Pain Management in Neurogenic Thoracic Outlet Syndrome – Pharmacologic Strategies

35

Marta J. Rozanski, Christopher Gilligan, and James P. Rathmell

Abstract

The diagnosis and management of thoracic outlet syndrome (TOS) is challenging and controversial. The symptoms seen in TOS patients depend on which structures are affected in the thoracic outlet. The most common form of TOS is the neurogenic TOS (NTOS), which frequently can cause neuropathic pain (NP). Treatment strategies for NTOS patients include minimally invasive therapies, muscle relaxants, anti-inflammatories and analgesics, trigger point injections or surgery. Treatment for NP will also include medications that target peripheral and central nerves or different cytokines affecting the sensitivity of sensory neurons to painful stimuli. The pharmacological treatment is challenging and patients often need to be treated with more than just one medication. Antidepressants, alpha-2-delta calcium-channel ligands, and topical lidocaine are considered as first-line treatments for NP in recent evidence-based recommendations. Tricyclic antidepressants (TCA) are established to be efficacious for several different types of NP and the antidepressant effect may be beneficial, because depression is a common concomitant disease in patients with chronic pain. Selective serotonin reuptake inhibitors are better tolerated than TCA's, they are superior to placebo, but show only a weak analgetic effect. Anticonvulsants are a further important group. Carbamazepine, a sodium-channel blocker, has shown efficacy in the treatment of some forms of NP. Gabapentin is approved by the U.S. Food and Drug Administration for the treatment of postherpetic neuralgia (PHN).

M.J. Rozanski, MD • C. Gilligan, BA, MPhil, MD, MBA
J.P. Rathmell, MD (✉)
Department of Anesthesia,
Critical Care and Pain Medicine,
Massachusetts General Hospital
Center for Pain Medicine,
Boston, MA 02114, USA
e-mail: mrozanski@partners.org;
cgilligan@partners.org; jrathmell@partners.org

K.A. Illig et al. (eds.), *Thoracic Outlet Syndrome*,
DOI 10.1007/978-1-4471-4366-6_35, © Springer-Verlag London 2013

The pain relieving effects of pregabalin have been demonstrated in randomized controlled trials. Lidocaine patches are used as supplemental therapy. The benefits of opioids have been proven in RCT's in central and peripheral NP. Pharmacological treatment of NP associated with TOS is challenging. Combination therapy appears useful and pain relief in NP patients is often achieved at the expense of unwanted systemic side effects. Clinical trials looking at pharmacological treatment of NP in patients with NTOS are lacking.

Thoracic Outlet Syndrome

The etiology, diagnosis, and management of thoracic outlet syndrome (TOS) is challenging and controversial. One of the most important complaints of NTOS patients is pain. Pain reduction is therefore the primary goal in NTOS treatment. Treatment strategies include minimally invasive therapies (physiotherapy, ergonomic and postural correction or work limitation), medications such as muscle relaxants, anti-inflammatories and analgesics, trigger point injections or surgery [1]. Typically, the treatment will also include medications targeting neuropathic pain. Entrapment syndromes, such as TOS, frequently cause NP [2]. NP is defined as "pain arising as a direct consequence of a lesion or disease affecting the somatosensory system" [3]. The temporal characteristics of the pain (continuous, paroxysmal) and quality (i.e., heat and cold intolerance, burning, shooting) vary a considerable amount. Due to the nerve injury, an up- or down-regulation of numerous receptors and ion channels in the peripheral nerves and the spinal cord neurons are encountered. These targets are sodium and calcium channels, as well as heat-, cold-, histamine, adrenergic, and GABA-receptors. Patients' complaints of a specific quality of pain may correlate with which receptors are affected. For example, patients suffer from heat or cold hyperalgesia when thermal receptors are upregulated. Similar actions are seen in adrenergic or histamine receptors. Another pathologic mechanism is an injury induced inflammatory reaction, which causes an activation of macrophages releasing cytokines that increases the sensitivity of sensory neurons to painful stimuli.

Understanding these mechanisms may provide a better rationale for choice among various treatment possibilities [4]. Pharmacological treatment is the most important option for NP [5], yet treatment is difficult and there is no single agent that shows good efficacy for all patients. Treatment must be individualized, considering comorbidities and their treatment, individual risk of drug use, possible drug overdose or abuse, and cost [6].

There are several guidelines and reviews on pharmacological treatment of NP developed among others from the International Association for the Study of Pain, Neuropathic Pain Special Interest Group [7], the Canadian Pain Society [8], and the European Federation of Neurological Societies Task Force [9]. These recommendations are based on randomized controlled trials (RCT's) of neuropathic pain conditions. Most large RCT's included patients with diabetic peripheral neuropathic pain (DPNP) and postherpetic neuralgia (PHN), and only a few smaller studies explored other conditions. There is scant direct scientific evidence regarding the treatment of NP associated with NTOS, and the recommendations in this chapter stem from extrapolating treatment results from the more well-studied NP conditions.

These recent evidence-based recommendations consider antidepressants (tricyclic antidepressants, norepinephrine and serotonin reuptake inhibitors), alpha-2-delta calcium-channel ligands (gabapentin and pregabalin), and topical lidocaine (lidocaine patch 5 %) as first-line treatments for NP [10, 11]. In the next section, we give a short overview of these recommendations.

Antidepressants

Tricyclic antidepressants (TCA) are established to be efficacious for several different types of NP [12]. They inhibit the presynaptic neuronal reuptake of amines, such as norepinephrine and serotonin, and block postsynaptic alpha-adrenergic, H1-histaminergic and muscarinic cholinergic receptors, leading to an increased bioactive availability of these neurotransmitters and resulting in their increased inhibitory effects on the nociceptive pathway. The tertiary amines (i.e. imipramine) have a broader spectrum of activity than the secondary amines (i.e. desipramine and nortryptiline). Different TCA agents have in addition different effects on monoamine reuptake. The number needed to treat (NNT) (i.e., the number of patients that need to be treated to reduce 50 % of the pain intensity in one patient in a clinical trial) for TCA in NP ranges from 2 to 4 [13]. The antidepressive effect does not impair the analgesic properties and may be beneficial, because depression is a common concomitant disorder in patients with chronic pain.

Because TCA's interact with multiple transmitter systems, they also have diverse side effects. Amitriptyline and other tertiary amines show more side effects than nortriptyline and other secondary amines. Therefore secondary amines are the favored TCA when side effects are a predominant concern. Frequent adverse events are mostly due to the anticholinergic properties and are described in Table 35.1. Fewer side effects are seen when patients are started on a low dose and titrated to higher doses [14, 15].

Selective serotonin reuptake inhibitors (i.e. fluoxetine) seem to be better tolerated than TCA's but there are only small studies of this agent in patients with NP, mostly in DPNP, low back pain and fibromyalgia. In relieving NP they are superior to placebo but show only a weak analgesic effect [16].

The efficacy of selective serotonin/norepinephrine reuptake inhibitors such as venlafaxine for treating neuropathic pain is controversial. Potential for analgesia is suggested by its mechanism of action. NNT of 3.1 for pain relief in NP is described in a single trial [17], but other RCT's including various peripheral, central, and post-mastectomy NP states show inconsistent or even negative outcomes [18, 19]. A lower dosage may be associated with less pain relief due to a reuptake inhibition of only serotonin, whereas higher dosage inhibits both serotonin and norepinephrine reuptake providing better pain relief [20].

Duloxetine is a potent inhibitor of both serotonin and norepinephrine reuptake. It shows a balanced affinity for serotonin and norepinephrine transporters which is in contrast to venlafaxine [15]. Duloxetine is approved by the Food and Drug Administration for some chronic pain-related diseases including fibromyalgia and DPNP. It has been studied in three RCT's with DPNP patients [21–23]. The NNT was 5.1 [24], and significantly lower pain scores were seen in comparison with patients receiving placebo. Response was noted within days of starting therapy and this has been attributed to this agent's activation of both receptors [25, 26].

Anticonvulsants

The unfavorable adverse effect profile of TCA's has elevated gabapentin to be used commonly as a first-choice treatment for NP [27]. Anticonvulsant drugs are used for NP because neuronal hyperexcitability and corresponding molecular changes in NP show similarities to the changes in certain forms of seizure disorder. Clinical trials have shown the efficacy of carbamazepine, a **sodium-channel blocker**, in the treatment of trigeminal neuralgia, DPNP and postherpetic neuralgia [28]. It has a NNT of 1.7 [29]. But this older agent is associated with frequent drug-related toxicity, including bone marrow suppression and hepatic toxicity. Gabapentin, a gamma-aminobutyric acid (GABA) analogue, was developed as an antiepilepsy drug. Despite its structural similarity to GABA, it does not have a relevant GABA-related binding site [30]. Rather, it binds to the **alpha-2-delta** subunit of voltage-gated **calcium-channels** leading to a blockade of the channels and inhibiting the release of norepinephrine, substance P, and glutamate [23, 30, 31]. This effects the transmission of nociceptive neuronal traffic

Table 35.1 Pharmacolocigal treatment of neuropathic pain, overview

Drugs by class	Name	Pharmacology	Dosage and doseinterval (maximum)	NNT	Adverse effect
Antidepressants					
Tricyclic antidepressants					
Secondary amine	Nortriptyline	Norepinephrine and serotonin reuptake inhibitor, negligible effects on dopamine reuptake, sodium channel block, NMDA receptor blockade, antagonistic effects at H1, 5-HT1, 5-HT2, alpha1-adrenergic, mACh receptors	10–25 mg p.o./day (200 mg/day)	2–4	Sedation, dry mouth, urinary retention, weight gain, balance problems, hypotension, cardiac events
	Desipramine	Norepinephrine and to a lesser extent serotonin reuptake inhibitor	10–25 mg p.o./day (1,300 mg/day)		Confusion, dry mouth, urinary retention, nightmares, numbness, other unusual sensations, tremors, cardiac events
Selective serotonin/norepinephrine uptake inhibitor	Duloxetine	Norepinephrine and serotonin reuptake inhibitor	30 mg p.o./day (120 mg/day)	5.1	Nausea, dry mouth, constipation, dizziness, weakness
	Venlafaxine	Norepinephrine and serotonin reuptake inhibitor	37.5 mg b.i.d. (225 mg/day)	3.1	Nausea
Anticonvulsants					
Alpha-2-delta calcium-channel ligands	Gabapentin	Calciumchannel alpha-ligand	300 mg p.o./day (3,600 mg/day)	5.1	Dizzines, somnolence, edema, cognitive impairments
	Pregabalin	Calciumchannel alpha-ligand	75 mg b.i.d. (600 mg/day)	4.2	Dizzines, somnolence, headache
Sodium channel blockers	Carbamazepine	Norepinephrine reuptake inhibitor, sodium channel block	100–300 mg p.o./day (1,500 mg/day)	1.7	Gastric irritations, sedation, nausea, hematologic abnormalities
	Oxcarbamazepine	Sodium channel block	75 mg (600–1,200 mg/day)	n.k.	Dizziness, somnolence, nausea, abnormal vision, hyponatremia

		Sodium channel block	1–3 patches (3 patches/day)	4.4	Skin reactions
Topical agents	5 % Lidocain patch				
Opioids				2.5–3.9	
	Tramadol	U-receptor agonism, norepinephrine and serotonin reuptake inhibitor	50 mg b.i.d. (400 mg/day)		Nausea, vomiting, constipation, dizziness
	Morphine, oxycodone, methadone, fentanyl	U-receptor agonism, oxycodone also k-receptor antagonist	10–15 mg morphine every 4 h		Nausea, vomiting, constipation, dizziness, pruritus, respiratory depression

p.o./day once per day, *NNT* Number needed to treat, *b.i.d.* twice daily, *n.k.* not known following tissue damage from peripheral receptors to the central nervous system where the neuronal impulses are converted to the sensation of pain. Large clinical trials since the mid-90s demonstrate the efficacy of gabapentin in reducing NP of various types [14]. Gabapentin has U.S. Food and Drug Administration approval for the treatment of postherpetic neuralgia (PHN). It is also effective in DPNP and mixed NP states. The NNT in NP of all conditions is in high and low dose 5.1 [14]. Gabapentin requires slow upward titration to minimize side effects, although it is generally safe. Importantly, it does not have relevant drug-drug interactions.

Pregabalin, also binds to calcium channels on central terminals of primary afferent nociceptors and has a NNT in patients with PHN and DPNP of 4.2 for daily doses ranging from 150 to 600 mg [14]. Its efficacy in pain relief has been demonstrated in RCT's in PHN [32, 33], in DPNP [34], and in relieving central NP [35]. The dose-dependent side effects are similar to those of gabapentin. As with gabapentin, the dose needs to be reduced in patients with renal impairment and in elderly patients. There are no comparative efficacy trials available to guide the choice of one agent over another.

Topical Agents

Pain relief in NP patients is often achieved at the expense of unwanted systemic side effects. Three types of topical preparations provide pain relief: Capsaicin, NSAID preparations and local anesthetics. The most often used are lidocaine-based topical medications. Lidocaine patches, creams and gels are peripherally acting topical analgesics without substantial systemic side effects. They should be applied to intact skin only. They nonspecifically block sodium channels on small damaged afferent fibers but do not interfere with normal conduction of impulses in large sensory fibers. They provide pain relief by producing local analgesia [36]. The 5 % lidocaine patch is approved for PHN, but is also used for peripheral neuropathy and myofascial pain. In patients with PHN and allodynia lidocaine patches have been shown to alleviate pain better than vehicle-controlled (placebo) patches [37]. The NNT as a supplemental therapy in patients with regional pain in various localizations of peripheral NP is 4.4 [14]. Lidocaine patches should be used carefully in patients treated with antiarrhythmic medication or with hepatic dysfunction.

Opioids

Opioids work as agonists at the pre- and postsynaptic opioids receptors. The benefits of opioids have been proven in RCT's in central and peripheral NP [7, 9]. Oral morphine has been shown to have a NNT in patients with PHN, DPNP and phantom limb pain of 2.5. NNT for oxycodone in DPNP and PHN patients is 2.6 and tramadol, a weak opioid that also inhibits serotonin and norepinephrine reuptake, was shown to have a NNT of 3.9 in PHN patients [14]. Similar reduction of pain was achieved with opioids when compared with antidepressants, but patients had greater satisfaction with opioids [38]. However, there have been more frequent side effects after treatment with opioids than with TCA's and anticonvulsants. Although opioids have been shown to relieve pain in patients with NP, they have not been shown to improve function [39]. Moreover, opioids are problematic in chronic pain conditions such as NP because patients develop tolerance and physical dependence to them, although they rarely develop overt addiction.

Combination Therapy for NP

The complexity of NP reflected in the variety of receptors involved offers different points of action for analgesic agents, thus combination therapy may be useful in those that fail to adequately respond to a single agent. The rank order of the processes leading to NP have not yet been determined, and patients often need to be treated with more than just one medication, although there have been few trials evaluating combination therapies. Combination therapy appears useful for gabapentin and morphine resulting in decreased pain intensity and improvement in physical activity and health-related quality of life in patients with PHN, DPNP and NP after spinal cord injury [2, 40, 41]. Combined gabapentin and nortriptyline demonstrates greater efficacy than either drug given alone for NP [42].

It is still unclear why some TOS patients develop NP. Risk factors such as age, gender, pain before and after the lesion, and emotional and cognitive status are just a few of the known risk factors. Pharmacological treatment of NP after TOS is, as in other chronic diseases, challenging. Clinical trials looking at pharmacological treatment of NP in patients with NTOS are needed, but the relative rarity of the condition makes recruiting adequate numbers of patients for such trials challenging.

References

1. Christo PJ, McGreevy K. Updated perspectives on neurogenic thoracic outlet syndrome. Curr Pain Headache Rep. 2010;15:14–21.
2. Raja SN, Haythornthwaite JA. Combination therapy for neuropathic pain–which drugs, which combination, which patients? N Engl J Med. 2005;352:1373–5.
3. Treede RD, Jensen TS, Campbell JN, et al. Neuropathic pain: redefinition and a grading system for clinical and research purposes. Neurology. 2008;70:1630–5.
4. Baron R. Mechanisms of disease: neuropathic pain – a clinical perspective. Nat Clin Pract Neurol. 2006;2:95–106.
5. Finnerup NB, Sindrup SH, Jensen TS. The evidence for pharmacological treatment of neuropathic pain. Pain. 2010;150:573–81.
6. Haanpaa ML, Gourlay GK, Kent JL, et al. Treatment considerations for patients with neuropathic pain and other medical comorbidities. Mayo Clin Proc. 2010;85:S15–25.
7. O'Connor AB, Dworkin RH. Treatment of neuropathic pain: an overview of recent guidelines. Am J Med. 2009;122:S22–32.
8. Moulin DE, Clark AJ, Gilron I, et al. Pharmacological management of chronic neuropathic pain – consensus statement and guidelines from the Canadian pain society. Pain Res Manag. 2007;12:13–21.
9. Attal N, Cruccu G, Baron R, et al. EFNS guidelines on the pharmacological treatment of neuropathic pain: 2010 revision. Eur J Neurol. 2010;17:1113–e88.
10. Dickinson BD, Head CA, Gitlow S, et al. Maldynia: pathophysiology and management of neuropathic and maladaptive pain – a report of the AMA council on science and public health. Pain Med. 2010;11:1635–53.
11. Dworkin RH, O'Connor AB, Audette J, et al. Recommendations for the pharmacological management of neuropathic pain: an overview and literature update. Mayo Clin Proc. 2010;85:S3–14.
12. Bryson HM, Wilde MI. Amitriptyline. A review of its pharmacological properties and therapeutic use in chronic pain states. Drugs Aging. 1996;8:459–76.
13. Dharmshaktu P, Tayal V, Kalra BS. Efficacy of antidepressants as analgesics: a review. J Clin Pharmacol. 2011;52(1):6–17.
14. Finnerup NB, Otto M, McQuay HJ, et al. Algorithm for neuropathic pain treatment: an evidence based proposal. Pain. 2005;118:289–305.
15. Dworkin RH, O'Connor AB, Backonja M, et al. Pharmacologic management of neuropathic pain: evidence-based recommendations. Pain. 2007;132:237–51.
16. Max MB, Lynch SA, Muir J, et al. Effects of desipramine, amitriptyline, and fluoxetine on pain in diabetic neuropathy. N Engl J Med. 1992;326:1250–6.
17. Saarto T, Wiffen PJ. Antidepressants for neuropathic pain: a Cochrane review. J Neurol Neurosurg Psychiatry. 2010;81:1372–3.
18. Tasmuth T, Hartel B, Kalso E. Venlafaxine in neuropathic pain following treatment of breast cancer. Eur J Pain. 2002;6:17–24.
19. Yucel A, Ozyalcin S, Koknel Talu G, et al. The effect of venlafaxine on ongoing and experimentally induced pain in neuropathic pain patients: a double blind, placebo controlled study. Eur J Pain. 2005;9:407–16.
20. Rowbotham MC, Goli V, Kunz NR, et al. Venlafaxine extended release in the treatment of painful diabetic neuropathy: a double-blind, placebo-controlled study. Pain. 2004;110:697–706.
21. Raskin J, Pritchett YL, Wang F, et al. A double-blind, randomized multicenter trial comparing duloxetine with placebo in the management of diabetic peripheral neuropathic pain. Pain Med. 2005;6:346–56.
22. Wernicke JF, Pritchett YL, D'Souza DN, et al. A randomized controlled trial of duloxetine in diabetic peripheral neuropathic pain. Neurology. 2006;67:1411–20.
23. Goldstein DJ, Lu Y, Detke MJ, et al. Duloxetine vs. Placebo in patients with painful diabetic neuropathy. Pain. 2005;116:109–18.
24. Bellingham GA, Peng PW. Duloxetine: a review of its pharmacology and use in chronic pain management. Reg Anesth Pain Med. 2010;35:294–303.
25. Pritchett YL, McCarberg BH, Watkin JG, et al. Duloxetine for the management of diabetic peripheral neuropathic pain: response profile. Pain Med. 2007;8:397–409.
26. Bymaster FP, Lee TC, Knadler MP, et al. The dual transporter inhibitor duloxetine: a review of its preclinical pharmacology, pharmacokinetic profile, and clinical results in depression. Curr Pharm Des. 2005;11:1475–93.

27. Tremont-Lukats IW, Megeff C, Backonja MM. Anticonvulsants for neuropathic pain syndromes: mechanisms of action and place in therapy. Drugs. 2000;60:1029–52.

28. Jensen TS. Anticonvulsants in neuropathic pain: rationale and clinical evidence. Eur J Pain. 2002;6(Suppl A):61–8.

29. Wiffen PJ, Derry S, Moore RA, et al. Carbamazepine for acute and chronic pain in adults. Cochrane Database Syst Rev. 2011;1:CD005451.

30. Taylor CP. Mechanisms of analgesia by gabapentin and pregabalin–calcium channel alpha-2-delta [Cavalpha2-delta] ligands. Pain. 2009;142:13–6.

31. Taylor CP. The biology and pharmacology of calcium channel alpha2-delta proteins Pfizer satellite symposium to the 2003 society for neuroscience meeting. Sheraton New Orleans hotel, New Orleans, LA November 10, 2003. CNS Drug Rev. 2004;10:183–8.

32. Dworkin RH, Corbin AE, Young Jr JP, et al. Pregabalin for the treatment of postherpetic neuralgia: a randomized, placebo-controlled trial. Neurology. 2003;60: 1274–83.

33. Sabatowski R, Galvez R, Cherry DA, et al. Pregabalin reduces pain and improves sleep and mood disturbances in patients with post-herpetic neuralgia: results of a randomised, placebo-controlled clinical trial. Pain. 2004;109:26–35.

34. Tolle T, Freynhagen R, Versavel M, et al. Pregabalin for relief of neuropathic pain associated with diabetic neuropathy: a randomized, double-blind study. Eur J Pain. 2008;12:203–13.

35. Siddall PJ, Cousins MJ, Otte A, et al. Pregabalin in central neuropathic pain associated with spinal cord injury: a placebo-controlled trial. Neurology. 2006;67: 1792–800.

36. Katz NP, Gammaitoni AR, Davis MW, et al. Lidocaine patch 5 % reduces pain intensity and interference with quality of life in patients with postherpetic neuralgia: an effectiveness trial. Pain Med. 2002; 3:324–32.

37. Galer BS, Rowbotham MC, Perander J, et al. Topical lidocaine patch relieves postherpetic neuralgia more effectively than a vehicle topical patch: results of an enriched enrollment study. Pain. 1999;80:533–8.

38. Raja SN, Haythornthwaite JA, Pappagallo M, et al. Opioids versus antidepressants in postherpetic neuralgia: a randomized, placebo-controlled trial. Neurology. 2002;59:1015–21.

39. Ballantyne JC, Mao J. Opioid therapy for chronic pain. N Engl J Med. 2003;349:1943–53.

40. Gilron I, Bailey JM, Tu D, et al. Morphine, gabapentin, or their combination for neuropathic pain. N Engl J Med. 2005;352:1324–34.

41. Barrera-Chacon JM, Mendez-Suarez JL, Jauregui-Abrisqueta ML, et al. Oxycodone improves pain control and quality of life in anticonvulsant-pretreated spinal cord-injured patients with neuropathic pain. Spinal Cord. 2011;49:36–42.

42. Gilron I, Bailey JM, Tu D, et al. Nortriptyline and gabapentin, alone and in combination for neuropathic pain: a double-blind, randomised controlled crossover trial. Lancet. 2009;374:1252–61.

Pain Management in NTOS – Advanced Techniques

36

Joshua Prager

Abstract

When thoracic outlet syndrome (TOS) causes chronic neuropathic pain, or in rare cases causes complex regional pain syndrome (CRPS), a wide variety of advanced therapies can be used to treat the chronic, debilitating pain of neurogenic thoracic outlet syndrome (NTOS). Chronic pain treatment algorithms typically begin with less invasive, reversible therapies and those that have few side effects. Thus, physical therapy and non-narcotic medications are used first, often in conjunction with behavioral therapy. These may be followed by more potent analgesics, nerve blocks, neurostimulation, or medication infusions into the spinal fluid by implantable pumps, and finally by neuroablation. Unlike neuroablation, neurostimulation (spinal cord stimulation, peripheral nerve stimulation, deep brain stimulation, and motor cortex stimulation), intrathecal drug delivery, and ketamine infusions spare nerve tissue and can be reversed or discontinued if necessary. Consistent definitions of pain types by the International Association for the Study of Pain (IASP) have allowed indications for these therapies to be refined. Continuing elucidation of the anatomy, physiology, and psychology of pain, as well as recommendations for best practices, have been the focus of study by The North American Neuromodulation Society and the International Neuromodulation Society. A host of technical advances in equipment also support pain practitioners in managing the pain of NTOS more effectively.

Introduction

When a delay in diagnosis or treatment of thoracic outlet syndrome (TOS) causes chronic neuropathic pain or, in rare cases, complex regional pain syndrome (CRPS), interventional pain specialists can choose from a variety of advanced therapies. Chronic pain treatment algorithms

J. Prager, MD, MS
Departments of Anesthesiology and Internal Medicine,
UCLA, 100 UCLA Medical Plaza, Suite 760,
Los Angeles, CA 90095, USA
e-mail: joshuaprager@gmail.com

K.A. Illig et al. (eds.), *Thoracic Outlet Syndrome*,
DOI 10.1007/978-1-4471-4366-6_36, © Springer-Verlag London 2013

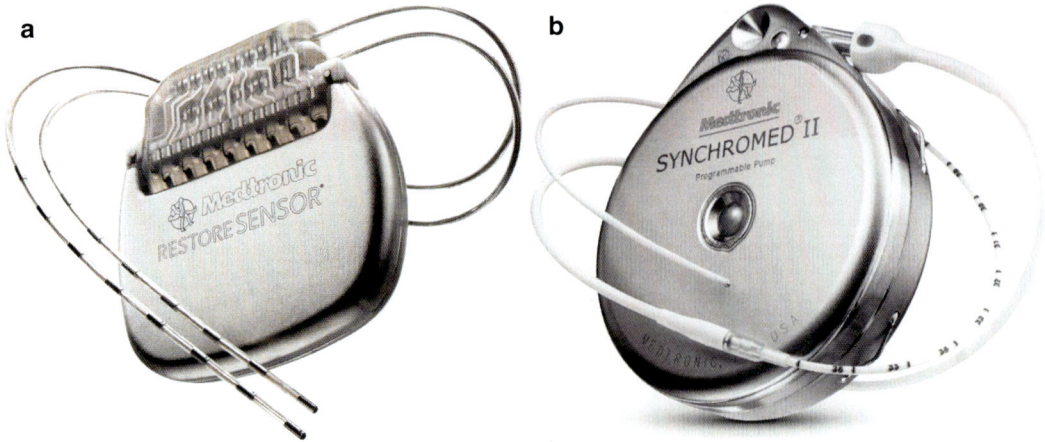

Fig. 36.1 Spinal cord stimulator and intrathecal drug delivery devices used in neuromodulation. (**a**) Spinal cord stimulator, RestoreSensor® Neurostimulator. Implantable pulse generators come in battery-operated or rechargeable models. Battery life is 2–5 years, depending on the stimulation level (Reprinted with the permission of Medtronic, Inc. © 2012). (**b**) Intrathecal Drug Delivery Device, Synchromed® II. Since 1981, more than 100,000 patients have been treated with intrathecal drug delivery (Reprinted with the permission of Medtronic, Inc. © 2012)

emphasize a step-wise approach to treatment, beginning with less invasive, reversible therapies and those that have few side effects. In this schema physical therapy and non-narcotic medications are used first, often in conjunction with behavioral therapy. These may be followed by more potent analgesics, nerve blocks, neurostimulation or medication infusions into the spinal fluid by implantable pumps, and finally by neuroablation, which is fraught with complications, irreversible, and not uniformly effective [1]. Unlike neuroablation, the therapies discussed here spare nerve tissue and can be reversed or discontinued if necessary. Consistent definitions of pain types by the International Association for the Study of Pain (IASP) have allowed indications for these therapies to be refined. The North American Neuromodulation Society and the International Neuromodulation Society serve as forums for continuing elucidation of the anatomy, physiology, and psychology of pain, as well as recommendations for best practices as successive technical improvements have been made. Collectively, neurostimulation and intrathecal drug delivery (IDD) are termed neuromodulation.

Neurostimulation

There are four forms of neurostimulation utilized for treating neuropathic pain: spinal cord stimulation (SCS, previously termed dorsal column stimulation; the more modern term reflects the fact that more than the dorsal columns in the spinal cord are stimulated), peripheral nerve stimulation (PNS), deep brain stimulation (DBS), and motor cortex stimulation (MCS).

Spinal Cord Stimulation

For more than 40 years, SCS has been used to treat chronic neuropathic pain with the technical goal of producing stimulation paresthesia at a subjectively tolerable (comfortable) level, concordant with a patient's topography of pain (Fig. 36.1) [2]. Clinical experience demonstrates that SCS more effectively curbs neuropathic or sympathetically mediated pain than nociceptive pain, and suppresses chronic pain but not acute pain. The most common indication for SCS in North America is to treat chronic neuropathic pain, [2, 3] whereas Europeans use SCS most often to treat cardiac ischemic pain [4]

Table 36.1 Patient selection criteria for spinal cord stimulation

Inclusion criteria

Established diagnosis of specific pain syndrome (peripheral neuropathic pain, peripheral vascular disease, complex regional pain syndrome)

Appendicular pain following at least one previous spine surgery

Informed consent

Clearance after psychological evaluation

Exclusion criteria

Surgical procedure within 6 months of screening trial

Evidence of active, disruptive psychiatric disorder; active drug abuse; personality disorders that might affect pain perception, compliance with intervention, or ability to evaluate therapy

Patients <18 years old

Patients who have not received an adequate course of nonsurgical care

Patients who have failed a previous SCS trial

Relative contraindications

An unresolved major psychiatric comorbidity

The unresolved possibility of secondary gain

An inappropriate dependency on pharmaceuticals (especially controlled substances)

Inconsistency among the patient's history, pain description, physical examination, and diagnostic studies

Abnormal or inconsistent pain ratings

Predominance of nonorganic signs (e.g., Waddell's signs)

Alternative therapies with a risk/benefit ratio comparable to that of SCS remain to be tried

Pregnancy

Occupational risk (e.g., employment requires climbing ladders or operating certain machinery)

Local or systemic infection

Presence of a demand pacemaker or cardiac defibrillator

Foreseeable need for an MRI

Presence of a major comorbid chronic pain syndrome

Anticoagulant or antiplatelet therapy

Absolute contraindications

Inability to control the device

Coagulopathy, immunosuppression, or other condition associated with an unacceptable surgical risk

Need for therapeutic diathermy (a contraindication for implantable devices)

Reprinted from Prager et al. [6]. With permission from Lippincott Williams & Wilkins

and peripheral vascular disease [5]. The potential benefits of SCS include pain relief, increased activity levels or function, reduced use of pain medication, improvement in quality of life, patient satisfaction, improved neurologic function, return to work for previously employed people, and reduced consumption of healthcare [2, 6].

Spinal cord stimulation is a minimally invasive procedure that should follow appropriate noninvasive therapies. By the same reasoning, SCS should precede ablative therapies (e.g., sympathectomies, dorsal root entry zone lesions, or dorsal root gangli-onectomy) or surgery. One advantage of SCS is that

patients can undergo a screening trial to evaluate pain relief before committing to therapy. Table 36.1 lists patient selection criteria as well as relative and absolute contraindications for SCS. Candidates may proceed to implantation if their pain is reduced by at least 50 %, the paresthesia is tolerable and covers the painful area, and analgesic intake remains stable or can be decreased [7]. Approximately one-third of candidates do not proceed with implantation after an SCS trial. Earlier practice utilized 50 % pain relief as the principal criterion to determine a successful trial. More current thinking reflects concern for patient quality of life, such as ability to walk, sleep, climb stairs, drive, participate in sexual relations and reduce analgesic consumption.

The potential risks of SCS relate to implantation complications (hematoma, hemorrhage, seroma, cerebrospinal fluid [CSF] leakage, infection and erosion), device-related complications (hardware malfunction or migration, pain at the implant site, allergic response, reoperation), or stimulation-induced complications (discomfort, loss of pain relief, chest wall stimulation).

The Neuromodulation Therapy Access Coalition conducted a comprehensive, evidence-based literature review of SCS in 2007, the most extensive examination to date of the likelihood of success with SCS for specific indications [2]. They found excellent evidence (A) for the efficacy of SCS in treating CRPS I and II, and good evidence (B) in treating peripheral neuropathic pain, root injury pain, and spinal cord injury/lesion.

Peripheral Nerve Stimulation

Peripheral nerve stimulation (PNS), using an implanted pulse generator or receiver with electrodes placed around a peripheral nerve and an external transmitter, delivers electrical impulses to induce paresthesias in a painful area. The technique has successfully relieved neuropathic pain for more than 40 years [8, 9]. Peripheral nerve field stimulation (PNFS) employs a subcutaneous lead to create a small electrical field that decreases nociceptive input. Despite reported success with PNS, [10, 11] randomized controlled trials and meta-analysis have not been conducted.

A recent report of five cases of PNS with 20-year follow-up suggests that the technique merits consideration [12]. Eleven patients with neuropathic pain who were treated with PNS in the 1980s had significantly reduced pain at 52-month follow-up. A comprehensive evaluation was conducted on five of these patients after 20 years of treatment. The PNS had no effect on tactile sensation, cool, warmth, cold pain and heat pain thresholds. Positron emission tomography (PET) revealed increased blood flow in the primary somatosensory cortex, the anterior cingulate and insular cortices of treated patients. All of the patients had experienced long-term pain relief with PNS. A prospective clinical study conducted more recently also supplied encouraging results [13]. Eight patients with carpal tunnel syndrome underwent lead implantation and 6 h of daily transdermal stimulation along the median nerve for 5 days. Pain was measured before, during and after treatment. Two patients experienced ≥30 % pain reduction for the entire time. Pain returned to baseline after explant, increasing by 37–46 %. Mean patient satisfaction was 96 %, and all of the patients indicated a preference for permanent implantation.

Deep Brain Stimulation

First used to treat refractory chronic pain in 1954, DBS using an internal power source and lead(s) has more recently been adopted to treat the dyskinesia and pain of advanced Parkinson disease [14, 15]. The pain relief experienced from sensory thalamic stimulation (STN) in one series of Parkinson patients at 24 months follow-up was similar to that from medication at baseline [16]. High-frequency stimulation mimics the functional effects of ablation in some brain structures, [17] which may explain why STN mitigates neuropathic pain. A meta-analysis of 13 studies and 1,114 patients with neuropathic or nociceptive pain found that 561 (50 %) had successful long-term relief from DBS [18, 19]. Of the 711 patients with neuropathic pain, 296 (42 %) had success at long-term follow-up, and success was more likely for patients who had cervical or brachial avulsion or peripheral neuropathy.

Intercranial hemorrhage is the most serious complication of DBS, with an incidence ranging from 1.9 to 4.1 % [18]. Mortality is rare (0–1.6 %) with three of four reported deaths resulting from intracranial hemorrhage. In addition, technical advances have reduced morbidity and mortality since the 1980s when the earliest studies in the meta-analysis were conducted. After more conservative therapies have failed, including less invasive neurostimulation, DBS offers hope for alleviating intractable neuropathic pain.

Motor Cortex Stimulation

As early as 1954, intracranial neurostimulation (including both DBS and MCS) was investigated for treating chronic neuropathic pain refractory to medical therapy. Beginning in the early 1990s, a series of case studies reported on the use of MCS to treat chronic pain, primarily for conditions such as trigeminal and post-stroke pain for which other treatments are lacking. Satisfactory results were reported in 40 to 75 % of cases [20]. A critical review of 14 unblinded, uncontrolled case studies and 210 patients conducted in 2009 found that approximately 55 % achieved ≥40 to 50 % pain relief postoperatively from MCS [20]. Forty-five percent of the 152 patients followed up a year later had maintained this level of pain relief. Response was good in 54 % of the 117 patients treated for central pain and in 68 % of the 44 patients treated for trigeminal pain. Ten of the 14 studies reported on adverse events associated with MCS [20]. The most common adverse event was infection (5.7 %, n = 157), followed by hardware-related problems (5.1 %). Seizures occurred in 12 % of patients (n = 19) during the early postoperative period, but chronic seizures did not ensue.

Although MCS appears to be relatively safe and effective in the treatment of chronic neuropathic pain, studies to date have been small, retrospective, and lack a control arm. Differences in surgical technique, electrode placement, and stimulation settings likely contributed to the varying results. Predictive factors for a good outcome are still being determined. Despite these shortcomings, some patients with severe and medically resistant pain have benefitted substantially, saying they would repeat the surgery even though they only reported a 10 to 39 % reduction in pain [21].

Intrathecal Drug Delivery

Since its introduction in 1981, more than 285,000 pumps have been implanted in patients with intractable pain (Fig. 36.1) [22]. The approved indications for intrathecal drug delivery (IDD) are "the chronic intrathecal infusion of preservative-free morphine sulfate sterile solution in the treatment of chronic intractable pain, or preservative-free ziconotide for the management of severe chronic pain" – in other words, no specific diseases or syndromes are indicated or contraindicated. Intrathecal infusion, by delivering drugs directly to opioid receptors, limits systemic exposure and decreases the opioid doses required for pain relief, generally reducing side effects [23]. Consensus statements regarding the intrathecal delivery of other medications have appeared periodically, [24, 25] with revisions to guidelines currently pending.

Analgesic response to IDD has been documented in patients with neuropathic, visceral, deafferentation, and mixed pain [26]. The safety and efficacy of IDD have been well documented in the peer-reviewed literature, [26, 27] although early mortality due to respiratory depression has occurred [28]. The safety issues stem primarily from inadequate monitoring, dosing errors, problems with pump fills or refills, and interaction between concomitant medications, especially opioids and benzodiazepines. Consequently, pumps should be implanted and managed by providers trained and skilled specifically in IDD.

Patients should have an accurate diagnosis of a specific pain state that would likely respond to IDD before undergoing physical, psychological and environmental evaluations and a screening trial. If comorbidities such as diabetes, coagulopathy, immunosuppressive disorders and sleep apnea exist, the conditions should be well-controlled before considering IDD. Doses must be titrated cautiously while monitoring for both efficacy and side effects. A recent and comprehensive review of IDD found that it was efficacious, fiscally neutral and appropriate when used judiciously in expert hands [29]. One caveat – pain practitioners may want to consider treating neuropathic pain with SCS before contemplating IDD.

Ketamine Infusions

Ketamine, an N-methyl-D-aspartate receptor antagonist, has been used for half a century for pain relief in the operating room (2 mg/kg for induction of anesthesia), and in the intensive care unit for patients with brain or spinal cord injuries [30]. Ketamine has also been used to treat refractory CRPS in both inpatient [31] and outpatient settings [32]. Unlike opioids, ketamine does not prolong sedation, depress respiration, or lower blood pressure. Some patients treated with ketamine experience hallucinations, but these can be effectively counteracted with midazolam (1–2 mg), clonidine or dexmedetomidine.

Complete recovery from rapidly progressing CRPS was reported in one case after treatment with anesthetic doses of ketamine (3–5 mg/kg/h) and midazolam administered for 5 days in the intensive care unit [33]. The patient maintained remission for 8 years. High-dose medically induced ketamine coma was initiated in 20 patients with refractory CRPS [34]. Significant pain relief ($P < 0.001$) was obtained at 1, 3 and 6 months following treatment, with complete remission in all patients (100 %) at 1 month, 17 patients (85 %) at 3 months, and 16 patients (80 %) at 6 months.

Still practiced in Germany and Mexico, high-dose ketamine therapy has been replaced in the U.S. by subanesthetic doses administered on an inpatient or outpatient basis. Protocols vary but typically begin with ten daily treatments of accelerating 50–500 mg doses per day over a 2-week period [35]. This may be followed by several months of periodic outpatient therapy. Results of a small pilot study of outpatient therapy were disappointing [35]; there was no change in pain measured by visual analogue scale (VAS). However, a double-blind placebo-controlled study of outpatient ketamine infusion is currently under way [36]. One of the participating investigators reports that between 66 and 80 % of patients have shown overall improvement measured by increased functional capacity, decreased pain medication, or both [37].

Ketamine clearly shows promise in relieving refractory pain, but treatment protocols are still evolving. Several cautions apply as well. Patients receiving ketamine infusions should be fully monitored (with blood pressure, pulse oximetry, ECG, and CO_2 end tidal measurement) by a physician experienced in anesthesiology and airway management. Although side effects are relatively rare and generally manageable, liver toxicity has been reported after high-dose infusions. Three patients developed hepatotoxicity when receiving the second of two intravenous 100-h ketamine infusions (10–20 mg/h) separated by 16 days [38]. Therapy was discontinued and liver enzymes returned to normal within 2 months. There is also some question about the durability of pain relief following subanesthetic infusions.

Complex Regional Pain Syndrome

Chronic nerve irritation or ischemia can produce CRPS. When evaluating a patient with arm pain and temperature change, CRPS may be in the differential diagnosis as well as NTOS. After a negative NTOS work-up, CRPS should be considered as a possible explanation of the patient's clinical signs [39]. Patients with CRPS may exhibit hyperhydrosis, tremor, dystonia or trophic changes, unlike NTOS patients. Treatment for CRPS follows a treatment algorithm set forth by the IASP and updated periodically (Fig. 36.2) [40]. This approach emphasizes functional rehabilitation utilizing various forms of progressive physical therapy, with adjuvant interventional pain management techniques, including neuromodulation when necessary, as well as behavioral treatment. The treatment algorithm can be used as a model of treatment for TOS patients who have suffered from severe debilitating pain to the point of losing function.

Summary

A steadily improving understanding of chronic neuropathic pain, accompanied by a host of technical advances, is supporting pain practitioners in deploying more effective pain management strategies.

Fig. 36.2 Treatment algorithm for complex regional pain syndrome. This multidisciplinary care continuum adapts the treatment plan to the patient's response. The plan emphasizes functional rehabilitation utilizing various forms of progressive physical therapy, with adjuvant interventional pain management techniques, including neuromodulation when necessary, as well as behavioral treatment. The algorithm is periodically updated by the International Association for the Study of Pain, with the newest recommendations to follow a conference in August 2012. (Adapted from Stanton-Hicks et al. [41]. With permission from John Wiley & Sons, Inc)

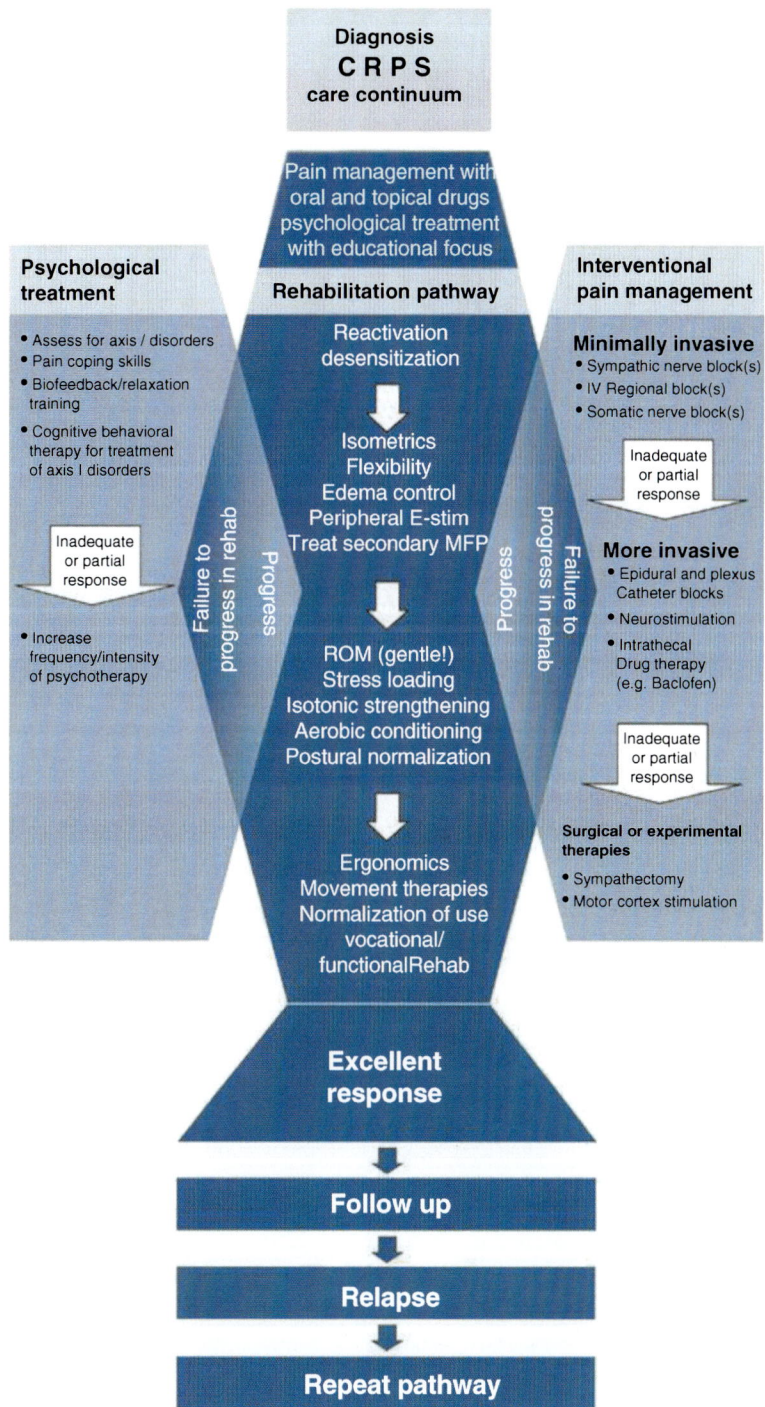

Diagnosis
C R P S
care continuum

Pain management with oral and topical drugs psychological treatment with educational focus

Psychological treatment

- Assess for axis / disorders
- Pain coping skills
- Biofeedback/relaxation training
- Cognitive behavioral therapy for treatment of axis I disorders

Inadequate or partial response

- Increase frequency/intensity of psychotherapy

Rehabilitation pathway

Reactivation desensitization

Isometrics
Flexibility
Edema control
Peripheral E-stim
Treat secondary MFP

ROM (gentle!)
Stress loading
Isotonic strengthening
Aerobic conditioning
Postural normalization

Ergonomics
Movement therapies
Normalization of use
vocational/
functionalRehab

Failure to progress in rehab / Progress

Interventional pain management

Minimally invasive
- Sympathic nerve block(s)
- IV Regional block(s)
- Somatic nerve block(s)

Inadequate or partial response

More invasive
- Epidural and plexus Catheter blocks
- Neurostimulation
- Intrathecal Drug therapy (e.g. Baclofen)

Inadequate or partial response

Surgical or experimental therapies
- Sympathectomy
- Motor cortex stimulation

Excellent response

Follow up

Relapse

Repeat pathway

References

1. Furlan AD, Lui PW, Mailis A. Chemical sympathectomy for neuropathic pain: does it work? Case report and systematic literature review. Clin J Pain. 2001;17(4): 327–36.

2. North RB, Shipley J. The neuromodulation therapy access coalition. Practice parameters for the use of spinal cord stimulation in the treatment of chronic neuropathic pain. Pain Med. 2007;8:S200–75.

3. Oakley JC, Weiner RL. Spinal cord stimulation of complex regional pain syndrome: a prospective study of 19 patients at two centers. Neuromodulation. 1999;2:47–50.

4. DeJongste MJL. Spinal cord stimulation for ischemic heart disease. Neurol Res. 2000;22:293–8.

5. Huber SJ, Vaglienti RM, Huber JS. Spinal cord stimulation in severe, inoperable, peripheral vascular disease. Neuromodulation. 2000;3:131–43.

6. Prager JP, Stanton-Hicks M. Neurostimulation. In: Cousins MJ, Bridenbaugh PO, Carr DB, et al., editors. Cousins and Bridenbaugh's neural blockade in clinical anesthesia and pain medicine. 4th ed. Philadelphia: Williams & Wilkins; 2010. p. 948–90.

7. Oakley JC. Spinal cord stimulation for the treatment of chronic pain. In: Follett KA, editor. Neurosurgical pain management. Philadelphia: Saunders; 2004. p. 131–44.

8. Campbell JN, Long DM. Peripheral nerve stimulation in the treatment of intractable pain. J Neurosurg. 1976;45(6):682–9.

9. Levy R. Differentiating the leaves from the branches in the tree of neuromodulation: the state of peripheral nerve field stimulation. Neuromodulation. 2011;14:201–5.

10. Stanton-Hicks M, Salamon J. Stimulation of the central and peripheral nervous system for the control of pain. J Clin Neurophysiol. 1997;14(1):46–62.

11. Hassenbusch SJ, Stanton-Hicks M, Schoppa D, Walsh JG, Covington EC. Long-term results of peripheral nerve stimulation for reflex sympathetic dystrophy. J Neurosurg. 1996;84:415–23.

12. Kupers R, Laere KV, Calenbergh FV, et al. Multimodal therapeutic assessment of peripheral nerve stimulation in neuropathic pain: five case reports with a 20-year follow-up. Eur J Pain. 2011;15(2):161.

13. Deer TR, Levy RM, Rosenfeld EL. Prospective clinical study of a new implantable peripheral nerve stimulation device to treat chronic pain. Clin J Pain. 2010; 26(5):359–72.

14. Kim HJ, Paek SH, Kim JY, et al. Chronic subthalamic deep brain stimulation improves pain in Parkinson disease. J Neurol. 2008;255(12):1889–94.

15. Kim HJ, Jeon BS, Paek SH. Effect of deep brain stimulation on pain in Parkinson disease. J Neurol Sci. 2011;310(1-2):251–5.

16. Kim HJ, Jeon BS, Lee JY, Kim DG. The benefit of subthalamic deep brain stimulation on pain in Parkinson disease: a 2-year follow-up study. Neurosurgery. 2011;70(1):18–23.

17. Breit S, Schulz JB, Benabid A-L. Deep brain stimulation. Cell Tissue Res. 2004;318(1):275–88.

18. Levy R, Deer TR, Henderson J. Intracranial neurostimulation for pain control: a review. Pain Physician. 2010;13:157–65.

19. Levy RM. Deep brain stimulation for the treatment of intractable pain. Neurosurg Clin N Am. 2003;14(3): 389–99, vi.

20. Fontaine D, Hamani C, Lozano A. Efficacy and safety of motor cortex stimulation for chronic neuropathic pain: critical review of the literature. J Neurosurg. 2009;110:251–6.

21. Nuti C, Peyron R, Garcia-Larrea L, et al. Motor cortex stimulation for neuropathic pain: four year outcome and predictors of efficacy. Pain. 2005;228:43–52.

22. Prager J, Bruel B, Buchser E, Caraway D, Cousins M, Deer T, et al. Best practices for intrathecal drug delivery. Neuromodulation. 2013 (in press).

23. Prager J. Neuraxial medication delivery: the development and maturity of a concept for treating chronic pain of spinal origin. Spine. 2002;27(22):2593–605.

24. Hassenbusch SJ, Portenoy RK, Cousins M, et al. Polyanalgesic consensus conference 2003: an update on the management of pain by intraspinal drug delivery – report of an expert panel. J Pain Symptom Manage. 2004;27:540–63.

25. Deer T, Krames ES, Hassenbusch SJ, et al. Polyanalgesic consensus conference 2007: recommendations of the management of pain by intrathecal (intraspinal) drug delivery: report of an interdisciplinary expert panel. Neuromodulation. 2007;10:300–28.

26. Deer TR, Smith HS, Cousins M, et al. Consensus guidelines for the selection and implantation of patients with noncancer pain for intrathecal drug delivery. Pain Physician. 2010;13:E175–213.

27. Krames E. Intrathecal infusional therapies for intractable pain: patient management guidelines. J Pain Symptom Manage. 1993;8(7):451–3.

28. Coffey RJ, Owens ML, Broste SK, et al. Mortality associated with implantation and management of intrathecal opioid drug infusion systems to treat noncancer pain. Anesthesiology. 2009;111(4):881–91.

29. Deer T. A critical time for practice change in the pain treatment continuum: we need to reconsider the role of pumps in the patient care algorithm. Pain Med. 2010;11:987–9.

30. Hijazi Y, Bodonian C, Bolon M, Salord F, Boulieu R. Pharmacokinetics and haemodynamics of ketamine in intensive care patients with brain or spinal cord injury. Br J Anaesth. 2003;90(2):155–60.

31. Correll GE, Maleki J, Gracely EJ, et al. Subanesthetic ketamine infusion therapy: a retrospective analysis of a novel therapeutic approach to CRPS. Pain Med. 2004;5:263–75.

32. Goldberg ME, Domsky R, Scaringe D, et al. Multiday low dose ketamine infusion for the treatment of CRPS. Pain Physician. 2005;8:175–9.

33. Kiefer RT, Roht P, Ploppa A, Altemeyer KH, Schwartzman RJ. Complete recovery from intractable complex regional pain syndrome, CRPS-type I, following anesthetic ketamine and midazolam. Pain Pract. 2007;7(2):147–50.

34. Kiefer RT, Rohr P, Ploppa A, et al. Efficacy of ketamine in anesthetic dosage for the treatment of refractory

complex regional pain syndrome: an open-label phase II study. Pain Med. 2008;9(8):1173–201.

35. Kiefer RT, Rohr P, Ploppa A, et al. A pilot open-label study of the efficacy of subanesthetic isomeric S(+)-ketamine in refractory CRPS patients. Pain Med. 2008;9(1):44–54.

36. Drexel University College of Medicine. Double blind placebo controlled study of outpatient intravenous ketamine for the treatment of CRPS. Available at: http://clinicaltrials.gov/ct2/show/NCT00579085. Accessed 8 May 2009.

37. Getson P. Update on low-dose ketamine infusions. RSDSA Rev. 2009;22(2):8–9.

38. Noppers IM, Miesters M, Aarts LP, et al. Drug-induced liver injury following a repeated course of ketamine treatment for chronic pain in CRPS type 1 patients: a report of 3 cases. Pain. 2011;152(9):2173–8.

39. Kemler MA, Barendse GA, van Kleef M, et al. Spinal cord stimulation in patients with chronic reflex sympathetic dystrophy. N Engl J Med. 2000;343:618–24.

40. Stanton-Hicks M, Janig W, Hassenbusch SJ, et al. Reflex sympathetic dystrophy: changing concepts and taxonomy. Pain. 1995;3:127–33.

41. Stanton-Hicks MD, Burton AW, Bruehl SP, et al. An updated interdisciplinary clinical pathway for CRPS: report of an expert panel. Pain Pract. 2002;2:1–16.

Psychosocial Factors in NTOS

37

Michelle M. Dugan

Abstract

Neurogenic thoracic outlet syndrome is a chronic pain syndrome that may take years to be diagnosed. Years of undiagnosed or undertreated chronic pain can lead to anger, confusion, frustration, depression, family strains, and financial difficulties. This may lead to social isolation, loss of social support, and loss of employment.

This chapter discusses the importance of incorporating psychosocial factors into treatment plans for neurogenic thoracic outlet syndrome. Psychosocial factors affect a patient's response to pain and treatment outcomes. Adequate social supports, treatment of depression, patient educational level, financial means, and encouraging return to work may improve patient's treatment course.

Introduction

Thoracic outlet syndrome (TOS) is defined as the occurrence of upper extremity symptoms due to compression of the neurovascular bundle by various structures in the area just above the first rib and behind the clavicle [1]. Adding the qualifier of neurogenic defines the structure of compression: NTOS is the compression of nerves by bony structures, soft tissue (muscles), or fibrocartilaginous bands in the region of the thoracic outlet or just beneath the pectoralis minor muscle [2]. This compression leads to headaches, arm numbness, and chest and neck pain and such symptoms are exacerbated by provocative maneuvers.

NTOS is a neuropathic chronic pain syndrome and a lifelong condition. Chronic pain is devastating and life-altering. The pain interrupts, interferes with, and alters ones identity [3]. Years of undiagnosed or undertreated chronic pain often leads to anger, confusion, frustration, depression, family strains, and financial difficulties, and these in turn may lead to social isolation, loss of social support, and loss of employment [4]. Patients have varying degrees of social support structures, coping skills, pain thresholds, and stamina. Age, gender, and stage of life also affect how one responds to pain.

M.M. Dugan, MSN, FNP-BC
Department of Neurosurgery,
University of Rochester Medical Center,
601 Elmwood Avenue, Box 670,
14642 Rochester, NY, USA
e-mail: michelle_dugan@urmc.rochester.edu

K.A. Illig et al. (eds.), *Thoracic Outlet Syndrome*,
DOI 10.1007/978-1-4471-4366-6_37, © Springer-Verlag London 2013

Diagnosis and Treatment of NTOS

In a majority of cases, a diagnosis of NTOS is not made correctly or in a timely manner. It may take 2–5 years for the diagnosis to be made [5, 6]. Failure to provide a proper diagnosis leads to initiation of inappropriate and incorrect treatment plans, which in turn exacerbate the psychological and social harm that results.

Delayed diagnosis and treatment is multifactorial. Factors that contribute to such delays include controversy over the diagnosis of NTOS by some, lack of a diagnostic gold standard, and lack of medical providers' awareness of the entity [1, 7–10]. There are few surgeons, providers, and therapists who are experienced in evaluating, diagnosing, and treating NTOS, and there are few medical centers specializing in this syndrome. Finally, opinions significantly differ regarding treatment plans [5, 11].

Both conservative therapy and surgical decompression are appropriate options in patients with NTOS, depending on the specific case. Conservative options consist of NTOS-directed pain management, occupational (OT), and/or physical therapy (PT). Alternative therapies for pain such as acupuncture, cognitive behavioral therapy (CBT), or hypnosis are advocated by some and can be encouraged in conjunction with traditional treatments. Surgical treatment is the decompression of the nerve structure by removing or revising bony structures, muscle, soft tissue, and or bands [6, 12].

Psychosocial Factors

Psychosocial factors have been investigated and correlated with treatment outcomes in many pain syndromes and surgical procedures [13–18]. For example, in patients with chronic back pain "yellow flag" psychosocial risk factors are assessed to determine increase risk for worsening chronic pain and disability [19], and some insurance companies require psychosocial screening and clearance prior to proceeding with operations such as spinal cord stimulator or intrathecal pump implantation for pain management.

Evaluation of pain syndromes should include assessment of depression, availability of social supports, motivation to get well, and the patient's ability to cope with the perception of or actual treatment failure [18]. Ideally a "patient at risk" should be assessed by a pain provider and/or pain psychologist to recommend and assist with chronic pain treatment [20].

Assessment of psychosocial factors in the management of NTOS probably occurs quite rarely, even in centers that concentrate on the diagnosis [12], and the literature is sparse in regards to the psychosocial needs of the NTOS patient. Much of the psychosocial discussion in this chapter is extrapolated from NTOS outcomes, chronic pain literature, and the author's anecdotal experience working in a NTOS clinic associated with a large academic center. When assessing psychosocial issues in patients with NTOS, it is convenient to separately consider social support, education level, depression, financial means, and return to work.

Social Support

Social support comes from a variety of sources. The patient's spouse, family and friends are generally the first line of helpful supports. Studies have shown NTOS patients without a spouse have greater disabilities at long term follow-up [21], a finding that parallels findings elsewhere in the chronic pain literature (especially muscular skeletal disorders and chronic low back pain) [22, 23].

When there is no "conventional" other reliable support, consider alternatives. Church groups can be an option for those whom are spiritually oriented or have limited financial resources. Counseling may be sought based on the patient preference, identified needs, and financial means. Unfortunately there are very few regions with physical NTOS support groups. There are many resources and support groups available on the internet. Examples of reputable sites are the American Thoracic Outlet Syndrome Association http://www.atosa.org, the National Pain Foundation, http://www.nationalpainfoundation.org/cat/18/thoracic-outlet-syndrome, and The American chronic pain association http://www.theacpa.org (See Chap. 96 for more information regarding this issue).

Depression

Depression can develop at any time during a chronic pain experience, and this will significantly impact response to treatment [24] (see Chaps. 8 and 38 for further discussion). NTOS patients with depression report higher pain scores, greater functional and job disability, and are less likely to experience a reduction in symptoms after surgery [21]. Depression is noted more often in treatment-resistant patients with NTOS [25] and decreases the chance of (and lengthens time to) return to work in a variety of studies. The presence of depression and anxiety should be determined prior to treatment initiation as it is highly predictive of success (or lack thereof). Providers with limited experience or comfort level in evaluating and treating depression or anxiety should consider asking for assistance from someone who has more (such as a pain specialist, psychiatrist, or psychologist).

Patient Education

Formal education (and financial means) affect patient pain response and treatment outcomes [21]. Patients with lower educational levels report higher pain scores and greater postoperative disability [21]. It may be that patients with higher educational levels have greater critical thinking skills, improved ability to navigate the health care system, or more effective interactions with the treatment team [26]. We are unable to change the patient's formal education or intellectual capacity but can acknowledge that these are factors and adjust approaches based on these issues.

Prior to patient and family teaching there should be an assessment of educational levels, beliefs, and expectations regarding chronic pain and treatments [24]. Pain relief may not be in the patient's immediate future and even after treatment may never be absolute [27], and especially if perceptions and expectations are unrealistic regarding the treatment course [28]. Alternative pain therapies may be of benefit when not presented to the patient as a last resort therapy.

A focus on the realistic expectations for conservative and surgical treatment with time frames for success should be present for all options. The patient should receive consistent and accurate education and information at every visit [29]. Even if pain is not immediately treatable, identification of the potential pain source and defining the diagnosis can be elating for a patient who has been in a prolonged, unidentified pain syndrome [27].

It is obviously essential to have continuity of care including, if possible, a multidisciplinary team specializing in NTOS (see Chap. 97, "Establishing a TOS-focused Practice"). The entire team needs to be aware of and updated on goals, timeframes and plan changes at each visit. There is some evidence of a beneficial practitioner/therapist effect in the treatment of low back pain [30] and patients with NTOS may well respond in a similar fashion.

Financial

Limited finances and poor (or no) medical insurance are associated with increased pain intensity and restriction of a patient's ability to access care and carry out treatment plans [26]. Out of pocket expenses are not insignificant and include copays for physician visits and physical or occupational therapy, medications, diagnostic tests, and other provider visits. Transportation costs, overnight stays, meals, uncovered medical equipment and service fees are also expenses created by physical ailments. Assistance or grants may be available to patients from chronic pain associations, medical associations, or pharmaceutical companies through such sites as NeedyMeds http://www.needymeds.org. Team Continuum may help with bills other than medical costs http://www.teamcontinuum.net. Social workers and public welfare agencies can help.

Work Status

Physical and psychosocial factors obviously impact work status as well as pain and recovery [31]. Depression and lower education levels have been linked with decreased rates of return to work [32]. Interestingly, resistant NTOS treatment has not been associated with work disability and workers compensation claims according to Jordan [25]. A premorbid vocation requiring over-the-head repetitive activities correlates negatively with success of surgical treatment [33]. Encourage patients to utilize employee assistance programs, request modification of work environment, or consider job change options and retraining. The longer a patient is out of work the chances of returning to the work force decreases [5]. Every effort should be made to encourage return to work for psychosocial, economic, and recovery purposes (see also Chap. 95, for further examination of this issue).

The Future

There are no prospective studies (much less randomized and blinded) evaluating the impact of psychosocial factors on pain interventions and other treatment for NTOS. There is a need to study the impact of psychosocial factors on these problems [26], and there should be consideration of and uniform agreement for a new or existing universal tools for the preoperative and postoperative assessment of psychosocial risk factors.

Summary

NTOS is a life-long chronic neuropathic pain disorder, and, as such, requires assessment of psychosocial evaluation and guidance to ensure that these needs are being met. Probably most important are a stable social support structure and adequate treatment of underlying depression. In addition to these factors, a clearly described diagnosis and establishment of realistic goals and timeframes for various treatment plans may enhance coping, shorten recovery, and improve long term outcomes. With appropriate resources, treatments, therapies, and modification; patients may return to a productive functional life.

References

1. Sanders RJ, Hammond SL, Rao NM. Diagnosis of thoracic outlet syndrome. J Vasc Surg. 2007;46(3):601–4 (Review. PubMed PMID: 17826254).

2. Sanders RJ, Rao NM. The forgotten pectoralis minor syndrome: 100 operations for pectoralis minor syndrome alone or accompanied by neurogenic thoracic outlet syndrome. Ann Vasc Surg. 2010;24(6):701–8 (Epub 14 May 2010. PubMed PMID: 20471786).

3. Morley S. Psychology of pain. Br J Anaesth. 2008;101(1):25–31 (Epub 28 May 2008. Review. PubMed PMID: 18511440).

4. Richardson JC. Establishing the (extra)ordinary in chronic widespread pain. Health (London). 2005;9(1):31–48.

5. Franklin GM, Fulton-Kehoe D, Bradley C, Smith-Weller T. Outcome of surgery for thoracic outlet syndrome in Washington state workers' compensation. Neurology. 2000;54(6):1252–7.

6. Sanders RJ, Hammond SL, Rao NM. Thoracic outlet syndrome: a review. Neurologist. 2008;14(6):365–73.

7. Hendler NH, Kozikowski JG. Overlooked physical diagnoses in chronic pain patients involved in litigation. Psychosomatics. 1993;34(6):494–501 (PubMed PMID: 8284339).

8. Hendler N, Bergson C, Morrison C. Overlooked physical diagnoses in chronic pain patients involved in litigation, part 2. The addition of MRI, nerve blocks, 3-D CT, and qualitative flow meter. Psychosomatics. 1996;37(6):509–17 (PubMed PMID: 8942201).

9. Samarasam I, Sadhu D, Agarwal S, Nayak S. Surgical management of thoracic outlet syndrome: a 10-year experience. ANZ J Surg. 2004;74(6):450–4.

10. Watson LA, Pizzari T, Balster S. Thoracic outlet syndrome part 1: clinical manifestations, differentiation and treatment pathways. Man Ther. 2009;14(6):586–95 (Epub 9 Sep 2009. Review. PubMed PMID: 19744876).

11. Landry GJ, Moneta GL, Taylor Jr LM, Edwards JM, Porter JM. Long-term functional outcome of neurogenic thoracic outlet syndrome in surgically and conservatively treated patients. J Vasc Surg. 2001; 33(2):312–7, discussion 317–9 (PubMed PMID: 11174783).

12. Fugate MW, Rotellini-Coltvet L, Freischlag JA. Current management of thoracic outlet syndrome. Curr Treat Options Cardiovasc Med. 2009;11(2): 176–83.

13. Dempsey PG, Burdorf A, Webster BS. The influence of personal variables on work-related low-back disorders and implications for future research. J Occup Environ Med. 1997;39(8):748–59 (Review. PubMed PMID: 9273879).

14. Block AR, Ohnmeiss DD, Guyer RD, Rashbaum RF, Hochschuler SH. The use of presurgical psychological screening to predict the outcome of spine surgery. Spine J. 2001;1(4):274–82.

15. Schultz IZ, Crook JM, Berkowitz J, Meloche GR, Milner R, Zuberbier OA, Meloche W. Biopsychosocial multivariate predictive model of occupational low back disability. Spine (Phila Pa 1976). 2002;27(23):2720–5 (PubMed PMID: 12461399).

16. Trief PM, Grant W, Fredrickson B. A prospective study of psychological predictors of lumbar surgery outcome. Spine (Phila Pa 1976). 2000;25(20):2616–21 (PubMed PMID: 11034646).

17. LaCaille RA, DeBerard MS, Masters KS, Colledge AL, Bacon W. Presurgical biopsychosocial factors predict multidimensional patient: outcomes of interbody cage lumbar fusion. Spine J. 2005;5(1):71–8 (PubMed PMID: 15653087).

18. Celestin J, Edwards RR, Jamison RN. Pretreatment psychosocial variables as predictors of outcomes following lumbar surgery and spinal cord stimulation: a systematic review and literature synthesis. Pain Med. 2009;10(4):639–53 (Review. PubMed PMID: 19638142).

19. van Tulder M, Becker A, Bekkering T, Breen A, del Real MT, Hutchinson A, Koes B, Laerum E, Malmivaara A. COST B13 working group on guidelines for the management of acute Low back pain in primary care. Chapter 3. European guidelines for the management of acute nonspecific low back pain in primary care. Eur Spine J. 2006;15 Suppl 2:S169–91 (PubMed PMID: 16550447).

20. Anderson PA, Schwaegler PE, Cizek D, Leverson G. Work status as a predictor of surgical outcome of discogenic low back pain. Spine (Phila Pa 1976). 2006;31(21):2510–5 (PubMed PMID: 17023863).

21. Axelrod DA, Proctor MC, Geisser ME, Roth RS, Greenfield LJ. Outcomes after surgery for thoracic outlet syndrome. J Vasc Surg. 2001;33(6):1220–5.

22. Badley EM, Ibañez D. Socioeconomic risk factors and musculoskeletal disability. J Rheumatol. 1994;21(3):515–22.

23. Schade V, Semmer N, Main CJ, Hora J, Boos N. The impact of clinical, morphological, psychosocial and work-related factors on the outcome of lumbar discectomy. Pain. 1999;80(1–2):239–49.

24. Turk DC, Audette J, Levy RM, Mackey SC, Stanos S. Assessment and treatment of psychosocial comorbidities in patients with neuropathic pain. Mayo Clin Proc. 2010;85(3 Suppl):S42–50 (Review. PubMed PMID: 20194148; PubMed Central PMCID: PMC2844010).

25. Jordan SE, Ahn SS, Gelabert HA. Differentiation of thoracic outlet syndrome from treatment-resistant cervical brachial pain syndromes: development and utilization of a questionnaire, clinical examination and ultrasound evaluation. Pain Physician. 2007;10(3): 441–52. Erratum in: Pain Physician. 2007;10(4):599 (PubMed PMID: 17525778).

26. Poleshuck EL, Green CR. Socioeconomic disadvantage and pain. Pain. 2008;136(3):235–8 (Epub 28 Apr 2008. Review. PubMed PMID: 18440703; PubMed Central PMCID: PMC2488390).

27. Castro AR, Siqueira SR, Perissinotti DM, Teixeira MJ, Siqueira JT. Emotional aspects of chronic orofacial pain and surgical treatment. Int J Surg. 2009;7(3):196–9 (Epub 2009 Mar 10. PubMed PMID: 19281877).

28. Klaber Moffett JA, Newbronner E, Waddell G, Croucher K, Spear S. Public perceptions about low back pain and its management: a gap between expectations and reality? Health Expect. 2000;3(3):161–8 (PubMed PMID: 11281925).

29. Novak CB, Collins ED, Mackinnon SE. Outcome following conservative management of thoracic outlet syndrome. J Hand Surg Am. 1995;20(4):542–8.

30. Lewis M, Morley S, van der Windt DA, Hay E, Jellema P, Dziedzic K, Main CJ. Measuring practitioner/therapist effects in randomised trials of low back pain and neck pain interventions in primary care settings. Eur J Pain. 2010;14(10):1033–9 (Epub 4 May 2010. PubMed PMID: 20444631).

31. Johnston V, Jull G, Souvlis T, Jimmieson NL. Interactive effects from self-reported physical and psychosocial factors in the workplace on neck pain and disability in female office workers. Ergonomics. 2010;53(4):502–13 (PubMed PMID: 20309746).

32. Ozegovic D, Carroll LJ, Cassidy JD. What influences positive return to work expectation? Examining associated factors in a population-based cohort of whiplash-associated disorders. Spine (Phila Pa 1976). 2010;35(15):E708–13 (PubMed PMID: 20535047).

33. Green RM, McNamara J, Ouriel K. Long-term follow-up after thoracic outlet decompression: an analysis of factors determining outcome. J Vasc Surg. 1991;14(6):739–45, discussion 745–6 (PubMed PMID: 1960804).

Psychiatric Considerations in NTOS

38

Beverly Field

Abstract

Depression and substance abuse are two psychiatric co-morbidities found in chronic pain populations. Because both can influence quality of life, pain perception, and response to treatment, they should regularly be evaluated and treated when present. Treatment for depression includes various antidepressants, some of which have analgesic properties, and psychotherapy. Patients actively abusing pain medications, alcohol or illicit drugs should be referred to a substance abuse treatment program. However, distinguishing between pain medication overuse/abuse and poorly controlled pain can be difficult, and over diagnosing pain medication abuse may result in pejorative labeling of patients and withdrawal of pain-relieving analgesics.

Introduction

In the transition from acute to chronic pain, psychiatric co-morbidities and psychosocial factors begin to play a more prominent role. Anxiety, depression, expectations, attributions, and reinforcement of pain behaviors can influence response to treatment, pain perception, and disability.

Depression not only affects a patient's quality of life, but can negatively impact treatment. A study by Axelrod et al. [1] found that, in patients undergoing decompression surgery for thoracic outlet syndrome (TOS), a co-existing diagnosis of major depression resulted in greater disability following surgery. Similarly, Jordan et al. [2] found major depression to be one of the factors that differentiated treatment-resistant from treatment-responsive patients following first rib resection or botulinum chemodenervation. Results from these two studies are similar to previous studies which found depression to be a predictor of disability [3] following surgery for lumbar spinal stenosis, and the combination of depression and anxiety to be predictive of less improvement in pain rating and daily functional capacity, and return to work [4] after spine surgery.

Substance abuse may also influence treatment outcomes as noted in a study by Spengler et al [5]. Of 30 patients for whom surgical approaches failed to provide improvement, 25 were found to

B. Field, PhD
Department of Anesthesiology,
Washington University School of Medicine,
660 South Euclid Avenue, Campus Box 8054,
St. Louis, MO 63110, USA
e-mail: fieldb@wustl.edu

K.A. Illig et al. (eds.), *Thoracic Outlet Syndrome*,
DOI 10.1007/978-1-4471-4366-6_38, © Springer-Verlag London 2013

have a history of medication and/or alcohol abuse. For patients prescribed opioid analgesics for pain, a current history of alcohol and/or illicit drug abuse has potentially fatal consequences.

Psychiatric Comorbidities

To date, there are few published studies that specifically address the prevalence of psychiatric co-morbidities in the population of patients with neurogenic thoracic outlet syndrome (NTOS) or the interrelationships between psychiatric co-morbidities and NTOS. However, NTOS may be considered under the broader definition of chronic pain syndromes, as patients can suffer for years with pain before receiving a diagnosis and treatments are not always effective in relieving pain [6, 7]. Chronic non-cancer pain is defined as pain that continues for longer than 6 months or beyond the expected time of healing, for which there has been no or inadequate response to treatment, and which may continue for a person's lifetime. Individuals with chronic pain often present with a number of physical and emotional problems, either as antecedent conditions or as a consequence of injury and pain. Depression and substance abuse are two co-morbidities found in the chronic pain population that should be recognized and treated when present, as they can influence response to treatment, pain perception and adaptive coping.

Depression

Depression is a common co-morbidity in the chronic pain population. Patients with chronic pain suffer not only from pain, but also with physical limitations and multiple losses. They may be unable to maintain employment and experience adverse economic changes, loss of daily activities, and a diminished sense of self-worth. Physical limitations often result in an inability to participate in sports and recreational activities and can even limit everyday activities and self-care. People who suffer with chronic pain may feel misunderstood by others, resulting in withdrawal from family and friends, and social isolation. Banks and Kerns present a diathesis-stress model outlining an association between pain and depression [8]. They suggest that individuals bring to the experience of chronic pain certain vulnerabilities, or diatheses. These diatheses are activated when the multiple stressors of chronic pain are experienced. A negative or helpless view of life, feelings of lack of control, or inadequate coping resources may produce feelings of hopelessness and despair, or trigger a major depressive episode. In this study, Banks and Kerns performed a meta-analysis based on selected studies using stringent criteria for major depression. Their results estimated the prevalence of depression in patients with chronic pain to be between 30 and 54 %. The impact of pain on life style and interpersonal relationships may certainly be a factor in the development, or worsening, of depression. However, pain and depression also share neurochemical pathways including serotonergic and noradrenergic neurotransmitters.

The *Diagnostic and Statistical Manual of Mental Disorders* (4th ed., text revision) (DSM-IV-TR) criteria for major depression include symptoms such as insomnia, fatigue, changes in appetite and/or weight, and changes in memory and concentration [9]. These symptoms may also be partially or entirely attributable to pain and/or to the medications used to treat pain. Because of overlapping symptoms, some authorities have recommended modifying the diagnostic criteria for major depression in medically ill patients. However, most such attempts have not improved the accuracy of diagnosis and/or have resulted in a high rate of false negatives. Thus, the DSM criteria are still recommended for diagnosing depression in the medically ill.

Evaluation and treatment of depression is important for several reasons. In the chronic pain population, depression is associated with poor adherence to treatment, greater pain intensity, poorer functioning, greater pain-related disability, and use of passive coping strategies [10]. In addition, completed suicides occur at a rate two to three times the rate of suicides in the general population [11]. Treatments for depression include medications (primarily antidepressants) and nonpharmacologic interventions, such as various modalities of psychotherapy. Tricyclic antidepressants (eg, amitriptyline and nortriptyline) and the newer serotoninnorepinephrine reuptake inhibitors (SNRIs; eg, duloxetine) have both antidepressant and analgesic properties. The selective serotonin reuptake inhibitors (SSRIs) are effective antidepressants but are less effective as analgesics.

Substance Abuse

High-risk behaviors, such as driving while intoxicated or under the influence of illicit drugs, can result in accidents from which patients sustain injuries resulting in NTOS and other chronic pain conditions. Although these painful conditions need to be adequately treated, for patients who are actively abusing alcohol and/or illicit drugs, pain medication can be potentially life threatening. If a patient is actively abusing substances, he or she should be referred to a substance abuse treatment program with follow up in a recovery program such as Alcoholics Anonymous (AA) or Narcotics Anonymous (NA). For patients with a history of substance abuse, it is possible to manage pain with pain medication if expectations regarding proper use of pain medications are clearly established, use is closely monitored with frequent follow up visits, and patients undergo random drug testing.

Addiction to opioids among patients prescribed opioid analgesics for pain is uncommon. Although the exact prevalence of addiction to opioids among chronic pain patients is not known, a 1992 study by Fishbain, Rosomoff and Rosomoff suggested that the prevalence ranged from 3 to 19 % [12]. Even defining what behaviors constitute addiction to opioids among patient prescribed opioids for pain is controversial. "Drug-seeking" behaviors, such as taking pain medications faster than prescribed, requesting an increase in dosage or obtaining pain medication from more than one doctor, may reflect nothing more than poorly controlled pain. "Pseudoaddiction", which often presents as "drug seeking" behavior, commonly resolves when pain is adequately managed.

Patients, their families, and their physicians may have different concerns about the patient's use of opioid analgesics for chronic pain. Physicians may fear litigation for alleged over- or under-prescriptions of opioids and patient diversion of prescribed pain medication, and have concerns about side effects and worsening pain from long-term use of opioids (opioid tolerance hyperalgesia). Patients and their families often fear addiction to opioids prescribed for chronic pain.

Although addiction to opioids occurs rarely in individuals who have no history of substance abuse, many patients prescribed opioid analgesics for pain have been diagnosed with opioid addiction based on the DSM-IV-TR criteria for Substance Dependence. Because tolerance and dependence, both of which occur with long-term administration of opioids, are two of three criteria needed for a diagnosis of opioid dependence, patients prescribed opioid analgesics for pain can easily meet these diagnostic criteria. In order to address the problem of unwarranted diagnoses of opioid addiction, the Liaison Committee on Pain and Addiction met in 2001 and developed the following definitions that more accurately reflect tolerance, dependence, and addiction in patients prescribed opioids for pain [13]. **Tolerance** is a state of adaptation in which exposure to a drug induces changes that result in a diminution of one or more of the drug's effects over time. **Physical dependence** is a state of adaptation that is manifested by a drug class-specific withdrawal syndrome that can be produced by abrupt cessation, rapid dose reduction, decreasing blood level of the drug, or administration of an antagonist. **Addiction** is a primary, chronic neurobiological disease with genetic, psychosocial, and environmental factors influencing its development and manifestations. It is characterized by behaviors that include one or more of the following: impaired control over drug use, compulsive use, continued use despite harm, and craving.

Although patients being considered for pain treatment with opioid analgesics should be assessed for the risk of abuse or addiction to opioids, no strong predictors of misuse and addiction have been identified. Michna et al. found that patient and family histories of substance abuse and histories of legal problems predicted behaviors such as multiple unsanctioned escalations in dose of pain medications, episodes of lost or stolen prescriptions, frequent unscheduled visits to the pain center or emergency room, excessive phone calls, concern expressed by a significant other about the patient's use of opioids, and unanticipated positive results in urine toxicology tests [14]. Because abuse of, and addiction to, opioids is potentially life threatening, a careful assessment should be made of a patient's substance use history. Although there are no established predictors of which patients might abuse pain medications, the presence of multiple risk factors suggests the need for careful monitoring.

References

1. Axelrod DA, Proctor MC, Geisser ME, Roth RS, Greenfield LF. Outcomes after surgery for thoracic outlet syndrome. J Vasc Surg. 2001;33(6):1220–5.
2. Jordan SE, Ahn SS, Gelabert HA. Differentiation of thoracic outlet syndrome from treatment-resistant cervical brachial syndromes: development and utilization of a questionnaire, clinical examination and ultrasound evaluation. Pain Physician. 2007;10: 441–52.
3. Sinikallio S, Aalto T, Lehto SM, Airaksinen O, Herno A, Kroger H, Viinamaki H. Depressivesymptoms predict post-operative disability among patients with lumbar spinal stenosis: a two year prospective study comparing two age groups. Disabil Rehabil. 2010;32(6): 462–8.
4. Trief PM, Grant W, Fredrickson B. A prospective study of psychological predictors of lumbar spine surgery outcome. Spine. 2000;25(20):2616–21.
5. Spengler DM, Freeman C, Westbrook R, Miller JW. Low back pain following multiple lumbar spine procedures: failure of initial selection? Spine. 1980;5(4):356–60.
6. Gruss JD. Thoracic outlet syndrome (TOS). Int Angiol. 2009;28(3):167–9.
7. Sanders RJ, Hammond SL, Rao NM. Thoracic outlet syndrome: a review. Neurologist. 2008;14(6):365–73.
8. Banks SM, Kerns RD. Explaining high rates of depression in chronic pain: a diathesis-stress framework. Psychol Bull. 1996;119(1):95–110.
9. American Psychiatric A. Diagnostic and statistical manual of mental disorders. 4th ed. Washington: American Psychiatric Association; 2000 (text rev).
10. Fisher BJ, Haythornthwaite JA, Heinberg LJ, Clark M, Reed J. Suicidal intent in patients with chronic pain. Pain. 2001;89:199–206.
11. Fishbain DA, Goldberg M, Rosomoff RS, Rosomoff H. Case reports: completed suicide in chronic pain. Clin J Pain. 1991;7(1):29–37.
12. Fishbain DA, Rosomoff HL, Rosomoff RS. Drug abuse, dependence and addiction in chronic pain populations. Clin J Pain. 1992;8:77–85.
13. Liaison Committee on Pain and Addiction. American Academy of Pain Medicine, American Pain Society, American Society of Addiction Medicine. Definitions related to the use of opioids for the treatment of pain. 2001. http://www.asam.org/advocacy/find-a-policy-statement/view-policy-statement/public-policy-statements/2011/12/15/definitions-related-to-the-use-of-opioids-for-the-treatment-of-pain-consensus-statement. Accessed 5 Apr 2012.
14. Michna E, Ross EL, Hynes WL, Nedeljkovic SS, Soumekh S, Janfaza D, Palombi D, Jamison RN. Predicting aberrant drug behavior in patients treated for chronic pain: importance of abuse history. J Pain Symptom Manage. 2004;28(3):250–8.

Assessment and Treatment of Recurrent NTOS

39

Stephen J. Annest and Richard J. Sanders

Abstract

Recurrent neurogenic thoracic outlet syndrome (TOS) is usually caused by scar tissue formation, which re-entraps and compresses the nerves of the brachial plexus. Other causes include missed diagnoses or inadequate surgical procedures. Symptoms and signs of recurrent neurogenic TOS are similar to those that preceded the initial operation. Treatment begins with evaluation for pectoralis minor syndrome. If nerve entrapment is present beneath the pectoralis minor muscle tendon, pectoralis minor tenotomy is an outpatient procedure with minimal risk that may be effective in many patients with recurrent neurogenic TOS. If pectoralis minor syndrome is not present or if pectoralis minor tenotomy has failed, other procedures to consider include (1) supraclavicular scalenectomy, if the previous operation was transaxillary first rib resection; (2) transaxillary first rib resection, if the previous operation was supraclavicular scalenectomy without rib resection; (3) brachial plexus neurolysis, if both supraclavicular scalenectomy and first rib resection have been performed; or (4) in the case of multiple failed operations, combined transaxillary and supraclavicular brachial plexus neurolysis combined with a latissimus dorsi muscle flap.

S.J. Annest, MD, FACS (✉)
Department of Vascular Surgery, Presbyterian
St. Luke's Medical Center, Vascular Institute
of the Rockies, 1601 East 19th Avenue,
Suite 3950, Denver, CO 80218, USA
e-mail: annest@vascularinstitute.com

R.J. Sanders, MD
Department of Surgery, HealthONE
Presbyterian-St. Lukes Hospital,
4545 E. 9th Ave #240, Denver, CO 80220, USA
e-mail: rsanders@ecentral.com

Introduction

There are no guarantees of success for any operation to relieve the symptoms of neurogenic TOS. Symptoms may recur even after postoperative improvement for many months, and are most often due to compression of the brachial plexus nerves by postoperative scar tissue in the operative area.

K.A. Illig et al. (eds.), *Thoracic Outlet Syndrome*,
DOI 10.1007/978-1-4471-4366-6_39, © Springer-Verlag London 2013

Etiology and Types

Surgery for neurogenic TOS rarely renders the patient completely symptom-free, and recurrent symptoms occur to at least some degree in as many as 30 % of patients. Only a small fraction of these patients will have symptoms severe enough to warrant reoperation. Most published recurrence rates are calculated not on the basis of all patients with recurrent symptoms, but only on the percentage of patients with symptoms that are deemed severe enough to warrant reoperation.

Recurrent neurogenic TOS is considered the redevelopment of symptoms after a period of notable relief following an initial thoracic outlet decompression procedure, whereas persistent neurogenic TOS is defined as failure to achieve any symptomatic improvement. Persistent neurogenic TOS is typically due to an incorrect diagnosis, an inadequate initial operation, or predominance of another diagnosis accompanying neurogenic TOS despite an adequate initial operation. Some patients with persistent neurogenic TOS may have had particularly severe and/or longstanding symptoms of brachial plexus compression prior to treatment, with failure to improve likely reflecting an advanced level of pre-existing neural injury and dysfunction. Whether it occurs spontaneously or following a specific injury, recurrent neurogenic TOS is usually caused by the development of scar tissue entrapping the brachial plexus nerve roots, and may also have osseous and or soft tissue contributions. Scar tissue may cause restrictive attachments to develop between the nerves and residual first rib, scalene muscle, or thickened extrapleura tissues somewhere along its course. These pathologic attachments subsequently interfere with and restrict normal nerve root mobility.

Time of Recurrence

Recurrence of neurogenic TOS may become manifest anywhere from 2 months to many years after initial surgical treatment. Over half of recurrences present within the first year and 80 % within 2 years. After that time, most instances of recurrence are associated with a new injury. Supraclavicular and transaxillary procedures seem to have similar incidences of recurrence [1].

Differential Diagnosis and Associated Conditions

Several peripheral nerve compression syndromes can co-exist with neurogenic TOS (e.g., the "double-crush" syndrome), [2] or they may represent the primary diagnosis. These conditions include cervical disc disease, cervical spine facet arthritis, ulnar nerve compression at the cubital tunnel or at Guyan's canal, and median nerve entrapment in the forearm or wrist [3]. Other conditions to consider in the differential diagnosis include cervical disc osteophyte(s), Pancoast tumors of the apical lung, nerve sheath tumors, brachial plexitis, syrinx, spinal cord tumors, Chiari malformation, primary shoulder (e.g., rotator cuff) pathology, fibromyalgia, multiple sclerosis, acute coronary syndromes, vasospastic disorders, and complex regional pain syndrome (CRPS) [4].

Symptoms

The symptoms of recurrent neurogenic TOS often mimic those seen prior to the initial operation. Complaints include radiating pain into the neck, trapezius, shoulder girdle and/or upper extremity; paresthesias in the arm, hand and/or fingers; interference with sleep; arm weakness; general fatigue; and aggravation of symptoms with use of the arm, particularly in an elevated position. Occipital headaches are common, and some patients report jaw and/or facial pain. Pain and/or tenderness in the anterior chest wall beneath the clavicle, as well as in the axilla, are common symptoms of brachial plexus compression at the level of the pectoralis minor tendon. Many patients will not mention these symptoms unless specifically asked about pain or tenderness in these areas. In a large series of patients seen for primary or recurrent neurogenic TOS, symptoms consistent with pectoralis minor syndrome were present in approximately 75 % [5, 6].

Physical Examination

The essential aspect of examination is the demonstration that stretching the brachial plexus reproduces the patient's symptoms, while compression of the brachial plexus causes tenderness. Tapping, massage, or thumb pressure over the scalene muscles in the supraclavicular space may elicit local discomfort, as well as complaints of dysesthesias in the arm, chest, back, or neck. Provocative maneuvers include neck rotation, lateral flexion, the elevated arm stress test and the modified upper limb tension test, all of which stretch the brachial plexus thereby eliciting symptoms [7].

Physical examination should include investigation for other sites of nerve compression that can accompany neurogenic TOS and may be associated with the "double-crush" phenomenon [2], or which may serve as the primary diagnosis. These maneuvers include Tinel's testing in the arm for median, radial, and/or ulnar nerve irritability. Further efforts to localize the area of nerve entrapment can be aided by median, ulnar and radial nerve stretches, as described by Elvey [8].

Another important component of the physical examination is the elicitation of tenderness to palpation in the areas below the clavicle at the coracoid process, and in the axilla, which may indicate the pectoralis minor muscle tendon as one site of nerve compression. One way to demonstrate involvement of the pectoralis minor muscle is to stretch the muscle by placing the arm in 90° shoulder abduction, 90° elbow flexion, 90° shoulder external rotation, and shoulder extension against resistance (Fig. 39.1).

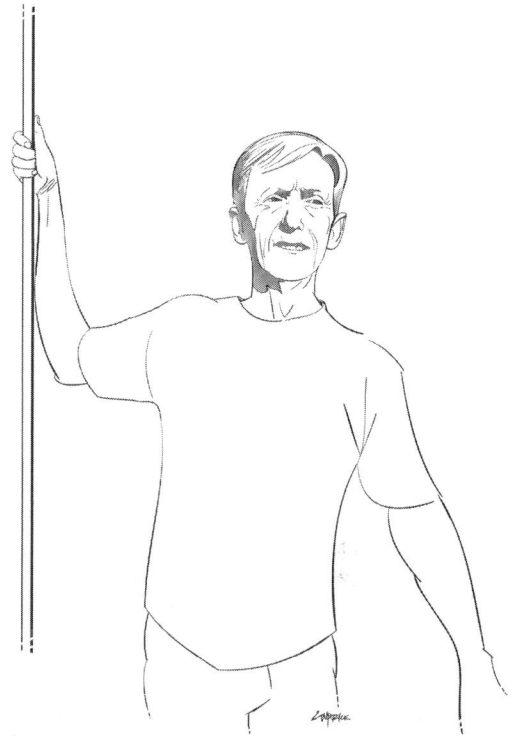

Fig. 39.1 Pectoralis minor muscle stretch. The pectoralis minor muscle can be selectively stretched by asking the patient to abduct and externally rotate the shoulder and then turn the torso in the opposite direction, while holding the affected arm against resistance. A positive response is reproduction of arm complaints and axillary discomfort (Courtesy of HealthONE Presbyterian/St. Lukes Hospital, Denver, Colorado by Wes Price)

neurogenic TOS if the previous surgical treatment included scalenectomy and pectoralis minor tenotomy.

Electrodiagnostic Studies

Standard upper extremity electromyography (EMG) and nerve conduction velocity (NCV) studies are usually normal in those with neurogenic TOS, but can occasionally reveal other sites of pathology. Additional neurodiagnostic measurements that are not typically performed during upper extremity EMG/NCV evaluation may support a diagnosis of neurogenic TOS and/or pectoralis minor syndrome. These include normal cervical paraspinous EMG measurements, which

Diagnostic Tests

Muscle Blocks

Local anesthetic blocks of the anterior scalene and/or pectoralis minor muscles can be valuable aides in confirming a diagnosis of brachial plexus nerve compression in the scalene triangle, subcoracoid space, or both [9]. Unfortunately, this approach is not applicable in evaluating recurrent point away from a central cause of pain, slowing of C8 nerve root conduction, which suggests thoracic outlet compression, and prolonged latency and/or reduced amplitude of medial antebrachial cutaneous sensory nerve action potentials, which have also been correlated with brachial plexus nerve compression either above or below the clavicle [10–12].

Imaging

Chest radiographs and four-view cervical spine X-rays can demonstrate rib anatomy and assess diaphragmatic function, and might identify the rare Pancoast tumor of the lung. Cervical magnetic resonance imaging (MRI) allows accurate recognition of cervical spine pathology, but conventional MRI has not yet been shown to be helpful in the diagnosis of neurogenic TOS. Repeat MRI in the absence of a specific cervical intervention or a new injury therefore has a high cost, without a distinct benefit.

Treatment of Recurrent Neurogenic TOS: Non-Operative Treatment

Attempt to Verify the Diagnosis

It is important to identify and treat any and all associated diagnoses first, before considering treatment specific to neurogenic TOS. Liberal use of consultants is thereby warranted, particularly from the specialties of cervical spine surgery, pain management, physical medicine and rehabilitation, rheumatology, orthopedic surgery, hand surgery, and neurology.

Physical Therapy

Physical therapy is the first choice of treatment in attempting to improve the symptoms of recurrent neurogenic TOS. By trial and experimentation, several different treatment regimens may prove beneficial. General conditioning, core body strengthening, and postural correction help to balance shoulder protractors with shoulder retractors, and thereby lessen muscle stress. The Feldenkreis technique is one tool by which to address these goals [13–16]. Flexibility and stretching exercises are beneficial if they stretch muscles without causing nerve irritation. The patient and therapist should be instructed to avoid, both during and after therapy, any specific exercises that cause dysaethesias, paresthesias, and uncomfortable sensations of "nerve pulling", "electric shocks", or coldness of the extremity. The use of therabands, resistance exercises and heavy weights is best avoided, whereas modalities such as heat, ice packs, therapeutic ultrasound, and electrical stimulation can help to relax chronically fatigued muscles and to combat the muscular component of extremity pain. Acupuncture and use of a transcutaneous nerve stimulator are other options that may be of benefit for some patients. At least 3 months of appropriate physical therapy should be tried before assessing the results and considering alternative forms of treatment.

Workplace and Lifestyle Alterations

Sometimes the activities which stimulate intolerable symptoms of neurogenic TOS can be altered or replaced with activities that are less likely to provoke symptoms. Job retraining, avoidance of aggravating exercise routines, improved workstation ergonomics, or the use of a different bed or pillow may allow adequate relief of symptoms to avoid the need for further interventional therapies.

Pain Management Regimens

In many individuals with recurrent neurogenic TOS, sophisticated assessment by pain management specialists may allow sufficient improvement to avoid having to consider reoperation. The use of pain blocks, trigger-point injections, botulinum toxin injections, and utilization of synergistic medication combinations may offer the hope of providing enough benefit to improve quality-of-life without the need for repeat surgery.

Treatment of Recurrent Neurogenic TOS: Surgical Treatment

In cases of persistent or recurrent neurogenic TOS, evaluation of the details and the adequacy of the first operation will help in decisions regarding the type of reoperation that might be most beneficial. Surgical treatment is considered when: (1) All associated diagnoses have been optimally treated, or their treatment is intended to follow brachial plexus surgery; (2) At least 3 months of conservative therapy targeted towards neurogenic TOS have been completed, without successful or sufficient improvement in symptoms; (3) Symptoms are interfering significantly with work, activities of daily living, or recreational activities important to the patient; and (4) Sufficient time has passed since the initial operation, since it may be preferred to wait at least 6–12 months to allow maturation of scar and to thereby reduce the elevated risk of complications associated with reoperation.

Choice of Operation

Pectoralis Minor Tenotomy

Pectoralis minor tenotomy is the first operation to consider if the patient has physical examination findings suggesting brachial plexus compression in the subcoracoid space and especially if there has been a good response to a pectoralis minor muscle block. If there is minimal improvement with a pectoralis minor muscle block and more improvement with an anterior scalene muscle block, pectoralis minor tenotomy can be easily added to the thoracic outlet decompression procedure. When performed alone, pectoralis minor tenotomy is a low-risk, outpatient procedure. A small axillary incision allows safe and complete pectoralis minor tenotomy and release of any constricting claviopectoral fascia. Performance of pectoralis minor tenotomy does not preclude further or additional operations, if symptom relief is found to be inadequate. The effectiveness of this procedure in the treatment of recurrent neurogenic TOS is well documented in the literature [5, 17].

Supraclavicular Scalenectomy Plus Exploration and Neurolysis of the Brachial Plexus

When re-operating on the brachial plexus, it is beneficial to enter a previously un-operated field. If the first procedure utilized a transaxillary approach, a supraclavicular approach is chosen for reoperation, with performance of anterior and middle scalenectomy and external neurolysis of the nerve roots and trunks of the brachial plexus. In performing neurolysis, emphasis is placed on freeing the brachial plexus from extrinsic scar tissue but care is taken not to enter the nerve sheath or to dissect nerve tissue at the epineural level. Excising scar may include resection of thickened apical pleura based on the appearance and feel of the floor of the supraclavicular field. Scar excision allows the surgeon to dissect, expose and free the nerves to the foramina of the C8 and T1 nerve roots. Any residual cervical or first rib, if not excised at the initial operation and thought to potentially contribute to nerve entrapment, can also be removed at the time of supraclavicular re-exploration.

Transaxillary First Rib Resection and Neurolysis of C8, T1, and Lower Trunk

If the initial procedure was a supraclavicular scalenectomy without first rib resection, transaxillary exposure allows entry through a previously un-operated field. The surgeon enters the pleural cavity at the upper border of the second rib, dissecting pleural scar from the subclavian vein, subclavian artery, and the lower trunk of the brachial plexus, primarily using blunt technique. The first rib (or residual portions of the first rib when the first operation included partial rib resection) is removed, and any scarred middle and anterior scalene muscle remnants are excised. The main goal is to visualize and release the C8 and T1 nerve roots and the lower trunk of the brachial plexus from fibrous tissue entrapment. Circumferential arterial dissection and control using a vessel loop can facilitate dissection of the two lower nerve roots and provides a measure of safety in the event that an arterial injury occurs.

Combined Transaxillary and Supraclavicular Brachial Plexus Exploration

Patients who have symptoms that suggest both upper and lower brachial plexus involvement may be best treated by combining the transaxillary and supraclavicular approaches. The transaxillary procedure is performed first and the C8 and T1 nerve roots are mobilized. The patient is then repositioned to lie supine with the head elevated at 20°–30°, with the neck slightly flexed and the chin anterior in position, to allow decompression of upper and middle trunks through the previously placed supraclavicular incision. The authors prefer this combined approach to the posterior thoracoplasty approach, because it avoids the risk of chronic chest pain known as the "posterior thoracotomy syndrome." Additionally, by using two separate fields of dissection, a much wider field of visualization is obtained of the subclavian artery, the five nerve roots and all three trunks of the brachial plexus, the suprascapular nerve, the phrenic nerve and rarely the dorsal scapular nerve.

Transaxillary and Supraclavicular Neurolysis Plus Latissimus Dorsi Muscle Transfer Flap

When multiple re-operations have been performed, the likelihood is great that the next reoperation will also result in localized scar formation potentially causing a later return of symptoms. To avoid this repeat scenario in those who have undergone multiple surgical procedures around the brachial plexus, the authors have utilized a latissimus dorsi muscle (LDM) flap transfer to cover the brachial plexus, after completing the combined transaxillary and supraclavicular neurolysis procedure. This approach is supported by earlier work in the literature on scarred peripheral nerves [18].

The procedure has three separate steps, two of which are complete scar excision via the transaxillary and supraclavicular routes. The third step is to mobilize the LDM and to wrap it around the brachial plexus. The patient is first placed in a lateral decubitus position with the arm on a mechanical arm holder, prepping from the anterior midline to the dorsal spine and from the angle of the jaw to below the iliac crest (Fig. 39.2). The transaxillary dissection is performed by dissecting along the superior border of the second rib, identifying the subclavian vein and artery as well as lower trunk of the brachial plexus, taking care not to injure the long thoracic nerve which lies on the posterior scalene muscle. The intercostal-brachial cutaneous nerve may be divided to prevent postoperative neuralgia. Any regenerated or remaining first rib is excised. The thickened pleural scar is entered along the superior edge of the second rib and bluntly dissected away from the subclavian vein, subclavian artery, and lower trunk of the brachial plexus, grasping the pleura with a long clamp and excising it. All structures of the thoracic outlet are identified, using a nerve stimulator in combination with a non-paralyzing anesthetic (Fig. 39.3). An attempt is made to carefully separate the lower nerve trunk from the subclavian artery and to visualize the T1 nerve root. Vascular injury is the greatest risk during the transaxillary portion of the procedure, whereas nerve injury is of greater concern during the supraclavicular phase.

Next, through a new oblique incision placed laterally over the ipsilateral scapula, the entire LDM is mobilized and based on the thoracodorsal vessels. The LDM is divided at its origin and is totally freed from the chest wall. The thoracodorsal nerve is divided while leaving the LDM insertion attached to the upper inner humerus [19–21]. The flap is then rotated and passed under the skin bridge between the back and axillary incisions, and placed into the axillary space (Fig. 39.4). The back incision is closed over a drain and a local anesthetic infusion catheter, and the axillary incision is temporarily closed with staples.

The patient is repositioned to a supine, beach-chair position and re-prepped with the axillary incision and the entire ipsilateral neck in the field for the supraclavicular dissection. This replicates the original supraclavicular technique,

Fig. 39.2 Surgical treatment of recurrent neurogenic TOS. Positioning of the patient and location of incisions for the latissimus dorsi rotational muscle flap procedure(Courtesy of HealthONE Presbyterian/St. Lukes Hospital, Denver, Colorado by Wes Price)

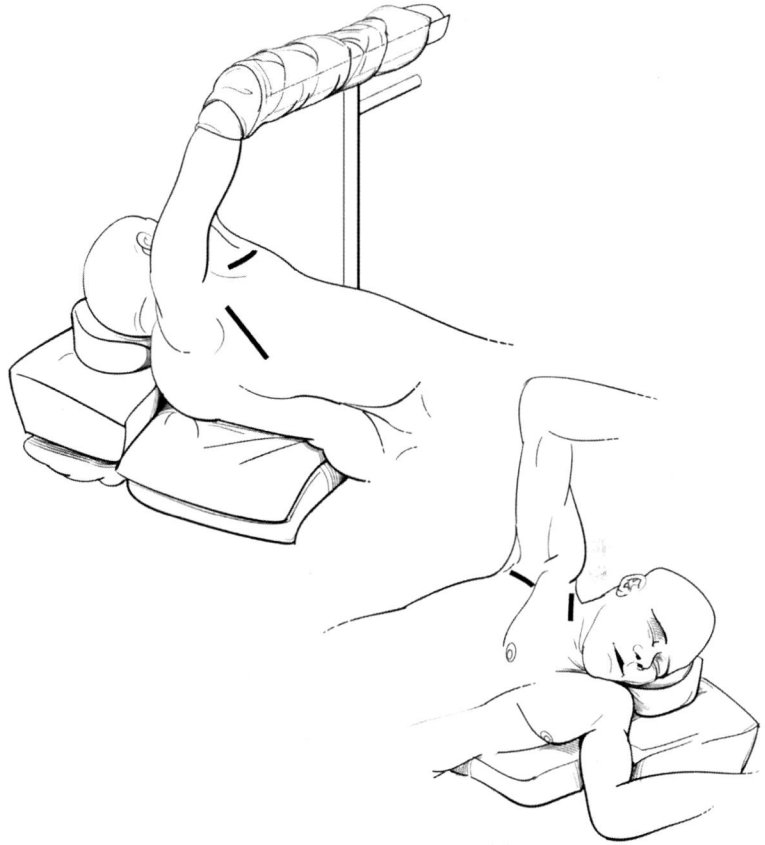

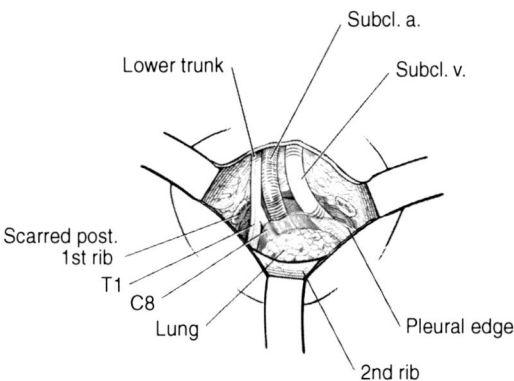

Fig. 39.3 Surgical treatment of recurrent neurogenic TOS. View of the transaxillary portion of the procedure after completion of apical pleurectomy, resection of any residual first rib, and dissection of the brachial plexus nerves, subclavian artery, and subclavian vein (Courtesy of HealthONE Presbyterian/St. Lukes Hospital, Denver, Colorado by Wes Price)

mobilizing and retracting medially the sterno-cleidomastoid muscle, dividing the scalene fat pad with a harmonic scalpel to decrease lymph leakage, and sectioning the omohyoid muscle if it is still intact. The C5 nerve root, lateral border of the upper brachial plexus and phrenic nerve are all identified at this time. A self-retaining retractor is used to facilitate the exposure. Careful, complete external neurolysis follows, mobilizing the five nerve roots and three trunks of the brachial plexus, as well as identifying and protecting the subclavian artery, phrenic nerve, long thoracic nerve and supra-scapular nerves. The dorsal scapular nerve and subclavian vein are rarely visualized.

After achieving complete neurolysis yet leaving the epineurium intact, the LDM flap is passed from the axilla over the second rib, dorsal and cephalad to the plexus, and in front of the long thoracic nerve (Fig. 39.5). The muscle flap is then dropped caudally, in front of the plexus, and its tail is tucked into the space between lower nerve trunk and artery (Figs. 39.6 and 39.7). A local anesthetic continuous-infusion catheter (0.2 % ropivacaine) is inserted for long-acting pain control, being placed inside the LDM wrap, and a drain is placed

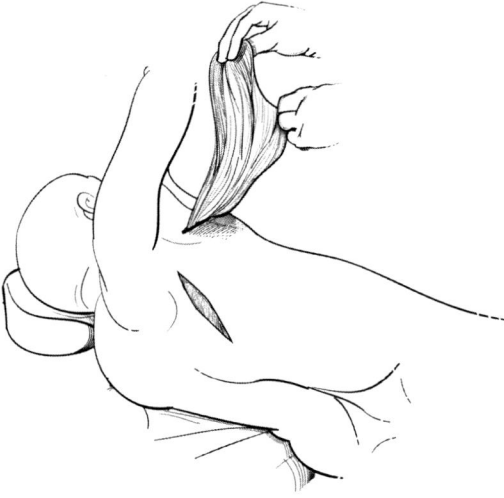

Fig. 39.4 Surgical treatment of recurrent neurogenic TOS. The latissimus dorsi muscle has been harvested and passed from the posterior to the axillary incision. Next, the posterior incision will be closed over a drain and a local anesthetic infusion catheter. The muscle will be tucked into the axilla and the axillary wound will be temporarily stapled closed (Courtesy of HealthONE Presbyterian/St. Lukes Hospital, Denver, Colorado by Wes Price)

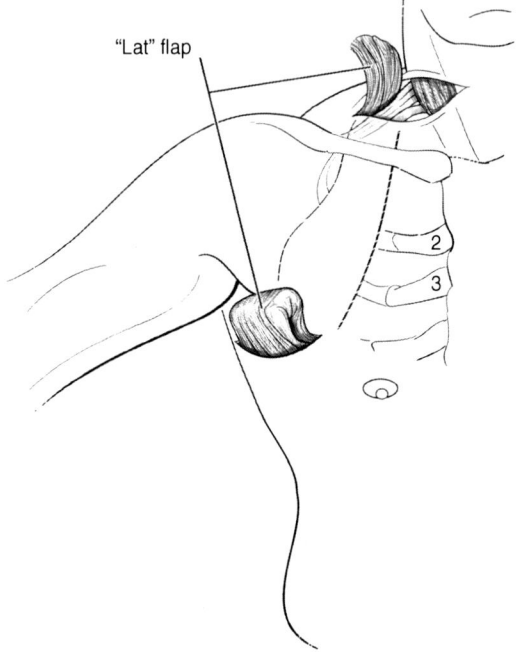

Fig. 39.5 Surgical treatment of recurrent neurogenic TOS. The supraclavicular brachial plexus neurolysis has been completed. The axillary wound is reopened and the muscle flap is passed over the second rib and behind the plexus, taking care to leave the arterial supply on the deep surface of the muscle. A 19 French channeled drain may be placed into the pleural cavity through a separate stab wound and positioned at this time (Courtesy of HealthONE Presbyterian/St. Lukes Hospital, Denver, Colorado by Wes Price)

into the apex of the pleural space thru a separate stab wound in the axilla. The supraclavicular and axillary wounds are closed in layers.

The purpose of the muscle flap is to provide a vascularized protective pad with a smooth glide surface on which the nerves can move. It provides a protective cushion and is designed to be a space-filler to help prevent ingrowth of scar tissue into the area of the brachial plexus nerve bundle. Neo-vascularization is also a possibility, extending from the well-vascularized muscle into the adjacent nerves [3–18].

The authors have performed neurolysis with a rotational LDM flap wrapped around the brachial plexus 36 times on 34 patients, 29 of whom were women. All had disabling neurogenic symptoms, many having had multiple previous attempts at neurolysis. Complications included one patient with postoperative anemia requiring transfusion, one wound infection, one pneumonia, one with significant atelectasis, one exacerbation of asthma, and one episode of postoperative atrial fibrillation. There were no injuries to the subclavian artery or vein, or to the phrenic nerve, long thoracic nerve

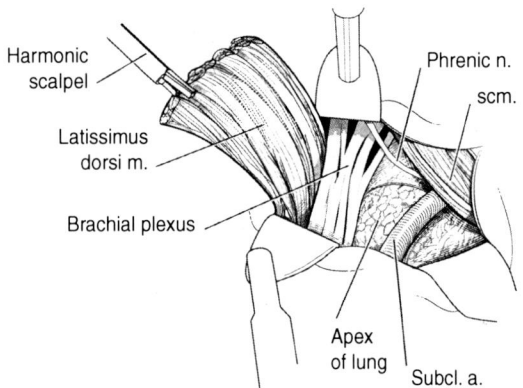

Fig. 39.6 Surgical treatment of recurrent neurogenic TOS. Excess muscle is trimmed using a harmonic scalpel so that the rotated muscle flap can be comfortably wrapped over the brachial plexus. A local anesthetic infusion catheter is placed over the plexus and under the flap (Courtesy of HealthONE Presbyterian/St. Lukes Hospital, Denver, Colorado by Wes Price)

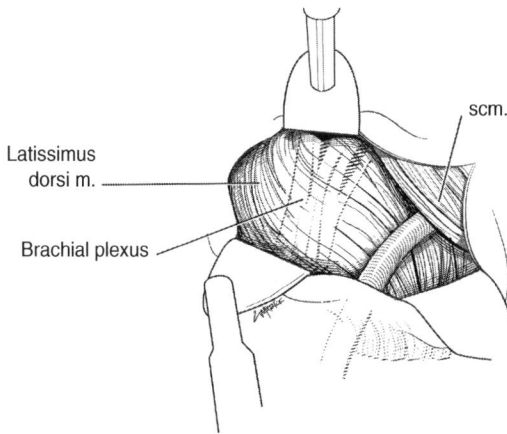

Fig. 39.7 Surgical treatment of recurrent neurogenic TOS. The muscle flap is inserted into the space between the brachial plexus nerves and the subclavian artery, and secured with sutures. The supraclavicular and axillary incisions are then closed (Courtesy of HealthONE Presbyterian/St. Lukes Hospital, Denver, Colorado by Wes Price)

or brachial plexus. Most patients remained hospitalized for 7 days following the procedure. Follow up data is available on 24 patients who have been contacted and questioned regarding outcomes, with a length of follow-up ranging from 6 months to 7 years after the procedure (mean, 43 months). One patient experienced no improvement in symptoms of recurrent neurogenic TOS. All other patients experienced a decrease in symptoms and improvement in arm function that ranged from 30 to 90 % by patient estimate, with the mean patient assessment of improvement being 60 %. These results have led us to consider use of the LDM flap in those patients suffering with severe neurogenic symptoms who have failed multiple previous attempts at surgical treatment.

References

1. Sanders RJ, Pearce WH. The treatment of thoracic outlet syndrome: a comparison of different operations. J Vasc Surg. 1989;10:626–34.
2. Upton ARM, McComas AJ. The double crush in nerve-entrapment syndromes. Lancet. 1973;2:359–62.
3. Mckinnon SE, Dellon AL. Multiple crush syndrome. In: Mackinnon SE, Dellon AL, editors. Surgery of the peripheral nerve. New York: Theime Medical Publishers; 1988. p. 347–92.
4. Huang JH, Zager E. Thoracic outlet syndrome. Neurosurgery. 2004;55:897–902.
5. Sanders RJ, Rao NM. The forgotten pectoralis minor syndrome: 100 operations for pectoralis minor syndrome alone or accompanied by neurogenic thoracic outlet syndrome. Ann Vasc Surg. 2010;24:701–8.
6. Sanders RJ. Recurrent neurogenic thoracic outlet syndrome stressing the importance of pectoralis minor syndrome. Vasc Endovascular Surg. 2011;45:33–8.
7. Sanders RJ, Hammond SL. Diagnosis of thoracic outlet syndrome. J Vasc Surg. 2007;46:601–4.
8. Elvey RL. The investigation of arm pain. In: Boyling JD, Palatonga N, Grieve GP, editors. Grieve's Modern manual therapy: the vertebral column. 2nd ed. Edinburgh: Churchill Livingstone; 1994. p. 577–85.
9. Jordan SE, Machleder HI. Diagnosis of thoracic outlet syndrome using electrophysiologically guided anterior scalene blocks. Ann Vasc Surg. 1998;12:260–4.
10. Machanic BI, Sanders RJ. Medial antebrachial cutaneous nerve measurements to diagnose neurogenic thoracic outlet syndrome. Ann Vasc Surg. 2008;22:248–54.
11. Murovic JA, Kim DH, Kim SH, Kline DG. Thoracic outlet syndrome, part II. Management and outcomes of 133 operative neurogenic thoracic outlet syndrome cases. Neurosurg Q. 2007;17:13–8.
12. Felice KJ, Butler KB, Druckemiller WH. Cervical root stimulation in a case of classic neurogenic thoracic outlet syndrome. Muscle Nerve. 1999;22:1287–92.
13. Ohman A, Astrom L, Malmgren-Olsson EB. Feldenkrais therapy as group treatment for chronic pain: a qualitative evaluation. J Bodyw Mov Ther. 2011;15:153–61.
14. Malmgren-Olsson EB, Branholm IB. A comparison between three physiotherapy approaches with regard to health-related factors in patients with non-specific musculoskeletal disorders. Disabil Rehabil. 2002;24:308–17.
15. Jain S, Janssen K, DeCelle S. Alexander technique and feldenkrais method: a critical overview. Phys Med Rehabil Clin N Am. 2004;15:811–25.
16. Ives JC. Comments on the feldenkrais method; a dynamic approach to changing motor behavior. Res Q Exerc Sport. 2003;74:116–26.
17. Ambrad-Chalela E, Thomas GI, Johansen KH. Recurrent neurogenic thoracic outlet syndrome. Am J Surg. 2004;187:505–10.
18. Jones NF, Shaw WW, Katz RG. Circumferential wrapping of a flap around a scarred peripheral nerve for salvage of end-stage traction neuritis. J Hand Surg. 1997;22A:527–35.
19. Bartlett S, May JW, Yaremchuk MJ. The latissimus dorsi muscle: a fresh cadaver study of the primary neurovascular pedicle. Plast Reconstr Surg. 1981;67:631–6.
20. Bostwick J, Nahai F, Wallace JG, Vasconez LO. Sixty latissimus dorsi flaps. Plast Reconstr Surg. 1979;63:31–41.
21. Tobin GR, Moberg AW, DuBou RH, Weiner LJ, Bland KI. The split latissimus dorsi myocutaneous flap. Ann Plast Surg. 1979;7:272–80.

Ying Wei Lum and Julie Ann Freischlag

Abstract

Surgical intervention remains the mainstay of therapy for the treatment of neurogenic thoracic outlet syndrome (NTOS). Evaluation of results and long term outcomes following surgical treatment has been difficult because there are no reliable, standardized or objective criteria to establish a diagnosis of NTOS and there is great variability in follow-up time and criteria for outcome. Various methods including subjective reporting, functional questionnaires, quality of life questionnaires, visual analogue scales and satisfaction scores have all been used to try to determine whether treatment has benefitted the patient. The etiology of the problem, patient demographics, the description and duration of symptoms, the response to the selective use of anterior scalene muscle blocks and surgical technique are amongst the major factors that have been studied in an attempt to predict outcome. Postoperative complications in most contemporary series cite relatively low complication rates, most of which are minor. Neurological injuries during surgical decompression demonstrate a much lower incidence in recent publications, at no more than 1 % or less.

In conclusion, few areas in surgery are as controversial as the topic of surgical therapy for NTOS. However, most who treat such patients believe that surgery remains an excellent option in properly selected patients with NTOS, particularly in those who have failed conservative treatment.

Introduction

Surgical intervention remains the mainstay of therapy for the treatment of neurogenic thoracic outlet syndrome (NTOS). Several different techniques (transaxillary, supraclavicular, transthoracic, posteriorly or subclavicular) are used for surgical decompression [1], with no obvious significant difference in success rates between the various surgical approaches. Evaluation of

Y.W. Lum, MD (✉)
Division of Vascular Surgery, John Hopkins
Hospital, 600 N. Wolfe Street, Harvey 611,
Baltimore, MD 21218, USA
e-mail: ylum@jhmi.edu

J.A. Freischlag, MD
Department of Surgery, Johns Hopkins
Medical Institutions, Baltimore, MD, USA

results and long term outcomes following surgical treatment has been difficult because there are no reliable, standardized or objective criteria to establish a diagnosis of NTOS and there is great variability in follow-up time and criteria for outcome. Furthermore, other pathologic conditions such as herniated cervical disk, rotator cuff injuries, peripheral nerve entrapment, chronic pain syndromes (such as chronic regional pain syndromes and fibromyalgia), as well as psychological conditions may mimic NTOS and affect long term results. It is this difficulty in diagnostic variability (in patient selection) and measurement of outcomes that accounts for the wide range of results achieved in the literature.

Assessment of Outcomes

While widely variable in the literature, early postoperative success for surgical treatment of NTOS has been reported to occur in as many as 90 % of cases [2]. Unlike venous or arterial TOS, there is no good objective test that has been firmly established to measure differences in baseline and post-therapeutic intervention levels. Subsequently, various methods including subjective reporting, [1, 3] functional questionnaires, [4–6] quality of life questionnaires, [7, 8] visual analogue scales and satisfaction scores [9, 10] have all been used to try to determine whether treatment has benefitted the patient. These scales integrate various subjective measurements of pain relief, ability to return to usual work or activities, reduction or freedom from narcotic pain medication usage, and freedom from re-intervention to determine outcome. Regardless of the method in assessing outcome, the early success rate has remained similar throughout the various studies.

Predictors of Surgical Outcomes

The etiology of the problem, patient demographics, the description and duration of symptoms, the response to the selective use of anterior scalene muscle blocks, and surgical technique are amongst the major factors that have been studied in an attempt to predict outcome.

One of the most well-established factors predicting outcome in patients with NTOS is the cause of the problem. Several investigators have documented that injury due to trauma or repetitive stress injuries in the work place are predictors of a worse outcome [3, 11–14]. It has been postulated that secondary gain factors such as economic compensation and litigation issues are the confounding factors that lead to this. Conversely, non-laborious positions are associated with better outcomes than laborious occupations [15, 16].

A longer duration of symptoms prior to surgical intervention has been associated with poorer outcome [3, 14, 17]. For example, Cheng found poorer surgical outcomes in patients whose symptom duration was greater than 24 months prior to treatment [17]. Some have postulated the possibility of repetitive stimulation of central pain pathways that result in autonomous pain generators over time, in a fashion similar to the situation in patients with chronic regional pain syndrome [4, 18]; this concept correlates well with the notion that vague symptomatology also has a negative effect on surgical outcomes. [5, 6] The exact duration of symptoms prior to surgical intervention that is likely to adversely affect outcome remains to be determined and is likely highly "fuzzy." A duration of symptom cutoff as long as 24 months was previously described [3, 17], but others have noticed delays as short as 6 months correlate with worsened outcomes [1]. One group has gone as far as excluding patients with symptoms greater than 12 months, which interestingly resulted in more durable long term outcomes [4]. Intuitively, a longer duration of symptoms could also translate into a higher number of prior interventions, which in turn has also been identified as a factor correlating with a lower rate of surgical success.[3]

There is evidence that the results of preoperative anterior scalene muscle blockade correlate with surgical outcome [4, 19–21] (See Chap. 27). The accuracy of these procedures to selectively inject the anterior scalene muscle can be further increased with the adjunctive use of electromyography [19], ultrasonography [22], and/or computerized tomography [23].

Demographic factors such as age [14] have been less well studied. One group found a higher rate of continued disability following surgery for NTOS in patients that were older at age of injury. Similarly, unpublished data at our institution derived from 159 first rib resection and anterior scalenectomy procedures show that surgery was more likely to relieve symptoms (at 12 months) in patients younger than 40 (90 % vs. 77.8 %, $p < 0.05$).

Surprisingly, the presence of a cervical rib as well as the necessity and extent of first rib resection itself are poor predictors of outcome. These topics are addressed in Chap. 13, "Cervical Ribs and NTOS," but in general the surgical success rates for patients with a cervical rib and NTOS are no better than for those without. [1, 11], which supports the view that the diagnosis of NTOS should be made clinically with little reliance on the presence or absence of a bony anomaly [24]. The very concept of first rib resection after scalenectomy has been questioned by some [17] (See Chap. 69). This notion does not correlate with the concept that various anatomic abnormalities such as fibrous bands are often present, however [10, 15]. Perhaps a plausible explanation could be that acceptable immediate results following scalenectomy can be achieved, but that these results may not be durable due to scarring and reattachment of the scalene muscles to the rib. Indeed, there is also evidence that the recurrence rates for NTOS are higher without adequate rib resection [6, 15, 25, 26].

Postoperative Complications

A factor that may delay surgery in patients with NTOS is the potential for complications [27, 28]. Such a delay will lead to an increased duration of symptom, which in turn will negatively affect surgical outcome. In reality, most contemporary series cite relatively low complication rates, most of which are minor. Overall complication rates (excluding intercosto-brachial numbness) usually range between 2 and 15 % [3, 6, 29]. Pneumothoraces, at 2–15 %, account for

the vast majority of complications, which are self-limiting and treated with tube decompression [30]. At our institution, tube decompression is performed using a pediatric chest tube placed intra-operatively and removed the following day with no delay in length of stay, and many other institutions treat such patients with observation alone. Other complications that have relatively low rates of incidence include chylothorax, seroma, wound infection, and suture granuloma. Short of major vascular injuries (which are very rare (<1 %) [15]), neurological complications are the most devastating potential complication of thoracic outlet decompression. Reported results vary widely. Although earlier reports described "brachial plexus nerve injury" rates of as high as 24 % [31], most recent reports demonstrate a much lower incidence, at no more than 1 % or less [1, 2, 10, 15, 29, 32]. Other potential neurologic injuries (rates depending upon surgical approach, procedure(s) performed, and levels of suspicion and investigational tools used) include phrenic nerve injuries in up to 12 % of patients, permanent long thoracic nerve injuries in less than 1 % (probably underreported), and Horner's syndrome (also in less than 1 %) [1, 33]. Overall, these data demonstrate that surgical decompression of the thoracic outlet can be safely performed. The surgeon's comfort with the anatomy and choice of surgical approach is of paramount importance in performing these procedures to ensure that the risk-benefit ratio of these procedures continue to justify operative intervention for NTOS.

Late Term Outcome

One of the main problems in the assessment of results following treatment for NTOS is the lack of a clear objective diagnostic standard. Obviously the most important factor influencing long-term results is the accuracy of this diagnosis [34]. Recurrent symptoms often occur following the initial surgery [35], which helps determine the patterns of failure and differences in early versus late outcomes. Even in series reporting the best possible early outcomes, such initial success has been reported to be followed by deterioration

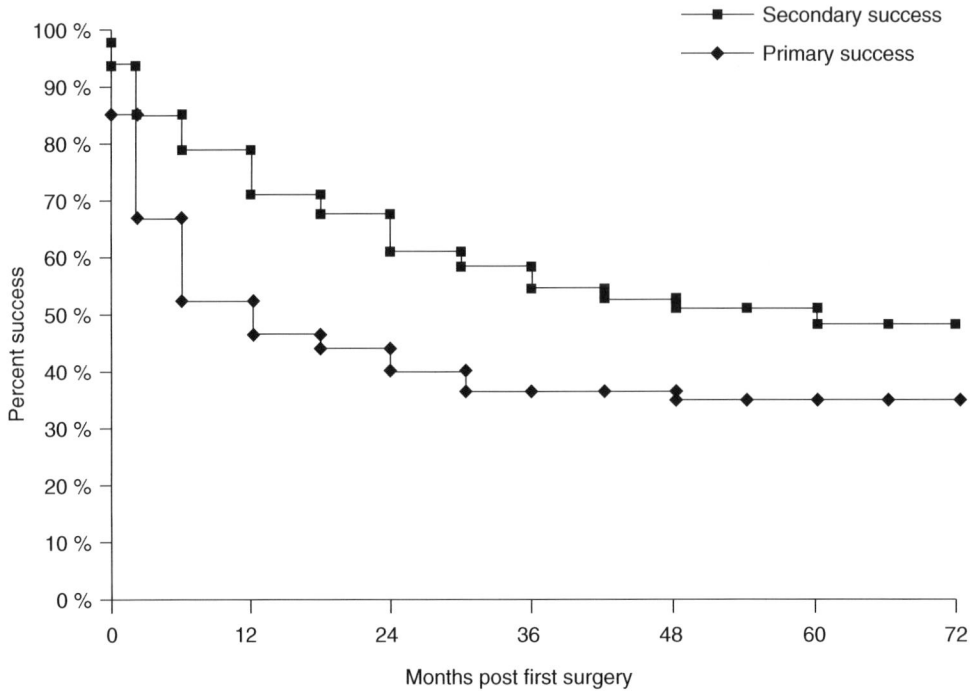

Secondary success

At risk	254	200	128	87	54	31	13
S.E.	0.000	0.025	0.034	0.041	0.049	0.065	0.097

Primary success

At risk	254	155	74	54	36	17	10
S.E.	0.000	0.029	0.039	0.040	0.050	0.070	0.091

Fig. 40.1 Life table analysis demonstrating pattern of failure over time (Reprinted from Altobelli et al. [3]. With permission from Elsevier)

after 12–18 months (Fig. 40.1) and as late as 5–10 years [7]. Outcomes in series with a minimum of 2 years follow up demonstrate overall success rates as low as 37 % [34] and as high as 95 % [15]. Most series seem to document medium- to long-term success, however, in 60–85 % of patients (Table 40.1).

Despite a less than optimal long term success rate, however, patients that do see a benefit from surgery for NTOS have a significant improvement in their quality of life. Chang et al. performed a quality of life study using two validated patient-reported quality of life instruments, the Disability of the Arm, Shoulder and Hand (DASH) and Short-Form 12 (SF-12) surveys.

Patients with NTOS had a significantly lower Physical Component Score (PCS) and Mental Component Score (MCS) at presentation compared to the normal population. A striking finding was that this score was even lower than the levels recorded in patients with chronic prostatitis, hypertension, or diabetes, and similar to those with chronic heart failure. Following surgery, however, these patients demonstrated improvements in returning to full time work or activity. Interestingly, in terms of quality of life, patients had quicker improvements in mental function (plateauing at 12 months following surgery) as compared to physical function (plateauing at 23 months following surgery) (Fig. 40.2) [8].

Table 40.1 Comparison of various TOS studies showing results

Series	Type of TOS					Follow-up (years)	Surgical approach			Excellent and good results
	Arterial (A-TOS)	Venous (V-TOS)	Neurogenic (N-TOS)	Combined (C-TOS)	Recurrent (R-TOS)		Transaxillary	Supraclavicular	Other	
Degeorges et al. [6]	38	27	15	96	–	7.5 (2–19)	107	69	–	84 %
Green et al. [36]	–	–	147	–	–	5	147	–	–	72–83 %
Jamieson [29]	29	12	368	–	–	4	93 %	7 %	–	72 %
Hempel et al. [37]	16	46	708	–	–	>2	–	770	–	86 %
Kieffer et al. [38]	38	–	–	–	–	3.6	–	33	–	86.8 %
Landry et al. [39]	–	–	79	–	–	4.2 (2–7.5)	19 (surgery)	–	64 (no operation)	66 % (no operation); 54 % (surgery)
Leffert [40]	–	–	282	–	–	4.6 (0.5–21.1)	282	–	–	69.2 %
Lindgren et al. [35]	3	2	146	24	–	2	175	–	–	59 %
Sanders et al. [41]	–	–	–	–	134	–	26	108	–	84 % (3 months); 59 % (second year); 41 % (10 years)
Sanders and Hamond [11]	–	–	46	–	8	<5	2	52	–	59 %
Urschel and Razzuk [42]	240	264	2,210	–	1,221	–	2,714	–	Posterior if R-TOS	77.6 % (V-TOS); 95 % (N-TOS)
Wood and Twito [43]	20	20	81	–	2	5.5	123	–	–	89 %

Reprinted from Degeorges et al. [6]. With permission from Elsevier

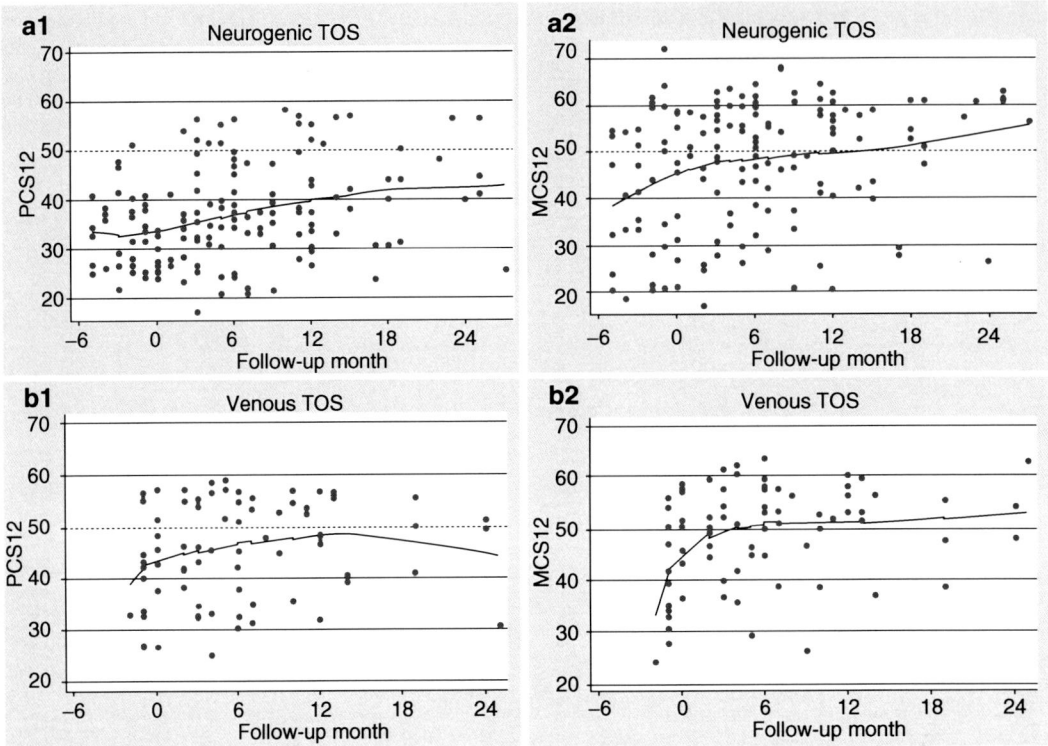

Fig. 40.2 Graphs demonstrating quality of life outcome of NTOS patients, with their (**a1**) Physical component scores (PCS) and (**a2**) Mental component scores (MCS). Comparisons were made to venous TOS patients with their (**b1**) Physical component scores (PCS) and (**b2**) Mental component scores (MCS) (Reprinted from Chang et al. [8]. With permission from Elsevier)

Similar benefits in long term outcomes have been demonstrated by others. [4] In a recent series reported by Scali, surgically treated patients demonstrated a decreased need for nonsteroidal anti-inflammatory drugs, muscle relaxants, physical therapy, and subsequent additional scalene blockade. There was a trend towards decreased narcotic use, although that did not reach statistical significance [4].

Conclusion

Few areas in surgery are as controversial (or as poorly studied) as the topic of surgical therapy for NTOS. Citing series showing dips in the success rates to 60 % several years following surgical intervention [3, 7]. A recent Cochrane review concluded that "there is currently no evidence demonstrating the beneficial effects of established operative or non-operative interventions compared with natural progression for pain relief in TOS" [44]. Furthermore, good results from conservative treatment alone with intensive

physical therapy alone [27, 45] or anterior scalene muscle block with botulinum toxin [20, 23] have been reported. However, most who treat such patients believe that surgery remains an excellent option in properly selected patients with NTOS, particularly in those who have failed conservative treatment [29, 46–48]. In addition, there is uncontrolled evidence that surgery may offer potential longer term benefits and significant improvement in quality of life over time [8]. It is stressed that well controlled, long-term studies of outcome with the varying treatment options available are badly needed in this area.

References

1. Toso C, et al. Thoracic outlet syndrome: influence of personal history and surgical technique on long-term results. Eur J Cardiothorac Surg. 1999;16(1):44–7.
2. Sanders RJ. Results of the surgical treatment for thoracic outlet syndrome. Semin Thorac Cardiovasc Surg. 1996;8(2):221–8.

3. Altobelli GG, et al. Thoracic outlet syndrome: pattern of clinical success after operative decompression. J Vasc Surg. 2005;42(1):122–8.

4. Scali S, et al. Long-term functional results for the surgical management of neurogenic thoracic outlet syndrome. Vasc Endovascular Surg. 2010;44(7):550–5.

5. Jordan SE, Ahn SS, Gelabert HA. Differentiation of thoracic outlet syndrome from treatment-resistant cervical brachial pain syndromes: development and utilization of a questionnaire, clinical examination and ultrasound evaluation. Pain Physician. 2007;10(3):441–52.

6. Degeorges R, Reynaud C, Becquemin JP. Thoracic outlet syndrome surgery: long-term functional results. Ann Vasc Surg. 2004;18(5):558–65.

7. Bosma J, et al. The influence of choice of therapy on quality of life in patients with neurogenic thoracic outlet syndrome. Br J Neurosurg. 2010;24(5):532–6.

8. Chang DC, et al. Surgical intervention for thoracic outlet syndrome improves patient's quality of life. J Vasc Surg. 2009;49(3):630–5, discussion 635–7.

9. Mackinnon SE. Thoracic outlet syndrome. Ann Thorac Surg. 1994;58(2):287–9.

10. Vogelin E, et al. Long-term outcome analysis of the supraclavicular surgical release for the treatment of thoracic outlet syndrome. Neurosurgery. 2010;66(6):1085–91, discussion 1091–2.

11. Sanders RJ, Hammond SL. Management of cervical ribs and anomalous first ribs causing neurogenic thoracic outlet syndrome. J Vasc Surg. 2002;36(1):51–6.

12. Poole GV, Thomae KR. Thoracic outlet syndrome reconsidered. Am Surg. 1996;62(4):287–91.

13. Ellison DW, Wood VE. Trauma-related thoracic outlet syndrome. J Hand Surg [Br]. 1994;19(4):424–6.

14. Franklin GM, et al. Outcome of surgery for thoracic outlet syndrome in Washington state workers' compensation. Neurology. 2000;54(6):1252–7.

15. Urschel Jr HC. Neurovascular compression in the thoracic outlet: changing management over 50 years. Adv Surg. 1999;33:95–111.

16. Goff CD, et al. A comparison of surgery for neurogenic thoracic outlet syndrome between laborers and nonlaborers. Am J Surg. 1998;176(2):215–8.

17. Cheng SW, et al. Neurogenic thoracic outlet decompression: rationale for sparing the first rib. Cardiovasc Surg. 1995;3(6):617–23, discussion: 624.

18. Birklein F, et al. The important role of neuropeptides in complex regional pain syndrome. Neurology. 2001;57(12):2179–84.

19. Jordan SE, Machleder HI. Diagnosis of thoracic outlet syndrome using electrophysiologically guided anterior scalene blocks. Ann Vasc Surg. 1998;12(3):260–4.

20. Jordan SE, et al. Selective botulinum chemodenervation of the scalene muscles for treatment of neurogenic thoracic outlet syndrome. Ann Vasc Surg. 2000;14(4):365–9.

21. Howard M, Lee C, Dellon AL. Documentation of brachial plexus compression (in the thoracic inlet) utilizing provocative neurosensory and muscular testing. J Reconstr Microsurg. 2003;19(5):303–12.

22. Jordan SE, Ahn SS, Gelabert HA. Combining ultrasonography and electromyography for botulinum chemodenervation treatment of thoracic outlet syndrome: comparison with fluoroscopy and electromyography guidance. Pain Physician. 2007;10(4):541–6.

23. Christo PJ, et al. Single CT-guided chemodenervation of the anterior scalene muscle with botulinum toxin for neurogenic thoracic outlet syndrome. Pain Med. 2010;11(4):504–11.

24. Donaghy M, Matkovic Z, Morris P. Surgery for suspected neurogenic thoracic outlet syndromes: a follow up study. J Neurol Neurosurg Psychiatry. 1999;67(5):602–6.

25. Mingoli A, et al. Long-term outcome after transaxillary approach for thoracic outlet syndrome. Surgery. 1995;118(5):840–4.

26. Ambrad-Chalela E, Thomas GI, Johansen KH. Recurrent neurogenic thoracic outlet syndrome. Am J Surg. 2004;187(4):505–10.

27. Lindgren KA. Conservative treatment of thoracic outlet syndrome: a 2-year follow-up. Arch Phys Med Rehabil. 1997;78(4):373–8.

28. Melliere D, et al. Severe injuries resulting from operations for thoracic outlet syndrome: can they be avoided? J Cardiovasc Surg (Torino). 1991;32(5):599–603.

29. Jamieson WG, Chinnick B. Thoracic outlet syndrome: fact or fancy? A review of 409 consecutive patients who underwent operation. Can J Surg. 1996;39(4):321–6.

30. Atasoy E. Combined surgical treatment of thoracic outlet syndrome: transaxillary first rib resection and transcervical scalenectomy. Hand Clin. 2004;20(1):71–82, vii.

31. Dale WA. Thoracic outlet compression syndrome. Critique in 1982. Arch Surg. 1982;117(11):1437–45.

32. Chang DC, et al. Reported in-hospital complications following rib resections for neurogenic thoracic outlet syndrome. Ann Vasc Surg. 2007;21(5):564–70.

33. Rigberg D, Freischlag JA. Complications of thoracic outlet surgery. In: Towne J, Hollier LH, editors. Complications in vascular surgery. New York: Marcel Dekker; 2004. p. 429–38.

34. Lepantalo M, et al. Long term outcome after resection of the first rib for thoracic outlet syndrome. Br J Surg. 1989;76(12):1255–6.

35. Lindgren SH, Ribbe EB, Norgren LE. Two year follow-up of patients operated on for thoracic outlet syndrome. Effects on sick-leave incidence. Eur J Vasc Surg. 1989;3(5):411–5.

36. Green RM, McNamara J, Ouriel K. Long-term follow-up after thoracic outlet syndrome decompression: an analysis of factors determining outcome. J Vasc Surg. 1991;14:739–46

37. Hempel KG, et al. 770 consecutive supraclavicular first rib resections for thoracic outlet syndrome. Ann Vasc Surg. 1996;10:456–63

38. Kieffer E, Jue-Denis P, Benhamou M. Complications artérielles du syndrome de la traversée thoracobrachiale. Chirurgie. 1983;109:714–22

39. Landry GJ, et al. Long-term functional outcome of neurogenic thoracic outlet syndrome in surgically and

conservatively treated patients. J Vasc Surg. 2001;34:760–1

40. Leffert RD. Thoracic outlet syndrome: results of 282 transaxillary first rib resection. Clin Orthop. 1999;368:66–79

41. Sanders RJ, Craig EH, Pearce WP. Recurrent thoracic outlet syndrome. J Vasc Surg. 1990;12:390–400

42. Urschel HC, Razzuk MA. Neurovascular compression in the thoracic outlet. Ann Surg. 1998;228: 609–17

43. Wood VE, Twito R. Thoracic outlet syndrome: the results of first rib resection in 100 patients. Orthop Clin North Am. 1988;19:131–46

44. Povlsen B, et al. Treatment for thoracic outlet syndrome. Cochrane Database Syst Rev. 2010;1: CD007218.

45. Wishchuk JR, Dougherty CR. Therapy after thoracic outlet release. Hand Clin. 2004;20(1):87–90, vii.

46. Martens V, Bugden C. Thoracic outlet syndrome: a review of 67 cases. Can J Surg. 1980;23(4):357–8.

47. Sheth RN, Campbell JN. Surgical treatment of thoracic outlet syndrome: a randomized trial comparing two operations. J Neurosurg Spine. 2005;3(5):355–63.

48. Sanders RJ, Pearce WH. The treatment of thoracic outlet syndrome: a comparison of different operations. J Vasc Surg. 1989;10(6):626–34.

Directions in Clinical Research on NTOS

Robert W. Thompson, Anna M. Wittenberg, and Francis J. Caputo

Abstract

Neurogenic thoracic outlet syndrome (NTOS) is a relatively uncommon condition caused by compression and irritation of the brachial plexus nerve roots. The location of nerve compression may be within the scalene triangle at the level of the first rib or in the subcoracoid space beneath the pectoralis minor muscle tendon. NTOS most frequently occurs in relatively young, active, and otherwise healthy individuals, often in association with previous neck and/or upper extremity injury, and the symptoms may progress to cause substantial disability. Despite several decades of debate regarding proper diagnosis and optimal treatment, NTOS continues to be poorly understood and understudied. Thus, there is a tremendous need and opportunity for productive clinical research related to NTOS, particularly with increased emphasis on evidence-based medicine. In this chapter we outline some of the areas that appear to be most fruitful for investigation, and several strategies by which to help move forward our understanding and management of NTOS.

R.W. Thompson, MD (✉)
Department of Surgery, Section of Vascular Surgery,
Center for Thoracic Outlet Syndrome,
Washington University, Barnes-Jewish Hospital,
Campus Box 8109/Suite 5101 Queeny Tower,
660 S Euclid Avenue, St. Louis, MO 63110, USA
e-mail: thompson@wudosis.wustl.edu

A.M. Wittenberg, MPH
Department of Internal Medicine/Cardiovascular
Division, Barnes-Jewish Hospital,
Campus Box 8109/Suite 5101 Queeny Tower,
660 S Euclid Avenue, St. Louis, MO 63110, USA

F.J. Caputo, MD
Division of Vascular and Endovascular Surgery,
Department of Surgery, Cooper University Hospital,
Camden, NJ 08103, USA

Introduction

Neurogenic thoracic outlet syndrome (NTOS) is a relatively uncommon condition caused by compression and irritation of the brachial plexus nerve roots. The site of neural compression is typically within the scalene triangle at the level of the first rib, but may also occur within the subcoracoid space underneath the pectoralis minor muscle tendon. NTOS most frequently occurs in relatively young, active, and otherwise healthy individuals, particularly those engaged in heavy lifting or repetitive overhead use of the upper extremity in recreational or occupational activities. NTOS is often associated with a history of neck and/or upper extremity injury, previous surgical and non-surgical treatment approaches intended to alleviate the presenting symptoms, and protracted delays in diagnosis.

The clinical presentation of NTOS is typified by symptoms of pain, numbness and paresthesias in the arm and/or hand, often accompanied by pain in the neck, chest, and/or upper back, with reproducible exacerbation by overhead positioning and use of the upper extremity. The symptoms of NTOS may be particularly important as they can progress to disability in young active persons in school or the prime of working life. A consistent constellation of physical examination findings includes localized tenderness to palpation over the supraclavicular and/or subcoracoid space with reproduction of radiating upper extremity symptoms, and exacerbation of symptoms during positional upper extremity maneuvers, such as the 3-min elevated arm stress test (EAST).

Conservative management based on physical therapy is the mainstay of initial treatment for NTOS, along with muscle relaxants, anti-inflammatory agents and adjustments in workplace ergonomic factors. Unfortunately, physical therapy alone may not improve symptoms in patients with substantial and/or longstanding disability. Surgical treatment for NTOS may be recommended in this setting but its role has often been controversial, due in part to differences in diagnostic criteria, variations in the efficacy of physical therapy, inconsistent indications for surgery, and diversity in the patient populations treated. The role of surgery has also been difficult to define due to the use of different surgical approaches, techniques and adjuncts, the relatively small clinical volumes and short-term follow-up in reported studies, and a limited application of defined outcome metrics by which to quantitatively assess results, making the factors determining outcomes for surgical treatment of NTOS incompletely understood. Upon this background it is evident that NTOS remains one of the most controversial conditions in clinical medicine and that there is a great need and opportunity for clinical research related to this disorder. In his chapter we outline some of the most

needed and promising directions for clinical research on NTOS.

Incidence, Etiology, and Pathophysiology of NTOS

Several fundamental questions about NTOS remain to be resolved, related to the incidence, etiology and pathophysiology of this condition. As highlighted throughout this textbook, it is no longer sufficient to state that NTOS is "rare," that its existence is "controversial," or that its cause is "idiopathic." The following areas need to be addressed to obtain better data-driven understanding of the various risk factors and variables that might influence the development of NTOS.

• There is a fundamental need for more detailed information regarding the actual incidence of NTOS in the general population, as well as within certain groups potentially at elevated risk for developing this condition (e.g., manual laborers, office workers involved in repetitive motion tasks). Use of information derived from population databases is a considerable challenge for NTOS, given variations and inaccuracies in diagnostic coding and incomplete data. The most likely approach to help resolve this question will be through development of condition-specific registries, driven by physicians, therapists, clinical investigators, and health care administrators. This effort will in turn require multidisciplinary consensus regarding the most appropriate criteria for diagnosis and patient classification.

• Variations in anatomy surrounding the brachial plexus nerve roots are often considered a key factor in the development of NTOS. It is important to develop a better understanding of the pathophysiology of NTOS as related to congenital variations such as cervical ribs, first rib anomalies, and soft tissues (e.g., scalene minimus muscle, ligamentous and fibrous bands).

• Development of NTOS is also frequently associated with head, neck or upper extremity injury, and several studies have demonstrated microscopic alterations in the scalene muscles removed from patients that have undergone surgery for NTOS. It would be particularly valuable to obtain more rigorous information on the type and extent of scalene muscle trauma, and the pathological sequence of changes that occur within these muscles, as related to the development and progression of NTOS. Obtaining additional information on the types of injury that precipitate scalene muscle injury would also be a valuable direction.

- Postural and functional alterations in use of the neck and upper extremity are common in patients with NTOS, but it is not always clear if these changes occur before the onset of symptoms, coincident with neural compression, or as a secondary consequence to compensate for brachial plexus compression. Further investigation is therefore needed to evaluate the specific roles of repetitive motion injury, postural alterations, and imbalances in shoulder girdle muscle mechanics in the etiology of NTOS.

- Many patients with NTOS experience a long and frustrating history of symptom progression, but others appear to have symptoms that readily improve without extensive or invasive treatment approaches. It would be valuable to achieve a better understanding of the "natural history" of NTOS as it relates to the progression and regression of symptoms over time in the absence of treatment, how symptoms are affected by various activities and other factors, and the potential for permanent or sustained nerve injury or dysfunction in those that have had prolonged symptoms.

Diagnosis and Functional Assessment in NTOS

The diagnosis of NTOS is typically based on clinical pattern-recognition, often suggested by a stereotypical history and description of symptoms, coupled with the exclusion or identification of other conditions which might produce overlapping symptoms and physical exam findings. It remains a considerable challenge to distinguish

NTOS from such other conditions and there are to date no single definitive diagnostic tests that can accurately establish the presence or absence of NTOS. It is also apparent that patients with NTOS exhibit a wide range in the extent and severity of symptoms, and that the functional effects of NTOS vary considerably from one individual to another. Investigations to address the following areas will be particularly important to improve the diagnosis and functional assessment of NTOS.

- Future progress in the field is dependent on defining more consistent protocols for the clinical evaluation of patients suspected to have NTOS and the most appropriate and productive approaches by which to establish or exclude this condition. It is important that protocols include standardized aspects of the history and physical examination as related to both NTOS and potentially overlapping or coexisting neurogenic conditions (e.g., cervical spine and/or peripheral nerve compression syndromes), the potential coexistence of NTOS with either arterial or venous forms of TOS, and to avoid aspects of evaluation found to be unproductive, confusing, and unnecessarily expensive.

- There is a vital need to develop more clear, rigorously validated, objective diagnostic criteria for NTOS. It is clear that this effort will be more similar to that used to define conditions requiring sets of diagnostic criteria, such as rheumatological diseases, as opposed to the identification of a single diagnostic test. The effort to develop criteria of this nature may involve studies from individual centers but will be most effectively achieved by a multidisciplinary consensus process that takes into account the diversity of approaches used by different specialists. Additional investigations will be subsequently needed to validate such diagnostic criteria against other coexisting criteria and against outcomes-based measures, to help understand the importance of individual factors in reaching a diagnosis and in predicting outcomes.

- In conjunction with the development of standardized approaches to clinical evaluation and definition of diagnostic criteria for NTOS, it will be helpful to identify specific clinical characteristics that might more effectively stratify individual patients and/or better predict outcomes of treatment. This effort, similar to the development of "staging" systems for other disorders, will be especially useful in facilitating comparative effectiveness research to evaluate optimal approaches to treatment for patients across a spectrum of severity.

• In recent years, one of the most frequently used approaches to the diagnosis of NTOS has been the use of scalene muscle blocks with local anesthetic. This approach has been developed and refined, particularly by Jordan and colleagues, to establish optimal methods for the techniques for localizing the anesthetic injection, use of different imaging modalities, spectrum of muscle targets to be injected, and interpretation of results; use of scalene muscle blocks with botulinum toxin has also been examined as a mode of treatment for NTOS. Further studies are therefore needed to continue defining the most effective use of scalene muscle blocks for diagnostic, prognostic, and treatment purposes in patients with NTOS.

• A number of radiographic studies have been utilized as part of the diagnostic approach to NTOS, both to help exclude potential overlapping or coexisting conditions (e.g., cervical spine MRI for degenerative disc disease) or to help demonstrate brachial plexus compression and/or functional abnormalities (ranging from plain cervical spine radiographs to demonstrate the presence or absence of cervical ribs to functional MR "neurography" to detect nerve root impingement and perineural inflammation or edema). To date, such imaging studies have not been widely accepted as either sufficient or necessary for the diagnosis of NTOS. Additional investigations are thereby needed to more rigorously evaluate the role of specific types of imaging that might prove useful in the diagnosis of NTOS and potentially in guiding treatment decisions and optimal approaches.

• The role of electrophysiological testing in the diagnosis of NTOS has been examined for many years, yet it is generally recognized that overt abnormalities on conventional electromyography (EMG) and nerve conduction velocity (NCV) studies are not usually present in most patients otherwise considered to have a sound diagnosis. A number of explanations have been offered for the lack of objective findings on EMG/NCV in NTOS, yet some physicians insist that the diagnosis is flawed in the absence of electrophysiological abnormalities. In addition, more recent investigations have suggested that some forms of NCV testing, focused on the medial antebrachial cutaneous nerve, can have a particularly high sensitivity and specificity in patients with NTOS, and may even demonstrate normalization following treatment. Much more study is needed to define the validity of electrophysiological testing in NTOS, both as an adjunct to clinical diagnosis and as a means to predict outcomes of treatment.

• In addition to diagnosis, the evaluation of patients with NTOS typically involves an assessment of functional disability attributable to the condition. This is usually conducted by an informal assessment of activities and positions that aggravate symptoms, and by evaluating the ability of the patient to perform specific tasks. Functional assessment is important in stratifying the severity of NTOS in individual patients, to make treatment decisions, and to estimate the potential for improvement and/or return to work following treatment. It is thereby crucial to develop better and more specific tools to measure functional activity and disability in patients with NTOS, including potentially more objective measures such as those that might be obtained through focused activity surveys, performance-based testing, and use of arm motion monitors and other technical approaches.

Treatment Approaches to NTOS and Evaluation of Clinical Outcomes

Conservative treatment with physical therapy and pharmacological pain management is recommended as initial management for virtually all patients with NTOS, but there remain few studies documenting the overall response to and effectiveness of this approach. Valid comparisons between conservative treatment and surgical approaches are unlikely, given that these treatments are generally recommended sequentially and in different clinical situations, for different patient populations, and at different stages of disability. Thoracic outlet decompression may be effective and safely performed by either transaxillary or supraclavicular approaches, but valid comparisons between different operations are complicated by substantial variations in technique, as well as a lack of consistent criteria for reporting results, and there is presently no high-quality evidence indicating any significant differences in early or long-term outcomes. Limited observations indicate that reoperations for recurrent NTOS can be equally effective, but the optimal approach to recurrent and persistent symptoms must be individualized based on the previous procedure(s) performed and other patient-specific factors. From a limited number of studies using quality-of-life endpoints, it appears that the long-term results of surgical treatment for NTOS are probably considerably better than commonly understood or described in the literature, but this is dependent on relatively long periods of recovery and ongoing patient management. The following topics thereby offer a spectrum of potential directions for clinical research to address these various considerations.

- There remains a significant need to identify better pharmacological approaches and protocols for pain management appropriate for patients with NTOS, including judicious use of opiate narcotic analgesics, muscle relaxants, neuromodulators, antidepressants, pain management interventions, and psychological and psychiatric support.
- Focused studies are needed to determine the optimal forms of physical therapy for NTOS and how individualized treatment might be optimally devised and translated to wider patient populations at various stages of disability.
- Further investigations are needed toward the improvement of surgical techniques and adjuncts, along with approaches to postoperative care, to provide more thorough and durable

results of treatment for NTOS. This in turn will depend on better understanding of the causes and mechanisms of persistent and recurrent NTOS. Efforts to identify optimal postoperative physical therapy and rehabilitation regimens, as well as goal-directed return-to-work protocols, are important toward improving surgical outcomes.

- It will remain valuable to identify and examine "best approaches" from treatment centers specializing in the management of patients with NTOS and to prospectively evaluate how approaches unique to such centers might be most effectively translated to other centers where NTOS might be treated less frequently. Similarly, it will be valuable to explore the clinical outcomes and implications of regionalization of specialist care for NTOS and how this has been implemented in different areas of the country.
- Treatment approaches to NTOS utilizing scalene/pectoralis muscle injection with botulinum toxin injections have been explored in recent years, but the results of this approach remain uncertain and likely temporary at best. Use of botulinum toxin would nonetheless appear to have promise in some clinical settings. Better definition of the role for botulinum toxin in the treatment of at least some subsets of patients with NTOS would therefore be a fruitful area for further study.
- It will remain crucial to better characterize current short- and long-term outcomes for the treatment of NTOS and to establish which outcomes measures are optimal for assessing results for this condition. It is clear from recent studies that the application of current quality-of-life instruments is feasible and valid for longitudinal assessment in this patient population and can be expected to yield a great deal of new information regarding the long-term outcomes of patients with NTOS. This effort will be best achieved through development of one or more large registries by which patient outcomes can be accurately tracked.
- The best management of patients with persistent and recurrent symptoms of NTOS following surgical intervention remains to be defined,

along with the application of various topical medications and adjunctive interventional techniques, such as trigger-point (muscle) injections and spinal cord stimulators. The role of reoperations for NTOS also remains an understudied area, as is the role of various treatment options for disorders that often coexist with NTOS, such as complex regional pain syndrome (CRPS).

Conclusion

In summary, despite the recognition that there are substantial variations in the diagnosis and treatment of NTOS between various specialists and across the country, this disorder continues to be poorly understood and understudied. There is a tremendous need and opportunity for productive clinical research related to NTOS, particularly with an increasing emphasis on evidence-based medicine. While the topics described in this chapter offer some of those appearing most fruitful for further investigation, there will undoubtedly be other important areas yet to be discovered. The importance of sound clinical research efforts and novel investigative strategies cannot be overstated, as a vital means by which to advance our understanding and management of NTOS.

Part V

Neurogenic TOS: Controversies in NTOS

The title of this section: "Controversies in NTOS" is almost redundant, as NTOS is arguably one of the most controversial conditions in medicine. Practitioners involved with NTOS patients invariably have opinions regarding the optimal method for diagnosis and treatment of this condition, but comparative clinical trials are lacking. In this section, experienced TOS clinicians discuss their viewpoints regarding the pathophysiology, diagnosis and surgical treatment of NTOS.

Establishing a correct diagnosis of NTOS is paramount to a successful treatment outcome, and controversies in establishing this diagnosis are addressed in two of the chapters in this section. Dr. Johansen discusses the role of laboratory studies in diagnosing NTOS, and outlines the advantages and limitations of the various diagnostic modalities. Dr. Urschel and colleagues discuss the difficult question of whether the diagnosis of NTOS is over or under-utilized.

The role that inflammation plays in the pathophysiology of NTOS symptoms is discussed by Dr. Ellis. He also outlines a strategy for treating NTOS by modulating the inflammatory response both locally and systemically.

There is no consensus on the ideal surgical treatment of NTOS. The two most common approaches, the transaxillary and the supraclavicular, are discussed by Dr. Green. He discusses his recommendations for the ideal scenario for each surgical approach. Dr. Sanders, with his extensive experience performing scalenectomy with and without first rib resection, discusses the necessity of removing the first rib during thoracic outlet surgery. Finally, thoracic outlet surgery is performed by a variety of subspecialists including vascular, thoracic, neuro, orthopedic and plastic surgeons. Dr. Donahue reviews the various technical nuances that each surgical subspeciality brings to the operating room in performing thoracic outlet decompression.

Controversies in NTOS:
Is Laboratory Testing Necessary
in Patients with NTOS?

42

Kaj H. Johansen

Abstract

The diagnosis of neurogenic thoracic outlet syndrome (NTOS) is made on clinical grounds and affirmed by a positive response to a properly performed scalene muscle block. Numerous laboratory evaluations – including electrodiagnostic, non-invasive vascular, and cross sectional imaging studies – have been used in the assessment of patients potentially harboring neurogenic TOS. However, none has a sensitivity and specificity to a degree that is dependable in making the diagnosis of the condition. Instead, such laboratory tests are useful in ruling out the alternative conditions with which neurogenic TOS may initially be confused.

Introduction

All involved in the management of patients potentially harboring neurogenic thoracic outlet syndrome (NTOS) agree that this condition is diagnosed predominantly on clinical grounds, i.e. on the basis of the patient's injury history, symptomatology, physical examination – including various provocative maneuvers – and clinical course over time, including the patient's response to various conservative measures such as rest or physical therapy. The role of various scalene (or other) skeletal muscle denervation tests, considered by many to be crucial confirmatory evaluations for the diagnosis of NTOS, is discussed in

Chap. 20. Is there a role for additional testing in confirming, refining or ruling out the diagnosis of NTOS?

Three broad categories of laboratory examinations – imaging studies, noninvasive vascular laboratory assessment, and electrodiagnostic modalities – have been utilized in patients thought possibly to harbor NTOS. The accuracy and relevance of such studies continues to be debated, to a substantial degree because of an ongoing lack of complete certainty about the underlying pathophysiology of NTOS.

Medical Imaging Studies

Numerous different types of medical imaging studies can provide excellent definition of the anatomy of the thoracic outlet, both in normal subjects as well as in patients who may harbor NTOS [1]. Some may also have a role to play in

K.H. Johansen, MD, PhD
Department of Vascular Surgery,
Swedish Heart and Vascular Institute,
1600 E. Jefferson St. #101, Seattle,
WA 98122, USA
e-mail: kaj.johansen@swedish.org

K.A. Illig et al. (eds.), *Thoracic Outlet Syndrome*,
DOI 10.1007/978-1-4471-4366-6_42, © Springer-Verlag London 2013

demonstrating (or at least suggesting) pathophysiologic changes characteristic of NTOS in the
brachial plexus or the structures which surround
it, although correlation between imaging and outcomes have not been thoroughly studied (see
Chap. 18).

Plain radiography can upon occasion provide
useful insights in patients whose clinical picture
suggests the presence of NTOS. An obvious
example is the demonstration, on a cervical
spine or apical lordotic chest x-ray, of the presence of a cervical rib, a displaced or ectopic first
thoracic rib, or a past or current clavicular fracture. Bony erosion in this region may indicate
the presence of an apical pulmonary (Pancoast)
or other malignancy, invasion of which into the
brachial plexus results in the patient's NTOS
symptoms.

Standard gray-scale ultrasonography has been
utilized for assessment of the anatomy of the thoracic outlet [2]. Such studies can demonstrate
scalene muscle hypertrophy, a constant finding in
patients with NTOS.

Computerized tomographic (CT) scanning has
less commonly been utilized for anatomic assessment of the structures of the thoracic outlet.
Particularly when contrast-enhanced, CT scanning provides excellent detail of various anatomic
relationships, both normal and abnormal, at this
level [3], but data are sparse in this regard.

Magnetic resonance (MR) imaging has been
extensively utilized in the evaluation of the anatomic relationships within and around the thoracic outlet. Because of this modality's capability
to characterize normal and abnormal tissue
densities representative of various forms of
pathophysiology in the region, MR has provided
real insights into this condition. For example,
abnormal scalene muscle structure (edema,
hypertrophy, scarring, inflammation) can be demonstrated with exquisite detail on MR imaging of
the thoracic outlet and its structures [4]. However,
whether MR (or other) imaging studies can provide diagnostic results which are of a high enough
sensitivity and specificity to be utilized as a "gold
standard" for the diagnosis of NTOS remains
elusive.

Noninvasive Vascular Laboratory Evaluation

Various vascular ultrasonographic modalities
have been utilized in the assessment of patients
thought possibly to be harboring NTOS. Most
commonly, vascular laboratory studies, both
direct (by focused duplex scanning [5]) and indirect (by digital plethysmography [6]), have been
utilized to attempt to demonstrate extrinsic compression of the subclavian artery (or vein) within
or near the thoracic outlet. Because the subclavian artery travels through the thoracic outlet in
close proximity to the brachial plexus, it is felt by
some that the same extrinsic compression which
results in the symptoms of NTOS should also
impinge upon the subclavian artery at this site.
Indeed, presuming that such extrinsic compression is part of the actual pathophysiology of
NTOS, the negative predictive value of a normal
subclavian artery duplex scan (i.e. unchanged
with the arm in provocative postures) is likely
high. However, because at least 30 % of the normal asymptomatic population demonstrate
extrinsic compression of the subclavian artery
with the arm in the same provocative postures
[7], the positive predictive value of an abnormal
subclavian duplex scan in a patient thought to be
harboring NTOS is so low as to make such a
finding nondiagnostic.

Electrodiagnostic Studies

It would seem logical that a condition such as
NTOS caused by neural compression at the level
of the thoracic outlet would be characterized by
consistent electrodiagnostic abnormalities. While
this is indeed the case in the event of cases resulting from direct blunt or penetrating brachial
plexus trauma [8], the vast majority of patients
with nonspecific NTOS have normal (or at least
inconclusive) results of standard electrodiagnostic studies [9, 10]. Indeed, when such patients'
studies show an abnormal result, the abnormality
is almost uniformly indicative of nerve impingement either centrally at the cervical spine or at

more peripheral sites such as the carpal or cubital tunnels (see Chap. 19).

In NTOS patients, routine electrodiagnostic testing demonstrates neither nerve conduction abnormalities at the site of brachial plexus compression nor neuromuscular disturbances more peripherally, probably for three separate reasons. First, the site of nerve compression – at the level of the scalene triangle – is too medial for placement of a "control" electrode for measurement of nerve conduction abnormalities across the site of nerve impingement [11]. Second, standard electrodiagnostic studies are too insensitive, i.e. do not have adequate resolution, to detect the nerve or muscle membrane changes relevant to the brachial plexus compression that occurs in the usual form of NTOS. Finally, NTOS is a dynamic condition in which pathophysiologic compression of the brachial plexus usually occurs only with the arm in provocative postures: Extrinsic impingement on the brachial plexus is not constantly present.

Pilot studies of newer and more sensitive electrodiagnostic techniques – for example, that of the median antebrachial sensory nerve conduction velocity [12, 13] – have been introduced but have yet to be validated. Further, such studies appear to have substantial variability based upon operator skill and persistence.

Other Laboratory Studies

Histopathologic evaluation of scalene muscle removed at the time of thoracic outlet decompression surgery has demonstrated a predictable alteration of such muscle, including a markedly increased collagen deposition and a wholesale change in skeletal muscle fiber type [14]. Such findings are currently *ex post facto* only – they simply help confirm that the condition being treated was indeed NTOS – but their consistency suggests the possibility that some as-yet undetermined new imaging or electrophysiologic study might be demonstrated to be adequately sensitive and specific for use in diagnosing NTOS during a preoperative evaluation.

Discussion

As noted above, the diagnosis of NTOS depends to a significant degree upon the patient's clinical presentation and course. A critical aspect of making the diagnosis of NTOS, however, is the satisfactory *exclusion* of alternative diagnoses which might share a similar clinical presentation to that of NTOS, such as abnormalities of the cervical spine or nerve roots, shoulder pathology, myofascial or rheumatologic conditions such as fibromyalgia or polymyalgia rheumatic, or a peripheral nerve compression syndrome. Many of these conditions can be ruled in or out, thereby narrowing the differential diagnosis, by means of the various laboratory or imaging studies discussed above. MR or CT scanning of the shoulder joint can accurately demonstrate the presence or absence of a rotator cuff tear; electrodiagnostic or medical imaging studies can demonstrate the presence of cervical spine or neural foraminal abnormalities; and EMG and/or NCV studies are highly sensitive and specific in finding the presence of carpal or cubital tunnel syndrome.

Accordingly, perhaps the greatest role to be played by the performance of various laboratory studies in assessing patients thought potentially to be harboring NTOS is to rule out alternative competing conditions. If cervical spine, nerve root, shoulder and peripheral nerve compression problems have been satisfactorily excluded, the likelihood that NTOS is the actual diagnosis rises markedly. The profusion of diagnostic tests promoted to evaluate patients who might be harboring NTOS is proof positive of the unhappy truth that none is adequately sensitive or specific to confirm or eliminate that diagnosis, but such evaluations remain valuable for excluding other potential diagnoses.

References

1. Demondion X, Herbinet P, Van Sint Jan V, et al. Imaging assessment of thoracic outlet syndrome. Radiographics. 2006;26:1735–50.

2. Demondion X, Herbinet P, Boutry N, et al. Sonographic mapping of the normal brachial plexus. AJNR Am J Neuroradiol. 2003;24:1303–9.

3. Remy-Jardin M, Remy J, Masson P, et al. Helical CT angiography of thoracic outlet syndrome: functional anatomy. AJR Am J Roentgenol. 2000;174:1667–74.

4. Demondion X, Bacqueville E, Paul C, et al. Thoracic outlet: assessment with MR imaging in asymptomatic and symptomatic populations. Radiology. 2003;227: 461–8.

5. Longley DG, Yedlicka JW, Molina JE, et al. Thoracic outlet syndrome: evaluation of the subclavian vessels by color duplex sonography. AJR Am J Roentgenol. 1992;158:623–30.

6. Baxter BT, Blackburn D, Payne K, et al. Noninvasive evaluation of the upper extremity. Surg Clin N Am. 1990;70:87–97.

7. Juvonen T, Satta J, Laitala P, et al. Anomalies at the thoracic outlet are frequent in the general population. Am J Surg. 1995;170:33–7.

8. Dubuisson A, Nguyen Khac M, Scholtes F, et al. Gilliatt-Sumner hand or true neurogenic thoracic

outlet syndrome. A report on seven operated cases. Neurochirurgie. 2011;57:9–14.

9. Ferrante MA, Wilbourn AJ. Electrodiagnostic approach to the patient with suspected brachial plexopathy. Neurol Clin. 2002;20:423–50.

10. Rousseff R, Tzvetzanov P, Valkov I. Utility (or futility?) of electrodiagnosis in thoracic outlet syndrome. Electromyogr Clin Neurophysiol. 2005;45:131–3.

11. Tender GC, Thomas J, Thomas N, et al. The Gilliatt-Sumner hand revisited: a 25-year experience. Neurosurgery. 2004;55:883–90.

12. Seror O. Medial antebrachial cutaneous nerve conduction study, a new tool to demonstrate mild lower brachial plexus lesions. A report of 16 cases. Clin Neurophysiol. 2004;115:2316–22.

13. Machanic B, Sanders RJ. Medial antebrachial cutaneous nerve measurements to diagnose neurogenic thoracic outlet syndrome. Ann Vasc Surg. 2008; 22:248–54.

14. Sanders RJ, Jackson CGR, Baushero N, et al. Scalene muscle abnormalities in traumatic thoracic outlet syndrome. Am J Surg. 1990;159:231–6.

Controversies in NTOS: Inflammation and Symptom Formation in NTOS

43

Wladislaw Ellis

Abstract

NTOS frequently becomes chronic with spreading and migrating sensory, motor and autonomic dysfunction that is poorly understood. Intraoperative thermography, microscopy, and cytokine staining revealed "innervated fibrosis" of brachial plexus nerve trunks leading to the local presence of pro-inflammatory cytokines. Because similar abnormal, actively secreting growths have been reported in a wide variety of chronic, painful disorders, suggesting a common etiology, we propose a model involving potentially de-differentiated neurites and Schwann cells as well as activated mast cells, macrophages, and fibroblasts to account for symptom formation, progression, and intransigence. This conceptual structure suggests new strategies for better symptom control, including thorough brachial plexus neurolysis at the time of operation, perineural anti-inflammatory treatment, and systemic anti-inflammatory modulation.

Any practitioner who treats patients with neurogenic Thoracic Outlet Syndrome (NTOS) for any length of time is aware of the wide variety, spread, and intermittency of reported symptoms. In addition, many patients with apparently optimal thoracic outlet decompression and non-operative therapy do not improve. Inflammation has been implicated in an increasing number and wide variety of problems in the human body. For all these reasons we have explored the potential role of inflammation in patients with NTOS.

We have closely analyzed the small foci of adherent fibrous tissue shown to be neurologically active using intra-operative thermography and examination of specimens removed during neurolysis of the brachial plexus and cervical roots in patients being operated on for NTOS. Histological examination showed that these fibrous foci were richly innervated with both myelinated and unmyelinated nerve fibers. Many of these were immature and secreting calcitonin, gene related peptide, and Substance P, all proinflammatory neuropeptides involved in pain, hyperesthesia, and autonomic dysfunction, and existing in an extracellular matrix richly populated by macrophages, mast cells and fibroblasts [1]. This finding of such cellular and molecular substrates may help explain the evolution and spread

W. Ellis, MD
Private Practice, Neurology/Psychiatry,
1220 Oxford St, Berkeley, CA 94709, USA
e-mail: wladislawellis@gmail.com

of painful, disabling symptomatology in NTOS [2, 3]. Interestingly, this same perpetuating mechanism of "innervated fibrosis" spreading both locally and distantly via neurogenic inflammatory mechanisms is operant in multiple other disorders ranging from endometriosis to varieties of migraine [4, 5].

Events that initiate NTOS are thought to be those that directly traumatize the brachial plexus, most commonly a seatbelt, flexion-extension, or acute stretch trauma during a motor vehicle accident (MVA) [6]. The consequent inflammatory edema activates neuropeptides and cytokines initiating a plethora of various growth and inflammation stimulating cascades (cytokine, interleukin, chemokine, many growth factors, and, importantly, a minimal arachidonic acid cascade limiting steroid effectiveness) with potential long term consequences [7, 8]. This situation leads to an environment suitable for the initiation of recurrent neurogenic inflammation caused by Schwann cell activation resulting neurite ingrowth from nervi nervorum (perhaps from or associated with investing fibrosis) at first intra and then perineurally becoming macroscopic "innervated fibrosis" over time [9]. Mechanosensitivity of both neural and glial (Schwann) cells, probably due to continued neuritic de-differentiation, leads to further generation of inflammatory and trophic factors perpetuating and extending the pathology and creates the groundwork for double, triple crush injuries as well as scalene hypertrophy and fibrous interdigitations [10, 11]. De-differentiation explains not only the continued hyperesthesia and paresthesias but also easy re-injury, therapeutic unresponsiveness, spread, continued disability and an excellent response to terminal differentiation as induced by erythropoietin.

A second proposed major category of initiating events for NTOS is constant mechanical tension (for example: repetitive work injury) of the brachial plexus and its rami [12]. The primary problem seems to lie not with the nerve itself but with the supporting Remak Schwann cells which, in response to tension or ischemia, initiate local neuronal sprouting and neurite ingrowth by decreasing myelin associated glycoprotein expression [13]. Continued mechanosensitivity

facilitates the progression of the innervated fibrosis described above leading to the evolution of general, shared symptoms over time, despite varied initial presentations. Why some, mainly women, become affected with chronic, progressive symptoms while others recover remains unanswered but there are hints that the genome could provide some answers [14].

In over half of these patients, initial symptoms are pain in the shoulder arm and hand. Following initial injury symptoms originate locally and then spread both distally and centrally, driven by the released cytokines [15]. Patients with repetitive work injury usually develop hand pain initially followed by proximal spread of symptoms. Many of these patients therefore receive carpal tunnel decompressions with no benefit, but then do receive significant relief from thoracic outlet decompressions, underscoring the importance of the brachial plexus lesion being the underlying cause of the referred pain in the forearm, wrist, and hand.

Headaches, especially those suboccipital, radiating, and migranoid in nature, have been long recognized as a presenting sign of NTOS [16]. Ulnar paresthesias, severe episodic left chest and arm pain, cold sensitivity, hyperhidrosis, varied gastrointestinal and genitourinary symptoms, and episodes of hyperesthesia or allodynia can all precede clinical diagnosis of NTOS or accompany its development [17].

It is likely that the products of nerve driven inflammation not only change the involved nerves themselves but also diffuse to involve nearby structures such as the stellate ganglion, vagus, laryngeal or phrenic nerves. In addition this process could affect the dorsal root ganglion, spinal dorsal horn, producing motor symptoms that seem unrelated but are, in fact, driven by the basic pathophysiology of NTOS [18–20]. Central sensitization and mirror symptomatology occur with time after repeated re-injuries of the already sensitized nerves and account for much of the subsequent spread and additional dysfunction [21].

In summary, evidence suggests that trauma, overt or subtle, leads to small intra and per-neural foci of inflammation and neural ingrowth as part of the fibrosis around the brachial plexus and adjacent structures. This leads to a wide variety of pain and sensory symptoms, but also explains autonomic and motor disturbances depending on the location, combination, and concentration of inflammatory substances expressed. Recurrent and or self-perpetuated activation of this process, driven probably by immature neuro-glial elements, results in spreading pathology and symptoms for what is, essentially, aberrant wound healing.

This formulation, although conjectural, explains the varied clinical and tissue findings, and lack of response to many therapies. In addition, it suggests new interventions. Most importantly it implies that aggressive neurolysis of the brachial plexus during operation may be of benefit, coupled with directed local or systemic pharmacologic interventions, one of which, erythropoietin, acts by inducing terminal differentiation in immature neurites and Schwann cells [22, 23].

References

1. Ellis W, Cheng S. Intraoperative thermographic monitoring during neurogenic thoracic outlet decompressive surgery. Vasc Endovasc Surg. 2006;40(3):251–4.
2. Zimmerman M. Pathobiology of neuropathic pain. Eur J Pharmacol. 2001;429:23–37.
3. Bridges D, Thompson S, Rice A. Mechanisms of neuropathic pain. Br J Anesth. 2001;87(1):12–26.
4. Anal V, et al. Hyperalgesia, nerve infiltration and nerve growth factor expression in deep adenomyotic nodules, peritoneal and ovarian endometriosis. Hum Reprod. 2002;17(7):1895–900.
5. Gepetti P, et al. CGRP and migraine: neurogenic inflammation revisited. J Headache Pain. 2005;6:61–70.
6. Sanders R, Haug C. Thoracic outlet syndrome: a common sequela of neck injuries. Philadelphia: Lippincott; 1991. p. 21–8.
7. Watkins L, Maier S. Beyond neurons: evidence that immune and glial cells contribute to pathological pain states. Physiol Rev. 2002;82:981–1011.
8. Neuwelt E, et al. Engaging neuroscience to advance translational research in brain barrier biology. Nat Rev Neurosci. 2011;12:169–82.
9. Gupta R, Steward O. Chronic nerve compression induces concurrent apoptosis and proliferation of Schwann cells. J Comp Neurol. 2003;461:174–86.
10. Tapadia M, Mozaffar T, Gupta R. Compressive neuropathies of the upper extremity: update on pathophysiology, classification, and electrodiagnostic findings. J Hand Surg. 2010;35(4):668–77.
11. Golovchinsky V. Relationship between damage of cervical nerve roots or brachial plexus and development of peripheral entrapment syndromes in Upper extremities (double crush syndrome). J Neurol Orthop Med Surg. 1995;16:61–9.
12. Breig A. Adverse mechanical tension in the central nervous system, an analysis of cause and effect. Stockholm: Almqvist & Wiksell International; 1978. p. 122–7.
13. Gupta R, Rummler L, Steward O. Understanding the biology of compressive neuropathies. Clin Orthop Relat Res. 2005;436:251–60.
14. Nair H, et al. Genomic loci and candidate genes underlying inflammatory nociception. Pain. 2011;152: 599–606.
15. Myers R, Campana W, Shubayev V. The role of neuroinflammation in neuropathic pain: mechanisms and therapeutic targets. Drug Discov Today. 2006;11(1–2): 8–20.
16. Raskin N, Howard M, Ehrenfeld W. Headache as the leading symptom of the thoracic outlet syndrome. Headache. 1985;25(4):208–10.
17. Wang H, et al. Chronic neuropathic pain is accompanied by global changes in gene expression and shares pathobiology with neurodegenerative diseases. Neuroscience. 2002;114(3):529–46.
18. Delmas P, Hao J, Radat-Despoix L. Molecular mechanisms of mechanical transduction in mammalian sensory neurons. Nat Rev Neurosci. 2011;12:139–54.
19. Meggs W. Neurogenic switching: a hypothesis for a mechanism for shifting the site of inflammation in allergy and chemical sensitivity. Environ Health Perspect. 1995;103(1):54–6.
20. Richardsaon J, Vasko M. Cellular mechanisms of neurogenic inflammation. J Pharmacol Exp Ther. 2002;302(3): 839–45.
21. Milligan E, et al. Spinal glia and proinflammatory cytokines mediate mirror-image neuropathic pain in rats. J Neurosci. 2003;23(3):1026–57.
22. Xiaoqing L, Gonis S, Camana M. Schwann cells express erythropoietin receptor and represent a major target for Epo in peripheral nerve injury. Glia. 2005;51(4):254–65.
23. Bartesaghi S, et al. Erythropoietin: a novel neuroprotective cytokine. Neurotoxicology. 2005;26:923–8.

Controversies in NTOS: Transaxillary or Supraclavicular First Rib Resection in NTOS?

44

Richard M. Green

Abstract

Most believe that proper treatment of neurogenic thoracic outlet syndrome (NTOS) requires excision of the first rib and adequate scalenectomy. The supraclavicular approach allows most thorough scalene muscle excision and brachial plexus neurolysis, while the transaxillary approach is most cosmetic and seems to decompress the thoracic outlet very nicely. Large series utilizing either approach show excellent and equivalent results. I believe that the patient with upper plexus symptoms, cervical tenderness, a broad bony cervical rib and/or a history of trauma is best treated by supraclavicular first rib excision. By contrast, those patients with clear-cut lower plexus (ulnar nerve) symptoms in the absence of trauma should be offered transaxillary resection.

There are large series of patients from reputable centers demonstrating that neurologic thoracic outlet syndrome (NTOS) can be safely and successfully treated by both transaxillary and supraclavicular [1–3]. I believe that both procedures are complimentary and that anyone treating patients with NTOS should be facile in each. The choice for me largely depends on the patient's presenting symptoms, the body habitus, and the presence of bony anomalies.

Whether or not NTOS exists remains a matter of debate [4]. As my own practice has evolved I am recommending operative decompression in fewer patients while utilizing therapy and conditioning as my first and best option unless an accompanying anatomic abnormality is identified or the patient presents with a significant neurologic impairment [5]. Nonoperative therapy consists of correcting any muscular imbalance in the cervicoscapular region by increasing mobility, strength (endurance) and range of motion all with the goal of decreasing compression on the brachial plexus. In addition to traditional physical therapy, postural training to correct drooping or sagging shoulders is essential. When aggressive nonoperative management fails in a compliant patient there is usually a fixed anatomic abnormality such as a fibromuscular band that requires decompression.

A review of our experience with NTOS at the University of Rochester in 136 patients was conducted to determine what factors affected outcome after transaxillary first rib resection [6].

R.M. Green, MD
Department of Surgery, Lenox Hill Hospital,
130 East 77th St, New York, NY 10075, USA
e-mail: rgreen@nshs.edu

The mean follow-up was 60 ± 7 months. Secondary supraclavicular operations were required in 20 patients. This rather high recurrence rate has been noticed by others [7]. The quality of the operative result was determined by whether the patient was able to return to pre-illness activities and whether the patient would undergo operation again if the same result would be obtained. The most important determinant of result was a history of trauma precipitating the neurologic symptoms, particularly in women. Only 25 of the 53 patients (47 %) with a history of trauma returned to pre-illness activities compared to 65 of the 83 patients (78 %) without such a history. Overall patient satisfaction was not affected by trauma. Thirty-eight of the 53 patients with trauma (72 %) and 69 of the 83 patients (83 %) without trauma were satisfied. When the men and women were analyzed separately men were found to have better results after trauma than did women. Other factors with a negative impact on operative results were the need to return to an activity that required repetitive arm movements, coverage under a worker's compensation insurance policy, and fixed joint abnormalities or neurologic findings in the upper extremity. The presence of an anatomic abnormality had no effect on operative results. These factors should all be considered before recommending first rib resection to a patient with NTOS.

The decision to recommend the transaxillary or supraclavicular approach should be made on the basis of the patient's presentation. Patients with upper plexus symptoms (C5, C6 or C7) or those with broad cervical ribs are best treated with a supraclavicular approach. Patients with upper plexus compression present with sensory changes in the first three fingers and pain in the anterior chest, deltoids and parascapular area as well as down the outer arm to the extensor muscles of the forearm. Patients with lower plexus compression (C8 and T1) exhibit sensory changes in the fourth and fifth digits with muscle pain or weakness anywhere from the rhomboid area to the intrinsic muscles of the hand. Patients with long narrow cervical ribs usually present with lower plexus symptoms and can be treated with a transaxillary approach. Whereas the supraclavicular approach allows division of each of the scalene muscles and visualization of the plexus and any anomalous fibrous band as well as removing the first rib, the transaxillary approach allows removal of the rib and release of all the muscular attachments but yields a less complete decompression. Despite what appears to be a clear-cut distinction between the two forms of NTOS, the transaxillary approach can relieve upper plexus symptoms, probably because most muscles and ligaments that compress the upper plexus attach to the first rib. In addition, anatomic studies show that the median nerve usually implicated in the upper plexus syndrome receives fibers from C8 and T1.

The pathophysiology of NTOS is most often a combination of an anatomic predisposition to plexus pressure plus an injury to the scalene muscles [8]. The predisposition can be a congenital band, ligament, or cervical rib that narrows the scalene triangle, or it can be a variation in anatomic relationships whereby the cords of the brachial plexus emerge at a point high in the scalene triangle where the anterior and middle scalene muscles are very close. Injury to the scalene muscles result in muscle fibrosis and mild plexus compression by tightened or spastic anterior and middle scalene muscles.

One of the strongest arguments for the supraclavicular approach is a study showing that 83 % of patients with TOS had the nerves of the brachial plexus emerge from the scalene triangle in a high position where there is no space, compared to an incidence of only 40 % in cadaver controls [9]. Scalene muscle involvement has been given increased credibility by recent histologic studies of scalene muscles in patients with NTOS, which have revealed a consistent pattern of abnormal fiber type change (type 1 predominance and type 2 atrophy) plus an increase in connective tissue to an average of 35 % (controls were under 15 %). The positive correlation of improvement after scalene muscle block and after scalenectomy or rib resection gives validity to implicating the scalene muscles as the site of disease. Since TAFRR only disconnects these muscles from the first rib, it may be an inadequate procedure when the scalene muscles are involved in this pathologic process.

In conclusion, while both approaches can lead to excellent results, I believe that the patient with upper plexus symptoms, cervical tenderness, a broad bony cervical rib and/or a history of trauma is best treated by supraclavicular first rib excision. By contrast, those patients with clear-cut lower plexus (ulnar nerve) symptoms in the absence of trauma should be offered transaxillary resection.

References

1. Urschel H, Kourlis H. Thoracic outlet syndrome: a 50-year experience at Baylor University Medical Center. Proc (Bayl Univ Med Cent). 2007;20:125–35.
2. Roos DB. Thoracic outlet syndrome. Arch Surg. 1966;93:71–4.
3. Sanders RJ. Results of the surgical treatment for thoracic outlet syndrome. Semin Thorac Cardiovasc Surg. 1966;8:221–8.
4. Wilbourn AJ. Thoracic outlet syndrome: a neurologist's perspective. Chest Surg Clin N Am. 1999;9: 821–39.
5. Novack CB. Conservative management of thoracic outlet syndrome. Semin Thorac Cardiovasc Surg. 1996; 8:201–7.
6. Green RM, McNamara J, Ouriel K. Long-term follow-up after thoracic outlet decompression: an analysis of factors determining outcome. J Vasc Surg. 1991;14: 739–46.
7. Sanders RJ, Monsour JW, Gerber FG, Adams WRA, Thompson N. Scalenectomy versus first rib resection for treatment of the thoracic outlet syndrome. Surgery. 1979;85:109–21.
8. Sanders RJ, Pearce WH. The treatment of thoracic outlet syndrome: a comparison of different operations. J Vasc Surg. 1989;10:626–34.
9. Sanders RJ, Raymer S. The supraclavicular approach to scalenectomy and first rib resection: description of technique. J Vasc Surg. 1985;2:751–6.

Richard J. Sanders

Abstract

The first rib may not always require excision in NTOS. It has been shown that the pathology is in the scalene muscles (fibrosis), not in the rib. Scalenectomy alone has as good a long-term improvement rate as first rib resection, and rib resection results in more complications and morbidity. However, if when performing scalenectomy, the lower trunk of the brachial plexus is found to lie touching the first rib, it should be excised.

Introduction

Most clinicians today believe that the first rib should be excised in essentially all patients with NTOS, but there are both theoretical and empirical data to suggest that this does not always need to be performed.

The Pathology is in the Scalene Muscles

It has been well documented that in most patients with neurogenic thoracic outlet syndrome (nTOS) the pathology lies mainly in the scalene muscles,

R.J. Sanders, MD
Department of Surgery,
HealthONE Presbyterian-St. Lukes Hospital,
4545 E. 9th Ave #240, Denver, CO 80220, USA
e-mail: rsanders@ecentral.com

primarily anterior but also middle. Supporting this point of view are the following:

1. Histologic demonstration of a threefold increase in the amount of scar tissue in the scalene muscles of nTOS patients [1] (See Fig. 6.2).
2. Histologic demonstration of an increase in slow twitch muscle fibers (Type 1) and decrease, atrophy, and anisocytosis of fast twitch fibers (Type 2) [1, 2] (See Fig. 6.2).
3. The observation that scalene muscle block with lidocaine relaxes the anterior scalene muscle and relieves most symptoms within 120 seconds [3, 4].
4. And, most importantly, the observation that scalenectomy without first rib resection has as good a success rate as scalenectomy with first rib resection [5, 6].

Although first rib resection is the most common operation for relief of symptoms of nTOS, we suggest that it is successful not because the

Fig. 45.1 (a) Almost vertical first rib which rests against the lower trunk of the brachial plexus and is excised. (b) Curved first rib which usually lies free of the lower trunk and is not removed (Reprinted from Sanders [9]. With permission from Elsevier)

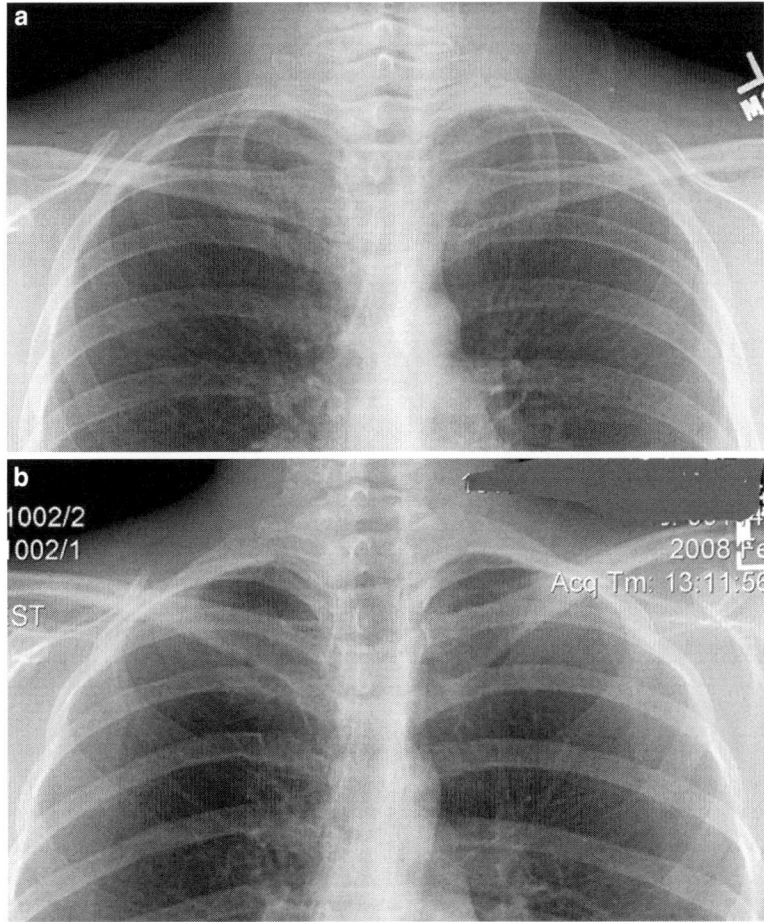

first rib has been removed but rather because to remove the rib anterior and middle scalenotomy must be performed.

It should be noted that some nTOS patients who undergo scalenectomy without first rib resection do not improve and a second operation to remove the rib is required. While identifying these patients is difficult, we have found that at the time of performing supraclavicular anterior and middle scalenectomy the relationship of the lower trunk of the brachial plexus and first rib can easily be observed. If the nerve is in contact with the rib, the rib is removed; otherwise the rib remains. In following this protocol we found that only about 30 % of patients require first rib resection while 70 % require scalenectomy alone, with the overall success rate in both groups being the same [5–8].

In a retrospective review of chest x-rays in patients who did or did not have their first ribs excised patients in whom the rib was excised had a vertical, straight first rib on chest x-ray (Fig. 45.1a) while most patients who had no first rib removal had a wide curve in their first ribs (Fig. 45.1b). The chest x-ray can be used to predict who will need first rib excision, but because this is not totally accurate, the final decision of who needs their first rib excised must still be made on observations in the operating room.

Advantage of Sparing the First Rib

Complications are more frequent with rib resection compared to scalenectomy without rib resection. In an analysis of complications in 740 primary TOS operations (301 scalenectomies alone and 439 rib resections, both transaxillary and supraclavicular), the incidence of plexus injuries, long thoracic nerve injuries, and major hemorrhage each occurred in between 1 and 2 % of patients after rib resection versus zero to 0.3 % for those undergoing scalenectomy alone [10]. Furthermore, recovery time is shorter and morbidity less when the first rib is spared.

Conclusion

Several authors have noted that the results of scalenectomy without first rib resection are the same as scalenectomy with first rib resection. In our hands, the decision to remove or spare the first rib is determined by observing the relationship of the first rib to the lower trunk of the brachial plexus after the scalene muscles have been excised while the supraclavicular incision is still open. If the nerve trunk is touching the first rib the rib is excised, but if there is at least 2–3 mm of space between nerve and rib it is left alone. Finally, the shape of the first rib on the preoperative chest x-ray can usually predict who will need first rib excision on this basis – a rib that runs in a vertical direction is often removed, while first ribs that have a wide curve on x-ray usually are not.

References

1. Sanders RJ, Jackson CGR, Banchero N, Pearce WH. Scalene muscle abnormalities in traumatic thoracic outlet syndrome. Am J Surg. 1990;159:231–6.
2. Machleder HI, Moll F, Verity A. The anterior scalene muscle in thoracic outlet compression syndrome: histochemical and morphometric studies. Arch Surg. 1986;121:1141–4.
3. Jordan SE, Machleder HI. Diagnosis of thoracic outlet syndrome using electrophysiologically guided anterior scalene blocks. Ann Vasc Surg. 1998;12:260–4.
4. Sanders RJ, Haug CE. Thoracic outlet syndrome: a common sequela of neck injuries. Philadelphia: Lipppincott; 1991. p. 91–3.
5. Sanders RJ, Pearce WH. The treatment of thoracic outlet syndrome: a comparison of different operations. J Vasc Surg. 1989;10:626–34.
6. Cheng SWK, Reilly LM, Nelken NA, Ellis WV, Stoney RJ. Neurogenic thoracic outlet decompression: rationale for sparing the first rib. Cardiovasc Surg. 1995;3:617–23.
7. Thomas GI. Diagnosis and treatment of thoracic outlet syndrome. Perspect Vasc Surg. 1995;8:1–28.
8. Martin GT. First rib resection for the thoracic outlet syndrome. Br J Neurosurg. 1993;7:35–8.
9. Sanders RJ. Thoracic outlet syndrome: general considerations. In: Cronenwett JL, Johnston KW, editors. Rutherford's vascular surgery. 7th ed. Philadelphia: Saunders; 2010. p. 1867.
10. Sanders RJ, Haug CE. Thoracic outlet syndrome: a common sequela of neck injuries. Philadelphia: Lipppincott; 1991. p. 162.

Controversies in NTOS: Is NTOS Overdiagnosed or Underdiagnosed?

46

Harold C. Urschel Jr.[†], Charles R. Crane, J. Mark Pool, and Amit N. Patel

Abstract

The topic of this chapter is to address the rhetorical question, "Is neurogenic thoracic outlet syndrome (TOS) overdiagnosed or underdiagnosed," and the answer depends a great deal on the experience of a given physician, medical center, or geographic location. The necessity of a multi-disciplinary team to improve the diagnosis and treatment of this difficult condition renders a variety of situations with regard to the question at-hand. For example, if a physician is in solitary practice or isolated geographically, it is very unlikely that they will "overdiagnose" neurogenic TOS unless they happen to know a great deal about it (from some form of unique previous exposure in training or practice), have it themselves, or something similar. On the other hand, if he or she is a member of a large primary care or multidisciplinary group, or one of several referring specialties (such as thoracic surgery, cardiovascular surgery, neurology or neurological surgery, orthopedic surgery or sports medicine, physical medicine and rehabilitation, pain management medicine, psychiatry, cardiology, internal medicine or general practice), the diagnosis of neurogenic TOS may well have been regularly considered in a differential diagnosis and this condition may even have been even "overdiagnosed."

[†]Deceased

H.C. Urschel Jr., MD (✉)
Department of Cardiovascular and Thoracic Surgery,
Baylor University Medical Center,
University of Texas Southwestern Medical School,
3600 Gaston Ave, Ste. 1201, Dallas, TX 75246, USA
e-mail: drurschel@me.com

C.R. Crane, MD
Department of Certified Pain Management, American
Board of Physical Medicine and Rehabilitation,
American Board of Electrodiagnositic Medicine,
P.O. Box 550337, Dallas, TX 75355, USA

J.M. Pool, MD
Department of Cardiac, Vascular
and Thoracic Surgical Associates,
Texas Health Presbyterian Hospital of Dallas,
8230 Walnut Hill Lane, Suite 208,
Dallas, TX 75231, USA

A.N. Patel, MD
Department of Cardiothoracic Surgery,
School of Medicine, The University of Utah,
30 North, 1900 East, Suite 3C127,
Salt Lake City, UT 84132, USA

K.A. Illig et al. (eds.), *Thoracic Outlet Syndrome*,
DOI 10.1007/978-1-4471-4366-6_46, © Springer-Verlag London 2013

Introduction

The topic of this chapter is to address the rhetorical question, "Is neurogenic thoracic outlet syndrome (TOS) overdiagnosed or underdiagnosed," and the answer depends a great deal on the experience of a given physician, medical center, or geographic location. The necessity of a multidisciplinary team to improve the diagnosis and treatment of this difficult condition renders a variety of situations with regard to the question at-hand. For example, if a physician is in solitary practice or isolated geographically, it is very unlikely that they will "overdiagnose" neurogenic TOS unless they happen to know a great deal about it (from some form of unique previous exposure in training or practice), have it themselves, or something similar. On the other hand, if he or she is a member of a large primary care or multidisciplinary group, or one of several referring specialties (such as thoracic surgery, cardiovascular surgery, neurology or neurological surgery, orthopedic surgery or sports medicine, physical medicine and rehabilitation, pain management medicine, psychiatry, cardiology, internal medicine or general practice), the diagnosis of neurogenic TOS may well have been regularly considered in a differential diagnosis and this condition may even have been even "overdiagnosed."

One illustrative example of these differences is at our institution, Baylor University Medical Center in Dallas, Texas, where three physicians (Dr. Edward M. Krusen, Jim Caldwell and Charles Crane) were all very experienced with the techniques involved in the diagnosis of neurogenic TOS. They evaluated over 8,000 patients per year for upper extremity neuromuscular symptoms, and made the diagnosis of neurogenic TOS in 3,000 patients a year. Most of these individuals (approximately 90 %) were treated without surgery. Ours is a large urban medical center with three vascular surgery groups, three cardiac surgery groups, and several orthopedic surgery and neurosurgical groups, so there were a large number of surgeons who could operate on patients with TOS when necessary, in contrast to more remote, non-urban, medical centers or institutions

where there were few physicians with experience in treating neurogenic TOS. Indeed, a patient with neurogenic TOS seen in the past (e.g., during the late 1940s and 1950s) at centers such as the Massachusetts General Hospital (Boston) or the Queen's Square Neurologic Hospital (London), would likely have been markedly "underdiagnosed," because the diagnosis of neurogenic TOS was rarely considered and frequently the condition was thought "not to exist" by the neurological staff and trainees in both institutions (this subsequently changed with greater experience).

One element of the growing understanding and acceptance of neurogenic TOS in many centers is that if physicians recognized that there were arterial and venous components of TOS, they might also accept the possibility that there could be compression of neural structures, and might therefore be more inclined to look carefully for that possibility during clinical examination. Similarly, if physicians understood that a cervical rib can produce an aneurysm of the axillary-subclavian artery, they might be more likely to recognize and accept that the brachial plexus nerves could also be compressed, either in cases presenting with vascular compression or even in patients with similar symptoms but the absence of an axillary-subclavian artery aneurysm.

The failure of many physicians in general practice and internal medicine to recognize the diagnosis of neurogenic TOS led to a large number of such patients being referred to psychiatrists after "objective" studies failed to demonstrate any abnormality. One of the most difficult parts of recognizing neurogenic TOS is in taking a careful history, which is critical for the diagnosis. There are also situations where certain test results, such as the presence of obvious vascular insufficiency (either arterial or venous), serves to "tip-off" the physician that the patient might also have neurogenic TOS. The same is true of people that present with chest pain. If the patient initially had arm pain, hand pain, and numbness, they might be considered to have neurogenic TOS, whereas if all of the symptoms are referred to the chest, the evaluating physician might focus entirely on cardiac diagnoses and completely

Table 46.1 Nerve conduction velocities across the thoracic outlet

Category	Velocity measured (m/s)	Treatment
Normal	>85	None
Abnormal	60–85	Usually improved with PT
Abnormal	<60	Might require surgery

neglect the possibility of neurogenic TOS (even when results of all cardiac testing are normal).

In many situations, if the physician eliminates other diseases that might give rise to similar or overlapping symptoms, they can accurately make the diagnosis of neurogenic TOS by exclusion. In other words, rule-out other diagnoses (e.g., multiple sclerosis, cervical spine pathology, etc.), leaving one with the possible diagnosis of neurogenic TOS remaining in the differential. There have also been longstanding efforts to identify specific testing procedures that can be used to positively support the diagnosis of neurogenic TOS. This is important because if a person is dealing with a large number of patients with suspected neurogenic TOS, similar history and physical signs (such as a positive Adson's test) may be present in normal patients and it would therefore be extremely helpful to be able to objectively determine whether a patient's pain or symptoms are related to an objective test finding in making a diagnosis. Electrodiagnostic testing with somatosensory evoked potentials (SSEPs) was described by various physicians, including Dr. Machleder and colleagues at UCLA, who found that in a group of 80 patients with neurogenic TOS, 74 % had abnormal SSEPs [1]. Use of objective electrophysiological tests was also initiated by Caldwell, Krusen and Crane, involving nerve conduction velocity (NCV) studies across the thoracic outlet [2]. Although it is easy to measure NCVs across the carpal tunnel at the wrist or cubital tunnel at the elbow because there is plenty of space above the site to place the stimulator, Erb's point (analogous to the apex of the brachial plexus) is just a few millimeters or no more than a centimeter, above the clavicle. This makes it very difficult to locate this point in order to initiate the electric signal that has to be slowed down across the thoracic outlet, which is between the clavicle and the shoulder. The specific techniques for reliably demonstrating altered NCVs

(ulnar and median nerves) are therefore critical in substantiating the diagnosis of neurogenic TOS (Table 46.1). Moreover, this is even more important in patients with recurrent symptoms after previous treatment for neurogenic TOS, which might involve decisions whether or not to perform a reoperation because of the recurrent scarring in the area of the previous thoracic outlet surgery [3].

Finally, the experience and expertise of those directing the conservative management of neurogenic TOS may influence the degree to which this condition might be "overdiagnosed" or "underdiagnosed" in a particular practice setting. It is important that the appropriate physical therapy be performed in care of patients with neurogenic TOS, involving improvements in posture, strengthening the shoulder girdle, and loosening and stretching the relevant muscles of the neck. In many situations, therapists with minimal exposure to TOS may perform "inadequate" or "inappropriate" physical therapy, such as vigorous cervical stretching, muscle strengthening, or other techniques that might normally be used for cervical spine or shoulder disorders. It is recognized that such exercises will actually act to exacerbate symptoms of neurogenic TOS, rather than relieve them, and this failure to improve with physical therapy may lead to a perception that the diagnosis of neurogenic TOS does not apply [4].

In conclusion, no general answer can be accurately given regarding whether neurogenic TOS is "overdiagnosed" or "underdiagnosed," as this is highly dependent on the local environment and practice setting in which a given patient might be seen, the experience and expertise of the evaluating physicians, and the availability of specific testing procedures. Indeed, there is no doubt that this question will continue to prompt vigorous debate and discussion, as knowledge regarding neurogenic TOS and its optimal treatment continue to evolve over time.

Acknowledgement The authors appreciate the contributions of Mrs. Rachel Montano and Mrs. Brenda Knee for their dedication and commitment to the research and completion of this publication.

References

1. Machleder HJ, Moll F, Nuwer M, Jordan S. Somatosensory evoked potentials in the assessment of thoracic outlet compression syndrome. J Vasc Surg. 1987;6:177–84.

2. Caldwell JW, Crane CR, Krusen EM. Nerve conduction studies, an aid in the diagnosis of the thoracic outlet syndrome. South Med J. 1971;64:210–2.

3. Urschel Jr HC, Razzuk MA, Albers JE, Wood RE, Paulson DL. Reoperation for recurrent thoracic outlet syndrome. Ann Thorac Surg. 1976;21(1):19–25.

4. Urschel Jr HC, Razzuk MA. Current management of thoracic outlet syndrome. N Engl J Med. 1972; 286:21.

Controversies in NTOS: Is TO Decompression a Vascular, Thoracic, or Neurosurgical Procedure?

47

Dean M. Donahue

Abstract

Thoracic outlet decompression is performed by a variety of surgical specialties including vascular, thoracic, neurologic, orthopedic, plastic, and general surgeons. A well-trained surgeon in any of these specialties should be able to properly care for patients with thoracic outlet syndrome, and each brings a unique perspective to this area. The specific technical skills required for thoracic outlet decompression should be mastered by anyone performing surgery for TOS, whatever their specialty is.

Introduction

The specialties represented by the contributing authors of this textbook reflect the broad range of practitioners involved in the diagnosis and management of thoracic outlet syndrome (TOS). This creates both advantages and challenges of having multiple points of view directed at treatment of patients this condition, with each specialty bringing a somewhat unique perspective to the table.

Thoracic outlet decompression is performed by physicians trained in a variety of surgical specialties. A recent report by Lee, Illig and colleagues reviewed a national inpatient database over a 10-year period between 1998 and 2007. Of 25,642 operations performed for TOS, vascular surgeons were responsible for 52.8 %, thoracic surgeons for 19.7 %, neurosurgeons for 7.2 %, and orthopedic surgeons for 6.1 % [1]. Plastic surgeons and general surgeons also perform thoracic outlet decompression surgery and likely accounted for most of the remaining 14 % or so. The question of which specialty performs the most effective decompression procedure is rhetorical, but there are technical skills that each specialty provides that should be mastered by each surgeon involved in TOS. Rather than reviewing which specialty is best suited to surgically treat TOS, the question should be: what can we learn from each other?

Specialty-Specific Surgical Principles

Thoracic outlet decompression can be performed through a variety of approaches. Regardless of the exposure used to decompress the thoracic outlet, basic surgical principles common to all specialties must first be strictly adhered to. Successful surgery requires a detailed knowledge

D.M. Donahue, MD
Department of Thoracic Surgery,
Massachusetts General Hospital,
Blake 1570, 55 Fruit Street, Boston, MA 02114, USA
e-mail: donahue.dean@mgh.harvard.edu

K.A. Illig et al. (eds.), *Thoracic Outlet Syndrome*,
DOI 10.1007/978-1-4471-4366-6_47, © Springer-Verlag London 2013

of the anatomy of the thoracic outlet, including the numerous anatomic variations that may be present. During the dissection to delineate a patient's anatomy, the tissues must be handled in an atraumatic manner to minimize local injury. This must be performed with minimal traction placed on the local nerves and blood vessels, yet still performing a full release of tissues causing impingement on these structures.

While symptoms of vascular compression account for less than 5 % of thoracic outlet decompression operations performed nationally [1], vascular surgeons play a leading role in the surgical management of TOS. Vascular TOS has more objective clinical findings, and diagnosis is more straightforward. The ability to employ endovascular diagnostic and treatment techniques allows the vascular surgeon a primary role in these patients. Their experience with vascular TOS can transfer to the operative management of neurologic TOS (NTOS). Vascular surgeons routinely perform technical skills such as vascular mobilization, exposure for proximal and distal vessel control and arterial and venous grafting. Other specialties involved in TOS surgery have training in the technical skills required in safely handling blood vessels, but these are routinely practiced by vascular surgeons and must be understood by all other TOS surgical specialties.

Thoracic surgeons bring the unique perspective of performing other, occasionally more radical, surgical procedures in the thoracic outlet region. Thoracic surgeons routinely treat superior sulcus (Pancoast) tumors which invade the lower trunk of the brachial plexus, and upper chest wall requiring radical resection including disarticulation of the first thoracic rib at the spine. They also treat a variety of sarcomas of the clavicle, upper chest wall and manubrium requiring similar surgical exposure. Video thoracoscopy can be used at the apex of the chest for sympathectomy, or resection of nerve sheath tumors involving the sympathetic trunk. Surgically treating these conditions provides the thoracic surgeon with a unique anatomic perspective of the thoracic outlet region.

Neurosurgeons and orthopedic subspecialists are experienced in many conditions that can mimic TOS, including cervical spine disease and peripheral nerve entrapment conditions. Neurosurgeons are the most experienced TOS surgeons in handling nerve tissue during nerve mobilization or neurolysis. These skills are also practiced by upper extremity orthopedic and plastic surgeons. The experience that these specialties have, particularly in deciding the correct plane for a thorough neurolysis, is critical for all TOS surgical practitioners to acquire. Successful release of adjacent scar tissue without devascularizing the spinal nerves and brachial plexus trunks is frequently required for a successful outcome.

Perhaps more important than a surgeon's particular specialty is their experience with thoracic outlet decompression and, not trivially, their interest in TOS as a disease entity. Similar to what has been documented for many other major surgical procedures, complication rates for TOS surgery are directly related to surgical volume: hospitals that performed more than 15 TOS decompression procedures yearly had significantly lower complication rates than lower-volume centers [1].

A "Hybrid" TOS Surgeon

Surgeons involved in the care of TOS patients should become familiar with the technical skills that each specialty provides. This includes the proper handling of nerves and blood vessels, as well as techniques for disarticulating the first rib from the spine. Understanding the proper plane required to remove scar tissue from a nerve without concurrent devascularization is critical. In addition to surgical techniques, each specialty brings experience with a variety of conditions that can mimic TOS thus improving diagnostic accuracy. Thoracic outlet decompression should be analyzed and approached in a multidisciplinary fashion, with cooperation among the different specialties in developing skills specific to thoracic outlet decompression. In the era of telecommunications and improved intraoperative imaging, collaboration regarding surgical techniques should be employed more frequently.

Reference

1. Lee JT, Dua MM, Chandra V, et al. Surgery for thoracic outlet syndrome: a nationwide perspective. Presented at Society of vascular surgeons meeting, Chicago, IL, June 2011.

Venous thoracic outlet syndrome (VTOS) describes a group of symptoms that occur when the subclavian vein becomes compressed during passage between the clavicle and first rib at the costoclavicular junction. VTOS is the second most common form of thoracic outlet syndrome, constituting 2–3 % of TOS cases in most series but occurring much more commonly in many TOS-focused practices. VTOS most commonly presents with frank axillosubclavian vein thrombosis ("effort thrombosis" or Paget-Schroetter syndrome), but can also present as intermittent compression of the subclavian vein (McCleery's syndrome). Patients with VTOS demonstrate a range of clinical sequelae, depending on the degree of intrinsic damage to the vein and duration of insult. The classic patient with Paget-Schroetter syndrome describes the rapid onset of discoloration, swelling, congestion, and pain on the side of the dominant hand, accompanied by collateral development across the shoulder and lateral pectoral areas; 60–80 % report prior engagement in vigorous or repetitive upper extremity activity. VTOS may also present more chronically as residual obstruction from prior total or partial thrombus causes persistent symptoms. Finally, patients with intermittent non-thrombotic (almost always positional) venous compression describe symptoms only when position or activity leads to impaired venous flow; of all VTOS patients treated at Johns Hopkins Medical Institutions from 2003 to 2011, only 11 % have presented with intermittent compression.

No prospective randomized trial has been performed to define treatment of VTOS, and standard practice has largely been shaped by case reports, reviews, and opinion papers. Over the past few decades, VTOS treatment has evolved from anticoagulation alone, to thrombolytic therapy in the late 1970s, and finally decompression of the thoracic outlet by first rib resection and scalenectomy. Modifications to this paradigm include shortening the duration of anticoagulation and employing alternative surgical approaches, such as supra-, para-, or infraclavicular rib resection. Standard treatment for chronic occlusion in VTOS relies less heavily on aggressive thrombolytic therapy, since chronic clots are resistant to thrombolysis, and involves surgical decompression only if the patient is symptomatic. Treatment of VTOS patients presenting with intermittent compression similarly involves surgical decompression to correct the structural abnormality. Finally, very reasonable (albeit minority) voices point out that first rib resection itself might not even be needed in many patients.

The following section will explore this subject in detail, and present conventional and alternative points of view for each step in the treatment of these patients. Particularly important are the thoughts on where we should go next. Precisely because so little high level research has been done in this area it is critically important to understand what we do because it is right, and what we do because of habit – and how to differentiate between the two when it really matters.

Adam J. Doyle and David L. Gillespie

Abstract

This chapter serves as an introduction and overview of axillo-subclavian vein thrombosis in general, an occurrence, when primary (actually caused by extrinsic bony compression of the vein at the junction of the clavicle and first rib) is called venous thoracic outlet syndrome (VTOS). Although the risk of pulmonary embolus is low, patients who are untreated or treated with anticoagulation alone have a significant chance of lifelong disability. Conversely, modern treatment algorithms (with the goal being to lyse the acute clot and then relieve the external bony compression on the vein and at times fix residual endovenous problems) are associated with lifetime patency and symptom-free status in 90 % or more of patients. For both of these reasons it is critical that any patient with a swollen arm and no obvious cause for venous thrombosis be referred to a physician specializing in thoracic outlet syndrome, or the window of opportunity for successful treatment may be lost.

Introduction

The generic term "Thoracic Outlet Syndrome," or TOS, is often used to describe patient with neurogenic (NTOS), venous (VTOS), and arterial (ATOS) symptomatology related to compression of nerves, vein, and/or arteries as they traverse the thoracic outlet. In the case of VTOS, pathology in and surrounding the axillo-subclavian vein is accountable for development of upper-extremity symptoms. Upper extremity deep-vein thrombosis (DVT) is thought to account for approximately 10 % of all DVTs, with an incidence estimated at 0.4–1 case per 10,000 people per year [1–3]. VTOS is composed, in turn, of two distinct problems: intermittent positional obstruction (with an open vein), and primary axillo-subclavian vein occlusion, also called effort thrombosis or Paget-Schroetter syndrome.

Axillo-subclavian vein thrombosis can be broken down into primary and secondary forms. The majority of cases are secondary to catheter injury, infection, or other causes, whereas primary thrombosis, the most common form of VTOS, is a rare condition believed to occur at a rate of approximately 1/50,000–1/100,000

A.J. Doyle, MD • D.L. Gillespie, MD (✉)
Department of Surgery,
University of Rochester Medical Center,
601 Elmwood Ave, Rochester, NY 14642, USA
e-mail: adam_doyle@urmc.rochester.edu;
david_gillespie@urmc.rochester.edu

Table 48.1 Primary and secondary Axillo-subclavian vein thrombosis

Type	Onset and timing of symptoms	Severity	Pathologic mechanism
Primary (venous TOS)			
Intermittent positional obstruction	Chronic positional usually with exertion	Mild-moderate	Positional obstruction of axilosubclavian vein at the thoracic outlet, limited symptoms when not provoked
Partial obstruction	Chronic waxing/waning usually with exertion	Mild-moderate	Repetitive compression with partial to complete thrombosis and recanalization leading to a fixed intrinsic venous stenosis
Acute thrombosis	Acute constant, usually following exertion	Mild-severe	Following repetitive or strenuous activity that compresses the axilosubclavian vein inducing acute thrombosis
Chronic occlusion	Chronic with exertion	None-moderate	End-stage sequelae the above pathologies with resultant complete obstruction and development of collateral circulation. Symptoms likely the result of collateral compression or venous insufficiency with increase arterial blood flow of activity
Secondary			
Medical implant associated (central venous catheter, pacemaker/defibrillator leads)	Acute following catheter insertion	None-severe	Catheter induced venous injury with reduced/obstructed blood flow leading to stasis and thrombosis, usually in the setting of other risk factor for thrombosis[a]
Cancer-associated thrombosis	Acute	None-severe	Cancer-related coagulation abnormalities, chemotherapy-induced coagulation abnormalities, indwelling catheter as above, vein compression or invasion from tumor mass, radiation injury
Iatrogenic/traumatic	Acute following event	None-severe	Direct injury or compression of the axilosubclavian vein from improper positioning, or stasis related to prolonged immobilization
Hypercoagulable disorder	Acute	None-severe	Thrombosis related to acquired or congenital hypercoagulable disorder
Dialysis related	Progressive following placement of ipsilateral A-V access	None-severe	Venous insufficiency from stenosis (likely a result of prior central venous catheter which cause damage to the vein and subsequent stenosis) in the setting of increased venous return when A-V access is place

Based on data from Kucher [10]

[a]**Patient related risk factors**: Post-surgery, cancer, trauma, repetitive activity, vigorous exertion, pregnancy, congenital hypercoagulable state, acquire hypercoagulable state. **Treatment related risk factors**: Radiation therapy to the chest, bolus chemotherapy, TPN, oral contraceptives, ovarian hyper stimulation. **Catheter related risk factors**: catheter malposition, left-sided placement, multiple placement attempts, larger size, prior central venous catheter, open-ended catheter, central line infection, polyvinylchloride or polyethylene material10

people per year [4–6]. Patients suffering primary VTOS are reported to be in the early 30's, with males outnumbering females at a rate of 2–1. The right side is most commonly affected, and a history of recent strenuous use of the upper extremity is present in 60–80 % of patients [6–9]. Patients with secondary thrombosis tend to be older and have more co-morbid conditions. Primary thrombosis (VTOS) is thought to be due to anatomic compression of the axilosubclavian vein at the costoclavicular junction with subsequent venous obstruction and eventual thrombosis, whereas secondary VTOS is felt to be the result of a distinct inciting factor (Table 48.1).

A closely related entity is that of venous outflow obstruction associated with dialysis, which can be secondary to catheter-induced venous injury or can arise from costoclavicular junction injury (See Chap. 51).

The spectrum of presenting signs and symptoms of axillo-subclavian vein thrombosis can range from none to limb-threatening venous gangene [11, 12]. Often there is little correlation between the severity of symptoms and the extent of the underlying obstruction. As a result the clinician must have a low index of suspicion to rule out this diagnosis as it is easily treated, treatment carries with it long-term success rates approaching 100 %, and axillo-subclavian vein thrombosis of any etiology can result in significant long-term morbidity if left untreated.

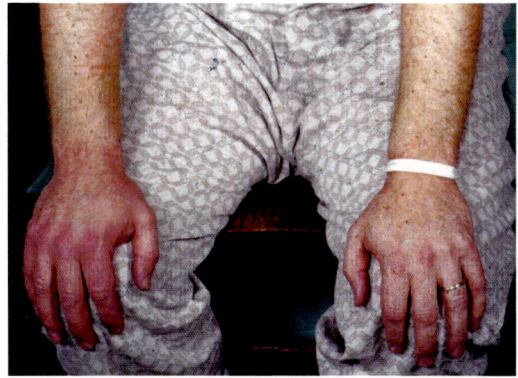

Fig. 48.1 Physical exam findings of VTOS, which includes *red/purplish* discoloration of the right hand with concomitant non-pitting edema (Courtesy Drs. James T. Adams and James A. DeWeese)

Natural History of VTOS

The literature surrounding VTOS (primary axillo-subclavian vein thrombosis) is difficult to interpret, as selection bias relating to physician and surgeon referral is unusually prevalent. Early reports of *untreated* VTOS suggest that significant long-term morbidity can occur in a significant number of patients, up to 75 % in some series [7, 11, 13]. Even patients treated with anticoagulation alone develop persistent symptoms and disability at rates ranging between 41–91 % and 29–68 %, respectively [7, 9, 13–18]. Modern therapy has evolved to include preliminary anticoagulation therapy, catheter-directed thrombolysis, and decompressive surgery for most patients, and such multimodal algorithms produce long-term symptomatic relief in 84–95 % of patients [19–21].

History, Physical Exam Findings, and Presenting Symptoms

In patients with acute severe symptomotology, VTOS should be very high on the differential diagnosis if an obvious secondary cause (such as a catheter) is not present. Patients will generally report a purple-red discolored swollen extremity

with concurrent non-pitting edema (Fig. 48.1). Many will complain of dull aching pain and the sensation of arm heaviness of the affected extremity. Occasionally patients will have concurrent paresthesias and/or weakness. Patients with partial, positional, or chronic occlusions will often present with the same symptoms, but with report relapsing symptoms with exertion, and remission with rest [22]. The vast majority of patients with primary axillo-subclavian vein thrombosis will report a history of recent upper extremity use with the development of symptoms within the following day; this symptom pattern is common enough to have led to the alternative term "effort thrombosis" for this diagnosis.

On physical exam these patients will almost uniformly have a pattern of visible dilated superficial collateral veins across their shoulder, back, chest, and neck within the first several days of symptom onset [7, 19, 23–25]. Figure 48.2a demonstrates the radiographic findings of VTOS with distended collateral veins, and Fig. 48.2b is an example of chest wall collateral veins in a patient with VTOS. Discoloration of the skin with concomitant non-pitting edema may also be present. Table 48.2 lists the physical exam findings, symptoms, and risk factors for VTOS.

A recent study examined and validated the pretest prediction score of certain factors

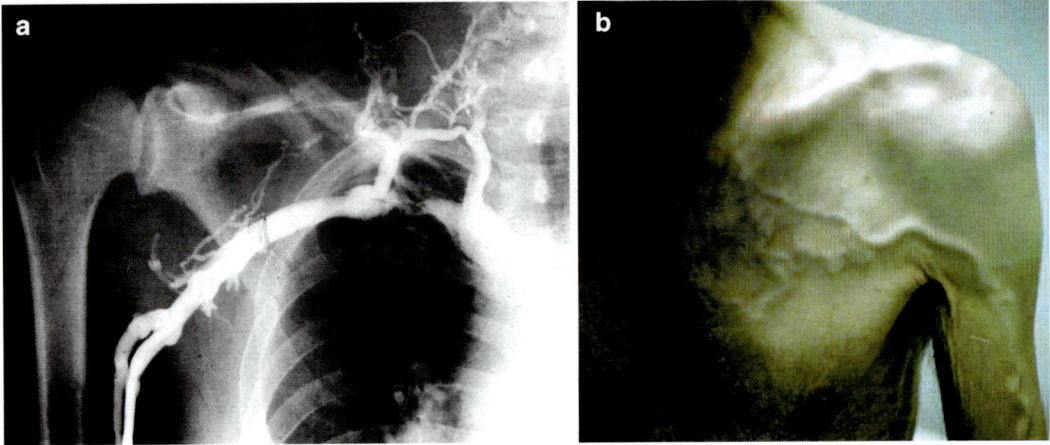

Fig. 48.2 (**a**) Venogram demonstrating VTOS and distended collateral veins which are usually evident on physical exam (Courtesy Drs. James T. Adams and James A. DeWeese). (**b**) Photograph demonstrating distended collateral veins on the chest wall which are usually evident on physical exam. These collateral pathways usually exist on either the anterior or posterior chest wall, in addition to being found at the base of the neck

Table 48.2 Physical exam findings, symptoms, and risk factors for Axillo-subclavian venous occlusion 10

Physical exam findings	Common: Distended superficial veins on neck/chest/back, skin discoloration, non-pitting edema, pain with palpation above or below the clavicle, pallor
	Occasional: Ecchymosis, paresthesias, weakness, poikilothermia
	Rare: Decreased or absent arterial pulse, and facial swelling
Symptoms	Common: Ach or pain of arm/neck/chest/back, heaviness of arm
	Occasional: Numbness of arm, weakness of arm, cool extremity
	Rare: shortness of breath, headache
Patient related risk factors	Post-surgery, cancer, trauma, repetitive activity, vigorous exertion, pregnancy, congenital hypercoagulable state, acquire hypercoagulable state
Treatment related risk factors	Radiation therapy to the chest, bolus chemotherapy, TPN, oral contraceptives, ovarian hyper stimulation
Catheter related risk factors	Catheter mal-position, left-sided placement, multiple placement attempts, larger size, prior central venous catheter, open-ended catheter, central line infection, polyvinylchloride or polyethylene material

Based on data from Kucher [10]

associated with axillo-subclavian vein occlusion [26]. Patients were assigned one point for a central venous catheter or pacemaker, pain, and/or edema, and one point was subtracted if there was a likelihood of an alternative diagnosis. Upper extremity DVT was found in the validation cohort at rates of 13, 38, and 69 % for patients with scores of 0 or less, 1, and 2 or more, respectively. Other tests such as D-dimer have shown little utility in aiding the diagnosis of VTOS [27]. Generally speaking one should have a low threshold to pursue additional diagnostic imaging in the setting of an acutely swollen arm.

Initial Evaluation, Diagnostic Testing, and Referral

When patients present with a history, signs or symptoms suggestive of axillo-subclavian vein thrombosis, further diagnostic testing is warranted regardless of potential etiology. In the setting of a catheter-related thrombosis, the catheter should be removed if feasible, although removal is not always needed [28]. If clinical suspicion is high enough, one could consider starting empiric anticoagulation with low molecular weight heparin injections (LMWH), in appropriately selected patients, prior to pursuing further imaging. The risk of pulmonary embolism is low so the value of diagnosis is to allow proper and expeditious treatment.

If a patient has a swollen arm, urgent duplex ultrasound (DUS) of the axillo-subclavian venous complex should be obtained. Overall, this test is highly sensitive and specific in the diagnosis of VTOS, with numbers approaching 97 % (95 % confidence interval (CI), 90–100 %), and 96 % (95 % CI, 87–100 %), respectively [29]. This yields positive predictive values of 96 % and negative predictive values of 97 %. All patients with a positive DUS result should be started on anticoagulation and referred to a vascular surgeon for evaluation. Almost all practitioners who treat patients with VTOS feel that the sooner these patients undergo treatment the higher the likelihood of success. Based on some data in VTOS patients [19] and extrapolated from the arterial literature, a goal of 14 days from the onset of symptoms is used by many. Some reports extend this, however, to as long as 6 weeks [30], and good results have been obtained by some using alternative algorithms with time to evaluation and treatment averaging as long as 8 months [31]. Despite the conflicting data, most agree that in the setting of acute onset of symptoms, urgent referral (hours to a day or so) to a surgeon who treats patients with VTOS should follow. If the DUS is negative or non-diagnostic for DVT, if suspicion is high the patient should still be referred to a TOS surgeon as specialized imaging may be needed to diagnose positional or partial obstruction. For patients with a negative DUS and minimal symptoms no further axial imaging such as CT and MRI is necessary.

Conclusion

Axillo-subclavian vein occlusion, whether secondary to a definable cause or due to costoclavicular junction compression (VTOS) presents by causing arm swelling. Although the risk of pulmonary embolus is low, patients who are untreated or treated with anticoagulation alone have a significant chance of lifelong disability. Conversely, modern treatment algorithms (with the goal being to lyse the acute clot and then relieve the external bony compression on the vein and at times fix residual endovenous problems) are associated with lifetime patency and symptom-free status in 90 % or more of patients. For both of these reasons it is critical that any patient with a swollen arm and no obvious cause for venous thrombosis be referred to a physician specializing in thoracic outlet syndrome, or the window of opportunity for successful treatment may be lost.

References

1. Isma N, Svensson PJ, Gottsater A, Lindblad B. Upper extremity deep venous thrombosis in the population-based Malmo thrombophilia study (MATS). Epidemiology, risk factors, recurrence risk, and mortality. Thromb Res. 2010;125(6):e335–8.
2. Joffe HV, Kucher N, Tapson VF, Goldhaber SZ. Upper-extremity deep vein thrombosis: a prospective registry of 592 patients. Circulation. 2004;110(12):1605–11.
3. Munoz FJ, Mismetti P, Poggio R, et al. Clinical outcome of patients with upper-extremity deep vein thrombosis: results from the RIETE registry. Chest. 2008;133(1):143–8.
4. Hurley WL, Comins SA, Green RM, Canizzaro J. Atraumatic subclavian vein thrombosis in a collegiate baseball player: a case report. J Athl Train. 2006;41(2):198–200.
5. Illig KA, Doyle AJ. A comprehensive review of Paget-Schroetter syndrome. J Vasc Surg. 2010;51(6):1538–47.
6. Lindblad B, Tengborn L, Bergqvist D. Deep vein thrombosis of the axillary-subclavian veins: epidemiologic data, effects of different types of treatment and late sequelae. Eur J Vasc Surg. 1988;2(3):161–5.
7. Adams JT, DeWeese JA. "Effort" thrombosis of the axillary and subclavian veins. J Trauma. 1971;11(11):923–30.
8. Horattas MC, Wright DJ, Fenton AH, et al. Changing concepts of deep venous thrombosis of the upper extremity – report of a series and review of the literature. Surgery. 1988;104(3):561–7.
9. Tilney N, Griffiths H, Edwards E. Natural history of major venous thrombosis of the upper extremity. Arch Surg. 1970;101:792–6.
10. Kucher N. Deep-vein thrombosis of the upper extremity. N Engl J Med. 2011;364(86):861–9.
11. Adams J, McEvoy R, DeWeese J. Primary deep venous thrombosis of upper extremity. Arch Surg. 1965;91:29–42.
12. Sullivan VV, Wolk SW, Lampman RM, Prager RL, Hankin FM, Whitehouse Jr WM. Upper extremity venous gangrene following coronary artery bypass. A case report and review of the literature. J Cardiovasc Surg (Torino). 2001;42(4):551–4.

13. Hughes E. Venous obstruction upper extremity: review of 320 cases. Int Abstr Surg. 1949;88:89–127.
14. AbuRahma AF, Sadler D, Stuart P, Khan MZ, Boland JP. Conventional versus thrombolytic therapy in spontaneous (effort) axillary-subclavian vein thrombosis. Am J Surg. 1991;161(4):459–65.
15. Becker DM, Philbrick JT, Walker FB. Axillary and subclavian venous thrombosis. Prognosis and treatment. Arch Intern Med. 1991;151(10):1934–43.
16. Heron E, Lozinguez O, Emmerich J, Laurian C, Fiessinger JN. Long-term sequelae of spontaneous axillary-subclavian venous thrombosis. Ann Intern Med. 1999;131(7):510–3.
17. Monreal M, Lafoz E, Ruiz J, Valls R, Alastrue A. Upper-extremity deep venous thrombosis and pulmonary embolism. A prospective study. Chest. 1991; 99(2):280–3.
18. Urschel Jr HC, Razzuk MA. Paget-Schroetter syndrome: what is the best management? Ann Thorac Surg. 2000;69(6):1663–8, discussion 1668–9.
19. Doyle A, Wolford HY, Davies MG, et al. Management of effort thrombosis of the subclavian vein: today's treatment. Ann Vasc Surg. 2007;21(6):723–9.
20. Lee JT, Karwowski JK, Harris EJ, Haukoos JS, Olcott C. Long-term thrombotic recurrence after nonoperative management of Paget-Schroetter syndrome. J Vasc Surg. 2006;43(6):1236–43.
21. Urschel Jr HC, Razzuk MA. Neurovascular compression in the thoracic outlet: changing management over 50 years. Ann Surg. 1998;228(4):609–17.
22. Adams J, DeWeese J, Mahoney E, Rob C. Intermittent subclavian vein obstruction without thrombosis. Surgery. 1968;68:147–65.
23. Inahara T. Surgical treatment of "effort" thrombosis of the axillary and subclavian veins. Am Surg. 1968; 34(7):479–83.
24. Prandoni P, Bernardi E. Upper extremity deep vein thrombosis. Curr Opin Pulm Med. 1999;5(4):222–6.
25. Sharafuddin MJ, Sun S, Hoballah JJ. Endovascular management of venous thrombotic diseases of the upper torso and extremities. J Vasc Interv Radiol. 2002;13(10):975–90.
26. Constans J, Salmi LR, Sevestre-Pietri MA, et al. A clinical prediction score for upper extremity deep venous thrombosis. Thromb Haemost. 2008;99(1): 202–7.
27. Merminod T, Pellicciotta S, Bounameaux H. Limited usefulness of D-dimer in suspected deep vein thrombosis of the upper extremities. Blood Coagul Fibrinolysis. 2006;17(3):225–6.
28. Kearon C, Kahn SR, Agnelli G, Goldhaber S, Raskob GE, Comerota AJ. Antithrombotic therapy for venous thromboembolic disease: American college of chest physicians evidence-based clinical practice guidelines (8th edition). Chest. 2008;133(6 Suppl):454S–545s.
29. Di Nisio M, Van Sluis GL, Bossuyt PM, Buller HR, Porreca E, Rutjes AW. Accuracy of diagnostic tests for clinically suspected upper extremity deep vein thrombosis: a systematic review. J Thromb Haemost. 2010;8(4):684–92.
30. Urschel Jr HC, Patel AN. Surgery remains the most effective treatment for Paget-Schroetter syndrome: 50 years' experience. Ann Thorac Surg. 2008;86(1): 254–60, discussion 260.
31. Guzzo JL, Chang K, Demos J, Black JH, Freischlag JA. Preoperative thrombolysis and venoplasty affords no benefit in patency following first rib resection and scalenectomy for subacute and chronic subclavian vein thrombosis. J Vasc Surg. 2010;52(3):658–63.

Anatomy and Pathophysiology of VTOS

Harold C. Urschel Jr.[†], J. Mark Pool, and Amit N. Patel

Abstract

Acute axillosubclavian vein thrombosis is a disorder of the anterior thoracic outlet, and is always associated with an abnormally lateral insertion of the costoclavicular ligament. This is a low pressure system associated with extrinsic compressive forces, and conventional intraluminal therapy designed to treat atherosclerotic arterial lesions is not appropriate in this situation. In our experience of over 600 extremities with this condition, prompt thrombolysis followed by thoracic outlet decompression leads to excellent results in over 95 % of patients, especially if treatment is instituted soon after thrombosis occurs.

Introduction

Venous thoracic outlet syndrome (VTOS) refers to the spectrum of problems caused by compression of the subclavian vein at the costoclavicular junction in the thoracic outlet. Rarely, patients can present with intermittent obstruction (worse with raising the arms overhead), but most commonly with frank thrombotic occlusion of the vein. Paget-Schroetter syndrome, also called "effort thrombosis" of the axillosubclavian vein, is, by definition, secondary to a costoclavicular junction problem. It occurs in patients with excessive arm activity combined with the presence of one or more compressive elements in the thoracic outlet. The syndrome was described independently by Von-Schroetter [1] in 1884 in Vienna and by Paget [2] in 1875 in London. For many years, therapy included elevation of the arm with anticoagulants and subsequent return to work [3]. If symptoms recurred, the patient was considered for first rib resection with or without thrombectomy.

When the congenital lateral insertion of the costoclavicular ligament was recognized as the underlying pathological cause, prompt

H.C. Urschel Jr., MD (✉)
Department of Cardiovascular and Thoracic Surgery,
Baylor University Medical Center,
University of Texas Southwestern Medical School,
3600 Gaston Ave, Ste. 1201, Dallas, TX 75246, USA
e-mail: drurschel@me.com

J.M. Pool, MD
Department of Cardiac, Vascular and Thoracic Surgical
Associates, Texas Health Presbyterian
Hospital of Dallas, 8230 Walnut Hill Lane,
Suite 208, Dallas, TX 75231, USA

A.N. Patel, MD
Department of Cardiothoracic Surgery,
School of Medicine, The University of Utah,
30 North, 1900 East, Suite 3C127, Salt Lake City,
UT 84132, USA

[†]Deceased

transaxillary rib resection was employed immediately following thrombolysis [4]. Availability of thrombolytic agents [5–7], combined with prompt surgical neurovascular decompression of the thoracic outlet [4], have reduced morbidity and substantially improved clinical results, including the return to work.

Anatomy

The axillosubclavian vein traverses the tunnel formed by the clavicle anteriorly, the scalenus anticus muscle laterally, the first rib inferiorly, and the costoclavicular ligament medially (Fig. 49.1). In patients with the Paget-Schroetter Syndrome, the costoclavicular ligament is thought to insert further laterally than normal (Fig. 49.2). When the scalenus anticus muscle, lateral to the vein, becomes hypertrophied through recurrent activity and exercise, the vein is significantly narrowed [8]. This is not the case when the costoclavicular ligament inserts in a normal place much more medially on the first rib, even when significant scalenus anticus muscle hypertrophy occurs. It should be noted that many "normal" people have significant compression seen on stress venography (arms elevated) but never develop VTOS [9], supporting the idea that there is an anatomic abnormality in the patients who

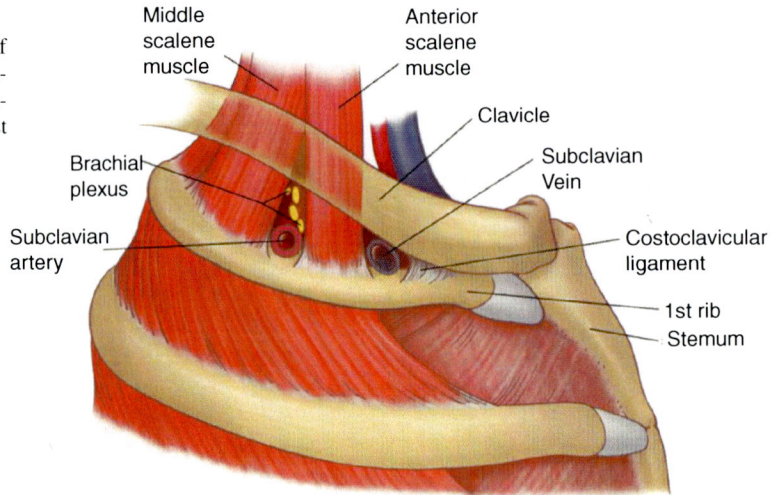

Fig. 49.1 Normal anatomy of the thoracic outlet with conventional insertion of the costoclavicular ligament on the first rib

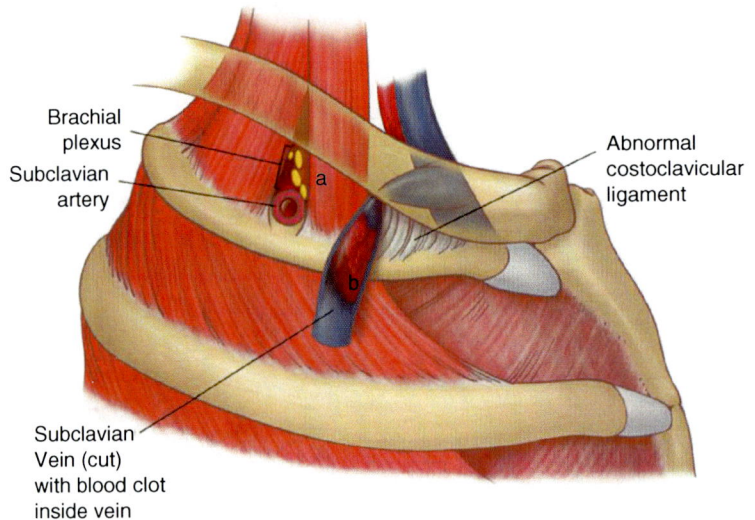

Fig. 49.2 Congenital abnormal lateral insertion of the costoclavicular ligament on the first rib with: (**a**) hypertrophy of the scalenus anticus muscle lateral to the vein; (**b**) thrombosis of axillary-subclavian vein (Paget-Schroetter Syndrome)

do. This costoclavicular ligament abnormality was recognized in 1986 and published initially in 1991 [4], and in our experience every patient (over 500) with Paget-Schroetter Syndrome has demonstrated this anomaly [10]. It should be stressed that this is a disorder of the *anterior* thoracic outlet, and the structures at the sternum, primarily the hypertrophied and abnormally inserted costoclavicular ligament are well underneath the clavicle and must be treated [11, 12].

Pathophysiology

When the axillosubclavian vein clots secondary to thoracic outlet syndrome, Paget-Schroetter Syndrome is present. It is usually associated with a severe inflammatory reaction in the area of the thoracic outlet [13]. This markedly handicaps the surgical dissection and often obscures the location of the first rib, as well as the anatomy of the thoracic outlet. In addition to the inflammation, there is a loss of the usual blue color of the vein because of the lack of blood flowing through it. This removes one of the best anatomical landmarks, further increasing the difficultly for the surgeon in the acute and subacute phase of the syndrome [14, 15].

The finding of increased venous collateral around the shoulder (Urschel's sign) usually suggests total obstruction of the axillary subclavian vein [16, 17]. Other significant pathophysiological observations result in the PSS because the axillosubclavian vein is a "low pressure" system. Therapeutic techniques which are usually successful in the "high pressure" arterial system almost uniformly fail in this "low pressure" venous system, particularly when the abnormal insertion of the costocliclar ligament is not recognized and not removed [18, 19].

When the vein initially occludes, thrombolysis is usually successful if the clot is treated soon after it forms. If successful, a "tight constriction" of the vein is often present. This is quite often secondary to the abnormal external costoclavicular ligament, but may be misread as an intravenous stenosis and dilated as a "balloon angioplasty" through a catheter. Failing to recog-

nize the low venous pressure and managing it as a "high pressure arterial lesson", the "stenosis" is dilated multiple times. Its failure to remain dilated (because of the unrecognized external compression from the abnormal costoclavicluar ligament) may prompt the insertion of an internal venous stent. Because this is a "low pressure" system, the stents uniformly clot [20].

Following thrombosis of the stent or in patients who had failure of thrombolysis, saphenous vein bypass grafts have been placed in 18 patients referred to our hospital, all of who have subsequently occluded (again, because it is a "low pressure" system) [12]. Finally, thrombectomy, if performed, also uniformly fails in this "low-pressure" system [10].

Another complication of the pathological inflammation in PSS is the failure to recognize the first rib because of obliteration of the many anatomical landmarks, which serve as guides to the correct recognition of this structure [19]. To date, 232 patients have been referred to our hospital who have had the second rib mistakenly removed. Malpractice lawsuits frequently ensue.

Results

We recently reviewed our experience over the past four decades in patients with effort thrombosis [10, 12, 15], which includes treatment of 626 extremities in 608 patients. The series includes 307 females and 301 males with a mean age of 32 (ranging from 16 to 51). 432 patients had unusual occupations that involved excessive, repetitive muscular activity of the shoulder, arm, and hand. Potentially aggravating occupations included such sports as golf, tennis, baseball, football, weight lifting, cheerleading, and drill team members, or vocations such as painters, beauticians, and linotype operators. The symptoms were usually exacerbated by working overhead, cold temperatures, or having the arm hang down for long periods of time.

In all 626 extremities, swelling or venous distention over the chest, arm, or hand was present, initially suggesting the clinical diagnosis of venous obstruction. Elevation of the arm or hand did not seem to change the configuration of the veins or swelling acutely. Bluish discoloration was observed in 544 arms, and aching pain, which was increased by exercise, occurred in 520. Cervical ribs were noted in 62 instances. Bilateral thrombosis occurred in 18 patients (12 females and 6 males), simultaneously in 2 (one with previous bilateral clavicular fractures) and sequentially in 16. In 24 patients, only minimal symptoms were present.

One hundred percent of the extremities demonstrated a positive Adson's sign, hyperabduction sign, or some other compressive sign related to thoracic outlet compression in general. Diagnostic tests performed included venous ultrasound studies, venous scintillation scans, venography, plethysmography, temperature studies of the extremity, and bilateral upper extremities nerve conduction velocities including both the median and ulnar nerves.

The diagnosis was established by clinical history, physical examination, ultrasound studies, and venography performed through a medial antecubital vein. Substantial narrowing or occlusion of the axillosubclavian vein in the area of the first rib and clavicle was observed in all patients. Some collateral circulation was evident in 621 extremities, although it was obviously not adequate if swelling were present. The pathways for the most efficient collateral communication were between the cephalic, transverse cervical, transverse scapular, and tributaries of the internal jugular veins producing an increased subcutaneous venous plexus around the shoulder (Urschel's sign).

Prompt transaxillary first rib resection, neurovascular decompression, and resection of the "abnormal" costclavicular was the therapy of choice [21]. In a few cases with fracture of the clavicle and large callous formation, total clavicalectomy was performed [22].

Results were evaluated as good, fair, or poor according to the criteria in Table 49.1 and the results are summarized in Table 49.2. Of patients seen less than 6 weeks after thrombosis and

Table 49.1 Evaluation of results

	Pain relief	Employment	Limited recreation
Good	Complete	Full	None
Fair	Partial	Limitation	Moderate
Poor	None	No return	Severe

Table 49.2 Results

	No. of patients	Good	Fair	Poor
Optimal Rx <6 weeks	502	493	9	0
Optimal Rx (total)	626	599	25	2

Table 49.3 Results of PTVA + Stent

	No. of patients
PTVA + Stent	47
Occlusion	47 (100 %)

treated, 486 of 506 extremities had good results. Those seen after 6 weeks from thrombosis did not fare as well. Coumadin did not seem to improve results. Of the 47 patients evaluated from other centers who had received intravenous stents, all 47 were occluded (Table 49.3) [20]. There was no mortality in any group and no observed evidence of pulmonary embolism.

Summary

Acute axillosubclavian vein thrombosis is a disorder of the anterior thoracic outlet, and is always associated with an abnormally lateral insertion of the costoclavicular ligament. This is a low pressure system associated with extrinsic compressive forces, and conventional intraluminal therapy designed to treat atherosclerotic arterial lesions is not appropriate in this situation. In our experience of over 600 extremities with this condition, prompt thrombolysis followed by thoracic outlet decompression leads to excellent results in over 95 % of patients, especially if treatment is instituted soon after thrombosis occurs.

Acknowledgment The contribution of Mrs. Rachel Montano and Mrs. Brenda Knee are of immeasurable value for her dedication and commitment to the research and completion of this publication.

References

1. Von-Schroetter L. Erkrandungen der Gefossl. In: Nathnogel Handbuch der Pathologie und Therapie. Wein: Holder; 1884.
2. Paget J. Clinical lectures and essays. London: Longmans Green; 1875.
3. De Weese JA, Adams JT, Gaiser DI. Subclavian venous thrombectomy. Circulation. 1970;16 Suppl 2:158–70.
4. Urschel Jr HC, Razzuk MA. Improved management of the Paget-Schroetter syndrome secondary to thoracic outlet compression. Ann Thorac Surg. 1991; 52:1217–21.
5. Zimmerman R, Marl H, Harenberg J, et al. Urokinase therapy of subclavian axillary vein thrombosis. Klin Wochenschr. 1981;59:851–7.
6. Taylor LM, McAllister WR, Dennis DL, et al. Thrombolytic therapy followed by first rib resection for spontaneous subdavian vein thrombosis. Am J Surg. 1985;149:644–7.
7. Drury EM, Trout HH, Giordonon JM, et al. Lytic therapy in the treatment of axillary and subclavian vein thrombosis. J Vasc Surg. 1985;2:821–9.
8. Urschel HC Jr. Anatomy of the thoracicoutlet. In: Ferguson MK, Deslauriers J, editors. Thoracic surgery clinics, vol 17, no 4. Philadelphia: Elsevier; 2007. p. 511–20.
9. Urschel Jr HC. Paget-Schroetter syndrome. Ital J Vasc Endovasc Surg. 2008;15(4):265–71.
10. Urschel Jr HC, Patel AN. Surgery remains the most effective treatment for Paget-Schroetter syndrome: 50 Years' experience. Ann Thorac Surg. 2008;86: 254–60.
11. Urschel HC Jr. Treatment of deep venous thrombosis in the upper extremity. Advances in venous therapy, vol 188. 15th European Vascular Course (EVC), Maastricht; 2011. p. 131–37.
12. Urschel Jr HC, Kourlis Jr H. Thoracic outlet syndrome: a 50-year experience at Baylor University Medical Center. Bayl Univ Med Cent Proc. 2007;20:125–35.
13. Urschel Jr HC, Razzuk MA. Management of the thoracic outlet syndrome. N Engl J Med. 1972;286: 1140–3.
14. Urschel Jr HC, Razzuk MA. Thoracic outlet syndrome. In: Sabiston Jr DC, Spencer FC, editors. Gibbon's surgery of the chest. 6th ed. Philadelphia: WB Saunders; 1995. p. 536–53.
15. Urschel Jr HC, Razzuk MA. Neurovascular compression in the thoracic outlet: changing management over 50 years. Transactions of the American Surgical Association 1998. Ann Surg. 1999;141.
16. MacKinnon SE, Patterson GA, Urschel Jr HC. Thoracic outlet syndromes. In: Pearson FG, editor. Thoracic surgery. New York: Churchill Livingstone; 1995. p. 1211–35.
17. Urschel HC Jr. The John H. Gibbon Jr. Memorial lecture thoracic outlet syndromes. Presented at the annual meeting of the American College of Surgeons, San Frandsco, 10–15 Oct 1993.
18. Urschel Jr HC, Razzuk MA. The failed operation for thoracic outlet syndrome: the difficulty of diagnosis and management. Ann Thorac Surg. 1986;42:532–8.
19. Urschel Jr HC, Patel AN. Reoperation for recurrent thoracic outlet syndrome through the posterior thoracoplasty approach with dorsal sympathectomy. In: Pearson FG et al., editors. Thoracic surgery, vol. 1. 3rd ed. Philadelphia: Churchill Livingstone, Elsevier; 2008.
20. Urschel Jr HC, Patel AN. Paget Schroetter syndrome therapy: failure of intravenous stents. Ann Thorac Surg. 2003;75:1693–6 (Presented at STSA meeting, Miami, 8 Nov 2002).
21. Urschel Jr HC, Cooper JD. Atlas of thoracic surgery. New York: Churchill Livingstone; 1995.
22. Lord JW, Urschel Jr HC. Total claviculectomy. Surg Rounds. 1988;11:17–27.

Clinical Presentation and Patient Evaluation in VTOS

50

Richard L. Feinberg

Abstract

This chapter traces the historical development of our current understanding of the pathophysiology of TOS and discusses the specific anatomic relationships at the thoracic outlet pertinent to venous TOS (VTOS). The clinical presentation of patients with VTOS is described, and the diagnostic evaluation is outlined. A unified, multi-modal approach to Paget-von Schroetter syndrome is discussed, which includes catheter-directed lytic therapy, surgical thoracic outlet decompression, endovenous intervention for intrinsic venous disease, and systemic anticoagulation. Several possible clinical scenarios are discussed and treatment algorithms presented.

In virtually all series describing the subject, the venous form of thoracic outlet syndrome (VTOS) constitutes just 2–3 % of all cases of TOS which come to medical attention [1]. Despite its relatively low incidence, however, VTOS remains an important clinical entity because of the unusual degree of health and vigor of the patient population affected, the often dramatic and unmistakable clinical presentation, the considerable morbidity which results when the condition is neither promptly diagnosed nor properly treated, and the excellent long-term outlook when a proper treatment algorithm is applied. These factors make VTOS an extremely successful and rewarding category of TOS for the surgeon to manage.

Background

Our current understanding of the anatomy and pathophysiology at work in the various forms of thoracic outlet syndrome has evolved over time: from an early emphasis on the importance of a cervical rib, later shifting to the primacy of the scalenus anticus muscle, and finally to a more multi-faceted understanding of the interplay among the many structures which comprise the small space that is the thoracic outlet.

Galen, in the second century A.D., first identified the presence of a cervical rib, later confirmed by the anatomic studies of Vesalius in the 1700s. Sir Astley Cooper correlated the occurrence of arm symptoms with the presence of a cervical rib in 1818 [2], and for nearly the next 100 years cervical

R.L. Feinberg, MD
Department of Vascular Surgery,
John Hopkins University School of Medicine,
11065 Little Patuxent Parkway, Suite 150,
Columbia, MD 21044, USA
e-mail: rfeinbe4@jhmi.edu

ribs were thought to be the primary cause of TOS (which was considered one entity and throughout that time referred to as the "cervical rib syndrome"). In 1861, Coote performed the first cervical rib resection for relief of upper extremity symptoms of neurovascular compression [3]. In a shift of emphasis, Bramwell, in 1903, incriminated the first rib as a cause of symptomatic neurovascular compression [4], and 7 years later Murphy reported the first instance of first rib resection for the management of neurogenic TOS [5]. Two decades later, Naffziger and Grant [6], and Ochsner et al. [7], in separate reports, posited the importance of the scalene muscles in producing symptoms of neurovascular compression, and after reporting successful relief of symptoms with scalene muscle division coined the term, "scalenus syndrome". Falconer, in 1943, added further to the understanding of this entity by highlighting the role of compression by the costoclavicular ligament as a component of the scalenus syndrome [8], and in 1956 Peet consolidated much of this acquired understanding by suggesting the adoption of the more inclusive term "thoracic outlet syndrome" to encompass the roles played by the numerous structures in and around the thoracic outlet in producing symptomatic neurovascular compression [9]. The modern era in the treatment of thoracic outlet compression can be traced to the seminal report by Roos in 1966 describing transaxillary first rib resection for the relief of neurovascular compromise [10].

Anatomy

A clear understanding of the anatomic relationships within the thoracic outlet is important to understand the pathophysiology of VTOS and appreciate the differences between the manifestations of the various forms of compression at this location (see Chap. 3). Venous thoracic outlet syndrome is distinct from both the arterial and neurogenic forms of TOS by virtue of the fact that the axillo-subclavian vein runs anterior to the anterior scalene muscle, and is adjacent to and intimately involved with the junction of the first rib and clavicle and associated structures (see

Chap. 6). Thus comprised, this antero-medial sub-compartment of the costoclavicular space through which the subclavian vein passes is, under the best of circumstances, a very tight space with little room to spare. Any combination of predisposing anatomic factors creating an abnormally small space, or aggravating acquired factors (e.g., muscular hypertrophy within this space or scarring as a result of repetitive motion trauma) serve to encroach on the vulnerable subclavian vein and can initiate a cycle of irritation, inflammation and fibrosis which, in turn, can lead to venous stenosis and thrombosis ("effort thrombosis" or Paget-von Schroetter syndrome).

Clinical Presentation

The clinical presentation of patients with VTOS is, in the majority of cases, straightforward and unmistakable. The vast majority of patients are young, healthy, well-developed and usually engaged in the pursuit of vigorous upper extremity physical activities. The classic example is that of a weightlifter, but any young or middle-aged person with well-developed upper body musculature who frequently performs repetitive overhead arm exertion sufficient to result in hypertrophy of the subclavius and scalene muscles (e.g., swimming, pitching, arduous mechanical labor, etc.) can develop symptomatic VTOS. Both radiologic and anatomic studies have demonstrated that arm abduction (such as an auto mechanic might employ while working on a vehicle on an overhead lift) results in compression of the neurovascular structures within the thoracic outlet and a closing off of the already narrow costoclavicular space in many people without symptoms [11, 12]. The repetitive nature of many of the aforementioned precipitating activities promotes a recurring cycle of stretching and the application of frictional forces to the subclavian vein, initiating the cycle of inflammation and fibrosis.

Symptomatic VTOS disproportionately affects males – most likely as a result of gender-based differences in the architecture of the normal thoracic outlet, combined with the more frequent overdevelopment of upper extremity musculature in men [13]. The dominant arm is most often affected. The symptoms of VTOS are those of venous hypertension in the affected extremity. Patients may present with symptoms of intermittent, exercise-induced, non-thrombotic venous obstruction, or they may manifest the sudden onset of severe and sustained arm swelling due to occlusive subclavian vein thrombosis. It is important to note that, even in cases presenting as sudden "unheralded" subclavian vein thrombosis, detailed questioning frequently reveals an antecedent history of more subtle episodic symptoms of intermittent venous obstruction related to arm exercise. Less obvious symptoms can include a sensation of fullness, pressure, heaviness, fatigue and engorgement of the affected arm following exercise, while some patients may report a variety of paraesthesiae in the fingers, hand and forearm. Arm pain is usually quite minimal and, if present, reflects the increased pressure due to passive venous congestion. More intense pain, if present, is usually localized to the axilla and is a direct consequence of the pain of the local phlebitic process at the site of the venous thrombosis.

In patients with effort thrombosis, the physical findings include pronounced unilateral arm swelling, plethora, and engorgement of the superficial veins of the arm. A prominent network of collateral draining veins rapidly appears about the shoulder and chest, and the development of these collateral drainage pathways is often followed by marked improvement (and sometimes complete resolution) of the initial arm swelling. Despite this apparent "resolution" most patients will report some degree of venous claudication – a sensation of fullness, heaviness or discomfort – with any degree of sustained arm activity, especially if in a position of "stress" (either overhead or in abduction). In patients with non-thrombotic VTOS (intermittent positional obstruction), the physical findings at the time of examination may be minimal. Subtle findings may include an unusual prominence of superficial veins of the arm, or the reproduction of subjective symptoms of fullness, pressure or paraesthesiae with provocative maneuvers such as simple arm abduction or the performance of the elevated arm stress test

(EAST). Initially described by Roos [14], the EAST consists of having the patient place the arms in the "stick'em up" position for 3 min while clenching and unclenching the fists. While this is not an "objective" test and is somewhat controversial in that a lack of specificity has been reported, we have found that a reproduction of the patient's subjective symptoms with this test helps to raise the index of suspicion for VTOS in the appropriate clinical setting. Other physical maneuvers originally posited to be pathognomonic for TOS (e.g., the Adson maneuver) are notoriously inaccurate and have generally fallen into disuse [15].

Diagnostic Testing

The diagnosis of VTOS is largely made on clinical grounds at the time of initial presentation. In the typical instance of sudden painful arm swelling and engorgement in an otherwise healthy, muscular young male engaged in overhead arm activity who has a prominent network of collateral veins about the shoulder, the diagnosis of effort thrombosis is quite straightforward and can be made simply on the basis of the history and physical findings. Nevertheless, diagnostic testing plays a supporting role in a number of cases and may be especially useful in the setting of non-thrombotic venous thoracic outlet obstruction, in which the physical findings at the time of examination may be minimal. As already mentioned, provocative maneuvers designed to elicit signs of neurovascular impingement during physical examination are notoriously inaccurate, with both a lack of specificity and sensitivity amply documented. Such tests have little role in the modern evaluation and management of TOS and are mentioned more for their historical interest than for their utility. Adson's test, first described in 1927, consists of chin elevation, neck extension, and rotation of the head *toward* the affected side. With deep inspiration, the loss of a palpable radial artery pulse indicates a "positive" result [16]. The historical importance of this test consists primarily in its implicit acknowledgement of the importance of the scalenus anticus muscle

Fig. 50.1 Duplex scan, longitudinal view, demonstrating absence of flow within the subclavian vein in a 40 year old male patient with effort thrombosis. Note patency of external jugular vein (*EJV*) providing collateral pathway to the innominate vein. *SUBCL* subclavian; *V* vein; *INNOM* innominate

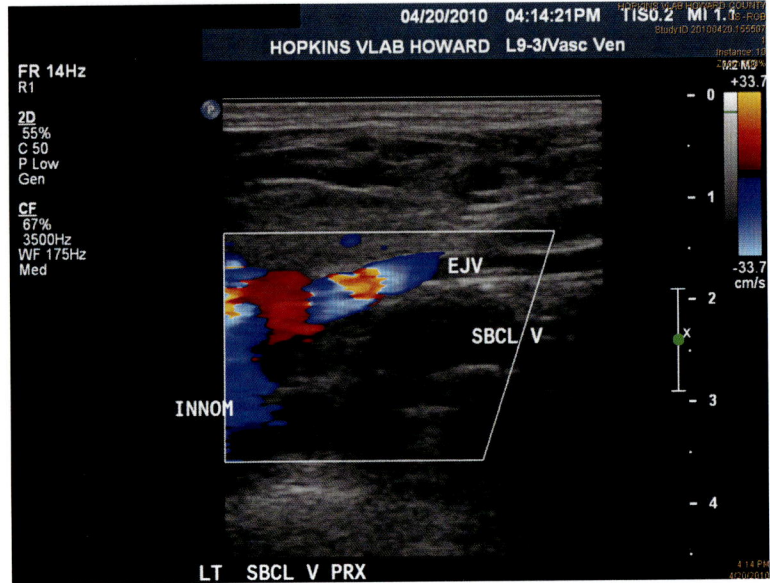

in thoracic outlet pathology, as the Adson position accentuates tension within the anterior scalene muscle. Unfortunately, this test is non-specific in that a "positive" result is found in a large number of "normal" individuals, and points more to pathology (if present) in the arterial/neurogenic triangle. Similarly, the costo-clavicular maneuver, described by Falconer in 1943, consisting of the backward and downward bracing of the shoulders, lacks both specificity and sensitivity. As already mentioned earlier in this chapter, the elevated arm stress test also lacks objective reproducibility, although we find this can be mildly useful in reproducing subjective symptoms in some patients with non-thrombotic VTOS. Most of these tests, finally, are "positive" in the setting of neurogenic TOS.

Venous plethysmography – either impedance or air – can be performed both before and after stress positioning as a non-invasive means of obtaining some objective confirmation of increased venous obstruction at the thoracic outlet. These tests are cumbersome, however, and are no longer commonly utilized.

The dominant non-invasive test currently employed in the diagnostic evaluation of vascular TOS is duplex ultrasonography [17–19]. It is important to emphasize that the particular examination should focus specifically on the

structures (arterial or venous) pertinent to the specific variety of TOS in consideration. Thus, when evaluating a potential case of VTOS, complete duplex evaluation of the axillary and subclavian veins is essential. This includes full grey-scale imaging of the subclavian vein in both transverse and longitudinal section, as well as Doppler spectral waveform analysis – both at rest (arm in full adduction, at the patient's side) and during stress positioning (arm abduction at 90 and 180°) . In cases of Paget-Schroetter syndrome, the duplex findings are unequivocal: complete thrombotic occlusion of the axillo-subclavian venous segment is readily identified (See Figs. 50.1 and 50.2). In contrast, in cases of non-thrombotic venous thoracic outlet obstruction, positive findings can include the presence of a fixed, visible stenosis of the subclavian vein seen on high-resolution B-mode imaging, normal venous anatomy at rest but narrowing of the vein evident during stress positioning, and marked dampening or complete cessation of Doppler flow within the axillary and subclavian veins – or increased-velocity flow within the subclavian vein at a locus of visible constriction – while in the stress position (see Figs. 50.3 and 50.4).

Despite the widespread availability of duplex ultrasonography and its nearly universal acceptance as the pivotal initial imaging study for assessing

Fig. 50.2 Transverse view in the same patient, showing non-compressibility and the presence of echogenic thrombus within the subclavian vein. *A* artery; *V* vein

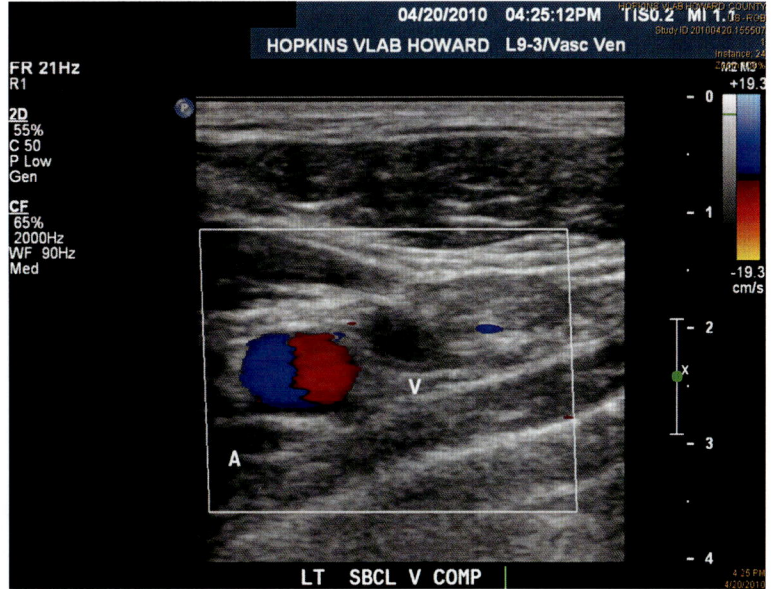

patients with possible VTOS, contrast venography continues to occupy a critical position in the evaluation and treatment of these patients. In the modern era, most patients come to venography with a diagnosis of VTOS having already been established by prior ultrasonography. The utility of venography resides primarily in its use as a portal for venous intervention – either for the initiation of lytic therapy in patients with acute effort thrombosis or for the performance of subsequent venous intervention (i.e., venous angioplasty). Initial access is typically obtained via either the basilic or the brachial vein in the mid-to-distal upper arm using a 4 or 5 Fr micropuncture kit and ultrasound guidance (the cephalic vein enters the deep system too centrally for full intervention in many cases and is a poor choice for access for this reason). In cases of non-thrombotic VTOS, contrast injection and visualization of the axillo-subclavian venous segment is performed first with the arm adducted and subsequently with the arm in abduction. In the setting of thrombotic occlusion of the subclavian vein (i.e., Paget-von Schroetter Syndrome), definitive visualization of the venous anatomy in the region of the thoracic outlet is not possible as a result of non-opacification of the thrombosed venous structures. In such cases, a hydrophilic guidewire is used to probe the thrombus, and a multi-sidehole infusion catheter (e.g., UniFuse ®,

AngioDynamics) is embedded within the thrombus to enable initiation of intra-clot thrombolytic therapy with t-PA (Alteplase ®, Genentech) (see Chap. 84). If thrombolysis is successful, follow-up venography allows full characterization of any residual intrinsic venous stricture as well as any foci of extrinsic compression of the subclavian vein within the costoclavicular space. When venous intervention is to be performed (usually after the thoracic outlet has been decompressed), a larger access sheath may be required.

Treatment

Once diagnosed, the definitive treatment of VTOS requires mechanical decompression of the thoracic outlet. In cases of effort thrombosis, the use of lytic therapy followed by anticoagulation alone, without the performance of definitive mechanical decompression, has been shown to yield unacceptably high rates of recurrent thrombosis and long-term morbidity [20]. As our understanding of the anatomic and pathophysiologic considerations at the root of TOS have evolved over the decades, a consensus has taken shape regarding the essential elements for proper mechanical decompression. It is fairly uniformly accepted that full decompression of the costoclavicular

Fig. 50.3 (**a** and **b**) Duplex images of the left axillary and subclavian veins (*longitudinal* view) in a 32 year old male patient with episodic symptoms of non-thrombotic VTOS. These images, taken in the neutral position, demonstrate wide patency of both veins and normal phasic venous flow patterns

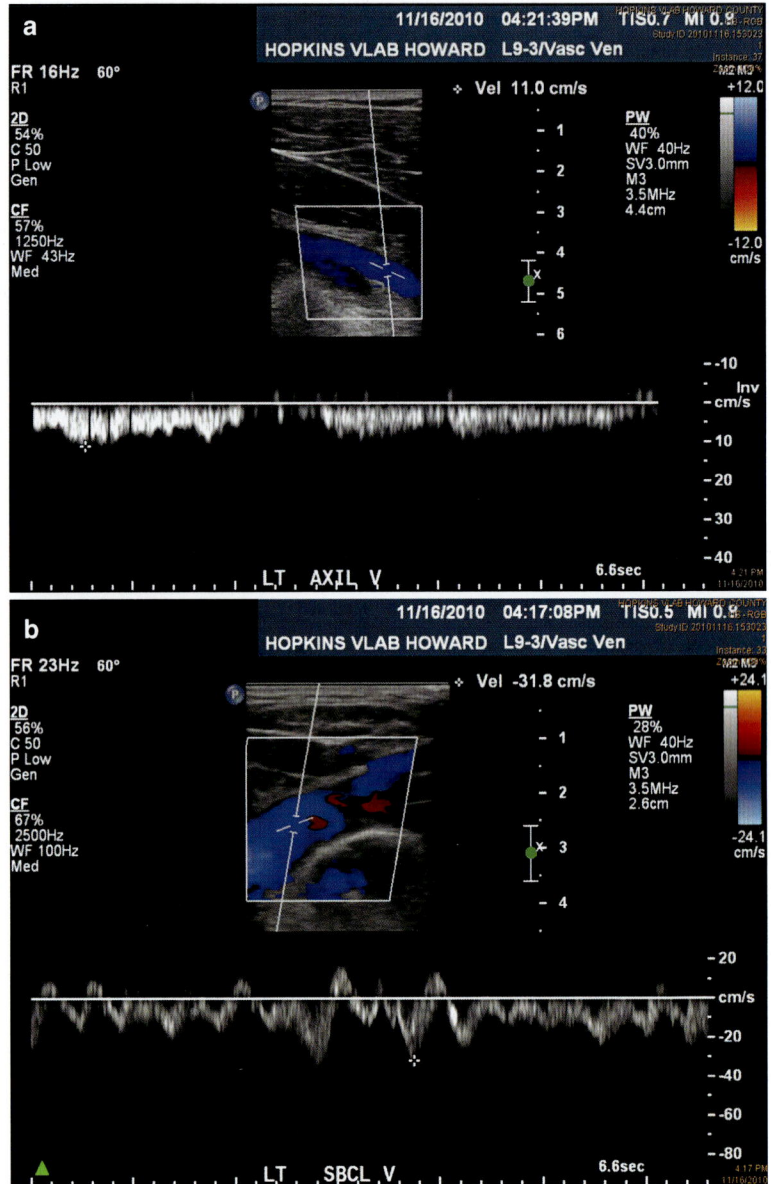

space requires: (1) resection of the first rib, as far anteriorly as its confluence with the sternum medially; (2) resection of the anterior scalene muscle; and (3) venolysis: division of all fibrous bands and associated scar tissue surrounding the subclavian vein. This can be accomplished by either a trans-axillary, a supra-clavicular or an infra-clavicular approach. The advantages of trans-axillary first rib resection include excellent exposure of the anterior extent of the first rib (facilitating wide decompression) and excellent cosmetics, as the scar is hidden in the axillary skin creases (no small consideration in this young and otherwise healthy patient population). Alternatively, supra- or infra-clavicular first rib resection or even claviculectomy affords better visualization of the subclavian vein in the event that surgical repair or replacement is felt to be necessary. It is important to note, however, that endovascular intervention has reduced the need for open venoplasty or bypass,

Fig. 50.4 (**a** and **b**) Duplex images of the same patient with the arm abducted 180°. Note the complete absence of venous Doppler flow signals in both the axillary and subclavian veins during stress positioning

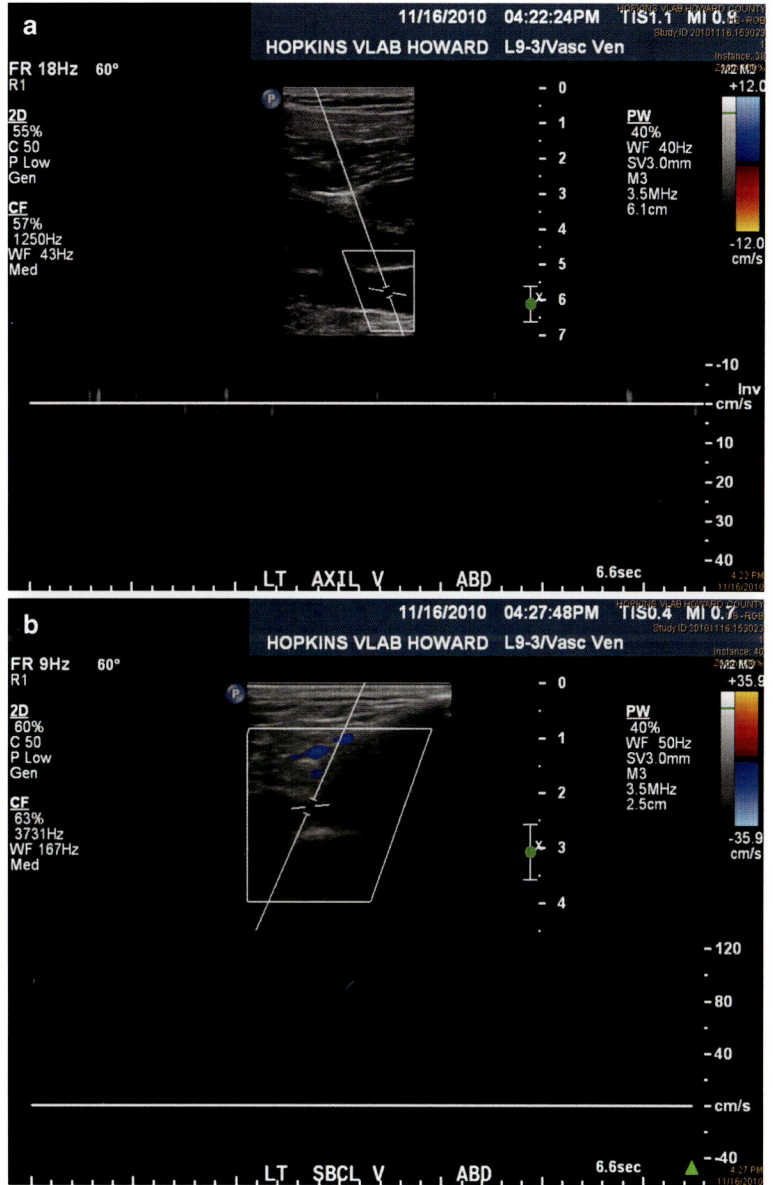

Clinical Scenarios

With the foregoing as background, it is clear that a few distinct presenting clinical scenarios will be encountered, each with its own specific diagnostic and management schema. The most thus negating this theoretical advantage of the supra-clavicular approach.

fundamental initial distinction to be made is that between patients with thrombosis of the subclavian vein (i.e., Paget-von Schroetter syndrome) versus those with symptoms of non-thrombotic obstruction of the vein due to intermittent recurring mechanical compression at the thoracic outlet. Among patients with thrombosis, the next most important distinction is that between those with acute thrombosis and those with longstanding, chronic occlusion.

The most common presenting scenario is that of classic acute effort thrombosis: a young, otherwise healthy individual presenting with acute painful swelling of the arm following a period of strenuous upper extremity physical exertion. Because symptoms almost always become manifest within 24 h of the thrombosis, these patients usually present for evaluation without undue delay, and the diagnostic work-up must be carried out expeditiously so as to enable initiation of prompt catheter-directed thrombolysis. Thrombolysis is likeliest to be successful if performed within 2 weeks of the onset of symptoms, although we and other authors have noted instances of successful thrombolysis even when lytic therapy has been instituted as much as 3 months (or longer) after the thrombotic event. Following thrombolysis, it is essential that the thoracic outlet be fully decompressed and any residual intrinsic venous pathology be corrected. The algorithm originally proposed by Kunkel and Machleder in 1989 consists of thrombolysis followed by 3 months of anticoagulant therapy (warfarin), after which trans-axillary first rib resection and scalenectomy (FRRS) is performed and any residual venous stenosis is treated [21]. However, the 3 month window from the time of lysis to eventual thoracic outlet decompression represents a period during which patients are potentially at-risk for re-thrombosis, and several authors [22–24] have attempted to reduce or even close this window, and many surgeons now advocate thoracic outlet decompression during the same admission [25].

A second clinical scenario is that of the patient with effort thrombosis in whom there has been sufficient delay in diagnosis and treatment that thrombolytic therapy either cannot be undertaken or has been attempted unsuccessfully. In patients with recalcitrant chronic subclavian vein occlusions such as this, we have found that anticoagulation alone – with FRRS performed at a variable time interval after diagnosis – allows spontaneous recanalization of the subclavian vein in a significant percentage of patients, and patency and symptomatic relief have been sustained at intermediate-term follow-up [26, 27].

Finally, in patients presenting with episodic symptoms of non-thrombotic venous obstruction due to mechanical impingement at the thoracic outlet, the management schema is much less time-sensitive, and the diagnostic work-up and treatment can be conducted in a more elective fashion. These patients undergo full upper extremity venous duplex examination in both resting and stress positions as the initial diagnostic study. If this confirms significant impingement of the subclavian vein within the costoclavicular space, elective FRRS is performed. Follow-up venography is performed 2 weeks post-operatively, and any residual venous pathology is treated percutaneously at that time [28].

Conclusions

As discussed later in this section, Level 1 evidence for much of what we do to treat patients with VTOS simply does not exist, and thus within the broad outlines of the treatment algorithms described above there remains considerable room for individual variation in practice. Such issues as the optimal surgical approach for decompression (transaxillary versus supraclavicular), the degree of aggressiveness with lytic therapy or with endovascular interventions, and the duration of post-treatment anticoagulant regimens all remain unsupported by controlled randomized data. It is, therefore, important to remember that recommendations regarding strategies for "best management" are merely guidelines within which the practitioner has ample room to navigate. Nevertheless, a few fundamental tenets warrant reiteration: (1) all patients with symptomatic VTOS (thrombotic and non-thrombotic) benefit from thoracic outlet decompression, and this is an essential component in the management of virtually every case; (2) patients with acute effort thrombosis benefit from early (within 14 days if possible) initiation of thrombolytic therapy and can usually be restored to their pre-morbid clinical status following successful lysis and surgical decompression; (3) patients with subacute or chronic subclavian vein occlusions may not benefit from aggressive attempts at pharmaco-mechanical recanalization and do quite well with thoracic outlet decompression and anticoagulation alone; and (4) in patients hospitalized with acute effort thrombosis, surgical decompression of the thoracic outlet can be safely and effectively performed immediately following thrombolysis, thereby allowing definitive treatment without undue delay.

References

1. Sanders RJ, Hammond SL, Rao NM. Thoracic outlet syndrome: a review. Neurologist. 2008;14:365–73.
2. Adson AW, Coffey JR. Cervical rib: a method of anterior approach for relief of symptoms by division of the scalenus anticus. Ann Surg. 1927;85:839–57.
3. Coote H. Pressure on the axillary vessels and nerves by an exostosis from a cervical rib; interference with the circulation of the arm; removal of the rib and exostosis, recovery. Med Times Gaz. 1861;2:108.
4. Bramwell E. Lesion of the first dorsal nerve root. Rev Neurol Psychiatry. 1903;1:236.
5. Murphy T. Brachial neuritis caused by pressure of first rib. Aust Med J. 1910;15:582–5.
6. Naffziger HC, Grant WT. Neuritis of the brachial plexus mechanical in origin: the scalenus syndrome. Surg Gynecol Obstet. 1938;67:722–30.
7. Ochsner A, Gage M, DeBakey M. Scalenus anticus (Naffziger) syndrome. Am J Surg. 1935;28:699.
8. Falconer MA, Weddell G. Costoclavicular compression of the subclavian artery and vein: relation to scalenus syndrome. Lancet. 1943;2:539–43.
9. Peet RM, Hendriksen JD, Anderson TP, Martin GM. Thoracic outlet syndrome: evaluation of the therapeutic exercise program. Proc Mayo Clin. 1956;31:281–7.
10. Roos DB. Transaxillary approach for first rib resection to relieve thoracic outlet syndrome. Ann Surg. 1966;163:354–8.
11. Colon E, Westdrop R. Vascular compression in the thoracic outlet: age dependent normative values in noninvasive testing. J Cardiovasc Surg. 1988;29:166–71.
12. Criado E, Berguer R, Greenfield L. The spectrum of arterial compression at the thoracic outlet. J Vasc Surg. 2010;52:406–11.
13. Freischlag J. Venous thoracic outlet syndrome: transaxillary approach. Op Tech Gen Surg. 2008;10(3):122–30.
14. Roos DB. New concepts of TOS that explain etiology, symptoms, diagnosis and treatment. Vasc Surg. 1979;13:313–21.
15. Sanders RJ, Hammond SL, Rao NM. Diagnosis of thoracic outlet syndrome. J Vasc Surg. 2007;46:601–4.
16. Adson AW. Surgical treatment for symptoms produced by cervical ribs and the scalenus anticus muscle. Surg Gynecol Obstet. 1947;85:687–700.
17. Wadhwani R. Color Doppler and duplex sonography in 5 patients with thoracic outlet syndrome. J Ultrasound Med. 2001;20:795–801.
18. Odderson IR. Use of sonography in thoracic outlet syndrome due to a dystonic pectoralis minor. J Ultrasound Med. 2009;28:1235–8.
19. Ouriel K. Non-invasive diagnosis of upper extremity vascular disease. Semin Vasc Surg. 1998;11(2):54–9.
20. Thompson JF, Winterborn RJ, Bays S, White H, Kinsella DC, Watkinson AF. Venous thoracic outlet compression and the Paget-Schroetter syndrome: a review and recommendations for management. Cardiovasc Intervent Radiol. 2011;34(5):903–10 (Epub ahead of print).
21. Kunkel JM, Machleder HI. Spontaneous subclavian vein thrombosis: a successful combined approach of local thrombolytic therapy followed by first rib resection. Surgery. 1989;106:114.
22. Urschel HC, Razzuk MA. Paget-Schroetter syndrome: what is the best management? Ann Thorac Surg. 2000;69:1663–9.
23. Angle N, Gelabert HA, Farooq MM, Ahn SS, Caswell DR, Freischlag JA. Safety and efficacy of early surgical decompression of the thoracic outlet for Paget-Schroetter syndrome. Ann Vasc Surg. 2001;15:37–42.
24. Molina EJ, Hunter DW, Dietz CA. Paget-Schroetter syndrome treated with thrombolytics and immediate surgery. J Vasc Surg. 2007;45:328–34.
25. Caparrelli DJ, Freischlag JA. A unified approach to axillosubclavian venous thrombosis in a single hospital admission. Semin Vasc Surg. 2005;18:153–7.
26. Guzzo JL, Chang K, Demos J, Black JH, Freischlag JA. Preoperative thrombolysis and venoplasty affords no benefit in patency following first rib resection and scalenectomy for subacute and chronic subclavian vein thrombosis. J Vasc Surg. 2010;52:658–63.
27. deLeon RA, Chang DC, Busse C, Call D, Freischlag JA. First rib resection and scalenectomy for chronically occluded subclavian veins: what does it really do? Ann Vasc Surg. 2008;22:395–401.
28. deLeon RA, Chang DC, Hassoun HT, Black JH, Roseborough GS, Perler BA, Rotellini-Coltvet L, Call D, Busse C, Freischlag JA. Multiple treatment algorithms for successful outcomes in venous thoracic outlet syndrome. Surgery. 2009;145:500–7.

VTOS in the Patient Requiring Chronic Hemodialysis Access

51

Carolyn Glass

Abstract

Central venous obstruction (CVO) is the most common cause of failure of Arteriovenous fistulae (AVF) and grafts (AVG) placed for dialysis access. In essentially all reports, including international consensus statements for management of such patients, all CVOs are lumped together, implicitly assuming that all should be treated first with endovascular means. We point out that while stenosis in veins surrounded by soft tissue are appropriate for endoluminal intervention, those that occur at the costoclavicular junction are identical in pathophysiology to and should be treated in a fashion similar to those in patients with "conventional" venous thoracic outlet syndrome. By aggressive use of thoracic outlet decompression in patients with dialysis access dysfunction caused by costoclavicular stenosis we have achieved fistula salvage in approximately two-thirds of patients who would otherwise have required ligation. This lesion should be considered "dialysis-dependent venous TOS" and treated aggressively.

Introduction

Over 350,000 persons have dialysis-dependent renal failure in the United States alone [1]. A fair number of these patients – 20–50 % – develop central venous obstruction (CVO) [2], defined as obstruction of the subclavian vein, innominate vein, or superior vena cava. Blood flow to the right atrium is restricted, resulting in significant arm or facial edema, prolonged fistula bleeding

(during cannulation and post-dialysis), inefficient dialysis, and eventual fistula failure [3].

The underlying pathophysiology of CVO in dialysis patients is multifactorial and complex. Catheter induced trauma is thought to be the most common cause of CVO in the dialysis population [4]. Approximately 60–80 % of dialysis patients at some point receive central venous catheterization for acute or long term access needs [2]. Catheter trauma induces venous endothelial denudation, subsequent subendothelial pericyte proliferation, increased secretion of tissue factor, and upregulation of cytokines and growth factors [5]. Thrombotic and inflammatory cascades are activated resulting in venous intimal hyperplasia and luminal

C. Glass, MD, MS.
Department of Vascular Surgery,
Strong Memorial Hospital,
601 Elmwood Avenue, Rochester, NY 146642, USA
e-mail: carolyn_glass@urmc.rochester.edu

obstruction [6]. The high flow through this area in patients with an ipsilateral fistula probably exacerbates or accelerates this cycle.

Dialysis-Associated Venous Thoracic Outlet Syndrome

Whether the central venous lesion is caused by an intrinsic problem (such as venous intimal hyperplasia) or extrinsic compression is imperative to select appropriate treatment for these patients [7]. Current literature of treatment options in dialysis patients with CVO only target correcting intrinsic causes, mainly venous intimal hyperplasia, and implicitly lump all CVO together as one entity. The National Kidney Foundation-K/DOQI guidelines recommend percutaneous transluminal venoplasty with or without stenting as the initial treatment for all CVO [8]. While endoluminal intervention is acceptable for central venous lesions associated with intimal hyperplasia and in vessels surrounded by soft tissue only, however, this is not the situation at the costoclavicular junction (Fig. 51.1). At this point the clavicle and first rib, joined together anteriorly by the costoclavicular ligament and their attachments to the sternum, apply a huge amount of force to the subclavian vein (which is the most anterior structure passing through this area). We believe that this "dialysis-associated venous thoracic outlet syndrome" should be treated exactly as we do any patient with VTOS, whether they have a fistula or not [7].

In an earlier paper from our institution, Bakken et al. reported a fistula salvage rate of only 54 % at 6 months when patients with CVO were treated with angioplasty and/orstenting [9]. Many of these patients, in retrospect, had lesions at the costoclavicular junction. Following this we made the mental connection between CVO at the costoclavicular ligament and VTOS, and began to apply VTOS treatment principles to these patients. We recently reported our experience with costoclavicular decompression in patients with fistula dysfunction [10]. All patients had prior unsuccessful balloon dilations (mean 2.3 attempts) with continued fistula dysfunction. Patients underwent surgical decompression with first rib resection or claviculectomy, the latter if reconstruction was anticipated. In this report six underwent transaxillary first rib resection and four medial claviculectomy, and in all patients aggressive external externalvenolysis was performed. A central venogram through the fistula was completed following surgical decompression and endovascular treatment performed if necessary. Fistula salvage was promising at 80 % with mean follow up 8.3 months. All patients reported complete relief of upper

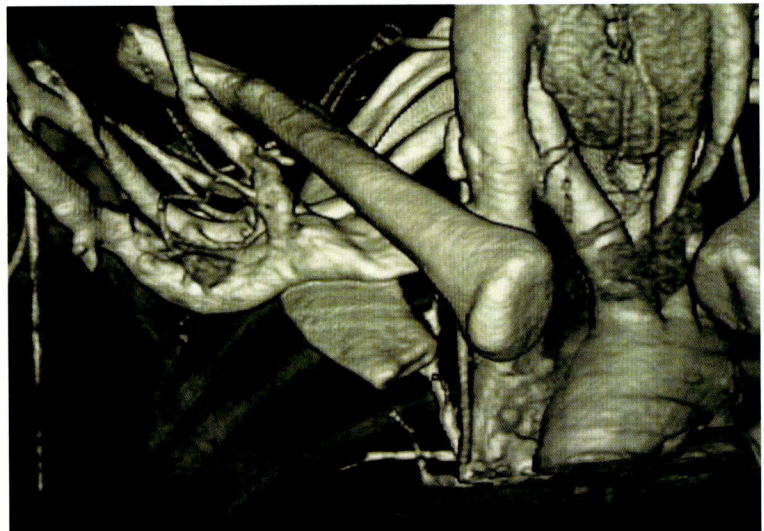

Fig. 51.1 CT reconstruction of a patient with venous thoracic outlet syndrome clearly showing the point of compression at the anterior thoracic outlet (the "void" above the vein is the nonvisualized subclavius muscle, illustrating the importance of this structure). Note that the arm is in a raised position (Courtesy Wallace Foster, MBBS, FRACS, Royal Brisbane and Women's Hospital, Brisbane, Australia)

Fig. 51.2 Fistulagram of a patient with an arteriovenous fistula and central vein obstruction at the costoclavicular junction – "dialysis-associated venous thoracic outlet syndrome." Venogram shows a focal stenosis beginning at the costoclavicular junction with normal vein peripherally (*solid arrow*), and extensive collateralization (*open arrow*)

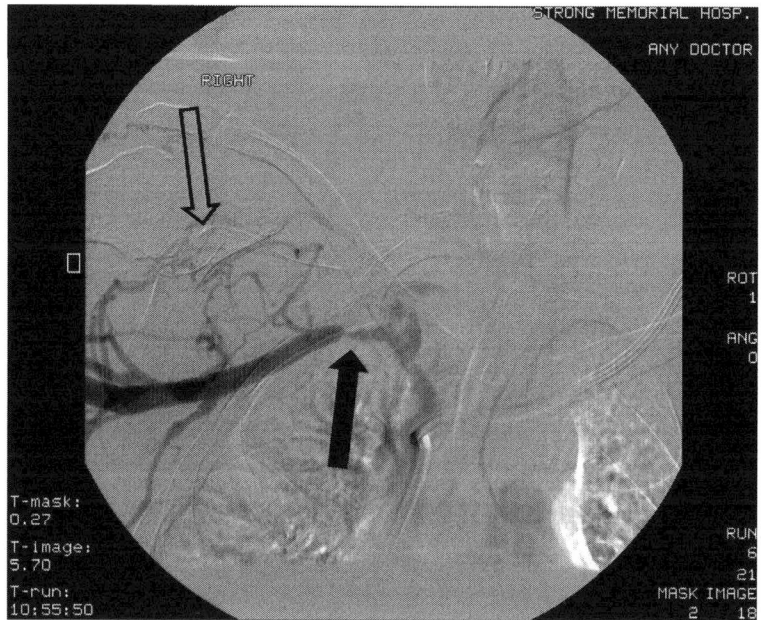

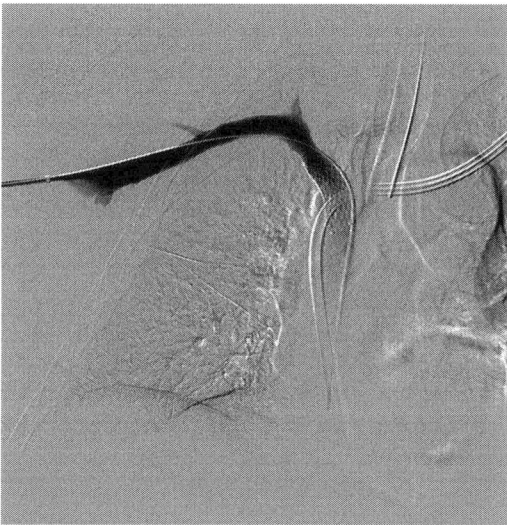

Fig. 51.3 The same patient after transaxillary first rib excision, external venolysis, and balloon angioplasty. Note the immediate absence of collateral flow. The lesion did not respond to venoplasty alone and required stenting

arm edema and pain. There was no mortality or significant morbidity. We now recommend transaxillary first rib resection in essentially all dialysis patients with costoclavicular lesions (Figs. 51.2 and 51.3).

Endoluminal Intervention

Kreienberg et al. showed short subclavian strictures in Paget-Schroetter patients could be safely treated with angioplasty and stenting *after* decompression with reasonable long term patency. All patients (N=23) underwent angioplasty immediately following supraclavicular thoracic inlet decompression, and 61 % required subclavian vein stenting for residual stenosis after angioplasty. Nine of 14 stented veins remained patent at mean follow-up of 3.5 years. It should be noted that while mall numbers precluded subgroup analysis, all of the patients in this series who occluded had been stented [11]. Five of the dialysis patients who underwent surgical decompression in our series later required central venoplasty (four subclavian, one innominate) and three had stents placed (two subclavian, one innominate). At 8 months all stents were functionally patent.

Intravascular ultrasound (IVUS) is a helpful adjunct when stenting the central venous system. Healthy vein is measured proximal and distal to the lesion to approximate appropriate stent size. Raju et al. championed the use of IVUS guided stenting for chronic iliocaval and iliofemoral occlusions [12], and Gillespie et al. extended the use of IVUS guided stenting in the innominate vein and superior vena cava [13], showing that dialysis patients with central venous stents placed using IVUS guidance had significantly larger stents compared to venographically-guided procedures (19.7±3.2 mm vs. 10.0±2.0 mm, p=0.003). IVUS guided stenting was also associated with an increase in fistula salvage rate.

Surgical Reconstruction

If the central lesion is occluded or cannot be crossed with a wire, alternatives include direct surgical reconstruction, "extraanatomic" HeRO catheter placement (Hemosphere, Eden Prarie, MN), bypass, or abandoning the fistula. If a patient is unfit for major surgery (e.g., median sternotomy) with limited life expectancy, the fistula should be ligated and another access site pursued. The contralateral arm or leg can be considered for new fistula creation. If the patient can tolerate direct surgical repair and has a reasonable life expectancy, superior vena cava reconstruction or bypass [14–16] can be considered. In an effort to avoid sternotomy, we recently treated a subset of dialysis patients with occluded central veins with a substernally tunneled subclavian to right atrial bypass. Patients treated in this fashion had an existing fistula with symptomatic venous hypertension, no other options in the contralateral arm, and failed leg fistulas. Claviculectomy was performed and a third intercostal space "minipericardiotomy" to the right atrial appendage was used. Eleven underwent surgery, and at 6 and 10 months, 66 and 33 % of the fistulas remained functional, respectively. While durability was not great, dialysis access was maintained for a length of time in those who had no other access options [16].

The most recent census from the National Kidney Foundation predicts the number of patients requiring long-term hemodialysis will only continue to rise [1], resulting in an inevitable increase of patients with central venous obstruction. We believe a significant number of patients with threatened AV access due to central venous stenosis have lesions attributable to compression at the costoclavicular junction (e.g. "dialysis-associated venous thoracic outlet syndrome"). Recognizing the lesion is the first step. The principles of venous thoracic outlet syndrome treatment, mainly surgical decompression by means of first rib or clavicular resection and thorough external venolysis, should then be applied.

References

1. Fistula First Data. http://www.fistulafirst.org/AboutFistulaFirst/FFBIData.aspx. Accessed May 2011.
2. Agarwal AK. Central vein stenosis: current concepts. Adv Chronic Kidney Dis. 2009;16:360–70.
3. Roy-Chaudhury P, Spergel LM, Besarab A, Asif A, Ravani P. Biology of arteriovenous fistula failure. J Nephrol. 2007;20:150–63.
4. Dosluoglu H, Harris LM. Hemodialysis access: non-thrombotic complications. In: Cronenwett JL, Johnston KW, editors. Rutherford's vascular surgery. 7th ed. Philadelphia: Saunders Elsevier; 2010. p. 1137–54.
5. Costa E, Rocha S, Rocha-Pereira P, Castro E, Reis F, Teixeira F, Miranda V, Do SameiroFaria M, Loureiro A, Quintanilha A, Belo L, Santos-Silva A. Cross-talk between inflammation, coagulation/fibrinolysis and vascular access in hemodialysis patients. J Vasc Access. 2008;9(4):248–53.
6. Fox EA, Kahn SR. The relationship between inflammation and venous thrombosis. A systematic review of clinical studies. Thromb Haemost. 2005; 94(2):362–5.
7. Illig K. Management of central vein stenoses and occlusions: the critical importance of the costoclavicular junction. Semin Vasc Surg. 2011;24(2):113–8.
8. NKF-K/DOQI clinical practice guidelines for vascular access 2000. Am J Kidney Dis 2001;37:s137–81.
9. Bakken AM, Protack CD, Saad WE, Lee DE, Waldman DL, Davies MG. Long-term outcomes of primary angioplasty and primary stenting of central venous stenosis in hemodialysis patients. J Vasc Surg. 2007;45:776–83.
10. Glass C, Dugan M, Gillespie D, Doyle A, Illig K. Costoclavicular venous decompression in patients with threatened arteriovenous hemodialysis access. Ann Vasc Surg. 2011;25(5):640–5.
11. Kreienberg PB, Chang BB, Darling 3rd RC, Roddy SP, Paty PS, Lloyd WE, et al. Long-term results in patients treated with thrombolysis, thoracic inlet decompression, and subclavian vein stenting for Paget-Schroetter syndrome. J Vasc Surg. 2001;33 Suppl 2:S100–5.
12. Neglén P, Raju S. Intravascular ultrasound scan evaluation of the obstructed vein. J Vasc Surg. 2002;35(4):694–700.

13. Glass C, Gillespie D. Intravascular ultrasound for innominate vein and superior vena cava stenting. Feb 2011 American venous forum (San Diego), abstract.

14. Kalra M, Gloviczki P, Andrews JC, Cherry Jr KJ, Bower TC, Panneton JM, et al. Open surgical and endovascular treatment of superior vena cava syndrome caused by nonmalignant disease. J Vasc Surg. 2003;38:215–23.

15. Yu SH, Dilley RB. Internal jugular vein turndown for subclavian vein occlusion. Techniques in the surgical and catheter based treatment of venous disorders. Operative Tech Gen Surg. 2008;10(3):149–53.

16. Glass C, Maevsky V, Massey T, Illig KA. Subclavian vein to right atrial appendage bypass without sternotomy to maintain AV access in patients with complete central vein occlusion: a new approach. Ann Vasc Surg. 2009;23(4):465–8.

VTOS in the Pediatric Age Group

52

Purandath Lall and Linda Harris

Abstract

VTOS in the pediatric patient is usually due to either positional obstruction or effort thrombosis. Children may present with acute symptoms of arm swelling and discomfort and some may present with chronic symptoms associated with dilated collateral veins. All patients should undergo hypercoagulable workup and duplex imaging of the axillo-subclavian vein to confirm the diagnosis. Further imaging of the thoracic outlet for soft tissue or osseous abnormalities should be also be performed. Those patients with acute thrombosis can undergo thrombolysis, followed by surgical decompression and anticoagulation. Patients who present with chronic symptoms should undergo decompressive surgery and adjunctive venolysis or repair followed by anticoagulation. Prognosis following decompression is superior to anticoagulation alone. Available evidence suggests a higher rate of bony abnormalities in this group, and that treatment should be identical to that of this condition in adults.

Venous TOS (VTOS) is used to describe either episodic positional compression or thrombosis of the axillo-subclavian vein at the costoclavicular junction. Primary thrombosis is relatively rare and is thought to occur at an annual incidence of about 2 patients per 100,000 population [1, 2]. Entrapment of the subclavian vein and/or extrinsic compression due to bony anomalies, muscular

P. Lall, MD
Department of Surgery, VA WNY Health Care System,
3495 Bailey Avenue, Buffalo, NY 14215, USA
e-mail: purandath.lall@va.gov

L. Harris, MD (✉)
Department of Surgery, Kaleida Health,
3 Gates Circle, Buffalo, NY 14209, USA
e-mail: lharris@kaledahealth.org

hypertrophy, or acquired functional factors in the small costoclavicular space causes cumulative chronic injury to the vein in this area. In the acute setting, patients typically complain of a swollen, discolored, painful upper extremity usually following a history vigorous activity, while those in whom occlusion is chronic usually present with heaviness, aching, and a prominent venous pattern of dilated superficial collaterals involving the shoulder region, neck and anterior chest wall.

Most patients typically present in their early 30's, but it is not unusual to see teenagers with this problem. It is difficult to truly document the number of children with VTOS as they are frequently included together with adults in most reports; [3] most publications specific to the pediatric population have been small case series and case reports. About 3–5 % of adults with TOS present with VTOS, but VTOS appears to be more common in pediatric patients with thoracic outlet issues. Unlike the adult population (where the condition affects twice as many males as females), there is an equal male to female ratio in children with VTOS [4, 5]. Furthermore, in reviews of competitive athletes with effort thrombosis, the age of presentation is markedly younger than the standard adult population with NTOS. In a report by Melby et al. [6], the average age of VTOS presentation in competitive athletes was 20.3 years of age, while 17 of the 32 patients were less than 20. The dominant side was affected in all 14 teenaged patients. In other words, VTOS tends to present at a younger age than does NTOS.

Several small recent reports discuss VTOS in patients younger than 20. Rigberg described 18 cases of TOS in teenagers [7]. Twelve patients had NTOS and 6 (33 %) venous, two thirds of whom were male. All patients operated for VTOS had resolution of symptoms, with no further surgical intervention needed. Maru described 12 young (age 12–20 year) patients with TOS and noted 66 % of patients had vascular symptoms, including 25 % with VTOS [8]. Vercellio described eight children with TOS, ranging in age from 8 to 16 years of age, 75 % of whom had VTOS [5]. Two of the children had effort thrombosis, while functional intermittent obstruction was seen in the remaining four. All patients with VTOS underwent surgery, and improved without signs of recurrence at a mean of 18 months of follow-up. An additional 2 patients had venous malformations and were treated conservatively. In Arthur's report of pediatric TOS [4], he found that 52 % of his patients had vascular TOS, with 11 (44 %) of the 25 having VTOS. Seven of these had effort thrombosis, with the remaining four having intermittent venous impingement. Three of the patients were found to have hypercoagulable states, with one having extensive thrombosis of the upper extremity, and did not undergo further intervention, and gender was equally divided

with 55 % male and 45 % of the VTOS being female.

There seems to be a relatively high proportion of musculoskeletal abnormalities seen in children with VTOS. One of Rigberg's six VTOS patients had a cervical rib [7]. O'Brien et al. [9] and Filis et al. [10] reported cases of VTOS secondary to first rib osteochondroma and clavicular exostosis respectively, and Vijaysadan et al. [11] described a 19 year old male who presented with effort thrombosis secondary to hypertrophy of the coracobrachialis and short head of the biceps (seen on MRI) due to strenuous exercises.

Hypercoagulability has traditionally been believed not to play a role in VTOS, but there are recent data that suggest otherwise. Cassada recently showed that up to 67 % of patients (all ages) may have an underlying thrombophilic condition [12], while Brandao noted that some measure of hypercoagulability may be present in up to 50 % of adolescents [13]. By contrast, Bruins reviewed 34 adolescents with Paget Schroetter syndrome and found only 2 (6 %) who were positive for a thrombophilic condition, but noted that in 50 % of patients testing was not performed or results not reported [14].

The current standard of care for the treatment of VTOS in adults is catheter-directed thrombolysis followed by definitive decompression and anticoagulation for 3–6 months. Whether or not this algorithm should be identical in children is unknown, but some data support that treatment should be similar. Brandao reported his group's experience with six children who had VTOS in 2006 [13]. All six had confirmed VTOS on duplex and venography and three had a documented thrombophilic condition. All patients were treated with anticoagulation but did *not* undergo thoracic outlet decompression. Patients were seen at 3, 6 and 12 month interval and recurrence was confirmed by clinical exam and imaging. Unfortunately, all patients were *symptomatic* at last follow up. Three patients were followed for more than 12 months, 2 with recurrence of thrombosis and another who underwent decompression. He concluded that adolescents diagnosed with VTOS and treated with anticoagulation alone have a poor outcome.

In most series of children with VTOS, the majority of patients underwent surgical intervention. Those with occlusion also underwent thrombolysis in several series, but this was not as universally applied. In Vercellio's series (eight patients), for example, patients with venous thrombosis did not undergo thrombolysis [5]. At a mean follow of 18 months one patient rethrombosed and had recurrent, nondebilitating edema. Conversely, in the series reported by Melby et al. [6], 9 of the 14 teenaged patients had thrombolytic therapy and all patients underwent subsequent surgical decompression (complete anterior and middle scalenectomy, brachial plexus neurolysis, excision of the subclavius muscle tendon, and resection of the entire first rib). All patients also had circumferential external venolysis extending from the axillary vein to the subclavian-jugular-innominate vein junction, four required subclavian vein bypass and one patch reconstruction (and, interestingly, seven also underwent radiocephalic AVF). All patients were anticoagulated for 12 weeks. At a median follow up was 3.6 years, all patients returned to unrestricted use and at least the equivalent athletic activity, although one patient had early bypass thrombosis that required thrombectomy with graft revision. Similarly Rigberg, in his series of six patients, treated all patients with thrombolysis followed by transaxillary first rib resection and anticoagulation [7]. Fifty percent required balloon angioplasty or additional lysis in the postoperative period, but none required venous reconstruction or additional scalenectomy. All patients were able to return to baseline activities. They noted no differentiating factors in treatment of adolescents VTOS from their adult counterparts.

In summary, children and adolescents seem to have a higher chance of presenting with VTOS when compared to the adult TOS population. Optimal treatment remains controversial, although most series that report the "adult" protocol of thrombolysis followed by surgical intervention and chronic (3–6 months') anticoagulation show very good long term results. The presence of hypercoagulable states has not been well established in this group, and needs further investigation. Overall we recommend treating these patients using the same algorithm as used in adults.

References

1. Illig KA, Doyle AJ. A comprehensive review of Paget-Schroetter syndrome. J Vasc Surg. 2010;51: 538–47.
2. Hughes ES. Venous obstruction in the upper extremity. Br J Surg. 1948;36:155–63.
3. Stone DH, Scali ST, Bjerk AA, et al. Aggressive treatment of idiopathic axillo-subclavian vein thrombosis provides excellent long-term function. J Vasc Surg. 2010;52:127–31.
4. Arthur LG, Teich S, Hogan M, Caniano DA, Smead W. Pediatric thoracic outlet syndrome: a disorder with serious vascular complications. J Pediatr Surg. 2008; 43(6):1089–94.
5. Vercellio G, Baraldini V, Gatti C, Coletti M, Ciopolat L. Thoracic outlet syndrome in pediatrics: clinical presentation, surgical treatment, and outcome in a series of eight children. J Pediatr Surg. 2003; 38(1):58–61.
6. Melby SJ, Vedantham S, Narra VR, Paletta GA, Khoo-Summers L, Driskill M, et al. Comprehensive surgical management of competitive athlete with effort thrombosis of the subclavian vein. J Vasc Surg. 2008;47:809–21.
7. Rigberg DA, Gelabert H. The management of thoracic outlet syndrome in teenaged patients. Ann Vasc Surg. 2009;23(3):335–40.
8. Maru S, Dosluoglu H, Dryjski M, et al. Thoracic outlet syndrome in children and young adults. Eur J Vasc Endovasc Surg. 2009;38:560–4.
9. O'Brien PJ, Ramsunder S, Cox MW. Venous thoracic outlet syndrome secondary to first rib osteochondroma in a pediatric patient. J Vasc Surg. 2011;53(3): 811–3.
10. Filis KA, Nguyen TQ, Olcott C. Subclavian vein thrombosis caused by an unusual congenital clavicular anomaly in an atypical anatomic position. J Vasc Surg. 2002;36:629–31.
11. Vijaysadan V, Zimmerman AM, Pajaro RE. Paget-Schroetter syndrome in the young and active. J Am Board Fam Pract. 2005;18:314–9.
12. Cassada DC, Lipscomb AL, Stevens SL, et al. The importance of thrombophilia in the treatment of Paget-Schroetter syndrome. Ann Vasc Surg. 2006;20: 596–601.
13. Brandao LR, Williams S, Kahr WH, et al. Exercise-induced deep vein thrombosis of the upper extremity. 2. A case series in children. Acta Haematol. 2006;115: 221–9.
14. Bruins B, Masterson M, Drachtman RA, et al. Deep venous thrombosis in adolescents due to anatomic causes. Pediatr Blood Cancer. 2008;51:125–8.

VTOS in the Competitive Athlete

Robert W. Thompson

Abstract

Axillary-subclavian vein (ASCV) effort thrombosis (Paget-Schroetter syndrome) is the acute manifestation of venous thoracic outlet syndrome (VTOS). While relatively uncommon, this condition is probably the most frequently encountered vascular disorder in the young, healthy, competitive athlete. Understanding VTOS is particularly important for vascular and thoracic surgeons caring for athletes, as well as orthopedic surgeons, emergency room physicians, and sports medicine specialists, since delayed diagnosis and/or incomplete treatment can prevent further participation in sports and recreational activities. Although the treatment options to be considered for VTOS are similar for all patients, competitive athletes often present special circumstances that need to be taken into account in the decision-making process. With early recognition, proper initial treatment, and definitive surgical care, most competitive athletes affected by VTOS can return to previous levels of performance within several months of diagnosis.

Venous thoracic outlet syndrome (VTOS) is caused by compression of the axillary-subclavian vein (ASCV) between the clavicle and first rib, as well as the surrounding musculature and soft tissues. Compressive injury to the ASCV stimulates localized tissue fibrosis within and around the vein wall, and during repetitive cycles of injury and repair, the site of vein compression eventually becomes surrounded by a collar of constricting scar tissue. This is usually asymptomatic due to simultaneous development of venous collaterals, but eventually, stagnant blood and turbulent flow within the narrowed segment of ASCV promotes thrombosis and occlusion. This results in the sudden symptoms that constitute the "effort thrombosis" (Paget-Schroetter) syndrome: substantial arm swelling, cyanotic discoloration, heaviness, pain and/or fatigue. Given the association between vigorous overhead use of the upper extremity and the development of VTOS, it is not surprising that VTOS is regularly seen in competitive athletes involved in frequent throwing or weight lifting regimens.

R.W. Thompson, MD
Department of Surgery, Section of Vascular Surgery,
Center for Thoracic Outlet Syndrome,
Washington University Barnes-Jewish Hospital,
660 S Euclid Avenue, Campus Box 8109/Suite 5101
Queeny Tower, St. Louis, MO 63110, USA
e-mail: thompson@wudosis.wustl.edu

K.A. Illig et al. (eds.), *Thoracic Outlet Syndrome*,
DOI 10.1007/978-1-4471-4366-6_53, © Springer-Verlag London 2013

Clinical Presentation, Diagnosis, and Initial Treatment

ASCV effort thrombosis should be suspected in any young, healthy, active individual that presents with the sudden onset of arm swelling, particularly those with a history of vigorous overhead activities or weightlifting, as well as in any young individual with otherwise unexplained pulmonary embolism. Physical examination reveals pronounced arm swelling, cyanotic discoloration and distention of subcutaneous veins around the upper arm, chest, and shoulder. The diagnosis may at times be mistaken for reaction to an insect bite on the upper extremity, an allergic reaction to topical medication, or a nonspecific musculoskeletal strain.

The diagnosis and initial treatment of ASCV effort thrombosis is described in detail elsewhere in this text. Briefly, it is important to emphasize that upper extremity Duplex ultrasound is relatively inaccurate for this condition and cannot be used to exclude the diagnosis, and that the definitive diagnosis requires conventional contrast venography. Contrast venography is also required for catheter-based thrombolysis, which has emerged as the preferred initial step in treatment. The goal of thrombolysis is to clear any recent clot from the ASCV and principal collaterals, which will usually result in a marked improvement in symptoms. There is usually a focal occlusion or high-grade residual stenosis of the proximal ASCV, representing underlying fibrous tissue at the level of the first rib. Attempts to treat this by balloon angioplasty are usually unsuccessful, and placement of stents in the ASCV should be completely avoided in the absence of venous decompression. Systemic anticoagulation in then continued while subsequent treatment options are rapidly explored.

Treatment Options

Following initial diagnosis and thrombolytic therapy, there are three principal treatment options to be considered: (1) Anticoagulation alone; (2) Surgical treatment by thoracic outlet decompression with observation and secondary interventional treatment of the ASCV; and (3) Surgical treatment by thoracic outlet decompression with immediate assessment and treatment of the ASCV.

Anticoagulation

Although treatment with long-term anticoagulation alone may be considered, this "conservative" approach is associated with a substantial incidence of recurrent thrombosis, persistent symptoms, and residual limitations in arm activity. Anticoagulation is also incompatible with athletic activities involving physical contact or the potential for head injury. There is little information available on the appropriate duration of anticoagulation for ASCV effort thrombosis, since the results of treatment for iliofemoral deep vein thrombosis cannot be extrapolated to this condition given the distinct pathophysiology underlying VTOS. Lifelong anticoagulation thereby often appears the most reasonable recommendation in the absence of thoracic outlet decompression to remove the cause of venous compression. Because the limitations of this approach are unacceptable for the competitive athlete hoping to return to their sport (as well as for the large majority of individuals affected by ASCV effort thrombosis), definitive surgical treatment is usually the best recommendation. It has also become clear over the past decade that optimal results are achieved when surgical treatment is performed within approximately 2–3 weeks of diagnosis and thrombolytic therapy [1–3]. Since delays in treatment while attempting conservative management may allow re-thrombosis, which may preclude certain therapeutic options, in most patients prompt referral for definitive surgical management is recommended at the time of initial diagnosis or thrombolytic therapy.

Surgical Treatment

Operative treatment of VTOS is centered upon two goals: (1) decompression of the ASCV and collateral venous pathways throughout the thoracic outlet, and (2) restoration and maintenance of normal blood flow through the ASCV. Thoracic outlet decompression is accomplished by first rib resection along with division or removal of the anterior scalene and subclavius muscles. These steps can be effectively performed through transaxillary, supraclavicular or infraclavicular (subclavicular) approaches, or combinations of these incisions.

The transaxillary approach to VTOS typically involves partial resection of the first rib and simple division of its scalene muscle attachments, but it is not feasible to expose or control the ASCV from this incision alone. For this reason, these operations are usually coupled with the use of intraoperative or postoperative venography and performance of balloon angioplasty and/or stent placement to deal with any residual stenosis in the ASCV [4–6]. From the information available, it appears that a residual ASCV stenosis is present in at least 50 % of patients treated with first rib resection alone; thus, this approach is coupled with a high frequency of secondary interventions that may not always resolve the venous pathology. In contrast, anterior (supraclavicular and/or infraclavicular) approaches to thoracic outlet decompression permit more thorough resection of the anterior scalene and subclavius muscles and more complete first rib resection, particularly the anteromedial first rib, which is directly adjacent to the ASCV and may harbor abnormalities, such as occult fractures (observed in approximately 40 % of patients with VTOS) [7, 8]. Anterior approaches also allow direct ASCV reconstruction, by either patch angioplasty or interposition bypass graft placement, with completion of all of the necessary steps during a single operative procedure. Some of the largest reported series in the literature on VTOS and those with the most successful results have been described with anterior approaches coupled with direct ASCV reconstruction [9, 10].

For the reasons stated above, in our institution we have preferred operative treatment for VTOS using a "paraclavicular" approach, which combines the advantages of both supraclavicular and infraclavicular incisions [11, 12]. In a reported experience drawing from more than 100 patients treated over a 10-year period, we treated 32 high-performance athletes (31 % high school, 47 % collegiate, and 22 % professional) [10]. The mean interval between symptoms and definitive venographic diagnosis in these patients was 20.2 ± 5.6 days (range 1–120), with catheter-directed subclavian vein thrombolysis performed in 26 (81 %). Surgical treatment consisted of anterior and middle scalenectomy and complete first rib resection, with no patient requiring division of the clavicle, disruption of the sternoclavicular joint, or partial sternotomy. With the excellent exposure of the ASCV afforded by the paraclavicular approach, immediate patency of the ASCV was restored by circumferential external venolysis alone (56 %) or by direct venous reconstruction (44 %, with venous bypass grafts in 11 and vein patch angioplasty in 3). Anticoagulation was maintained for 12 weeks after surgery and all 32 athletes resumed unrestricted use of the upper extremity, with a return to competitive sports at a median interval of 3.5 months (range 2–10 months). We found that the overall duration of management (from symptoms to a return to full athletic activity) was significantly correlated with the time interval from venographic diagnosis to operation, and longer in patients with persistent symptoms or rethrombosis prior to referral. We have concluded from this experience that optimal management of VTOS in the competitive athlete is dependent on early recognition by treating physicians, diagnostic venography and thrombolytic therapy; prompt referral for comprehensive surgical management based on paraclavicular thoracic outlet decompression with external venolysis and frequent use of subclavian vein reconstruction; and temporary postoperative anticoagulation integrated with care by a physical therapy team that has expertise in the management of all forms of TOS [13].

Special Considerations in the Competitive Athlete

The vascular surgeon, thoracic surgeon or other physician specializing in the management of TOS is often consulted for advice regarding the optimal treatment for a competitive athlete that has developed ASCV effort thrombosis. In evaluating the various treatment options for VTOS, the physician must obviously be closely familiar with the pros and cons of each treatment strategy. In addition, it is valuable to have an understanding of the demands of the individual athlete's sport, the timing and duration of the season and off-season schedule, and the particular nuances that may accompany competition at various levels. For example, the competitive high school athlete is sometimes driven by parental pressure to achieve a level of success sufficient to earn a college scholarship, in which case the timing of medical/surgical treatment must be juxtaposed with a desired return to sport during the school year, particularly the junior and senior years. Similar considerations apply to the collegiate athlete; however, some individuals are motivated to complete in a final year or two of sports without anticipation of a professional career, and may therefore have less ambitious plans for future participation in sports. For the professional athlete, the type and timing of treatment is often dictated by the point in the season or off-season at which ASCV effort thrombosis occurs. Whether or not the team is actively competing for a championship in that particular season or is a "rebuilding" phase, the role played by the individual athlete in that team effort versus the potential substitute(s) available, and the finances and stage of an individual athlete in their professional contract, may all influence the aggressiveness desired in achieving a rapid return to play. At times there is a temptation to offer partial or temporizing treatment to allow an athlete to complete play during a given season, planning for definitive treatment once the season has ended. However, the feasibility of this approach is limited with VTOS, since in most sports the patient cannot compete while on anticoagulation treatment, and an early resumption of athletic activity in the absence of anticoagulation can be expected to result in early rethrombosis. Thus, in patients who have undergone venographic diagnosis and thrombolytic therapy, the best option is almost always a consideration for prompt surgical treatment, ideally within several weeks of thrombolysis to allow for the most rapid recovery

and rehabilitation. With respect to the choice of operative treatment, the consulting physician should be familiar with the two principal approaches that are generally used to manage VTOS and their respective advantages and disadvantages, and be able to place these considerations into the context of the potential need for additional treatments and an anticipated return to athletics for the patient, family, athletic trainers, other team representatives, and agents (in the case of the professional athlete). It is not uncommon for the athlete, family, team and/or agent to request several different opinions; thus, it is helpful for the consulting physician to be aware of the specialists with greatest experience in treating patients with VTOS and to be able to facilitate additional referrals when necessary.

For the surgeon undertaking treatment of the competitive athlete with VTOS, it is crucial to recognize the impact that this condition has had, and will have, on the patient's participation in competitive sports, which in many cases is the patient's means to obtain or maintain a collegiate scholarship or is even their principal livelihood. An extra degree of attention is required with regard to close and open communication with the patient, family, and team representatives regarding expectations and progress at each step of care, along with close collaboration between the surgeon and other health care personnel, particularly the physical therapy team assisting with postoperative care. With a coordinated effort and well-established protocols, the surgeon can obtain excellent results with a high degree of patient satisfaction, along with a prompt and successful return of the athlete to competitive activity.

References

1. Molina JE. Need for emergency treatment in subclavian vein effort thrombosis. J Am Coll Surg. 1995; 181(5):414–20.
2. Urschel Jr HC, Razzuk MA. Paget-Schroetter syndrome: what is the best management? Ann Thorac Surg. 2000;69(6):1663–8.
3. Caparrelli DJ, Freischlag J. A unified approach to axillosubclavian venous thrombosis in a single hospital admission. Semin Vasc Surg. 2005;18(3):153–7.

4. Kreienberg PB, Chang BB, Darling 3rd RC, Roddy SP, Paty PS, Lloyd WE, Cohen D, Stainken B, Shah DM. Long-term results in patients treated with thrombolysis, thoracic inlet decompression, and subclavian vein stenting for Paget-Schroetter syndrome. J Vasc Surg. 2001;33(2 Suppl):S100–5.

5. Urschel Jr HC, Patel AN. Surgery remains the most effective treatment for Paget-Schroetter syndrome: 50 years' experience. Ann Thorac Surg. 2008;86:254–60.

6. Chang KZ, Likes K, Demos J, Black JH, Freischlag JA. Routine venography following transaxillary first rib resection and scalenectomy (FRRS) for chronic subclavian vein thrombosis ensures excellent outcomes and vein patency. Vasc Endovascular Surg. 2012; 46(1):15–20.

7. Thompson RW, Schneider PA, Nelken NA, Skioldebrand CG, Stoney RJ. Circumferential venolysis and paraclavicular thoracic outlet decompression for "effort thrombosis" of the subclavian vein. J Vasc Surg. 1992;16(5):723–32.

8. Sheng GG, Duwayri YM, Emery VB, Wittenberg AM, Moriarty CT, Thompson RW.

Costochondral calcification, osteophytic degeneration, and occult first rib fractures in patients with venous thoracic outlet syndrome. J Vasc Surg. 2012;55(5):1363–9.

9. Molina JE, Hunter DW, Dietz CA. Paget-Schroetter syndrome treated with thrombolytics and immediate surgery. J Vasc Surg. 2007;45(2):328–34.

10. Melby SJ, Vedantham S, Narra VR, Paletta Jr GA, Khoo-Summers L, Driskill M, Thompson RW. Comprehensive surgical management of the competitive athlete with effort thrombosis of the subclavian vein (Paget-Schroetter syndrome). J Vasc Surg. 2008; 47(4):809–20.

11. Thompson RW. Venous thoracic outlet syndrome: paraclavicular approach. Op Tech Gen Surg. 2008; 10(3):113–21.

12. Thompson RW. Comprehensive management of subclavian vein effort thrombosis. Semin Interv Radiol. 2012;29(1):44–51.

13. Thompson RW, Driskill MR. Neurovascular problems in the athlete's shoulder. Clin Sports Med. 2008;27: 789–802.

Advanced Imaging for Vascular TOS

54

Constantine A. Raptis, Kathryn Fowler,
and Vamsi Narra

Abstract

Noninvasive advanced imaging of vascular thoracic outlet syndrome is best performed with computed tomography (CT) and magnetic resonance imaging (MRI). Both modalities allow for dynamic imaging of the thoracic outlet and can demonstrate narrowing of the arteries or veins that is induced by positional changes. This chapter focuses on the technical aspects of CT and MR imaging of the thoracic outlet, with particular attention paid to the advantages and limitations of these techniques. In addition, case examples of both arterial and venous thoracic outlet syndrome diagnosed with CT or MRI are provided.

Imaging of the Vascular Thoracic Outlet

Multiple diagnostic imaging modalities are useful for evaluating the thoracic outlet, especially with regard to vascular (venous or arterial) pathology, including plain radiographs, duplex ultrasound, computed tomography (CT), magnetic resonance imaging (MRI), and digital subtraction angiography (DSA). The use of ultrasound for VTOS was reviewed in Chap. 50, "Clinical Presentation and Patient Evaluation in VTOS," and both ultrasound and angiography for ATOS are covered in the next section. This chapter will

C.A. Raptis, MD (✉) • K. Fowler, MD
V. Narra, MD, FRCR
Mallinckrodt Institute of Radiology,
Washington University School of Medicine,
510 South Kingshighway Boulevard,
St. Louis, MO 63110, USA
e-mail: raptisc@mir.wustl.edu

focus on CTA and MRI techniques [1–4], including their diagnostic value and limitations in the assessment of vascular thoracic outlet syndrome; because the techniques are so similar, both venous and arterial imaging will be covered.

Computed Tomographic Imaging of the Thoracic Outlet

CT of the thoracic outlet provides exquisite detail of the relationship between the subclavian artery and vein with the adjacent ribs and clavicle (Fig. 54.1). CT requires exposure to ionizing radiation, but newer algorithms and advancements in technology can help to limit the overall radiation dose. It is critically important to understand that the dynamic nature of vascular TOS necessitates scanning the patient in multiple positions with provocative maneuvers to illicit vascular compression. The typical approach involves

K.A. Illig et al. (eds.), *Thoracic Outlet Syndrome*,
DOI 10.1007/978-1-4471-4366-6_54, © Springer-Verlag London 2013

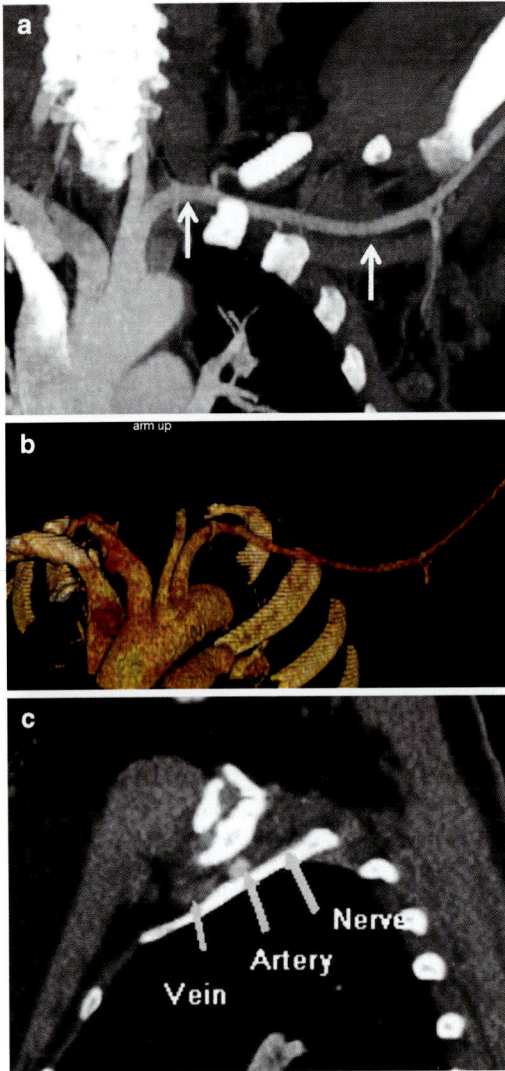

Fig. 54.1 Normal CTA. Images (**a**) (sub-volume maximum intensity projection CT) and (**b**) (volume rendered image) from the same patient. The subclavian artery is normal in caliber with arm in the abducted position (*arrows*). Note the depiction of the vascular and bony relationship in image (**c**) which is reformatted and displayed in sagittal orientation from a separate patient

acquiring images both with the patient's arms adducted to the side and abducted over their head. In the abducted position, the costoclavicular space and retropectoralis space become narrowed even in healthy volunteers. This narrowing, however, may be significant enough in symptomatic patients to lead to vascular (or neurologic) compression. The presence of luminal narrowing of

the subclavian vein or artery in the abducted position can thus support the diagnosis of thoracic outlet syndrome in a symptomatic patient (Fig. 54.2). When evaluating solely for venous disease, mild compression alone may be of questionable significance given that the subclavian vein may appear narrowed in healthy volunteers during provocative maneuvering. Although late manifestations, the presence of venous collaterals, thrombosis, or fixed stenosis of the subclavian vein regardless of position are much more specific signs of venous TOS (Fig. 54.2). Similarly, in evaluating arterial compression, post-stenotic dilatation or frank aneurysm formation as well the presence of collateral vessels support a diagnosis of arterial TOS.

Technique

Non-ionic intravenous contrast is required for visualization of the vessels on CTA. Clinical differentiation between arterial or venous etiology for thoracic outlet syndrome is often difficult on a single acquisition and hence both arterial and venous phases are typically obtained. Prior to the scan, a large bore intravenous catheter, capable of accommodating injection rates up to 4.5 ml/s should be placed on the contralateral or asymptomatic side in order to avoid extensive streak artifact from dense contrast in the subclavian vein obscuring visualization of the subclavian artery on the symptomatic side. Timing of the arterial phase of image acquisition may be achieved by using a set delay of 15–20 s (following monophasic injection at 4 ml/s), using a test bolus, or via bolus tracking. With the bolus tracking method, a region of interest is placed over the aorta and imaging commences either immediately or after a set delay once the region of interest enhances beyond a set threshold. Venous phase images are acquired following the arterial phase, usually 80–90 s after injection. Images are acquired in the transaxial plane with thin slices, allowing for the creation of multiplanar reconstructions, volume rendered images, and maximal intensity projections of the final data sets. If both

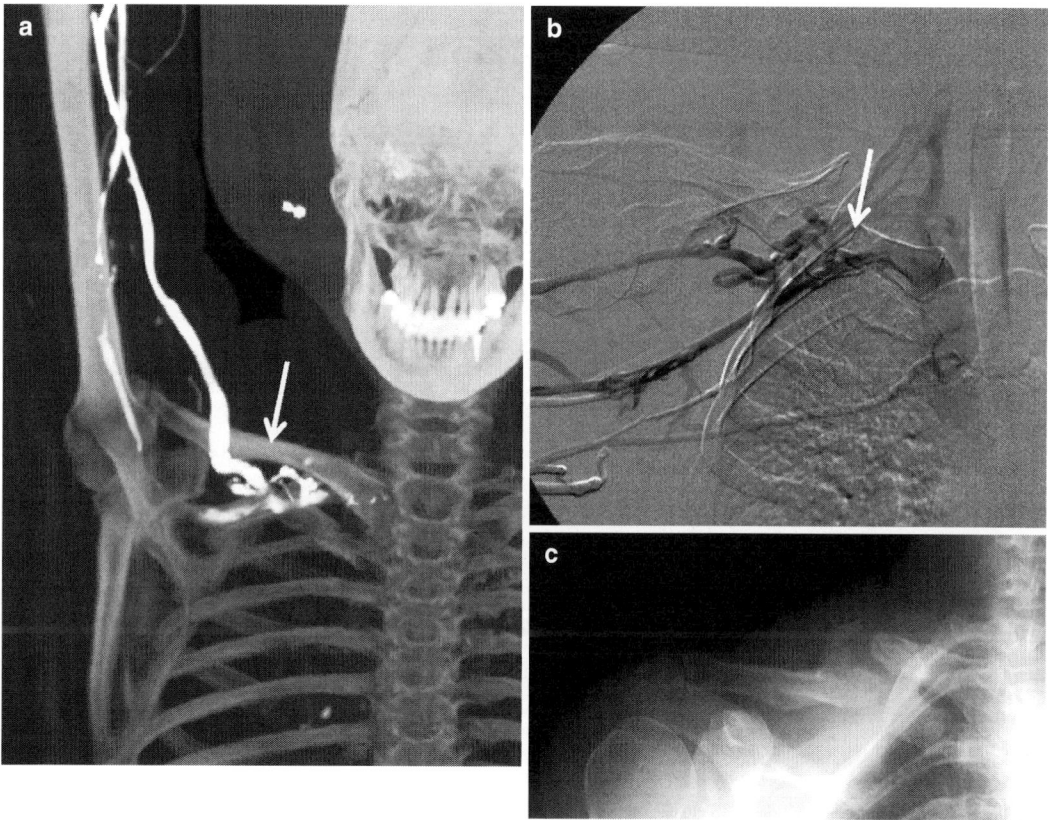

Fig. 54.2 CTA of right venous thoracic outlet syndrome. Image (**a**) (maximum intensity projection CT) demonstrates narrowing of the right subclavian vein (*arrow*) with enlarged venous collaterals. The maximum point of compression coincides with the location of a non-united clavicular fracture, also seen on digital subtraction angiography (**b**) and radiograph (**c**)

arms are to be evaluated, a split bolus injection (injected into both arms) should be used with a 5 min delay between injections to avoid venous contamination. If the primary concern is venous occlusion, additional scans can be performed while injecting at a lower rate (1–2 cc/s) on the symptomatic side with the patient in abduction and adduction. This allows for visualization of early collateral vessel filling.

Advantages of CT Scanning

The major advantage of CT scanning is that it provides superb visualization of blood vessels without catheter-directed injection. It also provides the best spatial resolution and anatomic detail of bony structures with the images acquired in a matter of seconds. It can, of course, be performed with contrast in patients who are on dialysis.

Limitation of CT Scanning

CT contrast agents should not be used in patients with renal insufficiency due to the potential risk of nephrotoxicity. Patients are usually screened on the basis of serum creatinine (with a typical cutoff of 1.6–1.8 mg/dl) or glomerular filtration rate (with typical lower threshold of 30 mg/dl/m^2). However, in the setting of acute renal insufficiency, creatinine and GFR should be taken in the context of the patient's normal baseline. In addition to the relative contraindication of renal insufficiency, prior contrast allergy may be a limiting factor in performing CTA. Pretreatment regimens including prednisone (or equivalent steroid) as well as antihistamines may be appropriate in patients with prior mild reactions such as hives or itching. However, prior anaphylactoid reaction to intravenous contrast is a contraindication to elective CTA despite pre-treatment. Finally, while CTA is especially useful in evaluating the bony anatomic boundaries of the thoracic outlet, it is suboptimal in evaluating the neurologic and soft tissue components due to limitations in achievable soft tissue contrast resolution; MRI is a better choice for these indications.

Magnetic Resonance Imaging of the Thoracic Outlet

MRI provides dynamic evaluation of the thoracic outlet without the use of ionizing radiation. Superior soft tissue contrast and anatomic detail of both vascular and neurologic components of the thoracic outlet make MRI an optimal imaging modality in young patients with suspected vascular compromise. Similar to CT, MRI is performed with the arms in the neutral adducted position as well as abducted over the head. MRI protocols may involve both anatomic sequences to evaluate the musculature and bony anatomy (usually T1 weighted images) as well as angiographic images. Diagnosis of vascular compression is similar to CT with observation of luminal narrowing, post-stenotic dilation, collaterals, and thrombosis (Figs. 54.3 and 54.4). Superior soft tissue resolution may allow for identification of fibrous bands or aberrant musculature at the level of vascular compression.

Technique

A comprehensive thoracic outlet MRI protocol provides evaluation of the vasculature as well as anatomic imaging of the bones, musculature, and brachial plexus. T1 and T2-weighted high resolution sagittal and axial images provide an anatomic overview of the thoracic outlet, allowing for diagnosis of cervical ribs, fibrous bands,

and aberrant musculature. Intravenous gadolinium contrast agents are used in acquiring MR angiographic images to produce bright signal within the vessels. When utilizing conventional extravascular gadolinium agents, two injections are typically performed, one with the arms adducted and then a second with the arms abducted. Although many techniques exist for acquiring arterial phase images, use of a test bolus to determine accurate arterial phase timing appears to be most reliable. Venous phase images are then typically obtained using a fixed time delay of approximately 80 s, but multiple delayed images can be obtained as desired. Angiographic images are obtained in a coronal plane using a 3D acquisition before and after contrast administration, which then allows for subtraction of the two data sets. The final images can also be displayed as maximal intensity projections, sub-volume maximum intensity projections, or using volume rendering techniques. The typical field of view usually allows for visualization from the aortic arch to the proximal-mid brachial artery with achievable field of view determined primarily by the patient's body habitus, size of the coil, and technical parameters of the MR scanner (Fig. 54.4). Additional coverage to include more distal vessels requires patient and coil repositioning.

With the recent addition of a new blood pool agent, Gadofosveset trisodium (Ablavar, Lanthues, Billerica, MA), to the MR contrast armamentarium, MR angiography techniques have become somewhat simpler. Gadofosveset trisodium allows for both first-pass angiographic imaging of the arteries as well as steady state imaging. During the steady state, arteries and veins both enhance and vascular imaging can be obtained for up to an hour after injection. Prolonged enhancement of the vasculature allows for dynamic imaging following a single injection, which is especially useful in the thoracic outlet where positional changes in vessel caliber are the hallmark of diagnosis.

While contrast enhanced MR evaluation provides superior and more reliable determination of vessel patency, non-contrast MRI techniques, such as time-of-flight and quiescent interval

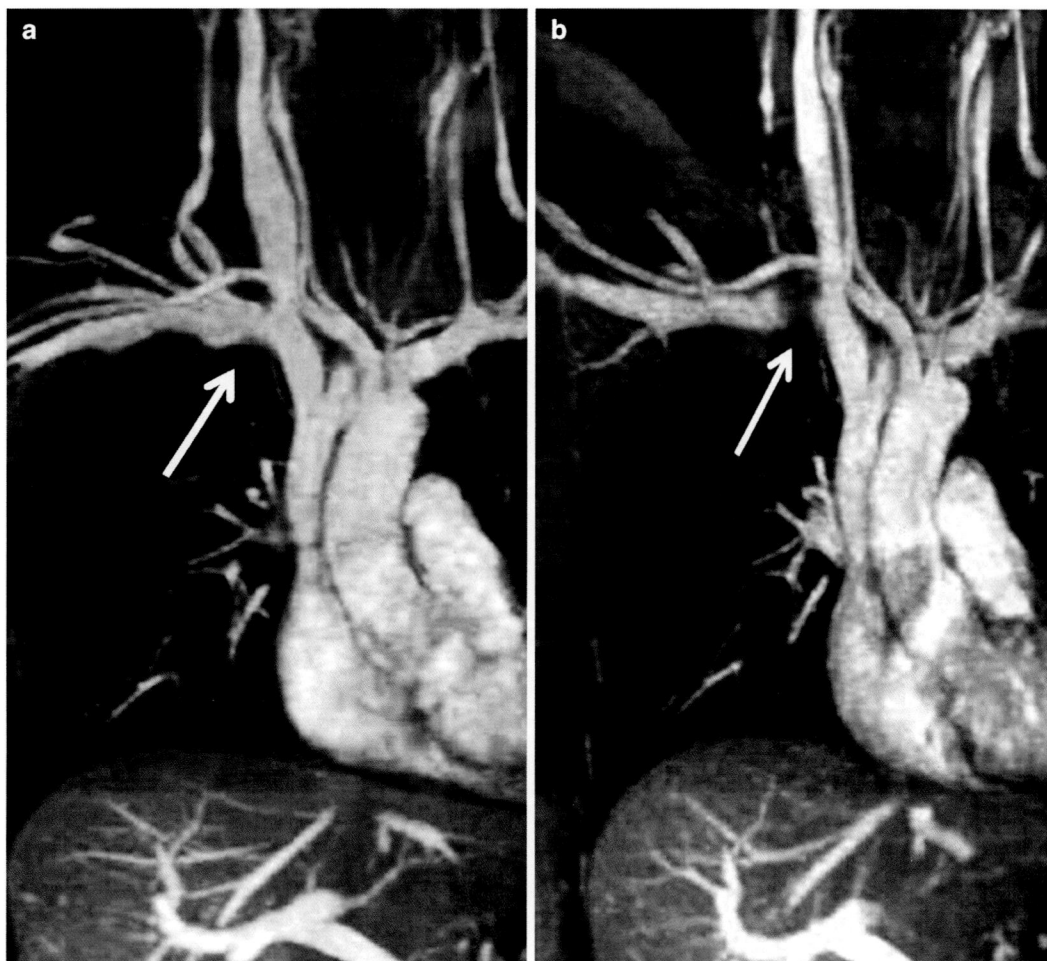

Fig. 54.3 MRI of right venous thoracic outlet syndrome. Image (**a**) (sub-volume maximum intensity projection MRI) in adducted position and Image (**b**) (maximum intensity projection MRI) in abducted position. The subclavian vein (*arrow*) demonstrates dynamic narrowing in the abducted position in this patient who subsequently underwent right thoracic outlet decompression

steady state imaging, may be an option in patients who receive contrast due to allergy or poor renal function. Time-of-flight techniques utilize repeated RF pulses to null background tissue signal in a single slice. When blood outside the slice flows into the nulled plane, it is bright, and thus angiographic images are produced. Saturation bands can be used in the direction of venous or arterial flow to avoid unwanted contamination. Because this technique relies on blood that is flowing through the plane of acquisition, vessels that are tortuous or flow horizontally within the slice may demonstrate artifactual lack of signal and appear as non-patent. Hence, caution should be used when interpreting areas of possible occlusion in vessels that are oriented parallel to the acquisition plane.

Advantages of MR Scanning

One major advantage is the absence of exposure to ionizing radiation, although severe renal insufficiency (see below) remains an issue. MRA/V provides excellent contrast-to-noise for vascular imaging, and dynamic imaging can be performed with the single injection of a blood

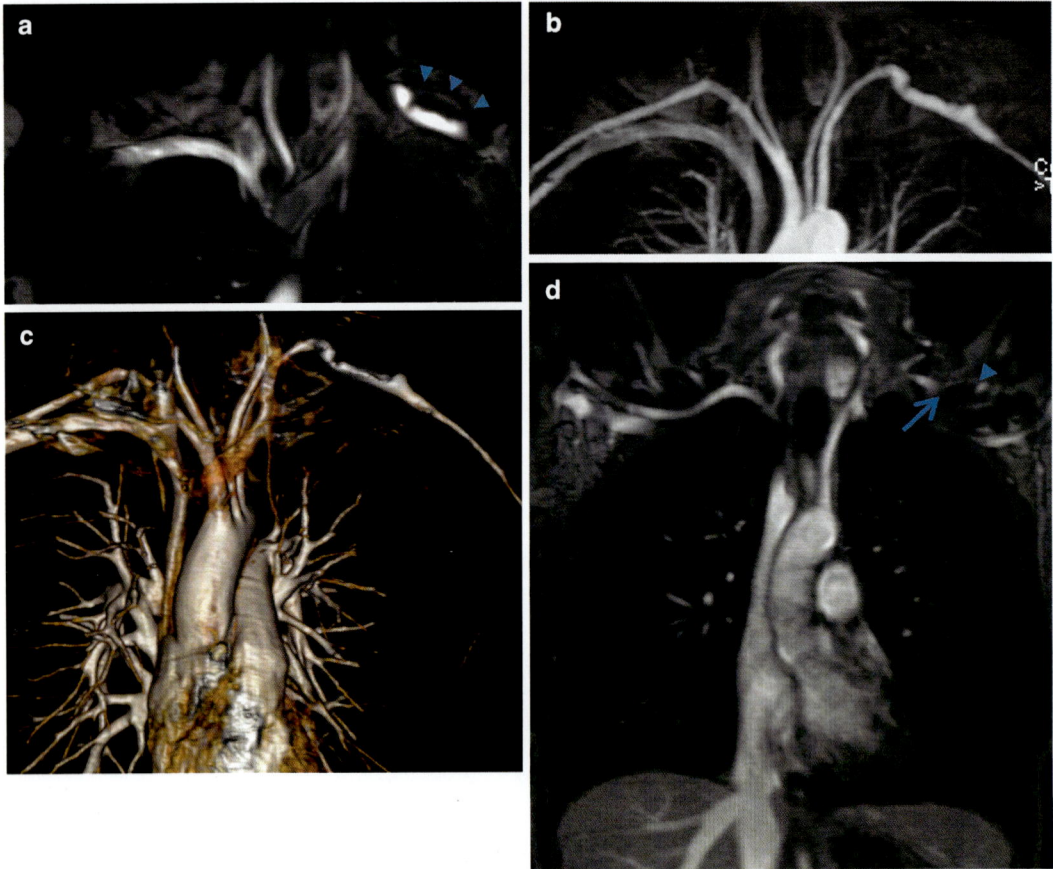

Fig. 54.4 MRI of left arterial thoracic outlet syndrome: With the arms adducted, coronal source (**a**), MIP (**b**), and 3D volume rendered images (**c**) demonstrate narrowing of the left subclavian artery at the thoracic inlet with a partially thrombosed post-stenotic aneurysm (*arrowheads*). In the equilibrium phase (**d**) with the arms up, there is complete occlusion of the left subclavian artery (*arrow*) as it passes below the left clavicle (*arrowhead*). This patient underwent surgery to repair the aneurysm and relieve the obstruction. This study was performed with only 6 ml of gadofosveset trisodium, a blood pool contrast agent

pool agent. MRI also offers the best contrast resolution allowing for visualization of fibrous bands, muscles, nerves, and vessels (see Chap. 18).

Limitations of MR Scanning

Because MR images are acquired with the use of a magnetic field, patients with some metallic devices (such as pacemakers or neurogenic stimulators) may not be able to undergo MRI examination safely. Screening of all patients is therefore necessary. Ferromagnetic metal may also be problematic from an imaging standpoint as it can result in extensive artifacts that may obscure

visualization of the vessels (Fig. 54.5). It should be noted that the majority of newer vascular stents do not result in significant artifact and MRI is usually still an option in these patients. Visualization and evaluation of the stent lumen is limited and one cannot use MRI to exclude an in-stent stenosis. Because MRI sequences are motion sensitive, breath-holding is often required for imaging the chest and region of the thoracic outlet. Hence, patients who are unable to hold their breath for 20 s may not be suitable candidates for MRI. Additionally, the bore or opening of the MRI magnet is often smaller than that of a CT scanner and claustrophobia or patient size may prohibit MRI, although open or large bore

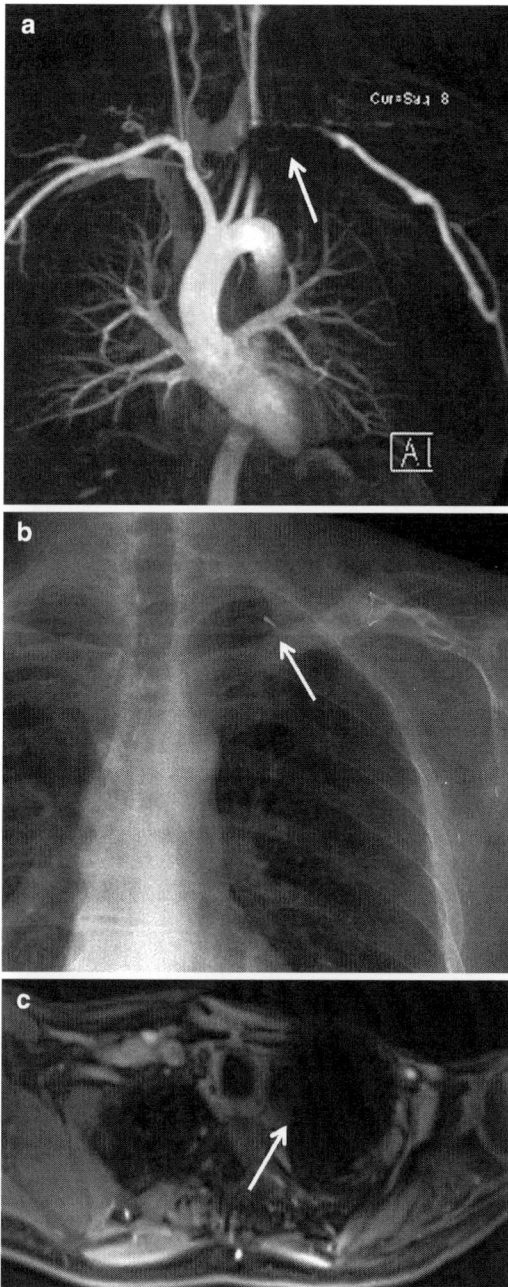

magnets allow for imaging larger patients and patients with less severe claustrophobia.

Finally, patients with severe renal insufficiency cannot receive gadolinium contrast agents due to the risk of nephrogenic systemic fibrosis (NSF). In patients with moderate renal insufficiency (glomerular filtration rates of 30–60 mg/dl/m^2), MRI contrast may be a better option than CT contrast as gadolinium is not nephrotoxic and the risk of NSF in these patients is very low to negligible.

References

1. Demondion X, Herbinet P, Van Sint Jan S, Boutry N, Chantelot C, Cotten A. Imaging assessment of thoracic outlet syndrome. Radiographics. 2006;26:1735–50.
2. Charon JPM, Milne W, Sheppard DG, Houston JG. Evaluation of MR angiographic technique in the assessment of thoracic outlet syndrome. Clin Radiol. 2004;59:588–95.
3. Demondion X, Bacqueville E, Paul C, Duquesnoy B, Hachulla E, Cotten A. Thoracic outlet: assessment with MR imaging in asymptomatic and symptomatic populations. Radiology. 2003;227(2):461–8.
4. Remy-Jardin M, Remy J, Masson P, Bonnel F, Debatselier P, Vinckier L, Duhamel A. Helical CT angiography of the thoracic outlet: functional anatomy. Am J Radiol. 2000;174(6):1667–74.

Fig. 54.5 Artifact obscuring the left thoracic outlet vasculature. Image (**a**) (maximum intensity projection MRI) in adducted position, Image (**b**) (radiograph), and Image (**c**) (transaxial volumetric interpolated breath held T1 weighted MRI). There is apparent nonvisualization of the left subclavian vessels (*arrow*) on the maximum intensity image. However, upon viewing the radiograph and the transaxial source images, the signal loss is actually related to metallic susceptibility artifact (*arrows*)

Differential Diagnosis, Decision-Making, and Pathways of Care for VTOS

55

Hugh A. Gelabert

Abstract

Venous thoracic outlet syndrome (VTOS) may presents with a variety of symptoms and at different stages of the disease process. Thrombolysis, angioplasty, stenting, and surgical decompression are appropriate for some presentations, but may not serve for others. Best results are obtained with the correct diagnosis, evaluation and treatment. This chapter focuses on the different presentations, the evaluation, and the care pathways which lead to best outcomes for patients presenting with VTOS.

Introduction

Venous thoracic outlet syndrome (VTOS) most often presents with the acute onset of arm swelling, discoloration, pain, and heaviness due to thrombotic occlusion of the axillosubclavian vein. It is a rare condition and is not the first one considered by most primary care physicians.

Best medical care for patients with VTOS requires familiarity with the range of presentations as well as the ability to quickly differentiate between VTOS and conditions which may be confused with it

H.A. Gelabert, MD
Division of Vascular Surgery,
UCLA David Geffen School of Medicine,
200 UCLA Medical Plaza, Ste 526,
Los Angeles, CA 90095-6904, USA
e-mail: hgelabert@mednet.ucla.edu

Venous TOS

Venous thoracic outlet syndrome refers to the constellation of symptoms and findings associated with extrinsic compression of the subclavian vein as it courses across the *anterior* thoracic outlet (see Chap. 49). This compression is caused by the junction of the first rib and clavicle along with associated muscles. This approximation is dynamic, and aided by contraction of the anterior scalene and subclavius muscle which raise the first rib. Compression is further accentuated by hypertrophy of the anterior scalene and subclavius muscles, and as these muscles enlarge the space between them will be reduced. This space is the normal domain of the subclavian vein, and impingement will reduce the venous lumen. Once venous lumen is reduced to a critical degree then venous blood flow is restricted and consequent congestive symptoms will result. While affected patients tend to be young (ages 20–30s are most common), age of the patient may vary. Similarly, while most patients have engaged in vigorous activities using their upper extremities, many VTOS patients are not very active or athletic.

Presentation

In general VTOS can present in one of four ways: acute upper extremity venous thrombosis, post-phlebitic stenosis, intermittent non-thrombotic compression, and chronic venous occlusion [1] (Table 55.1).

Acute upper extremity venous thrombosis: The most common manifestation of VTOS is that of acute upper extremity venous thrombosis, also called Paget-Schroetter syndrome or effort thrombosi. This commonly occurs in active individuals who are engaged in labor, sporting activities, or other occupations which require repeated vigorous use of the upper extremities, and this history of vigorous upper extremity activity provides a context upon which the diagnosis of VTOS may be more quickly suspected. The presenting history most often relates a rapid onset of congestion, swelling, discoloration and pain in the affected extremity. Most patients are motivated to seek attention by the dramatic nature of the presentation (Fig. 55.1).

When seen acutely, the limb may be dramatically congested and discolored with venous prominence, dramatic size discrepancy, and pain. This most dramatic presentation is often recognized as an acute deep vein thrombosis (DVT) by most physicians, although not all patients present with such dramatic symptoms. The diagnosis of an upper extremity DVT is very easily established with either duplex ustraounography or venography, but the dangers are that either the fact that this is VTOS (i.e., requires attention to the thoracic outlet) will be missed or that "conventional" DVT treatment alone (i.e., thrombolysis will not be considered) will be pursued.

Intermittent non-thrombotic venous compression: Some patients with VTOS do not have thrombotic occlusion. Such patients may complain of intermittent symptoms of congestion and swelling with a variety of arm positions or activities [2–5], but when not stressed by these activities the arm is normal. These intermittent symptoms may be

Table 55.1 Major presentations of vTOS

Major presentations of vTOS
Acute upper extremity DVT
Post-phlebitic vein with stenosis and extrinsic compression
Intermittent non-thrombotic compression at thoracic outlet
Chronic venous occlusion across thoracic outlet

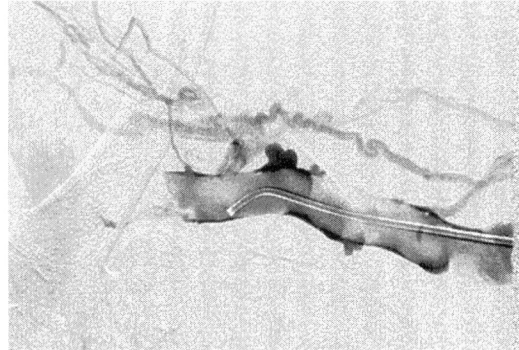

Fig. 55.1 Acute Axillo-subclavian vein occlusion. Note the intraluminal filling defects in the region of the catheter, the absence of flow centrally, and the pathognomonic collateral filling

challenging for physicians as they are not as common or extreme as those ariseing from an acute DVT. Initially described by Mc Cleery and associates in 1953, it is sometimes denoted McCleery's syndrome [2] but more generically referred to as intermittent non-thrombotic venous compression. It is critical to perform venography with the arm fully abducted in order to demonstrate positional compression (Fig. 55.2).

Post-phlebitic stenosis: Some patients present with post-phlebitic stenosis as a consequence of a prior acute DVT. These patients may have been treated initially with anticoagulation only and have been fortunate enough to recanalize their vein due to endogenous thrombolysis. Such a vein has features which identify it as post-phlebitic (in the proper clinical context): the walls are irregular and the diameter of the vein is reduced. An area of high-grade compression is seen at the thoracic outlet, usually accompanied by venous collateralization across the thoracic outlet. The symptoms which these patients suffer include swelling, heaviness and arm fatigue, again exacerbated by

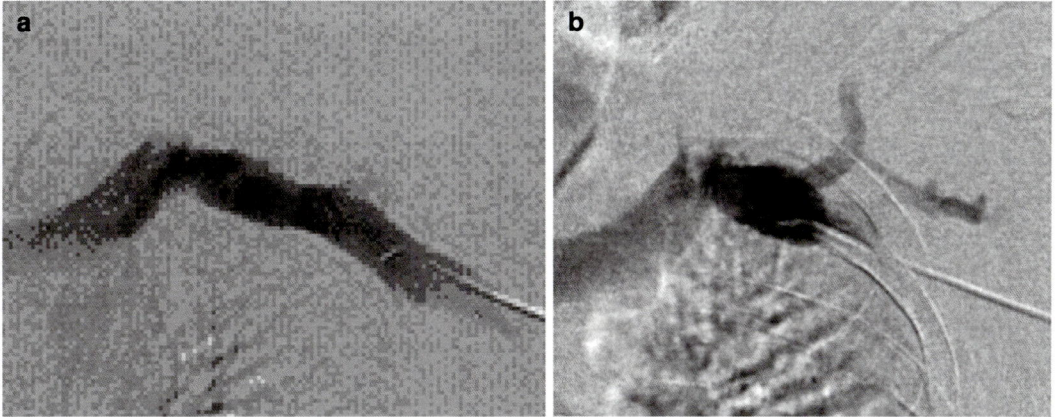

Fig. 55.2 Intermittent compression with position change. No collateral seen with arm in neutral position (**a**). Note the visible collateral when the arm is abducted (**b**)

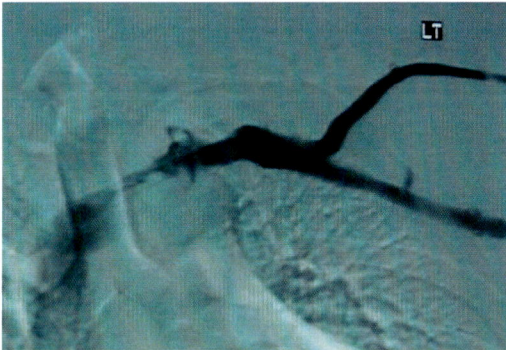

Fig. 55.3 Post-phlebitic vein with stenosis

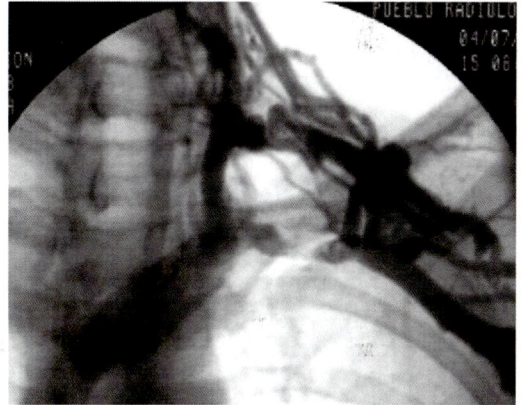

Fig. 55.4 Chronic occlusion

use or abduction of the extremity. Positional venography is diagnostic (Fig. 55.3).

Chronic venous occlusion: Finally, chronic venous occlusion occurs when a thrombosed subclavian vein fails to recanalize. The venous occlusion is usually the result of fibrous conversion of the thrombus within the vein following the initial DVT, and is readily distinguished from an acute DVT by the resistance of the thrombus to pharmacological or mechanical thrombolysis or even wire passage. Because of the chronicity and the degree of occlusion, ample venous collateralization is noted across the thoracic outlet (Fig. 55.4). The presenting symptoms are those of chronic venous congestion which exacerbates with use of the arm. Occasionally severe extrinsic compression without thrombosis or fibrosis can occur; such a "pseudo occlusion" is detected by gentle

passage of a guide wire across the occluded segment. Some patients with chronic occlusion can present with acute exacerbation of symptoms caused by loss of a critical collateral.

Differential Diagnosis

The differential diagnosis which must be entertained in patients with VTOS includes those conditions which result in upper extremity limb swelling, discoloration, and discomfort. The presentation may be subdivided according to acute and chronic presentations (Table 55.2).

Acute thrombosis can be secondary or primary ("spontaneous"). In this context, "spontaneous" indicates that no prior instrumentation of the vein

Table 55.2 Differential diagnosis of arm swelling

Primary venous thrombosis
  Acute axillo-subclavian vein thrombosis
  Paget Schroetter syndrome (PSS)
  Thoracic outlet compression
  Pancoast tumors
  Thrombophilia
Secondary venous thrombosis
  Venous catheters
  Pacemaker wires
Chronic causes of arm swelling
  Central venous stenosis and AV dialysis fistulas
  Lymphedema
  Klipple Treanay Syndrome (KTS)
  Chronic post phlebitic syndrome
Miscellaneous causes of arm swelling
  Rheumatological disorders (Raynaud's disease,
  scleroderma, systemic lupus erythematosus,
  dermatomyositis, polymyositis, mixed connective
  tissue disorder, cold agglutinin disease, rheumatoid
  arthritis, cryoglobinemia, vasculitis)
  Infections with cellulitis, allergic reactions, insect
  bites, and trauma
  Mass effect of adenopathy or aneurysms
  Metabolic causes: thyroid dysfunction with
  myxedma and anasarca, heart failure

has occurred, and in most instances, this presentation is considered synonymous with Paget-Schoroetter syndrome [6, 7]. Paget-Schoroetter syndrome is usually felt to be the acute form of VTOS, but some clinicians use this to refer to any thrombosis in this area. Conditions that can cause thrombosis include Pancoast tumors, thrombophilia, and trauma, and prior to embarking on treatment it is important to distinguish these conditions. In part this distinction is made by evaluation of the patient's coagulation profile, skeletal anatomy, and venous anatomy revealed by venography in conjunction with the clinical situation. Ideally, the thrombus within the vein should be cleared in order to allow evaluation of the subclavian vein at the thoracic outlet, and identification of the extrinsic compression of the subclaivan vein at the thoracic outlet at rest or with positional maneuvers is made.

Pancoast tumors are malignancies which involve the apex of the chest [8], either primary lung tumors or metastatic lesions which have established themselves in this location. They can present with distal neurologic symptoms including pain, paresthesias, and weakness if the brachial plexus is involved, and thrombosis of the subclavian vein if that structure is involved. This diagnosis is suspected by the presence of a mass or opacification of the apex of the chest, and computerized tomographic (CT) or magnetic resonance (MR) scanning provides optimal definition of the extent of the tumor and the involvement of neurovascular structures. The subclavian vein may thrombose in the face of a hypercoagulable condition [9], and the presence of a malignancy or previously diagnosed hyerpcoagulable condition may suggest the correct diagnosis. Ultimately these patients are identified by documentation of a normal (unimpinged) subclavian vein following thrombolysis along with thrombophillic factors identified by testing. Although data are sparse most agree that there is some overlap between "VTOS" and thrombophilia, as a significant number of patients with thrombosis at the thoracic outlet may demonstrate thrombophillia on testing (see Chap. 58).

Patients with secondary venous thrombosis have a history of instrumentation of the subclavian vein with venous catheters and/or wires [10], including central catheters placed for venous access, chemotherapy, TPN, or hemodialysis, or temporary or permanent cardiac pacemakers and defibrillators. The presence of a catheter or wire within the subclavian vein may cause an acute DVT. While there may be a coexistence between instrumented veins and thoracic outlet compression, these patients are managed according to the inciting event – the presence of the catheter or wire – and only occasionally require thoracic outlet decompression.

The second general class of conditions which should be considered as part of the differential diagnosis include those entities which produce *chronic swelling*. Included in this group are patients with central venous stenosis and AV fistulas, lymphedema, Klippel-Trenaunay-Weber syndrome (KTS), chronic post phlebitic syndrome, and metabolic causes of limb swelling.

Central venous stenosis in patients with an arteriovenous fistula or graft (AVF/AVG) is one of the most common causes of significant upper extremity swelling [11]. The diagnosis should be suspected in anyone with a functioning fistula in the affected limb, and is confirmed by venography. Such a lesion can be anywhere in the venous outflow tract, but if at the costoclavicular junction may well be a variant of VTOS (defined as most successfully managed by thoracic outlet decompression) [12].

Lymphedema can be primary or secondary to the combination of surgical lymphadenectomy and radiation therapy for breast cancer [13]. Unlike VTOS, such swelling is not usually accompanied by cyanosis, venous engorgement, or venous collateralization, and venography or ultrasonography will not show a venous abnormality. Treatment is based on compression therapy with use of compression wrapping, manual lymphatic drainage, elastic compression garments, and pulsatile pneumatic compression sleeves, as indicated, Klippel-Trenaunay-Weber syndrome is a condition which combines venous developmental anomalies, classically atresia of the deep system, with skeletal growth discrepancies [14]. Typically the syndrome includes the presence of port-wine skin marking, hemihypertrophy and limb length discrepancy, and anomalies of venous development, and patients present clinically with an enlarged limb and varices. Conventional or MR venography shows developmental anomalies (aplasia, hypoplasia, persistent fetal patterns) of the deep venous system. Like lymphedema, use of elastic compression is central to the management of the affected limb.

Chronic post phlebitic syndrome secondary to a previous primary or secondary thrombosis can affect an upper extremity [15], but, as discussed above, is classified by many as a form of VTOS itself (rather than an item on the differential diagnosis list). A history of prior venous thrombosis and occlusion is common, although the index event could have been missed clinically. In addition to swelling, pigmentation can be present, although ulceration is rare. Swelling can include the entire arm and hand, and in severe cases patients may be disabled. The diagnosis is established by venography with demonstration of occlusion of venous egress of the extremity, and

the differentiation from VTOS (depending on terminology) is based on history of catheterization and/or associated diagnoses such as chronic renal failure. Consideration should be given to thoracic outlet decompression, but initial treatment in a non-TOS patient is compression sleeve garments. Selected patients with severe symptoms may be candidates for venous reconstruction (see Chap. 65).

Finally, rheumatologic disorders such as Raynaud's disease, scleroderma, lupus, dermatomyositis, polymyositis, mixed connective tissue disorder, cold agglutinin disease, rheumatoid arthritis, cryoglobinemia, or nonspecific vasculitis, which should all be suspected on the basis of physical examination and laboratory testing and specifically identified by a rheumatologist. Cellulitis, allergic reactions, insect bites, and trauma should be easy to diagnose. Cervical lymphadenopathy or arterial aneurysms may occasionally compromise venous and lymphatic drainage of the arm and result in arm swelling. Finally, metabolic or global causes of limb swelling such as heart failure or myxedema, while systemic, can sometimes cause asymmetric arm swelling.

Decision-Making

Decision-making in a patient with VTOS includes several fundamental questions, most of which are discussed in more detail in the following chapters:
- What is the role of anticoagulation?
- What is the role of pre-operative thrombolysis?
- Is this a condition which benefits from surgery?
- Should this patient undergo operation or not?
- What operative approach is most effective?
- What elements should the operation consist of?
- When should angioplasty or stenting be considered?
- When should venous repair be offered?
- And what post-operative interventions are indicated?

Resolution of these questions is based on appreciation of the natural history of VTOS as well as the reported results of the various interventions. The natural history of VTOS remains poorly defined. While some patients will suffer recurrent thrombosis, others may not.

Acute Axillosubclavian Vein Thrombosis: The Role of Anticoagulation

The role of anticoagulation as part of the management of acute subclavian vein thrombosis is well established. Clinical reports dating to 1948 indicate the beneficial effect of anticoagulation in this situation [6, 7, 16], although, as discussed below, this is in the context of further intervention. The current ACC guidelines suggest anticoagulation for acute DVT for a period of 3 months, while recurrent thrombosis mandates life-long anticoagulation.

Is anticoagulation alone, however, enough? DeWeese described a series of 25 patients managed with rest and anticoagulation only in the 1950s and 1960s. Twelve percent of these patients developed pulmonary embolization, 18 % had persistent intermittent congestive symptoms, and 68 % had severe disabling persistent symptoms [17]. This experience was later (1971) updated by Adams, who described 85 % with recurrent and persistent symptomatic venous congestion and 11 % had recurrent pulmonary emboli [18]. Tilney described a series of 48 patients managed with anticoagulation who did not undergo surgical decompression, and were followed for a mean of 6.6 years. They noted that 17 % of patients developed recurrent thrombosis and 74 % had persistent symptoms [19]. Gloviczki analyzed 95 patients with axillosubclavian venous occlusion, and described permanent symptoms with mild exertion in 17 % and symptoms at rest in 12 % of their cohort [20]. Finally, Machleder described a series of 50 patients who were initially managed with anticoagulation and subsequently underwent surgery. Of these, 34 % suffered multiple thrombotic events prior to proceeding with surgical decompression [21]. Noting that we have not yet discussed thrombolysis, it is clear that anticoagulation alone yields dismal outcomes

The role of anticoagulation in the patient with VTOS not associated with acute thrombosis (post-phlebitic stenosis, intermittent non-thrombotic compression, and chronic venous occlusion) is less well established. While some of these patients have suffered a DVT and are presumably at risk of recurrent thrombosis or even PE, such patients do not have symptoms which would suggest ongoing acute thrombosis or clot extension, and current guidelines do not suggest such patients require anticoagulation unless there is evidence to suggest a recurrent acute thrombus.

Acute Axillosubclavian Vein Thrombosis: The Role of Thrombolysis

If anticoagulation alone is associated with such poor outcomes, can we offer the patient anything better? Thrombolysis in the management of acute presentations of VTOS has been shown to be a significant advancement over standard anticoagulation therapy. Early reports identified the benefits of thrombolysis: rapid resolution of symptoms, the ability to identify the cause of thrombosis, the ability to salvage venous patency, and, when combined with proper decompression of the thoracic outlet, superb symptom-free long-term results [22]. Most authors and clinicians agree that patients presenting with a recent (within 2–4 weeks) acute DVT should be offered thrombolysis. Unfortunately this is not universally appreciated and a significant number of patients are still (2011) managed with anticoagulation alone.

The role of thrombolysis in patients who present in a subacute or chronic fashion is poorly defined. Some authors advise a trial of thrombolysis in all patients regardless of the time interval from the acute thrombosis [23], while others feel there is no benefit in this [24].

Ultimately, Is VTOS a Surgical Disease, and Will Patients Benefit from Surgical Decompression?

Anticoagulation alone leaves patients with significant long-term morbidity, and while thrombolysis can dissolve fresh thrombus, ultimately this conditions is caused by extrinsic compression by the bones and muscles making up the venous (anterior) thoracic outlet. While alternative viewpoints exist (see Chap. 71) and certainly level 1 evidence does not, virtually all clinicians and authors agree that relief of the extrinsic compression – by surgical decompression of this area – is required for long-term "cure" of this condition, at least in patients in whom axillosubclavian patency can be reestablished.

As in all of surgery, however, the decision as to whether to chose surgical decompression or non-operative management in individual cases may relate to patient selection issues. The age of the patient, level of activity, occupation, presence of co-morbid conditions, and stamina all bear directly upon the decision of whether or not to proceed with surgery. It is clear that elderly, debilitated and chronically ill patients are poor candidates for surgery and probably should not be offered surgical decompression, but these patients seldom develop VTOS. The more important question is whether young, active, healthy persons should undergo decompression or not. While the non-operative approach may succeed in sedentary patients, it is less likely to be as successful in young active individuals, most frequently affected by venous TOS – because of their increased activity, these patients are more likely to remain symptomatic and ultimately require decompression.

The decision to proceed with surgery is the result of balancing the morbidity and success of an operation against the natural history of the disease process. Morbidity relates to the removal of the first rib: pain, bleeding, nerve injury, and the attendant period of disability which is required during recovery from surgery, but long-term success rates are superb (see Chap. 67). The natural history of the nondecompressed venous thoracic outlet seems to be that of recurrent thrombosis, pulmonary embolization, and post-phlebitic symptoms in the extremity. Because not all patients treated conservatively have poor outcomes, Lee and colleagues have suggested a selective surgical treatment algorithm. In a 2000 publication they described an algorithm whereby all patients underwent thrombolysis (and were anticoagulated), but only those who had persistent congestive symptoms or re-thrombosis were operated upon. They found that 9 of 22 patients (41 %)

did not require surgery during the study period (average follow up of 22 post-lysis) [25]. A later publication with an increased number of patients (total of 64), observed that after a mean follow up period of 51 months that 27 patients (42 %) did not require surgical decompression. They noted that younger, more active patients tended to develop recurrent symptoms or thrombosis when managed in an expectant manner, and that these younger patients were more likely to require surgery [26].

Should Thoracic Outlet Decompression be Performed in Patients with Chronic or Persistent Venous Occlusion?

While the rationale for surgical decompression in those instances where the subclavian vein is impinged upon yet remains patent (or has been recanalized) is evident, the same may not be true for those patients with persistently or chronically occluded veins. Despite this, many feel that decompression is indicated even in this situation (see Chap. 56). One rationale for this is to allow improved venous collateralization. In addition, come "occlusions" are the result of severe, fixed compression and do not reflect obliteration of the venous lumen, and removal this extrinsic compression allows the vein to open. A final reason for decompressing even chronically thrombosed and occluded veins is that some of these may recanalize and re-open following a prolonged period of anticoagulation [27].

A related issue is that of indications for surgery in cases where the subclavian vein is compressed but has not suffered thrombosis. Many such patients present with intermittent congestive symptoms, and venography, while often normal at rest, shows compression of the subclavian vein and newly filling collaterals with the arm in abduction. Surgery in these instances is planned with the intention of relieving congestive symptoms related to the intermittent compression. It is important to recognize that these indications are fundamentally different from operating to prevent recurrent thrombosis; this is a prophylactic operation to forestall the development of subclavian thrombosis.

What Approach Is Best?

The choice of which surgical approach is to be used for VTOS is greatly dependent on the surgical goals, and in choosing one over another it is worth keeping in mind the relative strengths and limitations of each option (See Chap. 73).

The transaxillary approach allows complete resection of the first rib from the costochondral junction to the articulation with the vertebral body's transverse process [28, 29]. The approach offers access to both the anterior scalene and subclavius muscles, although only the lower 2 cm or so of the anterior scalene can be resected, but exposure to the medial portion of the vein is difficult. The net effect is that transaxillary approach offers excellent ability to remove the compressive elements, but does not allow open surgical manipulation or reconstruction of the subclavian vein. The supraclavicular approach, by contrast, offers partial exposure of the subclavian vein (the medial portion is visible although partially obstructed by the clavicle) [30, 31]. The anterior scalene is readily exposed and may be resected entirely, but the anterior portion of the first rib and subclavius muscles are both obstructed by the clavicle and cannot be removed by this approach. For this reason the supraclavicular approach has been modified to become a 'paraclavicular' appraoach, adding an infraclavicular incision for exposure of the distal subclavian vein, the subclavius tendon, and the anterior portion of the first rib. This approach also allows open surgical repair of the subclavian vein, patch angioplasty and venous reconstruction. Finally, while not as commonly performed, claviculectomy provides excellent exposure of the subclavian vein, resection of the subclavius tendon and the anterior scalene muscle [32, 33]. The main limitation of this approach is the cosmetic deformity resultant from the resection of the clavicle. Additionally some patients will develop chronic pain resultant from the clavicular resection. In patients who need to carry objects over their shoulder (backpacks, straps, etc.), or who require vigorous use of the extremity, clavicular resection may not be ideal. Athletes should not undergo claviculectomy if they anticipate further competition.

What Are the Goals of Surgery?

The fundamental goal in patients with VTOS is to decompress the thoracic outlet and thereby relieve the persistent extrinsic compression of the subclavian vein. This requires excision of the first rib, but also partial resection of the subclavius and anterior scalene muscles [34]. Of importance is adequate resection of essentially the entire first rib, especially the anterior portion. This is the point where the subclavius and anterior scalene muscles insert and this is the fulcrum which effects the compression of the subclavian vein. As noted above, the chief limitation of the supraclavicular approach is inability to address the costoclavicular junction itself, and for this reason a paraclavicular incision must be added in patients with VTOS.

What are the Roles of Reconstruction, Venoplasty, Ballon Angioplasty, and Stenting?

The question of whether and how to perform open endophlebectomy or more complex reconstruction of the subclavian vein remains the subject of ongoing review. Molina has been the most avid proponent of reconstruction using endophlebecomty and patch angioplasty of the subclavian vein. He reported a series of 114 patients, 85 of whom underwent endophlebectomy with patch angioplasty, 12 of whom extended patch angioplasty with sternotomy, and 12 of whom were deemed inoperable due to chronic occlusion. The overall results were excellent with only one late occlusion in the 102 operated patients [23, 35]. Melby and associates, reported their preferred use of venous graft reconstruction of the subclavian vein in 2008. They analyzed 32 competitive athletes who presented with subclavian vein thrombosis. Of these, 14 underwent direct axillo-subclavian vein reconstruction (44 %) with a combination of techniques including panel graft bypass (eight patients), saphenous vein interposition (three patients) and patch angioplasty (three patients); all patients were able to resume athletic competition [36]. It should be noted that there is no randomized or level 1 evidence in this area, accordingly the guidelines for reconstruction or open venoplasty remain subjective.

The indications for intraoperative angioplasty or stenting is also poorly defined. There appears to be considerable institutional variance as to these practices: some authors seeming to advocate routine use of these techniques in all cases, and others not using them. Peri-operative angioplasty and stenting was described by Kreienberg in 2001. He reported a series of 23 patients who underwent preoperative thrombolysis and surgical decompression, followed by venoraphy. All 23 (100 %) of their patients underwent balloon angioplasty and 14 (61 %) required placement of a stent. Of the nine patients who underwent PTA only, all were patent at post-op follow up. Of the 14 patients who underwent PTA/stenting, 5 (35 %) were occluded on follow up exam [37].

Schneider routinely obtains intra-operative post-decompression imaging, and if a residual significant stenosis is present then angioplasty and stenting is performed. In their experience 64 % of patients required intra-operative intervention, and on follow up ultrasound exam only two patients (8 %) had subsequent thomrbosis [38]. Finally, the role of stenting in the postoperative patient remains unclear. While many advocate stenting on a routine basis [37], others have found stenting to be unnecessary and possibly counterproductive [22, 35, 38].

It is important to note the distinction between post-operative use of stenting (as discussed here) and stenting in the non-decompressed arm. Stenting in the non-decompressed thoracic outlet does not work: it is very poorly tolerated and should be condemned.

What Is the Role of Postoperative Imaging and Late Intervention?

There is a broad consensus that patients who are operated with the intention of achieving patency of their subclavian veins should undergo postoperative imaging with the consideration of repeat thrombolysis or endovascular intervention, should either be needed. Reviews of postoperative venograms indicate that about 30–45 % of patients will have residual stenosis which may

require angioplasty [39]. In addition, as many as 15 % of patients have been reported to have experienced interval occlusion in previously patent subclavian veins following decompression for acute subclavian vein thrombosis [39].

Pathways of Care

It is apparent that patients with VTOS can present in many different ways and that the timing of presentation and severity of symptoms can differ significantly. In our opinion, treatment of patients with VTOS can best be conceptualized by considering the four major ways in which patients can present: those with acute axillosubclavian thrombosis, those with postphlebitic venous stenosis, those with intermittent venous compression, and those with chronic occlusion. The following protocols generally describe the algorithms followed by the plurality of surgeons, but it is again stressed that very little level 1 evidence exists regarding what is truly best for such patients (Fig. 55.5).

Acute Axillosubclavian Thrombosis

Patients presenting with acute subclavian vein DVT are best managed with anticoagulation and early thrombolysis. Anticoagulation prevents clot

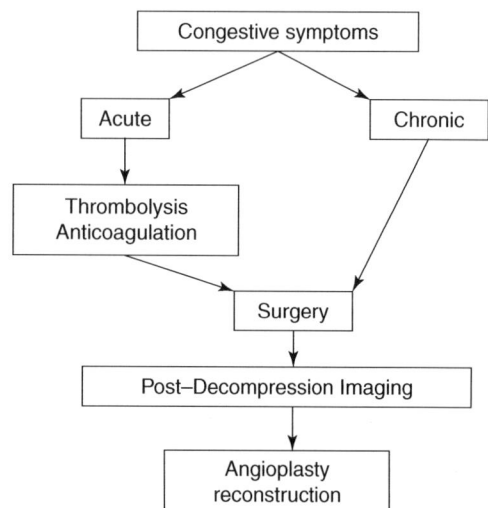

Fig. 55.5 Diagramatic representation of treatment algorithms

propagation, while thrombolysis allows rapid resolution of symptoms and definition of the cause of the thrombosis. Venous TOS is then confirmed when a point of extrinsic compression is identified at the thoracic outlet (with abduction films, if venography is normal at rest). In young active patients with confirmed VTOS, surgical decompression is most often advised, while in certain elderly or infirm patents expectant care with anticoagulation for a period of 3 months followed by observation may be appropriate. Active patients undergo decompression by means of first rib resection, subclavius muscle resection, and external venolysis, most effectively via a transaxillary approach if venous reconstruction is not required, and surgery should be performed "immediately" (i.e., during the same hospitalization). The use of adjunctive techniques such as venoplasty or venous reconstruction at the time of surgery depends on the findings of preoperative or intraoperative imaging, and the surgical approach is modified if reconstruction is felt to be needed. The use immediate post-decompression venography is advised as a significant number of patients will have residual stenosis which require treatment. Angiopalsty in these instances is recommended for significant (greater than 50 %) stenosis of the subclavian vein, but the role of stenting remains the subject of debate.

Post-phlebitic Stenosis

The finding of post phlebitic stneosis indicates that the thrombotic condition has been present and has partially resolved with anticoagulation and time. Such patients have chronic clot and/or fibrotic stenoses, and the use of anticoagulation in this context is thus based on the individual case considering the risks of anticoagulation versus recurrent thrombosis. Thrombolysis would not seem to be of benefit, but exception should obviously be made when the clinical situation suggest an acute change, even when chronic venous symptoms have been present. Surgical decompression is required, and the role of adjunctive measures such as venoplasty, reconstruction, or balloon angioplasty is critical. Post-operative venography and angiopaslty are required in this group as there is a significant likelihood of residual stenosis of the subclavian vein.

Intermittent Non-Thrombotic Compression

Non-thrombotic venous compression usually requires no anticoagulation or lysis, as the vein is, by definition, normal. Surgical decompression is essential component of care. In the absence of thombosis the subclavian vein is less likely to require venous reconstruction or venoplasty, but post decompression imaging is required to assess the possible need of intervention and to verify an intrinsically normal vein.

Chronic Occlusion

Most feel that patients with chronic venous occlusion will still benefit from surgical decompression. Whether or not an attempt at thrombolysis should be made is unresolved; some find no success beyond a few weeks' worth of symptoms while others advocated aggressive attempts at recanalization. Stents in this situation should, however, never be used. Whether to proceed with venous reconstruction at the time of decompression remains a point of debate. Experience suggests that not all patients require venous reconstruction, as many will experience symptomatic improvement following decompression or even recanalize. If recanalization or collateralization do not occur after a given period of time, venous reconstruction may be indicated, especially if the patients is highly symptomatic.

Conclusion

The management of patients with VTOS should be predicated on a thorough understanding of the pathology, presentation, and interventions which are applicable to each group. Treatment should be based on the best available data regarding outcomes for a given patient group. Ultimately the decision to proceed with a given course of intervention is based on assessing the risks and benefits of the care options. When the decision is made not to offer surgical decompression, it may expose a patient to risks of recurrent DVT, pulmonary embolization and chronic post-phlebitic syndrome. Thus a 'conservative' or non interventional decision may by itself present significant risk. Interventions themselves, however, obviously carry inherent risks, which may occur even when best care is offered.

When the fundamental pathology involves compression of the subclavian vein at the thoracic outlet, relief of the compression is essential to the goal of restoring normal venous function. Accordingly first rib resection is most often the treatment of choice, no matter what other interventions are performed. In the absence of rib resection, the risk of recurrent thrombosis, post phlebitic syndrome and pulmonary embolization remains significant. Given the high efficacy, low morbidity and low mortality of this procedure, surgical intervention is most often the best choice for care.

References

1. de León RA, Chang DC, Hassoun HT, Black JH, Roseborough GS, Perler BA, Rotellini-Coltvet L. Multiple treatment algorithms for successful outcomes in venous thoracic outlet syndrome. Surgery. 2009;145(5):500–7 (Epub 21 Mar 2009).
2. McCleery RS, Kesterson JE, Kirtley JA, Love RB. Subclavius and anterior scalene muscle compression as a cause of intermittent obstruction of the subclavian vein. Ann Surg. 1951;133(5):588–602.
3. Charrette EJ, Iyengar KS, Lynn RB, Challis TW. Symptomatic non-thrombotic subclavian vein obstruction. Surgical relief in six patients. Vasc Surg. 1973;7(4):220–31.
4. Sanders RJ, Hammond SL. Subclavian vein obstruction without thrombosis. J Vasc Surg. 2005;41(2):285–90.
5. Thakur S, Comerota AJ. Bilateral nonthrombotic subclavian vein obstruction causing upper extremity venous claudication. J Vasc Surg. 2010;52(1):208–11.
6. Hughes ESR. Venous obstruction in the upper extremity. Br J Surg. 1948;36:155–63.
7. Hughes ESR. Venous obstruction in the upper extremity; Paget-Schroetter's syndrome; a review of 320 cases. Surg Gynecol Obstet. 1949;88:89 (International abstracts of surgery).
8. Rusch VW. Management of pancoast tumours. Lancet Oncol. 2006;7(12):997–1005.
9. Cassada DC, Lipscomb AL, Stevens SL, Freeman MB, Grandas OH, Goldman MH. The importance of thrombophilia in the treatment of Paget-Schroetter syndrome. Ann Vasc Surg. 2006;20(5):596–601 (Epub 24 Jun 2006).
10. Luciani A, Clement O, Halimi P, Goudot D, Portier F, Bassot V, Luciani JA, Avan P, Frija G, Bonfils P. Catheter-related upper extremity deep venous thrombosis in cancer patients: a prospective study based on Doppler US. Radiology. 2001;220(3):655–60.
11. Glass C, Dugan M, Gillespie D, Doyle A, Illig K. Costoclavicular venous decompression in patients with threatened arteriovenous hemodialysis access. Ann Vasc Surg. 2011;25(5):640–5 (Epub 21 Apr 2011).
12. Illig KA. Management of central vein stenosis in the dialysis access patient. Semin Vasc Surg 2011;24(2):113–8.
13. Hack TF, Kwan WB, Thomas-Maclean RL, Towers A, Miedema B, Tilley A, Chateau D. Predictors of arm morbidity following breast cancer surgery. Psychooncology. 2010;19(11):1205–12. doi:10.1002/pon.1685.
14. Gloviczki P, Driscoll DJ. Klippel-Trenaunay syndrome: current management. Phlebology. 2007;22(6):291–8.
15. Persson LM, Arnhjort T, Lärfars G, Rosfors S. Hemodynamic and morphologic evaluation of sequelae of primary upper extremity deep venous thromboses treated with anticoagulation. J Vasc Surg. 2006;43(6):1230–5, discussion 1235.
16. Marks J. Anticoagulant therapy in the idiopathic occlusion of the axillary vein. Br Med J. 1956;1(4957):11–3.
17. Adams JT, McEvoy RK, DeWeese JA. Primary deep vein thrombosis of the upper extremity. Arch Surg. 1965;91:29–41.
18. Adams JT, DeWeese JA. Effort thrombosis of the axillary and subclavian veins. J Trauma. 1971;11:923–30.
19. Tilney NL, Griffiths HJG, Edwards EA. Natural history of major venous thrombosis of the upper extremity. Arch Surg. 1970;101:792–6.
20. Gloviczki P, Kazmier FJ, Hollier LH. Axillary-subclavian venous occlusion: the morbidity of a non-lethal disease. J Vasc Surg. 1986;4(4):333–7.
21. Machleder HI. Evaluation of a new treatment strategy for Paget-Schroetter syndrome: spontaneous thrombosis of the axillary-subclavian vein. J Vasc Surg. 1993;17(2):305–15, discussion 316–7.
22. Machleder HI. Thrombolytic therapy and surgery for primary axillosubclavian vein thrombosis: current approach. Semin Vasc Surg. 1996;9(1):46–9.
23. Molina JE, Hunter DW, Dietz CA. Paget-Schroetter syndrome treated with thrombolytics and immediate surgery. J Vasc Surg. 2007;45(2):328–34.
24. Guzzo JL, Chang K, Demos J, Black JH, Freischlag JA. Preoperative thrombolysis and venoplasty affords no benefit in patency following first rib resection and scalenectomy for subacute and chronic subclavian vein thrombosis. J Vasc Surg. 2010;52(3):658–62, discussion 662–3.

25. Lee WA, Hill BB, Harris Jr EJ, Semba CP, Olcott IV C. Surgical intervention is not required for all patients with subclavian vein thrombosis. J Vasc Surg. 2000;32(1):57–67.

26. Lee JT, Karwowski JK, Harris EJ, Haukoos JS, Olcott 4th C. Long-term thrombotic recurrence after nonoperative management of Paget-Schroetter syndrome. J Vasc Surg. 2006;43(6):1236–43.

27. de León RA, Chang DC, Busse C, Call D, Freischlag JA. First rib resection and scalenectomy for chronically occluded subclavian veins: what does it really do? Ann Vasc Surg. 2008;22(3):395–401.

28. Kashyap VS, Ahn SS, Machleder HI. Thoracic outlet neurovascular compression: approaches to anatomic decompression and their limitations. Semin Vasc Surg. 1998;11(2):116–22.

29. Roos DB. Transaxillary approach for first rib resection to relieve thoracic outlet syndrome. Ann Surg. 1966;163(3):354–8.

30. Duwayri YM, Emery VB, Driskill MR, Earley JA, Wright RW, Paletta Jr GA, Thompson RW. Positional compression of the axillary artery causing upper extremity thrombosis and embolism in the elite overhead throwing athlete. J Vasc Surg. 2011;53(5):1329–40 (Epub 26 Jan 2011).

31. Reilly LM, Stoney RJ. Supraclavicular approach for thoracic outlet decompression. J Vasc Surg. 1988; 8(3):329–34.

32. DeWeese JA, Adams JT, Gaiser DL. Subclavian venous thrombectomy. Circulation. 1970;41(5 Suppl): II158–64.

33. Green RM, Waldman D, Ouriel K, Riggs P, Deweese JA. Claviculectomy for subclavian venous repair: long-term functional results. J Vasc Surg. 2000;32(2): 315–21.

34. Urschel Jr HC, Patel AN. Surgery remains the most effective treatment for Paget-Schroetter syndrome: 50 years' experience. Ann Thorac Surg. 2008;86(1):254–60, discussion 260. Erratum in: Ann Thorac Surg. 2008 Nov; 86(5):1726.

35. Molina JE, Hunter DW, Dietz CA. Protocols for Paget-Schroetter syndrome and late treatment of chronic subclavian vein obstruction. Ann Thorac Surg. 2009;87(2):416–22.

36. Melby SJ, Vedantham S, Narra VR, Paletta Jr GA, Khoo-Summers L, Driskill M, Thompson RW. Comprehensive surgical management of the competitive athlete with effort thrombosis of the subclavian vein (Paget-Schroetter syndrome). J Vasc Surg. 2008;47(4):809–20, discussion 821 (Epub 14 Feb 2008).

37. Kreienberg PB, Chang BB, Darling 3rd RC, Roddy SP, Paty PS, Lloyd WE, Cohen D, Stainken B, Shah DM. Long-term results in patients treated with thrombolysis, thoracic inlet decompression, and subclavian vein stenting for Paget-Schroetter syndrome. J Vasc Surg. 2001;33(2 Suppl):S100–5.

38. Schneider DB, Dimuzio PJ, Martin ND, Gordon RL, Wilson MW, Laberge JM, Kerlan RK, Eichler CM, Messina LM. Combination treatment of venous thoracic outlet syndrome: open surgical decompression and intraoperative angioplasty. J Vasc Surg. 2004; 40(4):599–603.

39. Angle N, Gelabert HA, Farooq MM, Ahn SS, Caswell DR, Freischlag JA, Machleder HI. Safety and efficacy of early surgical decompression of the thoracic outlet for Paget-Schroetter syndrome. Ann Vasc Surg. 2001; 15(1):37–42.

Management of the Patient Who Presents Late After Thrombosis

56

Nancy L. Harthun

Abstract

Diagnosis of venous thoracic outlet syndrome can be delayed for many reasons or treatment of this condition can fail, all of which can lead to chronic occlusion of the subclavian vein. Treatment of these patients centers on surgical decompression of the thoracic outlet and limited post-operative percutaneous venous interventions. Stenting of the subclavian vein prior to surgical decompression or as a stand-alone treatment is contra-indicated. Late recanalization of the vein has been reported in some cases.

Prevalence

Venous thoracic outlet syndrome (Paget-Schroetter syndrome or effort thrombosis) comprises only 5 % of all cases of thoracic outlet syndrome. It is estimated that between one [1] and two [2] patients per 100,000 of population per year experience this syndrome. The natural history of this disorder is progression to chronic thrombosis with significant disability [3]. Anticoagulation improves outcomes when compared to the natural history of this disorder, but many patients still have chronic thrombus and experience residual symptoms [4, 5].

A variety of interventions have been developed and implemented with success, largely preventing late thrombosis and alleviating chronic disability. However, some patients do not seek treatment until after a significant time interval has elapsed. Some patients present when they first have symptoms but the diagnosis is not made in a timely fashion. Other patients do undergo timely treatment, but the treatment fails to resolve the thrombus or the clot resolves but then recurs later. These patients comprise a group of patients with venous thoracic outlet most at risk currently for long-term disability, so devoting separate consideration to their treatment is important.

Definition

There is no standard length of time that determines an axillo-subclavian vein occlusion as acute verses chronic. Many authors support "early" treatment, which means hospitalization and intervention at first presentation [6–8].

N.L. Harthun, MD, MS
Department of Surgery,
Johns Hopkins Bayview Medical Center,
4940 Eastern Ave, Baltimore, MD 21224, USA
e-mail: harthun@jhmi.edu

K.A. Illig et al. (eds.), *Thoracic Outlet Syndrome*,
DOI 10.1007/978-1-4471-4366-6_56, © Springer-Verlag London 2013

"Chronic" thrombosis, by contrast, was defined in one series as patients presenting for treatment at a mean of 22 weeks after diagnosis [9]. Somewhere between first presentation and 22 weeks later is an arbitrary line defining these two entities. Illig and Doyle define the distinction between acute and chronic thrombus at 2 weeks after initial symptoms due to the likelihood of success of attempted thrombolysis [1]. In addition, patients with recurrent venous occlusions can present as a result of failure of a variety of interventions including thoracic outlet decompressive surgery, venous thrombolysis with or without stenting, anticoagulation, or a combination of these interventions [10–14].

Acute Thrombus Management

In the ideal setting a patient will present very soon (hours to days) following thrombosis. Assuming the proper diagnosis has been made, the standard of care has evolved to be preliminary catheter-directed thrombolysis followed by decompression of the venous thoracic outlet after the clot has been lysed. This pathway has been determined without the benefit of any type of randomized controlled clinical trial (see Chap. 83). Differences of opinion exist as to timing of decompression and management of residual defects, but this general algorithm is the most commonly used. Thoracic outlet decompression in this situation is designed to keep an open vein open – i.e. to prevent recurrent thrombosis in a vein where patency has been restored. Many patients, for the reasons cited above, however, will have continued occlusion of the subclavian vein despite all efforts at recanalization.

Chronic Thrombus Management

Most authors agree that the primary factor in venous thoracic outlet syndrome is mechanical compression of the subclavian vein at the anterior aspect of the thoracic outlet where the vein passes posterior to the subclavius muscle and tendon and anterior to the anterior scalene muscle. This premise is true for both acute and chronic presentations of this disease. Therefore, it is important to focus on correcting this problem first, and not correcting the actual venous occlusion primarily. If the venous lesion can be traversed with a wire (but not otherwise corrected), it is tempting to try to "force" the vein open with a stent. This should be avoided because stenting prior to surgical thoracic outlet decompression has been found to be related to higher rates of venous occlusion in multiple series [10, 15]. The problem is extrinsic compression by relatively fixed bony structures, coupled with a very strong lever arm with movement of the arm. No stent can withstand these forces, and stent fragmentation, common in this situation, makes a bad situation even worse. Several studies suggest that even successful preoperative thrombolysis may not improve long-term subclavian venous patency and relief of symptoms in patients with "subacute" and "chronic" occlusions [14, 16].

Hopkins Protocol

A protocol has been developed at Johns Hopkins Hospital by Freischlag and associates that demonstrates this understanding of venous thoracic outlet syndrome pathophysiology. Patients that present late with subclavian vein thrombosis caused by thoracic outlet syndrome are first given injectable anticoagulation followed by oral warfarin. They are evaluated as outpatients by history, physical exam, and duplex ultrasound. Trans-axillary first rib resection is performed within weeks of evaluation. Two weeks after surgery, diagnostic venogram is performed which is accompanied by venoplasty, if indicated and technically feasible. If the vein remains occluded, or if it is patent and a percutaneous procedure is performed, oral anticoagulation is continued for 3 months. If the vein is patent and requires no intervention during the venogram, anticoagulation is discontinued. Physical therapy is begun 2 weeks after surgery, and is continued for 6–8 weeks. Recent data suggest that chronic venous occlusions that are resistant to postoperative percutaneous intervention may actually recanalize months to years following surgical decompression [9]. Follow-up imaging of the subclavian veins is obtained with venous duplex ultrasound.

These results support the hypothesis that decompression of the thoracic outlet is the critical step in treating chronic venous thoracic outlet syndrome, but does not provide specific clues about why this is true from a pathophysiologic standpoint. Potential theories include the interruption of chronic trauma to the subclavian vein, allowing it to recanalize. Another potential benefit of thoracic outlet decompression is to improve flow in collateral veins, which improves the venous hemodynamics of the upper extremity. Another factor could be the effect of anticoagulation. While not likely to change outcomes in isolation, anticoagulation in combination with surgical decompression may tip native antithrombotic processes enough to recanalize the vein in the long-term.

Imaging Techniques

Venography is the gold standard to demonstrate patency or occlusion of the subclavian vein. Duplex ultrasonography may not adequately differentiate between a recanalized subclavian vein and a large collateral vein adjacent to an occluded subclavian vein. However, in patients who are asymptomatic weeks to months after thoracic outlet decompression and venography, justifying an invasive procedure to make this differentiation is unfounded because it will not alter future treatment. In addition, serial duplex ultrasonography performed by technologists experienced with thoracic outlet syndrome diminishes the likelihood of inaccurate interpretation due to the ability to compare serial ultrasound images and venography images to prevent misidentification of a collateral vein.

Other Scenarios

Patients with recurrent thrombosis may have had subtotal thoracic outlet decompression, and thus require repeat surgery [17]. This can be performed safely and requires exhaustive attention to the adequacy of first rib resection. Patients who continue to be symptomatic and have continued subclavian vein occlusion following complete thoracic outlet decompression and postoperative venoplasty may be candidates for venous reconstruction. This can be performed with saphenous vein bypass or jugular venous turndown. These procedures typically require incisions above and below the clavicle and may even require partial claviculectomy. There is little data regarding these procedures mostly because the number of patients requiring this eventual intervention is quite low (see Chap. 65).

Outcomes

Many patients with chronic occlusion of the subclavian vein return to their baseline functional status, without major symptoms. The patency rates for the involved subclavian vein are slightly worse than the rate of patients who are symptom free in most series [4, 17, 18], implying that vein patency should always be the ultimate goal of treatment. Extensive collateral venous networks frequently develop around a subclavian vein thrombosis (see Fig. 56.1). These collaterals protect the patient from symptoms of upper extremity venous hypertension even if the subclavian vein remains occluded. When considering further invasive treatment for an occluded subclavian vein, the presence of venous collaterals and the potential for damaging them with further interventions needs to be carefully considered.

Fig. 56.1 Occluded right
subclavian vein with
extensive collateral veins

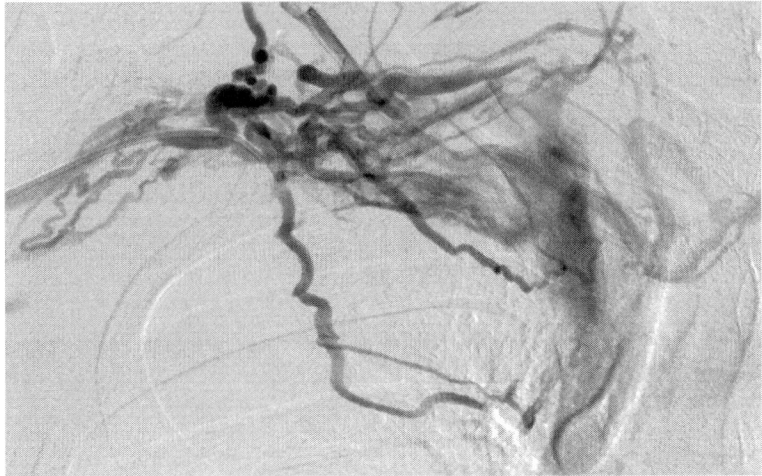

References

1. Illig KA, Doyle AJ. A comprehensive review of Paget-Schroetter syndrome. J Vasc Surg. 2010; 51:1538–47.
2. Lindblad B, Tengborn L, Bergqvist D. Deep vein thrombosis of the axillary-subclavian veins: epidemiologic data, effects of different types of treatment and late sequelae. Eur J Vasc Surg. 1988;2:161–5.
3. Tilney NL, Griffiths HJG, Edwards EA. Natural history of major venous thrombosis of the upper extremity. Arch Surg. 1970;101:792–6.
4. Urschel Jr HC, Patel AN. Surgery remains the most effective treatment for Paget-Schroetter syndrome: 50 years' experience. Ann Thorac Surg. 2008;86:254–60.
5. Lee WA, Hill BB, Harris Jr EJ, et al. Surgical intervention is not required for all patients with subclavian vein thrombosis. J Vasc Surg. 2000;32:57–67.
6. Lee MC, Grassi CJ, Belkin M, et al. Early operative intervention after thrombolytic therapy for primary subclavian vein thrombosis: an effective treatment approach. J Vasc Surg. 1998;27:1101–8.
7. Angle N, Gelabert HA, Farooq MM, et al. Safety and efficacy of early surgical decompression of the thoracic outlet for Paget-Schroetter syndrome. Ann Vasc Surg. 2001;15:37–42.
8. Caparrelli DJ, Freischlag J. A unified approach to axillosubclavian venous thrombosis in a single hospital admission. Semin Vasc Surg. 2005;18:153–7.
9. de Leon RA, Chang DC, Busse C, et al. First rib resection and scalenectomy for chronically occluded subclavian veins: what does it really do? Ann Vasc Surg. 2008;22:395–401.
10. Lee JT, Karwowski JK, Harris EJ. Long-term thrombotic recurrence after nonoperative management of Paget-Schroetter syndrome. J Vasc Surg. 2006; 43:1236–43.
11. de Leon RA, Chang DC, Hassoun HT, et al. Multiple treatment algorithms for successful outcomes in venous thoracic outlet syndrome. Surgery. 2009; 145:500–7.
12. Schneider DB, Dimuzio PJ, Martin ND, et al. Combination treatment of venous thoracic outlet syndrome: open surgical decompression and intraoperative angioplasty. J Vasc Surg. 2004;40:599–603.
13. Kreinenberg PB, Chang BB, Darling III RC, et al. Long-term results in patients treated with thrombolysis, thoracic inlet decompression, and subclavian vein stenting for Paget-Schroetter syndrome. J Vasc Surg. 2001;33:S100–5.
14. Doyle A, Wolford HY, Davies MG, et al. Management of effort thrombosis of the subclavian vein: today's treatment. Ann Vasc Surg. 2007;21:723–9.
15. Urschel Jr JC, Patel AN. Paget-Schroetter syndrome therapy: failure of intravenous stents. Ann Thorac Surg. 2003;75:1693–6.
16. Guzzo JL, Chang K, Demos J, et al. Preoperative thrombolysis and venoplasty affords no benefit in patency following first rib resection and scalenectomy for subacute and chronic vein thrombosis. J Vasc Surg. 2010;52:658–63.
17. Molina JE. Reoperations after failed transaxillary first rib resection to treat Paget-Schroetter syndrome patients. Ann Thorac Surg. 2011;91:1717–22.
18. Divi V, Proctor MC, Axelrod DA, et al. Thoracic outlet decompression for subclavian vein thrombosis. Arch Surg. 2005;140:54–7.

Conservative (Non-Operative) Treatment of VTOS

57

Kaj H. Johansen and Karl A. Illig

Abstract

Thoracic outlet decompression (generally by first rib resection) and, if necessary, subclavian venous reconstruction is commonly recommended for patients with venous TOS presenting as spontaneous subclavian vein thrombosis (effort thrombosis, Paget-Schroetter syndrome, or axillosubclavian vein thrombosis; ASVT). This recommendation arises from a widely-perceived risk of incapacitating symptoms of post-thrombotic syndrome in patients not so treated. Certain contemporary data, however, suggest that such patients, if treated with venous thrombolysis, balloon angioplasty of subclavian venous stenoses, and 3–6 months of anticoagulation *without first rib resection* may fare just as well as patients undergoing aggressive surgical reconstruction. Nonoperative, observational management may be a reasonable alternative to aggressive surgical intervention for subclavian venous thrombosis.

Introduction

Venous thoracic outlet syndrome (VTOS) refers to the condition arising from problems with the subclavian vein at the costoclavicular junction. VTOS can be associated with episodic obstruction to flow or frank subclavian deep venous thrombosis (DVT), best referred to as axillosubclavian vein thrombosis (ASVT): such thrombosis, in turn, can be either secondary to the presence of various foreign bodies (pacemaker leads or indwelling catheters, for example) or primary. It is widely held that the chronic post-thrombotic consequences of primary subclavian vein occlusion are frequent, predictable, and morbid, so that after initial venography and thrombolysis, thoracic outlet decompression (with or without subclavian venous reconstruction) should be performed. This has become so much of an established "fact" that debate currently revolves not around the necessity for surgical intervention for subclavian venous thrombosis but rather its timing – whether a certain period of time should be allowed to pass before operating or, alternatively,

K.H. Johansen, MD, PhD (✉)
Department of Vascular Surgery,
Swedish Heart and Vascular Institute,
1600 E. Jefferson St. #101, Seattle, WA 98122, USA
e-mail: kaj.johansen@swedish.org

K.A. Illig, MD
Department of Surgery, Division of Vascular Surgery,
University of South Florida, 2 Tampa General Circle,
STC 7016, Tampa, FL 33606, USA
e-mail: killig@health.usf.edu

whether immediate surgical decompression should be performed [1].

It is obligatory, however, that the choice of therapy for a particular disease state be based on a clear understanding of the natural history of that condition. It is vital from the decision-making perspective of both the patient and the physician that the relative risks and benefits of *all* therapeutic options – both operative and non-operative – be understood. Preferably such data would be derived from contemporary prospective randomized trials of various alternative treatments or, even better, meta-analyses of such reports. Large multicenter trials can be of use, and even single-center experiences have a role to play. What data underlie our current understanding of the natural history of subclavian DVT?

Historical Data

Reports regarding subclavian venous thrombosis have been published since the 1940s. Starting in the late 1960s a series of single-center reports suggested that 40–90 % of individuals who have suffered an episode of subclavian venous thrombosis would experience subsequent disabling upper extremity post-thrombotic symptoms (Table 57.1) [2–5]. These data, reflecting those for the development of symptoms of post-thrombotic syndrome following lower extremity DVT, influenced the decision-making of the current generation of senior vascular surgeons and led directly to the current aggressive surgical approach recommended by most in the management of primary subclavian venous thrombosis. That a substantial proportion – 80 % of primary subclavian venous thrombosis patients treated by first rib resection and, if necessary, venous reconstruction – appear to do well after surgical reconstruction is seen as a confirmation of this approach (Table 57.2) [1, 6–10].

Contemporary Natural History Data

The initial approach to a patient with acute ASVT currently includes immediate anticoagulation followed by upper extremity venography,

Table 57.1 Historical data regarding natural history of primary subclavian DVT

	Significant PTS symptoms (%)
Swinton et al. [2]	91
Tilney et al. [3]	74
Donayre et al. [4]	47
Gloviczki et al. [5]	40

VTOS venous thoracic outlet syndrome, *PTS* post-thrombotic syndrome

Table 57.2 Results of aggressive operative intervention for primary ASVT

	Persistent or recurrent PTS symptoms (%)
Machleder [6]	7
Lee et al. [7]	11
Urschel and Razzuk [8]	0
Schneider et al. [9]	8
Doyle et al. [10]	5
Molina et al. [11]	0
Stone et al. [12]	14
Guzzo et al. [13]	9

Table 57.3 Recent reports on the natural history of primary ASVT managed by thrombolysis (occasionally with venous angioplasty) and anticoagulation

	Persistent or recurrent PTS symptoms (%)
Heron et al. [14]	13
Sabeti et al. [15]	10
Martinelli et al. [16]	10
Elman and Kahn [17]	15
Sajid et al. [18]	17
Lechner et al. [19]	4

catheter-directed thrombolysis and, some would advocate, subclavian venous angioplasty. It should be noted, however, that the concept of, and techniques to carry out, catheter-directed thrombolysis and angioplasty were only introduced in the 1980s and were not part of the management of any of the historical series (some of which did not even systematically include anticoagulation) noted in Table 57.1.

Over the past 15 years several reports and reviews of patients treated by anticoagulation, venous thrombolysis and (where appropriate) subclavian venous angioplasty *but without operative intervention*, have been published (Table 57.3) – four observational single-center

Table 57.4 Recent surgical reports on the natural history of primary ASVT treated by endovascular means and anti-coagulation but withholding operation

	Persistent or recurrent PTS symptoms (%)
Hingorani et al. [20]	6
Lee et al. [21]	13
Lokanathan et al. [22]	10
Johansen	8

Table 57.5 Cordobes-Gual and colleagues [23] reported a series of patients operated upon for neurogenic or venous TOS and assessed pre- and post-operatively using a validated functional tool (Disabilities of the Arm, Shoulder and Hand, DASH) (American Academy of Orthopedic Surgeons, 1996):

	DASH pre-op	DASH post-op	p-value
Neurogenic TOS	54.0	17.8	0.01
Venous TOS	14.9	14.8	NSS

Reprinted from Cordobes-Gual et al. [23]. With permission from Elsevier

NSS not statistically significant

studies [14–16, 19] and two meta-analyses [17, 18]. These studies show that a large majority of such patients are either asymptomatic or only minimally hampered by post-thrombotic symptoms in the affected upper extremity at the time of follow-up. More recently several studies from a variety of surgical centers [20–22] have also suggested that the likelihood of chronic post thrombotic symptomatology in subclavian DVT patients who have not undergone surgical intervention is actually quite low (Table 57.4). Among 50 consecutive patients with subclavian vein thrombosis followed for 1–12 years (mean 4.7 years) after transcatheter thrombolysis, subclavian venous angioplasty and 3 months of oral anticoagulation, 92 % had no or minimal upper extremity post-thrombotic symptoms (Johansen, unpublished data).

Such results fuel skepticism about the necessity to carry out routine thoracic outlet decompression and venous reconstruction for acute subclavian DVT. A Spanish study [23] demonstrated that, in contradistinction to patients with *neurogenic* TOS (in whom pain and disability scores were initially substantially abnormal and were significantly improved following thoracic outlet decompression), patients with *venous* TOS had minimal symptomatology preoperatively and were unimproved by operation (Table 57.5). Observational studies of patients with *secondary* subclavian vein thrombosis (most commonly caused by the presence of a chronic catheters or pacemaker wires) reveal that virtually none have any significant ipsilateral upper extremity post-thrombotic symptoms.

Perhaps most persuasive for vascular specialists should be the observation of what happens with hemodialysis patients presenting with arm swelling due to an occluded subclavian vein central to a patent ipsilateral arteriovenous fistula or graft. One alternative is to salvage the fistula or graft by carrying out a first rib resection and subclavian venoplasty [24]. Alternatively, however, such patients' ipsilateral upper extremity congestive symptoms – which may be extreme – predictably *also* disappear with dismantling of the offending arteriovenous anastomosis. Vascular surgeons almost never see persistent arm swelling following AV fistula/graft ligation in ESRD patients with chronically-occluded central veins.

It is not completely straightforward to understand how clinicians' assessment of the apparent natural history of upper extremity venous thrombosis could have changed so markedly over the course of the past 50 years. A review of what is known about how the body responds to venous thrombosis (and its treatment), and how this pathophysiologic response differs between the upper and the lower extremities [19], may help clarify this question.

The Physiologic Consequences of Subclavian DVT and Its Treatment

Several stereotypical responses at the tissue and vessel level result are operative when venous thrombosis occurs. Venous collaterals develop, likely as a consequence both of the increased venous pressure gradient across the vascular occlusion, as well as (hypothetically) an alteration in vasculogenic factors arising from diminished pH or altered tissue metabolism resulting from the venous occlusion. Anticoagulation prevents propagation or extension of the venous thrombosis and prevents branch or tributary vessel thrombosis.

Exogenous thrombolysis, either systemically or by catheter-directed administration, partially or completely recanalizes the main venous channel, thereby increasing flow and diminishing flow through venous collaterals. With time, clot burden diminishes in size and partial or complete vein recanalization may occur. Exercise may have beneficial effects on the occluding venous thrombus, both by augmenting endogenous thrombolysis as well as by stimulating venous collateral formation.

A failure to clear a venous thrombosis completely results in the possibility that post-thrombotic changes will occur in the affected extremity. In the veins of the lower extremity, post-thrombotic syndrome occurs in at least a third of patients who have suffered an iliofemoral venous thrombosis. Such patients' symptoms arise consequent to both deep venous occlusion as well as venous valvular incompetence, but also crucially revolve around the substantial blood volume within the limb, the effects of gravity over the length of the limb as well as the extent of the venous thrombosis within it (it is an anatomic truism that the ability of venous collaterals to decompress a limb will be in inverse proportion to the length of the venous thrombosis itself).

In the upper extremity, on the other hand, limb blood volume is a small fraction of that within the lower extremity, gravity plays little or no role in sequestering blood in the extremity, venous valvular function is functionally irrelevant and the length of the subclavian venous thrombosis which must be "bypassed" by venous collateral development is very short – often only a few centimeters in length. For all these reasons the pathophysiology of the post-thrombotic syndrome which occurs following *lower* extremity venous thrombosis has little relevance to that which occurs following *upper* extremity venous thrombosis [19].

Comment

On historical grounds subclavian vein thrombosis has been thought to have a morbid and disabling natural history, a conclusion that has led to a widespread posture among specialists in the field that thoracic outlet decompression (at the least) and axillosubclavian venous reconstruction (if necessary) is obligatory in the management of this condition. Indeed, if contemporary patients continued to suffer the 40–90 % incidence of chronic or recurrent swelling, pain and limitation of motion documented in the earlier literature, such a conclusion would be entirely warranted.

However, more recent data appear to suggest that anticoagulation, thrombolysis, and subclavian venous angioplasty *without routine subsequent operative intervention* may result in long-term outcomes that are equivalent to those achieved when traditional thoracic outlet decompression is performed. Indeed, a comparison of several large series of subclavian DVT patients managed by observational, non-operative means (Tables 57.3 and 57.4) shows functional outcomes which are essentially equivalent to those of recent series of patients undergoing aggressive thoracic decompression and/or venous reconstruction (Table 57.2) – *without* the uncommon but occasionally severe complications that may accompany operative thoracic outlet decompression [25, 26].

It is possible that there exists a subset of patients – elite upper-extremity athletes, for example, or the young and vigorous – in whom thoracic outlet decompression (and/or venous reconstruction) is advantageous [27]. Unfortunately, no persuasive head-to-head comparative data are available to clarify this point. Instead, a sober analysis of available data invites the conclusion that the excellent results of thoracic outlet decompression and/or venous reconstruction reported by advocates of such an aggressive surgical approach (Table 57.2) may have less to do with the surgical technique employed and more to do with the fact that the underlying condition has an intrinsically benign outcome (Tables 57.3 and 57.4).

Conclusion

At the least, data presented in this Chapter suggest the non-inferiority of an initial observational, non-operative approach to subclavian DVT, and that a *selective*, rather than *routine*, surgical intervention in patients with subclavian DVT should be considered. Operating during the initial hospitalization in such patients, as has been suggested recently [1, 13], eliminates the very real possibility that many or most such patients might not need operation at all! If initial operative intervention were withheld, perhaps for 6–12 months following initial non-operative management, a substantial number of subclavian DVT patients, by now asymptomatic, might well avoid operation altogether. A randomized trial of such an approach would clarify this issue and is under discussion.

Editorial Note: *Conservative (nonoperative) management of axillosubclavian vein thrombosis*

Dr. Johansen here presents an excellent analysis of long-term results of various forms of treatment of axillosubclavian vein thrombosis (ASVT), the most severe form of venous TOS. He brings decades of experience to this field, and is a voice well worth paying attention to.

The views in this chapter, however, represent a minority opinion. Based on the perception of long-term disability if the first rib is not removed, most clinicians today advocate thoracic outlet decompression in virtually every patient with ASVT after clot dissolution, and many (see Chap. 56, for example) even in patients who remain chronically occluded. Dr. Johansen argues that this approach is not necessarily warranted, presenting results (Tables 57.2 through 57.4) that are roughly equivalent for thrombolysis alone versus the addition of first rib excision.

A close look at these data, however, must be performed. Eight series are presented in Table 57.2, showing long-term disability rates after thrombolysis and first rib resection ranging from 0 to 14 %, and ten series (nine published) in Tables 57.3 and 57.4, showing rates ranging from 4 to 17 % in patients undergoing thrombolysis *without* first rib excision. Roughly the same, but are these series equivalent? Taking into account size only, the answer is clearly no. By far the two largest series in

the "conventional treatment" group – rib excision after thrombolysis – are those of Urschel [8] and Molina [11] – and both describe long-term disability rates of *zero*. By contrast, the two largest "series" of results in patients *without* rib resection cited in Tables 57.3 and 57.4 – both meta-analyses [17, 18] – show disability rates of *15–17 %*.

Dr. Johansen's argument is valid, but our point is that all reports are not created equal, and that the specific series cited need to be examined in detail to best answer this question. Ultimately, his final point that a prospective randomized trial is needed is the absolutely correct conclusion. No analysis of past reports, all unrandomized and for the most part single center with variable follow up, can be relied on to set policy in any field of medicine, much less one so ill-controlled as TOS. By the same argument, one cannot conclude that first rib resection has been proven effective, or that it is unethical to withhold this within the context of a research trial. Many centers have enough volume to answer this question in a few years, but a multi-institutional trial would speed the process further. This is a high priority for Dr. Johansen and the editors of this volume, and we applaud him and the few others who have kept this issue in play!

References

1. Angle N, Gelabert H, Farooq MM, et al. Safety and efficacy of early surgical decompression of the thoracic outlet for Paget-Schroetter syndrome. Ann Vasc Surg. 2001;15:37–42.
2. Swinton Jr NW, Edgett Jr JW, Hall RJ. Primary subclavian axillary vein thrombosis. Circulation. 1968;38:737–45.
3. Tilney NL, Griffiths HJG, Edwards E. Natural history of major venous thrombosis of the upper extremity. Arch Surg. 1970;101:792–6.
4. Donayre CE, White GH, Mehringer SM, Wilson SE. Pathogenesis determines late morbidity of axillosubclavian vein thrombosis. Am J Surg. 1986;152:179–84.
5. Gloviczki P, Kazmaier FS, Hollier LH. Axillary-subclavian venous occlusion: the morbidity of a non-lethal disease. J Vasc Surg. 1986;4:333–7.

6. Machleder HI. Evaluation of a new treatment strategy for Paget-Schroetter syndrome: spontaneous thrombosis of the axillary-subclavian vein. J Vasc Surg. 1993;17:305–17.

7. Lee MC, Grassi CJ, Belkin M, et al. Early operative intervention after thrombolytic therapy for primary subclavian vein thrombosis: an effective treatment approach. J Vasc Surg. 1998;27:1101–8.

8. Urschel Jr HA, Razzuk MA. Paget-Schroetter syndrome: what is the best management? Ann Thorac Surg. 2000;69:1663–8.

9. Schneider DB, Dimuzio PB, Martin ND, et al. Combination treatment of venous thoracic outlet syndrome: open surgical decompression and intraoperative angioplasty. J Vasc Surg. 2004;40:599–603.

10. Doyle A, Wolford HY, Davies MG, et al. Management of effort thrombosis of the subclavian vein: today's treatment. Ann Vasc Surg. 2007;21(6):723–9.

11. Molina JE, Hunter DW, Dietz CA. Protocols for Paget-Schroetter syndrome and late treatment of chronic subclavian vein obstruction. Ann Thorac Surg. 2009;87:416–22.

12. Stone DH, Scali ST, Bierk AA, et al. Aggressive treatment of idiopathic axillosubclavian vein thrombosis provides excellent long-term function. J Vasc Surg. 2010;52:127–31.

13. Guzzo JL, Chang K, Demos J, et al. Preoperative thrombolysis and venoplasty affords no benefit in patency following first rib resection and scalenectomy for subacute and chronic subclavian vein thrombosis. J Vasc Surg. 2010;52:658–62.

14. Heron E, Lozingues O, Emmerich J, et al. Long-term sequelae of spontaneous axillary-subclavian venous thrombosis. Ann Intern Med. 1999;131:510–3.

15. Sabeti S, Schillinger M, Miekusch W, et al. Treatment of subclavian-axillary vein thrombosis: long-term outcome of anticoagulation versus systemic thrombolysis. Thromb Res. 2002;108:279–85.

16. Martinelli I, Battoglioli T, Bucciarelli P, et al. Risk factors and recurrence rate of primary deep venous thrombosis of the upper extremities. Circulation. 2004;110:566–70.

17. Elman EE, Kahn SP. The post-thrombotic syndrome after upper extremity deep venous thrombosis in adults: a systematic review. Thromb Res. 2006;117:609–14.

18. Sajid MS, Ahmed N, Desai M, et al. Upper limb deep vein thrombosis: a literature review to streamline the protocol for management. Acta Haematol. 2007;118:10–8.

19. Lechner D, Wiener C, Weltermatin A, et al. Comparison between idiopathic deep vein thrombosis of the upper and lower extremity regarding risk factors and recurrence. J Thromb Haemost. 2008;6:1269–74.

20. Hingorani A, Ascher E, Lorenson E, et al. Upper extremity deep venous thrombosis and its impact on morbidity and mortality rates in a hospital-based population. J Vasc Surg. 1997;26:853–60.

21. Lee WA, Hill BB, Harris EJ, et al. Surgical intervention is not required for all patients with subclavian venous thrombosis. J Vasc Surg. 2000;32:57–67.

22. Lokanathan R, Salvian AJ, Chen JC, et al. Outcome after thrombolysis and selective thoracic outlet decompression for primary axillary vein thrombosis. J Vasc Surg. 2001;33:783–8.

23. Cordobes-Gual J, Lozano-Vilardell P, Torreguitant-Mirada N, et al. Prospective study of the functional recovery after surgery for thoracic outlet syndrome. Eur J Vasc Endovasc Surg. 2008;35:79–83.

24. Glass C, Dugan M, Gillespie D, et al. Costoclavicular venous decompression in patients with threatened arteriovenous hemodialysis access. Ann Vasc Surg. 2011;25:640–5.

25. Melliere D, Becquemin JP, Etienne G, et al. Severe injuries resulting from operations for thoracic outlet syndrome: can they be avoided? J Cardiovasc Surg (Torino). 1991;32:509–603.

26. Chang DC, Lidor AO, Matsen SL, Freischlag JA. Reported in-hospital complications following rib resections for neurogenic thoracic outlet syndrome. Ann Vasc Surg. 2007;21:564–70.

27. Feugier P, Aleksic I, Salari R, et al. Long-term results of venous revascularization for Paget-Schroetter syndrome in athletes. Ann Vasc Surg. 2001;15:212–8.

58

Stephan Moll

Abstract

Which patient with upper extremity DVT should be tested for hypercoagulable states (thrombophilia) and what test should be obtained? No solid advice can be given due to a lack of clear data whether (a) thrombophilias contribute to DVT formation in patients with upper extremity DVT, and with VTOS in specific, (b) presence of a thrombophilia leads to differential outcome whether surgical/vascular intervention is done or not, and (c) treatment should be any different based on absence or presence of a thrombophilia. This chapter reviews the published data and, given the sparsity of clinical research data on this topic and the absence of a consensus statement, presents the author's approach to testing.

Thrombophilias – General Perspective

Much of what we know about thrombophilias (hypercoagulable states) as risk factors for venous thromboembolism (VTE) stems from studies of lower extremity DVT. A number of large and well performed studies over the years have established the following abnormalities as the most common and robust risk factors for VTE: the factor V Leiden and prothrombin G20210A (II20210) mutations, deficiency of protein C, S and antithrombin, antiphospholipid antibody syndrome (repeatedly positive lupus anticoagulant,

anticardiolipin IgG or IgM antibodies, and anti-β2-glycoprotein-I IgG and IgM antibodies), and elevated serum homocysteine levels. Elevated factor VIII levels are a risk factor for first VTE, but a number of testing caveats and the fact that elevated levels are not a risk factor for recurrence of VTE makes this test not useful in routine clinical practice. Meta-analyses show that methylene-tetra-hydro-folate reductase (MTHFR) C677T and A1298C polymorphisms are not risk factor for VTE in countries where food is supplemented with folic acid [1]. In view of conflicting or indecisive results regarding abnormalities in the fibrinolytic pathway and an association with VTE (PAI-1 and tPA levels and polymorphisms, etc.) such abnormalities cannot be viewed as clear thrombophilias [1]. A few uncommon thrombophilias of clinical relevance exist, such as the myeloproliferative disorders (essential thrombocytosis

S. Moll, MD
Department of Hematology,
University of North Carolina School of Medicine,
932 Mary Ellen Janes Bldg Campus Box 7035,
Chapel Hill, NC 27599-7035, USA
e-mail: smoll@med.unc.edu

and polycythemia vera) and paroxysmal nocturnal hemoglobinuria (PNH).

While relevant for research purposes, whether a
thrombophilia is a risk factor for a first episode of
VTE is not of relevance for the clinician and patient,
as the patient has already declared that he/she had a
thrombotic event – no matter whether a thrombophilia is present or not. The key question and the
main reason to consider testing in an individual with
VTE is whether presence of a thrombophilia leads to
a higher risk of *recurrent* VTE and should lead to
different treatment, i.e. longer-term anticoagulation
if a thrombophilia is present, versus shorter-term
treatment if none is found. In that context it is relevant to note that the heterozygous state for factor V
Leiden is only a mild risk factor for recurrent VTE in
the lower extremities, and the prothrombin G20210A
mutation does not increase the risk of recurrence [2].
Clinical management in lower extremity DVT and
PE – length of anticoagulation – is, therefore, typically independent of the presence or absence of
heterozygous factor V Leiden or the prothrombin
G20210A mutation [3, 4].

The thrombophilias that predict a higher risk
of VTE *recurrence* and are, therefore, considered
strong thrombophilias, are listed in Table 58.1.
The presence of one of these may be one of the
reasons to consider longer-term anticoagulation
in the patient with a first episode of lower extremity DVT or PE. Thus, testing for these thrombophilias in patients in whom additional information
is needed to make a decision on length of anticoagulation can be appropriate [4]. The tests the
author of this chapter considers appropriate in
this situation are listed in Table 58.2. However,
data on the role of thrombophilias in patients with
upper extremity DVT are much sparser.

VTOS, DVT and Thrombophilia

Are Thrombophilias Risk Factors for DVT in Patients with VTOS?

It is NOT known whether thrombophilias contribute to DVT in patients with external compression
of the axillo-subclavian vein. No case-control,
prospective or retrospective cohort, or population-
based cross-sectional study has been done to

Table 58.1 The strong thrombophilias

Factor V Leiden, homozygous
Prothrombin G20210A (II20210) mutation, homozygous
Double heterozygous state (Factor V Leiden PLUS II20210 mutation)
Protein C deficiency
Protein S deficiency
Antithrombin deficiency
Antiphospholipid antibody syndrome

Table 58.2 What to test in 2013

Antiphospholipid antibodies
Lupus anticoagulant (= inhibitor)
Anticardiolipin IgG and IgM antibodies
Anti-β_2-glycoprotein-I IgG and IgM antibodies
Factor V Leiden (to detect the homozygous state or the double heterozygous state of factor V Leiden plus prothrombin 20210 mutation)
Prothrombin 20210 mutation (to detect the homozygous state or the double heterozygous state with factor V Leiden)
Antithrombin activity (= functional antithrombin)
Protein C activity (= functional protein C)
Protein S activity (= functional protein S)

investigate an association between thrombophilia
and VTOS. Two studies have tried to address this
issue. A case series reported in 2004 examining 31
patients with primary upper extremity DVT found
that 75 % of patients without an anatomic abnormality had a thrombophilia, versus only 22.5 % in
patients with an abnormality (p=0.006), suggesting that thrombophilias play less of a role, if any,
in VTOS with DVT compared to upper extremity
DVT without anatomic abnormality [5]. Another
retrospective case series, reported in 2006, examining 18 patients with VTOS who had undergone
first rib resection with scalenectomy reported that
thrombophilias were relatively common in this
population: 10/15 patients tested (67 %) had what
the authors defined as a thrombophilia [6].
However, this report lacked clear definition of the
thrombophilias (lack of reporting of degree of
antiphospholipid antibody positivity and results of
follow-up testing, degree of protein S decrease and
homocysteine increase) and included thrombophilias that are nowadays often not considered to
be thrombophilias (MTHFR and PAI-1 polymorphisms). In addition, the study lacked a control

group. Thus, the conclusion from the study that "thrombophilia may play an important role in the pathogenesis of VTOS" remains speculation and the conclusion that "clotting disorders should be aggressively evaluated" lacks supportive data.

Does Knowing Whether the Patient Has a Thrombophilia Change Management?

It is NOT known whether knowledge that a patient has a thrombophilia or not should lead to different treatment, i.e. longer anticoagulation after a VTOS-associated DVT – no matter whether a decompressive intervention/surgery is performed or not. No prospective outcomes studies using presence or absence of thrombophilia for treatment decision making have been published.

While the 2006 publication discussed above reported that the majority of complications after rib resection with scalenectomy in the 18 patients operated on occurred in patients with a thrombophilia, the limitations of the definition of thrombophilias in the study and the nature of some of the adverse outcomes (hemothorax, neuropathy, recurrent or persistent edema without documented large vessel thrombosis) makes the study's conclusion that "thrombophilia may be a determinant of success of surgical compression" a hypothesis without supportive data at this point [6]. Finally, the design of the study – retrospective case series – and the lack of testing of different treatments based on presence or absence of a thrombophilia, does not allow the conclusions made that "knowledge that a patient has a clotting disorder can improve therapeutic outcome" [6].

Primary Upper Extremity DVT and Thrombophilias

Are Thrombophilias Risk Factors for Primary (Unprovoked, Idiopathic) Upper Extremity DVT?

It is NOT clear whether thrombophilias contribute to a first event of primary upper extremity DVT. Data from mostly small case series and case control studies have been conflicting. Some

studies have shown a low prevalence of thrombophilias in patients with upper extremity DVT or no increased risk for DVT in patients with thrombophilia compared to controls without [7–9]. Others have reported an increased prevalence of thrombophilias or increased risk of DVT if a thrombophilia was present [5, 10–12]. The largest study to date does suggest that thrombophilias are a risk factor for upper extremity DVT [11]. It also suggests, based on observation that the combination of inherited thrombophilia and oral contraceptive pill leads to a greater DVT risk than each risk factor by itself, that upper extremity DVT may be a multifactorial process.

Does Knowing Whether the Patient Has a Thrombophilia Change Management?

It is NOT known whether knowledge that a patient has a thrombophilia or not should lead to different treatment, i.e. longer anticoagulation in patients with upper extremity DVT. No prospective randomized trials have been done. However, very limited data suggest that the risk of recurrent upper extremity DVT after an initial 6 months of anticoagulation therapy is relatively low, even if a thrombophilia is present [11]. However, the number of patients with strong thrombophilias in that study were so low (3 of 115 patients) that no solid conclusion is possible.

A Personal Approach

In the patient with upper extremity DVT who has clear-cut VTOS requiring surgical intervention, this author tends to not order thrombophilia testing, as a clear other risk factor for the DVT has been detected. However, frequently the cause of the DVT is not fully clear and it is not clear whether external subclavian-axillary vein compression was a triggering factor. Thus, in the patient with upper extremity DVT not associated with central venous lines or cancer, the author does tend to perform a thrombophilia work-up, trying to find an explanation for the DVT and determining whether the patient has a strong thrombophilia (Table 58.1) that might influence the length of anticoagulation decision. Table 58.2 lists the tests that the author orders.

Conclusion

Who should be tested and what should be tested for? No solid advice can be given due to a lack of clear solid data whether (a) thrombophilias contribute to DVT formation in patients with upper extremity DVT in general, and with VTOS in specific, (b) presence of a thrombophilia leads to differential outcome whether surgical/vascular intervention is done or not, and (c) treatment should be any different based on absence or presence of a thrombophilia. However, if thrombophilia testing is done, care needs to be taken to appropriately interpret the tests, as a number of factors can lead to false positive and false negative results. In addition, counseling needs to take place as to what the finding of the thrombophilia means for the patient and his/her family members. Referral to a hematologist and/or genetic counselor might be appropriate, as well as provision of patient education materials (such as the information resource www.clotconnect.org).

References

1. Foy P, Moll S. Thrombophilia: 2009 update. Curr Treat Options Cardiovasc Med. 2009;11(2):114–28.

2. Segal JB, et al. Predictive value of factor V Leiden and Prothrombin G20210A in adults with venous thromboembolism and in family members of those with a mutation: a systematic review. JAMA. 2009;301(23): 2472–85.

3. Kearon C et al. Antithrombotic therapy of VTE disease. Antithrombotic therapy and prevention of thrombosis, 9th ed: American College of Chest Physicians evidence-based clinical practice guidelines. Chest 2012;141;141(2)(Suppl):e419S-e494S.

4. Moll S. Who should be tested for thrombophilia? Genet Med. 2011;13(1):19–20.

5. Hendler MF, et al. Primary upper-extremity deep vein thrombosis: high prevalence of thrombophilic defects. Am J Hematol. 2004;76(4):330–7.

6. Cassada DC, et al. The importance of thrombophilia in the treatment of Paget-Schroetter syndrome. Ann Vasc Surg. 2006;20(5):596–601.

7. Ruggeri M, et al. Low prevalence of thrombophilic coagulation defects in patients with deep vein thrombosis of the upper limbs. Blood Coagul Fibrinolysis. 1997;8(3):191–4.

8. Martinelli I, et al. Risk factors for deep venous thrombosis of the upper extremities. Ann Intern Med. 1997;126(9):707–11.

9. Baarslag HJ, et al. Long-term follow-up of patients with suspected deep vein thrombosis of the upper extremity: survival, risk factors and post-thrombotic syndrome. Eur J Intern Med. 2004;15(8):503–7.

10. Prandoni P, et al. Upper-extremity deep vein thrombosis. Risk factors, diagnosis, and complications. Arch Intern Med. 1997;157(1):57–62.

11. Martinelli I, et al. Risk factors and recurrence rate of primary deep vein thrombosis of the upper extremities. Circulation. 2004;110(5):566–70.

12. Linnemann B, et al. Hereditary and acquired thrombophilia in patients with upper extremity deep-vein thrombosis. Results from the MAISTHRO registry. Thromb Haemost. 2008;100(3):440–6.

Physical and Occupational Therapy for Patients with VTOS

59

Matthew R. Driskill

Abstract

While surgical treatment has an important place in the management of most patients with VTOS, physical therapists play a crucial role in helping patients attain optimal post-operative outcomes. Physical therapy should be focused on the individual needs of each patient with VTOS. The initial goals should be aimed at range of motion deficits, patient comfort, diaphragmatic breathing exercises and patient education on post-surgical precautions. Based upon symptoms, exercise tolerance, neurological deficits, and the protocol of the surgeon, the patient should gradually progress to strengthening activities. Postures, faulty movement patterns, habits and work duties which contribute to impairments for one individual may be different from another. Addressing the unique needs of each patient with VTOS is essential in order to achieve optimal recovery and long-term functional outcomes following surgical treatment.

Introduction

Venous thoracic outlet syndrome (VTOS) is a rare condition that can have a significant impact on the affected individuals. While surgical treatment has an important place in the management of most patients with VTOS, physical therapists play a crucial role in helping patients attain optimal post-operative outcomes. With knowledge of the anatomic path of the axillary-subclavian vein combined with a thorough history and objective evaluation of the patient, the physical therapist can formulate a detailed treatment plan that is focused on the needs of the *individual* patient. The focus of this chapter is on the principles of physical therapy for patients that have undergone surgical treatment for VTOS.

Initial Evaluation

Post-operative physical rehabilitation begins early after surgery. The patient should be initially seen by a physical therapist within the first day or two of the operation, prior to discharge from the hospital, in order to begin gentle cervical and upper extremity range of motion exercises (mostly for "generic" recovery from first rib

M.R. Driskill, MSPT
Department of Outpatient Musculoskeletal,
The Rehabilitation Institute of St. Louis,
4455 Duncan Ave. N/A, St. Louis, MO 63110, USA
e-mail: mrd1839@yahoo.com

K.A. Illig et al. (eds.), *Thoracic Outlet Syndrome*,
DOI 10.1007/978-1-4471-4366-6_59, © Springer-Verlag London 2013

excision at this point). Following hospital discharge, the patient should begin outpatient rehabilitation. Although initially this treatment will continue to focus on cervical and upper extremity range of motion and recovery from rib excision, a complete subjective history highlighting the symptoms and a thorough objective evaluation focused on *individual* impairments and the venous pathology itself are essential in guiding further treatment.

During this initial evaluation it is important to discuss with the patient any potential precipitating events that occurred prior to the development of VTOS as well as the timeframe of the initial onset of symptoms, previous treatments, and surgical care. It is important to review any hobbies and work-related activities in order to highlight potential contributing factors that are unique to the individual. It is also relevant to discuss specific signs and symptoms, as well as any previous injuries or co-morbid conditions that may influence further physical therapy and eventual recovery of full activity.

The subjective background will further guide the objective evaluation. The physical therapist should first assess general patient appearance, with particular attention to the surgical site. The surgical incision should be visually examined for any abnormal signs that would require referral back to the surgeon. The presence and extent of any neck or arm swelling, as well as any discoloration, should be specifically noted. The patient's posture and alignment are also evaluated. Areas of importance include the slope of the shoulder girdle, the angle of the clavicle, the position of the scapula on the thorax, the position of the humerus in the glenoid fossa, the alignment of the thoracic spine, and posturing of the head and neck.

Range of motion of the neck, shoulder, elbow, wrist, and hand are specifically measured, while carefully monitoring the body mechanics associated with each of these motions. The quality of motion may also highlight any potential neurological deficits following surgery which may influence the course of therapy. For example, it is essential to monitor scapular motion to highlight any potential dysfunction of the long thoracic nerve, since neuromuscular abnormalities in this region will likely affect the progression of treatment.

Initial Treatment

The initial focus of treatment should be on restoration of range of motion of the neck and affected upper extremity, pain control and optimal patient comfort, use of diaphragmatic breathing exercises, and management of any residual edema. In order to fully address the needs of the patient, it is essential for the physical therapist to continually monitor the signs and symptoms of the patient and to modify the treatment plan in accord with specific conditions and progress at each interval.

Range of motion exercises for the neck and upper extremity are initiated to restore full motion, to help prevent any further loss of motion, and to prevent the development of postoperative adhesions in the area of the surgery. The sternocleidomastoid muscle may be tender, firm and/or shortened due to muscle spasm, therefore limiting cervical range of motion. Initial exercises to address this should include active or passive cervical stretching. The patient should also begin shoulder range of motion exercises including active or active-assistive supine shoulder flexion, as well as supine medial and lateral rotation (Fig. 59.1). Initially, the supine position may promote better body mechanics and may be more tolerable to the patient.

Motions of the shoulder performed against gravity (sitting or standing flexion) should be closely monitored. First, increased swelling of the arm may put additional stress on the neck and shoulder (and should be brought to the attention of the surgeon). In addition, improper scapular motion may also be a concern when lifting the arm overhead against gravity. Long thoracic nerve dysfunction may affect the patient's shoulder range of motion and contribute to altered body mechanics: if the serratus anterior muscle isn't working sufficiently, the patient should avoid full overhead elevation of the shoulder in a sitting or standing

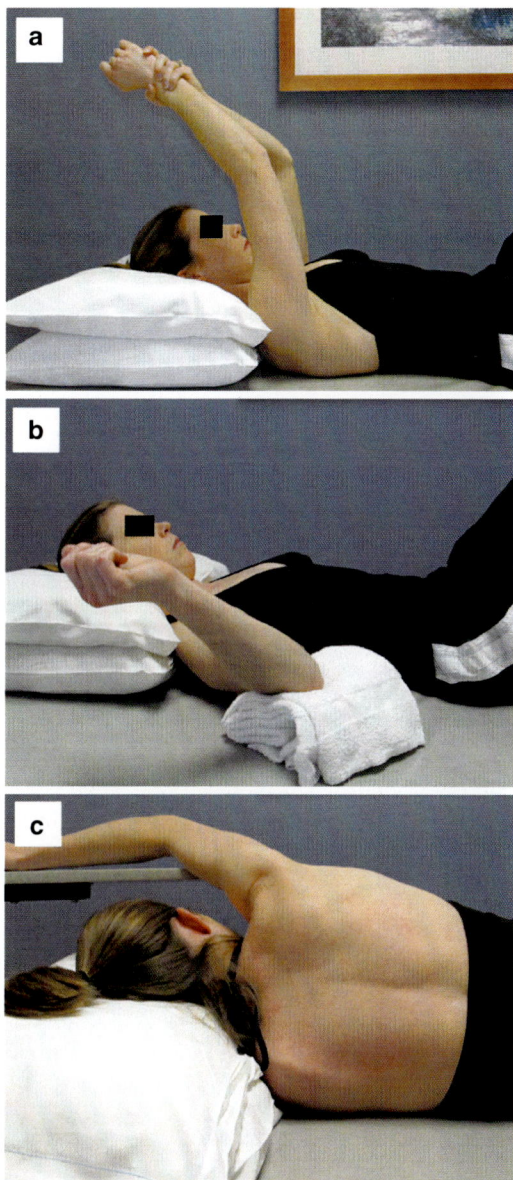

Fig. 59.1 Range-of-motion exercises for venous TOS. Exercises performed in the supine position including active-assisted shoulder flexion (**a**) and medial and lateral shoulder rotation (**b**). Sidelying shoulder flexion may also be performed as a gravity lessened position to facilitate improved body mechanics (**c**)

position. Such faulty body mechanics can lead to unwanted stress to the shoulder and surrounding tissues and need to be avoided until functional recovery of the long thoracic nerve has occurred. Active range of motion of the elbow, hand, and wrist should also be empha-

sized. These motions can help regain functional loss of motion of the affected upper extremity, and the active contraction of the muscles can assist with edema management. The use of ice can also assist with swelling in the surgical area.

Prolonged swelling of the arm can reduce range of motion, contribute to adhesions, and place additional stress on the shoulder due to the added weight of the extremity. Due to this potential added weight as well as discomfort associated with the surgery, the therapist should also instruct the patient in appropriate sitting and sleeping postures. When sitting, it may be beneficial to support the upper extremity on pillows or an armrest in order to unweight the arm. When lying supine, the patient may also use a pillow under the arm to help place it in the same plane as the glenoid fossa (Fig. 59.2a).

When appropriate, individual-based patient education should also include diaphragmatic breathing exercises, desensitization techniques for any potentially hypersensitive areas, scar management, and any protocols specific to the surgeon performing the original operative treatment. The patient may be on lifting restrictions and activity modifications for several weeks following surgery. Gentle and progressive strengthening will usually not begin for several weeks following surgery. The use of modalities and possibly aquatic therapy may be utilized to facilitate this gradual progression (Fig. 59.2b).

Treatment Progression

In general, the progression of exercises should be slow, in accord with the recommendations of the surgeon, and based on the individual's rate of healing and symptom resolution. Additionally, if the patient has any associated neurological deficits or other co-morbid conditions, the progression of rehabilitation may need to be modified. While all patients are encouraged to progress slowly through the healing process, the return to recreational activities and work-related duties needs to be based on the unique

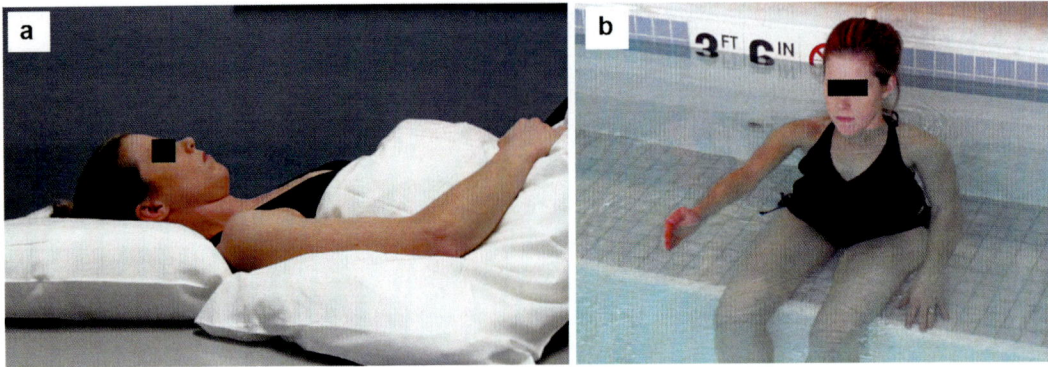

Fig. 59.2 Physical therapy for venous TOS. When lying supine, the patient may use a pillow under the arm to help place it in the same plane as the glenoid fossa; it may also be beneficial to support the upper extremity on pillows or an armrest when sitting, in order to help unweight the arm (**a**). Gentle and progressive strengthening will usually begin several weeks following surgery for VTOS, for which aquatic or pool therapy may be utilized to facilitate a gradual progression (**b**)

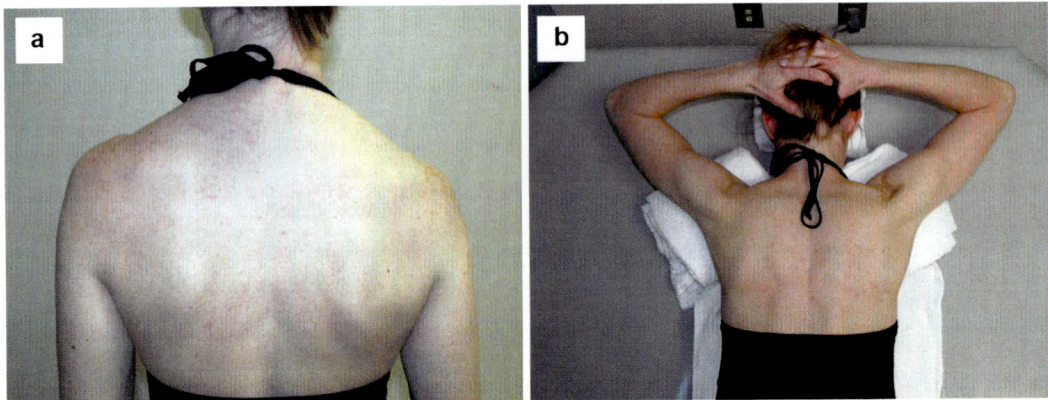

Fig. 59.3 Postural alterations and strengthening in venous TOS. Poor posture, as illustrated here by slumping of the shoulder girdle, may be a contributing factor in the development of VTOS (**a**). Active exercises to help correct postural alterations are an important component of postoperative physical therapy for patients with VTOS (**b**)

circumstances of the individual. For example, in the patient with dysfunction of the long thoracic nerve, overhead activities may be limited for several weeks to months while awaiting functional nerve recovery. It is also useful to consider that treatment should not only focus on the affected (surgical) side, but should take into account the conservative management of the contralateral side, in order to ensure optimal overall functional outcomes.

As the patient's range of motion gradually returns toward normal, any neurologic deficits subside, and general strength begins to improve, careful attention should be placed on posture, movement patterns of the spine and shoulder girdle, hobbies, and work-related duties which may have factored into the original compression of the neurovascular bundle. As the subclavian vein transverses the base of the neck through the thoracic outlet, poor posture may have contributed to its compression and should be addressed during post-operative care (Fig. 59.3). Dynamic patterns should also be analyzed and modified. The physical therapist should assess and address scapular mechanics and timing during upper extremity movements, precision of humeral motion within the glenoid cavity, and faulty movement patterns that may occur with various cervical and thoracic motions. Additionally, the sport, hobby or work activities that require any repetitive or overhead motion may need to be modified or discontinued.

Exercise routines should also be evaluated. Movements contributing to muscle imbalance, poor posture, and subsequent potential compression of the axillary-subclavian vein should be avoided. Exercises that may have contributed to scalene or pectoralis minor muscle hypertrophy may need to be modified or discontinued. Furthermore, strengthening of the latissimus dorsi muscle may have contributed to shoulder girdle depression and a narrowing of the costoclavicular space, and may also need to be limited. In addition, it may be important to evaluate a patient's breathing pattern. Patients who do not demonstrate a diaphragmatic breathing pattern may demonstrate increased use of the accessory muscles for breathing, which may contribute to muscle stiffness and spasm. Such patients may need to be instructed in more appropriate breathing patterns.

Additional Considerations

Although VTOS is a specific subset of TOS related to compression of the axillary-subclavian vein, the physical therapist should also take into consideration the nerves of the brachial plexus and the subclavian artery, as these structures also course through the anatomical passage of the thoracic outlet. Often the mechanisms that cause compromise for one structure will compromise the other parts of the neurovascular bundle, and surgery for one problem can create another. Effective treatment should thus be based on evidence regarding patients with any of the three types of TOS. Although the patient with VTOS may be seen primarily in the postoperative setting, approaches used in the conservative management of patients with other forms of TOS may be useful in guiding treatment, which is focused on improving body mechanics, posture, and activity modifications. Several treatment protocols and strategies have been suggested for conservative physical therapy for patients with neurogenic TOS, [1–7], and are further discussed in Chaps. 23 and 24, respectively.

Although several exercise programs and treatment strategies have been offered, it remains important to recognize that no individual protocol will be applicable to all patients. The reasons for the compression of the neurovascular bundle may vary between patients, and different individuals may have undergone different protocols for treatment of VTOS. The ongoing assessment of the individual will highlight the potential contributing factors to the compression of the neurovascular bundle which may be addressed with physical therapy.

In conclusion, physical therapy should be focused on the individual needs of each patient with VTOS. The initial goals should be aimed at range of motion deficits, patient comfort, diaphragmatic breathing exercises, edema management, and patient education on post-surgical precautions. Based upon symptoms, exercise tolerance, neurological deficits, and the protocol of the surgeon, the patient should gradually progress to strengthening activities. Postures, faulty movement patterns, habits and work duties that contribute to impairments for one individual may be different from the next. Upon the background of principles outlined here, addressing the unique needs of each patient with VTOS is essential toward achieving optimal recovery and long-term functional outcomes following surgical treatment.

References

1. Walsh MT. Therapist management of thoracic outlet syndrome. J Hand Ther. 1994;7(2):131–44.
2. Kenny RA, Traynor GB, Withington D, Keegan DJ. Thoracic outlet syndrome: a useful exercise treatment option. Am J Surg. 1993;165:282–4.
3. Novak CB. Conservative management of thoracic outlet syndrome. Semin Thorac Cardiovasc Surg. 1996; 8(2):201–7.
4. Watson LA, Pizzari T, Balster B. Thoracic outlet syndrome, part 2: conservative management of the thoracic outlet. Man Ther. 2010;15:305–14.

5. Lindgren KA. Conservative treatment of thoracic outlet syndrome: a 2-year follow-up. Arch Phys Med
   Rehabil. 1997;78(4):373–8.
6. Crosby CA, Wehbe MA. Conservative treatment for
   thoracic outlet syndrome. Hand Clin. 2004;20:43–9.
7. Edgelow P. Neurovascular consequences of cumulative
   trauma disorders affecting the thoracic outlet: a patient
   centered treatment approach. In: Donatelli R, editor.
   Physical therapy of the shoulder. New York: Churchill
   Livingston; 2004. p. 205–38.

Part VII

Venous TOS: Surgical Techniques

The majority of patients presenting with VTOS will require surgical intervention. The following chapters provide detailed descriptions of the wide range of surgical options that should be in the armamentarium of surgeons treating this patient population. Catheter-based pharmacological and mechanical thrombolysis are the first procedures most patients receive, and Dr. Darcy begins with an outline of the diagnostic and therapeutic options available.

All surgical techniques for treating VTOS involve resection of some or all of the first rib. This can be performed through a transaxillary approach, as well as a supraclavicular, infraclavicular or combined paraclavicular approach. In rare cases, a claviculectomy may be required to facilitate exposure.

The transaxillary approach described by Dr. Illig provides excellent exposure to the anterior thoracic outlet allowing access to resect the first rib and perform external venolysis with a cosmetically favorable incision. The infraclavicular approach outlined by Drs. Meltzer and Schneider allows resection of the anterior portion of the first rib as well as subclavian venolysis. This exposure can be extended by dividing the manubrium for vein reconstruction if necessary. Dr. Thompson discusses his extensive experience with his preferred technique: the paraclavicular approach. This provides access to the entire thoracic outlet, and allows for vein reconstruction when necessary. Dr. Sanders also adds his wealth of experience to the discussion on additional options for vein reconstruction. In unusual circumstances, claviculectomy may be used for exposure to the axillary, subclavian and innominate veins. Dr. Illig provides details and describes his experience with this surgical technique.

Surgical Techniques: Thrombolysis, IVUS, and Balloon Angioplasty for VTOS

60

Michael Darcy

Abstract

Venous thoracic outlet syndrome (VTOS) requires imaging to confirm the diagnosis and assess the extent of involvement and chronicity. In patients who present with acute effort thrombosis, thrombolysis is typically the first step. Tools for performing pharmacomechanical thrombolysis and strategies for their use will be discussed. Angioplasty and occasionally stenting are important techniques for managing residual stenoses after operative decompression of the thoracic outlet.

Introduction

Most patients with venous thoracic outlet syndrome (VTOS) present with an acutely occluded vein. Imaging in general is critical to confirm the diagnosis and assess the extent of involvement, as well as to try to determine duration of thrombus presence. In patients who present with acute effort thrombosis, it is uniformly agreed upon that thrombolysis is the first step. For both of these reasons a well-thought out strategy for both diagnosis and initial intervention is of critical importance.

Imaging

As discussed elsewhere, direct visualization of the venous system using duplex ultrasound is the first step in a patient with VTOS, because it is inexpensive, readily available, easy for the patient to tolerate, and totally non-invasive. However there are several disadvantages to ultrasound. Visualization of the vein as it passes beneath the clavicle may be difficult. If chronic occlusion is present it may be difficult to distinguish a large collateral vein from the subclavian vein. Compressing the subclavian may be difficult because of the overlying clavicle. Finally a high grade stenosis may slow flow so much that it can mimic thrombosis. For the above reasons it can be difficult to assess the length of the occlusion, and it may be difficult to distinguish acute from sub-acute thrombosis by ultrasound.

The sensitivity of ultrasound has been reported to be in the range of 71–100 % and specificity ranges from 82 to 100 % [1, 2]. The diagnostic capabilities of ultrasound may be a little more

M. Darcy, MD
Department of Radiology,
Mallinckrodt Institute of Radiology,
Barnes Jewish Hospital,
510 South Kingshighway Blvd, St. Louis,
MO 63110, USA
e-mail: darcym@mir.wustl.edu

K.A. Illig et al. (eds.), *Thoracic Outlet Syndrome*,
DOI 10.1007/978-1-4471-4366-6_60, © Springer-Verlag London 2013

413

limited in children: a study of upper extremity deep venous thrombosis in 66 children with acute lymphocytic leukemia revealed that the sensitivity of ultrasound was only 37 %, with all false negatives occurring in those with subclavian or central occlusion [3].

As discussed more thoroughly in Chap. 54, cross-sectional imaging (computed tomographic angiography (CTA), magnetic resonance imaging (MRI), and magnetic resonance venography (MRV)) have assumed greater roles in diagnosis of VTOS. Unlike ultrasound, both CT and MR are able to consistently visualize the subclavian vein under the clavicle. Both CT and MR can also readily define anatomy extrinsic to the vein that may be responsible for compression of the vein such as hypertrophy of the anterior scalene muscle. MR can be done without iodinated contrast and does not involve ionizing radiation. Also with MR it is possible to do provocative maneuvers (Fig. 60.1) to reveal subclavian compression not evident on standard images with the patient's arms at their side. MR has been reported to have a sensitivity of 100 % with a specificity of 97 % [4].

Since the diagnosis can be made non-invasively in the vast majority of patients, venography no longer has a role as a primary diagnostic test *per se*, but is nearly uniformly performed as a prelude to a catheter based intervention.

Is Thrombolysis Followed by Decompression Ever *Not* Indicated?

A variety of therapeutic strategies have been utilized in the years prior to the availability of thrombolytic techniques. 58–75 % of patients treated with anticoagulation alone will have persistent symptoms. Thrombolysis alone does not treat the underlying stenosis (Fig. 60.2). Although covered elsewhere (Chap. 71), series exploring thrombolysis alone are illustrative. In one, 25 patients were treated with thrombolysis, 12 of them with adjunctive PTA, while only two underwent operative decompression [5]. At 3 years of follow-up only 28 % were symptom free while 72 % had mild or severe symptoms. Another series of 35 patients treated non-operatively with

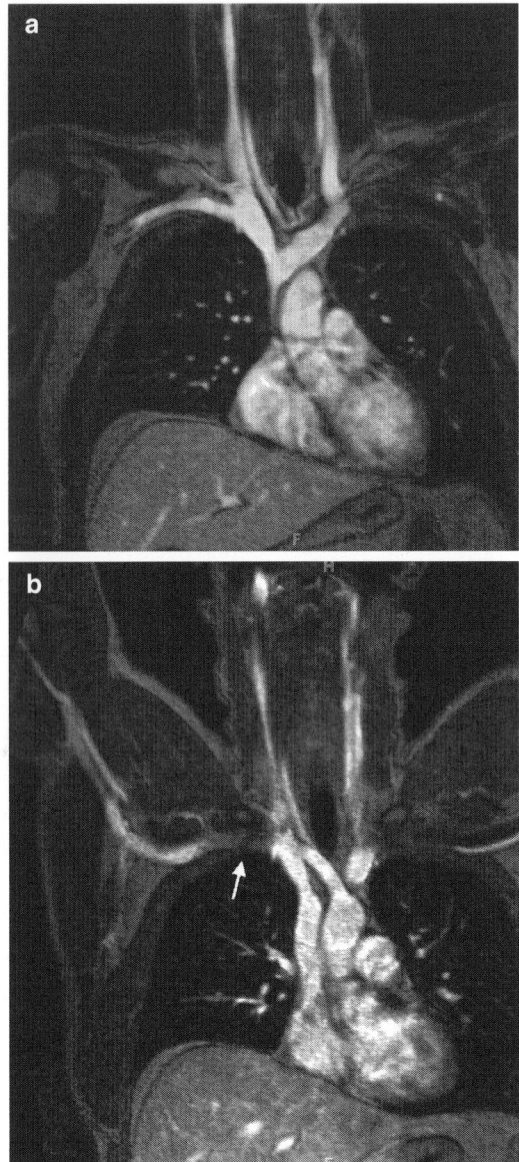

Fig. 60.1 (**a**) MR scan with the arms in neutral position at the side. The right subclavian vein appears to be normal. (**b**) Repeat MR after abducting and raising the arms shows narrowing (*arrow*) of the right subclavian vein

thrombolysis and anticoagulation resulted in a 23 % rate of recurrent thrombosis within 13 months post treatment [6].

Angioplasty without operative decompression is futile as the problem is *extrinsic* compression of the vein at the costoclavicular junction, which exerts massive leverage. Stenting the subclavian

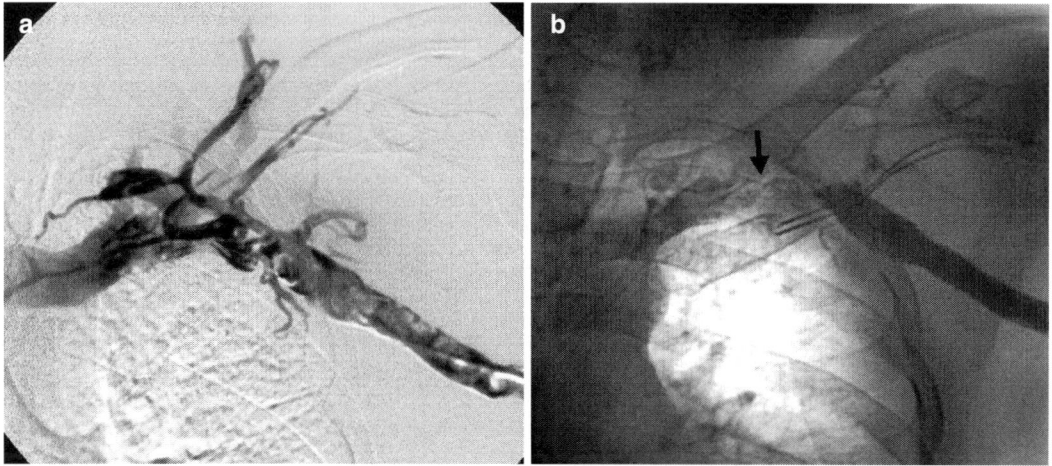

Fig. 60.2 (**a**) Venogram showing acute left subclavian and axillary vein thrombosis. (**b**) Venogram done after complete clot lysis reveals persistent subclavian vein stenosis (*arrow*)

vein without surgical decompression also generally fails, at rates approaching 100 % [7, 8]. Lee et al. showed that presence of a stent in the subclavian vein was an important contributor to rethrombosis after intervention [6], and the presence of a stent compromises the ability to surgically reconstruct the vein when the stent fails.

Thrombolysis Techniques

There are two main techniques for thrombolysis: catheter-directed infusion of a thrombolytic agent and pharmacomechanical thrombolysis (PMT). Catheter infusion is performed by placing a multi-side hole catheter into the clot and running thrombolytic agent through it for 6–48 h. This obviously requires that the thrombus be soft enough to traverse with the catheter; if the occlusion cannot be traversed, most interventionalists would abandon the attempt. However, a simple end-hole catheter can be embedded in the clot and lytic infusion started which occasionally will work. With the end-hole technique, more frequent catheter checks are required to keep advancing the catheter into the thrombus as the more peripheral thrombus dissolves.

No controlled trial has been done to identify which of the currently available drugs is optimal for VTOS lysis. Gelabert et al. [9] compared

urokinase and tissue plasminogen activator (tPA) in this situation, achieving complete clot lysis in 93 % of both groups. Urokinase, however, is no longer available, so by default tPA is most commonly used. The dose of tPA commonly used is 0.5–1 mg per hour. Before initiating thrombolysis it is vital that the patient be carefully interrogated for possible contraindications to thrombolysis such as an intracranial process like tumor or stroke or recent major intra-abdominal or intra-thoracic surgery.

The main advantage of catheter infusion is that it is simple, less labor intensive, and does not take much time in the angiography suite. The main disadvantage is that clot dissolution may take several days and the patient has to be monitored in an observation unit or ICU during this whole time. The likelihood of successful lysis depends on how old the thrombus is. While there are anecdotes of month old clot being successfully lysed, some have reported no success when the patient's symptoms indicated that the clot was present for over 2 weeks [10].

PMT is a generic term for use of a mechanical thrombolytic device in combination with infusion of a thrombolytic drug. The main benefit of using mechanical devices is that they can significantly speed up the process of clearing the entire clot. There are several mechanisms by which this occurs. First, most of the mechanical

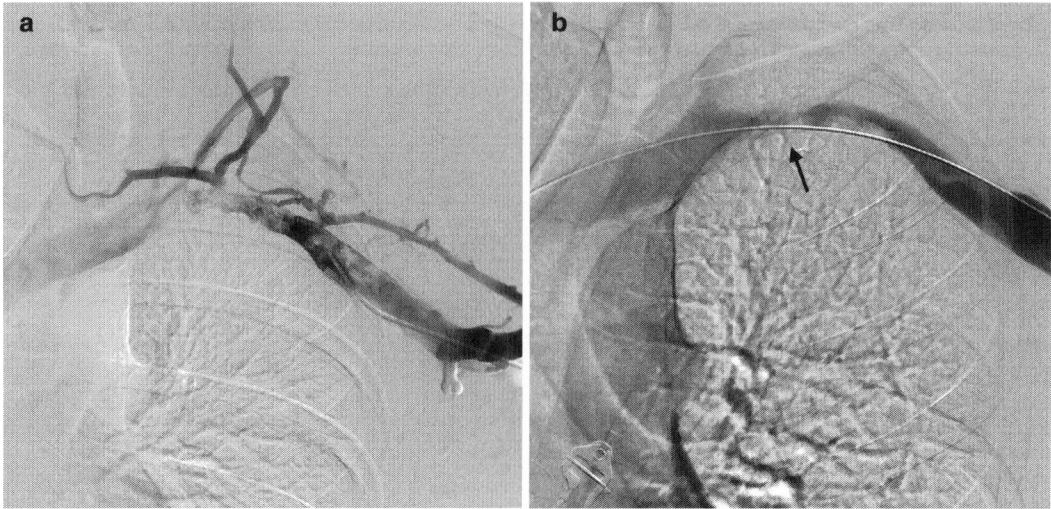

Fig. 60.3 (**a**) Pre thrombolysis left subclavian venogram showing thrombus and collaterals. (**b**) After thrombolysis the underlying stenosis (*arrow*) is present but the thrombus and collateral flow is no longer seen. This was accomplished in one 2-h session using an Angiojet device for pharmacomechanical thrombolysis

devices help disperse the lytic agent over a wider area and/or actually force lytic drug into the thrombus. Mechanical devices also cause fragmentation of thrombus, which carries with it two benefits: First, fragmentation can in some cases be efficient enough that the particles created are small enough to aspirate or safely pass into the pulmonary circulation, and, second, such fragmentation creates a greater surface area for lytic drug to work on and speeds the lytic effect.

The enhanced lysis speed allows lower overall doses of lytic drugs to be used. It also now makes it possible to sometimes lyse the thrombus in a single session (Fig. 60.3). Single session thrombolysis has several advantages. First it is potentially easier for the patient to tolerate as a prolonged indwelling infusion catheter is not needed. This also obviates the need to send the patient to a higher acuity observation unit or ICU since there is no prolonged infusion, and the risk of pericatheter bleeding, higher with prolonged infusion time, is virtually eliminated. The main disadvantage of single session thrombolysis is that these cases can take several hours, thus tying up proceduralist and interventional suite time.

Some interventionalists adopt a hybrid strategy where an infusion catheter is placed in the morning and the patient is infused in an observation unit for 4–6 h. They are then brought back to the angiography suite in the afternoon and the remaining clot is cleared with pharmacomechanical techniques. After several hours of thrombolytic infusion the thrombus is not only reduced in volume but is also generally softer and more readily fragmented with mechanical devices. This approach is a little less labor intensive but still generally accomplishes complete lysis in a single work-day.

Kim et al. [11] compared standard lytic infusions to PMT, and found that PMT yielded significantly shorter lysis treatment times (26.3 h versus 48 h for standard infusion). The total urokinase dose was significantly decreased (2.7 million units versus 5.6 million units), complete clot lysis was achieved more often (82 versus 73 %), and no increase in complications was seen.

Pharmacomechanical Devices

There are a number of devices that have been used for PMT. The Amplatz Thrombectomy Device (ATD) (EV3, Plymouth, MN) has an impeller that is housed in a cup at the end of the device (Fig. 60.4). This impeller creates a vortex that sucks clot into the impeller and fragments clot into micron sized pieces. There is no suction

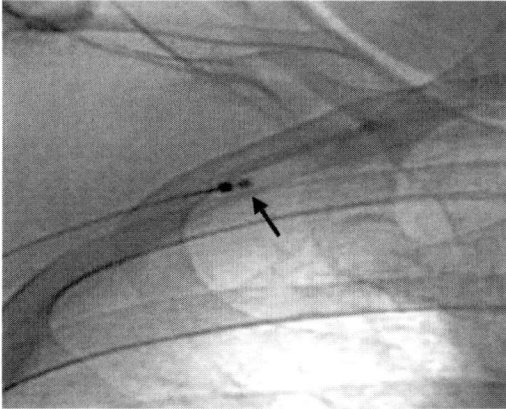

Fig. 60.4 Amplatz thrombectomy device being used to clear right axillary thrombus. The impeller that fragments the clot is housed in a cup (*arrow*) at the tip of the device

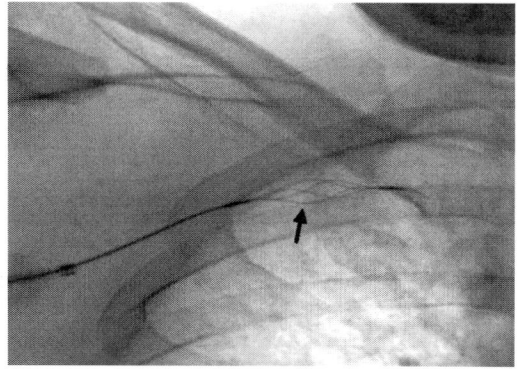

Fig. 60.5 The arrow percutaneous thrombectomy device being used in the subclavian vein. The *arrow* points to the rotating basket that macerates the clot

mechanism so the idea is to fragment the clot into small enough pieces that they can fully lyse and not cause major obstruction as they pass into the pulmonary circulation. Thrombolytic drug can be infused through a channel in the device. While very efficient at fragmenting clot, this device does not go over a wire and had minimal steerability so it is sometimes difficult to advance around curves or past side branches. Although great for debulking large amounts of clot, the company is reportedly no longer going to produce this device.

The Trerotola percutaneous thrombectomy device (PTD) (Arrow International, Reading, PA) also is a pure fragmentation device but of a different design. It consists of a motor driven rotating basket (Fig. 60.5) that acts somewhat like an egg-beater. Because the rotating basket has potential for wall contact this device could theoretically cause endothelial damage but this has not seemed to be an issue. This device does provide slightly more aggressive clot fragmentation and is sometimes useful when the thrombus is a little older and more organized. The PTD does come in an over-the-wire model so it can be more readily advanced around curves across which a guidewire has already been placed, although it requires a seven Fr sheath.

Several devices allow aspiration of lysed clot. The Angiojet System (Medrad, Inc. Warrendale, PA) uses a large pump system that works in several ways. In power-pulse mode the lytic agent is power injected into the clot leading to better penetration than can be accomplished by a standard IV infusion pump. In regular mode, saline is pumped in near the catheter tip while suction is applied to a more proximal port. The vortex created by this fluid circuit helps to macerate clot and facilitates aspiration through the suction lumen. There have been reports of bradyarrhythmias and even heart block when this device is used close to the heart [12, 13]. There are several theories regarding this, including activation of stretch receptors or release of excessive amounts of ATP from the lysed clot. Because of this it is recommended that the device be activated for short periods of time in susceptible patients.

The Trellis catheter (Bacchus Vascular, Santa Clara, CA) has two occlusion balloons that can be placed at both ends of the thrombosed vein segment (Fig. 60.6). The lytic agent is infused between the balloons which (at least theoretically) traps the lytic drug in that segment. A sinusoidal wire is then placed down the center guidewire lumen of the catheter. The sinusoidal wire is hooked to a drive motor which causes it to oscillate which disperses the lytic agent and thus homogenizes the clot which can then be removed through a separate aspiration lumen. One disadvantage of this device is that its design requires that the device can be advanced through the thrombus to the patent vein on the other side. If the thrombus is firm enough to prevent traversal, the Trellis cannot be

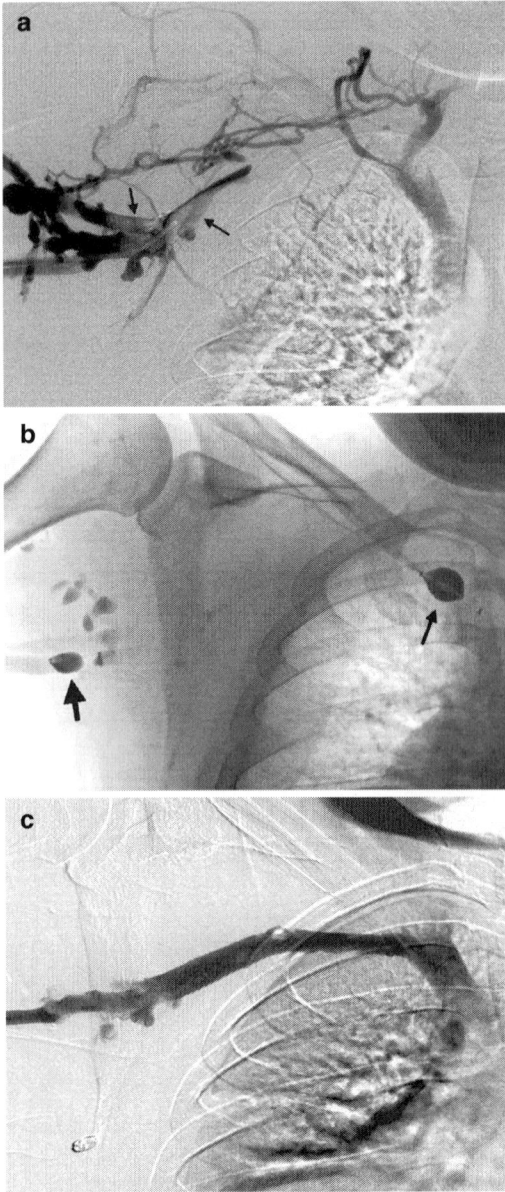

Fig. 60.6 (a) Right venogram showing acute axillo-sub-clavian vein thrombosis (*arrows*) with multiple collaterals. (b) The Trellis device has been positioned with the central balloon (*small arrow*) positioned just medial to the thrombus and the peripheral balloon (*large arrow*) positioned lateral to the thrombus. The tPA will be trapped between these balloons. The oscillating wire has not yet been advanced into the Trellis. (c) Patent veins after a single session of Trellis thrombectomy

used whereas the ATD, PTD, and Angiojet can all chip away at the thrombus and initial complete traversal is not required for their use.

A newer device called the Ekosonic Endovascular System (EKOS Corporation, Bothell, WA) works on a different principle. While the lytic agent is infused the EKOS wire generates ultrasound along the length of the device. This "sonication" increases the thrombolytic effect by increasing penetration of the lytic agent into thrombus [14]. There are several reported benefits to this approach, including penetration of lytic effect into difficult-to-reach places (such as behind valves) where a purely mechanical device might not reach, and reportedly allows diffuse penetration of the thrombus without causing macroscopic fragmentation of the clot that could lead to embolization. Since this process is not mechanical there is no damage to the vessel wall or valves and no red cell hemolysis [15]. Because of the lack of hemolysis, there is no adenosine release and thus no increased risk of arrhythmias, as well.

There have been no trials comparing the various devices so current usage is generally determined by the comfort level of the practitioner with individual devices.

Results

The success rates for thrombolysis are in the range of 62–84 % [10, 16]. However, the likelihood of successful lysis varies with the length of time the patient has symptoms prior to presenting for treatment. Molina et al. [17] described outcomes in 97 patients who presented for treatment within 2 weeks after the onset of symptoms. These patients had 100 % technical success with thrombolysis and 100 % patency on post op duplex imaging. In the same series were 17 patients first seen 2 week to 3 months after the onset of symptoms, and only five such patients (29 %) were able to undergo successful lysis and subsequent surgery. There are no firm guidelines regarding how long thrombolysis should be pursued before deciding that the thrombus will not lyse but one group [18] has suggested that if 20–25 mg of tPA have been given without substantial lysis then the procedure should be terminated.

The overall results of thrombolysis followed by surgical decompression are quite good. Primary and secondary patency rates at 1 year are 92 and 96 % respectively [19]. In a huge series of 506 extremities treated over the course of 50 years, 96 % of patients were improved during follow-up periods ranging from 1 to 32 years with an average follow-up of 7.2 years [8]. Several studies have reported that 100 % of athletes treated for VTOS were able to resume unrestricted use of the treated extremity [2, 20].

While pre-operative thrombolysis is generally considered to be beneficial, one recent report did contend that pre-operative thrombolysis provided no benefit [21]. In this retrospective study 45 patients underwent thrombolysis prior to first rib resection but 65 patients were treated with anticoagulation alone before the surgery. Both the lysis and heparinization groups had similar need for venoplasty when routine venograms were done 2 weeks after surgery. More importantly at follow-up, 91 % of both groups had patent veins and were free of symptoms regardless of which pre-operative treatment was used. Importantly, however, this series included a large number of patients who presented with subacute or even chronic thrombus, so these results must be applied only to this group.

A classic question is how soon after thrombolysis should decompressive surgery be done. Early investigators [22] recommended delaying operation for 2–3 months after thrombolysis to reduce the risk of bleeding, operating soon after lysis has become more common. The main advantage is that this approach avoids the chance of re-thrombosis caused by unrelieved stenosis of the subclavian vein. Melby et al. showed that as the time interval from diagnosis to operation increases the overall duration of management and time to full recovery also lengthen [2].

The major concern with early operation is the potential for bleeding, but most feel that this is not a major problem. Some authors report no major complications resulting from lysis. One study [18] of 60 patients only had minor complications in three patients (5 %). These consisted of one peri-catheter bleed, one minor hemoptysis, and one case of back pain, none of which caused

any long-term problems. In another study in which 23 patients were operated on within 24 h after thrombolysis, wound hematomas occurred in three patients (13 %), one of whom required thoracotomy for drainage [23]. Molina et al., however, reported only one bleeding complication in 97 cases in which early operation was performed [17].

Stenosis After VTOS Decompression Surgery

Because the chronic compression leads to fibrotic changes in the vein itself, the subclavian vein may remain stenotic despite complete surgical decompression. The reported incidence of this varies widely. Although Molina et al. [17] reported a 7 % incidence of stenosis after decompressive surgery, others feel this is much more common. Stone et al. [24] reported that 19 % of their patients required reintervention post-operatively, and Schneider et al. [19] identified residual stenoses on intra-operative venography immediately after decompressive surgery in 64 % of patients.

When a stenosis develops postoperatively, angioplasty (Fig. 60.7) should be the first approach. Angioplasty can be done easily as an outpatient procedure with local anesthesia and minimal sedation. The easiest access for this is ultrasound guided puncture into the basilic vein in the mid or lower upper arm. Given the size of the subclavian vein, larger diameter balloons, typically 10–14 mm, are needed. Post-operative stenoses are often very fibrotic and so high pressure non-compliant balloons are typically needed. Despite this, good results can be obtained. Schneider et al. [19] described patients treated with angioplasty alone after discovering stenoses on post surgical decompression venograms. At 1 year follow-up the primary and secondary patency rates were 92 and 96 %, respectively.

For stenoses that are resistant to balloon angioplasty the use of cutting balloons has been reported to be helpful [18]. Cutting balloons (Boston Scientific, Natick, MA) have micro-blades mounted on the balloon. As the balloon is inflated the small blades are pushed out against the fibrotic tissue

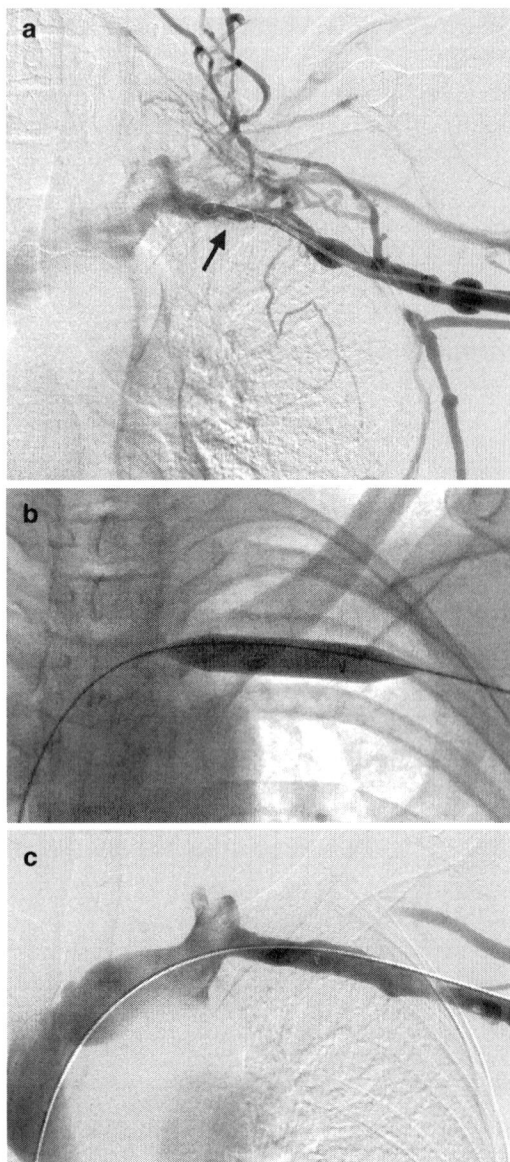

Fig. 60.7 (**a**) Left venogram done 3 weeks after surgery to decompress the thoracic outlet. There is significant residual subclavian vein stenosis (*arrow*) with multiple collaterals. (**b**) Angioplasty with a 12 mm diameter high pressure balloon. (**c**) Post PTA, the vein is patent and no collaterals are seen

For truly resistant stenoses, stent deployment is sometimes necessary, but it should again be emphasized that this should be considered only after bony decompression. Even after decompressive surgery, there is potential that a more rigid balloon expandable stent can be crushed by extrinsic forces, and self-expanding stents should be used. One group, in a series of patients undergoing PTA with stenting to follow in 30 %, described 1 and 5 year patency rates of 100 and 94 %, respectively [24]. Freedom from reintervention at those same time intervals was 100 and 74 %. In another study of selective stenting for patients with post-operative stenoses, those treated with angioplasty alone had 100 % patency whereas patency was only 64 % in those treated with stents [23]. While stents may be needed in some cases, routine use does not appear to be justified.

which is then cut. These balloons are low pressure balloons and, unfortunately, the largest available size is only 8 mm. For this reason, such stenoses generally need to be further dilated with a larger high pressure balloon. There are no studies evaluating the long term benefit of using cutting balloons.

References

1. Chin EE, Zimmerman PT, Grant EG. Sonographic evaluation of upper extremity deep venous thrombosis. J Ultrasound Med. 2005;24(6):829–38, quiz 39–40.
2. Melby SJ, Vedantham S, Narra VR, Paletta Jr GA, Khoo-Summers L, Driskill M, et al. Comprehensive surgical management of the competitive athlete with effort thrombosis of the subclavian vein (Paget-Schroetter syndrome). J Vasc Surg. 2008;47(4):809–20, discussion 21.
3. Male C, Chait P, Ginsberg JS, Hanna K, Andrew M, Halton J, et al. Comparison of venography and ultrasound for the diagnosis of asymptomatic deep vein thrombosis in the upper body in children: results of the PARKAA study. Prophylactic antithrombin replacement in kids with ALL treated with asparaginase. Thromb Haemost. 2002;87(4):593–8.
4. Chang YC, Su CT, Yang PC, Wang TC, Chiu LC, Hsu JC. Magnetic resonance angiography in the diagnosis of thoracic venous obstruction. J Formos Med Assoc. 1998;97(1):38–43.
5. Lokanathan R, Salvian AJ, Chen JC, Morris C, Taylor DC, Hsiang YN. Outcome after thrombolysis and selective thoracic outlet decompression for primary axillary vein thrombosis. J Vasc Surg. 2001;33(4):783–8.
6. Lee JT, Karwowski JK, Harris EJ, Haukoos JS, Olcott C. Long-term thrombotic recurrence after nonoperative management of Paget-Schroetter syndrome. J Vasc Surg. 2006;43(6):1236–43.
7. Maintz D, Landwehr P, Gawenda M, Lackner K. Failure of Wallstents in the subclavian vein due to stent damage. Clin Imaging. 2001;25(2):133–7.
8. Urschel Jr HC, Patel AN. Surgery remains the most effective treatment for Paget-Schroetter syndrome:

50 years' experience. Ann Thorac Surg. 2008;86(1): 254–60.

9. Gelabert HA, Jimenez JC, Rigberg DA. Comparison of retavase and urokinase for management of spontaneous subclavian vein thrombosis. Ann Vasc Surg. 2007;21(2):149–54.

10. Doyle A, Wolford HY, Davies MG, Adams JT, Singh MJ, Saad WE, et al. Management of effort thrombosis of the subclavian vein: today's treatment. Ann Vasc Surg. 2007;21(6):723–9.

11. Kim HS, Patra A, Paxton BE, Khan J, Streiff MB. Catheter-directed thrombolysis with percutaneous rheolytic thrombectomy versus thrombolysis alone in upper and lower extremity deep vein thrombosis. Cardiovasc Intervent Radiol. 2006;29(6):1003–7.

12. Dwarka D, Schwartz SA, Smyth SH, O'Brien MJ. Bradyarrhythmias during use of the AngioJet system. J Vasc Interv Radiol. 2006;17(10):1693–5.

13. Fontaine AB, Borsa JJ, Hoffer EK, Bloch RD, So CR, Newton M. Type III heart block with peripheral use of the angiojet thrombectomy system. J Vasc Interv Radiol. 2001;12(10):1223–5.

14. Francis CW, Blinc A, Lee S, Cox C. Ultrasound accelerates transport of recombinant tissue plasminogen activator into clots. Ultrasound Med Biol. 1995;21(3):419–24.

15. Soltani A, Singhal R, Garcia JL, Raju NR. Absence of biological damage from prolonged exposure to intravascular ultrasound: a swine model. Ultrasonics. 2007;46(1):60–7.

16. Beygui RE, Olcott C, Dalman RL. Subclavian vein thrombosis: outcome analysis based on etiology and modality of treatment. Ann Vasc Surg. 1997;11(3):247–55.

17. Molina JE, Hunter DW, Dietz CA. Paget-Schroetter syndrome treated with thrombolytics and immediate surgery. J Vasc Surg. 2007;45(2):328–34.

18. Thompson JF, Winterborn RJ, Bays S, White H, Kinsella DC, Watkinson AF. Venous thoracic outlet compression and the Paget-Schroetter syndrome: a review and recommendations for management. Cardiovasc Intervent Radiol. 2011;34(5):903–10.

19. Schneider DB, Dimuzio PJ, Martin ND, Gordon RL, Wilson MW, Laberge JM, et al. Combination treatment of venous thoracic outlet syndrome: open surgical decompression and intraoperative angioplasty. J Vasc Surg. 2004;40(4):599–603.

20. Feugier P, Aleksic I, Salari R, Durand X, Chevalier JM. Long-term results of venous revascularization for Paget-Schroetter syndrome in athletes. Ann Vasc Surg. 2001;15(2):212–18.

21. Guzzo JL, Chang K, Demos J, Black JH, Freischlag JA. Preoperative thrombolysis and venoplasty affords no benefit in patency following first rib resection and scalenectomy for subacute and chronic subclavian vein thrombosis. J Vasc Surg. 2010;52(3):658–62, discussion 62–3.

22. Machleder HI. Evaluation of a new treatment strategy for Paget-Schroetter syndrome: spontaneous thrombosis of the axillary-subclavian vein. J Vasc Surg. 1993;17(2):305–15, discussion 16–7.

23. Kreienberg PB, Chang BB, Darling 3rd RC, Roddy SP, Paty PS, Lloyd WE, et al. Long-term results in patients treated with thrombolysis, thoracic inlet decompression, and subclavian vein stenting for Paget-Schroetter syndrome. J Vasc Surg. 2001;33 (2 Suppl):S100–5.

24. Stone DH, Scali ST, Bjerk AA, Rzucidlo E, Chang CK, Goodney PP, et al. Aggressive treatment of idiopathic axillo-subclavian vein thrombosis provides excellent long-term function. J Vasc Surg. 2010;52(1): 127–31.

Karl A. Illig

Abstract

When treating a patient with venous thoracic outlet syndrome (VTOS), the most critical structures are the anterior part of the first rib, the anterior part of the clavicle, and the associated subclavius muscle and costoclavicular tendon connecting the two – the costoclavicular junction. The transaxillary exposure provides the best exposure of the *anterior* first rib, subclavius muscle, and costoclavicular tendon, yields excellent exposure of the entire subclavian vein to the level of the jugular vein, allows thorough circumferential external venolysis, and is most cosmetically attractive for patients, many of whom are in a young, active age group. When combined with thrombolysis and performed with proper technique for effort thrombosis, complications, most commonly hematoma, asymptomatic small pneumothorax, and temporarily troubling but temporary long thoracic nerve injury, should be rare, and long-term success achieved in over 90 % of patients treated.

Introduction

When treating a patient with venous thoracic outlet syndrome (VTOS), the most critical structures are the *anterior* part of the first rib, the *anterior* part of the clavicle, and the associated subclavius muscle and costoclavicular tendon connecting the two – the costoclavicular junction. As discussed elsewhere, the pathophysiology of VTOS is extrinsic compression caused by the

"nutcracker" effect of the first rib and clavicle held together by the fulcrum of the junction itself. As such, one of these bones must be removed. Moreover, we and others strongly feel that the vein should be freed of its external cicatrix, i.e., that external venolysis be routinely performed. For all of these reasons, we believe transaxillary exposure, first described by Roos in 1966 [1], is best in this situation. With regard to venous disease, this approach has the following advantages:

- It provides the best exposure of the *anterior* first rib, subclavius muscle, and costoclavicular tendon,
- It yields excellent exposure of the entire subclavian vein to the level of the jugular vein,

K.A. Illig, MD
Department of Surgery, Division of Vascular Surgery,
University of South Florida, 2 Tampa General Circle,
STC 7016, Tampa, FL 33606, USA
e-mail: killig@health.usf.edu

- It allows thorough circumferential external venolysis,
- It is most cosmetically attractive for patients, many of whom are in a young, active age group.

It should be noted that some investigators believe that most, if not all, veins in this case require formal reconstruction [2]. If so, another approach is needed, but in patients who do not need formal venous reconstruction the transaxillary route is, we believe, the best option. See also Thompson [3] for an excellent description of this approach applied primarily for neurogenic TOS.

Surgical Technique

No special preoperative preparation is needed. We ask all of our patients to wash their surgical site (in this case, the axillary region) with a surgical prep sponge the night before surgery. This area, with its rich supply of lymph nodes and sweat glands, is somewhat prone to infection, but this has not been a significant problem in our experience.

The operation is performed under general anesthesia (if a patient is too sick for general anesthesia, they probably should not be having this operation to start with). The patient is placed in full lateral decubitus position, with the affected side obviously upward. A "beanbag" is used to support the patient. An axillary roll is placed, the lower leg bent for stability, and a pillow placed between this and the straight upper leg. Tape is used to keep the patient upright, and the bean bag is molded to the patient and then "deflated." We find it helpful to have someone apply upward traction on the arm during positioning for added stability.

The arm must be elevated throughout the entire case, which can last an hour or more. Traditionally, an assistant has been used to hold the arm, traditionally by lifting it at the bent elbow (Fig. 61.1a). This can be quite difficult for the assistant, especially if the case is long, and provides variable degrees of exposure depending on strength, fatigue, and attention being paid.

Another option is to use a retractor developed at UCLA (Fig. 61.1b). This is a custom-made device and not widely available, although similar "home-made" options are easily created. The third option is a very simple technique that we developed after talking to our orthopedic surgeons. The arm is wrapped with a specially-made stockinette and secured by wrapping, and is then suspended by means of a weight over an overhead "shower curtain" assembly used for hip replacement surgery (Fig. 61.1c). We have performed approximately 80 transaxillary first rib excisions using this technique since 2006, and have had no patients suffer any apparent disability or harm because of this [5]. It provides superb and constant exposure, which incidentally can be regulated with a single hand by the surgeon. We recently discovered that what is probably a similar technique was briefly described by Urschel in 2000 [6].

We perform this operation with both surgeon and assistant wearing headlights; while good exposure is routinely obtained, there may not be enough room for both light and vision. In addition, if a television monitor headlight is available, this provides others in the room with a chance to follow the operation.

When exposure has been completed, the axillary region is prepped and draped. An incision is made relatively low in the axilla (a high incision provides no benefit and can simply lead one more directly to the lymph nodes). This incision does not have to be very large; the pectoralis major anteriorly and latissimus dorsi medially define but also limit exposure. The incision is first brought directly downward to the chest wall itself. The tissues superficial to this plane are then reflected upward, and the chest wall itself is followed up to the first rib. There are several small crossing vessels which need to be identified, controlled, and divided. The long thoracic nerve is vulnerable to retractor injury posteriorly, and the intercostobrachial cutaneous nerve, exiting between the first and second ribs, can sometimes be preserved but often must be sacrificed, leaving the patient with (usually temporary) axillary and inner upper arm numbness. Surprisingly good exposure can be obtained using two deep Weitlander retractors.

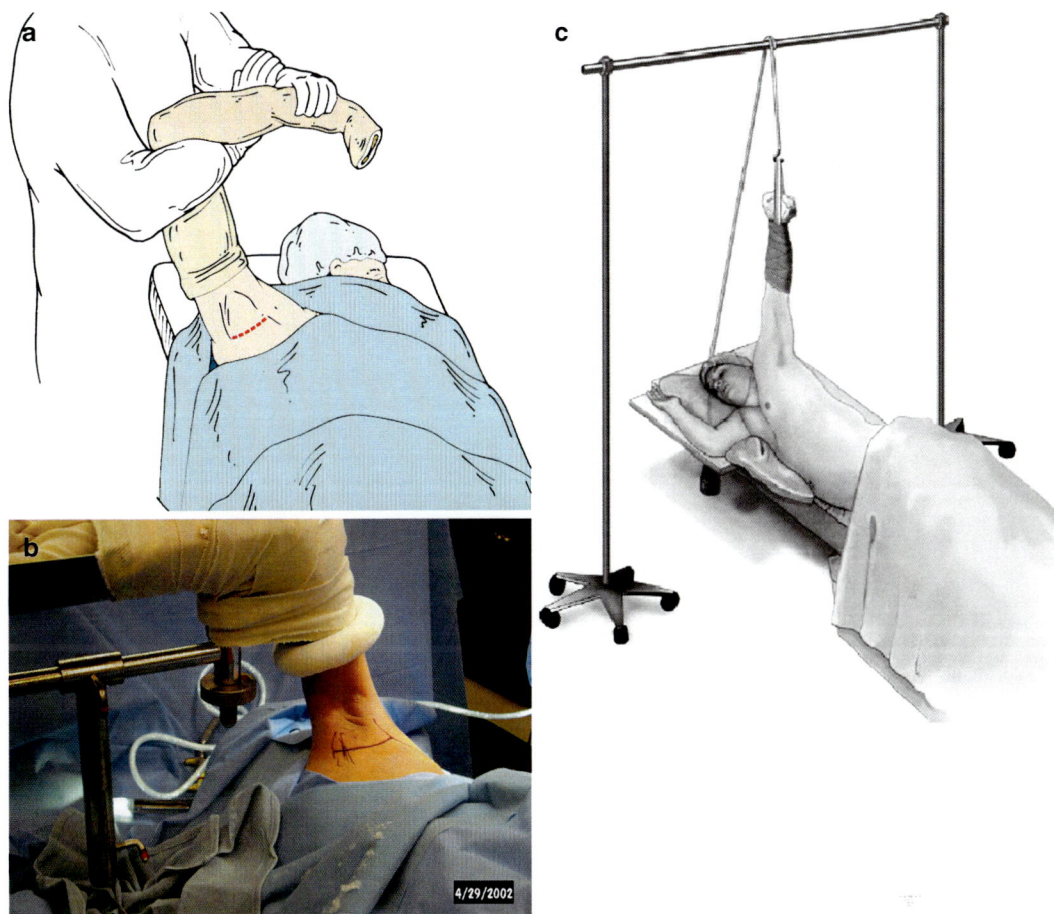

Fig. 61.1 Three methods of supporting the arm for transaxillary first rib resection. (**a**) The "traditional" approach – the arm is held upright by an assistant within the sterile field (Reprinted from Thompson and Driskill [4] with permission from Elsevier). (**b**) The "Machleder" retractor, developed by Herb Machleder at UCLA, also used at Johns Hopkins (Courtesy of Julie Ann Freischlag, MD). (**c**) The technique used at the University of Rochester (An apparently similar technique was briefly mentioned by Urschel in 2000; reference Schanzer and Messina [9] above). (Reprinted from Illig KA [5]. With permission from Elsevier)

To the novice thoracic outlet surgeon, the first rib can seem very high, but with experience it's fairly evident where this is. Second ribs have been removed by mistake. The absolute requirement for identifying the first rib is to note the insertion of the anterior scalene muscle, which should be very clearly seen, separating the subclavian artery (posterior) and vein (anterior) (Fig. 61.2).

At this point, the lateral border of the first rib is cleared. A useful trick is to take a metal instrument and place it on top of the first rib, with pressure directed downward, i.e., toward the chest, and bring it back out of the wound. When the edge of the rib is reached, the instrument will "fall down" into the soft area of intercostal muscles between the first and second rib. Leaving the instrument pushing the intercostals down, a cautery with a bent tip can then be used to incise the muscle and thus develop the lateral border of the rib. A periosteal elevator is then used to undermine the first rib (leaving the periosteum with the rib to be resected), and a right angle clamp is then be placed underneath it to be rotated upward when the medial border is reached. Gentle spreading at this point will provide a little bit of preliminary dissection without damaging any structures.

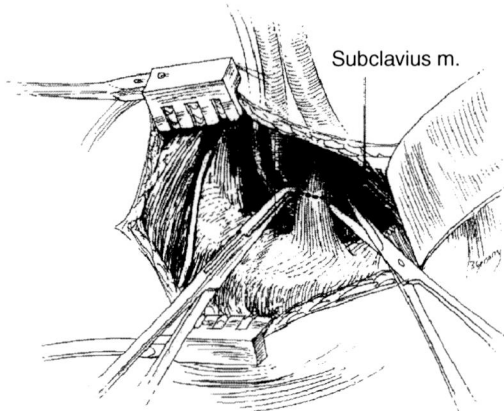

Subclavius m.

Fig. 61.2 For assurance that the first rib is actually being exposed, the operator *must* visualize the anterior scalene muscle arising from it and passing upwards. The axillary subclavian vein will be seen to lie immediately anterior to it, and the artery, immediately posterior. Note the long thoracic nerve posteriorly (*not labeled*) and the subclavius muscle under the clavicle anteriorly and superiorally (Reprinted from Thompson and Petrinec [3]. With permission from Elsevier)

At this point, using a combination of cautery and sharp and blunt dissection, the lateral and medial borders of the first rib are cleared from just posterior to the artery all the way to the costoclavicular junction. We and others strongly advocate full removal of the rib in all planes, as subperiosteal resection, at least in theory, increases the chance of regrowth. The rib is also cleared posteriorly, staying as close as possible to it to avoid injury to the long thoracic nerve. A straight or angled bone cutter is then used to cut the rib and it is removed from the field. At this point, a rongeur is used to bring the rib all the way back to the sternum itself; we persist until clear articular cartilage is seen. We do not aggressively pursue the rib posteriorly when resected for venous TOS. The rongeur is also useful to resect as much of the subclavius tendon as possible, and consideration is given to debulking the subclavius muscle, if large.

Attention is next directed to the vein itself, which should not be left alone. In patients with VTOS, there is almost always a very tough fibrotic "rind" surrounding the vein. With experience and gentle dissection, it's very easy to get within this cicatrix to expose native, relatively healthy, venous adventitia. This can then be further dissected and the cicatrix removed entirely.

In so doing the vein is mobilized 270–360° which completely frees it up from the subclavius muscle and costoclavicular ligament (which can also both be removed to provide even more room for the vein). With care and patience, this mobilization can be accomplished all the way down to the junction of the jugular vein, leaving the vein free and clear superiorly, anteriorly, and inferiorally (we tend to leave the posterior part of the vein undissected as there is minimal scar tissue, no obstructive structures, and the thoracic duct enters in this location). It should be noted that the phrenic nerve runs anterior to the vein in this location in approximately 90 % of cases but it can occasionally run posterior to it; this anomaly should be specifically sought out. External venolysis and subtotal mobilization can yield surprising benefits. Figure 61.3 shows venograms of a patient immediately before and immediately after this procedure, clearly illustrating that much of what is thought to be intrinsic disease may actually be extrinsic compression caused by the scar tissue. Such constriction will persist even if the bones are removed, and formal external venolysis should be a part of every operation for VTOS.

At this point, the operation is done. Pleural entry occurs in approximately 10 % of cases. This is usually not a problem, although if low grade bleeding is present hemothorax can occur. The wound is typically closed over #10 Jackson Pratt drain. If pleural entry is present, we cut side holes in a red rubber catheter, place it in the pleural space, attach it to suction, and, accompanied by a Valsalva maneuver, quickly remove it as the last fascial knot is cinched down. Again, if pleural entry is apparent, unusually close attention should be paid to hemostasis. The wound is closed cosmetically with the Jackson Pratt drain exiting through a separate stab incision.

Because the operation is uncomfortable for the patient of the short-term, we routinely prescribe patient controlled anesthesia (PCA) for the 1st day or 2. When patients are able to take oral medications they can be discharged. The drain is removed, if not chylous, on day 1. Rehabilitation strategies for the first month are focused simply on range of motion, with formal physical and occupational therapy, discussed elsewhere, started after the first postoperative visit.

Fig. 61.3 Pre (**a**) and postoperative (**b**) venograms in a patient with VTOS following thrombolysis and early first rib resection, illustrating the benefits of thorough external venolysis. "**a**" is the venogram after thrombolysis (performed at an outside institution) prior to rib resection, while "**b**" shows the situation after surgical decompression but without any additional endoluminal intervention. Note the dramatic improvement in flow and resistance (significantly diminished collateral flow) after external venolysis alone

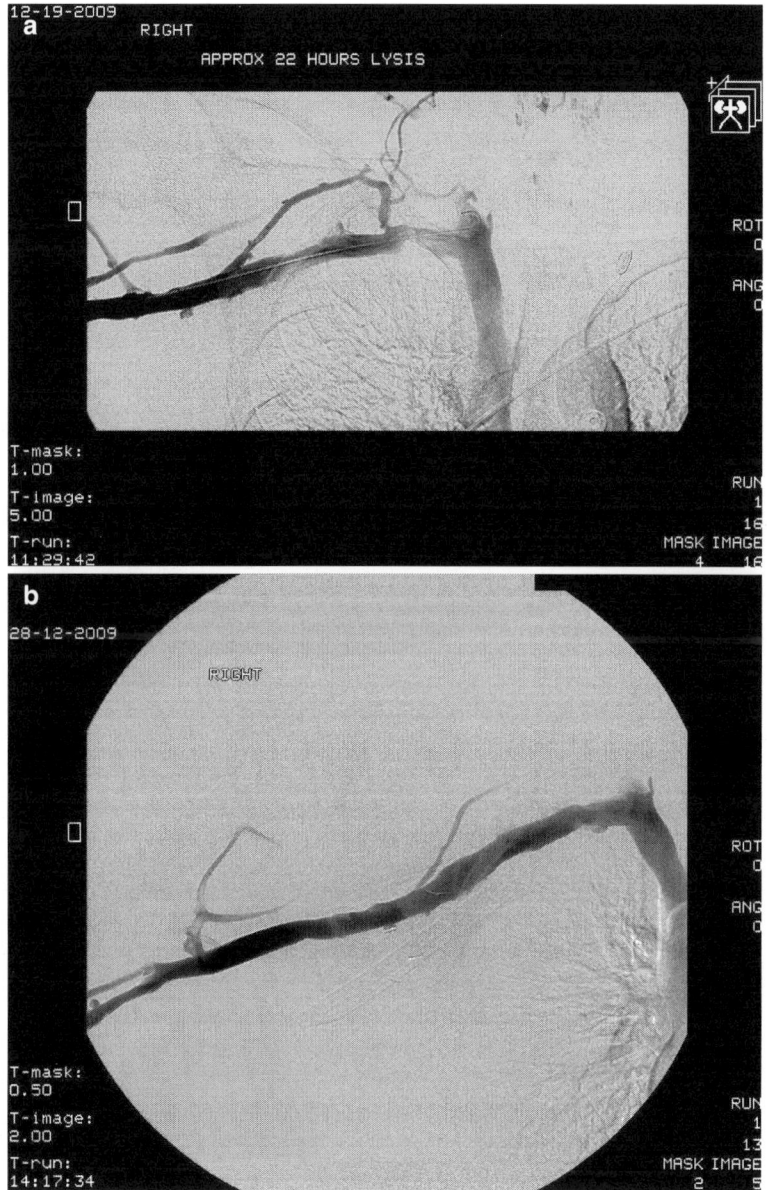

Complications

Complications are relatively infrequent. Pleural entry is discussed above. We routinely obtain chest X-ray in the recovery room. Occasionally, a low-grade pneumothorax can be seen, but we have never had to place a chest tube for this problem. Long thoracic nerve dysfunction with a winged scapula is occasionally seen. If present after transaxillary exposure it almost always indicates a stretch injury due to retraction and will usually resolve with time, although this may take up to a year. Certainly, inadvertent removal of the second rib is a significant complication; this can be eliminated by making sure that the anterior scalene muscle and true subclavian vessels are definitively identified. True chyle leak is quite rare. Prolonged lymphatic leak can occur because of the lymph nodes in this area, but will usually resolve with time. If a true thoracic duct injury is present, more advanced techniques (such as laparoscopic duct clipping) will have to be employed, as prolonged parenteral nutrition and bowel rest does not help very often.

Results

Drs. Kashyap, Ahn, and Machleder appropriately state that "A review of the literature would suggest that scientific judgment has given way to religious fervor regarding the issue of surgical management of TOS" [7], although this statement probably applies more to decompression for neurogenic rather than venous symptoms. In a seminal review of over 3,700 cases, Sanders reports "good" results after 83 % of transaxillary rib resections and 83 % after supraclavicular rib resections [8], although essentially all of these procedures were performed for neurogenic TOS. Reports of outcomes after transaxillary first rib resection for venous TOS, in almost all cases established Paget-Schroetter syndrome following thrombolysis, demonstrate "clinical success" in 93–100 % of cases with approximately 95 % patency at 5 years [6, 9–11].

True complication rates are difficult to determine because of the very low event rate (and likely publication bias). Chang recently analyzed this issue by means of a National Inpatient Sample query. Although they could not distinguish transaxillary from other approaches, becasuse the transaxillary approach is the most commonly performed method of rib resection this is probably a good approximation. This sample documented rates of brachial plexus and "vascular" injuries of 0.60 and 1.74 %, respectively [12], although note in their discussion multiple series by very experienced surgeons with no such injuries at all [13, 14], an experience with which we agree. We have had at least two patients with long thoracic nerve dysfunction in less than 100 venous cases over the past 5 years, yielding a rate of 3 % or so, but note that both patients fully resolved and thus suggest that both of these were due to traction and/or retraction injuries. We also point out that the rate of significant hematoma and/or hemothorax is not zero, especially when operating on

patients immediately after thrombolysis; the latter complication should be specifically sought out in any patient who has anemia and/or shortness of breath after transaxillary rib resection.

References

1. Roos DB. Transaxillary approach for first rib resection to relieve thoracic outlet syndrome. Ann Surg. 1966;163:354–8.
2. Molina JE, Hunter DW, Dietz CA. Protocols for Paget-Schroetter syndrome and late treatment of chronic subclavian vein obstruction. Ann Thorac Surg. 2009;87:416–22.
3. Thompson RW, Petrinec D. Surgical treatment of thoracic outlet compression syndromes: diagnostic considerations and transaxillary first rib resection. Ann Vasc Surg. 1997;11(3):315–23.
4. Thompson RW, Driskill M. Thoracic outlet syndrome: neurogenic. In: Cronenwett JL, Johnston KW, editors. Rutherford's vascular surgery. 7th ed. Philadelphia: Saunders/Elsevier; 2010. p. 1878–98.
5. Illig KA. An improved method of exposure for transaxillary first rib resection. J Vasc Surg. 2010;52: 248–9.
6. Urschel HC, Razzuk MA. Paget-Schroetter syndrome: what is the best management? Ann Thorac Surg. 2000;69:1663–9.
7. Kashyap V, Ahn S, Machleder H. Thoracic outlet neurovascular compression: approaches to anatomic decompression and their limitations. Semin Vasc Surg. 1998;11(2):116–22.
8. Sanders RJ. Results of the surgical treatment for thoracic outlet syndrome. Semin Thorac Cardiovasc Surg. 1996;8:221–8.
9. Schanzer A, Messina LM. Thoracic outlet syndrome: venous. In: Cronenwett JL, Johnston KW, editors. Rutherford's vascular surgery. 7th ed. Philadelphia: Saunders/Elsevier; 2010. p. 1907–17.
10. Illig KA, Doyle AJ. A comprehensive review of Paget-Schroetter syndrome. J Vasc Surg. 2010;51:1538–47.
11. de Leon RA, Chang DC, Hassoun HT, Black JH, Roseborough GS, Perler BA, et al. Multiple treatment algorithms for successful outcomes in venous thoracic outlet syndrome. Surgery. 2009;145:500–7.
12. Chang DC, Lidor AO, Matsen SL, Freischlag JA. Reported in-hospital complications following rib resections for neurogenic thoracic outlet syndrome. Ann Vasc Surg. 2007;21:564–70.
13. Green RM, McNamara J, Ouriel K. Long-term follow-up after thoracic outlet decompression: an analysis of factors determining outcome. J Vasc Surg. 1991; 14:739–45.
14. Leffert RD, Perlmutter GS. Thoracic outlet syndrome: results of 282 transaxillary first rib resections. Clin Orthop Relat Res. 1999;369:66–79.

Surgical Techniques: Operative Decompression Using the Infraclavicular Approach for VTOS

62

Andrew J. Meltzer and Darren B. Schneider

Abstract

The infraclavicular approach provides direct access to the costoclavicular space for focused treatment of VTOS. Using this approach complete first rib resection and subclavian venolysis can be performed without unnecessary exposure or manipulation of the brachial plexus or subclavian artery. Sacrifice of collateral veins that usually exist in the supraclavicular and axillary areas is also easily avoided with the infraclavicular approach. Residual venous stenoses may be directly addressed with patch angioplasty through the same exposure or by percutaneous angioplasty. Excellent results for the treatment of effort thrombosis and VTOS using the infraclavicular approach have been reported.

Introduction

The transaxillary, supraclavicular, and paraclavicular approaches are commonly used for thoracic outlet decompression and provide excellent access to the neurovascular structures within the interscalene space for treatment of neurogenic and arterial thoracic outlet syndromes. Many surgeons utilize the aforementioned techniques in the treatment of venous thoracic outlet syndrome as well, likely due to familiarity with these approaches. In the case of VTOS, however, the relevant anatomy and pathology (i.e., the subclavian vein) is found within the more anterior costoclavicular space. The costoclavicular space, first rib, and subclavian vein may be directly accessed via an infraclavicular approach and this has become our preferred approach for treatment of VTOS.

First described by Gol in the neurosurgical literature in 1968 for treatment of NTOS, the infraclavicular approach is best suited to treatment of VTOS by providing direct access to the subclavian vein and first rib within the costoclavicular space [1]. Potential advantages of the infraclavicular approach include minimal manipulation of the brachial plexus, phrenic nerve, and subclavian artery, which are not involved in VTOS.

A.J. Meltzer, MD • D.B. Schneider, MD (✉)
Division of Vascular and Endovascular Surgery,
Weill Cornell Medical College,
New York – Presbyterian,
Weill Cornell Medical Center,
525 East 68th St., New York, NY 10065, USA
e-mail: ajm9007@med.cornell.edu;
dschneider@med.cornell.edu

Collateral veins, which generally course through the supraclavicular space to enter the jugular veins or through the axilla to enter the chest wall, and may be interrupted by other surgical approaches, are avoided by the infraclavicular approach. Most importantly, the central portion of the subclavian vein can be directly visualized during the critical venolysis step of the procedure and, if needed, proximal exposure of the central veins can be gained by transmanubrial extension of the infraclavicular incision. For these reasons, we have found the infraclavicular approach to venous thoracic outlet syndrome to be an excellent choice. Limited utilization of the infraclavicular approach is most likely due to lack of familiarity with the technique, which is actually quite straightforward.

Technique

General endotracheal anesthesia is provided. The patient is positioned supine with the affected arm prepped into the field. The extremity is encircled with a sterile sling permitting mobility which facilitates exposure during the procedure, particularly during dissection along the posterior aspect of the first rib.

A transverse incision is made below the clavicle, overlying the first rib (Fig. 62.1). The incision extends from the lateral border of the munubrium to the deltopectoral groove. A plane is developed between fibers of the pectoralis major using a muscle-sparing approach and the more lateral pectoralis minor muscle is not divided. The anterior surface of the first rib is identified deep to the pectoralis major muscle (Fig. 62.2). The subclavius muscle is divided from its insertion onto the first rib. Working directly on the superior aspect of the first rib the attachments of the anterior and middle scalene muscles are divided with electrocautery; and along the inferior aspect of the rib the intercostal muscles are divided. A handheld renal vein retractor is placed alongside the first rib to facilitate exposure and to protect the neurovascular structures. Superior and anterior movement of the shoulder is extremely useful to facilitate exposure while the first rib is freed. Using a periosteal elevator, the pleura is cleared

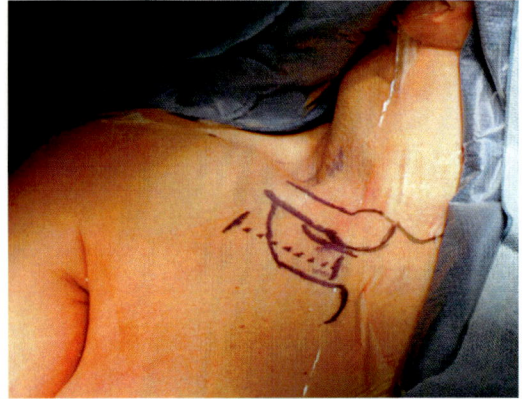

Fig. 62.1 A transverse incision is made overlying the first rib

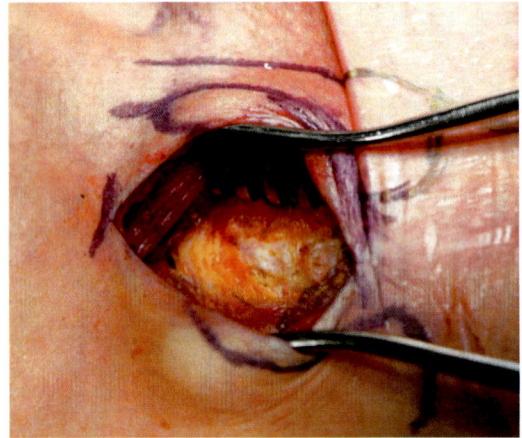

Fig. 62.2 After muscle-sparing division of the pectoralis fibers, the anterior surface of the first rib is encountered

from the deep surface of the rib. Cleared of it attachments, with the neurovascular structures protected, the first rib is then divided using either Kerison rongeurs or a rib cutter at the costomanubrial junction and close to the vertebral transverse process to facilitate complete removal. Residual fragments of the posterior rib can be removed using rongeurs.

A circumferential subclavian venolysis is then performed to remove fibrous tissue using sharp scissors dissection. Careful attention is paid to freeing the vein anteriorly as it courses behind costoclavicular ligament and the head of the clavicle and the manubrium (Fig. 62.3). Although others have reported routine patch angioplasty to address venous stenoses, our preferred method is to perform intraoperative venography following wound closure. Residual subclavian vein stenoses (>50 %) are treated with angioplasty using balloon diameters of 10–14 mm with inflation pressures up to 20 atm, when necessary (Fig. 62.4). Should more proximal exposure for surgical vein patch angioplasty prove necessary, the transmanubrial extension of the incision may be performed to expose the innominate veins; claviculectomy is unnecessary. The resection is done extra-

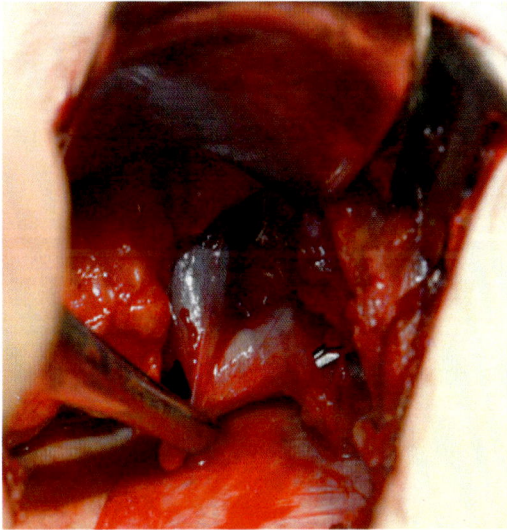

Fig. 62.3 Exposure facilitates an extensive subclavian venolysis

pleurally, and while it is not uncommon to create a rent in the pleura a thoracostomy tube is generally not needed. A drain is routinely placed in the bed of the resected first rib.

Postoperative Management

Intravenous ketorolac and narcotics are used for postoperative analgesia. Immobilization is unnecessary and gradual return to normal use of the upper extremity is encouraged. The drain is removed after output is less than 30 ml over a 24 h period. Postoperative anticoagulation is selectively used only for patients with residual non-occlusive chronic thrombus observed by intraoperative venography or duplex ultrasound after surgical decompression and angioplasty. Surveillance duplex ultrasonography is performed prior to hospital discharge and at 3, 6, and 12 months postoperatively.

Outcomes

Molina was the first describe an infraclavicular approach to venous thoracic outlet decompression [2]. Using an approach that consisted of immediate thrombolysis and urgent decompression via the infraclavicular technique, 100 %

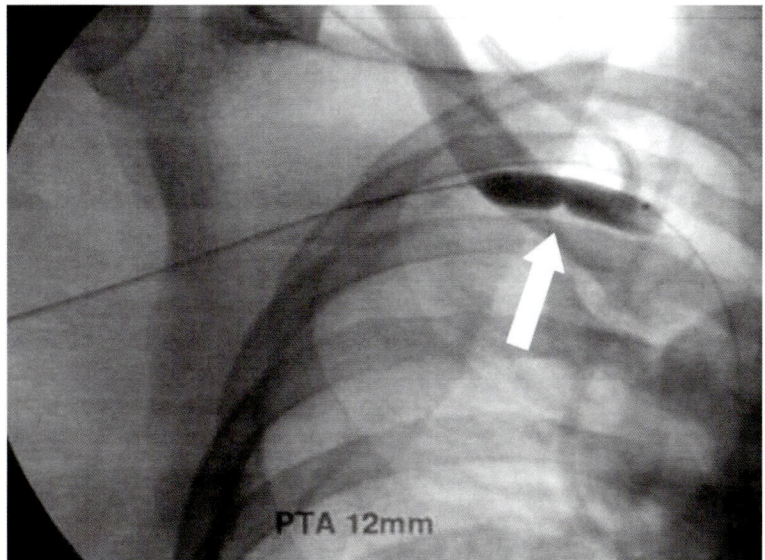

Fig. 62.4 Residual stenosis (*arrow*) is treated with balloon angioplasty

PTA 12mm

procedural success was achieved. Of 97 patients treated for VTOS and acute subclavian vein thrombosis, there was only one bleeding complication and two pneumothoraces that required tube thoracostomy. At short-term and long term follow-up (mean = 5.2 years, range 2–21 years) duplex assessed subclavian vein patency was 100 %. Arm function was noted to be normal in all patients.

Johnston et al. reported a 94 % primary patency and 100 % secondary patency in 21 patients treated for VTOS and acute subclavian vein thrombosis using the infraclavicular approach for rib resection and venolysis followed by intraoperative subclavian vein angioplasty to treat residual stenosis [3]. It should be noted that poorer results are typical for patients with chronic sub-

clavian thrombosis, especially when surgical reconstruction or replacement of the subclavian vein is needed, emphasizing the need for early identification and treatment of patients with effort thrombosis with catheter-directed thrombolysis.

References

1. Gol G, et al. Relief of costoclavicular syndrome by infraclavicular removal of first rib. J Neurosurg. 1968;28(1):81–4.
2. Molina JE, Hunter DW, Dietz CA. Paget-Schroetter syndrome treated with thrombolytics and immediate surgery. J Vasc Surg. 2007;45(2):328–34.
3. Johnston PC, et al. Focused infraclavicular first rib resection for direct and effective treatment of acute venous thoracic outlet syndrome. J Vasc Surg. (submitted).

Surgical Techniques: Operative Decompression Using the Paraclavicular Approach for VTOS

63

Robert W. Thompson

Abstract

Venous TOS is distinct from other forms of TOS with respect to pathophysiology, clinical presentation, and functional consequences for the patient. Optimal management of axillary-subclavian vein compression thereby requires different considerations and approaches from those applicable to either neurogenic or arterial TOS. The purpose of this chapter is to describe a comprehensive strategy to the surgical treatment of venous TOS based on paraclavicular thoracic outlet decompression. This approach combines the advantages of supraclavicular exposure with an infraclavicular exposure that permits complete resection of the medial first rib, as well as wide exposure of the subclavian vein to permit direct vascular reconstruction in the same setting. Use of this approach allows definitive surgical treatment to be offered to all patients with symptomatic venous TOS or recent effort thrombosis, regardless of the interval between initial diagnosis and referral, previous treatment, or adverse findings on contrast venography, with excellent early and long-term outcomes. This has led us to conclude that operative procedures based on paraclavicular exposure provide the most versatile, comprehensive, and safe approach to the treatment of venous TOS.

Introduction

Venous TOS (VTOS) is distinct from other forms of TOS with respect to pathophysiology, clinical presentation, and functional consequences for the patient, and optimal management of axillary-subclavian vein compression thereby requires different considerations and approaches from those applicable to either neurogenic or arterial TOS [1–3]. VTOS is due to extrinsic compression of the subclavian vein between the clavicle, first rib, subclavius muscle and costoclavicular ligament as they come together in the *anterior* portion of the thoracic outlet (costoclavicular junction), and treatment therefore requires that this area be specifically addressed.

Goals of Treatment

Surgical treatment provides definitive management for axillary-subclavian vein effort thrombosis and

R.W. Thompson, MD
Department of Surgery/Section of Vascular Surgery,
Center for Thoracic Outlet Syndrome,
Washington University, Barnes-Jewish Hospital,
Campus Box 8109/Suite 5101 Queeny Tower,
660 S Euclid Avenue, St. Louis, MO 63110, USA
e-mail: thompson@wudosis.wustl.edu

K.A. Illig et al. (eds.), *Thoracic Outlet Syndrome*,
DOI 10.1007/978-1-4471-4366-6_63, © Springer-Verlag London 2013

venous TOS and should be considered in almost all patients with this condition, although those with longstanding untreated subclavian vein occlusion or those that exhibit a long segment of residual venous occlusion extending into the axillary vein despite thrombolysis may require other approaches. The overall goals of operative treatment for venous TOS are three-fold:

1. Complete decompression of the subclavian vein and collateral venous pathways through the thoracic outlet by removal of the first rib and associated scalene and subclavius muscles;
2. Restoration and maintenance of normal blood flow through the axillary-subclavian vein by removing constricting scar tissue from around the vein, adjunctive balloon angioplasty, and/or direct venous reconstruction when necessary; and
3. Predictable recovery from operation within a reasonable period time with return to full unrestricted activity of the affected upper extremity, minimal risks of rethrombosis or long-term symptoms of venous congestion, and no need for ongoing treatment with anticoagulant or other medications.

Selection of Surgical Approach

As discussed in Chap. 55, several options exist for treatment of this problem. The most fundamental goal is treatment of the costoclavicular junction at the anterior part of the thoracic outlet, which is not easily accessible from the supraclavicular approach. In addition, most clinicians stress that the vein should be mobilized and external scar tissue removed, and many advocate an aggressive approach to reconstruction and immediate venography.

Transaxillary first rib resection typically involves partial resection of the first rib and division of its scalene muscle attachments, but because it is not feasible to fully expose or control the subclavian vein from the transaxillary approach, direct evaluation and/or reconstruction of the subclavian vein is not performed. Rather, transaxillary first rib resection is usually coupled with the subsequent use of intraoperative or postoperative venography and performance of balloon angio-

plasty and/or stent placement to deal with any residual stenosis in the subclavian vein [4]. Current estimates indicate that 40–50 % of patients will demonstrate a residual subclavian vein stenosis requiring balloon angioplasty, even several weeks after first rib resection. Because these lesions are typically composed of dense scar tissue within and around the wall of the vein, balloon angioplasty may be relatively ineffective in this setting, and for all these reasons we prefer more direct and thorough approaches to the management of patients with venous TOS.

In recent years wider use of anterior approaches to thoracic outlet decompression and direct operative reconstruction of the subclavian vein have been developed and analyzed [3, 5–11]. Molina and colleagues reported results with immediate surgery using subclavicular decompression and subclavian vein patch angioplasty in 114 patients [9]. Of 97 (85 %) patients treated within 2 weeks of symptoms, the outcomes were uniformly successful. However, of 17 (15 %) patients treated more than 2 weeks after the onset of symptoms, all had developed progressive subclavian vein fibrosis, with 12 (70 %) having postoperative restenosis and 5 (30 %) being considered inoperable.

Our group has long advocated use of paraclavicular thoracic outlet decompression that involves incisions above and below the clavicle [3, 5, 11]. This approach permits more complete first rib resection and more thorough venous decompression that can be obtained through alternative approaches, as well as optimal exposure to accomplish direct subclavian vein reconstruction when necessary. This approach also allows completion of these steps to be accomplished during a single operative procedure and hospital stay, with excellent functional outcomes in a large and ongoing clinical series.

Surgical Technique

Preparation

Anticoagulation is discontinued the evening prior to operation, and a 72-h scopolamine patch is prescribed to held diminish postoperative nausea related to the anesthetic. On the morning of surgery, a fresh intravenous catheter is placed into a forearm vein of the affected upper extremity and an additional route of intravenous access is placed in the contralateral upper extremity, but no central venous or intra-arterial monitoring lines are used. The patient is positioned supine on an operating table compatible with C-arm portable fluoroscopy, to permit intraoperative angiography with views of the shoulder and neck. After the induction of general endotracheal anesthesia, the head of the bed is elevated 30°, and the neck is extended and turned to the opposite side with a small inflatable cushion placed behind the neck. The neck, chest, and entire affected upper extremity are prepped into the field. The affected arm is wrapped in stockinet, to permit free range of movement during the operation and easy access to the forearm and wrist, and the arm is held in position across the abdomen. The ipsilateral thigh may be included in the sterile field to provide access to the greater saphenous vein.

Supraclavicular Exposure (Fig. 63.1)

Paraclavicular decompression for venous TOS begins with supraclavicular exposure. This has been previously describe in Chap. 29 and the most important points and those salient for VTOS will be described below.

A conventional supraclavicular incision is made (Fig. 63.1a) and the scalene fat pad exposed. The small supraclavicular cutaneous nerves crossing the operative field are divided if necessary to ensure adequate exposure. The omohyoid muscle is identified and its central portion is excised. One of the key elements in simplifying the supraclavicular exposure is proper mobilization and lateral reflection of the scalene fat pad. This begins with detachment of the scalene fat pad at the lateral edge of the internal jugular vein and along its inferior edge behind the clavicle, followed by gentle blunt dissection to progressively elevate the fat pad in a medial to lateral direction, exposing the surface of the anterior scalene muscle. The phrenic nerve is identified coursing in a superolateral to inferomedial direc-

tion upon the surface of the anterior scalene muscle, and the thoracic duct is usually observed at the medial edge of the scalene fat pad coursing toward the junction of the internal jugular and subclavian veins (more consistently present on the left side than the right) (Fig. 63.1b).

Attention is next turned to the insertion of the anterior scalene muscle upon the first rib, where the muscle is circumferentially dissected taking care to protect the phrenic nerve, the subclavian artery, and the brachial plexus nerve roots. The anterior scalene muscle is sharply divided from the bone under direct vision, using a scissors rather than the electrocautery, to avoid any inadvertent thermal injury to the adjacent structures (Fig. 63.1c). The inferior end is lifted superiorly and detached from the underlying subclavian artery, brachial plexus nerve roots, and extrapleural (Sibson's) fascia (Fig. 63.1d). A scalene minimus muscle anomaly is often observed at this stage, characterized by muscle fibers that pass between individual nerve roots of the brachial plexus, and these fibers are resected. The anterior scalene muscle is passed underneath the phrenic nerve to its medial side, and the dissection of the muscle is carried further superiorly to the C6 transverse process and removed.

At this stage it is now possible to identify all five nerve roots comprising the brachial plexus. In operations for VTOS the brachial plexus nerve roots are mobilized primarily to avoid injury, but in the event that they are found to be encircled by fibroinflammatory scar tissue a more complete external neurolysis is performed to help diminish the later development of neurogenic symptoms.

Medial retraction of the brachial plexus exposes the broad oblique attachment of the middle scalene muscle on the posterolateral first rib. The mid-portion of the muscle is penetrated by the long thoracic nerve, which is often represented by two or three branches at this level rather than a single nerve. The insertion of the middle scalene muscle is carefully divided from the top of the first rib initially using the electrocautery, and a periosteal elevator is used as the dissection proceeds more posteriorly along the surface of the first rib (Fig. 63.1e). The portion of the middle scalene muscle lying anterior to the long tho-

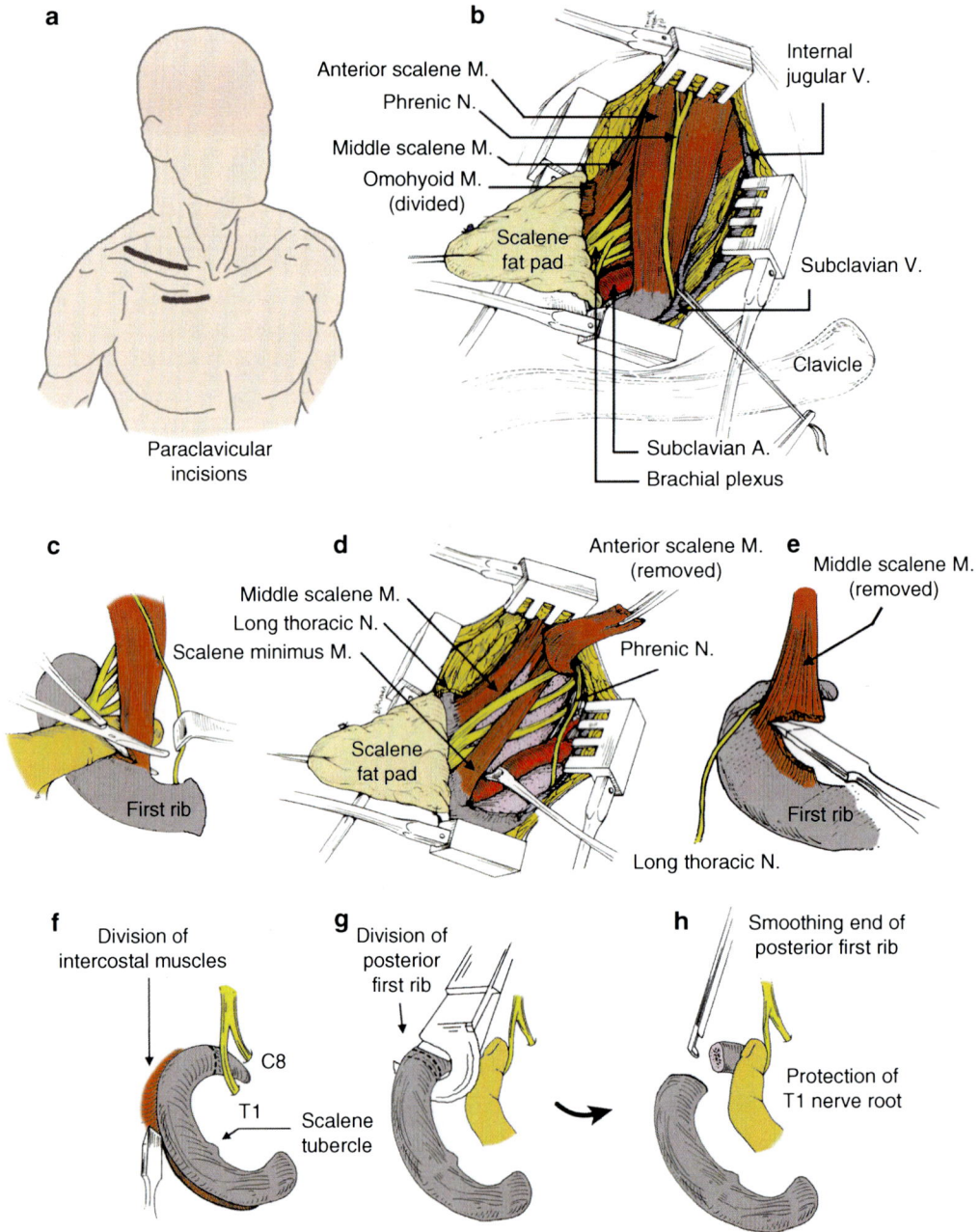

Fig. 63.1 Supraclavicular decompression for venous TOS. (**a**) Illustration of supraclavicular and infraclavicular incisions. (**b**) Initial supraclavicular exposure following mobilization and lateral reflection of the scalene fat pad, demonstrating the phrenic nerve, anterior scalene muscle, brachial plexus, middle scalene muscle. (**c**) Sharp division of the anterior scalene muscle from its insertion on the first rib. (**d**) Resection of the anterior scalene muscle, along with any additional scalene minimus muscle and/or aberrant fibrofascial bands. (**e**) Division of the middle scalene muscle from the upper surface of the posterolateral first rib. (**f**) Division of intercostal muscle along the lateral edge of the first rib. (**g**) Division of the posterior neck of the first rib. (**h**) Smoothing the posterior end of the divided first rib with a Kerrison rongeur

racic nerve is excised, and any remaining middle scalene muscle is detached from the posterior surface of the first rib. It is notable that cervical rib anomalies may be encountered at this stage, since they arise within the same tissue plane as the middle scalene muscle.

While protecting the brachial plexus and long thoracic nerve, the intercostal muscle along the posterolateral aspect of the first rib is divided with the electrocautery or periosteal elevator (Fig. 63.1f), a right-angle clamp passed underneath the rib is used to further detach intercostal muscles, and a modified Stille-Giertz rib cutter is used to divide and excise a small segment of the posterior first rib (Fig. 63.1g). A Kerrison bone rongeur is used to smooth the posterior end of the rib to a level immediately medial to the course of the underlying T1 nerve root, and the edge of the bone is sealed with bone wax (Fig. 63.1h). The free end of the divided first rib is elevated, and a fingertip is passed forward along the undersurface of the rib to bluntly separate additional extrapleural fascia and intercostal muscle attachments to the level of the anterior scalene tubercle. Although in operations for neurogenic and arterial TOS the first rib is next divided just medial to the scalene tubercle and removed, in operations for venous TOS the anterior portion of the first rib is not divided at this stage and the procedure is continued by moving to the infraclavicular portion of the operation.

Infraclavicular Exposure and First Rib Resection (Figs. 63.2 and 63.3)

Removal of the anterior portion of the first rib is crucial in the treatment of venous TOS, since the subclavian vein crosses underneath the clavicle and over the first rib very close to the junction of the rib with the sternum. However, the anteromedial portion of the first rib cannot be sufficiently exposed for resection solely through the supraclavicular approach. To accomplish this, a second transverse skin incision is made one fingerbreadth below the medial clavicle,

extending laterally from the edge of the sternum for approximately 6 cm (Fig. 63.2a). The incision is carried through the subcutaneous tissue to the level of the pectoralis major muscle fascia and subplatysmal flaps are developed (Fig. 63.3). A plane of separation is created between the upper and middle portions of the pectoralis major muscle, allowing exposure of the first rib without muscle division (Fig. 63.3c). The cartilaginous anterior portion of the first rib is identified by palpation, which is facilitated by applying downward pressure to the divided end of the posterior first rib with a finger placed into the previous supraclavicular incision (Fig. 63.2a). This places the attachments between the medial first rib and clavicle under tension, allowing the medial portion of the first rib to be more easily dissected from its soft tissue attachments through the infraclavicular incision (Fig. 63.3d). The subclavius muscle tendon, the costoclavicular ligament, and the muscles of the first intercostal space are divided from the surface of the first rib under direct vision, extending medially to the edge of the sternum, taking care to avoid the sternoclavicular joint (Fig. 63.2b). The cartilaginous portion of the first rib is then divided adjacent to the sternum using the cutting electrocautery, curved Mayo scissors, and/or a duckbilled rongeur. The first rib is then detached from any remaining soft tissues and removed from the operative field as a single specimen (Figs. 63.2c, 63.3e).

Exposure of the Subclavian Vein

The axillary-subclavian vein is initially identified as it passes underneath the midportion of the clavicle, as visualized through the lateral portion of the infraclavicular incision (Fig. 63.3f). The vein is carefully separated from the subclavius muscle moving toward the medial aspect of the surgical field, and any collateral vein branches that enter the subclavian vein are ligated and divided. Once the vein has been sufficiently separated from underneath the subclavius muscle,

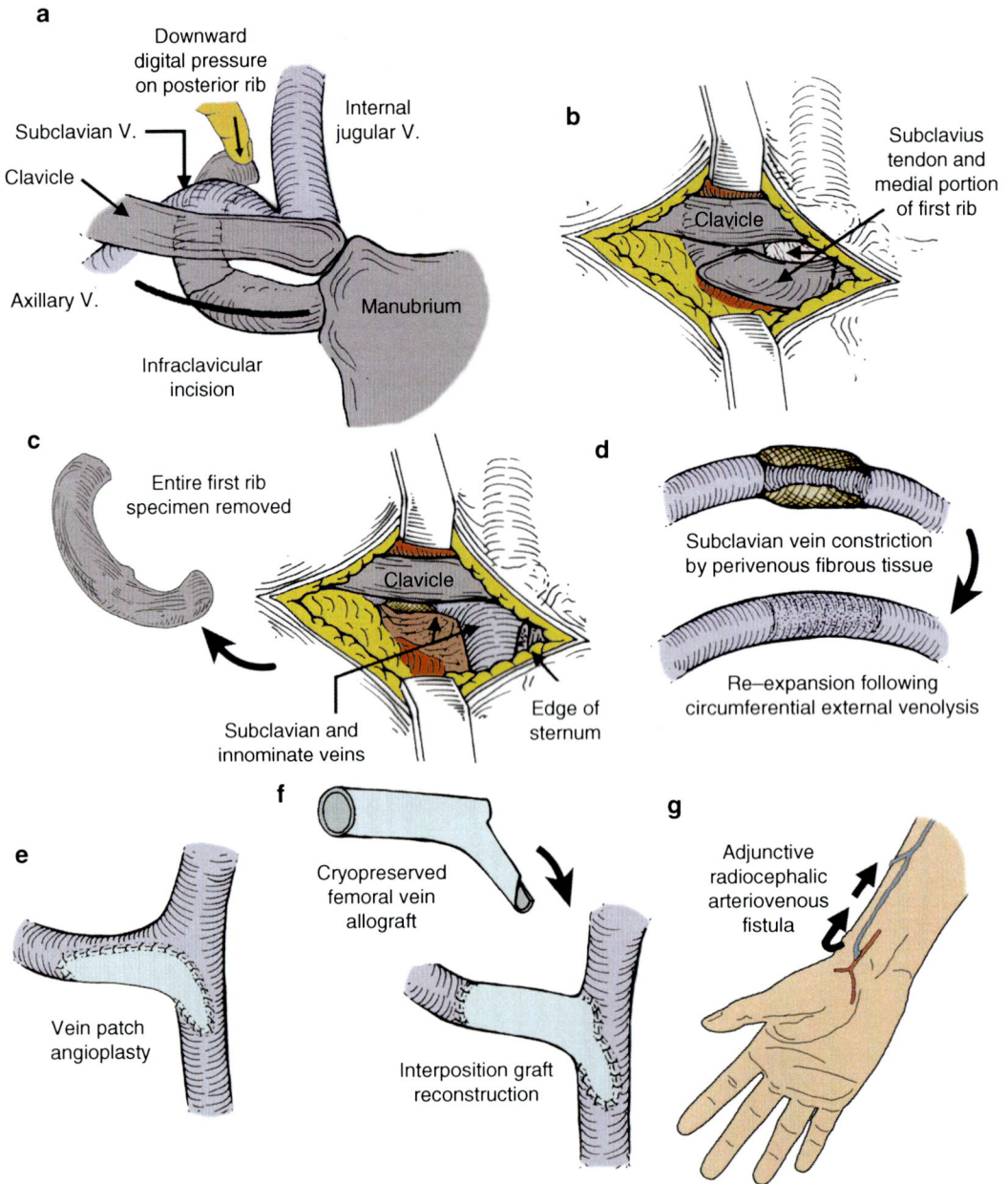

Fig. 63.2 Infraclavicular decompression for venous TOS. (**a**) A transverse infraclavicular incision is made directly over the palpable anterior first rib, which can be easily identified by motion felt when the posterior portion of the rib is pressed inferiorly with a fingertip in the supraclavicular incision. (**b**) The soft tissues attaching to the anteromedial first rib (subclavius muscle tendon and costoclavicular ligament) are divided and the rib is completely exposed. (**c**) The first rib is divided at its junction with the sternum and the entire specimen is removed. The axillary-subclavian vein can then be identified from the infraclavicular exposure and traced proximally (exposure of the proximal segment of the vein is accomplished through the supraclavicular exposure). (**d**) Resection of fibrous scar tissue from around the axillary-subclavian vein (external circumferential venolysis) may allow the vein to re-expand to a normal diameter, in which case further reconstruction may not be necessary. (**e**) Subclavian vein reconstruction by vein patch angioplasty, extending from the normal vein lateral to the stenosis to the innominate vein proximal to the stenosis. (**f**) Subclavian vein reconstruction by interposition bypass graft, placed from the distal subclavian (or axillary) vein to the innominate vein. (**g**) An adjunctive temporary radiocephalic arteriovenous fistula is created when axillary-subclavian vein reconstruction has been performed, to be ligated under local anesthesia 12 weeks after the initial operation

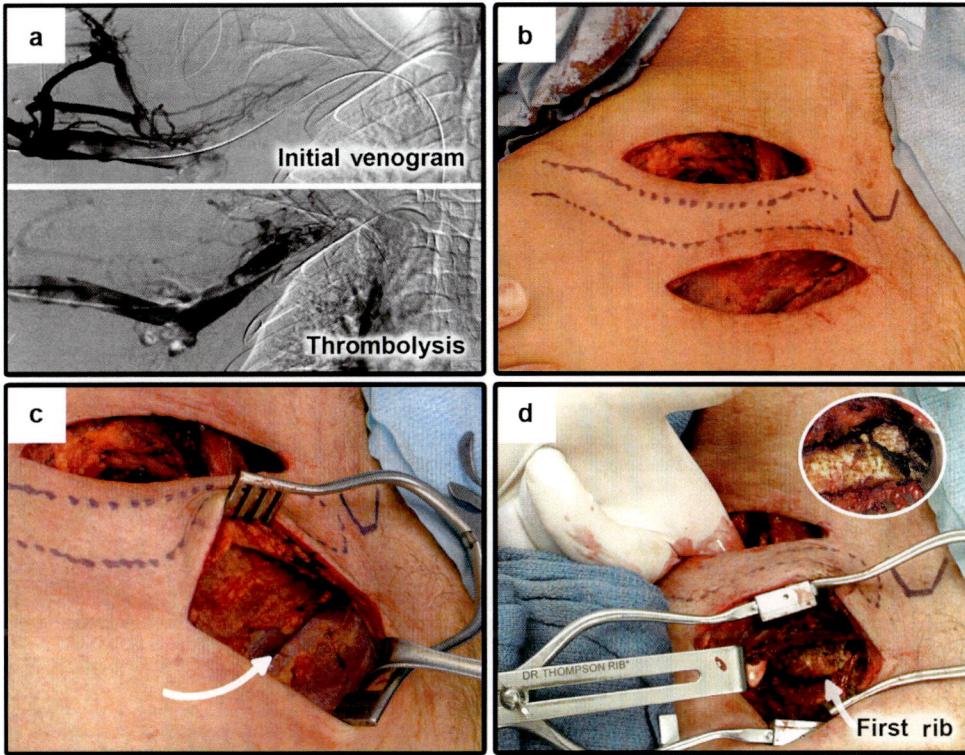

Fig. 63.3 Operative photographs depicting initial phase of paraclavicular decompression for venous TOS. (**a**): Preoperative venograms demonstrating thrombotic occlusion of the axillary-subclavian vein at initial presentation, with improvement following thrombolytic treatment. (**b**) Operative incisions following the initial supraclavicular decompression, at the start of the infraclavicular exposure. (**c**) Guided by palpation of the anterior first rib, the infraclavicular exposure is carried through a plane between the upper and middle portions of the pectoralis major muscle, without division of the muscle (*arrow*). (**d**) After exposure of the anterior first rib, a finger is passed from the supraclavicular exposure to the infraclavicular incision along the surface of the rib to protect the neurovascular bundle during resection of the remaining attachments to the rib. The inset demonstrates an area of calcification and a previous occult fracture in the anterior first rib. (**e**) The entire first rib specimen is resected and removed from the infraclavicular exposure. (**f**) The axillary-subclavian vein (*ASCV*) is initially identified and exposed through the infraclavicular exposure, just underneath the clavicle following resection of the subclavius muscle, where it is circumferentially dissected free of surrounding fibrous scar tissue. (**g**) The proximal portion of the axillary-subclavian vein (*ASCV*) is next dissected from the supraclavicular exposure and dissected to its junction with the internal jugular vein (*IJV*) and innominate vein (*InnV*). In this case there was fibrous wall thickening in the subclavian vein immediately past the jugular-innominate vein junction. (**h**) An intraoperative venogram is performed through an intravenous catheter previously placed in the forearm, to determine if subclavian vein reconstruction is needed

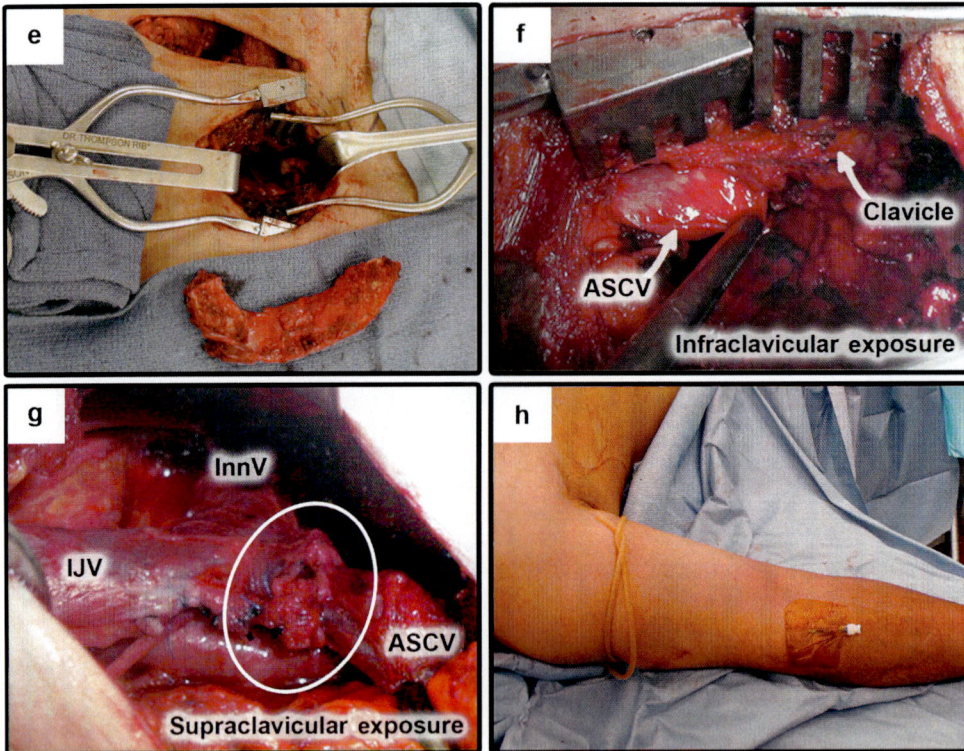

Fig. 63.3 (continued)

this muscle and its tendon are resected. Any fibrous scar tissue around the infraclavicular portion of the axillary-subclavian vein is resected and the underlying vein is assessed, taking note of its caliber, compressibility, and any palpable wall thickening or thrombotic obstruction. If the segment of the vein underneath the clavicle appears to be obstructed or if the patient is known to have a long-segment occlusion based on preoperative venograms, the axillary-subclavian vein is traced laterally until a more suitably soft and patent segment of the vein is identified. In this event it may be necessary to divide the pectoralis minor muscle close to its insertion on the coracoid process, oversewing the divided inferior edge of the muscle with interrupted silk sutures.

Further exposure of the proximal subclavian vein is best achieved through the previously established supraclavicular exposure. This is initiated along the portion of the subclavian vein that underlies the clavicle in the inferolateral aspect of the supraclavicular exposure, often in continuity with the exposure obtained through the infraclavicular incision, and it is continued medially along the course of the subclavian vein toward its junction with the internal jugular vein to form the innominate (brachiocephalic) vein (Fig. 63.3g). It is important to identify a large collateral vein that consistently arises from the top of the subclavian vein immediately underneath the clavicle; once this collateral vein has been satisfactorily ligated and divided, the subclavian vein will be able to fall away from the clavicle, allowing complete exposure to its junction with the internal jugular and innominate veins. The internal jugular vein is fully exposed for several centimeters above its junction with the subclavian vein, and the innominate vein is exposed for several centimeters beyond this junction into the upper mediastinum. During this dissection the course of the phrenic nerve into the upper mediastinum must be carefully noted, and the nerve protected where it passes underneath the subclavian vein. In some situations the phrenic nerve (or a more lateral accessory phrenic nerve) may be found to pass anterior to the subclavian vein, thereby contributing to venous obstruction; in this event the nerve is mobilized away from the subclavian vein but it is not divided.

External Subclavian Venolysis and Venography

At this stage in the procedure the pathological changes in the central portion of the subclavian vein can be fully assessed visually and by digital palpation. Although there may be no evidence of thrombotic luminal obstruction, particularly if the patient had undergone successful thrombolysis prior to surgery, the subclavian vein typically harbors a focal area of fibrous wall thickening resulting from chronic repetitive injury. Any residual scar tissue surrounding the proximal portion of the subclavian vein is therefore completely excised ("circumferential external venolysis"), which often results in re-expansion of the previously constricted segment of the vein (Fig. 63.2d). Indeed, if there is no focal reduction in the diameter of the vein following complete external venolysis, if the vein is soft and easily compressible to palpation, and if the vein shows evidence of rapid filling and emptying with respiratory variation, it is possible that no further venous reconstruction is necessary. In this event attention is turned to performance of an intraoperative venogram to confirm that the subclavian vein is widely patent, in which case the operation will be completed at this stage.

Upper extremity venography is performed using fluoroscopic visualization and digital subtraction technique, with injection of 20–30 mL of full-strength iodinated contrast through the previously-placed forearm vein, and a tourniquet placed gently around the upper arm to ensure that there is adequate contrast filling the deep veins rather than solely the cephalic vein (Fig. 63.3h). In our experience, decompression and external venolysis is sufficient to restore a widely patent axillary-subclavian vein in approximately 50 %

of patients with venous TOS, even in those with a long-segment stenosis or apparent occlusion prior to operation.

Subclavian Vein Reconstruction
(Figs. 63.2 and 63.4)

When external venolysis alone is insufficient to alleviate subclavian vein obstruction, or when the intraoperative venogram demonstrates a residual stenosis despite the apparent success of external venolysis (Fig. 63.4a), additional venous reconstruction is performed. A continuous infusion of Dextran (25 mL per hour) is started along with systemic anticoagulation with intravenous heparin (approximately 5,000 units). A "spoon" vascular clamp is placed across the innominate vein from the infraclavicular incision, taking care not to damage posterior collateral veins within the mediastinum and to exclude the phrenic nerve. From the supraclavicular incision a second clamp is placed across the internal jugular vein several centimeters above the jugular-subclavian junction, taking care to include the collateral veins that may enter this area on the medial side of the jugular vein. An angled DeBakey clamp is placed across the distal axillary-subclavian vein and any remaining collateral veins that enter the isolated segment of subclavian vein are controlled with separate bulldog clamps.

Vein Patch Angioplasty

As viewed best from the supraclavicular exposure, a longitudinal venotomy is initially created along the superior aspect of the proximal subclavian vein and the luminal surface is inspected (Fig. 63.4b). If there is only mild-moderate focal stenosis of the subclavian vein and the luminal surface is smooth and free of chronic thrombus or irregularity (following resection of any minimal intimal webs), a simple patch angioplasty is performed (Fig. 63.2e). In this event the venotomy is extended to span the entire length of the affected portion of subclavian vein, from a normal venous segment laterally into the anterior aspect of the

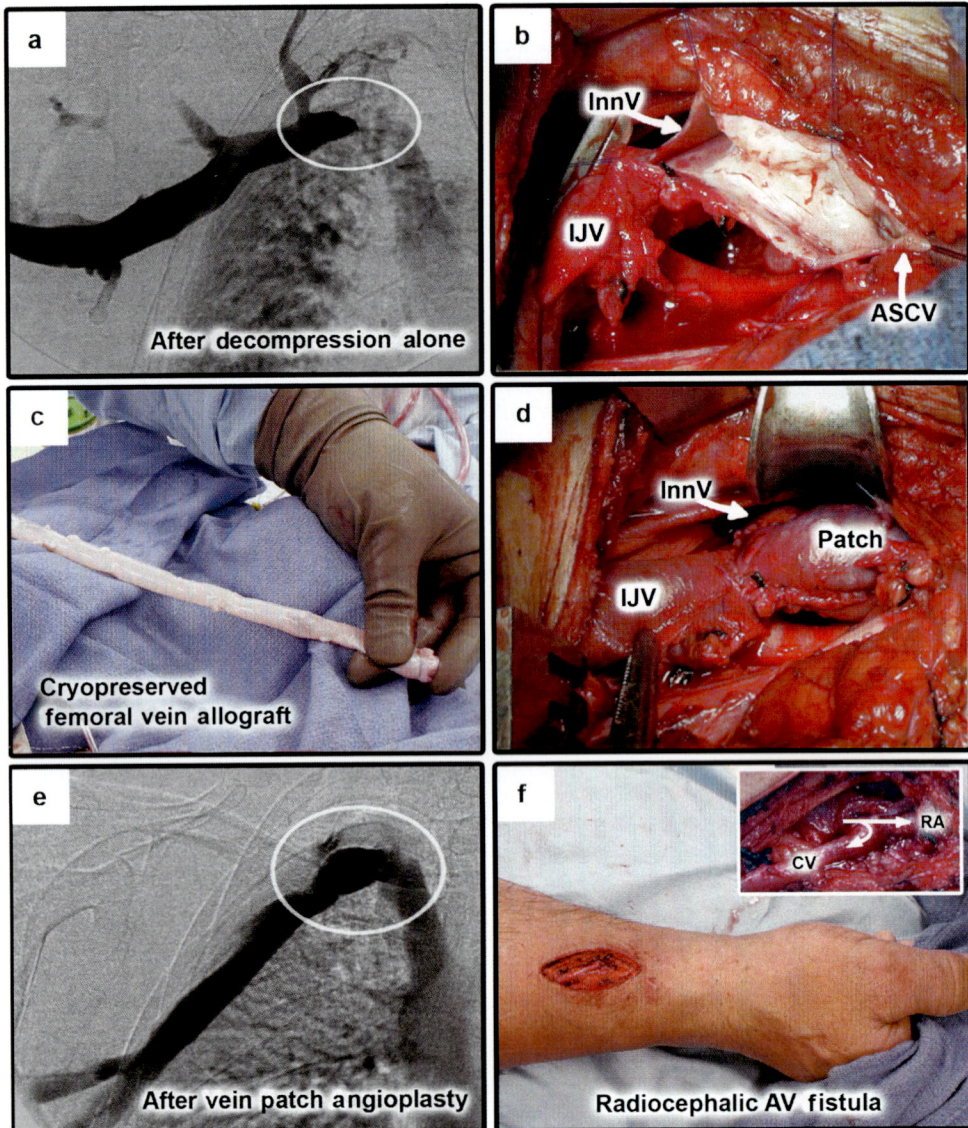

Fig. 63.4 Operative photographs depicting subclavian vein reconstruction for venous TOS. (**a**) Intraoperative venogram following paraclavicular first rib resection and external axillary-subclavian venolysis, demonstrating a residual focal high-grade stenosis of the proximal subclavian vein. (**b**) As viewed from the supraclavicular exposure, a long venotomy is created in the proximal subclavian vein and carried through the junction with the internal jugular vein (*IJV*) into the anterior wall of the innominate vein (*InnV*). After resection of several fibrous webs the intraluminal surface appears smooth and free of thrombus, indicating its suitability for vein patch angioplasty. (**c**) A cryopreserved femoral vein is thawed and prepared. The vein graft will be opened longitudinally to provide a wide segment for patch angioplasty. (**d**) After completion of the patch angioplasty and removal of the vascular clamps, the subclavian vein is quickly distended with venous blood, the suture lines are intact, and the vein is soft and easily compressible to palpation. (**e**) A completion venogram demonstrating a widely patent axillary-subclavian vein following patch angioplasty reconstruction. (**f**) When axillary-subclavian vein reconstruction is performed, an adjunctive radiocephalic arteriovenous fistula is created at the wrist. (**g**) Prior to wound closure two multihole perfusion catheters are placed within the operative field and attached to an osmotic minipump, to provide several days of continuous perineural administration of local anesthetic (0.5 % bupivacaine) as an adjunct to postoperative pain management. (**h**) A closed-suction drain is placed within the operative field with the tip extending into the pleural space, and the paraclavicular wounds are closed

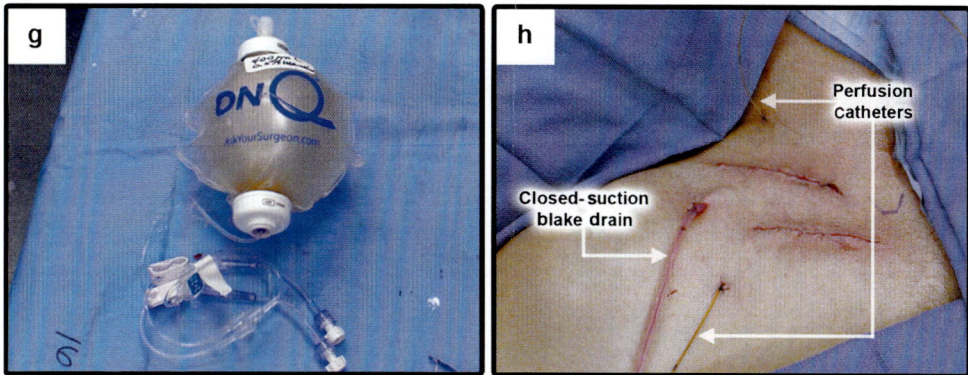

Fig. 63.4 (continued)

innominate vein (we have previously extended this venotomy along the lateral aspect of the internal jugular vein, but now prefer an inferior extension into the innominate vein to improve the geometry of the reconstruction). The vein patch angioplasty is constructed with a segment of cryopreserved femoral vein measuring approximately 10–14 mm in diameter (opened longitudinally with the valves lysed prior to use), which provides a readily available conduit with sufficient size to expand the subclavian vein (we have previous constructed vein patches of this type with autogenous saphenous vein, but have frequently found this to be of insufficient caliber for a satisfactory reconstruction) (Fig. 63.4c). The vein patch is attached with running 5–0 polypropylene utilizing numerous "stay" sutures to optimize the geometry, and to avoid obstructive kinking of the patched segment of vein once it is distended under physiological conditions in the upright position (Fig. 63.4d). A completion venogram is performed to verify that the subclavian vein reconstruction is satisfactory, with a widely patent lumen, rapid venous flow into the innominate vein, and the absence of collateral vein filling (Fig. 63.4e).

Vein Graft Bypass

When there is a chronic subclavian vein occlusion or an obstructed indwelling stent, dense fibrosis remaining within the wall of the subclavian vein despite external venolysis, or another obvious abnormality upon inspection of the luminal surface of the opened vein, the affected segment of the subclavian vein is replaced by an interposition bypass graft (Fig. 63.2f). The proximal subclavian vein is excised from an opening in the lateral edge of the jugular-innominate vein junction, extending the venotomy into the anterior wall of the innominate vein (as visualized through the supraclavicular incision), and the distal subclavian vein is divided on a long bevel at a location where there is a normal segment of axillary-subclavian (visualized through the infraclavicular incision), and the intervening segment of the native subclavian vein is removed. As noted above, we prefer the use of a cryopreserved femoral vein as the conduit for subclavian vein bypass, since the autologous saphenous vein is of insufficient size and would require construction of a "panel" graft for use. The proximal anastomosis is performed first to ensure optimal visualization of the opening in the innominate vein, and its construction is most easily accomplished through the supraclavicular incision. An end-to-side anastomosis is created with a long bevel using running 5–0 polypropylene suture. The clamps are then released from the innominate and jugular veins to restore flow and an atraumatic vascular clamp is replaced onto the vein bypass graft near the proximal suture line. The vein bypass graft is passed underneath the clavicle, taking care to avoid any kinking or twisting, and is brought into comfortable apposition with the distal segment of axillary-subclavian vein. The distal anastomosis is most easily constructed by visualization through the infraclavicular incision, and is constructed in an end-to-end manner to the unaffected distal subclavian vein. Venous flow is restored after removal of all clamps, the suture lines are inspected, and the geometry of the vein graft is observed throughout its course. Finally, a completion intraoperative venogram is performed to confirm a satisfactory subclavian vein reconstruction.

Adjunctive Arteriovenous Fistula

For many years our operative approach to venous TOS has included the construction of a temporary radiocephalic arteriovenous (AV) fistula whenever an axillary-subclavian vein reconstruction has been performed (patch angioplasty or interposition bypass graft), as an adjunct intended to increase upper extremity venous blood flow during the first several months after operation (Fig. 63.2g). This is constructed using a short incision in the wrist of the affected extremity for exposure of the distal radial artery and cephalic vein (Fig. 63.4f). This AV fistula is subsequently ligated under local anesthesia 12 weeks after the initial surgical treatment, at which time a final follow-up contrast venogram is also performed to evaluate the axillary-subclavian vein reconstruction.

Closure, Postoperative Care, and Recovery (Fig. 63.4)

Upon completion of the procedure the pleural apex is opened to facilitate postoperative drainage of fluid into the chest cavity. A #19 Blake closed-suction drain is placed within the superior operative field lying posterior to the brachial plexus, with its tip extending into the pleura. Two small multihole perfusion catheters connected to an osmotic pump (On-Q, Kimberly-Clark Healthcare, Inc.) are placed into the operative field and positioned near the brachial plexus and bed of the resected first rib, for continuous postoperative infusion of local anesthetic (0.5 %

bupivacaine for 3 days), which we have found to substantially improve early pain control (Fig. 63.4g). The scalene fat pad is restored to its anatomic position and held in place with several tacking sutures. The platysma layer is closed with interrupted sutures and the skin is closed with subcuticular stitches (Fig. 63.4h).

Postoperative care includes ample use of intravenous and oral pain medications, muscle relaxants, and anti-inflammatory agents. The potential complications of surgery are similar to those considered in other operations for TOS, as well as those related to venous reconstruction (Table 63.1). Chest radiographs are obtained for several days to monitor any collection of pleural fluid, which typically resolves over the course of the first week. The expected hospital stay is 4–5 days, with the closed-suction drain removed in the outpatient setting approximately 7 days after operation.

Therapeutic anticoagulation is initiated several days after operation with intravenous heparin (with or without the addition of aspirin or clopidogrel), followed by low molecular weight heparin and conversion to warfarin. Anticoagulant and antiplatelet agents are maintained until 12 weeks after operation then discontinued. For patients with venous TOS and a patent AV fistula, followup imaging studies are not performed in the absence of any symptoms of venous obstruction. These individuals then undergo outpatient ligation of the AV fistula under local anesthesia

Table 63.1 Potential complications of surgical treatment for venous TOS

Subclavian artery injury/intraoperative hemorrhage
Subclavian vein injury/intraoperative hemorrhage
Brachial plexus nerve injury or postoperative paresis
Phrenic nerve injury or postoperative paresis
Long thoracic nerve injury or postoperative paresis
Pneumothorax or pleural effusion
Postoperative lymph leak
Residual subclavian vein obstruction or early postoperative re-thrombosis
Postoperative bleeding/wound hematoma/excessive anticoagulation
Late postoperative axillary or subclavian vein obstruction or re-thrombosis

12 weeks after the primary operation, at which time followup contrast venography can also be performed.

Inpatient physical therapy is started the day after operation to maintain range of motion, with postoperative rehabilitation then overseen by a physical therapist with expertise in the management of TOS, usually in conjunction with a physical therapist located near the patient. Activity is gradually increased over the first 4–6 weeks after operation, with patients able to return to most sedentary activities, and restrictions on upper extremity activity are progressively lifted between 6 and 12 weeks. For manual laborers and athletes, recovery is typically considered fully complete within 12 weeks of operation and a full return to previous levels of function can usually be expected.

Conclusions

As described in this chapter, our approach to the treatment of venous TOS involves a comprehensive strategy based on paraclavicular thoracic outlet decompression [3]. This approach to the surgical treatment of venous TOS combines the advantages of the supraclavicular exposure used for neurogenic and arterial forms of TOS with an infraclavicular exposure that permits complete resection of the medial first rib, as well as wide exposure of the subclavian vein to permit vascular reconstruction. In a surgical experience that now exceeds several hundred procedures using this approach, we have been able to offer definitive surgical treatment to virtually all patients with symptomatic venous TOS or recent effort thrombosis, regardless of the interval between initial diagnosis and referral, previous treatment, or adverse findings on contrast venography. A recent review of our results in competitive athletes with effort thrombosis, a particularly challenging population, verifies that this strategy of surgical treatment can result in excellent early and long-term

outcomes [10]. This has led us to conclude that operative procedures based on paraclavicular exposure provide the most versatile, comprehensive, and safe approach to the treatment of venous TOS [10, 11].

References

1. Sanders RJ. Thoracic outlet syndrome: a common sequelae of neck injuries. Philadelphia: J. B. Lippincott Company; 1991.
2. Urschel Jr HC. The transaxillary approach for treatment of thoracic outlet syndromes. Semin Thorac Cardiovasc Surg. 1996;8(2):214–20.
3. Thompson RW, Petrinec D, Toursarkissian B. Surgical treatment of thoracic outlet compression syndromes. II. Supraclavicular exploration and vascular reconstruction. Ann Vasc Surg. 1997;11(4):442–51.
4. Urschel Jr HC, Razzuk MA. Paget-Schroetter syndrome: what is the best management? Ann Thorac Surg. 2000;69(6):1663–8; discussion 1668–9.
5. Thompson RW, Schneider PA, Nelken NA, Skioldebrand CG, Stoney RJ. Circumferential venolysis and paraclavicular thoracic outlet decompression for "effort thrombosis" of the subclavian vein. J Vasc Surg. 1992;16(5):723–32.
6. Molina JE. Surgery for effort thrombosis of the subclavian vein. J Thorac Cardiovasc Surg. 1992; 103(2):341–6.
7. Molina JE. Need for emergency treatment in subclavian vein effort thrombosis. J Am Coll Surg. 1995;181(5):414–20.
8. Azakie A, McElhinney DB, Thompson RW, Raven RB, Messina LM, Stoney RJ. Surgical management of subclavian vein "effort" thrombosis secondary to thoracic outlet compression. J Vasc Surg. 1998;28:777–86.
9. Molina JE, Hunter DW, Dietz CA. Paget-Schroetter syndrome treated with thrombolytics and immediate surgery. J Vasc Surg. 2007;45(2):328–34.
10. Melby SJ, Vedantham S, Narra VR, Paletta Jr GA, Khoo-Summers L, Driskill M, Thompson RW. Comprehensive surgical management of the competitive athlete with effort thrombosis of the subclavian vein (Paget-Schroetter syndrome). J Vasc Surg. 2008;47(4):809–20.
11. Melby SJ, Thompson RW. Supraclavicular (paraclavicular) approach for thoracic outlet syndrome (chapter). In: Pearce WH, Matsumura JS, Yao JST, editors. Operative vascular surgery in the endovascular era. Evanston: Greenwood Academic; 2008. p. 434–45.

Karl A. Illig

Abstract

Removal of the clavicle yields superb exposure of the entire axillary-subclavian-inominate vein complex, and leads to the most complete exposure possible for venous reconstruction, bypass, or replacement. At least two-thirds of the clavicle should be resected to avoid problems from the residual lateral segment; if this is done, long-term functional outcome is excellent.

Introduction

While supraclavicular exposure provides excellent access to the middle and posterior part of the first rib and transaxillary exposure to the anterior part, neither provides exposure to the subclavian vein itself. Various techniques have been described, including Molina's "sternal flap" (essentially disarticulating the clavicle, but leaving the junction intact) [1] and infra/supraclavicular ("paraclavicular") exposure popularized by Thompson [2], but neither provide consistent, continuous exposure to the vein itself with room to perform any intervention needed. Claviculectomy opens this area in its entirety, is surprisingly well tolerated, and

should be considered for patients in whom complex venous resection is required.

Technique

Claviculectomy itself is relatively straightforward. An incision is made over the clavicle, and cautery is used to expose the bone itself. The operation is classically described as a "medial claviculectomy," but we and others stress that at least two-thirds of the clavicle needs to be removed [3, 4]. Leaving too much clavicle in place produces a very mobile bone, which can either stick up and be cosmetically unattractive and painful, or worse, can be forced downward, creating a secondary thoracic outlet syndrome of any variety. Resecting as much of the bone as possible eliminates this problem.

Once the bone is identified, it is cleaned using a periosteal elevator. A large right-angle clamp can be used to get around the midportion of the bone circumferentially, and this can then be moved medially and laterally to divest the bone from the

K.A. Illig, MD
Department of Surgery, Division of Vascular Surgery,
University of South Florida,
2 Tampa General Circle, STC 7016,
Tampa, FL 33606, USA
e-mail: killig@health.usf.edu

underlying subclavius muscle. There is fear sometimes at this point that the vein is close enough to be injured, but in actuality the subclavian muscle and a significant amount of soft tissue remains, and the vein is quite safe with this maneuver.

At this point, an oscillating saw is used to divide the bone at least two-thirds of the way toward the shoulder. The bone is then elevated and dissection continued toward the costaclavicular junction. Especially inferiorly and medially, attachments can be tight, and this can be a surprisingly difficult part of the operation. Perseverance is the best tool. The goal is to formally disarticulate the clavicle from the sternum itself; no clavicle should be left behind medially but articular cartilage does not need to be removed.

At this point the bed of the clavicle is exposed. As described above, the vein is still deep to this. The subclavius muscle is the main structure remaining, although it is often indistinguishable from the surrounding tissue. The muscle and associated soft tissue should be resected, with attention paid to the vein at this point. The vein can be surprisingly hard to find, especially if obliterated in a patient with chronic stenosis or occlusion. A useful technique is to find a tributary vein (such as the cephalic) and follow it deeply until the main vein can be found. Large collateral veins can, at times, be mistaken for the subclavian vein, and dissection should be thorough enough to clearly identify normal axillary-subclavian vein peripherally and normal innominate vein centrally. Obviously, enough vein should be cleared at both locations for adequate clamping. If jugular transposition/turndown is contemplated, a separate incision is required as significant length of vein is needed.

Using this technique, superb exposure of as much of the axillary-subclavian-innominate vein family as is needed can be obtained. Reconstruction, covered elsewhere, may include patch venoplasty with internal venolysis, jugular vein turndown, or even interposition grafting with paneled saphenous vein, femoral vein, or, occa-

sionally, prosthetic. The clavicle should be discarded; trying to reattach this risks chronic malunion and long-term pain. It should be noted that the first rib can easily be resected once the clavicle is out, but this is not needed as the thoracic outlet is fully decompressed already (we have one patient with staged first rib and clavicle excisions who is symptom free several years after his last procedure).

Results

Clavicular resection is surprisingly well tolerated, even in healthy, competitive athletes. We have performed approximately 20 medial claviculectomies over the past two decades. Green reported our first decade's experience in 2000 [3]. Eleven patients were operated on, all for venous TOS, and followup occurred (in all 11) at a mean of 6 years (range 3–9 years). All patients (all young) returned to their preoperative vocation, four of which involve heavy labor. No patient describes any limitation of shoulder function, all 11 consider their operation "completely successful" from a functional standpoint, and only two are bothered by the cosmetic results. All reconstructed veins were patent, and only one patient had slight swelling with exertion.

An illustrative case is a patient with highly symptomatic VTOS who was operated on at our institution approximately 7 or 8 years ago. After clavicular resection (and jugular transposition), he went on to be Captain of his Ski Team at his Ivy League college and was named a Division I All-American. Currently a vascular surgery resident, he remains quite physically active and reports absolutely no functional problems from the claviculectomy.

As described above, at least two-thirds of the clavicle must be removed, as an overly-long lateral segment can be cosmetically unsightly (Fig. 64.1) at best, and protrude downward into the thoracic outlet, creating secondary problems, at worst. There are several reports of total

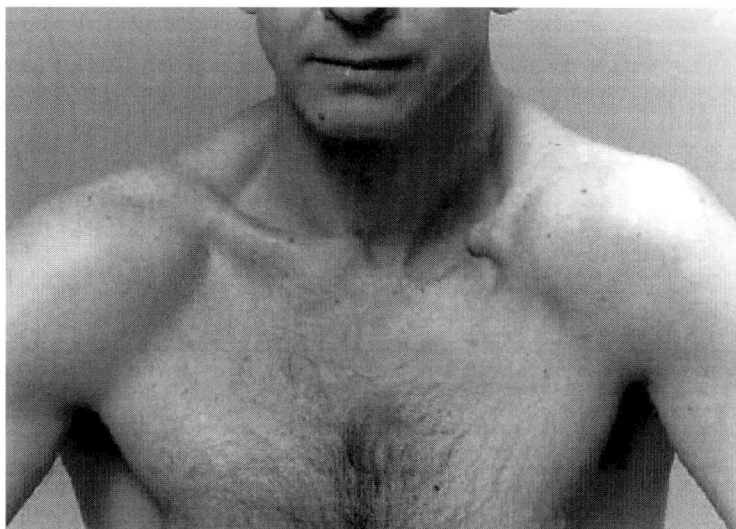

Fig. 64.1 A patient with a residual, lateral mobile clavicular segment illustrating the drawbacks of leaving too much clavicle in place (Reprinted from Green et al. [3] with permission from Elsevier)

claviculectomy in the orthopedic literature, and, although a bit dated, show that function is excellent [5, 6]. Patients, for example, can play golf, swim, and hunt. A 1947 paper, in fact, describes a family with 9 members who were born without clavicles and perform manual labor (farming) without problems [7].

Summary

While clavicular resection is not the first choice in dealing with VTOS, it provides superb exposure of as much vein as needed for reconstruction and is quite well tolerated. It should be stressed that at least two-thirds of the clavicle should be resected to avoid problems from the residual lateral segment; if this is done, long-term functional outcome is excellent.

Conflicts of Interest None

References

1. Molina JE, Hunter DW, Dietz CA. Protocols for Paget-Schroetter syndrome and late treatment of chronic subclavian vein obstruction. Ann Thor Surg. 2009;87:416–22.
2. Thompson RW, Schneider PA, Nelkin NA, Skioldebrand CG, Stoney RJ. Circumferential venolysis and paraclavicular thoracic outlet decompression for "effort thrombosis" of the subclavian vein. J Vasc Surg. 1992;16:723–32.
3. Green RM, Waldman D, Ouriel K, Riggs P, DeWeese JA. Claviculectomy for subclavian venous repair: long-term functional results. J Vasc Surg. 2000;32:315–21.
4. Sanders RJ, Haug CE. Thoracic outlet syndrome: a common sequela of neck injuries. Philadelphia: Lippincott; 1991. p. 255.
5. Lord JW, Wright IS. Total claviculectomy for neurovascular compression in the thoracic outlet. Surg Gynecol Obstet. 1993;176:609–12.
6. Wood VE. The results of total claviculectomy. Clin Orthop Relat Res. 1986;207:186–90.
7. Gurd FB. Surplus parts of the skeleton, a recommendation for excision of certain portions as a means of shortening the period of disability following trauma. Am J Surg. 1947;74:705–20.

Richard J. Sanders

Abstract

Following subclavian vein thrombosis, even when thrombolysis and thoracic outlet decompression have been successful, some patients may still be symptomatic and require some type of venous reconstruction. The procedures available include endovenectomy and patch graft, interposition replacement graft, and jugular vein turndown (also called jugular transposition). The addition of a temporary arteriovenous fistula will increase blood flow through the venous repair to reduce the incidence of postoperative thrombosis.

Introduction

Even after successful thrombolysis and thoracic outlet decompression, many patients will still require some form of venous reconstruction. Authors' and clinicians' attitudes vary widely as to the number of patients who will need this (literally from zero to every patient) and it should be stressed that no randomized comparisons exist.

Indications

Reconstruction may be performed early, immediately following thrombectomy, or in a delayed fashion. If after thrombolytic therapy there is

R.J. Sanders, MD
Department of Surgery,
HealthONE Presbyterian-St. Lukes Hospital,
4545 E. 9th Ave #240, Denver, CO 80220, USA
e-mail: rsanders@ecentral.com

significant residual stenosis or if lytic therapy has failed, some surgeons perform open thrombectomy and endovenectomy at the time of first rib resection to decompress the subclavian vein. Thus, the external (ligaments, muscles, and first rib that surround the vein) and internal (fibrosis and organized thrombus) factors causing subclavian vein thrombosis are treated simultaneously [1].

Other surgeons defer surgery following successful or even unsuccessful lytic therapy and follow the patient on anticoagulants. Surgery may be performed a few weeks later while some physicians will only perform surgery for persistent symptoms.

For chronic subclavian vein occlusion, or when occlusion persists in spite of treatment and when symptoms present significant disability, subclavian vein reconstruction is available. However, reconstruction should not be considered until several months have passed after occlusion occurred. The reason for this is collateral

K.A. Illig et al. (eds.), *Thoracic Outlet Syndrome*,
DOI 10.1007/978-1-4471-4366-6_65, © Springer-Verlag London 2013

circulation can develop during the first 6–12 months following occlusion. In the majority of patients symptoms subside to the point where they are no longer disabling and the residual symptoms are mild enough that surgery is not needed.

If reconstruction is indicated three approaches are available: jugular vein turndown, endovenectomy, or replacement with vein graft or prosthesis.

Incision

All subclavian vein reconstructions are performed through one of two incisions: Claviculectomy or infraclavicular. There are advantages and disadvantages to each. Claviculectomy provides the best exposure but at the risk of some complications from removing one of the supports of the shoulder girdle (see Chap. 64). In a minority of patients instability of the shoulder girdle may cause some impairment particularly for young active people who do heavy lifting with their arms [2], although the majority of patients who have received claviculectomy are happy with the end result and experience no disability [3].

Infraclavicular incisions preserve the clavicle but the exposure is not as good and the procedure is more difficult, especially in large patients.

Claviculectomy

Claviculectomy is covered in more detail in Chap. 64, but a few points are worth emphasizing. Excision of the clavicle provides the best exposure for all patients, but especially in the obese. As much as possible of the clavicle should be removed(at least two-thirds to three-quarters); removing a shorter length carries a risk of the medial end of remaining clavicle dropping onto the neurovascular bundle causing symptoms of venous obstruction or brachial plexus compression, and from a disability point of view there is no difference between excision of a short or long segment of clavicle. The periosteum should be removed to avoid regeneration of what could

become weak bone, and the clavicular head is disarticulated at the sternum [3, 4].

Infraclavicular Incision

The infraclavicular incision is used far more often than claviculectomy. An 8–10 cm transverse incision is made just lateral to the sternum and 2 cm below the clavicle. Pectoralis major is split in the direction of its fibers, and the subclavian and axillary veins are dissected free. Depending on the type of reconstruction to be done, the pectoralis minor muscle may be divided for better exposure of the axillary vein. The anterior two-thirds of the first rib should be excised prior to performing endovenectomy or replacement graft but the first rib need not be removed for a jugular vein turndown. First rib resection includes release of the anterior scalene and middle scalene muscles. The posterior part of the first rib is difficult to excise through this incision but when possible, enough rib is removed to leave the lower trunk of the brachial plexus free of the posterior rib stump.

Sternal Split

When the thickened portion of subclavian vein extends proximally beneath the sternum, the proximal subclavian vein is exposed by carefully freeing the vein from the back of the sternum by blunt dissection. When enough soft vein cannot be freed to apply a proximal vascular clamp, better exposure can be obtained by splitting the sternum to the first interspace as described by Molina (this is also an alternative to claviculectomy for access to the infraclavicular subclavian vein) [5]. The medial corner of the skin incision is retracted medially to expose the sternal notch. It may be necessary to extend the skin incision medially to see the notch. The periosteum of the sternum is incised and by finger dissection the underside of the sternum is freed down to the first interspace. More blunt dissection is added under the first rib interspace until the two dissections meet. A sternal knife or saw splits the sternum vertically

Fig. 65.1 Sternal flap for exposure of subclavian, innominate, and jugular veins (Reprinted from Molina [5] with permission from Elsevier)

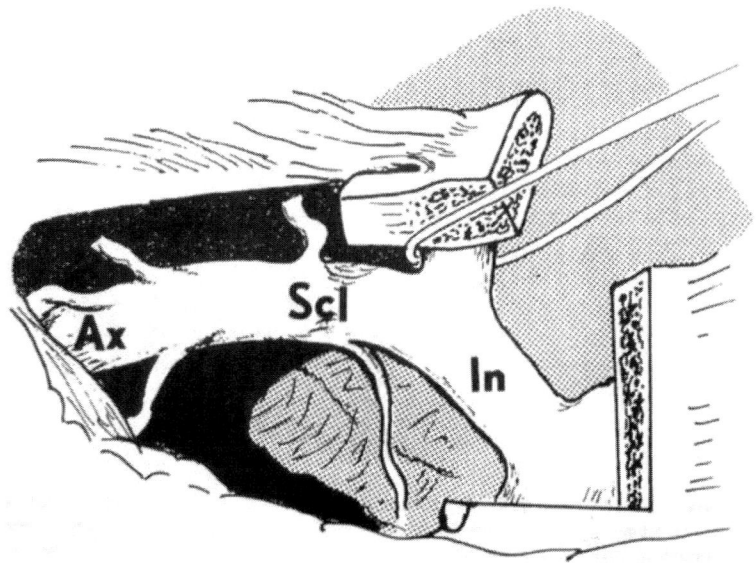

down to the first interspace and horizontally through the first interspace until the two cuts meet. After controlling hemorrhage from the bone edges with bone wax, the freed piece of sternum is retracted upwards, held by a self-retaining retractor, and the entire venous system including innominate, subclavian, axillary, and jugular veins are nicely exposed (Fig. 65.1) [5].

Once the vein repair is complete and hemostasis achieved, the sternum is repaired with 3 or 4 heavy braided Dacron or wire sutures inserted through predrilled holes. Although the original description of the sternal closure used only two wire sutures, we have found adding an additional one or two sutures makes the closure more secure. Postoperatively, the patient is instructed to restrict use of the arm for 6–8 weeks but also to gently raise the arm each day to 180° to avoid a frozen shoulder.

Subclavian Endovenectomy and Interposition Graft

These techniques are used in situations where "significant" (variously and subjectively defined) intraluminal stenosis or complete occlusion are present, and require exposure as above. Again, definitive proof is lacking; some advocate

reconstruction in virtually all patients and some only in those who are highly symptomatic.

Preoperative Evaluation

A venogram is essential to confirm adequate inflow from the brachial vein as well as to define the extent of axillosubclavian vein stenosis or occlusion. The procedure can't be performed if inflow is inadequate, and accurate assessment of a normal central vessel for outflow is critically important.

Technique

Following claviculectomy or infraclavicular exposure and first rib resection, the subclavian vein is dissected circumferentially as far distally as necessary to find soft axillary vein. Branches are preserved and controlled with vessel loops. By lifting the vein on a right angle clamp to identify absence of intraluminal material the distal and proximal points of the venotomy can be determined. To find soft vein proximally it is often necessary to carefully dissect the vein beneath the sternum, and if soft vein cannot be reached centrally, the sternum is split as described above.

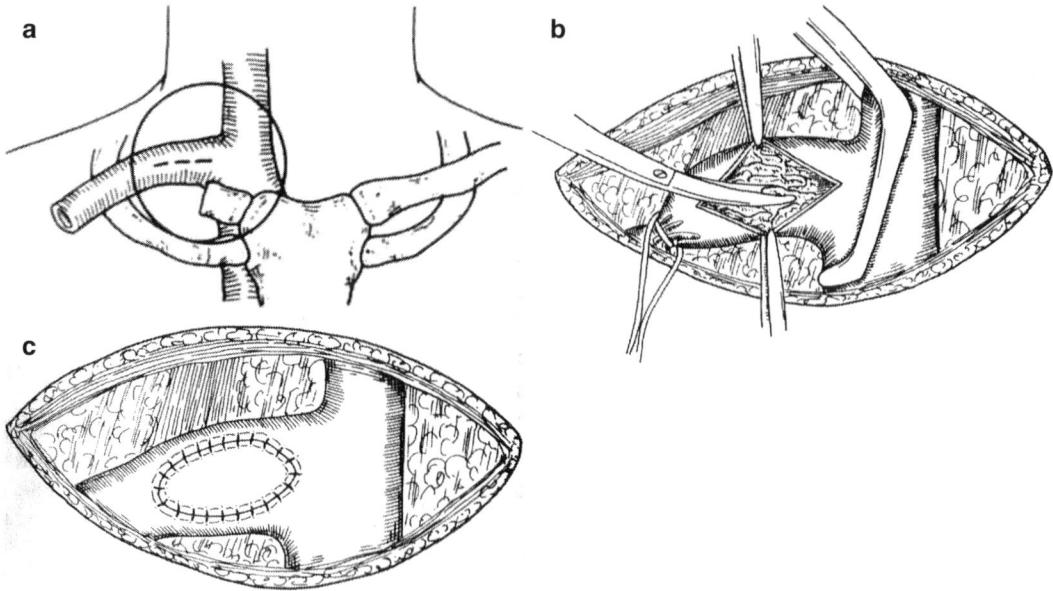

Fig. 65.2 Endovenectomy. (**a**) Location of incision in vein. (**b**) Scissors excision of scarred intima. (**c**) Vein patch graft (Reprinted from Sanders and Haug [7], p. 252 with permission from Lippincott Williams & Wilkins)

Endovenectomy

The patient is heparinized and the section of vein to be opened is isolated between vascular clamps. Venotomy is performed and a patent channel sought. Organized thrombus and scarred intima are excised (Fig. 65.2). It should be stressed that there are no dissection planes between intima and adventitia as in arterial endarterectomy; endovenectomy is a totally different operation. The scarred material inside the vein wall is excised with a sharp scissors taking care to avoid getting too close to the adventitia and perforating the vein wall, and a rim of firmly attached rough-surfaced intima or organized clot, 1–2 mm thick, is left inside the vein wall. A patch of saphenous vein or homograft vessel is used to close the venotomy.

Replacement Graft

If the vein is too badly scarred or fibrosed so that a reasonable channel cannot be identified and developed, the obliterated segment is excised and replaced with a 10–14 mm graft, such as

cryopreserved aortic homograft or a saphenous vein panel graft; prosthetic is not recommended in this situation. The graft is sewn proximally and distally with monofilament permanent suture (Prolene or similar).

If the wound is dry the heparin need not be neutralized. The patient is started on warfarin immediately and after 24 h is started on intravenous heparin or subcutaneous low molecular weight heparin. Low molecular weight Dextran is started during surgery and continued for 24–48 h postoperatively. Once the warfarin has reached therapeutic levels (INR = 2–3) the heparin is stopped. Anticoagulation with warfarin is continued for 3–6 months postoperatively.

Jugular Turndown (Jugular Vein Transposition)

If the length of occlusion is 5–6 cm long or less, a jugular vein turndown is possible [6]. Longer occlusions cannot be managed with a jugular turndown because the jugular vein won't stretch any further. This procedure requires a normal jugular vein on the ipsilateral side and an open jugular vein on the contralateral side.

Preoperative Evaluation

As for endovenectomy, a preoperative venogram is necessary to confirm adequate inflow and to determine the length of the total occlusion (again, an occlusion over 6 cm long will usually not be a candidate for a jugular turndown). Ultrasound is used to determine patency of the ipsilateral and contralateral jugular veins.

Incision

Either an infraclavicular incision or claviculectomy as described above is used to begin the operation. A moist sponge is placed in the wound while the jugular v. is prepared.

The internal jugular v. is dissected free through two 5 cm transverse incisions in the neck, one 2 cm above the clavicle and the other 3–4 cm below the mandible (Fig. 65.3a). Beginning in the lower incision, the internal jugular v is found by splitting muscle fibers of sternocleidomastoid to expose the vein. The vein is dissected circumferentially and surrounded with a quarter inch Penrose drain. From this point the vein is mobilized completely down to the clavicle and up as high as possible. Proximal dissection is then continued through the upper incision continuing to free the vein, first distally to meet the dissection from the lower incision and then cephalad to the base of the skull. The facial vein is ligated and divided.

Before dividing the vein, a tunnel is created by blunt dissection from the axillary vein, under the clavicle, and into the supraclavicular space. The tunnel is enlarged by dividing the subclavius muscle. In the supraclavicular space the tunnel is extended to the internal jugular vein just above the clavicle.

The proximal jugular v. is marked with a suture on its upper surface to avoid twisting when pulled through the tunnel. Proximally, the vein is suture ligated close to the base of the skull and the jugular

vein transected. The vein is pulled distally through the open vein bed and completely freed as distally as possible below the clavicle while paying attention to keep the marking suture upright. A valve in the vein prevents back bleeding so it is usually unnecessary to clamp the vein. Using a kidney pedicle clamp the jugular vein is pulled through the tunnel, again observing vein orientation to prevent twisting (Fig. 65.3b). One way to check for twisting is to pass a size 20–24 Fr. catheter up the jugular v. and into the SVC which should pass with ease; if not, the vein should be reoriented until the catheter does pass easily.

The axillary vein is occluded with vascular clamps or vessel loops and the jugular vein sewn end-to-side or end-to-end into it (Fig. 65.3c). Flow through the jugular vein is evaluated and the graft followed through its supraclavicular path releasing any kinks (Fig. 65.3d). The wounds are closed with subcutaneous and subcuticular absorbable sutures [7, 8].

Arteriovenous Fistula (AVF)

Because venous reconstructions are low pressure systems, they may thrombose more readily than arterial reconstructions. It has been demonstrated that this can be prevented by increasing flow and pressure across the suture line with a temporary arteriovenous fistula (AVF) [9–13]. This can be done with a Teflon reinforced PTFE prosthesis between the axillary artery and axillary vein distal (peripheral) to the axillary suture line which is looped to lie in the subcutaneous tissue making taking down the fistula fairly easy by dividing the prosthesis in the subcutaneous tissue and tying each end [12, 13]. Alternatively, an AVF can be created in the arm or forearm. The fistula is closed in 6–12 weeks.

We advocate constructing a temporary AVF after any of the venous reconstructions described above. While good results are obtainable without an AVF, data suggest that the added security of temporarily increasing flow across the fresh suture lines makes adding the AVF a worthwhile procedure [9–11].

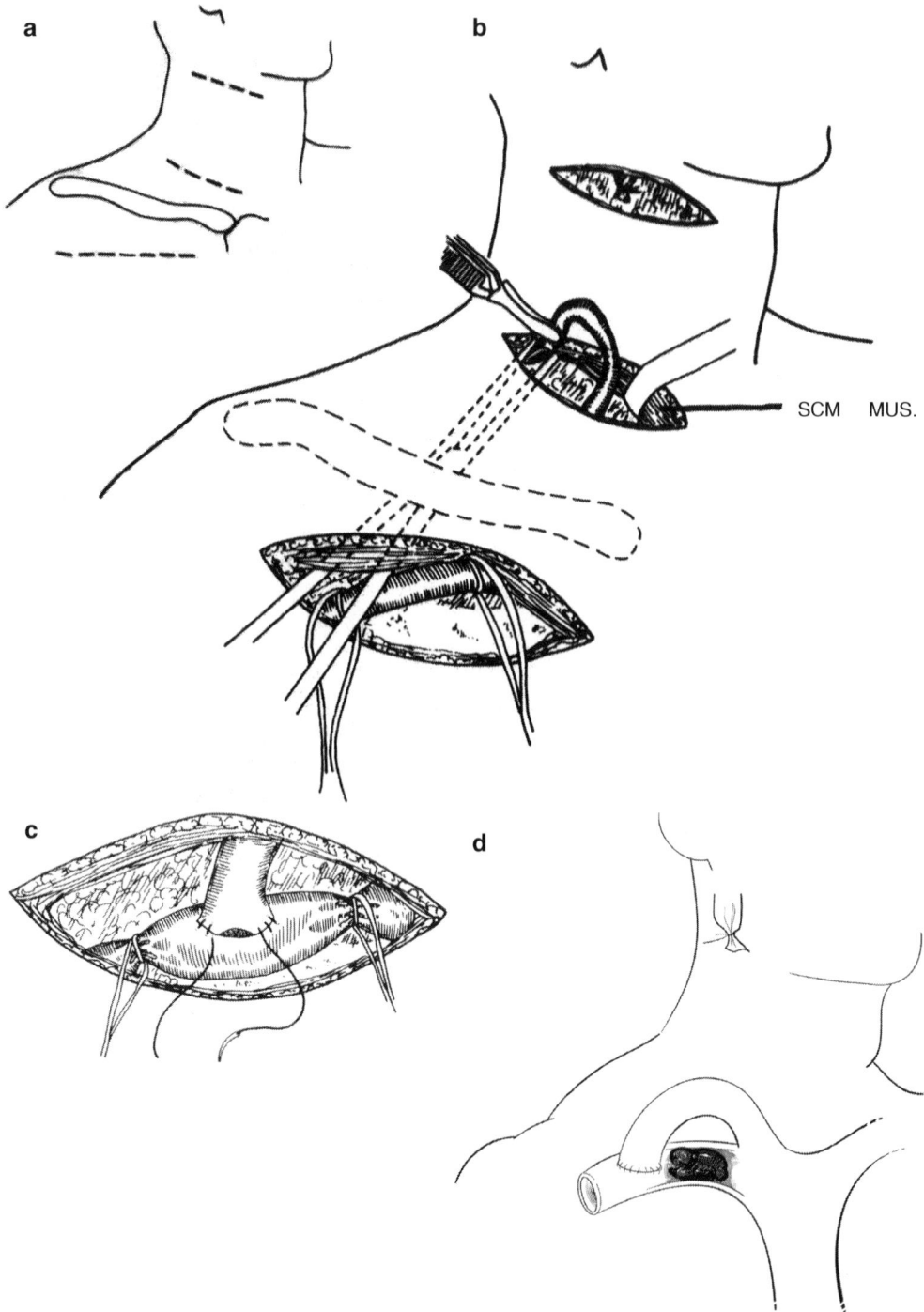

Fig. 65.3 Jugular vein turndown. (**a**) Location of incisions. (**b**) Jugular vein being passed through tunnel under clavicle. (**c**) Completed jugular-subclavian vein anastomosis. (**d**) Completed turndown (Reprinted with permission from Sanders and Haug [14] with permission from Elsevier)

References

1. Molina JE. Need for emergency treatment in subclavian vein effort thrombosis. J Am Coll Surg. 1995;181:414–20.
2. Pairolero PC, Walls JT, Payne WS, Hollier LH, Fairbairn JF. Subclavian-axillary artery aneurysms. Surgery. 1981;90:757–63.
3. Green RM, Waldman D, Oriel K, Riggs P, DeWeese JA. Claviculaectomy for subclavian venous repair. Long term functional results. J Vasc Surg. 2000;32:315–21.
4. Sanders RJ, Haug CE. Thoracic outlet syndrome: a common sequela of neck injuries. Philadelphia: Lippincott; 1991. p. 255.
5. Molina JE. A new surgical approach to the innominate and subclavian vein. J Vasc Surg. 1998;27:576–81.
6. Witte CL, Smith CA. Single anastomosis vein bypass for subclavian vein obstruction. Arch Surg. 1966;93:664–6.
7. Sanders RJ, Haug CE. Thoracic outlet syndrome: a common sequela of neck injuries. Philadelphia: Lippincott; 1991. p. 258.
8. Sanders RJ, Haug C. Subclavian vein obstruction and thoracic outlet syndrome: a review of etiology and management. Ann Vasc Surg. 1990;4:397–410.
9. Kunlin J. Le reestablissment de la circulation veineuse par graffe en cas d'obliteration traumatique ou thrombophlebetique. Mem Acad Chir. 1953;79:109–10.
10. Levin PM, Rich NM, Hutton Jr HC, et al. Role of arteriovenous shunt in venous reconstruction. Am J Surg. 1971;122:183–91.
11. Johnson V, Eiseman B. Evaluation of arteriovenous shunt to maintain patency of venous autograft. Am J Surg. 1969;118:915–20.
12. Eklof B, Albretique IJ, Einarsson E, et al. The temporary arteriovenous fistula in venous reconstructive surgery. Int Angiol. 1985;4:455–62.
13. Sanders RJ, Rosales C, Pearce WH. Creation and closure of temporary arteriovenous fistulas for venous reconstruction or thrombectomy: description of technique. J Vasc Surg. 1987;6:504–5.
14. Sanders RJ, Haug CE. Management of subclavian vein obstruction. In: Bergan JJ, Kistner RL, editors. Atlas of venous surgery. Philadelphia: WB Saunders; 1992. p. 255–72.

VTOS: Postoperative Care

66

David C. Cassada

Abstract

Surgery for venous thoracic outlet syndrome (TOS) may be required for symptoms ranging from severe recalcitrant arm swelling to acute axillo-subclavian vein thrombosis. The etiology appears to be multi-factorial, involving not only mechanical compression of the subclavian vein between the anterior scalene muscle, first rib, clavicle, subclavius muscle and costoclavicular ligament, but also hematological factors such as acquired and hereditary thrombophilia. Although the visible incisions appear rather small, a sizeable operation is often required to effectively decompress the subclavian vein after clot dissolution. Such surgery and the associated need for postoperative anticoagulation carry a number of risks and considerations. Attention to the many details of successfully helping a patient recover through first rib resection and postoperative care is required for an ultimately successful outcome. This chapter is intended to describe the general approach used in our institution for venous TOS and includes historical considerations and data supporting some of the surgical and medical decision-making.

Introduction

Thoracic outlet decompression for venous TOS is arguably the most technically and strategically challenging of the thoracic outlet operations [1–3]. History and physical examination may reveal that the etiology is purely a mechanical one, such as observed in a high-functioning athlete who might repetitively exert the arms and develop thick musculature of the shoulders and neck. Venous TOS with subclavian vein thrombosis can also be combined with occult or overt clotting abnormalities, especially in patients with seemingly fewer behavioral risk factors [4, 5]. There are significant diagnostic and planning issues relating to venous clot burden, thrombolysis, and surgical strategy when subclavian vein compression is found by imaging studies. The technique of thoracic outlet decompression is discussed in other sections of this textbook;

D.C. Cassada, MD, FACS
Division for Vascular Surgery, Stroobants Heart Center,
Centra Lynchburg General Hospital,
1901 Tate Springs Road, Lynchburg, VA 24501, USA
e-mail: david.cassada@centrahealth.com

K.A. Illig et al. (eds.), *Thoracic Outlet Syndrome*,
DOI 10.1007/978-1-4471-4366-6_66, © Springer-Verlag London 2013

Table 66.1 Identified causes of thrombophilia and complications in patients undergoing surgical treatment for venous TOS

Thrombophilia disorder	# of patients	Interval venoplasty	# of complications	Residua thrombusl	Residual swelling
PAI-1 mutation	5	3	6	3	2
MTHFR mutation	1	0	0	0	0
Protein S deficiency	1	0	0	0	1
Anticardiolipin antibody	2	1	1	0	0
Hyperhomocysteinemia	3	0	1	0	0
Lupus anticoagulant	1	0	1	0	0
Normal coagulation	5	3	2	1	2

Adapted from Cassada et al. [5]. With permission from Elsevier
Abbreviations: *MTHFR* methyltetrahydrofolate reductase, *PAI* plasminogen activator inhibitor-1

however, technical points of the operation and postoperative concerns are often intertwined during this discussion.

There is controversy in the literature over the timing of surgery, and to some even whether an operation is always needed in venous TOS with subclavian vein effort thrombosis [5–9]. Some clinicians contend that venous TOS is simply the upper extremity variant of deep vein thrombosis (DVT) as more commonly seen in the leg and pelvis, which responds favorably to treatment with anticoagulation alone. Part of the nonsurgical care that should be applied to all patients includes serological testing for thrombophilia (Table 66.1). Planar radiographic imaging is also valuable to exclude apical thoracic compressive disease due to neoplasm, infection and other processes exerting a mass effect [10–12]. Since venous TOS is relatively rare, it is essential to exclude intrathoracic disease that would not benefit from the same therapy.

In the absence of another disease process to explain spontaneous arm swelling and cyanosis, the majority of surgeons caring for patients with venous TOS view the process as an acquired veno-compressive condition with chronic trauma to the vein. Compressive trauma causes endothelial denudation and exposure of medial collagen, chronic vein wall healing with exuberant intimal thickening, and ultimately venous thrombosis. In this latter explanation, clot removal and surgical decompression, with or without vein repair, is the mainstay of treatment.

The various operative approaches and treatment strategies that are currently used for venous TOS are described in Chaps. 60, 61, 62, 63, 64, and 65.

In-Hospital Postoperative Care

The main tenants of patient care following thoracic outlet decompression operations include: pain control, pulmonary physiotherapy and support, anticoagulation decisions and surveillance for bleeding and thrombosis. Postoperative chest X-rays are taken at regular intervals, starting in the recovery room and every 24 h thereafter, to detect hemothorax, pneumothorax, or hematoma in the area of surgical dissection. The chest cavity can quietly accrue up to 5 l of blood, allowing a simple venous trickle to potentially turn catastrophic, as tachycardia and hypotension may only be present after loss of 30 % of the blood volume due to hemorrhage. For this reason, a urinary Foley catheter is left in place to monitor urine output for 24–72 h after surgery, to serve as an early warning for a drop in intravascular volume.

We have generally allowed 24–48 h after surgery before beginning anticoagulation, except in the most fulminant of clotting disorders. Treatment with intravenous heparin allows direct control of the activated partial thromboplastin time (aPTT) and avoids the tendency to "overshoot" that can occur with single-dosing regimens of low molecular weight heparin (LMWH). A surgical closed-suction drain is left in the operative field, above the pleural reflection, and brought out through a separate stab incision. Although this type of drain cannot evacuate all blood, drain output may provide an indicator of bleeding during the effort to optimize postoperative anticoagulation, and having a drain in place can help manage lymphatic leaks or seroma formation. The drain is removed as early as possible after surgery, using parameters such as less than 30 mL output per shift as a reasonable endpoint for removal (typically 5–7 days after operation).

Good postoperative pain control is essential for pulmonary care and patient participation in early range-of-motion physical therapy exercises. Some patients with venous TOS may have previously taken narcotic analgesics to help manage ambient pain, in which case adjustments have to be made to allow for opiate receptor upregulation. Intravenous patient-controlled analgesia (PCA) through a self-administered dosing regimen with morphine, hydromorphone or fentanyl is helpful to keep up with pain medication requirements for the first 24–72 h; however, rapid conversion to oral oxycodone compounds should be attempted because of the disparity between half-lives in these drugs.

We prefer to use a sling to manage pain that might occur on incidental motion or bumping of the arm when the patient is in the upright posture. We also recommend a snug sling with waist fixation and an abduction pillow to help patients have a comfortable posture while standing or riding in a motor vehicle. This device is applied in the hospital in anticipation of a long car ride home, and is recommended for the first 3 weeks of recovery, until more vigorous physical therapy is possible as an outpatient. Patients are discouraged from being totally dependent on the sling, but rather, to do range of motion exercises at least three times daily, with pain being a guide to intensity. Long-range physical therapy begins at 3 weeks and lasts at least to 6 weeks, whereby the patient is taught how to engage in home exercises done on their own. The physical therapy includes gentle movements to encourage tissue compliance and nerve gliding, along with an emphasis on diaphragmatic breathing. A patient and gentle approach to postoperative physical therapy is important, because more vigorous use of isometrics, rubber bands and heavy strength workouts can quickly diminish the postoperative result by irritating the brachial plexus and aggravating muscle spasm.

Postoperative Complications

Pneumothorax occurs in 2–5 % of patients undergoing first rib resection. Many surgeons intentionally or incidentally open the pleura during thoracic outlet decompression, allowing drainage of blood, serum or lymph away from the surgical field, where it can be expected to undergo resorption from the pleural space within days to several weeks. In contrast, we take efforts to bluntly dissect the parietal pleura from the underside of the first rib to keep the pleural space intact, with the view that this will potentially help limit pain, pulmonary compromise, and any subsequent need for interval drainage. The principal problem that can occur is when there has been inadvertent operative injury to the lung, which can create tension pneumothorax or failure of resolution of lung collapse even in the presence of a tube thoracostomy. The latter problem may be seen particularly in patients with emphysema and apical pleural bleb disease.

Infection is rare following surgery for venous TOS, due in part to the robust blood supply of the dissected tissues. Surgery for venous TOS may carry a slightly higher rate of infection than other thoracic outlet procedures, due to blood accumulation and potential inoculation of thrombus. Surgical site cellulitis occurs at a rate consistent with other sterile surgical procedures; however, deeper space infections occur commensurate with blood accumulation. Again, frequent physical examination, chest x-rays and blood laboratory work can help reveal an infectious process early in its course and determine the need for surgical drainage or antibiotic therapy.

Pulmonary embolism (PE) is fortunately a rare occurrence in patients with venous TOS. For bland arm DVTs that go untreated, there has been a cited rate of up to 13 % PE found by imaging studies [6]. Fortunately, the clot burden sustained in the arm veins is relatively low, and because there are few reported incidences of life-threatening PE derived from the arm, there is no sound rationale for superior vena cava filter interruption. In our experience of 68 patients surgically managed for venous TOS with subclavian vein thrombosis, we found only one patient to have compromised pulmonary function. In this example, there was an incidental lower extremity DVT that prompted inferior vena cava filter placement. There have been no randomized or prospective observational studies to estimate the rate of subclinical PE in patients with venous TOS.

Because the thoracic duct joins the venous system near the junction of the internal jugular and subclavian veins, it is susceptible to injury during mobilization of the scalene fat pad and other aspects of surgery for venous TOS. Postoperative lymph leaks can occur even when there was no visible indication of lymphatic injury at the time of the primary operation, and may become apparent only several days after surgery (particularly once the patient has resumed a regular diet). If there is an enlarging pleural effusion or persistent output of lymphatic fluid into the closed-suction drain (e.g., more than 250 mL/day), particularly when this is chylous in appearance and on the left side, a clear liquid diet is maintained along with administration of octreotide (100 µg every 8 h, subcutaneous) to reduce the volume of lymph flow, and removal of the closed-suction drain is deferred until the leak has subsided. Early supraclavicular reexploration is recommended for persistent high-volume lymph leaks (more than 500 mL/day for more than 5 days) or those resulting in chylothorax (Fig. 66.1). When a lymphatic leak is observed during the course of the reoperative procedure, the site of the leak is identified and oversewn with a pledgeted polypropylene suture, and a topical hemostatic/fibrin tissue sealant is applied to the site before wound closure.

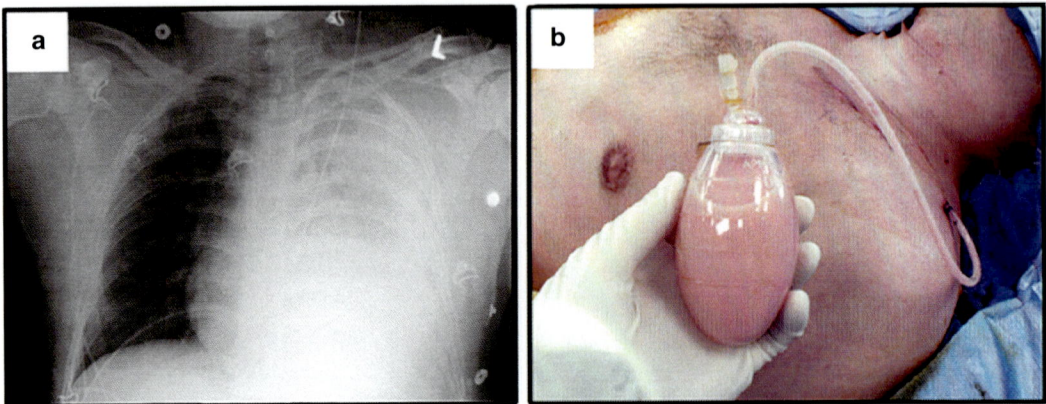

Fig. 66.1 Postoperative lymph leak. A young man underwent left-sided thoracic outlet decompression for venous TOS using a paraclavicular approach. (a) Postoperative chest x-ray 7 days after surgery demonstrating a large left pleural effusion. (b) There was high-volume output of cloudy lymph fluid into the closed-suction drain for several days, despite conversion to a clear liquid diet and treatment with octreotide. (c) Re-exploration through the supraclavicular incision revealed chylous lymph fluid from the area of the thoracic duct. This approach also allowed evacuation of several liters of lymph fluid from the pleural space. (d) The source of lymph leak was identified at the site of the thoracic duct, underneath the edge of the internal jugular vein. (e) Repair of the disrupted lymph vessel is best accomplished with a mattress suture technique using Dacron felt pledgets, to help "sandwich" the site of the leak. (f) Appearance of the site of lymph leak after mattress suture repair. (g) Topical application of a issue sealant (FloSeal) to the site of the lymph leak may also promote fibrous healing to prevent recurrence. (h) Chest x-ray the day after reoperation illustrating complete resolution of the left pleural effusion (Courtesy of Robert W. Thompson, MD (Washington University, St. Louis))

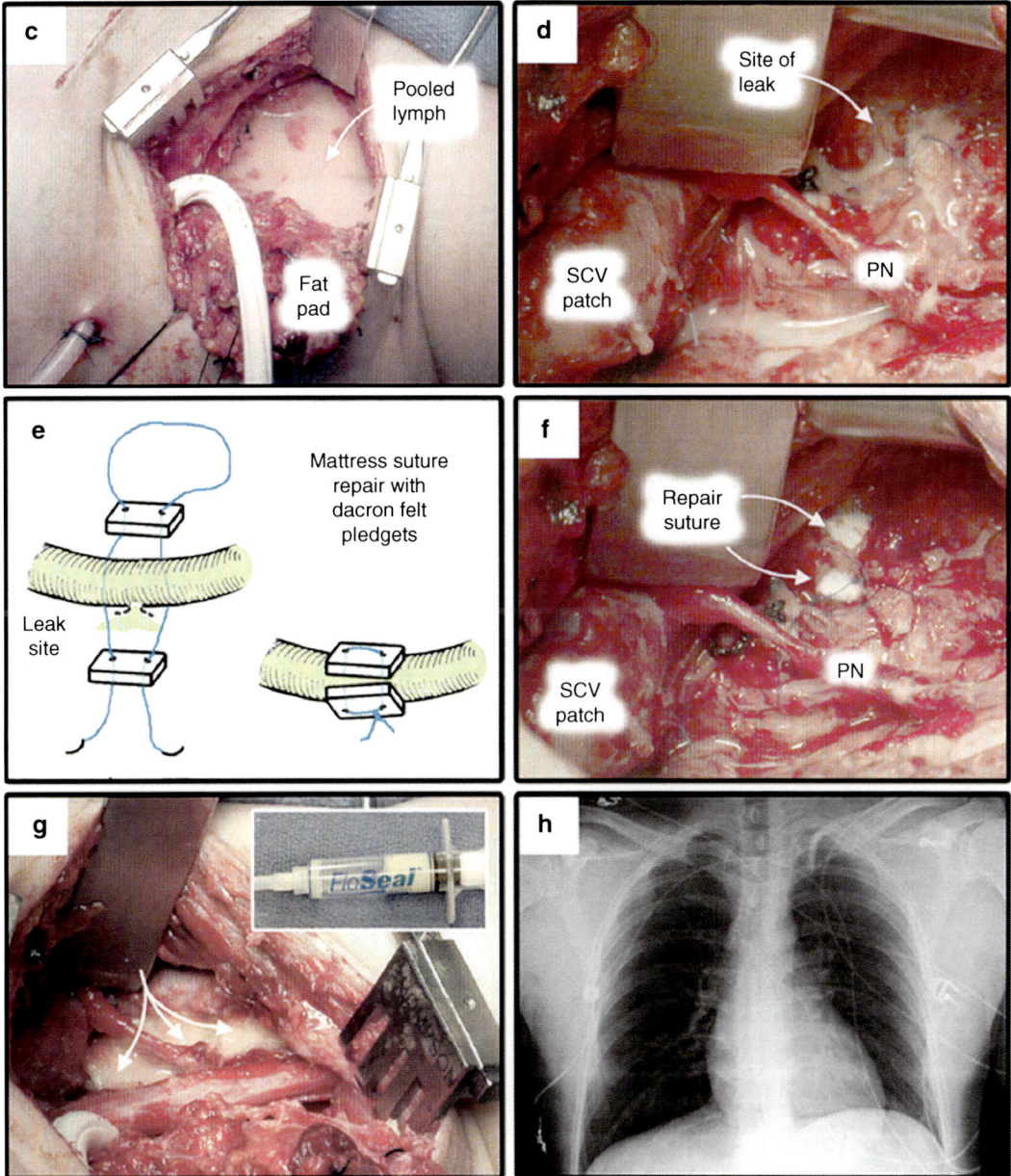

Fig. 66.1 (continued)

Adjunctive Approaches to Maintain Subclavian Vein Patency

Recently there has been literature about the fate of the damaged subclavian vein after surgical thoracic outlet decompression, and whether the native vein can spontaneously re-open or if expanded collateral vessels are sufficient to promote arm decompression [13]. Regardless of the mode of surgery or medical therapy, or the surgical procedure selected for venous TOS after initial diagnosis, ongoing evaluation is often required to help patients achieve optimal results of treatment. Techniques for imaging, including digital subtraction

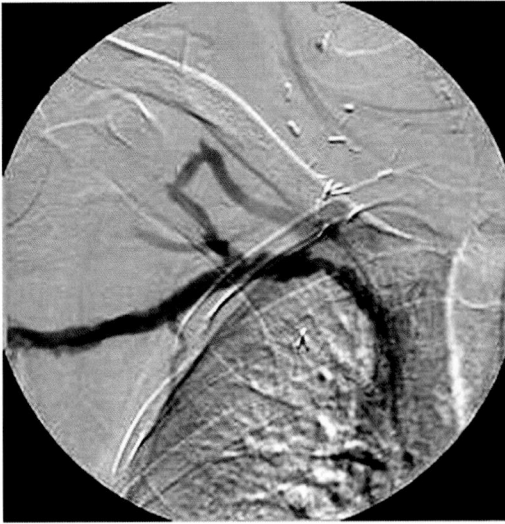

Fig. 66.2 Post-operative upper extremity venography. Right upper extremity contrast venogram performed 1 month after thoracic outlet decompression for venous TOS. There is an area of residual high-grade stenosis in the subclavian vein at the level of the first rib resection. A large suprascapular collateral vein is observed, draining from the axillary vein to the internal jugular vein

angiography (DSA), computerized tomographic angiography (CTA), magnetic resonance angiography (MRA), and intravascular ultrasound (IVUS) can all help determine vein patency, vascular wall thickening, intraluminal trabeculations, and residual thrombus (Fig. 66.2). The use of these tools can assist the decision for subclavian vein balloon angioplasty during or after surgery. Alternatively, some clinicians advocate direct subclavian vein reconstruction as part of the primary operation, when there is severe subclavian vein damage or chronic occlusion. Reconstructive techniques in this setting include subclavian vein patch angioplasty, axillo-subclavian vein bypass, and internal jugular vein turn-down bypass, with high reported primary patency rates and resolution of symptoms [2, 4, 14]. The use of endovascular stents in the dynamic region of the subclavian vein is strongly discouraged, due to the propensity of metal fracture with stress fatigue over a prolonged period and the young age of the typical patient, but there may be a role for endovascular stents in settings where first rib resection has already been completed.

Anticoagulation

Historically, post-decompressive anticoagulation has been managed variably, but often in a manner similar to that used in treating a DVT of the arm, or for up to 3–6 months after surgery. This treatment interval is influenced by the presence or absence of any underlying medical clotting disorders. The presence of pathological clotting is generally detected after at least 2 weeks of stopping a warfarin regimen. A strong family history of clotting problems can lead to persistent suspicion for a clotting disorder, even in the presence of completely negative coagulation panel results [5, 6]. Also, relying upon a positive coagulation panel test may depend upon waiting for a polymerase chain reaction or ELISA result, which can take weeks for a single patient. In general, knowing the precise etiology of any clotting tendency is useful for both patient and family counseling regarding the risk for thromboembolic events during surgery or illness and during the peripartum period. If there is no obvious family history, and a clear behavioral risk for subclavian vein effort thrombosis, then the use of strong anti-thrombotic agents might be limited to a shorter period of time or avoided altogether after surgery. At our institution, we advocate serological testing for concomitant blood disorders when a clear period of anticoagulation holiday is established (at least 14 days after discontinuing warfarin).

The decision for post-surgical anticoagulation should result in a "safe" interval relative to the risk of bleeding. Output from a closed-suction drain or tube thoracostomy (if present) may serve as an indicator of bleeding, when the patient is started on intravenous heparin and in the process of converting to oral anticoagulation with warfarin. During the first 48 h, a urinary catheter, heart monitor, frequent chest x-rays, and serial hemoglobin levels may help detect failure of hemostasis. If excessive bleeding occurs, anticoagulation is reversed and blood transfusion considered to stabilize the hemoglobin level. In a rare situation with severe hemorrhage, chest tube placement, chest exploration by video-assisted thoracoscopic surgery (VATS), or open thoracotomy might be needed. Although postoperative bleeding problems are rarely of concern after operations for neurogenic TOS, there should be heightened concern following operations for venous TOS due to the relatively early use of heparin, low molecular weight heparin (LMWH) and warfarin.

Some surgeons choose to restart anticoagulation with intravenous heparin 48–72 h after operation, with a transition to warfarin over the next several days; LMWH may also be used as a potential alternative to intravenous heparin. It is our practice to avoid LMWH due to the supratherapeutic or subtherapeutic levels that can occur with single dose regimens. Once administered, a single subcutaneous injection of LMWH blocks the intrinsic clotting system for up to 16 h, and lacks the responsiveness of simply turning off a heparin drip for rapid normalization of clotting. During the transition to long-term anticoagulation, many will use heparin for at least 48 h before adding warfarin; however, others will start warfarin at the same time as heparin given that it will take several days to achieve anticoagulant effects.

Temporary Arterio-Venous (AV) Fistulas

Due to the possibility of early re-thrombosis after a complex operation that might include direct axillary-subclavian vein reconstruction, many surgeons consider creating a minor arterio-venous fistula at the wrist to augment flow through the damaged region of the subclavian vein [15–17]. This has the additional effect of driving creation of hypertrophic collaterals that can further decompress venous hypertension in the arm. Surgical ligation of the fistula (or embolization) is generally performed between 3 and 6 months, after a stable endothelial lining of the subclavian vein is established. Upper extremity venography can also be performed at the time of planned AV fistula ligation, allowing the possibility of performing balloon angioplasty dilatation of any residual subclavian vein or anastomotic stenoses that might have developed during the postoperative period of healing.

Residual Subclavian Vein Obstruction

Failure of resolution of arm swelling or a delayed return to normal arm girth is not uncommon following thrombolysis and operations for venous TOS. This typically reflects one of two situations: the first is when there is a residual high-grade subclavian vein stenosis at the level of the first rib (or site of first rib resection), and the second is when there is complete subclavian vein occlusion, usually chronic in nature, with venous return provided solely by robust collaterals. Approximately 90 % of patients in the first group can be successfully treated in the postoperative period by venography and balloon angioplasty (sometimes employing a cutting and/or noncompliant balloon). This is usually performed 2–3 weeks after the principal operation, but some surgeons advocate intraoperative balloon angioplasty immediately upon completion of the surgical procedure, in a combined single-step surgical and endovascular strategy [18, 19]. In contrast, patients in the second group are optimally treated by an operative approach that permits subclavian vein bypass graft reconstruction (usually with creation of an adjunctive AV fistula) [20]. In the absence of direct vein reconstruction of this type, most patients with persistent symptoms and chronic subclavian vein occlusion should be treated with long-term anticoagulation to help prevent further thrombosis and loss of critical collaterals. In the rare patient with persistent arm swelling where there is no identifiable subclavian vein stenosis or occlusion, lymphedema can also be an etiological factor related to surgical dissection and post-surgical inflammation. This form of arm swelling can be managed with massage therapy and garment fitting to control fluid accumulation and symptoms of arm heaviness.

Follow-up Care

Patients are typically discharged from the hospital 3–4 days after uncomplicated operations for venous TOS, but hospital stay can be extended if full anticoagulation is desired prior to discharge. In addition to the steps described above, hospital

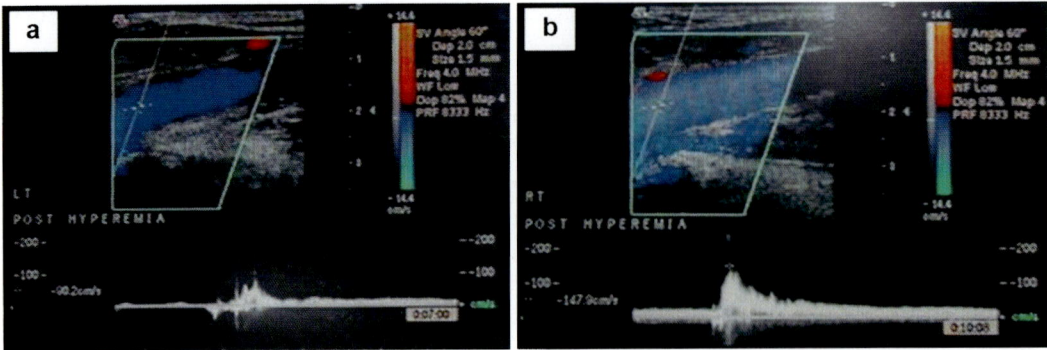

Fig. 66.3 Post-hyperemia venous duplex to detect residual subclavian vein obstruction. Duplex examination was performed 6 weeks after left-sided first rib resection for venous TOS. Pressure was placed over the mid-humerus level (brachial and basilic veins) of each arm for approximately 1 min until hyperemia was apparent. After release of the pressure, the patient was asked to inhale to equilibrate intrathoracic pressure with the arm, and Duplex images, waveforms, and peak velocity measurements were obtained. (**a**) Left-sided post-hyperemia Duplex image and waveform, demonstrating attenuation that likely reflects residual venous thrombus, intraluminal trabeculations, or venous stenosis that was not resolved by surgical treatment. This type of finding suggests the potential need for venography and possible balloon angioplasty. (**b**) Right-sided post-hyperema Duplex image and waveform, demonstrating high-flow consistent with a widely patent axillary-subclavian vein on the asymptomatic unaffected side

care is directed toward pulmonary care, avoiding atelectasis through incentive spirometry, and progressive activity. Patients are encouraged to ambulate by the second day after surgery and at least three times daily thereafter. Physical therapy is initiated the day after surgery to help maintain upper extremity range of motion. Release to home is considered when the patient has no fever, is tolerating pain well with oral narcotics, and is able to ambulate without assistance. After discharge the patient is seen within 2 weeks and then monthly until maximal medical improvement is determined. If the patient travels a long distance, follow up with a physical therapist is sought near the hometown.

Some form of monitoring of the status of the subclavian vein is often used during follow-up evaluation. Duplex ultrasound can be used to help identify upper extremity extremity thrombus and to track clot accumulation or resolution over time [21]. However, ultrasound examination of the subclavian vein is technically limited due to difficulties visualizing the vein beneath the clavicle and misinterpretation of flow through enlarged collaterals, and can therefore not be used to exclude subclavian vein stenosis or even focal occlusion. If complete imaging evaluation is desired, CT, MR or catheter-based contrast venography is needed. We have recently developed a novel method to enhance the information obtainable by Duplex examination, involving a brief period of venous hyperemia followed by release of blood flow [22]. By measuring the peak velocity of venous return and waveform quality during these maneuvers and comparing them to the normal contralateral extremity, we are able to create a dynamic picture that can detect central venous obstruction in areas otherwise inaccessible to direct ultrasound imaging (Fig. 66.3).

Progression of Activity

In our institution occupational therapy has taken an interest in the postoperative rehabilitation of patients with TOS. The main tenants of care are to teach the patient to engage in active or assisted-passive range of motion in all planes of the gleno-humeral joint, and to maintain mobility of serratus anticus by raising the arm overhead, but only to the point of pain. The goals of these instructions are to lightly maintain and improve compliance of the soft tissues while not inducing tissue damage or nerve irritation. After 3 weeks, the patient is seen in the office and prescribed a course of physical therapy based upon the theories of Peter Edgelow, PT, PhD. An arm sling is provided for longs periods of travel or standing, which has the characteristics of waist fixation and 30° shoulder abduction. The patient is encouraged to reduce dependency of the arm over the first 3 weeks following surgery to prevent edema.

Timing of Return to Work and Athletics

There is tremendous variation in the pace by which patients are able to return to occupational and recreational activities. Determinants include the type of work, athletics or play; the severity of underlying neuropathic pain; and psychological overlay. In addition, the presence of an active legal case that is contingent upon the patient having a certain level of disability is often an impasse to full recovery. These patients are, nonetheless, pushed to their threshold of activity under the supervision of surgeon and physical or occupational therapist.

No strengthening exercises are recommended prior to 3–6 weeks after surgery, with more aggressive strengthening exercises gradually introduced between 6 and 12 weeks to progress toward future intended activities. Failure to maintain postoperative improvement in these early stages is a poor prognosticator for future work capacity; however, a full year should occur prior to any consideration of reoperation for persistent symptoms. When ongoing pain management is required for optimal activity 3 months or longer after surgical recovery, it is our practice to refer patients to a specialist in techniques and pharmacology for chronic pain control.

Summary

In summary, venous TOS complicated by subclavian vein effort thrombosis is predominantly a surgical condition. Like other forms of TOS, a multi-modality approach among the clinicians

from various specialties is ideal for optimal outcomes. Based upon the goals of complete first rib resection and various approaches to establish a patent subclavian vein, the operations performed for venous TOS are necessarily complex. Attention to the details and many aspects of postoperative care is important to minimize the risk of early and late complications, and to reduce the potential for poor outcomes.

References

1. Divi V, Proctor MC, Axelrod DA, Greenfield LJ. Thoracic outlet decompression for subclavian vein thrombosis: experience in 71 patients. Arch Surg. 2005;140:54–7.
2. Sanders RJ, Hammond SL. Venous thoracic outlet syndrome. Hand Clin. 2004;20:113–8.
3. Illig KA, Doyle AJ. A comprehensive review of Paget-Schroetter syndrome. J Vasc Surg. 2010;51: 1538–47.
4. Sanders RJ, Haug C. Subclavian vein obstruction and thoracic outlet syndrome: a review of etiology and management. Ann Vasc Surg. 1990;4:397–410.
5. Cassada DC, Lipscomb AL, Stevens SL, Freeman MB, Grandas OH, Goldman MH. The importance of thrombophilia in the treatment of Paget-Schroetter syndrome. Ann Vasc Surg. 2006;20(5):596–601.
6. Kommareddy A, Zoroukian MH, Houssouna HI. Upper extremity deep vein thrombosis. Semin Thromb Hemost. 2002;28:89–99.
7. Lee WA, Hill BB, Harris Jr EJ, Semba CP, Olcott CI. Surgical intervention is not required for all patients with subclavian vein thrombosis. J Vasc Surg. 2000; 32:57–67.
8. Lee JT, Karwowski JK, Harris EJ, Haukoos JS, Olcott C. Long-term thrombotic recurrence after non-operative management of Paget-Schroetter syndrome. J Vasc Surg. 2006;43:1236–43.
9. Urschel Jr HC, Patel AN. Surgery remains the most effective treatment for Paget-Schroetter syndrome: 50 years' experience. Ann Thorac Surg. 2008;86: 254–60.
10. Hasanadka R, Towne JB, Seabrook GR, et al. Computed tomography angiography to evaluate thoracic outlet neurovascular compression. Vasc Endovascular Surg. 2007;41:316–21.
11. O'Brien PJ, Ramasunder S, Cox MW. Venous thoracic outlet syndrome secondary to first rib osteochondroma in a pediatric patient. J Vasc Surg. 2011; 53:811–3.
12. Chilihara K, Niwa H. Surgical treatment for tumors in the superior sulcus. Kyobu Geka. 2010;63:712–8.
13. de Leon R, Chang DC, Busse C, Call D, Freischlag JA. First rib resection and scalenectomy for chroni-

cally occluded subclavian veins: what does it really do? Ann Vasc Surg. 2008;22:395–401.

14. Melby SJ, Vedantham S, Narra VR, Paletta Jr GA, Khoo-Summers L, Driskill M, Thompson RW. Comprehensive surgical management of the competitive athlete with effort thrombosis of the subclavian vein (Paget-Schroetter syndrome). J Vasc Surg. 2008;47:809–20.

15. Sanders RJ, Rosales C, Pearce WH. Creation and closure of temporary arteriovenous fistulas for venous reconstruction or thrombectomy: description of technique. J Vasc Surg. 1987;6:504–5.

16. Thompson RW, Schneider PA, Nelken NA, Skioldebrand CG, Stoney RJ. Circumferential venolysis and paraclavicular thoracic outlet decompression for "effort thrombosis" of the subclavian vein. J Vasc Surg. 1992;16:723–32.

17. Thompson RW. Venous thoracic outlet syndrome: paraclavicular approach. Op Tech Gen Surg. 2008;10: 113–21.

18. Kunkel JM, Machleder HI. Treatment of Paget-Schroetter syndrome. A staged, multidisciplinary approach. Arch Surg. 1989;124:1153–7.

19. Schneider DB, Dimuzio PJ, Martin ND, Gordon RL, Wilson MW, Laberge JM, Kerlan RK, Eichler CM, Messina LM. Combination treatment of venous thoracic outlet syndrome: open surgical decompression and intraoperative angioplasty. J Vasc Surg. 2004;40: 599–603.

20. Thompson RW, Petrinec D, Toursarkissian B. Surgical treatment of thoracic outlet compression syndromes. II. Supraclavicular exploration and vascular reconstruction. Ann Vasc Surg. 1997;11:442–51.

21. Ouriel K. Noninvasive diagnosis of upper extremity vascular disease. Semin Vasc Surg. 1998;11:54–9.

22. Lebow MEJ, Nagarsheth KJ, Cassada D, Goldman M. Duplex derived maximal venous outflow velocity (MVOV) of the common femoral veins is asymmetric in normal women. J Vas Ultrasound. 2009;33:13–5.

Adam J. Doyle

Abstract

The study of venous thoracic outlet syndrome (VTOS), while apparently as objective an entity as any within this family of disorders, suffers from a lack of objectivity when results are reported. The literature is not consistent regarding how VTOS is diagnosed or results are described. VTOS is a spectrum of clinical problems, some representing acute issues and others chronic disease states. Most reports lump all patients together, there is little consistency with regard to outcomes reporting, and there are no prospective randomized studies. As a result, there is lack of consensus on how to treat these patients and no high-level evidence-based recommendations for care. This chapter attempts to describe outcomes within these constraints, but it is stressed that to truly understand this syndrome we must agree on criteria for diagnosis, acceptable methods of treatment, and consistent standards for reporting outcomes.

Introduction

The study of venous thoracic outlet syndrome (VTOS), while apparently as objective an entity as any within this family of disorders, suffers from a lack of objectivity when results are reported. The literature is not consistent regarding how VTOS is diagnosed or results are described. VTOS is a spectrum of clinical problems, some representing acute issues and others chronic disease states. Most reports lump all patients together, there is little consistency with regard to outcomes reporting, and there are no prospective randomized studies. As a result, there is lack of consensus on how to treat these patients and no high-level evidence-based recommendations for care. This chapter attempts to describe outcomes within these constraints, but it is stressed that to truly understand this syndrome we must agree on criteria for diagnosis, acceptable methods of treatment, and consistent standards for reporting outcomes. This chapter will present the outcomes of modern published reports relating to the treatment of primary VTOS and conclude with a suggested treatment algorithm.

A.J. Doyle, MD
Department of Surgery,
University of Rochester Medical Center,
601 Elmwood Ave, Box SURG,
Rochester, NY 14642, USA
e-mail: adam_doyle@urmc.rochester.edu

K.A. Illig et al. (eds.), *Thoracic Outlet Syndrome*,
DOI 10.1007/978-1-4471-4366-6_67, © Springer-Verlag London 2013

Methods

Outcomes can be reported on the basis of symptomatology or patency. Few studies have quantified these outcomes consistently, probably as a consequence of the rarity of the disease and the lack of standardized nomenclature and reporting standards. Treatment strategies that have been so developed represent clinical pathways used at each individual institution. Each step in any clinical pathway can be analyzed independently, although it must be recognized that doing this neglects the individual patient selection and judgment used at each institution. Finally, it must be emphasized that significant reporting bias exists within the literature surrounding VTOS (as it does with any rare disease). Specifically, patients referred to surgeons generally have more severe symptoms then those that are not and published results are dominated by those with large clinics and academic interests, and thus most of the results reported likely do not apply to less severe manifestations of VTOS.

For this chapter a systematic review of the literature was undertaken from 1996 to present. If multiple reviews had been published from any one institution, the most recent institutional review where VTOS was considered independently of ATOS and NTOS was used. Each paper was reviewed for specifics relating to patient factors, timing of presentation, modalities of treatment, adjuvant treatments, and outcomes. Although arbitrary, 6 weeks from onset of symptoms to initial treatment was used as a cutoff between acute and chronic presentation of VTOS. Each institutional series was categorized by the original intention to treat. Analyzed outcomes included percent of patients who were asymptomatic, vein patency, and length of followup. Asymptomatic status was especially emphasized as it should be considered the gold standard for successful functional treatment outcome, just as patency is the gold standard of anatomic surgical outcome. Results were pooled and reported as weighted averages when applicable. A summary of all studies considered for inclusion in this analysis is summarized in Table 67.1.

No Treatment and Anticoagulation Alone in VTOS

Although largely of historical interest, the natural history of truly untreated VTOS (literally no treatment at all) is important to know because lack of proper care led to significant long-term morbidity in the large majority of patients [1]. Even after the advent of oral anticoagulation patient outcomes were poor. In one early series, 78 % of patients treated with anticoagulation alone were left with persistent symptoms secondary to extremity venous obstruction [2], and in subsequent series persistent symptoms and significant disability were reported to occur in 41–91 % and 39–68 % of patients, respectively [1–7]. In modern reports "negligible symptoms" or "excellent to good long-term results" are found in only 46 and 29 % of patients, respectively, treated with anticoagulation alone [5, 8]. This treatment algorithm can probably be definitively condemned based on the weight of historical experience alone.

The Role of Decompressive Surgery in VTOS

In the mid-1960s and early 1970s several authors described surgical decompression of the thoracic outlet with or without adjuvant open thromboembolectomy for the treatment of effort thrombosis and reported good results in the majority of patients [2, 9–13]. Since that time most have accepted surgical decompression as standard of care. No prospective randomized data exists, however, comparing the current clinical pathway to other treatment modalities, and there are several algorithms that have been shown to provide adequate thoracic outlet decompression, relief of symptoms, and long-term patency [14–20].

What may be in common to all such options is that regardless of operative approach all such techniques require that the subclavian vein be completely decompressed and freed from adherent scar tissue.

Pre-decompression Catheter-Directed Interventions

First successfully used for the treatment of effort thrombosis in the late 1970s and early 1980s, catheter-directed thrombolysis for acute subclavian vein clot has become the standard of care for this problem, as it quickly and safely removes the occluding clot [21–24]. Combining the results of experience above, decompression of the bony thoracic outlet is recommended as the next and necessary step, but initially there was not consistent standard regarding the timing of such surgery. Thrombolysis can be expected to be successful in some patients up to 6 weeks following thrombosis (Table 67.2). Older series report decreasing rates of success if intervention occurred in patients with symptoms of more than 14 days, but newer series report more promising results [14, 24–26]. In general, thrombolysis probably has a limited role in chronic VTOS (defined variably) owing to low success rates [8, 14, 27]. Factors associated with either increased clot burden or clot chronicity have been associated with thrombolysis failure [28, 29].

Following thrombolysis a significant number of patients are found to have obvious intrinsic venous defects [14, 28, 29]. Although tempting to treat, there is probably no role for preoperative venoplasty in patients with any form of VTOS as success rates are low (Table 67.3). Endovascular intervention should probably be limited to the decompressed thoracic outlet; preoperative venoplasty, although tempting, may actually worsen outcomes [30, 31]. Finally, numerous centers have reported abysmal outcomes of stents placed in non-decompressed thoracic outlets, with failure rates approaching 100 %! [17, 30, 32–34].

When viewed in comparison to decompressive surgery, stent placement can be viewed as potentially causing harm.

Institutional Treatment Algorithms

Following the observation that surgical decompression had better outcomes than anticoagulation alone and that a high percentage of patients re-thrombose the subclavian vein if no decompression surgery is performed despite anticoagulation, decompression following thrombolysis became the standard of care at most centers. Although initially a delay was felt to be safer [17], over the past two decades it has been recognized that thoracic outlet decompression immediately following thrombolytic administration is safe and effective [14, 18, 35, 36]. A push for complete treatment within one hospitalization arose from the observation that one third to one half of patients re-thrombose within this original 1–3 month interval and that a "same admission" algorithm was safe [8, 37–40]. Several subsequent treatment algorithms have been developed to help guide care of these patients [14, 16, 17, 41–45].

There is no consensus regarding the best operative approach to thoracic outlet decompression (see Chap. 73) [15, 28, 46–48]. Each is well described, and in the hands of an experienced surgeon, is performed with low rates of morbidity. Success rates are nearly uniform with all and are reported to be greater than 90 % [14, 20, 42, 49]. The literature lacks uniform reporting of outcomes and long-term follow-up in these patients, and the short-term morbidity versus long-term outcomes are poorly compared.

Surprisingly, there are no prospective data to justify thrombolytic therapy. In fact, some practitioners question the need for thoracic outlet decompression in patients following successful thrombolysis as the majority of these patients will not re-thrombose. Data from Stanford reported recurrence (defined as requiring decompression)

Table 67.1 Summary of modern VTOS literature

Author (year) [Ref]	Institution	Subjects	Interval from Dx to tx	Type of VTOS	Preop management	Interval from lysis to decomp
Hempel (1996) [54]	Baylor	47	NR	Effort thrombosis (100 %) by venogram	Anticoagulation and/or thrombolysis (100 %), lysis success rate NR	1–2 weeks
Sheeran (1997) [44]	UCONN and Brown	14, mean age 34, 69 % right-sided, 43 % male	3.9 days	Effort thrombosis (100 %) by venogram	Thrombolysis and anticoagulation in 100 %, lysis success 93 % (13/14)	1 week to 7 months
Adelman (1997) [25]	NYU	17, mean age NR, 50 % right-sided, 33 % male	Within 8 days 82 % (14/17), greater than 8 days in 18 % (3/17)	Effort thrombosis (100 %) by venogram	Thrombolysis and anticoagulation in 100 %, lysis success 82 % (12/17)	6 weeks
Lee (1998) [30]	Brigham and Women's Hospital	11, mean age 30, side NR, 64 % (7/11) male	24 h to 2.5 weeks	Effort thrombosis (100 %) by venogram	Thrombolysis and anticoagulation in 100 %, lysis success 82 % (9/11), pre-op venoplasty 45 % (5/11), venoplasty success before decompression 0 % (0/5)	Within 5 days
Azakie (1998) [55]	UCSF and Washington University St. Louis, MO	21, mean age 26, 67 % (14/21) right-sided, gender NR	Less than 2 weeks	Effort thrombosis (100 %) by venogram	Thrombolysis and anticoagulation in 81 % (17/21), lysis success 100 % (17/17), pre-op venoplasty 29 % (6/21), venoplasty success before decompression 0 % (0/6), pre-op venoplasty + stent 5 % (1/21), Venoplasty + stent success before decompression 0 % (0/1)	Within 1 week

Mode of decomp	Venous reconstruction required	Adjuvant treatment	Recurrence rate	Post-op Anticoag	Morbidity and mortality	Outcome
Supraclavicular first rib resection and scalenectomy in 100 %	No	None	0 %	NR	None	100 % (47/47) asymptomatic, F/U NR
Method NR, immediate FRR or venous recon in 36 % (5/14), delayed FRR in 29 % (4/14)	7 % (1/14)	Venoplasty in 36 % (5/14)	0 % in lysis and immediate decompression group 44 % in lysis alone group	3 months of coumadin	None	44 % (4/9) asymptomatic if lysis with delayed FRR if recurrence @ 28 months mean F/U 80 % (4/5) asymptomatic with lysis and immediate FRR or venous recon @ 16 months mean F/U
first rib resection and scalenectomy in 92 % (11/12) following successfult lysis	0 %	0 %	8 % (1/12) of patients successfully Lysed	ASA alone	50 % (5/10) pneumothorax with rib resection	100 % (11/11) patency for successful thrombolysis + decompression @ 21 months mean F/U 100 % (11/11) asymptomatic for successful thrombolysis + decompression @ 21 months mean F/U 0 % (0/5) asymptomatic in patients with failed thrombolysis and no decompression @ 21 months mean F/U
Decompression in 100 % (11/11) by varied techniques, (3/11) transaxillary first rib resection and scalenectomy, (8/11) supraclacicular or paraclavicular with scalenotomy, Venolysis or reconstruction/ bypass in 100 % (11/11)	45 % (5/11) patch venoplasty in (3/11), IJ-SCV bypass in (2/11)	None	18 % (2/11)- re-operations for incomplete decompression, both with subsequent restoration of patency and relief of symptoms	3–6 months of coumadin	NR	100 % (6/6) patency for successful thrombolysis + decompression @ 1 to 6 months F/U 82 % (9/11) asymptomatic for successful thrombolysis + decompression @ 24 months mean F/U
Decompression in 100 % (21/21) by varied techniques, mainly supra/ paraclavicular first rib resection with scalenectomy, and circumfrential venolysis in 100 %	14 % (3/21) SCV-IJ bypass (1), thrombec-tomy and vein patch venoplasty (2)	19 % (4/21) required venoplasty post-decompres-sion, 100 % (4/4) success rate	5 % (1/21) for entire series, with RTOR for with successful restoration of patency	NR	15 % (5/34), for entire series (1 RTOR for bleeding, RTOR for re-thrombo-sis, 1 RTOR for lymph leak, 2 nerve injuries)	100 % (21/21) patency @ between 1 week and 3 months F/U 95 % (20/21) asymptomatic @ 31 months average F/U

(continued)

Table 67.1 (continued)

Author (year) [Ref]	Institution	Subjects	Interval from Dx to tx	Type of VTOS	Preop management	Interval from lysis to decomp
Azakie (1998) [55]	UCSF and Washington University St. Louis, Mo	8, mean age 32, 88 % (7/8) right-sided, gender NR	NR	Chronic occlusion (100 %) by venogram	Multiple prior failed decompression surgeries	NR
Azakie (1998) [55]	UCSF and Washington University St. Louis, Mo	4, mean age 49, 100 % (4/4) right-sided, gender NR	NR	High-grade symptomatic stenosis (100 %) by venogram	None	NR
Angle (2001) [35]	UCLA	9, mean age 36, side NR, 33 % (3/9) male	NR	Effort thrombosis (100 %) by venogram	Thrombolysis with anticoagulation 100 % (9/9), lysis success 100 % (9/9)	87 day median
Angle (2001) [35]	UCLA	9, mean age 27, side NR, 33 % (3/9) male	NR	Effort thrombosis (100 %) by venogram	Thrombolysis with anticoagulation 100 % (9/9), lysis success 89 % (8/9)	3 day median
Feugier (2001) [56]	Edouard Herriot Hospital, Lyon, France	11, mean age 33.6, 60 % right-sided, 80 % male	5.2 days	Effort thrombosis (100 %) by venogram	Anticoagulation alone 36 % (4/11), anticoagulation success 75 % (3/4), thrombolysis with anticoagulation 64 % (7/11), lysis success 71 % (5/7)	9 days to 12 months
Kreienberg (2001) [53]	Albany	23, mean age 30.3, 48 % right-sided, 48 % male	9.4 days	Effort thrombosis (100 %) by venogram	Thrombolysis and anticoagulation in 100 %, lysis success 91 % (21/23)	Immediate

Mode of decomp	Venous reconstruction required	Adjuvant treatment	Recurrence rate	Post-op Anticoag	Morbidity and mortality	Outcome
Decompression in 100 % (8/8) by varied techniques, mainly supra/paraclavicular first rib resection with scalenectomy, and circumfrential venolysis in 100 %	NR	NR	NR	NR	See above	0 % (0/8) asymptomatic @ 31 months average F/U 50 % (4/8) improved post decompression @ 31 months average F/U
Decompression in 100 % (4/4) by varied techniques, mainly supra/paraclavicular first rib resection with scalenectomy, and circumfrential venolysis in 100 %	NR	NR	NR	NR	See above	100 % (4/4) asymptomatic @ 31 months average F/U
Decompression in 100 % (9/9) by Transaxillary first rib resection with scalenectomy and venolysis	0 %	22 % (2/9) required venoplasty post-decompression, 100 % (2/2) success rate	11 % (1/9) rethrombosis, 100 % (2/2) successfully treated with thrombolysis	3 of coumadin	None	100 % patent (9/9) @ 2 weeks F/U 100 % asymptomatic (9/9) @ 51 days median F/U
Decompression in 100 % (9/9) by Transaxillary first rib resection with scalenectomy and venolysis	0 %	33 % (3/9) required venoplasty post-decompression, 100 % (3/3) success rate	22 % (2/9) rethrombosis, 100 % successfully treated with thrombolysis	3 of coumadin	None	100 % patent (9/9) @ 2 weeks F/U 100 % asymptomatic (9/9) @ 51 days median F/U
FRR by varied approaches in 91 % (10/11), claviculectomy in 9 % (1/11), combined with scalenectomy 82 % (9/11), and circumfrential venolysis in 73 % (8/11)	36 % (4/11)	Thrombectomy in 18 % (2/11)	0 %	NR		100 % patency (5/5) and 86 % (6/7) asymptomatic in patients who underwent lysis+decompression, @ 39 months mean F/U 100 % patency (3/3) and 50 % (2/4) asymptomatic in patients who underwent anticoagulation+decompression @ 35 months mean F/U
Scalenectomy and venolysis alone in 30 % (7/23), FRR and scalenectomy and venolysis in 70 % (16/23)	0 %	Venoplasty in 39 % (9/23)	0 % in patients that received lysis/decompression/venoplasty	6 to 18 months of coumadin		100 % patency (9/9) and 100 % asymptomatic in patients who underwent lysis+decompression+venoplasty @ 48 months mean F/U
		Venoplasty and stenting in 61 % (14/23)	36 % (5/14) in patients that received lysis/decompression/venoplasty+stent			64 % patency (9/14) and 57 % asymptomatic (8/14) in patients who underwent lysis+decompression+venoplasty+stent @ 36 months mean F/U

(continued)

Table 67.1 (continued)

Author (year) [Ref]	Institution	Subjects	Interval from Dx to tx	Type of VTOS	Preop management	Interval from lysis to decomp
Coletta (2001) [57]	Naval Medical center San Diego	19, mean age 26, 55 % right-sided, 76 % male	Hours to 10 months	Effort thrombosis (100 %) by venogram	Anticoagulation alone in 5 % (1/19), thrombolysis and anticoagulation in 95 % (18/19), lysis success rate NR	5 days to 3 weeks
Lokanathan (2001) [58]	University of British Columbia	28, mean age 36, 82 % dominant side, 71 % male	5.5 days	Effort thrombosis (100 %) by venogram	Anticoagulation alone in 11 % (3/28), anticoagulation and thrombolysis in 89 % (25/28), lysis success rate 88 % (22/25)	3–4 months
Schneider (2004) [19]	UCSF and Thomas Jefferson University	25, median age 30, side NR, 36 % (9/25) male	Less than 4 weeks	Effort thrombosis in 92 % (23/25), severe subclavian vein stenosis in 8 % (2/25), both diagnosed by venogram	Anticoagulation alone in 8 % (2/25), anticoagulation success rate 100 % (2/2) anticoagulation and thrombolysis in 84 % (21/25), lysis success rate 100 % (21/21)	Immediated

Mode of decomp	Venous reconstruction required	Adjuvant treatment	Recurrence rate	Post-op Anticoag	Morbidity and mortality	Outcome
Transaxillary first rib resection in 95 % (18/19)	No	Venoplasty alone in 11 % (2/18)	None	3 months of coumadin		Patency not reported
		Venoplsty + stent in 33 % (6/18)				100 % (10/10) asymptomatic in patients who underwent thrombolysis + anticoagulation + decompression
						100 % (2/2) asymptomatic in patients who underwent thrombolysis + anticoagulation + decompression + venoplasty
						83 % (5/6) asymptomatic in patients who underwent thrombolysis + anticoagulation + decompression + venoplasty + stent
						0 % (0/1) asymptomatic in the patient managed with anticoagulation alone
Transaxillary first rib resection in 4 % (1/28), claviculectomy in 4 % (1/28)	No	Venoplasty alone in 46 % (13/28), success = less than 50 % residual stenosis in 46 % (6/13)	27 % (3/11) in patients with follow-up imaging	3 months of coumadin minimum		73 % (8/11) patency at 3 - 17 months of follow-up
						28 % (6/21) asymptomatic @ 35 months mean F/U
						46 % (13/21) mild symptoms (DASH scores < 20) @ 35 months mean F/U
paraclavicular first rib resection in 92 % (23/25), infraclavicular first rib resection in 8 % (2/25), 100 % (25/25) with anterior and middle scalenectomy, venolysis on a cas-by-case basis	None	Venoplasty alone in 64 % (16/25), success = less than 30 % residual stenosis in 100 % (16/16)	8 % (2/25) rethrombosis with RTOR in both and thrombolysis, 50 % (1/2) lysis success	ASA in 84 % (21/25), Coumadin in remaining 16 % (4/25) cases of rethrombosis or non-occlusive thrombus on DUS	16 % (4/25), hematoma requiring RTOR in 3 patients	92 % primary patency @ 12 months by life table analysis
						96 % secondary patency @ 12 months by life table analysis
						96 % asymptomatic @ 12 months F/U

(continued)

Table 67.1 (continued)

Author (year) [Ref]	Institution	Subjects	Interval from Dx to tx	Type of VTOS	Preop management	Interval from lysis to decomp
Lee (2006) [16]	Sanford	64, mean age 32, 67 % dominant side, 66 % right-sided, 48 % male	NR	Axillosubclavian vein thrombosis 100 % (64/64), diagnosed by DUS and/or venogram	Anticoagulation alone in 9 % (6/64), anticoagulation success rate 100 % (6/6), anticoagulation and thrombolysis in 80 % (51/64), lysis success rate 78 % (40/51)	Re-evaluation at 1 month in 100 % (64/64)
Molina (2007) [18]	University of Minnesota	117, mean age 30, 75 % right-sided, 58 % male	Group I (97) = Less than 2 weeks, mean of 5.6 days	Group I: Effort thrombosis in 100 % (97/97), 87 % (85/97) <2 cm stenosis, 13 % (85/97) >2 cm stenosis diagnosed by venogram	Group I: Anticoagulation and thrombolysis in 100 % (97/97), lysis success rate 100 % (97/97)	4 h average
			Group II (17) = Greater than 2 weeks, mean of 34 days	Group II: Effort thrombosis in 100 % (17/17), 100 % (17/17) >2 cm stenosis diagnosed by venogram	Group II: Anticoagulation and thrombolysis in 100 % (17/17), lysis success rate 100 % (17/17)	

Mode of decomp	Venous reconstruction required	Adjuvant treatment	Recurrence rate	Post-op Anticoag	Morbidity and mortality	Outcome
Supraclavicular first rib resection in 45 % (29/64) for recurrent sx in 31 % (20/64), recurrent thrombosis in 8 % (5/64), or venous wall thickening in 6 % (4/64)	None	Venoplasty in 45 % (29/64), mechanical thrombectomy in 17 % (11/64), stent placement in 5 % (3/64)	0 % (0/29) in patients treated with lysis + anti-coagula-tion + decompres-sion, 23 % (8/35) in patients reated with Lysis + anticoagu-lation	3 months of coumadin	5 % (3/64), three small self resolving pneumotho-rax	96 % (28/29) Patency @ mean F/U of 51 months asymptomatic in patients who underwent thrombolysis + anticoagulation + early decompression 93 % (27/29) asymptom-atic@ mean F/U of 51 months asymptomatic in patients who underwent thrombolysis + anticoagula-tion + early decompression 80 % (28/35) Patency @ mean F/U of 54 months asymptomatic in patients who underwent thromboly-sis + anticoagula-tion + decompression for recurrence 100 % (35/35) asymptom-atic@ mean F/U of 41 months asymptomatic in patients who underwent thrombolysis + anticoagula-tion + decompression for recurrence 66 % (2/3) Stent patency at 11 months of F/U
Group I: Infraclavicular first rib resection, subclavius tendon resection, anterior and middle sclenectomy, and saphenous vein patch in 87 % (85/97)	100 % (103/103) of all who underwent an operation	Group I: Venoplasty and stent placement in 7 % (7/97)	Group I: 0 %	8 weeks of couma-din + plavix	5 % (5/97), 1 hematoma with RTOR, 2 pneumotho-rax requiring chest tubes, 2 lymphoceles requiring sclerotherapy	Group I: 100 % (97/97) patency @ 62 months average F/U
Same approach + extended hemi-sternotomy, and extended saphenous vein patch in 13 % (12/97)						100 % (97/97) asymptom-atic @ 62 months average F/U 100 % (7/7) stent Patency @ NR mean F/U (up to 14 years)
Group II: Infraclavicular first rib resection with extended hemi-sternotomy, subclavius tendon resection, anterior and middle sclenectomy, and extended saphenous vein patch in 29 % (15/17)		Group II: Venoplasty and stent placement in 60 % (3/5)	Group II: 0 %			Group II; 80 % (4/5) patency @ NR mean F/U 0 % (0/12) asymptomatic @ NR mean F/U

(continued)

Table 67.1 (continued)

Author (year) [Ref]	Institution	Subjects	Interval from Dx to tx	Type of VTOS	Preop management	Interval from lysis to decomp
Doyle (2007) [14]	University of Rochester	34, mean age 33, 72 % right-sided, 76 % male	Group I (26) = Less than 2 weeks, mean of 5.5 days	Group I (26): Effort thrombosis in 100 % (26/26) diagnosed by venogram	Group I: Anticoagulation + thrombolysis + venoplasty in 35 % (9/26), lysis success rate 44 % (4/9)	1–2 days
					Anticoagulation + thrombolysis 65 % (17/26), lysis success rate 71 % (12/17)	
					Residual lesions in 56 % (9/16)	
			Group II (8) = Greater than 4 weeks, mean NR	Group II (8): suclavian vein occlusion in 100 % (8/8) diagnosed by venogram	Group II: Anticoagulation in 75 % (6/8)	
					Anticoagulation + venoplasty in 25 % (2/8)	
					Venoplasty in 42 % (11/26)	
					Venoplasty success before decompression 11 % (1/9)	
Urschel (2008) [20]	Baylor University Medical Center, Dallas	608, mean age 32, side NR, 49.5 % male	Group I (36) = within 6 weeks of thrombosis	Substantial narrowing or occlusion on venogram in 100 % of extremities (626/626)	Group I = 100 % (36) managed with coumadin alone	Group I = delayed decompression in 72 % (26/36) with recurrent symptoms
			Group II (42) = no time interval NR		Group II = 100 % (42/42) managed with heparin and thrombolysis	Group II = 60 % (25/42) immediate decompression in
			Group III (506) = within 6 weeks of thrombosis		Group III = 100 % (506/506) managed with heparin and thrombolysis	Group III = 100 % (506/506) immediate decompression
			Group IV (42) = Greater than 6 weeks of thrombosis		Group IV = 100 % (42/42) managed with heparin and thrombolysis	Group IV = 100 % (42/42) immediate decompression

Mode of decomp	Venous reconstruction required	Adjuvant treatment	Recurrence rate	Post-op Anticoag	Morbidity and mortality	Outcome
Group I: Decompression in 92 % (24/26)	47 % (16/34) of all comers	Group I: Venoplasty in 4 % (1/26)	Group I: Lysis+decompression (1/11)	6 months of coumadin	15 % (5/34) overall requiring intervention, 6 % (2/34) hematoma with RTOR, 9 % (3/34) with pneumothorax requiring chest tube placement	Group I: 100 % (13/13) patency, 92 % (12/13) asymptomatic @ 33 months average F/U with Lysis+decompression+reconstruction
Transaxillary first rib resection in 42 % (11/26), claviculectomy and venous reconstruction in 50 % (13/26), with external venolysis, subclavius tendon resection, anterior sclenectomy in 100 % (26/26)			Lysis+decompression+reconstruction 0 % (0/13)			82 % (9/11) patency, 91 % (10/11) asymptomatic @ 33 months average F/U with Lysis+decompression 0 % (0/2) patency, 0 % (0/2) asymptomatic @ 33 months average F/U with Lysis+anticoagulation
Group II: Transaxillary first rib resection in 62.5 % (5/8), claviculectomy in 37.5 % (3/8), with external venolysis, subclavius tendon resection, anterior sclenectomy in 100 % (8/8)		Group II: Venoplasty in 13 % (1/8)	Group II: Lysis+decompression (0/5)			Group II;100 % (3/3) patency, 100 % (3/3) asymptomatic @ 33 months average F/U with decompression+reconstruction
		Venoplasty and stent placement in 13 % (1/8)	Lysis+decompression+reconstruction 0 % (0/3)			80 % (4/5) patency, 80 % (4/5) asymptomatic @ 33 months average F/U with decompression 100 % (1/1) stent patency @ 12 months F/U
Transaxillary first rib resection+subclavius tendon resection+anterior sclenectomy in over 99 % (597/599) Additional supraclavicular incision used in less than 1 % (2/599) Thrombectomy performed in 8 % (48/599)		Group I = none	Group I = NR	Group I: Coumadin	0 % mortality, morbidity NR	Patency NR for any group Group I = 44 % (16/36) good to excellent results
		Group II = none	Group II = NR	Group II/III/ IV: none		Group II = 100 % (25/25) good to excellent results if treated with thrombolysis and immediate surgery 0 % good to excellent results if treated with thrombolysis alone
		Group III = none	Group III = NR			Group III = 96 % (486/506) good to excellent results
	Group IV = 7 % (3/42) venous reconstruction	Group IV = 7 % (3/42) (roto-rooter treatment)	Group IV = NR			Group IV = 57 % (24/42) good to excellent results

(continued)

Table 67.1 (continued)

Author (year) [Ref]	Institution	Subjects	Interval from Dx to tx	Type of VTOS	Preop management	Interval from lysis to decomp
Guzzo (2010) [27]	The Johns Hopkins Hospital	103, mean age 31, side NR, 51 % male	Group I (45): 5.4 months	DUS, venography, CT, or MR in 100 % (110/110)	Group I=87 % (39/45) managed with anticoagulation Thrombolysis in 100 % (45/45) Preoperative venoplasty in 44 % (20/45)	Group I (45): 5.4 months
			Group II (65): 8.3 months		Group II=65 % (42/65) anticoagulation alone	Group II (65): 8.3 months

Table 67.2 Results of thrombolysis in VTOS

Author (year) [Ref]	Institution	Interval from Dx to tx	Attempted thrombolysis	Successful thrombolysis
Sheeran (1997) [44]	UCONN and Brown	3.9 days	14	13
Adelman (1997) [25]	NYU	Within 8 days 82 % (14/17), greater than 8 days in 18 % (3/17)	17	12
Lee (1998) [30]	Brigham and Women's Hospital	Less than 2.5 weeks	11	9
Azakie (1998) [55]	UCSF and Washington University St. Louis, Mo	Less than 2 weeks	17	17
Feugier (2001) [56]	Edouard Herriot Hospital, Lyon, France	5.2 days	7	5
Kreienberg (2001) [53]	Albany	9.4 days	23	21
Lokanathan (2001) [58]	University of British Columbia	5.5 days	25	22
Schneider (2004) [19]	UCSF and Thomas Jefferson University	Less than 4 weeks	21	21
Molina (2007) [18]	University of Minnesota	5.6 days	97	97
		34 days	17	17
Doyle (2007) [14]	University of Rochester	5.5 days	26	16
Stone (2010) [45]	Dartmouth-Hitchcoc Medical Center	12 days	30	30
		Overall	**305**	**280/305 = 92 % success**

Table 67.3 Results of Venoplasty prior to TOS decompression

Author (year) [Ref]	Institution	Pre-decompression venoplasty	Pre-decompression venoplasty success
Lee (1998) [30]	Brigham and Women's Hospital	5	0
Azakie (1998) [55]	UCSF and Washington University St. Louis, Mo	6	0
Doyle (2007) [14]	University of Rochester	9	1
	Overall	**20**	**(1/20) = 5 % success**

Mode of decomp	Venous reconstruction required	Adjuvant treatment	Recurrence rate	Post-op Anticoag	Morbidity and mortality	Outcome
Transaxillary first rib resection + sub-clavius tendon resection + anterior sclenectomy in over 100 % (110/110)	None	Group I: venoplasty in 47 % (21/45)	Group I: in 4 % (2/45)	Coumadin for 6 months or until patency was restored	NR	Group I: 91 % (41/45) patency and 96 % (43/45) asymptomatic @ 20 months mean F/U
		Group II: venoplasty in 56 % (36/65)	Group II = 5 % (3/65)			Group II: 91 % (59/65) patency and 98 % (64/65) asymptomatic @ 15 months mean F/U

in only 23 % of patients treated with thrombolysis and anticoagulation alone [16]. This series and others, however, neglect the morbidity of those observed who subsequently require surgery, and reduced rate of long-term "perfect" outcomes with this algorithm. Quality of life and functional assessments following initial decompressive surgery for VTOS are excellent [50, 51].

Many VTOS patients present relatively late after onset of symptoms. The Hopkins group has an unusually large experience with this population, and have shown excellent functional outcomes and restoration of patency in what would traditionally be considered chronic VTOS patients [27].

Post-decompression Angioplasty, Stenting, and Reconstruction

The use of venoplasty following thoracic outlet decompression has been reported to have excellent long-term outcomes (Table 67.4), although no prospective comparison trials have been performed. Selective stent placement has been shown variable rates of success in decompressed thoracic outlets (Table 67.5) [45, 49, 52, 53]. It should be stressed that a recalcitrant venous lesion that may require stenting (after failed venoplasty) as a marker of an only partially decompressed thoracic outlet. Caution should be

used with stenting the thoracic outlet as even those with a perfect result will fail at a certain rate, and will then require a much larger operation. We suggest the use of angioplasty whenever possible, with a conservative attitude toward stenting. There are only limited long-term data comparing stents in the thoracic outlet to venous reconstruction, which has excellent long-term efficacy and patency when performed at centers of excellence (Table 67.6) [14, 18, 28].

Intention to Treat Analysis of VTOS Treatment Algorithms

Figure 67.1 describes the outcome of 964 patients with VTOS who present within 6 weeks of symptom onset, divided by initial treatment modality, anticoagulation or thrombolysis. Those who are initially treated with anticoagulation alone are divided by whether they undergo thoracic outlet decompression or no further treatment, and those who undergo thrombolysis by those who undergo delayed first rib resection (FRR), immediate FRR, FRR and stenting, or no immediate treatment (with FRR reserved for recurrent symptoms).

Overall, the best results are seen in those who undergo thrombolysis and immediate first rib resection. Patients managed with anticoagulation alone regardless of subsequent treatment did worse than any other group. Patency and

Table 67.4 Results of venoplasty following TOS decompression

Author (year) [Ref]	Institution	Venoplasty	Outcome
Sheeran (1997) [44]	UCONN and Brown	36 % (5/14)	80 % (4/5) asymptomatic with lysis and immediate FRR or Venous recon @ 16 months mean F/U
Azakie (1998) [55]	UCSF and Washington University St. Louis, Mo	19 % (4/21), 100 % (4/4) success rate	100 % (21/21) patency @ between 1 week and 3 months F/U, 95 % (20/21) asymptomatic @ 31 months average F/U
Angle (2001) [35]	UCLA	22 % (2/9), 100 % (2/2) success rate	100 % patent (9/9) @ 2 weeks F/U, 100 % asymptomatic (9/9) @ 51 days median F/U
Angle (2001) [35]	UCLA	33 % (3/9), 100 % (3/3) success rate	100 % patent (9/9) @ 2 weeks F/U, 100 % asymptomatic (9/9) @ 51 days median F/U
Kreienberg (2001) [53]	Albany	39 % (9/23)	100 % patency (9/9) and 100 % asymptomatic in patients who underwent lysis + decompression + venoplasty @ 48 months mean F/U
Coletta (2001) [57]	Naval Medical center San Diego	11 % (2/18)	Patency not reported, 100 % (2/2) asymptomatic in patients who underwent Thrombolysis + anticoagulation + decompression + venoplasty
Schneider (2004) [19]	UCSF and Thomas Jefferson University	64 % (16/25), success = less than 30 % residual stenosis in 100 % (16/16)	92 % primary patency @ 12 months by life table analysis, 96 % secondary patency @ 12 months by life table analysis, 96 % asymptomatic @ 12 months F/U
Lee (2006) [16]	Sanford	45 % (29/64)	96 % (28/29) Patency, 93 % (27/29) asymptomatic @ mean @ mean F/U of 51 months in patients who underwent Thrombolysis + anticoagulation + early decompression
Guzzo (2010) [27]	The Johns Hopkins Hospital	Group I: 47 % (21/45)	Group I: 91 % (41/45) patency and 96 % (43/45) asymptomatic @ 20 months mean F/U
		Group II: 56 % (36/65)	Group II: 91 % (59/65) patency and 98 % (64/65) asymptomatic @ 15 months mean F/U
Stone (2010) [45]	Dartmouth-Hitchcoc Medical Center	3 % (1/36)	94 % patency @ 60 months by life table analysis, 86 % asymptomatic @ NR interval

Table 67.5 Results of venous stents following TOS decompression

Author (year) [Ref]	Institution	Post-decompression stenting	Outcome
Kreienberg (2001) [53]	Albany	Venoplasty and stenting in 61 % (14/23)	64 % patency (9/14) and 57 % asymptomatic (8/14) in patients who underwent lysis + decompression + venoplasty + stent @ 36 months mean F/U
Coletta (2001) [57]	Naval Medical center San Diego	Venoplsty + stent in 33 % (6/18)	Patency not reported, 83 % (5/6) asymptomatic in patients who underwent Thrombolysis + anticoagulation + decompression + venoplasty + stent
Lee (2006) [16]	Sanford	Stent placement in 5 % (3/64)	66 % (2/3) Stent patency at 11 months of F/U
Molina (2007) [18]	University of Minnesota	Venoplasty and stent placement in 7 % (7/97)	100 % (7/7) stent Patency @ NR mean F/U (up to 14 years)
Doyle (2007) [14]	University of Rochester	Venoplasty and stent placement in 13 % (1/8)	100 % (1/1) stent patency @ 12 months F/U
Stone (2010) [45]	Dartmouth-Hitchcoc Medical Center	Stent placement in 31 % (11/36)	Stent patency NR

Table 67.6 Results of venous reconstruction for VTOS

Author (year) [Ref]	Institution	Venous reconstruction required	Outcome
Molina (2007) [18]	University of Minnesota	100 % (103/103) of all who underwent an operation	99 % (102/103) patency, 95 % (98/103) asymptomatic @ 62 months average F/U
Doyle (2007) [14]	University of Rochester	47 % (16/34) of all comers	100 % (16/16) patency, 94 % (15/16) asymptomatic @ 33 months average F/U with Lysis + decompression + reconstruction

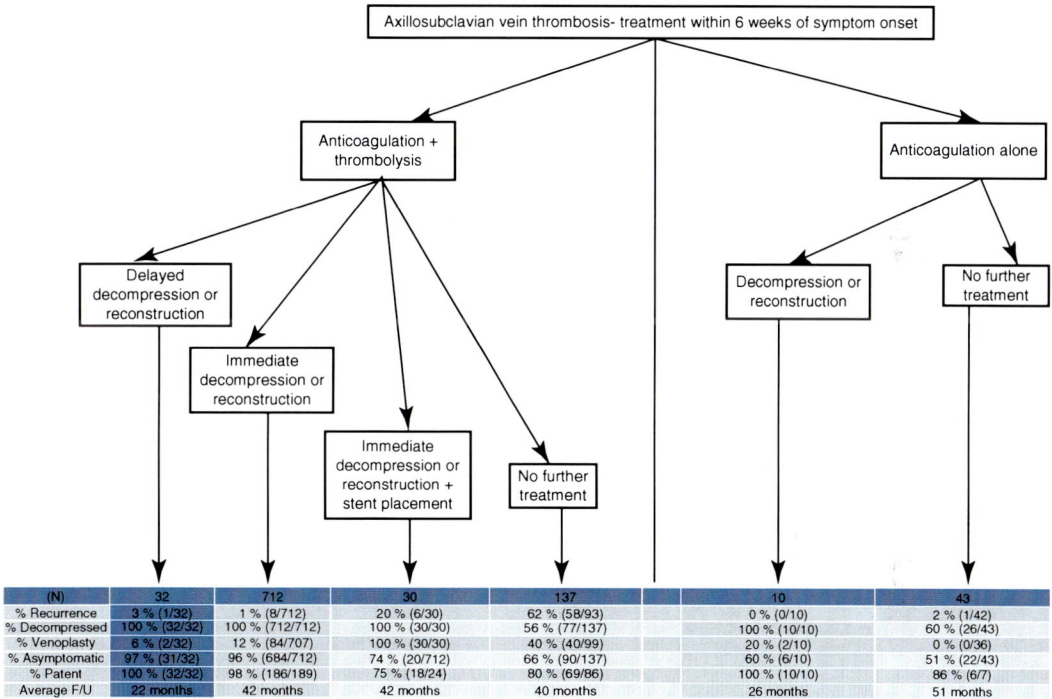

(N)	32	712	30	137	10	43
% Recurrence	3 % (1/32)	1 % (8/712)	20 % (6/30)	62 % (58/93)	0 % (0/10)	2 % (1/42)
% Decompressed	100 % (32/32)	100 % (712/712)	100 % (30/30)	56 % (77/137)	100 % (10/10)	60 % (26/43)
% Venoplasty	6 % (2/32)	12 % (84/707)	100 % (30/30)	40 % (40/99)	20 % (2/10)	0 % (0/36)
% Asymptomatic	97 % (31/32)	96 % (684/712)	74 % (20/712)	66 % (90/137)	60 % (6/10)	51 % (22/43)
% Patent	100 % (32/32)	98 % (186/189)	75 % (18/24)	80 % (69/86)	100 % (10/10)	86 % (6/7)
Average F/U	22 months	42 months	42 months	40 months	26 months	51 months

Fig. 67.1 Treatments outcomes in acute VTOS

asymptomatic status following thrombolysis and FRR are better than following thrombolysis followed by FRR and stent placement, or thombolysis followed by no further treatment.

The results of algorithms applied to those with VTOS who present with symptoms of more than 6 weeks are presented in Fig. 67.2. One hundred and seventy-seven patients were divided by initial treatment modality, anticoagulation versus thrombolysis. Patients initially treated with thrombolysis have better outcomes than those with no further treatment. Patients initially treated with anticoagulation and thoracic outlet decompression appear to have similar results to those treated with thrombolysis and decompression. No modern studies report outcomes for anticoagulation alone in chronic VTOS. Historical studies report significantly lower rates of patency and asymptomatic status in similarly managed patient cohorts [9].

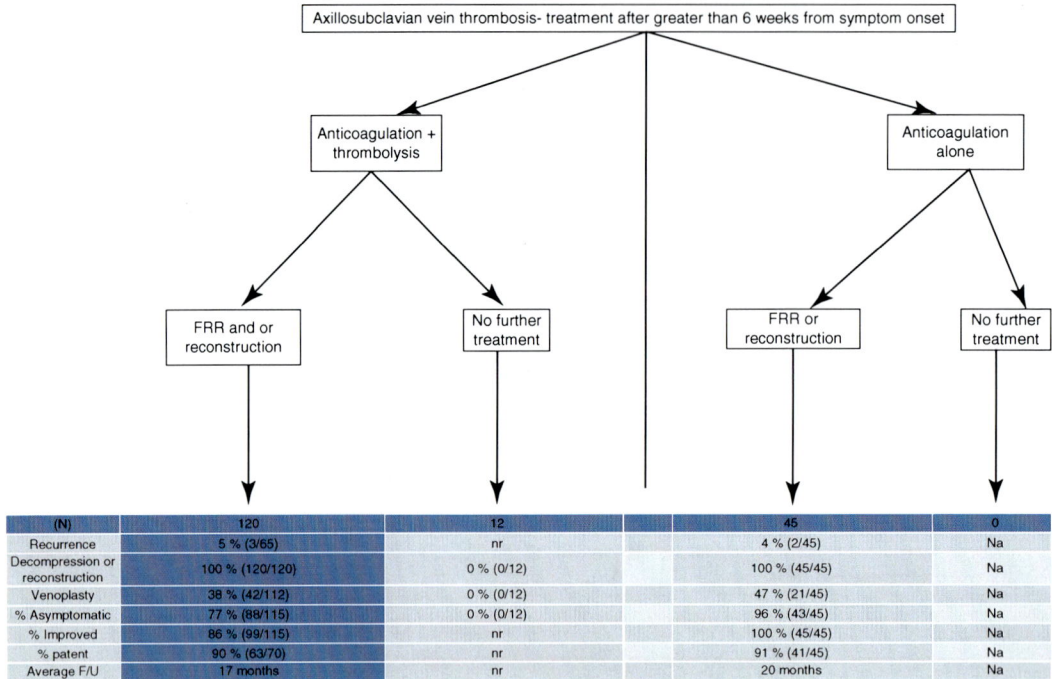

(N)	120	12		45	0
Recurrence	5 % (3/65)	nr		4 % (2/45)	Na
Decompression or reconstruction	100 % (120/120)	0 % (0/12)		100 % (45/45)	Na
Venoplasty	38 % (42/112)	0 % (0/12)		47 % (21/45)	Na
% Asymptomatic	77 % (88/115)	0 % (0/12)		96 % (43/45)	Na
% Improved	86 % (99/115)	nr		100 % (45/45)	Na
% patent	90 % (63/70)	nr		91 % (41/45)	Na
Average F/U	17 months	nr		20 months	Na

Fig. 67.2 Treatments outcomes in chronic VTOS

Suggested Treatment Algorithm

Figure 67.3 is a treatment algorithm for VTOS that integrates the results of modern literature and existing evidence-based recommendations [14, 18, 20, 27].

Conclusion

Current treatment of VTOS involves multimodal and often tailored treatment, and the data surrounding long-term outcomes of the varying institutional treatment algorithms are often difficult to accurately interpret. While no prospective randomized trials have been reported, the bulk of available data suggest that patients who present with acute subclavian vein thrombosis should be managed with thrombolysis followed by immediate first rib resection. Even if presentation is delayed, surgical decompression is of benefit. Figure 67.3 represents a treatment algorithm that takes into account the reporting and selection biases in the surgical literature and incorporates other evidence-based recommendations. Hopefully in the near future multi-institution prospective collaborations will be possible and allow further clarification of the natural history and optimal treatment for patients with VTOS.

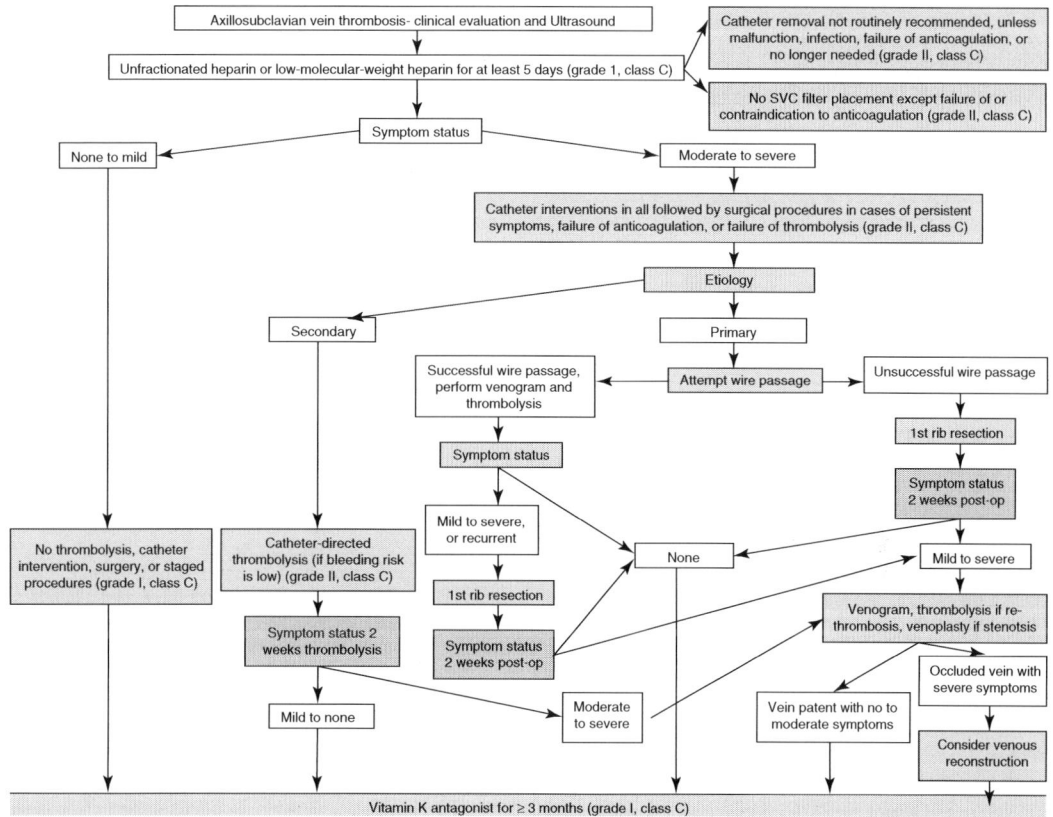

Fig. 67.3 VTOS treatment algorithm

References

1. Hughes E. Venous obstruction upper extremity: review of 320 cases. Int Abst Surg. 1949;88:89–127.
2. Adams JT, DeWeese JA. "Effort" thrombosis of the axillary and subclavian veins. J Trauma. 1971;11:923–30.
3. AbuRahma AF, Sadler D, Stuart P, Khan MZ, Boland JP. Conventional versus thrombolytic therapy in spontaneous (effort) axillary-subclavian vein thrombosis. Am J Surg. 1991;161:459–65.
4. Becker DM, Philbrick JT, Walker FB. Axillary and subclavian venous thrombosis. Prognosis and treatment. Arch Intern Med. 1991;151:1934–43.
5. Heron E, Lozinguez O, Emmerich J, Laurian C, Fiessinger JN. Long-term sequelae of spontaneous axillary-subclavian venous thrombosis. Ann Intern Med. 1999;131:510–3.
6. Monreal M, Lafoz E, Ruiz J, Valls R, Alastrue A. Upper-extremity deep venous thrombosis and pulmonary embolism. A prospective study. Chest. 1991;99:280–3.
7. Tilney N, Griffiths H, Edwards E. Natural history of major venous thrombosis of the upper extremity. Arch Surg. 1970;101:792–6.
8. Urschel Jr HC, Razzuk MA. Paget-Schroetter syndrome: what is the best management? Ann Thorac Surg. 2000;69:1663–8; discussion 8–9.
9. Adams J, McEvoy R, DeWeese J. Primary deep venous thrombosis of upper extremity. Arch Surg. 1965;91:29–42.
10. Roos DB. Transaxillary approach for first rib resection to relieve thoracic outlet syndrome. Ann Surg. 1966;163:354–8.
11. Inahara T. Surgical treatment of "effort" thrombosis of the axillary and subclavian veins. Am Surg. 1968;34:479–83.

12. Swinton Jr NW, Edgett Jr JW, Hall RJ. Primary sub-clavian-axillary vein thrombosis. Circulation. 1968; 38:737–45.

13. DeWeese JA, Adams JT, Gaiser DL. Subclavian venous thrombectomy. Circulation. 1970;41:II158–64.

14. Doyle A, Wolford HY, Davies MG, et al. Management of effort thrombosis of the subclavian vein: today's treatment. Ann Vasc Surg. 2007;21:723–9.

15. Freischlag J. Venous thoracic outlet syndrome: transaxillary approach. Oper Tech Gen Surg. 2008;10:122–30.

16. Lee JT, Karwowski JK, Harris EJ, Haukoos JS, Olcott C. Long-term thrombotic recurrence after nonopera-tive management of Paget-Schroetter syndrome. J Vasc Surg. 2006;43:1236–43.

17. Machleder HI. Evaluation of a new treatment strategy for Paget-Schroetter syndrome: spontaneous throm-bosis of the axillary-subclavian vein. J Vasc Surg. 1993;17:305–15; discussion 16–7.

18. Molina JE, Hunter DW, Dietz CA. Paget-Schroetter syndrome treated with thrombolytics and immediate surgery. J Vasc Surg. 2007;45:328–34.

19. Schneider DB, Dimuzio PJ, Martin ND, et al. Combination treatment of venous thoracic outlet syn-drome: open surgical decompression and intraopera-tive angioplasty. J Vasc Surg. 2004;40:599–603.

20. Urschel Jr HC, Patel AN. Surgery remains the most effective treatment for Paget-Schroetter syndrome: 50 years' experience. Ann Thorac Surg. 2008;86:254–60; discussion 60.

21. Becker GJ, Holden RW, Rabe FE, et al. Local throm-bolytic therapy for subclavian and axillary vein throm-bosis. Treatment of the thoracic inlet syndrome. Radiology. 1983;149:419–23.

22. Perler BA, Mitchell SE. Percutaneous transluminal angioplasty and transaxillary first rib resection. A multidisciplinary approach to the thoracic outlet syndrome. Am Surg. 1986;52:485–8.

23. Taylor Jr LM, McAllister WR, Dennis DL, Porter JM. Thrombolytic therapy followed by first rib resection for spontaneous ("effort") subclavian vein thrombo-sis. Am J Surg. 1985;149:644–7.

24. Zimmermann R, Morl H, Harenberg J, Gerhardt P, Kuhn HM, Wahl P. Urokinase therapy of subclavian-axillary vein thrombosis. Klin Wochenschr. 1981;59:851–6.

25. Adelman MA, Stone DH, Riles TS, Lamparello PJ, Giangola G, Rosen RJ. A multidisciplinary approach to the treatment of Paget-Schroetter syndrome. Ann Vasc Surg. 1997;11:149–54.

26. Wilson JJ, Zahn CA, Newman H. Fibrinolytic therapy for idiopathic subclavian-axillary vein thrombosis. Am J Surg. 1990;159:208–10; discussion 10–1.

27. Guzzo JL, Chang K, Demos J, Black JH, Freischlag JA. Preoperative thrombolysis and venoplasty affords no benefit in patency following first rib resection and scalenectomy for subacute and chronic subclavian vein thrombosis. J Vasc Surg. 2010;52:658–63.

28. Green RM, Waldman D, Ouriel K, Riggs P, Deweese JA. Claviculectomy for subclavian venous repair: long-term functional results. J Vasc Surg. 2000; 32:315–21.

29. Molina JE. Need for emergency treatment in subcla-vian vein effort thrombosis. J Am Coll Surg. 1995; 181:414–20.

30. Lee MC, Grassi CJ, Belkin M, Mannick JA, Whittemore AD, Donaldson MC. Early operative intervention after thrombolytic therapy for primary subclavian vein thrombosis: an effective treatment approach. J Vasc Surg. 1998;27:1101–7; discussion 7–8.

31. Sundqvist SB, Hedner U, Kullenberg HK, Bergentz SE. Deep venous thrombosis of the arm: a study of coagulation and fibrinolysis. Br Med J (Clin Res Ed). 1981;283:265–7.

32. Bjarnason H, Hunter DW, Crain MR, Ferral H, Miltz-Miller SE, Wegryn SA. Collapse of a Palmaz stent in the subclavian vein. AJR Am J Roentgenol. 1993; 160:1123–4.

33. Meier GH, Pollak JS, Rosenblatt M, Dickey KW, Gusberg RJ. Initial experience with venous stents in exertional axillary-subclavian vein thrombosis. J Vasc Surg. 1996;24:974–81; discussion 81–3.

34. Urschel Jr HC, Patel AN. Paget-Schroetter syndrome therapy: failure of intravenous stents. Ann Thorac Surg. 2003;75:1693–6; discussion 6.

35. Angle N, Gelabert HA, Farooq MM, et al. Safety and efficacy of early surgical decompression of the tho-racic outlet for Paget-Schroetter syndrome. Ann Vasc Surg. 2001;15:37–42.

36. Caparrelli DJ, Freischlag J. A unified approach to axillosubclavian venous thrombosis in a single hospi-tal admission. Semin Vasc Surg. 2005;18:153–7.

37. Urschel Jr HC, Razzuk MA. Neurovascular compres-sion in the thoracic outlet: changing management over 50 years. Ann Surg. 1998;228:609–17.

38. Druy EM, Trout 3rd HH, Giordano JM, Hix WR. Lytic therapy in the treatment of axillary and subcla-vian vein thrombosis. J Vasc Surg. 1985;2:821–7.

39. Machleder HI. Thrombolytic therapy and surgery for primary axillosubclavian vein thrombosis: current approach. Semin Vasc Surg. 1996;9:46–9.

40. Strange-Vognsen HH, Hauch O, Andersen J, Struckmann J. Resection of the first rib, following deep arm vein thrombolysis in patients with thoracic outlet syndrome. J Cardiovasc Surg (Torino). 1989;30:430–3.

41. Altobelli GG, Kudo T, Haas BT, Chandra FA, Moy JL, Ahn SS. Thoracic outlet syndrome: pattern of clinical success after operative decompression. J Vasc Surg. 2005;42:122–8.

42. de Leon RA, Chang DC, Hassoun HT, et al. Multiple treatment algorithms for successful outcomes in venous thoracic outlet syndrome. Surgery. 2009;145:500–7.

43. Illig KA, Doyle AJ. A comprehensive review of Paget-Schroetter syndrome. J Vasc Surg. 2010;51:1538–47.

44. Sheeran SR, Hallisey MJ, Murphy TP, Faberman RS, Sherman S. Local thrombolytic therapy as part of a multidisciplinary approach to acute axillosubclavian vein thrombosis (Paget-Schroetter syndrome). J Vasc Interv Radiol. 1997;8:253–60.

45. Stone DH, Scali ST, Bjerk AA, et al. Aggressive treatment of idiopathic axillo-subclavian vein thrombosis provides excellent long-term function. J Vasc Surg. 2010;52:127–31.

46. Illig KA. An improved method of exposure for transaxillary first rib resection. J Vasc Surg. 2010;52:248–9.

47. Thompson RW. Venous thoracic outlet syndrome: paraclavicular approach. Oper Tech Gen Surg. 2008; 10:113–21.

48. Molina JE. Approach to the confluence of the subclavian and internal jugular veins without claviculectomy. Semin Vasc Surg. 2000;13:10–9.

49. Molina JE, Hunter DW, Dietz CA. Protocols for Paget-Schroetter syndrome and late treatment of chronic subclavian vein obstruction. Ann Thorac Surg. 2009;87:416–22.

50. Berzaczy D, Popovic M, Reiter M, et al. Quality of life in patients with idiopathic subclavian vein thrombosis. Thromb Res. 2010;125:25–8.

51. Chang DC, Rotellini-Coltvet LA, Mukherjee D, De Leon R, Freischlag JA. Surgical intervention for thoracic outlet syndrome improves patient's quality of life. J Vasc Surg. 2009;49:630–5; discussion 5–7.

52. Hall LD, Murray JD, Boswell GE. Venous stent placement as an adjunct to the staged, multimodal treatment of Paget-Schroetter syndrome. J Vasc Interv Radiol. 1995;6:565–9; discussion 9–70.

53. Kreienberg PB, Chang BB, Darling 3rd RC, et al. Long-term results in patients treated with thrombolysis, thoracic inlet decompression, and subclavian vein stenting for Paget-Schroetter syndrome. J Vasc Surg. 2001;33:S100–5.

54. Hempel GK, Shutze WP, Anderson JF, Bukhari HI. 770 consecutive supraclavicular first rib resections for thoracic outlet syndrome. Ann Vasc Surg. 1996; 10:456–63.

55. Azakie A, McElhinney DB, Thompson RW, Raven RB, Messina LM, Stoney RJ. Surgical management of subclavian-vein effort thrombosis as a result of thoracic outlet compression. J Vasc Surg. 1998;28:777–86.

56. Feugier P, Aleksic I, Salari R, Durand X, Chevalier JM. Long-term results of venous revascularization for Paget-Schroetter syndrome in athletes. Ann Vasc Surg. 2001;15:212–8.

57. Coletta JM, Murray JD, Reeves TR, et al. Vascular thoracic outlet syndrome: successful outcomes with multimodal therapy. Cardiovasc Surg. 2001;9:11–5.

58. Lokanathan R, Salvian AJ, Chen JC, Morris C, Taylor DC, Hsiang YN. Outcome after thrombolysis and selective thoracic outlet decompression for primary axillary vein thrombosis. J Vasc Surg. 2001;33:783–8.

Assessment and Treatment of Recurrent VTOS

Robert W. Thompson

Abstract

Patients that have undergone treatment for venous TOS generally have excellent clinical outcomes, but a small proportion of individuals may present with persistent or recurrent upper extremity symptoms. The purpose of this chapter is to outline the spectrum of conditions that should be considered in evaluation of such patients and a systematic approach to address these problems. It can be expected that with comprehensive evaluation and appropriate treatment, the majority of patients with persistent or recurrent venous TOS can experience decreased symptoms and restoration of normal upper extremity function.

Introduction

Patients that have undergone treatment for venous TOS generally have excellent clinical outcomes, with the majority experiencing a decrease in symptoms and restoration of normal upper extremity function [1–4]. However, there remain a small proportion of patients who have persistent symptoms despite previous treatment, or who subsequently develop recurrent symptoms after a variable symptom-free interval. Evaluation and treatment of such patients is a substantial challenge and it requires careful delineation of the nature and time-course of the symptoms

described, consideration of the type and results of previous procedures, and performance of accurate imaging studies by which to guide treatment decisions. The initial treatment options for patients presenting with venous TOS are summarized in Table 68.1 and discussed in detail elsewhere in this text.

Clinical Characterization of Symptoms

The first step in evaluation is to accurately determine the nature of the original symptoms for which previous treatment was undertaken and to characterize how they relate to the current symptoms (Table 68.2). Patients that have been treated for venous TOS will typically describe an episode of spontaneous upper extremity swelling and discoloration characteristic of axillary-subclavian vein effort thrombosis (Paget-Schroetter syndrome), but may have had symptoms of more

R.W. Thompson, MD
Department of Surgery, Section of Vascular Surgery, Washington University Center for Thoracic Outlet Syndrome, Barnes-Jewish Hospital, Campus Box 8109/Suite 5101 Queeny Tower, 660 S Euclid Avenue, St. Louis, MO 63110, USA
e-mail: thompson@wudosis.wustl.edu

K.A. Illig et al. (eds.), *Thoracic Outlet Syndrome*,
DOI 10.1007/978-1-4471-4366-6_68, © Springer-Verlag London 2013

chronic intermittent arm swelling and cyanosis suggesting non-thrombotic positional axillary-subclavian vein obstruction [5, 6]. In either case, it is likely that the previous diagnosis was guided by findings of axillary-subclavian vein obstruction on venography. If patients that have had these symptoms are being evaluated for similar upper extremity symptoms dominated by swelling and discoloration, it is likely that this represents authentic persistent/recurrent venous TOS.

In contrast, some patients that were previously treated for venous TOS may describe original symptoms that included or were dominated by upper extremity and/or neck pain, with numbness and paresthesias in the arm or hand. These symptoms suggest the presence of neurogenic TOS due to brachial plexus compression and irritation [7],

which may have been present along with venographic findings of axillary-subclavian vein obstruction. In these situations it is important to consider if the nature of the original symptoms might have actually represented neurogenic TOS, for which the treatment provided may have had little effect if directed solely toward the venographic findings. Other patients may have initially undergone appropriate treatment for authentic venous TOS, but have subsequently developed different symptoms more characteristic of neurogenic TOS, perhaps as a result of extended local inflammatory responses surrounding the occluded subclavian vein, leading to scalene muscle spasm and brachial plexus irritation. It is therefore crucial to accurately evaluate the nature of the current symptoms in order to determine the most appropriate steps to be taken in further diagnosis and consideration of treatment options.

The second step in evaluation is to characterize the time-course of the current symptoms in relation to the previous treatment for venous TOS (Table 68.2). For example, if the original symptoms merely included arm swelling and discoloration but were dominated by findings suggesting neurogenic TOS, and were unaltered by the treatment provided, the patient is considered to have **persistent primary neurogenic TOS** that was either present initially as the dominant problem (if the evidence for venous TOS appears to have been weak) or was present as a co-existing but undetected condition along with venous TOS. Even if the original symptoms were dominated by arm swelling and discoloration and resolved following previous treatment, if the current symptoms are dominated by pain, numbness and paresthesias the patient is considered to have **secondary neurogenic TOS** that has either progressed since the original treatment or

Table 68.1 Initial treatment options for venous TOS

Anticoagulation
  Alone as primary treatment
  As a bridge to surgical treatment following thrombolysis
Interventions
  Catheter thrombolysis (TPA Infusion)
  Catheter thrombectomy (Pharmacomechanical)
    ± Balloon angioplasty
    ± Stent placement
Surgery
  Transaxillary first rib resection (subtotal or complete)
  Infraclavicular first rib resection (subtotal)
    ± Direct subclavian vein reconstruction (patch angioplasty)
  Paraclavicular first rib resection (complete)
    ± Direct subclavian vein reconstruction (patch angioplasty or vein bypass)
  Intraoperative balloon angioplasty ± stent placement
  Follow-up venography/balloon angioplasty/stent placement

Table 68.2 Characterization of persistent/recurrent venous TOS

Dominant original symptoms	Outcome of initial treatment for VTOS	Dominant current symptoms	Clinical classification
Arm pain/paresthesias	No resolution	Arm pain/paresthesias	Primary NTOS
Arm swelling/cyanosis	Resolution >6 weeks	Arm pain/paresthesias	Secondary NTOS
Arm swelling/cyanosis	No resolution	Arm swelling/cyanosis	Persistent VTOS
Arm swelling/cyanosis	Resolution >6 weeks	Arm swelling/cyanosis	Recurrent VTOS

Abbreviations: *NTOS* neurogenic TOS, *VTOS* venous TOS

Table 68.3 Evaluation and treatment options for persistent/recurrent venous TOS

Classification	Previous treatment	Evaluations needed	Treatment options
Primary NTOS	Surgical or	PhysRx, ASM/PM Block,	PhysRx
	Non-surgical	Venogram, CT/MRI	Operation
Secondary NTOS	Surgical or	PhysRx, ASM/PM Block,	PhysRx
	Non-surgical	Venogram, CT/MRI	Operation
Persistent VTOS	Non-surgical	Venogram	Anticoagulation
			Intervention
			Operation
Persistent VTOS	Surgical	Venogram, CT/MRI	Anticoagulation
			Intervention
			Operation
Recurrent VTOS	Surgical	Venogram, CT/MRI	Anticoagulation
			Intervention
			Operation

Abbreviations: *NTOS* neurogenic TOS, *VTOS* venous TOS, *PhysRx* physical therapy, *ASM* anterior scalene muscle, *PM* pectoralis minor muscle, *CT* computed tomography, *MRI* magnetic resonance imaging

has developed as a subsequent dominant problem despite successful previous treatment for axillary-subclavian vein obstruction. If the original symptoms were dominated by arm swelling and discoloration and this was not substantially altered by the previous treatment, the patient is considered to have *persistent venous TOS*. This may occur if the initial treatment was inadequate to relieve subclavian vein obstruction and collateral vein expansion has been insufficient to prevent venous congestion. Finally, if the original symptoms were dominated by arm swelling and discoloration with resolution for a period of at least 6 weeks following the previous treatment, but the patient now exhibits symptoms that are similar to those originally present, the patient is considered likely to have *recurrent venous TOS*. This may occur as a result of inadequate previous subclavian vein decompression, distal extension of previous thrombus, or de novo rethrombosis within the axillary or subclavian veins, causing obstruction of either the axillary-subclavian vein and/or principal venous collaterals. Based on the preceding evaluation, each patient can be classified with respect to the most likely cause of the current symptoms (Table 68.2). This will then help guide the further studies that may be needed to develop an appropriate treatment plan (Table 68.3).

Further Evaluation and Treatment Options

Persistent Primary and Secondary Neurogenic TOS

For patients with current symptoms that are dominated by upper extremity pain, numbness and paresthesias, physical examination should focus on defining if these symptoms can be best explained by the presence of neurogenic TOS [8, 9]. Confirmatory findings include a history of positional exacerbation of neural symptoms in the absence of overt arm swelling, localizing tenderness to palpation over the scalene triangle and/or subcoracoid space, and reproduction of symptoms during positional maneuvers, such as the 3-min elevated arm stress test (EAST), particularly when this occurs without significant arm swelling. More specific evaluation to assess neurogenic TOS may include anterior scalene muscle and/or pectoralis minor muscle anesthetic blocks, especially if previous treatment did not include a scalenectomy [10].

As in other situations involving the possibility of central subclavian vein obstruction, Duplex ultrasound studies are not sufficiently accurate to be of significant value, and would only be useful if positive for the presence of chronic axillary-subclavian vein occlusion. In most instances it is helpful to perform a contrast venogram, with variations in arm position to determine the presence or absence of subclavian vein obstruction. This is done with the recognition that venography may be negative in these clinical circumstances, and will thereby serve only to confirm the clinical diagnosis as related to neurogenic TOS. Contrast-enhanced CT and MRI studies are also useful for delineating the vascular and bony anatomy related to the previous operation and the current status of the central vessels, and may preclude the need for catheter-based venography if performed appropriately.

In the event that a diagnosis of persistent primary or secondary neurogenic TOS is confirmed, the initial steps in treatment are focused on TOS-specific physical therapy and other non-operative measures (Table 68.3). If this does not result in a sufficient improvement in symptoms, operative or reoperative treatment may be considered. The optimal surgical approach used in these circumstances will depend on the operative approach that was used in the previous operation, as well as the degree of familiarity and comfort of the surgeon with reoperative procedures for neurogenic TOS.

Persistent/Recurrent Venous TOS

In patients with current symptoms that are dominated by arm swelling and discoloration, either at rest or with upper extremity activity, further evaluation is targeted toward defining the presence, extent and cause of axillary-subclavian vein obstruction. As noted above, Duplex ultrasound studies of the subclavian vein are not sufficiently accurate to exclude central subclavian vein obstruction, and may thereby lead to false assurance that the subclavian vein is patent in those with recurrent symptoms. CT- or MR-based angiography is a valuable alternative as an initial step in this regard, as both studies can be performed with positional maneuvers and provide sufficiently accurate imaging of the subclavian vein to exclude central obstruction. In most cases, a catheter-based upper extremity venogram will be necessary to accurately visualize the entire axillary vein, subclavian vein, and collateral venous pathways. If there is a residual obstruction of the subclavian vein, either at rest or with arm elevation, the diagnosis of persistent/recurrent venous TOS is confirmed. In this event, plain radiographs and CT studies (with bone windows and 3-dimensional reconstruction) may also be a useful adjunct to visualize the bony structures related to the previous operation and to facilitate further treatment planning.

As with patients initially presenting with subclavian vein effort thrombosis, the treatment options for persistent/recurrent venous TOS revolve around the use of chronic anticoagulation, use of compression garments and other conservative measures, versus catheter-based interventions and various forms of reoperation (Table 68.3). Chronic anticoagulation may be a useful option if the symptoms are relatively mild and solely present with upper extremity exertion, and if the patient is not dependent on active use of the upper extremity for occupational or recreational purposes. This approach is limited by some degree of risk for the subsequent extension of thrombus or development of rethrombosis, even with maintenance of satisfactory anticoagulation. Furthermore, the appropriate duration of anticoagulation for such patients is unknown, and may need to be considered for years or even as lifelong treatment in some patients. Although it has been suggested that long-term anticoagulation may be associated with recanalization of the chronically occluded axillary-subclavian vein, this has not been demonstrated by direct venographic studies; [11–13] rather, it is more likely that patients with longstanding subclavian vein occlusion tend to continue developing increased collateral vein capacity over time along with a gradual reduction in symptoms (Fig. 68.1).

Initial intervention for persistent/recurrent venous TOS may include catheter-based procedures, particularly if venographic studies have demonstrated a patent axillary vein and a short-segment subclavian vein obstruction. In this circumstance balloon angioplasty may be considered as a first step to determine the physiological significance of the observed lesion, by assessing if the patient experiences an improvement in symptoms following resolution of the venous

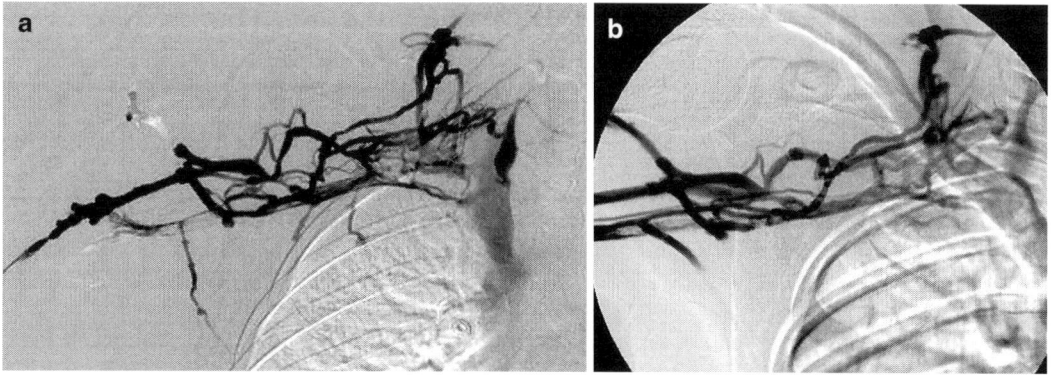

Fig. 68.1 Conservative management of persistent venous TOS. A patient with persistent symptoms of venous TOS presenting 6 weeks after an infraclavicular first rib resection for subclavian vein effort thrombosis. (**a**) A right upper extremity venogram demonstrates a long-segment axillary-subclavian vein occlusion with dense collateral veins. Reoperative treatment was not advised given that a complete resection of the anterior first rib had been performed and the lack of a suitable inflow vein for bypass graft reconstruction. The patient was maintained on oral anticoagulation and experienced a gradual decrease in symptoms. (**b**) A follow-up venogram 6 months later demonstrated persistent occlusion of the axillary-subclavian vein with a moderate enlargement of the collateral vein pathways

stenosis. It is recognized that balloon angioplasty is often technically limited in this situation, especially if there is fibrous scarring within and around the subclavian vein, thereby precluding complete balloon expansion, and rapid elastic recoil is often observed immediately after balloon angioplasty, thereby predicting early recurrence. Although placement of indwelling venous stents is not advocated in patients during initial treatment of venous TOS, this may be an alternative consideration in situations where a thoracic outlet decompression procedure with first rib resection has already been performed. Nonetheless, there is little experience with long-term use of venous stents in the axillary-subclavian vein and in most situations a reoperative strategy is more likely to be favored. In addition, it is notable that chronic occlusion of a long segment of the subclavian vein, particularly extending into the axillary vein at the level of the shoulder, will preclude the potential use of interventional techniques.

Reoperations for Venous TOS

Reoperation for persistent/recurrent venous TOS is a feasible option and will most often appear to be the approach of choice for patients with these complicated conditions. The principal goals of such reoperative procedures are to ensure complete decompression of the musculoskeletal anatomy of the thoracic outlet and to obtain a patent axillary-subclavian vein, either by external venolysis (excision of fibrous scar tissue from the outside of the vein, permitting re-expansion when the underlying vein is normal) or by direct reconstruction with patch angioplasty or bypass grafting when the underlying vein harbors residual fibrous wall thickening, chronic occlusion, or a previously-placed venous stent. Preoperative delineation of the bony anatomy is important to determine if there is a residual remnant of the first rib that should be removed during reoperative decompression, and examination of the venographic studies should demonstrate that there is an inflow vein of sufficient caliber upon which to base a bypass graft if venous reconstruction is to be considered. In selected circumstances where there is extensive chronic occlusion of the axillary-subclavian vein, reoperation may be exceptionally difficult and restoration of a patent subclavian vein not feasible even with bypass grafting. While decompression alone may still improve collateral vein function, in these circumstances continued anticoagulation is recommended to prevent additional extension of thrombus, while in the hope that there will be a progressive increase in collateral vein capacity over time (Fig. 68.1).

Table 68.4 Reoperations for venous thoracic outlet syndrome, 2008–2011

Age, sex	Side	Previous operation	Time interval	TOS Dx	Reoperative approach	Bone pathology	Treatment for SCV
19 M	R	IC FRR	1 year	RV	Paraclavicular	FR Remn	Graft bypass, AVF
22 M	R	PC FRR	7 month	RV	Infraclavicular	FR Remn	Graft bypass, AVF
38 F	L	PC FRR	2 year	RV	Paraclavicular	FR Remn	Graft bypass, AVF
19 M	L	TAx FRR	6 month	PV	Paraclavicular	FR Remn	Venolysis
23 F	R	TAx FRR	6 month	PV + SN	Paraclavicular	FR Remn	Vein patch, AVF
41 F	R	SC	5 year	RV + SN	Paraclavicular	FR Remn/Fx	Vein bypass, AVF
30 F	L	TAx FRR	1 year	PV + SN	Paraclavicular	FR Remn/Fx	Vein bypass, AVF
20 M	R	PC FRR	2 year	RV + SN	Paraclavicular	FR Remn	Venolysis

All patients were referred to Washington University Center for Thoracic Outlet Syndrome at Barnes-Jewish Hospital (St. Louis) after initial operations performed elsewhere. Time interval refers to the period of time from the initial operation for venous TOS to the current presentation with persistent/recurrent symptoms

Abbreviations: *IC* infraclavicular, *PC* paraclavicular, *SC* supraclavicular, *TAx* transaxillary, *FRR* first rib resection, *Remn* remnant, *Fx* fracture (occult), *AVF* arterio-venous fistula (radiocephalic, temporary), *PV* persistent venous TOS, *RV* recurrent venous TOS, *PN* persistent neurogenic TOS, *SN* secondary neurogenic TOS

Reoperations for persistent/recurrent venous TOS are exceptionally rare and technically challenging, and should be performed only after careful consideration of all alternatives and by those with ample experience in the operative management of all forms of TOS. It is notable that even with an active practice centered upon TOS in our institution, we have encountered only 8 patients requiring reoperations of this type over the past 3 years, representing 5.7 % of the operations performed for venous TOS during this interval (Table 68.4). Several examples of patients that have undergone reoperative procedures for persistent/recurrent venous TOS are illustrated in Figs. 68.2, 68.3, and 68.4.

Regardless of the surgical approach that was used in the initial operation, we have come to believe that the paraclavicular approach provides the most comprehensive exposure for reoperations for venous TOS and that it allows the greatest flexibility in managing the various abnormalities that might be encountered [14–19]. Most frequently, we have found that there is a remaining remnant of the first rib, particularly in the anteromedial segment close to the subclavian vein, and frequently a portion of the anterior scalene muscle, often tightly reattached to the first rib remnant. In some cases we have observed the presence of occult stress fractures of the anterior first rib, similar to our observations in patients undergoing operation for primary venous TOS [20]. The initial steps in decompression thereby involve complete resection of the first rib and scalene muscles, with adequate mobilization and protection of the brachial plexus nerve roots, followed by exposure of the entire axillary-subclavian vein and excision of surrounding fibrous scar tissue (external venolysis). Once this has been accomplished, an intraoperative venogram is performed and the need for any further venous reconstruction is determined. Vein patch angioplasty is performed for short focal stenotic lesions of the subclavian vein, but bypass graft construction is used when there are serial stenoses or a long segment occlusion, similar to the approaches we have used in operations for primary venous TOS (see Chap. 63). In addition, for patients undergoing subclavian vein reconstruction we frequently employ construction of a temporary radiocephalic arteriovenous fistula (AVF), as an adjunct to augment postoperative upper extremity venous flow, and thereby diminish any propensity toward early thrombosis. All patients are also treated with anticoagulation for a period of 12 weeks following operation, with a gradual increase in upper extremity activity. Following these approaches it has been our experience that successful reoperations for venous TOS can regularly result in durable patency to the axillary-subclavian vein and restoration of normal upper extremity function.

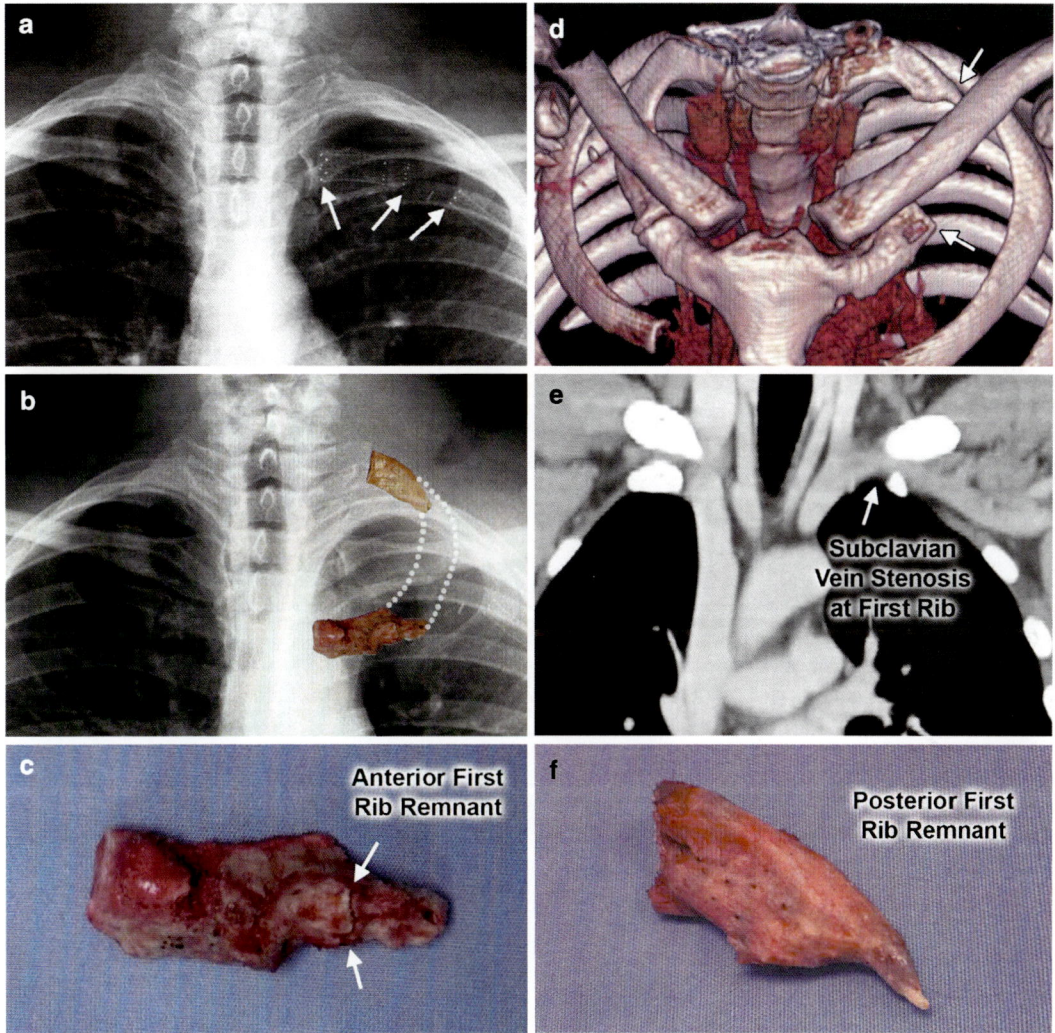

Fig. 68.2 Reoperative procedures for persistent venous TOS. (**a–c**) A patient with left-sided persistent venous TOS that had a previous transaxillary first rib resection and stents placed in the subclavian and axillary veins 1 year previously. A chest radiograph prior to reoperation (**a**) shows the location of the stents (*arrows*), compared with a postoperative chest radiograph (**b**) showing the superimposed specimens of residual first rib that were resected during paraclavicular decompression, followed by vein reconstruction with an axillary-to-innominate vein bypass graft. The anterior first rib specimen (**c**) demonstrates complete calcification and an occult fracture (*arrows*). (**d–f**) A patient with persistent left-sided venous TOS 6 months following a transaxillary first rib resection. CT image with bone windows and 3-dimensional reconstruction showing the residual anterior and posterior remnants of the first rib (**d**, *white arrows*), with maximal intensity projection (MIP) images from the contrast-enhanced study demonstrating compressive subclavian vein stenosis at the level of the residual anterior first rib (**e**, *white arrows*). Reoperation was performed by a paraclavicular approach with resection of the anterior and posterior first rib remnants (**f**), but further reconstruction of the subclavian vein was not necessary following external venolysis alone (Adapted from Sheng et al. [20]. With permission from Elsevier)

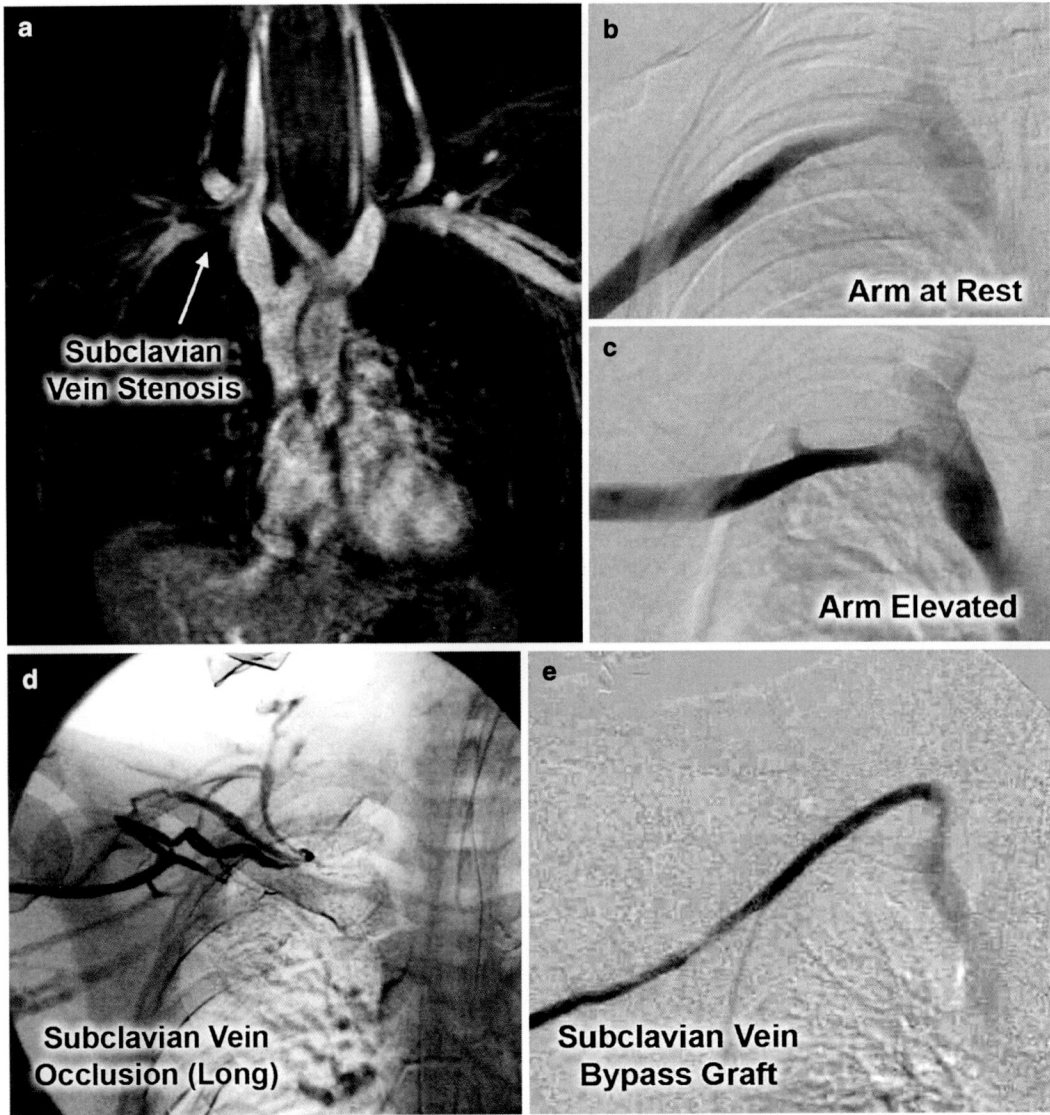

Fig. 68.3 Reoperative procedures for recurrent venous TOS. (a–c) A patient with right-sided recurrent venous TOS (and secondary neurogenic TOS) that developed 2 years after a paraclavicular first rib resection. An MR angiogram prior to reoperation shows a high-grade subclavian vein stenosis at the level of an anterior first rib remnant. (a) Following reoperative paraclavicular decompression with resection of the anterior first rib remnant and external venolysis, an intraoperative venogram demonstrates a widely patent subclavian vein and no collateral vein filling, both with the arm at rest (b) and in lateral vein filling, both with the arm at rest (b) and in elevation. (c) (d-e) A patient with recurrent right-sided venous TOS that developed 1 year following an infraclavicular first rib resection. A right upper extremity venogram prior to reoperation demonstrates a long-segment occlusion of the axillary-subclavian vein due to chronic thrombosis, with dense collateral vein filling. (d) Reoperation was performed using a paraclavicular approach, with resection of first rib remnant and direct subclavian vein reconstruction using an axillary-to-innominate vein bypass graft. An intraoperative completion venogram demonstrates a widely patent bypass graft with no filling of collateral veins (e)

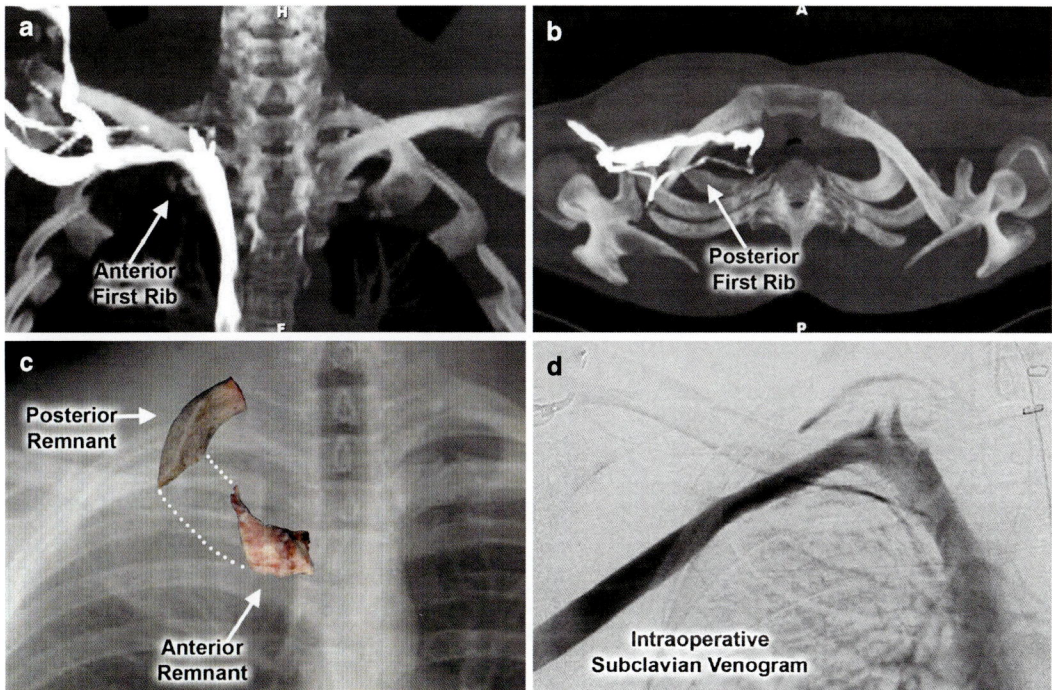

Fig. 68.4 Paraclavicular approach for reoperative treatment of venous TOS. A patient with symptomatic right-sided recurrent venous TOS and secondary neurogenic TOS, presenting 2 years after undergoing a paraclavicular first rib resection and repeated attempts at subclavian vein balloon angioplasty. (**a**) Maximal intensity projection (MIP) images from a contrast-enhanced CT study demonstrating a persistent focal stenosis in the proximal right subclavian vein during arm elevation, located adjacent to a small remnant of the anterior first rib (*arrow*). (**b**) Transverse MIP images demonstrating expanded collateral venous pathways passing through the thoracic outlet adjacent to a remnant of the posterior first rib (*arrow*). (**c**) Operative specimens of the anterior and posterior first rib remnants removed during reoperative paraclavicular decompression, superimposed on the plain chest radiograph (*arrows*). (**d**) Intraoperative contrast venogram obtained following external venolysis, demonstrating a widely patent subclavian vein with no filling of collateral venous pathways (Adapted from Thompson [19]. With permission from Thieme)

References

1. Illig KA, Doyle AJ. A comprehensive review of Paget-Schroetter syndrome. J Vasc Surg. 2010;51(6):1538–47.
2. Melby SJ, Vedantham S, Narra VR, Paletta Jr GA, Khoo-Summers L, Driskill M, Thompson RW. Comprehensive surgical management of the competitive athlete with effort thrombosis of the subclavian vein (Paget-Schroetter syndrome). J Vasc Surg. 2008;47(4):809–20.
3. Molina JE, Hunter DW, Dietz CA. Paget-Schroetter syndrome treated with thrombolytics and immediate surgery. J Vasc Surg. 2007;45(2):328–34.
4. Sanders RJ, Haug C. Subclavian vein obstruction and thoracic outlet syndrome: a review of etiology and management. Ann Vasc Surg. 1990;4:397–410.
5. Hughes ESR. Venous obstruction in the upper extremity (Paget-Schroetter's syndrome). Int Abstr Surg. 1949;88:89–127.
6. Sanders RJ, Hammond SL. Venous thoracic outlet syndrome. Hand Clin. 2004;20(1):113–8.
7. Thompson RW, Driskill M. Thoracic outlet syndrome: neurogenic. In: Cronenwett JL, Johnston KW, editors. Rutherford's vascular surgery. 7th ed. Philadelphia: Elsevier; 2010. p. 1878–98.
8. Emery VB, Rastogi R, Driskill MR, Thompson RW. Diagnosis of neurogenic thoracic outlet syndrome. In: Eskandari MK, Morasch MD, Pearce WH, Yao JST, editors. Vascular surgery: therapeutic strategies. Shelton: People's Medical Publishing House-USA; 2010. p. 129–48.
9. Sanders RJ, Hammond SL, Rao NM. Diagnosis of thoracic outlet syndrome. J Vasc Surg. 2007;46(3):601–4.

10. Jordan SE, Machleder HI. Diagnosis of thoracic outlet syndrome using electrophysiologically guided anterior scalene blocks. Ann Vasc Surg. 1998;12(3):260–4.

11. de Leon R, Chang DC, Busse C, Call D, Freischlag JA. First rib resection and scalenectomy for chronically occluded subclavian veins: what does it really do? Ann Vasc Surg. 2008;22(3):395–401.

12. de Leon RA, Chang DC, Hassoun HT, Black JH, Roseborough GS, Perler BA, Rotellini-Coltvet L, Call D, Busse C, Freischlag JA. Multiple treatment algorithms for successful outcomes in venous thoracic outlet syndrome. Surgery. 2009;145(5):500–7.

13. Chang KZ, Likes K, Demos J, Black JH, Freischlag JA. Routine venography following transaxillary first rib resection and scalenectomy (FRRS) for chronic subclavian vein thrombosis ensures excellent outcomes and vein patency. Vasc Endovascular Surg. 2012;46(1):15–20.

14. Thompson RW, Schneider PA, Nelken NA, Skioldebrand CG, Stoney RJ. Circumferential venolysis and paraclavicular thoracic outlet decompression for "effort thrombosis" of the subclavian vein. J Vasc Surg. 1992;16(5):723–32.

15. Thompson RW, Petrinec D, Toursarkissian B. Surgical treatment of thoracic outlet compression syndromes. II. Supraclavicular exploration and vascular reconstruction. Ann Vasc Surg. 1997;11(4):442–51.

16. Melby SJ, Thompson RW. Supraclavicular (paraclavicular) approach for thoracic outlet syndrome. In: Pearce WH, Matsumura JS, Yao JST, editors. Operative vascular surgery in the endovascular era. Evanston: Greenwood Academic; 2008. p. 434–45.

17. Thompson RW. Venous thoracic outlet syndrome: paraclavicular approach. Op Tech Gen Surg. 2008; 10(3):113–21.

18. Emery VB, Thompson RW. Axillary-subclavian vein effort thrombosis: surgical care. In: Lumsden AB, Davies MG, editors. Venous thromboembolic disease: contemporary endovascular management series, vol. 2. Minneapolis: Cardiotext Publishing; 2011. p. 163–78.

19. Thompson RW. Comprehensive management of subclavian vein effort thrombosis. Sem Intervent Radiol. 2012;29(1):44–51.

20. Sheng GG, Duwayri YM, Emery VB, Wittenberg AM, Moriarty CT, Thompson RW. Costochondral calcification, osteophytic degeneration, and occult first rib fractures in patients with venous thoracic outlet syndrome. J Vasc Surg. 2012;55(5): 1363–9.

Adam J. Doyle

Abstract

This chapter summarizes some of the steps that should be taken to facilitate future clinical research in venous thoracic outlet syndrome (VTOS). Standardization of nomenclature and classification of disease are a first priority. An example of possible classification scheme is proposed. This could then be followed by with multi-institutional observational data collection to solidify our understanding of the disease process. Following this, specific questions that remain unclear could be answered by undertaking prospective randomized study. Lastly, with a more thorough understanding of VTOS, rational basic science research could be performed.

Introduction

The study of venous thoracic outlet syndrome (VTOS) is made difficult by a surprising lack of reliable data, and virtually no knowledge has been derived from randomized trials. As a result there is limited evidence-based data about VTOS. Many feel that treatment for VTOS is standard and widely accepted. Upon close examination of the literature, however, it is clear that there is a surprising lack of consensus about how to classify, treat, and report outcomes surrounding VTOS. There is significant need for agreed-upon reporting standards, rigorous prospective study, and eventually multiple randomized trials.

A.J. Doyle, MD
Department of Surgery,
University of Rochester Medical Center,
601 Elmwood Ave, Box SURG, Rochester,
NY 14642, USA
e-mail: adam_doyle@urmc.rochester.edu

A recent Cochrane review identified a total of 301 articles, but only 33 were judged of sufficient quality to reviewed based on selection criteria and only two randomized controlled trials were identified [1]. As a starting point, this chapter will propose common nomenclature and reporting standards, specifically in this context to establish a framework for clinical investigation and ideally to make multi-institution prospective collaboration possible. Once the natural history of VTOS can truly be described, areas of uncertainty can be identified and prospectively studied in multi-institution randomized trials.

Nomenclature and Reporting Standards

The Society for Vascular Surgery has published reporting standards on virtually every aspect of vascular surgery except Thoracic Outlet

Table 69.1 Primary VTOS types and characteristics

Type of VTOS	Onset and timing of symptoms	Severity	Initial venographic findings	Post-thrombolysis venographic findings
Intermittent positional obstruction w/o thrombosis	Chronic positional with exertion	Mild-moderate	Normal vein at rest with varying degree of collateral pathways with provocative maneuvers	0 % stenosis
Intermittent positional obstruction w/ thrombosis	Acute	Moderate to severe	Complete occlusion with varying degree of collateral pathways	0 % stenosis
Partial obstruction w/o thrombosis	Chronic positional with exertion	Mild-moderate	Partial occlusion with multiple collateral pathways that compress with provocative maneuvers	1–99 % stenosis of varying length
Partial obstruction w/thrombosis	Acute worsening of prior symptoms	Moderate-severe	Complete occlusion with multiple collateral pathways with thrombosis	1–99 % stenosis of varying length
Chronic occlusion w/o thrombosis	Chronic with exertion	None – moderate	Complete occlusion with multiple collateral pathways	100 % stenosis of varying length
Chronic occlusion w/thrombosis	Acute worsening of prior symptoms	Moderate-severe	Complete occlusion with multiple collateral pathways with thrombosis	100 % stenosis of varying length

Syndrome, and such a document is, we feel, sorely needed. Reporting standards for patients with VTOS (and all of TOS in general) should include the following:

- Exact classification of the disease,
- Criteria for consistent description of the individual problem
- Categorization of intervention, and
- Criteria for posttreatment improvement, deterioration, failure, and complications (with grades for severity or outcome).

Classification of the Disease and Criteria for Consistent Description of the Problem

VTOS is divided into several somewhat overlapping entities by various authors: Intermittent positional obstruction, chronic partial obstruction, and complete occlusion, chronic or acute. While some patients present with chronic symptoms but no thrombosis, patients in any one of these can progress to acute axillo-subclavian vein thrombosis. Table 69.1 describes the different types of VTOS and the various associated characteristics. These processes likely overlap and together make up a spectrum of disease, each

potentially with varying rates of success to certain treatments. To reduce confusion and the subjective nature, VTOS should be considered as one diagnosis and subsequently reported according to the most relevant manifestation at the time of diagnosis and treatment. It may be that a simplified version of this (with subcategories) will be most useful.

Venous stenoses can be described in a fashion similar to the way lesions in the arterial system are described. Table 69.2 illustrates a possible division and description scheme by acuity, clinical symptoms, etiology, anatomic location, percent stenosis, and length of stenosis. All patients require pre-operative venography in order to accurately classify the underlying pathologic process. Finally, Table 69.3 describes a possible grading system to describe VTOS patients' clinical symptoms with objective criteria.

Categorization of Operation and Intervention

Any procedure performed in patients with VTOS needs to be reported in a consistent fashion. Each intervention/procedure should be

Table 69.2 VTOS classification scheme

Acuity	Clinical description	Etiology	Location	% stenosis (following thombolysis if acute thrombosis)	Length of stenosis
# Hours/days/ months/years	Asymptomatic/mild claudication/moderate to severe claudication/ rest pain	Thrombosis/ stenosis/positional obstruction	Subclavian vein/ axillary vein/ Innominate vein	0–100 %	0–20 cm

Table 69.3 Objective criteria for clinical description of VTOS

Grade	Clinical description	Objective criteria
0	Asymptomatic	No symptoms with moderate exertion
1	Mild claudication	Non-lifestyle-limiting symptoms develop after 5 min of moderate exercise, and are quickly relieved with rest
2	Moderate-severe claudication	Life-style-limiting symptoms develop within 5 min of moderate exercise, and slowly resolved with rest
3	Rest pain	Unrelenting symptoms at rest

Symptoms include: arm/scapular/axillary/base of neck/chest wall pain, non-pitting edema of arm, arm weakness, sensory changes

Table 69.4 Scale for changing change in clinical status in VTOS

+2	Asymptomatic
+1	Mild to moderate improvement, still symptomatic with exertion, but improved by at least one category
0	No change in symptoms or category
−1	Mild to moderately worse symptoms with no change in category
−2	Severe symptoms, one category worse, or major complication

reported independent of the overall treatment strategy, although possibly the combination of thrombolysis followed by planned first rib excision should be reported as one intervention (with specific description of events in the situations where interval re-occlusion or failure to complete the entire planned intervention occurs and "intent-to-treat" analysis made). Each intervention should have patency and associated change in clinical status or QOL reported (as below) when possible. The timing of such interventions should be described relative to either initial presentation and to other treatments modalities applied. Descriptions of an endovascular interventions should obviously include agent used, including dose and duration, a description of the underlying lesion (occlusion, stenosis, length of treated segment, vessel diameter), a detailed description of technique, including size and length of balloons or stents, method of access, and adjunctive measures to maintain patency, and any complications that occur.

Criteria for Improvement, Deterioration, and Failure

Various outcomes can be measured after treatment including patency, clinical status, and quality of life. All outcomes regardless of timing should be reported as 30 day outcomes and subsequently followed and reported using life table analysis for as long a duration as possible. The criteria for defining various outcomes should be clearly established. Patency must be based upon objective data and caution must be used when using ultrasound for this purpose as large collaterals can be mistaken for a patent vein. Anatomic patency and symptom status should be separately recorded.

Reporting changes in clinical status in patients with VTOS after treatment has been perhaps the most poorly described factor in most reports. Table 69.4 is a proposed scale to describe changes in clinical outcomes. Dr. Freischlag's group at Johns Hopkins has lead the way by prospectively obtaining and reporting functional and quality of life (QOL) data in patients with VTOS [2]. Both instruments used were previously validated questionnaires and included the Disability of the Arm, Shoulder and Hand (DASH) and the Short-Form 12 (SF-12). Improvements were noted in both instruments in patients treated for VTOS. Either, both, or a new instrument derived and validated from aspects the DASH and SF-12 could be used in the future to report QOL outcomes in VTOS.

Overall Strategy

After establishing standardized nomenclature, classification of disease, and reporting standards for interventions, and outcomes, the infrastructure would be established to allow collaborative study. Prospective randomized trials are always the gold standard, but because this is a relatively rare disease alternatives should be carefully considered. The simplest proposition is to create a standard protocol based on agreed-upon criteria as outlined above – perhaps best accomplished by the development of a TOS module within the Society for Vascular Surgery quality improvement initiative registry.

Research Directions

After multi-institutional collaboration and data collection has occurred the natural history of VTOS should become more clear. In addition, with the research infrastructure in place, multi-institution randomized control trials could be attempted. The following is a list of steps:
1. Establish and agree on reporting standards
2. Set up unified registry that allows for multi-institutional data collection and analysis
3. Collect observational data and solidify knowledge of natural history

4. Identify areas of research and conduct prospective randomized trials, ideally multi-institutional, with long-term follow-up and precise functional outcomes determined. For example:
   (a) First rib removal or not after thrombolysis?
   (b) Aggressive treatment of residual defects (endoluminal versus operative) after thrombolysis?
   (c) Intervene or observe for intermittent positional obstruction?
   (d) Prophylactic intervention or observe asymptomatic contralateral side?
   (e) Duration of anticoagulation after treatment?
   (f) Best method to approach the first rib?
5. Basic science research in genetics and pathophysiology of VTOS and potential nonoperative therapies or preventive strategies

Summary

The literature surrounding VTOS is often difficult to interpret as a result of a lack of standardized reporting standards. This chapter provides a brief framework for the steps that need to be taken to facilitate meaningful future clinical research in VTOS. By standardizing reporting and centralizing multi-institutional data collection much of the ambiguity surrounding VTOS would be removed and specific questions could be answered through thoughtfully preformed control trials.

References

1. Povlsen B, Belzberg A, Hansson T, Dorsi M. Treatment for thoracic outlet syndrome. Cochrane Database Syst Rev. 2010; (1):CD007218.
2. Chang DC, Rotellini-Coltvet LA, Mukherjee D, De Leon R, Freischlag JA. Surgical intervention for thoracic outlet syndrome improves patient's quality of life. J Vasc Surg. 2009;49(3):630–5; discussion 635–7.

Despite all our knowledge (or what we think is knowledge) about VTOS, questions arise as to the details of treatment at all stages and significant dissenting voices exist. This is due, to a significant extent, to the lack of prospective randomized trials. Though there is general consensus on a basic protocol, the best approach to almost every step in the treatment of these patients is debated.

For instance, while thrombolysis is routinely performed prior to thoracic outlet decompression by most, a recent review from the Johns Hopkins group demonstrated no advantage of preoperative thrombolysis compared to anticoagulation alone in patients with thromboses more than a few weeks old [1]. Richard Green addresses this topic below, noting that the age of the clot is one of the most important factors to consider when making this decision (see Chap. 70). By contrast, others argue the opposite point – that once the vein is reopened, not everyone needs first rib resection. This argument is nicely made by Kaj Johansson, whose experience with this algorithm spans several decades. If the rib is to be removed after thrombolysis, when should this occur? Early in our experience a delay of several months was advocated, while most modern series favor immediate resection. This issue, as well as the risks and benefits of each option, is explored by Jason Lee, while Richard Green analyzes the factors favoring one approach to the first rib over another specifically in patients with VTOS. Disagreement as to the postoperative management of VTOS largely concerns the use of stents and anticoagulation. David Gillespie analyzes what role, if any, stents play in treating this entity, while Hugh Gelabert discusses the data surrounding postoperative anticoagulation. Finally, VTOS is caused to a significant degree by anatomic factors, whether as a direct cause or a predisposition to later problems when the environment has added its input. As such, bilateral risk is not unreasonable to assume, and Adam Doyle analyzes this poorly-studied issue.

No matter how firm we all are in our opinions regarding treatment of VTOS, it is indisputable that essentially no prospective randomized data exist. Well-supported, thoughtful opinion from those with extensive experience in this field is critical to include in any discussion of treatment options for this problem.

Reference

1. Guzzo JL, et al. Preoperative thrombolysis and venoplasty affords no benefit in patency following first rib resection and scalenectomy for subacute and chronic subclavian vein thrombosis. J Vasc Surg. 2010;52(3):658–63.

Controversies in VTOS: Is Lysis
Always Required in Patient with
Effort Thrombosis?

70

Richard M. Green

Abstract

The treatment of subclavian venous thrombosis due to thoracic outlet
compression has been significantly altered over the past few decades due
to the advent of percutaneous therapies. Most believe that the combination
of venous thrombolysis followed by thoracic outlet decompression is safe
and effective, and best for most patients. The only cases that thrombolysis
is not used are those with subacute or chronic occlusions, those patients
with limited symptoms and functional needs, and those with significant
medical contraindications.

With increasing awareness that axillosubclavian
vein thrombosis is not just an "upper extremity
DVT," early diagnosis and aggressive treatment
have become the standard of care. The goals of
treatment include the elimination of symptoms,
prevention of long-term disability, and the avoidance of long-term anticoagulation. Untreated or
treatment with anticoagulant therapy alone is
suboptimal, resulting in some degree of chronic
disability and persistent symptoms of upper
extremity venous obstruction in anywhere from
25 to 75 % of affected patients [1, 2]. The contemporary management of acute effort thrombosis includes all the following elements: the
restoration of venous patency, the elimination of
any extrinsic compression and the correction of
any residual venous stenosis.

The paradigm that utilizes early catheter-
directed thrombolytic therapy as the initial therapy provides the best chance for complete clot
dissolution in the acute setting [3]. Whether or
not every patient requires complete clot dissolution for symptomatic relief is not certain. This
choice is in part made by the severity of the arm
swelling and the functional needs of the individual patient. Usually those patients with symptoms
following thrombosis will have functional
requirements that make clot dissolution important. The degree of success is largely dependent
on the duration of the thrombosis. Recently, after
a retrospective review of cases from Johns
Hopkins the effectiveness of thrombolysis was
questioned as it appears not to have improved
long-term vein patency for those patients with
sub-acute presentations [4].

Treatment with thrombolysis alone results in
rethrombosis rates of >50 %; treatment without
thoracic outlet decompression has high rates of
both rethrombosis and stent fracture. Therapy

R.M. Green, MD
Department of Surgery, Lenox Hill Hospital,
130 East 77th Street, New York, NY 10075, USA
e-mail: rgreen@nshs.edu

K.A. Illig et al. (eds.), *Thoracic Outlet Syndrome*,
DOI 10.1007/978-1-4471-4366-6_70, © Springer-Verlag London 2013

that includes early thrombolysis, thoracic outlet decompression and adjunctive treatment of residual venous stenoses achieves long-term patency rates of 92–100 % in multiple series.

Machleder [5] indicated that a period of time approaching 6 weeks should elapse between thrombolysis and rib removal. The prevailing current opinion is that thrombolytic therapy should be immediately followed by operative first-rib resection. The use of adjunctive catheter-based intervention of any underlying venous abnormality at the costo-clavicular space uncovered during thrombolysis is controversial. The potential advantages of such an aggressive strategy are that the risk for recurrent thrombosis is reduced and the patients are more likely to escape the consequences of major venous obstruction on the affected arm [6].

Thrombolysis

The results of catheter-directed thrombolytic therapy for axillo-subclavian venous thrombosis, regardless of etiology, are mostly dependent on the chronicity of the thrombus. Most contemporary series report rates of near-complete thrombus clearance when prompt treatment is initiated. Delayed thrombolysis, even if partially successful, often leaves areas of stenotic webs that may require operative repair. These chronic lesions may even be present when thrombolysis is performed immediately because the process is thought to be an acute manifestation of a chronic condition.

We would like to emphasize several technical caveats about thrombolysis. First, it is important to cannulate the median antecubital vein, not the cephalic vein. The latter is a mistake and will result in the guide wire entering the subclavian vein central to the thrombus. We will often use access from a femoral vein when the arm is swollen and the basilic vein is obscured. Second, we are reluctant to continue thrombolytic therapy when no immediate benefit is achieved and almost always stop treatment after 24 h. Rarely, thrombolysis will not be effective either physiologically or anatomically even when the thrombus can be crossed with a wire and catheter directed drug administration is possible. We may reluctantly recanalize the occluded vein with a self-expanding stent prior to operative decompression but this is not a long-term solution as the stents are subject to compression between the clavicle and first rib, fracture and recurrent thrombosis [7].

Management After Thrombolysis

There is a short-term recurrence rate approaching 30 % when the underlying condition responsible for the venous occlusion is neglected [8]. While it was once acceptable to delay therapy after thrombolysis in order to assess the residual venous abnormality and the effect it has on the patient, the treatment algorithm has clearly changed to earlier intervention in young, active patients. Some patients, particularly those who are elderly or sedentary, will remain asymptomatic even if their vein re-occludes and no further intervention is often a reasonable choice. In this setting our preference is not to use thrombolysis unless the arm is painfully swollen.

Our preferred approach at this time is to recommend first rib resection in the same hospitalization immediately after thrombolysis. Our preference for these patients is the transaxillary approach as it offers direct visualization and exposure of the costoclavicular space and the site of venous compression. It also allows the operator to perform an external venolysis when necessary in the presence of extrinsic venous compression. Urschel and Kourlis [9] challenged the wisdom of waiting to remove the rib and divided a group of patients with subclavian vein thrombosis into those treated with anticoagulation following thrombolysis and those treated with immediate operative decompression of the thoracic outlet. Almost two-thirds of the nonoperative group developed recurrent symptoms during a 6-week period of follow-up. In contrast, 89 % of those treated with immediate first rib decompression following thrombolysis were able to return to work free of symptoms but the follow-up period was only 6 weeks.

We now perform decompression while the patient is fully heparinized, typically place a large suction drain in the axillary space and have not had to re-operate for hematoma. Once the rib is removed we proceed with another venogram in the neutral and shoulder abducted position. A few patients will have no abnormalities of the subclavian vein in either position and they should be treated with a 3–6 month course of oral anticoagulation. Any extrinsic compressive lesion should have been eliminated by the operative procedure but the majority of patients will have an intrinsic lesion of the subclavian vein in the costoclavicular space. The pivotal question that must be addressed in patients with intrinsic lesions is whether the subclavian vein needs to be treated. We try to individualize our recommendations and those patients with persistent signs of venous obstruction, active life styles and physically demanding vocations should have venous intervention after successful thrombolysis. There are no studies comparing the long-term results of these procedures with less aggressive therapies however [10].

In conclusion, the treatment of subclavian venous thrombosis due to thoracic outlet compression has gone through a major change with the advent of percutaneous therapies. We currently believe that the combination treatment of venous thrombolysis followed by thoracic outlet decompression is safe and effective. The only cases that thrombolysis is not used are those with subacute or chronic occlusions, those patients with limited symptoms and functional need and those with medical contraindications. While we may in the immediate post-operative elect to perform a balloon angioplasty for a severe intrinsic lesion and persistent arm swelling, we feel that stent placement is rarely indicated.

References

1. Hughes ESR. Venous obstruction in the upper extremity (Paget-Schroetter's syndrome): a review of 320 cases. Int Abstr Surg. 1949;88:89–127.
2. Tilney NL, Griffiths HJG, Edwards EA. Natural history of major venous thrombosis of the upper extremity. Arch Surg. 1970;101:792–6.
3. Druy EM, Trout III HH, Giordano JM, Hix WR. Lytic therapy in the treatment of axillary and subclavian vein thrombosis. J Vasc Surg. 1985;2:821–7.
4. Guzzo JL, Chang K, Demos J, et al. Preoperative thrombolysis and venoplasty affords no benefit in patency following first rib resection and scalenectomy for subacute and chronic subclavian vein thrombosis. J Vasc Surg. 2010;52:658–62.
5. Machleder HI. Upper extremity venous occlusion. In: Ernst CB, Stanley JC, editors. Current therapy in vascular surgery. 3rd ed. St. Louis: Mosby-Year Book Inc.; 1995. p. 958–63.
6. Lee C, Grassi CJ, Belkin M, et al. Early operative intervention after thrombolytic therapy for primary subclavian vein thrombosis: an effective treatment approach. J Vasc Surg. 1998;27:1101–8.
7. Lee J, Karwowski J, Harris EJ, et al. Long-term thrombotic recurrence after nonoperative management of Paget-Schroetter syndrome. J Vasc Surg. 2006;43:1236–43.
8. Stange-Vognsen III HH, Hauch O, Anderson J, Struckmann J. Resection of the first rib following deep arm vein thrombolysis in patients with thoracic outlet syndrome. J Cardiovasc Surg. 1989;30:430–3.
9. Urschel HC, Kourlis H. Thoracic outlet syndrome: a 50-year experience at Baylor University Medical Center. Proc (Bayl Univ Med Cent). 2007;2:125–35.
10. Kreienberg PB, Chang BB, Darling 3rd RC, et al. Long-term results in patients treated with thrombolysis, thoracic inlet decompression, and subclavian vein stenting for Paget-Schroetter syndrome. J Vasc Surg. 2001;33(2 Suppl):S100–5.

Controversies in VTOS: Is Costoclavicular Junction Decompression Always Needed in VTOS?

71

Kaj H. Johansen

Abstract

Extrinsic compression of the subclavian vein as it traverses the costoclavicular space is postulated as the cause of venous thoracic outlet syndrome, and many believe that costoclavicular space decompression – by first rib resection or by claviculectomy – is required to treat this condition as well as to prevent its recurrence. Alternative therapeutic approaches include bypass of the obstructed vein, usually to (or utilizing) the ipsilateral internal jugular vein, or, alternatively, withholding operative intervention and instead allowing axillosubclavian vein thrombolysis and recanalization and venous collateralization to decompress the congested ipsilateral upper extremity.

Introduction

Contemporary management of venous thoracic outlet syndrome (VTOS) presenting as frank subclavian vein thrombosis often includes an initial effort at venous thrombolysis. When this is successful it is commonplace for the completion venogram to demonstrate a high-grade subclavian venous stenosis at the level of the costoclavicular junction (between the clavicle and first rib). Such a finding, associated with chronic intimal damage and neointimal hypertrophy within the vein at this site, suggests that extrinsic venous compression has resulted in a thrombogenic surface which has led in turn to the development of thrombosis. It is also commonplace to find significant scarring around the outside of the subclavian vein at this site at the time of operative exploration. Because it is widely held that this extrinsic compression results from the proximity of the bony bounds of the costoclavicular space, it has followed that opening of the costoclavicular space is recommended to prevent recurrent VTOS.

Arguments Favoring Decompression of the Costoclavicular Space

That extrinsic bony compression between the clavicle and the first rib is the cause of the subclavian venous stenosis and perivenous scarring commonly found in these patients is difficult to refute. Numerous clinical reports seem to suggest

K.H. Johansen, MD, PhD
Department of Vascular Surgery,
Swedish Heart & Vascular Institute,
1600 E. Jefferson St. #101, Seattle, WA 98122, USA
e-mail: kaj.johansen@swedish.org

K.A. Illig et al. (eds.), *Thoracic Outlet Syndrome*,
DOI 10.1007/978-1-4471-4366-6_71, © Springer-Verlag London 2013

that decompression of the costoclavicular space, either by first rib resection [1–3] or alternatively by claviculectomy [4], significantly diminishes the likelihood of recurrent VTOS. Some have also argued that opening the costoclavicular space results in favorable outcomes even when the subclavian vein is chronically occluded [5]. Even the observation that subclavian venous angioplasty, in comparison to thrombolysis alone, often results in improved outcomes [6], supports the conclusion that a structural problem exists at this site, relief of which is important in avoiding recurrent venous thrombotic complications.

While angioplasty may have a useful role to play for the treatment of the venous stenosis commonly seen in the subclavian vein at the level of the costoclavicular space, venous stenting has been associated with an unacceptably increased incidence of stent fracture [7]. However, venous stenting appears to be both effective and durable at other sites in the body devoid of bony extrinsic compression (for example, in failing arteriovenous access [8] and May Thurner syndrome [9]), and thus a further argument in favor of costoclavicular space decompression in VTOS is that subsequent subclavian venous stenting can be performed without concern for resulting stent fracture.

Certainly those who favor an aggressive surgical approach to VTOS would argue that failure to pursue such an option, particularly early in the course of the condition, results in a "loss of opportunity" to undergo definitive repair. If the patient returns later with a chronically occluded axillosubclavian vein, these advocates would argue that the patient's therapeutic options have been significantly limited by the prior failure to perform timely thoracic outlet decompression by means of a simple first rib resection (or claviculectomy).

Arguments Favoring Alternative Approaches to the Management of VTOS

Anatomically *all* of us have the anatomic potential for extrinsic compression of the subclavian vein at the costoclavicular space. Indeed, significant extrinsic subclavian vascular compression occurs with the arm held in provocative postures in a substantial proportion of asymptomatic individuals [10]. However, despite this anatomic truism, few of us develop VTOS. A substantial proportion – in my experience up to a third – of individuals undergoing thrombolysis for acute VTOS are found to have little or no angiographic evidence for a persistent intimal defect at the suggested site of extrinsic compression once acute thrombus has been cleared. In addition, an increased prevalence of one or another of the thrombophilic states – obviously an issue entirely independent of the venous anatomy within the costoclavicular space – has been documented in patients with VTOS [11] and may be an alternative risk factor for the development of venous TOS.

Accordingly, several alternatives to costoclavicular space decompression for the definitive management of VTOS have been proposed. The first, detailed elsewhere (see Chap. 57) is based on the assertion that the natural history of VTOS is benign in the vast majority of patients and that, if such individuals are simply treated by initial thrombolysis, balloon angioplasty (if feasible) and 3–6 months of anticoagulation, their ultimate outcomes will be no less favorable than those reported in patients undergoing first rib resection and subclavian venolysis or venoplasty or other such aggressive surgical interventions. In other words, this argument suggests observational care may be associated with results which are not inferior to those in VTOS patients undergoing a major operation.

An alternative to costoclavicular space decompression in patients with symptomatic VTOS focuses on the use of various forms of bypass of the congested upper extremity venous system *around* the site of venous stenosis or occlusion. This can be carried out either by an ipsilateral autogenous venous reconstruction (see Chap. 65) or alternatively by the interposition of a biologic or prosthetic bypass graft from the axillobrachial vein to (usually) the ipsilateral internal jugular vein [12]. Such patients commonly require long-term antithrombotic medication, and also may have an adjunctive arteriovenous fistula constructed to try to maintain bypass graft patency. Bypass procedures for the treatment of VTOS have been uncommonly performed and few data are available regarding their long-term success rates.

Comment

It is possible, although it is not proven, that extrinsic bony compression of the subclavian vein at the costoclavicular space results in both an intrinsic intimal defect as well as extrinsic adventitial scarring of the vein, all of which result in VTOS. If this is true it seems prudent to relieve this extrinsic compression at the same time subclavian venous patency is restored. The fact that 100 % of us have subclavian veins which pass through the costoclavicular space, as well as the fact that up to a third of us have significant extrinsic compression of the subclavian vein with our arms held in provocative postures yet never develop VTOS, suggests a more complex etiology for VTOS than a simple mechanical extrinsic compression at the costoclavicular space. Evidence that a substantial number of individuals who have suffered an episode of VTOS appear to do well without any surgical intervention at all suggests, at the least, that costoclavicular space decompression for VTOS patients should be selective rather than automatic. Consideration of observational care, perhaps for 6–12 months, with costoclavicular space decompression and either direct venous reconstruction or bypass at that point in those individuals still unacceptably symptomatic would seem to be an optimal approach.

References

1. Taylor LM, McAllister WR, Dennis DL, et al. Thrombolytic therapy followed by first rib resection for spontaneous ("effort") subclavian vein thrombosis. Am J Surg. 1985;149:644–7.
2. Kunkel JM, Machleder HI. Treatment of Paget-Schroetter syndrome. Arch Surg. 1989;124:1153–8.
3. Adelman MA, Stone DH, Riles TS, et al. A multidisciplinary approach to the treatment of Paget-Schroetter syndrome. Ann Vasc Surg. 1997;11:149–54.
4. Green RM, Waldman D, Ouriel K, et al. Claviculectomy for subclavian venous repair: long-term functional results. J Vasc Surg. 2000;32:315–21.
5. de Leon RA, Chang DC, Busse C, et al. First rib resection and scalenectomy for chronically-occluded subclavian veins: what does it really do? Ann Vasc Surg. 2008;22:395–401.
6. Glanz S, Gordon DH, Lipkowitz GS, et al. Axillary and subclavian vein stenosis: percutaneous angioplasty. Radiology. 1988;168:371–3.
7. Bjornason H, Hunter DW, Crain MR, et al. Collapse of a Palmaz stent in the subclavian vein. AJR Am J Roentgenol. 1993;160:1123–4.
8. Haskal ZJ, Trerotola S, Dolmatch B, et al. Stent graft versus balloon angioplasty for failing dialysis-access grafts. N Engl J Med. 2010;362:494–503.
9. Neglen P, Hollis KC, Olivier J, Raju S. Stenting of the venous outflow in chronic venous disease: long-term stent-related outcome, clinical and hemodynamic result. J Vasc Surg. 2007;46:979–90.
10. Juvonen T, Satta J, Laitala P, et al. Anomalies at the thoracic outlet are frequent in the general population. Am J Surg. 1995;170:33–7.
11. Cassada DC, Lipscomb SL, Stevens S, et al. The importance of thrombophilia in the treatment of Paget-Schroetter syndrome. Ann Vasc Surg. 2006;20:596–601.
12. Sanders RJ, Cooper MA. Surgical management of subclavian vein obstruction, including six cases of subclavian vein bypass. Surgery. 1995;118:856–63.

Controversies in VTOS: Timing of First Rib Resection After Thrombolysis

72

Jason T. Lee

Abstract

Thrombosis of the subclavian vein, or Paget-Schroetter syndrome, is an infrequent condition but one that leads to significant morbidity if not managed appropriately and initially aggressively. Over the last 20 years, a treatment paradigm has gained acceptance that rests on two principles: (1) the elimination (or at least reduction) of the thrombus load to re-establish venous patency; and (2) subsequent decompression of the "venous" thoracic outlet (costoclavicular junction). Catheter-directed thrombolysis should be considered standard of care to reduce clot burden, and response to this and a short course of anticoagulation can help determine the best candidates for operative intervention. An obligate short (3–4 week) period of operative delay allows the selection of those patients that may not require first rib resection. While younger patients who are potentially more active and might engage more rapidly in strenuous activities in the near future are perhaps the sub-group that should be offered surgical decompression, we believe it is unlikely that ALL patients must undergo operative decompression.

Introduction

Since the initial descriptions by Paget [1] and von Schroetter [2] over a century ago, the optimal therapy of effort-related primary subclavian vein thrombosis (the most common presentation of venous thoracic outlet syndrome; TOS) has been debated. While Paget-Schroetter Syndrome (PSS)

occurs infrequently and only accounts for about 1–4 % of all deep vein thromboses [3] and only about 3 % of all TOS patients [4], afflicted patients are often young and otherwise healthy. Major morbidity can develop in this patient population and lead to long-term disability if PSS is not promptly diagnosed and treated.

The major advance in treatment of PSS in the past two decades involved the recognition that early thrombolysis and then in most cases operative decompression, usually involving first rib resection and scalenectomy, is the best treatment option [5–8]. Further refinements of therapy include hybrid procedures with endovascular

J.T. Lee, MD
Department of Surgery, Stanford University Medical Center, 300 Pasteur Drive, Suite H3600, Stanford, CA 94305, USA
e-mail: jtlee@stanford.edu

K.A. Illig et al. (eds.), *Thoracic Outlet Syndrome*,
DOI 10.1007/978-1-4471-4366-6_72, © Springer-Verlag London 2013

techniques and open venous reconstruction to improve long-term vein patency [9, 10]. What remains controversial is the timing of surgery after successful thrombolysis, which is the topic of debate in this chapter.

Timing of First Rib Resection

Assuming successful thrombolysis, meaning that the majority of the thrombus load has been cleared and patient is symptomatically improved, the timing of operative decompression is the next major tree in the treatment algorithm. The decisions range from the most aggressive approach of immediate surgery during the same hospitalization to the most conservative approach of no surgery at all. While it would be convenient that there be Level I evidence showing one algorithm most superior in a well-designed prospective randomized trial, what we are faced in the literature with are non-controlled retrospective single institution series, albeit often with quite excellent results. Advantages of the most aggressive approach, namely operation during the same hospitalization, include a single hospital stay, the minimal amount of time to be on warfarin, the least chance of thrombotic recurrence from mechanical obstruction, the least amount of time away from work, sport, or school, and the knowledge that one can resume full activity in the shortest amount of time. The least aggressive approach would be to recommend no surgery at all, which would obviously have the advantage of avoiding an operation and all its attendant potential complications and disability. Reported operative complications such as brachial plexopathies, phrenic nerve paresis, subclavian arterial injuries, and lymphatic leaks, have summative incidences ranging from very low to as high as 20 % [11].

Like many clinical conditions, a semi-aggressive (or semi-conservative) approach involves selective operative decompression after successful thrombolysis. This strategy allows individual patient selection to dictate the final operative decision, and does not obligate the patient to a sole treatment method. Advantages of this approach, particularly if there is some delay until

surgery regardless, include the resolution of the surrounding inflammation immediately after a clot, allowing the patient to return to some moderately normal activity while scheduling the procedure, converting an urgent operation into an elective one, and being able to make arrangements for time off given that many of these patients are working or still in school. Obvious disadvantages to this approach include the of recurrent thromboembolism and the possibility that we are simply delaying inevitable upcoming surgery.

At our institution we have taken a middle-of-the-road approach, and found it to be particularly applicable to a wide range of patients, young and old, athletic and spontaneous, as well as risk averse and risk aggressive. Patients with resolution of symptoms after initial thrombolytic therapy and a short period of anticoagulation do not immediately undergo thoracic outlet decompression. Indications for early surgery after thrombolysis and the trial of outpatient anticoagulation include: (1) the persistence or recurrence of venous hypertensive symptoms; (2) any evidence for recurrent or new thrombus; (3) obstruction of peri-venous collaterals with abduction/external rotation in the face of subclavian vein occlusion; and (4) evidence of persistent or recurrent vein injury, as evidenced by significant wall thickening, which in our series led to 45 % of the patients undergoing early operative decompression [12].

For those that don't undergo early intervention, we determined retrospectively (through a 23 % thrombotic recurrence rate by 24 months) which risk factors led to a higher chance of recurrence. Stated another way, we determined factors if present would indicate poor candidacy for conservative treatment. We now offer younger patients <28 years old immediate surgery and agree with most other authors on the avoidance of stents prior to rib resection [13]. Our success rates of 93 % at a followup time of over 4 years with all returning to work parallel the other large series that recommend aggressive immediate operative decompression, as well as those groups that call for conservative methods.

Urschel's unparalleled experience with 294 patients over 30 years highlights the paradigm shift towards expeditious thrombolytic therapy followed by prompt first rib resection to obtain optimal results [7]. Many other institutions have employed this treatment algorithm of same hospitalization thoracic outlet decompression with high rates of symptom resolution and freedom from recurrence [6, 8]. Perhaps the fact that so many different approaches all yield excellent results means that a well-thought out algorithm at each individual institution likely will provide the best results. Even in the previously mentioned large series of patients that underwent obligate and immediate thoracic outlet decompression, there were always a few patients that refused surgery or were not operated upon, and follow-up on those patients echo our results in that many of them do remarkably well with low rates of recurrence. In Machleder's series, five patients underwent successful thrombolysis but avoided surgery by either refusing or failing to meet criteria [5]. They all did well in follow-up, with no recurrent thromboses, minimal to no symptoms, and returned to full activity.

No Decompression at All?

If there is an algorithm that is losing momentum, it would likely be the non-surgical route supported by Kaj Johansen (see Chaps. 57 and 71). His yet unpublished data continues to claim that in a series of 50 patients not decompressed, 82 % have no symptomatology out to 4 years of followup. While it is indisputable that group avoided the potential problems with an operation, the only other large series of non-operative therapy that is published is from Lokanathan et al. They reported results in 28 consecutive patients of whom only two underwent first rib resection in follow-up [14]. Re-thrombosis occurred in three (11 %) patients at 8, 16, and 17 months post initial thrombotic event, and only 6 out of 21 that they followed with a long-term questionnaire had complete resolution of symptoms, with 62 % still having mild symptoms. We feel the non-operative route is too conservative, and having no timing for surgery is likely not the optimal therapy.

Summary

In summary, Paget-Schroetter syndrome is an infrequent condition, but one that leads to significant morbidity if not managed appropriately and initially aggressively. Over the last 20 years, a treatment paradigm has gained acceptance that rests on two principles: (1) the elimination (or at least reduction) of the thrombus load to re-establish venous patency; and (2) subsequent decompression of the "venous" thoracic outlet (costoclavicular junction). Catheter-directed thrombolysis should be considered standard of care to reduce clot burden, and response to this and a short course of anticoagulation can help determine the best candidates for operative intervention. An obligate short (3–4 week) period of operative delay allows the selection of those patients that may not require first rib resection. During this time period there is potential reduction in inflammation around the vein, perhaps making the operation slightly safer. Younger patients who are potentially more active and might engage more rapidly in strenuous activities in the near future are perhaps the sub-group that should be offered surgical decompression. It is unlikely that ALL patients must undergo operative decompression, so we must use our clinical judgment and results from large series to help determine which patients should undergo operative therapy, and when that operation should occur.

References

1. Paget J. Clinical lectures and essays. London: Longman Green; 1875.
2. Von Schroetter L. Erkrankungen der Gefasse. In: Nothangels Handbuch der Speciellen Pathologie und Therapie, vol. 15. Vienna: Holder; 1899. p. 533–5.
3. Hurlbert SN, Rutherford RB. Basic data underlying clinical decision making—primary subclavian-axillary vein thrombosis. Ann Vasc Surg. 1995;9:217–23.
4. Lee JT, Dua MM, Hernandez-Boussard TM, Illig KA. Surgery for TOS: a nationwide perspective. J Vasc Surg. 2011;53:100S–1.
5. Machleder HI. Evaluation of a new treatment strategy for Paget-Schroetter syndrome: spontaneous thrombosis of the axillary-subclavian vein. J Vasc Surg. 1993; 17:305–17.

6. Lee MC, Grassi CJ, Belkin M, Mannick JA, Whittemore AD, Donaldson MC. Early operative intervention after thrombolytic therapy for primary subclavian vein thrombosis: an effective treatment approach. J Vasc Surg. 1998;27:1101–7.

7. Urschel HC, Razzuk MA. Paget-Schroetter syndrome: what is the best management? Ann Thorac Surg. 2000;69:1663–9.

8. Angle N, Gelabert HA, Farooq MM, Ahn SS, Caswell DR, Freschlag JA, et al. Safety and efficacy of early surgical decompression of the thoracic outlet for Paget-Schroetter syndrome. Ann Vasc Surg. 2001;15:37–42.

9. Kreienberg PB, Chang BB, Darling RC, Roddy SP, Paty PSK, Lloyd WE, et al. Long-term results in patients treated with thrombolysis, thoracic inlet decompression, and subclavian vein stenting for Paget-Schroetter syndrome. J Vasc Surg. 2001;33:S100–5.

10. Schneider DB, Dimuzio PJ, Martin ND, Gordon RL, Wilson MW, Laberge JM, et al. Combination treatment of venous thoracic outlet syndrome: open surgical decompression and intraoperative angioplasty. J Vasc Surg. 2004;40:599–603.

11. Lee WA, Hill BB, Harris EJ, Semba CP, Olcott C. Surgical intervention is not required for all patients with subclavian vein thrombosis. J Vasc Surg. 2000; 32:57–67.

12. Lee JT, Karwowski JK, Harris EJ, Haukoos JS, Olcott C. Long-term thrombotic recurrence after non-operative management of Paget-Schroetter syndrome. J Vasc Surg. 2006;43:1236–43.

13. Urschel HC, Patel AN. Paget-Schroetter syndrome therapy: failure of intravenous stents. Ann Thorac Surg. 2003;75:1693–6.

14. Lokanathan R, Salvian AJ, Chen JC, Morris C, Taylor DC, Hsiang YN. Outcome after thrombolysis and selective thoracic outlet decompression for primary axillary vein thrombosis. J Vasc Surg. 2001;33:783–8.

Controversies in VTOS:
What Is the Best Approach
to the First Rib in VTOS?

73

Karl A. Illig

Abstract

The critical consideration in planning treatment for patients with VTOS is that if decompression is performed, it must include the *anterior* part of the first rib. This area can be approached and resected very easily via the transaxillary approach, and this is our preferred option if no further reconstruction needs to be done. If the vein is not felt to need reconstruction, we advocate simply resecting the rib as above along with aggressive external venolysis; again, the transaxillary approach serves well. If the vein requires reconstruction, however – it is very badly diseased and the patient is symptomatic – direct and thorough exposure must be obtained. The two primary choices in this situation are the paraclavicular approach (with full mobilization of the vein from above) or rotation of the clavicle upwards ala Molina. Either approach, with the patient in the supine position, also makes completion venography very easy (and preserves the ability to correct any problems so found). Many feel there is benefit to decompressing the venous thoracic outlet even if the vein is chronically occluded. Finally, if the patient is highly symptomatic and reconstruction cannot be accomplished, jugular transposition (probably with some form of thoracic outlet decompression) is highly effective.

Introduction

Anatomic considerations are obviously important in understanding any form of thoracic outlet syndrome (TOS), but are absolutely critical for decision making in a person with venous problems

K.A. Illig, MD
Department of Surgery, Division of Vascular Surgery,
University of South Florida, 2 Tampa General Circle,
STC 7016, Tampa, FL 33606, USA
e-mail: killig@health.usf.edu

(VTOS). As discussed in Chap. 49, the subclavian vein runs past the junction of the first rib and clavicle anteriorally, and is usually intimately attached to the costoclavicular ligament and subclavius muscle (Fig. 73.1). VTOS arises as the result of damage to this area of the vein, and, as such, decompression must involve the *anterior* part of the first rib and associated structures.

Most believe that the venous thoracic outlet must be decompressed, almost always by means of first rib resection, in essentially all patients with VTOS. The primary surgical goal is thus

K.A. Illig et al. (eds.), *Thoracic Outlet Syndrome*,
DOI 10.1007/978-1-4471-4366-6_73, © Springer-Verlag London 2013

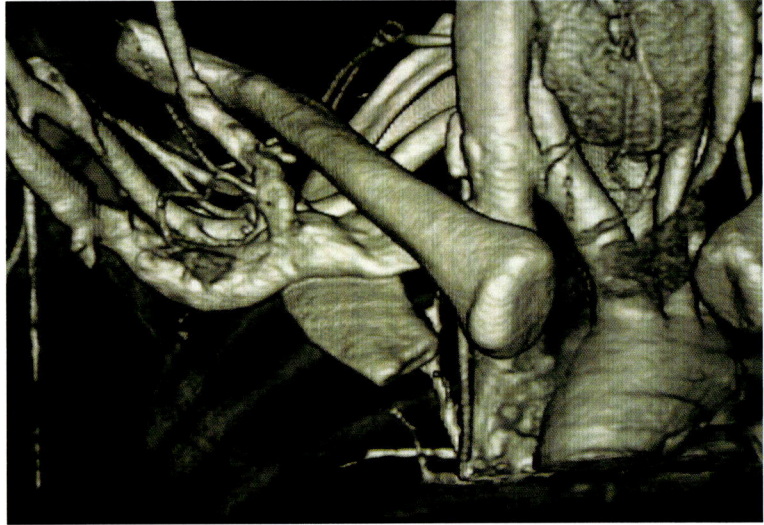

removal of the *anterior* part of the first rib. In the majority of cases there is also intrinsic damage to the vein (resulting from the chronic extrinsic compression), and the secondary issue is thus whether or not the vein must be reconstructed (or alternative drainage provided). These two factors determine the best surgical approach.

It is most convenient to divide patients with VTOS into three categories, once all possible preliminary tests and interventions (i.e., thrombolysis) have been performed: A patient with a normal vein, a patient with a diseased but patent (or very short segment occlusion) vein, and a patient with a chronically occluded vein that cannot be opened (Fig. 73.2).

The Patient with a Normal Vein

This is most often a patient with intermittent positional obstruction (seen early, before damage has occurred) – even after thrombolysis, few patients with effort thrombosis will have normal veins. In this case, the minimum goal is simply to decompress the anterior part of the thoracic outlet. While some believe that lysis or debridement of the external cicatrix surrounding the vein is helpful, essentially by definition this material is not a problem if the vein is still normal and this is not required. Transaxillary first rib excision (see Chap. 61) allows excellent exposure and removal of the rib up to the cartilaginous

insertion into the sternum, along with full visualization that the entire undersurface of the vein is free of external compression, and is thus our procedure of choice in this situation.

The Patient with a Diseased Vein

Most patients who present with effort thrombosis will have some degree of damage to the vein which will be obvious on venography after all thrombus has been removed. The first principle of therapy, decompression of the anterior part of the first rib, remains paramount, but two other goals are now potentially in play: Removal of the external scar tissue or "cicatrix," and reconstruction (or bypass) of the stenotic vein segment.

There is almost always external scar tissue in these cases, and the vein is always intimately attached to the subclavius muscle and costo-clavicular ligament. Removal of the scar tissue to the level of the inominate vein and mobilization of the vein off of these structures can fairly easily be accomplished via the transaxillary approach (recognizing that the phrenic nerves and thoracic duct (on the left) are in play). Many times a vein that is felt to be intrinsically damage will look surprisingly good after external venolysis (Fig. 73.3). The transaxillary approach, however, does not lend itself well to obtaining venography, so if this is felt necessary, another approach is needed.

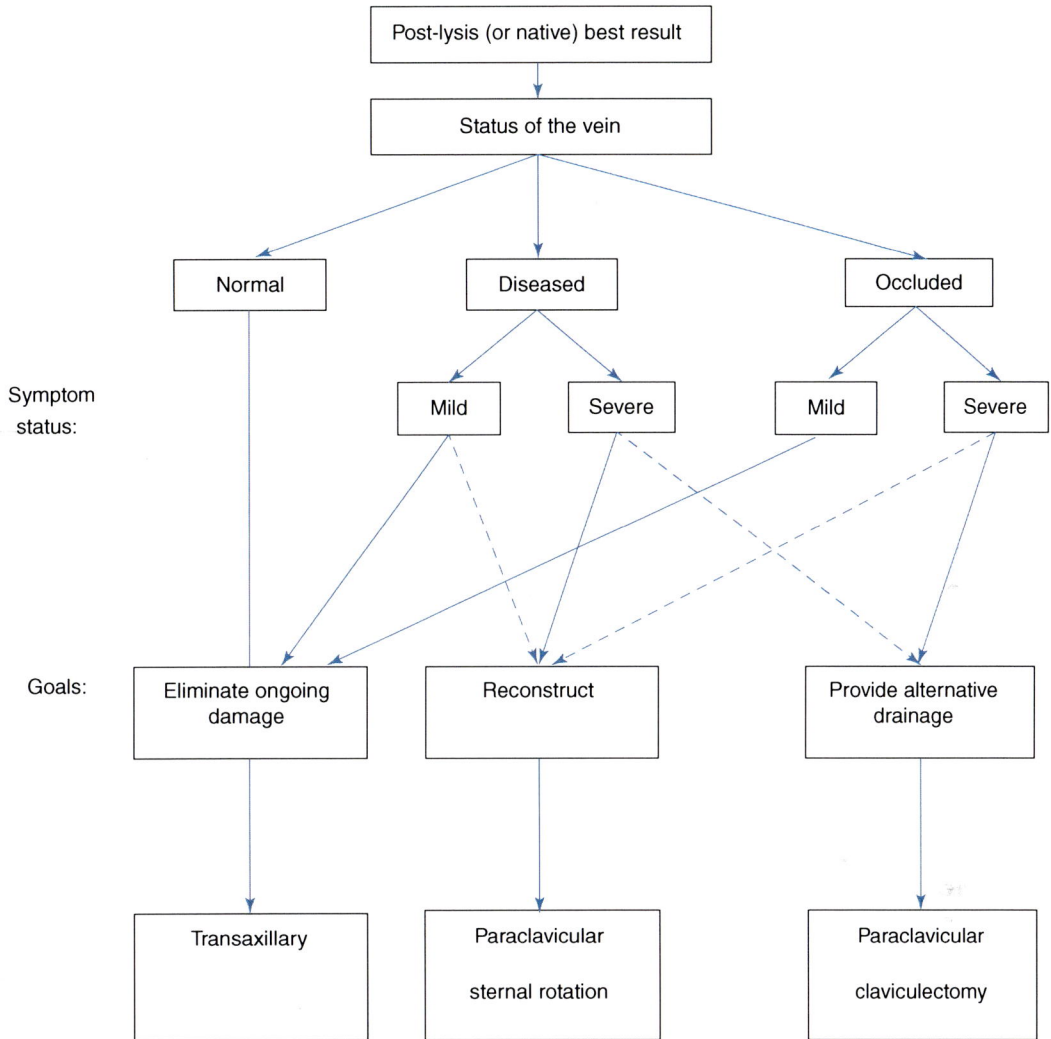

Fig. 73.2 Flowchart illustrating the general decision-making process in a patient who presents with complete thrombosis of the subclavian vein due to venous TOS. *Shaded boxes* indicate the key decision points; *dotted lines* indicate less common alternatives/preferences. If the vein is open the goal is simply to decompress the anterior part of the venous thoracic outlet, and transaxillary first rib resection is an excellent option. If the vein remains diseased after clot is removed, treatment depends on symptoms – if mild, decompression as above is probably adequate, but if severe, venous reconstruction (open or endovascular) requires exposure of the vein and the supine position, so the paraclavicular approach or upward rotation of the clavicle is needed. Finally, if the vein is occluded, decompression alone (transaxillary) is felt to allow recanalization, while a highly symptomatic patient may need extensive reconstruction or alternative drainage provided by means of jugular transposition

If the vein is severely diseased by venography, a decision must be made as to whether it requires reconstruction. Some authors advocate reconstruction in nearly every case [1], while we and others advise a selective approach. Our decision is guided by the patient's history, symptoms, and the events surrounding thrombolysis. If a patient with a significant intrinsic venous abnormality was highly symptomatic prior to thrombosis, remains more than minimally symptomatic after all acute thrombus has been removed, or rethrombosis after initially successful thrombolysis, we feel that the lesion itself (over and above the extrinsic compression, which will be corrected) is hemodynamically significant and that reconstruction is required. Reconstruction cannot be

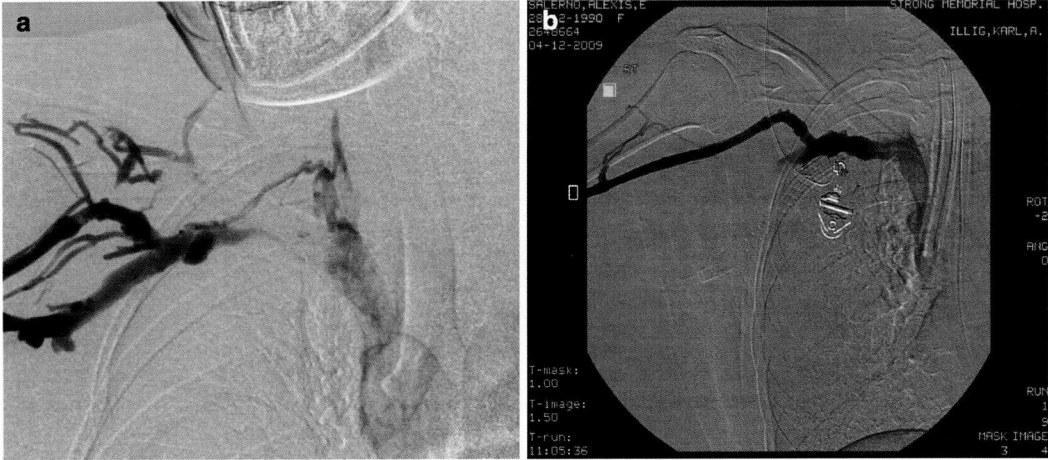

Fig. 73.3 A case illustrating the benefit that can be obtained by external venolysis without direct reconstruction. (**a**) Angiographic appearance after thrombolysis. It was assumed that venous reconstruction would be needed. (**b**) The patient underwent transaxillary first rib excision with extensive debridement of surrounding scar tissue; the vein was mobilized circumferentially to the level of the jugular and innominate veins. She was then placed supine, and a venogram was obtained prior to planned endovascular therapy. However, the vein was apparently undiseased and the collaterals disappeared. She was not further treated and remains asymptomatic at 2-1/2 years after surgery

thoroughly or safely accomplished via the transaxillary approach, and venography is frequently helpful in these situations, and thus a direct approach (with the patient supine) must be used. Two options are available in this situation – a paraclavicular approach (Chap. 63) or partial sternal division with upward mobilization of the clavicle ala Molina (Chap. 64) [2]. The former allows full mobilization of the subclavian vein to the level of the inominate vein from above in most cases, while the latter, albeit more invasive, allows superb visualization and access of the entire vein in essentially all cases (Fig. 73.3). Claviculectomy accomplishes the same goal, but is more radical and hence not usually needed unless specific clavicular pathology is present (Fig. 73.4). In all these cases reconstruction is best accomplished by means of local venotomy, internal debridement ("pseudo-endovenotomy"), and vein patch closure.

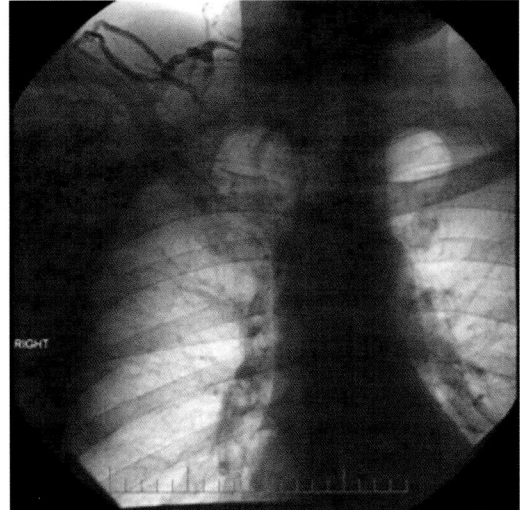

Fig. 73.4 A patient with a pathologic fracture of his clavicle following radiation therapy for cancer a decade ago. He presented with subclavian vein occlusion and arm swelling, but also had subtle neurogenic symptoms. After claviculectomy alone his neurologic symptoms were gone in the recovery room, and he was asymptomatic (and very grateful) at his first postoperative visit

The Patient with an Occluded Vein

If the vein is fully occluded (wire passage is unsuccessful or they present with chronic obstruction), the situation also depends upon the symptomatic status of the patient. If the patient is asymptomatic or minimally symptomatic, they can simply be left alone. As the vein is already occluded, in theory no decompression needs to be done. However, some, notably the Hopkins group, believe that the vein can sometimes recanalize after bony decompression [3], and, anecdotally, others believe that even if the subclavian vein remains occluded, first rib resection will decompress existing and potential collaterals. Many thus will remove the rib even if the vein is chronically occluded. In this case, as no reconstruction is required, the transaxillary approach is excellent. If the patient is highly symptomatic, however, an alternative route for blood flow will be needed. Long-segment reconstruction can be carried out, although as actual replacement is usually needed and exposure often extensive, this more often requires claviculectomy or at least swinging the clavicle up along with femoral vein harvest. A somewhat less invasive option in this case is jugular vein transposition/turndown (Chap. 65), which can be performed with or without claviculectomy (although it seems prudent to remove the first rib to avoid any secondary compression).

Summary

The critical consideration in planning treatment for patients with VTOS is that if decompression is performed, it must include the *anterior* part of the first rib – at least well into cartilage, if not to the sternum itself. This area can be approached and resected very easily via the transaxillary approach, and this is our preferred option if no further reconstruction needs to be done. If the vein is not felt to need reconstruction – it is not terribly diseased and/or the patient is not highly symptomatic – we advocate simply resecting the rib as above along with aggressive external venolysis; again, the transaxillary approach serves well. If the vein requires reconstruction, however – it is very badly diseased and the patient is symptomatic – direct and thorough exposure must be obtained. The two primary choices in this situation are the paraclavicular approach (with full mobilization of the vein from above) or rotation of the clavicle upwards ala Molina. Either approach, with the patient in the supine position, also makes completion

venography very easy (and preserves the ability to correct any problems so found). Many feel there is benefit to decompressing the venous thoracic outlet even if the vein is chronically occluded. Finally, if the patient is highly symptomatic and reconstruction cannot be accomplished, jugular transposition (probably with some form of thoracic outlet decompression) is highly effective.

It is important to recognize (and is a continuing theme of this book) that essentially no comparative data, much less prospectively obtained, exists to support any part of this algorithm. Among others, questions to answer include:

- The fate of the diseased and decompressed, but not reconstructed, vein
- Who needs reconstruction
- Whether decompression is needed in everyone
- The natural history of the decompressed versus nondecompressed thoracic outlet in a patient with chronic occlusion
- The fate of stents in the *decompressed* thoracic outlet

Happily, the vast majority of patients (95–100 %) with VTOS do very well after any form of (aggressive) treatment [4, 5], making this entity a pleasure to see. What treatment exactly is best for each patient, and perhaps who can be left alone, has yet to be determined.

References

1. Molina JE, Hunter DW, Dietz CA. Paget-Schroetter syndrome treated with thrombolytics and immediate surgery. J Vasc Surg. 2007;45(2):328–34.
2. Molina JE. A new surgical approach to the innominate and subclavian vein. J Vasc Surg. 1998;27:576–81.
3. de Leon R, Chang DC, Busse C, et al. First rib resection and scalenectomy for chronically occluded subclavian veins: what does it really do? Ann Vasc Surg. 2008;22:395–401.
4. Urschel Jr HC, Patel AN. Surgery remains the most effective treatment for Paget-Schroeter syndrome: 50 years' experience. Ann Thorac Surg. 2008;86:254–60.
5. Melby SJ, Vedantham S, Narra VR, Paletta Jr GA, Khoo-Summers L, Driskill M, Thompson RW. Comprehensive surgical management of the competitive athlete with effort thrombosis of the subclavian vein (Paget-Schroetter syndrome). J Vasc Surg. 2008; 47(4):809–20.

Controversies in VTOS: Is There Ever a Role for Venous Stents in VTOS?

74

Carolyn Glass and David L. Gillespie

Abstract

The bony venous thoracic outlet creates significant extrinsic force upon the subclavian vein, and intravascular stents in this location thus perform very poorly. There is some literature supporting the use of stents after decompression, but no level I evidence exists. At present the use of stents in venous thoracic outlet syndrome should not be considered until the bony thoracic outlet has been decompressed, and even then should be reserved for isolated cases with thorough followup.

The bony limitations of the venous thoracic outlet provide a particular challenge in managing patients with upper extremity deep venous thrombosis. While percutaneous angioplasty and stenting have become commonplace in the iliofemoral venous system for the treatment of venous outflow obstruction, the same is not true for upper extremity lesions [1, 2]. Venous thoracic outlet syndrome (TOS) is caused by extrinsic compression of the subclavian vein as it exits the chest and enters the upper extremity. The subclavian vein is bounded by the costoclavicular ligament medially,

C. Glass, MD, MS
Department of Vascular Surgery,
Strong Memorial Hospital,
601 Elmwood Avenue, Rochester, NY 14642, USA
e-mail: carolyn_glass@urmc.rochester.edu

D.L. Gillespie, MD (✉)
Department of Surgery,
University of Rochester Medical Center,
601 Elmwood Ave, Box 652,
Rochester, NY 14642, USA
e-mail: david_gillespie@urmc.rochester.edu

the anterior scalene muscle laterally, the clavicle and subclavius muscle superiorly, and the first rib inferiorly. Hypertrophy of the muscular components or aberrant cervical rib or callus formation after bony fracture also cause encroachment on what is already a narrow and very dynamic space [3].

While stents placed in central venous segments away from bony structures may be beneficial, those deployed in subclavian lesions without decompression of the thoracic outlet commonly result in stent deformation and eventual fracture. This causes further damage to the subclavian vein and often thrombosis. The published literature seems clear; percutaneous stent placement for venous TOS without initial surgical decompression is not effective and is in fact detrimental to our patients. Urschel and Patel reported on 22 patients referred to their institution with stents placed in the thoracic outlet without surgical compression. Each of the patients had the diagnosis made less than 6 weeks after vein occlusion, received previous thrombolytic

K.A. Illig et al. (eds.), *Thoracic Outlet Syndrome*,
DOI 10.1007/978-1-4471-4366-6_74, © Springer-Verlag London 2013

therapy, and post-stent anticoagulants. All 22 patients reoccluded their axillo-subclavian vein within 6 weeks upon their presentation, were retreated with thrombolytic therapy and required first rib resection. Ten remained patent and 12 remained occluded but developed adequate collateral circulation. The study concluded there was no indication for use for stents in patients with Paget-Schroetter syndrome [4].

Current literature supports the concept that, the predominant indication for stent placement in venous TOS is a residual lesion (>30 %) as demonstrated by venography, with or without continued symptoms following surgical decompression and angioplasty. In our experience, patients often have residual defects after thrombolysis and surgical decompression on completion venography and intravascular ultrasound (IVUS). Detection of these defects is aided by the use of either multiplanar venography or cross sectional imaging using IVUS. The literature supports the observation that IVUS provides a higher sensitivity for visualizing intrinsic defects such as webs, endothelial irregularities and residual thrombus [5, 6]. Neglen et al. found that venous IVUS appears to be superior to single-plane venography for the morphologic diagnosis of venous outflow obstruction and is an invaluable assistance in the accurate placement of venous stents after venoplasty [7]. Similarly we have found IVUS to be very useful for recognition of lesions in the upper extremity central venous system. In our review, 16 proximal central venous lesions (8 SVC, 8 innominate) were identified and confirmed by both IVUS and contrast venography [8]. Forty two percent of the central lesions were reported as "questionable" after venography alone. Subsequent IVUS exam of the "questionable lesions" identified 60 % of them as "moderate" lesions which prompted intervention, and the remaining "questionable" lesions showed no pathology, avoiding further intervention.

It should be noted that there is currently no consensus regarding treatment of a residual venous TOS defect after surgical decompression. Many treatment algorithms exist for residual venous lesions following presumed successful thrombolysis, surgical decompression, and thorough external venolysis. Some support observation and anticoagulation, recognizing the vein may remodel on its own after surgical decompression and anticoagulation alone [9]. Others recommend thrombolysis, surgical decompression, followed by a brief period (weeks) of endothelial recovery prior to angioplasty and stenting. Lastly, the most aggressive school of thought recommends thrombolysis, surgical decompression, and angioplasty and stenting during the same operative setting [10–12].

A recent study of Paget-Schroetter patients who *did not* receive thrombolysis and managed medically with anticoagulation alone after first rib resection reported the incidence of residual subclavian stenosis requiring angioplasty was 55 %. Ten patients (16 %) had subclavian vein occlusions. However, 80 % of occluded patients were reported to recanalize on anticoagulation alone after first rib resection (mean 4 months out) demonstrated by duplex exam. In this anticoagulation-alone group, 75 % remained on warfarin for an average of 3 months [13].

Kreienberg et al. evaluated the long term outcomes of balloon angioplasty alone versus additional stenting immediately following thrombolysis and surgical decompression in patients with effort thrombosis. Thrombolysis was administered approximately 10 days after the initial onset of symptoms. After surgical decompression, all patients underwent balloon venoplasty. Fourteen patients had residual stenosis (>50 %) after venoplasty requiring stenting of the subclavian vein. At 4 year follow up, patency was 100 % in patients who required angioplasty alone versus only 64 % at 3.5 years in those who also had stents placed. In the stenting group, two patients occluded within 2 days, two within 1 year and seven within 3 years. Three patients with occluded stents were later diagnosed with Factor V Leiden [14]. Based on this data, some have concluded patients do better with balloon venoplasty alone rather than stenting long term. It should be noted, however that there is a bias given those who required stenting had more difficult lesions that were minimally responsive to venoplasty alone.

The Dartmouth group recently reviewed their long term outcomes in patients with idiopathic axillo-subclavian vein thrombosis after aggressive surgical and endovascular treatment [11]. Catheter-directed thrombolysis was performed in 83 % with mean treatment time of 12 days from initial onset of symptoms. All 36 patients were treated with surgical decompression. Thirty one percent of patients had stents placed for residual venous stenosis. Overall patency at 1 and 5 years was reported as 100 and 94 %, respectively with mean follow up of 65 months. Greater than 85 % of patients returned to work and had sustained functional improvement. The study concluded patients should expect durable patency with sustained freedom from reintervention after aggressive combined surgical decompression and endovascular intervention, with selective stent placement for residual stenosis after angioplasty. Furthermore these authors felt that stenting for the treatment of residual medial stenoses was beneficial since it obviates the need for any surgical division of the sternum and open patch venoplasty as described by Molina [15].

Pupka et al. described 23 patients with Paget-Schroeter syndrome who underwent thrombolysis, anticoagulation, first rib resection, and venous angioplasty with intravascular stenting [16]. Patients underwent either delayed (3–4 months) or early (median 8 days) surgical decompression with stent placement after thrombolysis. No statistical difference was found between the two groups. This study concluded multimodal treatment of athletes with Paget-Schroeter syndrome using thrombolysis, early thoracic outlet decompression, and intravascular stents resulted in rapid return to the athlete's baseline capabilities.

Although stents are not commonly placed in our primary venous TOS patients with residual venous lesions, we have recognized an increasing number of hemodialysis patients with central venous lesions in or near the thoracic outlet. This clinical entity has been termed "dialysis-associated venous thoracic outlet syndrome" [17]. In addition to the usual symptoms of venous TOS, dialysis patients also suffer from prolonged fistula bleeding (during cannulation and post-dialysis), inefficient dialysis and eventual fistula failure of the ipsilateral upper extremity. We recently reported our experience with costoclavicular decompression in patients with fistula dysfunction [18]. Six underwent transaxillary first rib resection and four had medial claviculectomy. A central venogram through the fistula was completed following surgical decompression and endovascular treatment (angioplasty and/or stent) performed for residual lesions. Fistula salvage was promising at 80 % with mean follow up 8 months. In this special population, long term patency with stent placement was beneficial in extending functional dialysis time.

In summary, current evidence supports mixed opinions on whether stents are beneficial for venous TOS after surgical decompression. By evidence based medicine standards we would give it a grade of 2B. Our current treatment algorithm is to perform early first rib resection for patients with symptomatic venous thoracic outlet syndrome. Our preferred technique for first rib resection is transaxillary combined with intraoperative venography and venoplasty. For any patients with significant residual stenosis following venoplasty intravascular ultrasonography is performed. In those patients with a >50 % residual defect stenting would be considered. All patients are anticoagulated for 3–6 months and followed with ultrasound.

References

1. Gutzeit A, Zollikofer CL, Dettling-Pizzolato M, Graf N, Largiadèr J, Binkert CA. Endovascular stent treatment for symptomatic benign iliofemoral venous occlusive disease: long-term results 1987–2009. Cardiovasc Intervent Radiol. 2011;34:542–9.
2. Rosales A, Sandbaek G, Jørgensen JJ. Stenting for chronic post-thrombotic vena cava and iliofemoral venous occlusions: mid-term patency and clinical outcome. Eur J Vasc Endovasc Surg. 2010;40(2):234–40.
3. Illig KA, Doyle A. A comprehensive review of Paget-Schroetter syndrome. J Vasc Surg. 2010;51:1538–47.
4. Urschel Jr HC, Patel AN. Paget Schroetter syndrome therapy: failure of intravenous stents. Ann Thorac Surg. 2003;75:1693–6.
5. Canales JF, Krajcer Z. Intravascular ultrasound guidance in treating May-Thurner syndrome. Tex Heart Inst J. 2010;37(4):496–7.
6. Forauer AR, Gemmete JJ, Dasika NL, Cho KJ, Williams DM. Intravascular ultrasound in the diagnosis and

treatment of iliac vein compression (May-Thurner) syndrome. J Vasc Interv Radiol. 2002;13(5):523–7.

7. Neglén P, Raju S. Intravascular ultrasound scan evaluation of the obstructed vein. J Vasc Surg. 2002; 35(4):694–700.

8. Glass C, Gillespie D. Intravascular ultrasound for innominate vein and superior vena cava stenting. San Diego: American Venous Forum; 2011.

9. Freischlag J. Venous thoracic outlet syndrome: transaxillary approach. Oper Tech Gen Surg. 2008; 10:122–30.

10. Schneider DB, Dimuzio PJ, Martin ND, Gordon RL, Wilson MW, Laberge JM, Kerlan RK, Eichler CM, Messina LM. Combination treatment of venous thoracic outlet syndrome: open surgical decompression and intraoperative angioplasty. J Vasc Surg. 2004; 40(4):599–603.

11. Stone DH, Scali ST, Bjerk AA, Rzucidlo E, Chang CK, Goodney PP, Nolan BW, Walsh DB. Aggressive treatment of idiopathic axillo-subclavian vein thrombosis provides excellent long-term function. J Vasc Surg. 2010;52(1):127–31. Epub 2010 Apr 10.

12. Doyle A, Wolford HY, Davies MG, Adams JT, Singh MJ, Saad WE, Waldman DL, Deweese JA, Illig KA. Management of effort thrombosis of the subclavian vein: today's treatment. Ann Vasc Surg. 2007; 21(6):723–9. Epub 2007 Oct 17.

13. Guzzo JL, Chang K, Demos J, Black JH, Freischlag JA. Preoperative thrombolysis and venoplasty affords no benefit in patency following first rib resection and scalenectomy for subacute and chronic subclavian vein thrombosis. J Vasc Surg. 2010;52(3):658–62; discussion 662–3.

14. Kreienberg PB, Chang BB, Darling 3rd RC, Roddy SP, Paty PS, Lloyd WE, Cohen D, Stainken B, Shah DM. Long-term results in patients treated with thrombolysis, thoracic inlet decompression, and subclavian vein stenting for Paget-Schroetter syndrome. J Vasc Surg. 2001;33(2 Suppl):S100–5.

15. Molina JE. A new surgical approach to the innominate and subclavian vein. J Vasc Surg. 1998; 27(3):576–81.

16. Pupka A, Szyber PP, Garcarek J, Szyber P. The use of intravascular nitinol stents in the treatment of subclavian vein compression for thoracic outlet syndrome. Polim Med. 2007;37(2):51–5.

17. Illig K. Management of central vein stenoses and occlusions: the critical importance of the costoclavicular junction. Semin Vasc Surg. 2011;24(2):113–8.

18. Glass C, Dugan M, Gillespie D, Doyle A, Illig K. Costoclavicular venous decompression in patients with threatened arteriovenous hemodialysis access. Ann Vasc Surg. 2011;25(5):640–5. Epub ahead of print.

Controversies in VTOS: How Long Should Anticoagulation Be Used in VTOS?

75

Hugh A. Gelabert

Abstract

Anticoagulation is an important element in the management of most patients with VTOS. The use of anticoagulation should be tailored to the specific form of VTOS present, however, and modified according to the condition of the individual patient. In general, patients with non-thormbotic positional venous compression requires no anticoagulation. Those with acute axillosubclavian vein thrombosis require anticoagulation to prevent propagation of thrombus, reduce the risk of pulmonary embolus, and to reduce the risk of rethrombosis while awaiting decompression, and following this should be anticoagulated for 3 months. Patients with chronic venous occlusion do not require anticoagulation for safety, but long-term anticoagulation may be associated with spontaneous recanalization and thus can be considered.

Introduction

The rationale for anticoagulation after treatment of axillosubclavian vein thrombosis is based on experience with lower extremity deep vein thrombosis (DVT) and empirical experience with management of venous thoracic outlet syndrome (VTOS). The goals of anticoagulation are the relief of symptoms, the prevention of propagation of thrombus, and the prevention of pulmonary embolization. In the setting of VTOS

H.A. Gelabert, MD
Division of Vascular Surgery, Vascular Surgery Division,
UCLA David Geffen School of Medicine,
200 UCLA Medical Plaza, Ste 526, Los Angeles,
CA 90095-6904, USA
e-mail: hgelabert@mednet.ucla.edu

anticoagulation also plays a significant role in protecting patients from recurrent thrombosis until their thoracic outlet compression may be surgically relieved.

Goals

A major goal of anticoagulantion in patients with VTOS is the moderation of presenting symptoms. Symptoms from venous compression at the thoracic outlet result from reduced blood flow through the subclavian vein. Hydrostatic pressure within the venous system may be painful and give rise to congestive symptoms. The presence of a thrombus within a vein may give rise to an inflammatory reaction which can also result in pain. By inhibiting propagation and allowing

K.A. Illig et al. (eds.), *Thoracic Outlet Syndrome*,
DOI 10.1007/978-1-4471-4366-6_75, © Springer-Verlag London 2013

endogenous thrombolytic resolution of thrombus, anticoagulation will reduce symptoms due to venous congestion as well as those due to inflammation. Clinical reports dating to 1948 indicate the beneficial effect of anticoagulation on the course of acute subclavian vein thrombosis and relief of the symptoms of acute DVT [1, 2].

Recurrent thrombosis of the axillosubclavian vein is well recognized. Adams described 28 VTOS patients managed with anticoagulation, rest, and arm elevation alone [3]. Of these, 85 % had recurrent and persistent symptoms of venous congestion (and 11 % pulmonary embolization). Tilney and associates similarly described 48 patients managed with anticoagulation who did not undergo surgical decompression who were followed for a mean of 6.6 years, and noted that 17 % developed recurrent thrombosis [4]. Machleder described a series of 50 patients who were initially managed with anticoagulation and subsequently presented for surgery [5]. Seventeen (34 %) suffered multiple thrombotic events prior to proceeding with surgical decompression.

The incidence of pulmonary embolization (PE) in upper extremity DVT has been reported to be significant. As above, the historical Rochester experience documented a rate of 11 % in patients anticoagulated alone [3]. Kooij and colleagues noted in a retrospective review of all upper extremity DVTs an overall incidence of 12 %; in the 16 patients with primary upper extremity DVT, the rate was 6 % [6]. When studied prospectively by Monreal and associates, the incidence of PE in patients presenting with upper extremity catheter-related DVT was 13 % [7]. While series criteria and treatment varied, the rate of PE in patients with upper extremity DVT treated conservatively seems to be around 10 %.

Chest Guidelines

The most widely accepted guidelines for the management of acute deep vein thrombosis was published in 2008 in a supplementary issue of *Chest*. These guidelines are based on extensive review of current literature and are grouped according to the strength of published data which

underlies each recommendation. The recommended treatment of acute deep vein thrombosis is at least 3 months of anticoagulation with a target INR of 2.5. More prolonged administration of anticoagulants may be warranted based on a history of clotting, the presence of procoagulable factors, and ability to safely use anticoagulants [8]. Recurrent deep vein thrombosis is an indication for life-long anticoagulation. The presence of thrombophillic conditions is an indication for anticoagulation – at the very least during periods of increased DVT risk, and occasionally for life-long duration.

The principal exception to these guidelines, however, is if a condition which promotes thrombosis is removed. In such instances long-term anticoagulation may not be indicated. In cases of VTOS, extrinsic compression of the axillo-subclavian vein is the condition which promoted thrombosis. Surgical decompression of the thoracic outlet will alleviate the pro-thrombotic event and would thus in theory allow cessation of anticoagulation.

Duration of Therapy in Patients with VTOS

The duration of anticoagulation for venous TOS will thus be based on several factors: the presentation (acute upper extremity DVT, chronic post-thrombotic occlusion, post-phlebitic stenosis, and intermittent non-thrombotic venous compression), the underlying causes for thrombosis, and the condition of the vein following decompression.

Imaging

Venography and thrombolysis may offer significant insights into the casue of axillo-subclavian vein thrombosis. Venography will identify the presence of venous thrombosis or venous stenosis at the thoracic outlet. Venography will define the condition of the subclavian vein as either normal, post-phlebitic, or occluded. Venography will help define the chronicity of the venous compromise: the presence of large, mature, well developed venous collaterals speaks to the longstanding nature of the venous compression, the inability to traverse the occlusion with a guidewire will confirm the dense fibrosis of the occlusion. If venography indicates the presence of significant extrinsic compression at the thoracic outlet, then anticoagulation is indicated until the compression is resolved.

If venography uncovers a pre-occlusive stenosis anticoagulation is required to prevent re-thrombosis. Anticoagulation is maintained until such time as the stenosis can be repaired. Failure to employ anticoagulants may result in recurrent thrombosis. Following thrombolysis anticoagulation allows healing of the venous endothelium, it allows more rapid resolution of the endovenous inflammatory processed and thus reduced recurrent thrombosis of the vein. The protocol promoted by Machleder required a period of 3 months of anticoagulation following thrombolysis and prior surgical decompression of the thoracic outlet [5, 9]. The rationale for this was to allow a period of time for the venous endothelium to heal and the inflammation to recede following the acute DVT.

A report by Angle and colleagues comparing early and delayed surgical decompression made incidental note of interval thrombosis of the subclavian vein [10]. About 20 % of patients were noted to re-thrombose their subclavian veins when they were removed from anticoagulants in order to undergo first rib resection. This experience underscores the importance of anticoagulation in maintaining vein patency following thrombolysis in the face of high-grade extrinsic venous compression. The authors recommended resumption of anticoagulation following surgery for a period of 3 months post-op.

Finally, venography may occasionally revear a subclavian vein with no evidence of extrinsic compression. The venous thrombosis is not due to mechanical compressive elements and additional reasons for coagulation should be sought. Particular attention is given to the evaluation of hyper-coagulable conditions and malignancies. Anticoagulation in these patients is then based on the primary thrombophillic or malignant condition.

Thrombophilia

Hypercoagulable conditions may add further impetus to the growth and extent of the thrombus. Pro-thombophilic elements such as the use of exogenous steroids (OCP) and smoking will favor the development of thrombus. Vaya and colleagues notes that exogenous steroid use in the form of oral contraception increased the risk of upper extremity DVT [11]. This was further exacerbated by the presence of a hyper-coagulable condition with a synergistic increase in the risk of upper extremity DVT. This synergistic effect of thrombophilia and OCP use was also noted by Martinelli in a 2005 study of 115 primary upper extremity DVTs [12].

Other hematological conditions may add to the pro-thrombotic milieu. Heron and colleagues reported the incidence of hyper-coagulable findings (protein C and protein S deficiencies, anti-phospholipid syndrome, factor V mutations, and gene G20210A mutations) in patients with effort related upper extremity DVT to be about 15 %, whereas non-effort related DVTs were associated with a 42 % incidence of abnormal coagulation testing [13]. More recently, Casada and colleagues reported a series of 18 patients presenting with acute axillo-subclvian vein DVT related to TOS. They discovered that 67 % of patients were found to found to have relatively common coagulation disorders [14]. The presence of common thrombophyllic conditions such as protein C and protein S deficiencies, anti-thrombinb III deficiency, anti-phospholipid syndrome, factor V Leyden mutations, and gene G20210A mutations in the association with acute venous thrombosis require use of anticoagulation. Certain thrombophillic conditions may warrant prolonged or life-long anticoagulation.

Condition of the Axillosubclavian Vein Following Decompression

An additional consideration is the condition of the subclavian vein following surgical decompression. Most authors advise post-decompression venography to assess the

Table 75.1 Clinical indications for use of anticoagulation in axillo-subclavian vein thrombosis

Acute axillo-subclavian vein thrombosis

(a) With no planned thrombolysis: anticoagulantionis indicated for at least 3 months and until symptoms resolve

(b) Post-thrombolysis, with planned initial period of non-surgical management for mild to moderate residual venous stenosis: anticoagulation is indicated for at least 3 months and until the venous symptoms resolve

(c) Post-thrombolysis, with planned surgical decompression for residual pre-occlusive venous stenosis: anticoagulation is indicated for at least 3 months and until the venous stenosis is resolved

Post-phlebitic axillo-subclavian vein stenosis

(a) If no thrombotic event within a period of 6 months, anticoagulation may not be indicated

(b) If thrombosis is believed to have recurred within 6 months, then anticoagulation is indicated for at least 3 months and until the venous stenosis is resolved

Chronic post-thrombotic axillo-subclavian vein occlusion

(a) If within 3 months of thrombotic event- anticoagulation is indicated for at least 3 months, possibly up to 6 months

(b) If beyond 6 months from date of thrombosis – no anticoagulation indicated

(c) Post-decompression: If residual occlusion related congestive symptoms persist: anticoagulation may be indicted for a period up to 1 year in selected cases

Intermittent non-thrombotic axillo-subclavian vein compression

(a) Anticoagulation is not indicated

condition of the subclavian vein. Some authors perform this assessment in the course of the decompression operation. Other authors favor venography for post-operative evaluation at a later time. If persistent narrowing of the subclavian vein is identified, then venoplasty or venous reconstruction may be indicated. More recently balloon angioplasty and stenting has been used as the final step in restoring the subclavian vein to normal caliber and patency. Between 35 and 64 % of patients undergoing thoracic outlet decompression surgery for venous TOS after successful thrombolysis will require post-operative angioplasty [10, 15]. These patients have a persistent high grade stenosis of their subclavian vein due to fibrosis in reaction to the venous thrombus. Because the high grade stenosis presents the opportunity for recurrent thrombosis, anticoagulation is indicated. The duration of anticoagulation would be until such time as the stenosis is corrected.

Recommendations Based on Presentation

Four common presentations of vTOS are commonly noted: acute upper extremity DVT, chronic post-thrombotic occlusion, post-phlebitic stenosis, and intermittent non-thrombotic venous compression (Table 75.1)

A patient with **acute upper extremity DVT** (Paget-Schroetter syndrome) is best managed with *anticoagulation and thrombolysis in the acute period* (preferably within 10–14 days of the thrombotic event). Thrombolysis offers the advantages of rapid and more efficient clearing of the clot, and the ability to assess the condition of the axillo-subclavian vein. Thrombolysis is then followed by a period of anticoagulation and, when indicated, surgical decompression. *Based on the general guidelines for DVT these patients are managed with at least 3 months of anticoagulation* [8]. Further anticoagulation is indicated based on the response to initial therapy, the findings after thrombolysis, and the surgical management. If the post-thrombolytic vein is widely patent or mild to moderate residual stenosis is seen, anticoagulation should be continued for only 3 months (unless a significant hyper-coagulable condition is present).

Patients presenting with **chronic post-thrombotic occlusion** are not candidates for thrombolysis. These patients will often have a history of long-lasting venous congestive symptoms and a remote thrombotic event may be noted. If symptomatic, these patients can be offered thoracic outlet decompression in hopes of allowing improved collateralization across the area of occlusion, and possibly recanalization of the decompressed vein. Additional venous reconstruction may be warranted. *Anticoagulation is not needed in these patients due to the chronicity of the venous occlusion.*

There is some recent evidence that a course of long-term anticoagulation is associated with recanalization of some occlusions following surgical decompression. de Leon described a small group of patients who presented 12–34 weeks following thrombosis and were shown to have chronically occluded veins. Following surgical decompression, they were maintained on anticoagulation for up to 1 year and reimaged. In all four instances the subclavian veins were found to have recanalized on careful ultrasound exam, and in a later series, identical results were seen in 13 of 17 similar patients [9, 10]. *Based on this, they advise long-term post-operative anticoagulation in patients with chronic venous occlusion who have undergone thoracic outlet decompression.* The duration of the anticoagulation is "until the subclavian vein was demonstrated to be patent". It should be noted, however, that no evidence directly tied anticoagulation, per se, to recanalization; the two coexisted but causality was not proven and these results have not yet been replicated.

A distinct subgroup of VTOS patients will present with **post-phlebitic symptoms**. These patients will often present many months to years following a thrombotic event, with the delay often related to difficulty in establishing the diagnosis and/or identifying a physician who is able to manage their condition. Venography demonstrates a patent but irregular, recanalized subclavian vein with evident compression at the thoracic outlet. If symptomatic, these patients should be offered thoracic outlet decompression with the goal of restoring patency of the axillo-subclavian vein and improving venous outflow from the arm. *As these patients present months to years following their acute thrombosis, the role of anticoagulation is ambiguous.* In the absence of recent events which may suggest thrombosis, anticoagulation may not be necessary. In some instances where recurrent thrombosis is a significant concern of the patient or the physicians, anticoagulation may be justified given the well documented recurrent nature of axillo-subclavian venous thrombosis in VTOS [3–5]. By this reasoning anticoagulation could used to prevent recurrent thrombosis until such time as the thoracic outlet compression may be resolved and the vein restored to optimal patency.

Finally, **non-thombotic or positional venous compression** of the subclavian vein most commonly presents with congestive symptoms related to upper extremity exertion or positional changes. Venography will often be normal at rest, but reveal collaterals with elevation. *In the absence of acute venous thrombosis anticoagulation is not required* [11–15], although many or most investigators and clinicians recommend elective first rib resection.

Conclusions

Anticoagulation is an important element in the management of most patients with VTOS. The use of anticoagulation should be tailored to the specific form of VTOS present, however, and modified according to the condition of the individual patient. In general, patients with non-thormbotic positional venous compression requires no anticoagulation. Those with acute axillosubclavian vein thrombosis require anticoagulation to prevent propagation of thrombus, reduce the risk of pulmonary embolus, and to reduce the risk of rethrombosis while awaiting decompression, and following this should be anticoagulated for 3 months. Patients with chronic venous occlusion do not require anticoagulation for safety, but long-term anticoagulation may be associated with spontaneous recanalization and thus can be considered.

References

1. Marks J. Anticoagulant therapy in the idiopathic occlusion of the axillary vein. Br Med J. 1956;1(4957): 11–3.
2. Marks J, Truscott BM, Withycombe JF. Treatment of venous thrombosis with anticoagulants; review of 1135 cases. Lancet. 1954;267(6842):787–91.

3. Adams JT, De Weese JA. Effort thrombosis of the axillary and subclavian veins. J Trauma. 1971;11:923–30.

4. Tilney NL, Griffiths HJG, Edwards EA. Natural history of major venous thrombosis of the upper extremity. Arch Surg. 1970;101:792–6.

5. Machleder HI. Evaluation of a new treatment strategy for Paget-Schroetter syndrome: spontaneous thrombosis of the axillary-subclavian vein. J Vasc Surg. 1993;17(2):305–15; discussion 316–7.

6. Kooij JD, van der Zant FM, van Beek EJ, Reekers JA. Pulmonary embolism in deep venous thrombosis of the upper extremity: more often in catheter-related thrombosis. Neth J Med. 1997;50(6):238–42.

7. Monreal M, Lafoz E, Ruiz J, Valls R, Alastrue A. Upper-extremity deep venous thrombosis and pulmonary embolism. A prospective study. Chest. 1991;99(2):280–3.

8. Kearon C, Kahn SR, Agnelli G, Goldhaber SZ, Raskob G, Comerota AJ. Antithrombotic therapy for venous thromboembolic disease: ACCP evidence-based clinical practice guidelines (8th edition). Chest. 2008;133:454S–545.

9. Kunkel JM, Machleder HI. Treatment of Paget-Schroetter syndrome. A staged, multidisciplinary approach. Arch Surg. 1989;124(10):1153–7; discussion 1157–8.

10. Angle N, Gelabert HA, Farooq MM, Ahn SS, Caswell DR, Freischlag JA, Machleder HI. Safety and efficacy of early surgical decompression of the thoracic outlet for Paget-Schroetter syndrome. Ann Vasc Surg. 2001;15(1):37–42.

11. Vayá A, Mira Y, Mateo J, Falco C, Villa P, Estelles A, Corella D, Fontcuberta J, Aznar J. Prothrombin G20210A mutation and oral contraceptive use increase upper-extremity deep vein thrombotic risk. Thromb Haemost. 2003;89(3):452–7.

12. Martinelli I, Battaglioli T, Bucciarelli P, Passamonti SM, Mannucci PM. Risk factors and recurrence rate of primary deep vein thrombosis of the upper extremities. Circulation. 2004;110(5):566–70. Epub 2004 Jul 19.

13. Héron E, Lozinguez O, Alhenc-Gelas M, Emmerich J, Fiessinger JN. Hypercoagulable states in primary upper-extremity deep vein thrombosis. Arch Intern Med. 2000;160(3):382–6.

14. Cassada DC, Lipscomb AL, Stevens SL, Freeman MB, Grandas OH, Goldman MH. The importance of thrombophilia in the treatment of Paget-Schroetter syndrome. Ann Vasc Surg. 2006;20:596–601.

15. Schneider DB, Dimuzio PJ, Martin ND, Gordon RL, Wilson MW, Laberge JM, Kerlan RK, Eichler CM, Messina LM. Combination treatment of venous thoracic outlet syndrome: open surgical decompression and intraoperative angioplasty. J Vasc Surg. 2004;40(4):599–603.

Controversies in VTOS: What to Do About the Contralateral Side?

76

Adam J. Doyle

Abstract

Very little information is available regarding the natural history of the contralateral side in patients with venous TOS (VTOS). Despite the sparse data, some conclusions can be drawn – patients with VTOS do appear to be at an increased risk of developing contralateral VTOS, and abnormal venographic findings on the contralateral side are common in patients with VTOS. Asymptomatic venous stenosis with positional obstruction can progress to symptomatic venous obstruction, but the rate at which this occurs is not known. Screening for contralateral pathology is reasonable in patients with VTOS (interviews alone, with imaging reserved for only those with active symptoms), prophylactic surgery on the contralateral side is not indicated, and, lastly, the same principals used in treating primary VTOS should be applied when considering VTOS on the contralateral side.

Introduction

VTOS is a disorder of the anterior part of the thoracic outlet, where the subclavian vein passes by the intersection of the clavicle and first rib. It is unclear whether an anatomically smaller costoclavicular space, resulting from either hypertrophied muscle (scalenus anterior or subclavius) or abnormal bone morphology (clavicle or first rib) is required or whether this condition can simply occur without a defined abnormality. Regardless of which anatomic structure is thought to be abnormal, compression of the subclavian vein with movement by any one structure alone or in combination is felt to be responsible for VTOS (1–7). It is reasonable to assume that because anatomic factors, whether acquired or congenital, play such a large role in this disorder, patients who present with VTOS may be at risk for similar pathology on the contralateral side.

Adams and DeWeese demonstrated in normal patients that when the arm is hyper-abducted, or the shoulder caudally depressed, or externally rotated, or the neck hyper-extended, the subclavian vein is compressed within the costoclavicular space [1]. In addition, only 10 % of cadavers

A.J. Doyle, MD
Department of Surgery,
University of Rochester Medical Center,
601 Elmwood Ave Box SURG, Rochester,
NY 14642, USA
e-mail: adam_doyle@urmc.rochester.edu

were found to have what is considered normal anatomy in one study [2], and in another, the brachial plexus and subclavian artery were found to be compressed in half of normal specimens using the Wright position (maximum shoulder abduction and external rotation) [3]. Together these findings suggest that the structures contained in the thoracic outlet are likely routinely compressed to some extent during certain maneuvers in nearly all people. What separates patients who experience symptoms with provocative maneuvering from those that do not experience symptoms is unknown. Finally, It is unclear if VTOS develops as a consequence of a single event of effort, or the cumulative effects of repetitive compression of the subclavian vein with resultant damage and eventual stenosis/thrombosis.

Intermittent Positional Obstruction

Mc Cleery first described intermittent positional obstruction in his 1951 paper [4]. Intermittent positional obstruction occurs during certain provocative positioning or with muscular exertion, and results in bony and muscular structures compressing and obstructing the subclavian vein. This induces venous hypertension and subsequent symptoms, which subside with termination of exertion/positioning and rest. Surprisingly little is known about the natural history of this disorder. Adams and DeWeese described a phenomenon in their 1968 paper where certain patients develop venous compression with provocative maneuvers with subsequent symptomatic swelling and discoloration [1]. While many (or most) asymptomatic patients can be stressed enough to partially occlude their subclavian vein, this finding in a patient who complains of an intermittently swollen and discolored arm with exertion has significant therapeutic implications [5, 6]. These patients will often have venograms that are normal at rest but abnormal (varying degrees of extrinsic compression with "new" venous collaterals) with the arm abducted. These symptoms are felt to be the result of venous insufficiency with inadequate collateral drainage for the increase blood return from the active arm, leading to venous hypertension and

symptoms when either the venous outflow is obstructed. At the time of surgery, no thrombosis or venous injury is present.

Another observation is that almost all patients who progress to full thrombosis have vein compression with arm abduction seen after lysis [7–10] and/or recent vigorous use of the affected extremity [11–13]. These observations together have lead some to believe that patients diagnosed with intermittent positional obstruction are in the early stages of the pathologic process that ultimately leads to venous thrombosis [14]. Although the natural history of these patients is unclear, many patients with intermittent positional obstruction of the subclavian vein are often considered as having "VTOS" in the literature and offered decompressive surgery.

VTOS: The Contralateral Side Review of Literature

The modern literature surrounding bilateral VTOS is sparse and summarized in Table 76.1 [6, 15–31]. Only 22 of 1,266 patients in series reported from 1996 to 2011, or 2.2 %, underwent surgery for bilateral VTOS. This is substantially higher that the estimated rate of 1/50,000–1/100,000 people per year for primary VTOS [13, 32, 33]. The higher incidence may be the result of selection bias, in that patients diagnosed and treated by a physician who concentrates on VTOS are more likely to have contralateral venous imaging and undergo decompressive surgery, but could also be due to an increased anatomic risk for bilateral risk.

The largest case series in the literature reports 18 cases of contralateral VTOS [27]. In this series 16 of the 18 patients with bilateral disease had sequential development of symptoms, while only two patients presented with concurrent bilateral VTOS. A recent report documents the progression from asymptomatic contralateral subclavian vein stenosis to symptomatic stenosis [30]. Combining the observations of this case report and Urschel's series, it is evident that asymptomatic stenosis can progress over time to symptomatic stenosis.

Table 76.1 Modern literature on contralateral venous thoracic outlet syndrome

Author (year) (Ref)	Institution	Subjects	Contralateral compression on venogram	Concurrent VTOS requiring surgery	Sequential VTOS requiring surgery
Hempel (1996) [16]	Baylor	47	0	0	0
Sheeran (1997) [18]	UCONN and Brown	14	0	0	0
Adelman (1997) [17]	NYU	17	0	0	0
Lee 1998 [19]	Brigham and Women's Hospital	11	0	0	0
Azakie (1998) [6]	UCSF and Washington University St. Louis, MO	33	9	0	0
Angle (2001) [20]	UCLA	18	0	0	0
Feugier (2001) [7]	Edouard Herriot Hospital, Lyon, France	10	6	0	0
Kreienberg 2001 [22]	Albany	23	0	0	0
Coletta (2001) [21]	Naval Medical center San Diego	19	2	0	0
Lokanathan (2001) [23]	University of British Columbia	28	2	0	0
Schneider (2004) [24]	UCSF and Thomas Jefferson University	25	0	0	0
Lee (2006) [25]	Sanford	64	0	0	0
Molina (2007) [26]	University of Minnesota	114	0	0	0
Urschel (2008) [27]	Baylor University Medical Center, Dallas	608	18	2	16
Guzzo (2010) [28]	The Johns Hopkins Hospital	103	7	0	7
Stone (2010) [29]	Dartmouth-Hitchcock Medical Center	36	0	0	0
Thakur (2010) [30]	University of Michigan and Toledo Hospital	1	1	0	1
Doyle (2011) [31]	University of Rochester Medical Center	95	2	0	2
Overall		**1,266**	**3.7 %** (**47/1,266**)	**0.2 %** (**2/1,266**)	**2.1 %** (**26/1,266**)

In studies where the contralateral side was imaged as routine, venous compression or stenosis was found in between 27 and 60 % of patients [6, 21, 34]. In some of these case series patients were offered prophylactic decompression – all with good outcomes – although none were symptomatic. In the series by Azakie et al., 9 of 33 patients were found to have high-grade asymptomatic stenosis and positional occlusion of the contralateral subclavian vein by imaging. Interestingly, the eight patients who were managed without prophylactic surgery all remained completely asymptomatic at follow-up ranging

from 4 months to 6 years, (median 18 months). This appears to be the largest cohort of patients followed for this disease process. Overall the natural history of asymptomatic contralateral VTOS appears benign in the majority.

Summary and Recommendations

VTOS is the result of subclavian vein compression by any variety of anatomic structures as it traverses the thoracic outlet. Patients with VTOS are likely at an increased risk of developing contralateral VTOS – although this risk is relatively low in an absolute sense, it is clearly higher than in the general population. The literature does clearly show that abnormal venographic findings on the asymptomatic contralateral side are common when specifically looked for in patients with VTOS [6, 21, 34]. It is known that asymptomatic venous stenosis with positional obstruction can progress to symptomatic venous obstruction [30]. However, the rate at which asymptomatic lesions progress to symptomatic lesions is not known.

It is reasonable to have an index of suspicion for contralateral VTOS in all patients with VTOS. This can be pursued through patient interviews, but additional diagnostic imaging is probably not necessary unless patients report symptoms consistent with VTOS. In addition patients should be counseled with regard to symptomatic recurrence on either side, and instructed to have a low tolerance for recurrent symptoms on either side. The same principals used in treating primary VTOS should be applied when considering the contralateral side. As a result asymptomatic patients should be observed and not offered prophylactic surgery as a matter of routine. In the instance of contralateral VTOS excellent outcomes can be expected with little long-term morbidity if modern treatment paradigms are applied.

References

1. Adams J, McEvoy R, DeWeese J. Primary deep venous thrombosis of upper extremity. Arch Surg. 1965;91:29–42.
2. Falconer M, Weddell G. Costoclavicular compression of subclavian artery and vein. Lancet. 1943;2:539.
3. Gould P, Patey D. Primary thrombosis of axillary vein: study of eight cases. Br J Surg. 1928;16:208.
4. McCleery RS, Kesterson JE, Kirtley JA, Love RB. Subclavius and anterior scalene muscle compression as a cause of intermittent obstruction of the subclavian vein. Ann Surg. 1951;1335:588–602.
5. Sampson J, Saunders JB, Capp CS. Compression of the subclavian vein by first rib and clavicle. Am Heart J. 1940;19:292.
6. Azakie A, McElhinney DB, Thompson RW, Raven RB, Messina LM, Stoney RJ. Surgical management of subclavian-vein effort thrombosis as a result of thoracic outlet compression. J Vasc Surg. 1998;28(5): 777–86.
7. Feugier P, Aleksic I, Salari R, Durand X, Chevalier JM. Long-term results of venous revascularization for Paget-Schroetter syndrome in athletes. Ann Vasc Surg. 2001;15(2):212–18.
8. Urschel Jr HC, Razzuk MA. Improved management of the Paget-Schroetter syndrome secondary to thoracic outlet compression. Ann Thorac Surg. 1991; 52(6):1217–21.
9. Adams J, DeWeese J, Mahoney E, Rob C. Intermittent subclavian vein obstruction without thrombosis. Surgery. 1968;68:147–65.
10. Juvonen T, Satta J, Laitala P, Luukkonen K, Nissinen J. Anomalies at the thoracic outlet are frequent in the general population. Am J Surg. 1995;170(1):33–7.
11. Tanaka Y, Aoki M, Izumi T, Fujimiya M, Yamashita T, Imai T. Measurement of subclavicular pressure on the subclavian artery and brachial plexus in the costoclavicular space during provocative positioning for thoracic outlet syndrome. J Orthop Sci. 2010;15(1): 118–24.
12. Heron E, Lozinguez O, Emmerich J, Laurian C, Fiessinger JN. Long-term sequelae of spontaneous axillary-subclavian venous thrombosis. Ann Intern Med. 1999;131(7):510–13.
13. Urschel Jr HC, Razzuk MA. Paget-Schroetter syndrome: what is the best management? Ann Thorac Surg. 2000;69(6):1663–8; discussion 1668–9.
14. Illig KA, Doyle AJ. A comprehensive review of Paget-Schroetter syndrome. J Vasc Surg. 2010;51(6): 1538–47.
15. Green RM, Waldman D, Ouriel K, Riggs P, Deweese JA. Claviculectomy for subclavian venous repair: long-term functional results. J Vasc Surg. 2000;32(2): 315–21.
16. Hempel GK, Shutze WP, Anderson JF, Bukhari HI. 770 consecutive supraclavicular first rib resections for thoracic outlet syndrome. Ann Vasc Surg. 1996;10(5): 456–63.
17. Adelman MA, Stone DH, Riles TS, Lamparello PJ, Giangola G, Rosen RJ. A multidisciplinary approach to the treatment of Paget-Schroetter syndrome. Ann Vasc Surg. 1997;11(2):149–54.
18. Sheeran SR, Hallisey MJ, Murphy TP, Faberman RS, Sherman S. Local thrombolytic therapy as part of a multidisciplinary approach to acute axillosubclavian vein thrombosis (Paget-Schroetter syndrome). J Vasc Interv Radiol. 1997;8(2):253–60.
19. Lee MC, Grassi CJ, Belkin M, Mannick JA, Whittemore AD, Donaldson MC. Early operative intervention after thrombolytic therapy for primary subclavian vein thrombosis: an effective treatment approach. J Vasc Surg. 1998;27(6):1101–7; discussion 1107–8.
20. Angle N, Gelabert HA, Farooq MM, et al. Safety and efficacy of early surgical decompression of the thoracic outlet for Paget-Schroetter syndrome. Ann Vasc Surg. 2001;15(1):37–42.
21. Coletta JM, Murray JD, Reeves TR, et al. Vascular thoracic outlet syndrome: successful outcomes with

multimodal therapy. Cardiovasc Surg. 2001;9(1): 11–5.

22. Kreienberg PB, Chang BB, Darling 3rd RC, et al. Long-term results in patients treated with thrombolysis, thoracic inlet decompression, and subclavian vein stenting for Paget-Schroetter syndrome. J Vasc Surg. 2001;33(2 Suppl):S100–5.

23. Lokanathan R, Salvian AJ, Chen JC, Morris C, Taylor DC, Hsiang YN. Outcome after thrombolysis and selective thoracic outlet decompression for primary axillary vein thrombosis. J Vasc Surg. 2001;33(4): 783–8.

24. Schneider DB, Dimuzio PJ, Martin ND, et al. Combination treatment of venous thoracic outlet syndrome: open surgical decompression and intraoperative angioplasty. J Vasc Surg. 2004;40(4):599–603.

25. Lee JT, Karwowski JK, Harris EJ, Haukoos JS, Olcott C. Long-term thrombotic recurrence after nonoperative management of Paget-Schroetter syndrome. J Vasc Surg. 2006;43(6):1236–43.

26. Molina JE, Hunter DW, Dietz CA. Paget-Schroetter syndrome treated with thrombolytics and immediate surgery. J Vasc Surg. 2007;45(2):328–34.

27. Urschel Jr HC, Patel AN. Surgery remains the most effective treatment for Paget-Schroetter syndrome: 50 years' experience. Ann Thorac Surg. 2008;86(1): 254–60; discussion 260.

28. Guzzo JL, Chang K, Demos J, Black JH, Freischlag JA. Preoperative thrombolysis and venoplasty affords no benefit in patency following first rib resection and scalenectomy for subacute and chronic subclavian vein thrombosis. J Vasc Surg. 2010;52(3):658–63.

29. Stone DH, Scali ST, Bjerk AA, et al. Aggressive treatment of idiopathic axillo-subclavian vein thrombosis provides excellent long-term function. J Vasc Surg. 2010;52(1):127–31.

30. Thakur S, Comerota AJ. Bilateral nonthrombotic subclavian vein obstruction causing upper extremity venous claudication. J Vasc Surg. 2010;52(1): 208–11.

31. Doyle A. Venous thoracic outlet syndrome. Rochester: University of Rochester Medical Center; 2011.

32. Hurley WL, Comins SA, Green RM, Canizzaro J. Atraumatic subclavian vein thrombosis in a collegiate baseball player: a case report. J Athl Train. 2006;41(2):198–200.

33. Lindblad B, Tengborn L, Bergqvist D. Deep vein thrombosis of the axillary-subclavian veins: epidemiologic data, effects of different types of treatment and late sequelae. Eur J Vasc Surg. 1988;2(3):161–5.

34. Machleder HI. Evaluation of a new treatment strategy for Paget-Schroetter syndrome: spontaneous thrombosis of the axillary-subclavian vein. J Vasc Surg. 1993;17(2):305–15; discussion 316–7.

Arterial thoracic outlet syndrome (ATOS) is clearly the rarest form of the problem; the combined experience of the editors (one with extensive experience in high performance athletes) over the past three decades suggests a rate of only 1–3 % of all that present with any form of TOS. While many patients with neurogenic TOS will have evidence of sympathetic overactivity and/or positional arterial compression (and, indeed, many if not most asymptomatic people can be found to have loss of pulses with extreme maneuvers), the diagnosis of ATOS is reserved for those with symptoms truly referable to fixed arterial lesions caused by damage to the subclavian artery as it passes over the first rib. In a manner analogous to the relationship of pectoralis minor syndrome to neurogenic TOS, lesions of the humoral circumflex arteries, most commonly seen in athletes, while not strictly in the same family, are also treated by ATOS specialists and are considered below.

ATOS really consists of two things – the problem at the first rib, and the distal sequelae. The original problem is repetitive damage to the subclavian artery as it crosses the rib. Such damage can be either aneurysm formation or vessel occlusion due to damage. In turn, the distal problem can be either ischemia – if the patient is lucky – or embolization with fixed occlusion. The former is very easily treated by fixing the proximal problem, but if fixed small vessel lesions are present, even perfect therapy can fail to relieve the problem.

The classic patient with ATOS presents with distal ischemia of the upper extremities. Not much can cause this, and if the patient is very young, especially if an athlete, the diagnosis may be obvious. However, if older, conventional atherosclerosis or an inflammatory arteriopathy may be assumed to be the problem, and definitive treatment delayed until too late. Luckily, the diagnosis of ATOS is the easiest of the three forms of the syndrome, and treatment most obvious. However, as mentioned above, if fixed lesions due to embolization exist, outcomes may be no better, and, indeed, at times worse, than those after treatment of NTOS.

The following section will explore this subject in detail, and present conventional and alternative points of view for each step in the treatment of these patients. There is less controversy (or uncertainty) in the treatment of these patients than in other forms of TOS, but surgery can be more challenging and results not always as clean as one would expect. These are young, healthy patients, and proper understanding of the syndrome and proper care absolutely critical.

Richard J. Sanders

Abstract

The anatomy and pathophysiology of ATOS is centered on cervical and anomalous first ribs. These ribs lie just inferior to the subclavian artery causing the artery to constantly beat against the rib. This results in damage to the inferior wall of the artery which becomes fibrotic and eventually stenotic. If the degree of stenosis elicits vibrations in the range of audible sound, post-stenotic dilatation and aneurysm formation develop in the subclavian artery. Both stenosis and aneurysms can produce non-occlusive arterial thrombosis which is the source of distal emboli and subsequent digital ischemia or even gangrene.

Introduction

Arterial thoracic outlet syndrome (ATOS) is hand and digital ischemia produced by emboli from subclavian artery aneurysms or stenosis secondary to arterial compression by cervical ribs or anomalous first ribs. Arterial pathology resulting from the compression leads to thrombi forming either distal to a stenosis in the artery or as mural thrombi in an aneurysm. Patients are usually asymptomatic while the pathology is developing but become symptomatic when emboli are released.

Etiology

Arterial thoracic outlet syndrome (ATOS) is the diagnosis made when compression of the subclavian artery producing stenosis with or without aneurysm formation and subsequent emboli to the upper extremity is found. ATOS is uncommon, occurring in less than 5 % of all TOS patients in some series [1] and less than 1 % in others [2]. The term ATOS applies only when there has been a complication from compression of the subclavian artery, as many patients can be shown to have asymptomatic positional obstruction without any apparent problems. This compression is usually due to an osseous abnormality, a cervical rib, or anomalous first rib (see Chaps. 3 and 81). ATOS tends to be associated with objective, structural, defined abnormalities to a much greater extent than VTOS or NTOS, making diagnosis a bit easier, but occasionally it is due to a (radiolucent) tight band or muscle compressing

R.J. Sanders, MD
Department of Surgery,
HealthONE Presbyterian-St. Lukes Hospital,
4545 E. 9th Ave #240, Denver, CO 80220, USA
e-mail: rsanders@ecentral.com

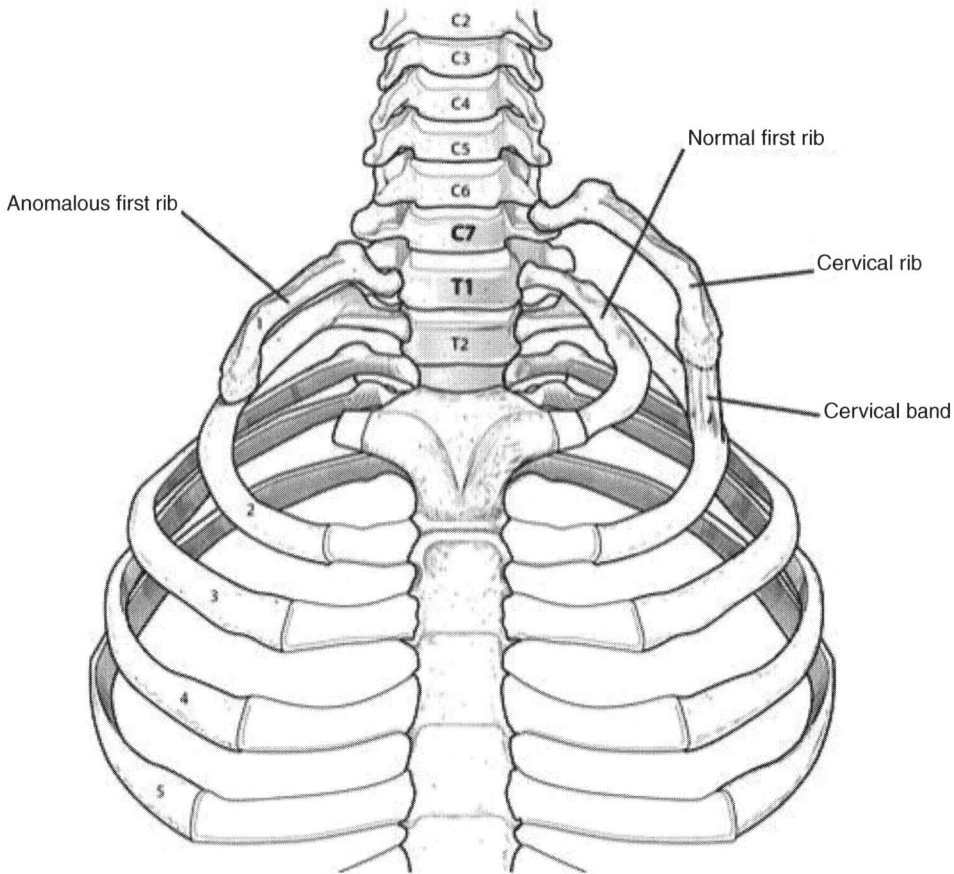

Fig. 77.1 Anomalous first rib and cervical rib. *Right side*: An anomalous first rib inserting into the midportion of the right second rib. Note there is no anterior portion of the right first rib to insert at the sternum as the normal left first rib is doing. Note too that the reason this is anomalous first rib is that it arises from the transverse process of T1. *Left side*: A cervical rib originating from the transverse process of C7. This is attaching to the midportion of the second rib via a congenital band. All incomplete cervical ribs attach to either the first of second rib by such a band

the artery. Although most cervical and anomalous first ribs are asymptomatic throughout life, a few cause arterial complications capable of producing severe disability and even limb loss.

Anatomy

Over 90 % of patients with ATOS have either a cervical rib or anomalous first rib. If a patient has an abnormal rib on one side there is greater than 50 % chance that there is a similar abnormality on the other side.

When an abnormal high lying rib is seen above the second rib, it is sometimes hard to determine if it is a cervical or anomalous first rib. By comparing the rib origin at the transverse process with the transverse process of the opposite side where there is a normal first rib, the origin of the abnormal high rib can be determined: T1 means an anomalous first rib, while C7 obviously means a cervical rib (Figs. 77.1 and 77.2) (see also Fig. 3.5). It should be noted, however, that this distinction is almost always of academic interest only and does not alter clinical management. Finally, even if a cervical rib is incomplete by radiographic imaging, it is almost always associated with a very tough fibrous band which runs from its tip to the first rib and elevates the structures within the scalene triangle.

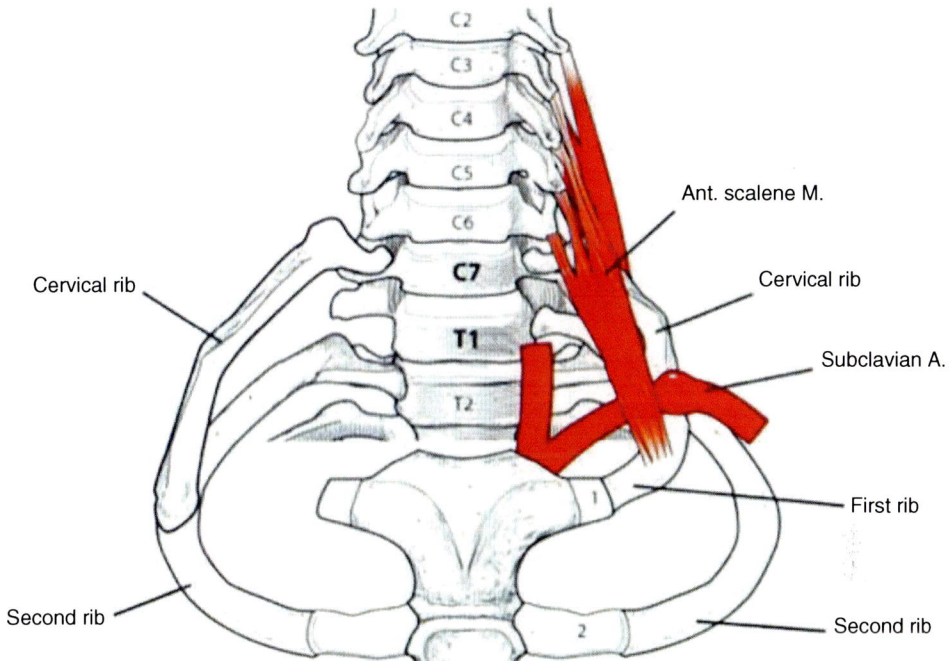

Fig. 77.2 Variations in cervical rib insertion and post-stenotic subclavian artery dilatation. Cervical ribs may insert on either the first rib as shown on the *left side* or second rib as shown on the *right side*. On the *right side* the first rib is absent which can lead to calling the cervical rib an anomalous first rib. The only difference is point of origin from either C7 versus T1. On the *left side* the cervical rib is inserting into a normal first rib sandwiching the subclavian artery between the rigid cervical rib and a tight anterior scalene muscle. This causes stenosis in the artery which in some patients leads to post-stenotic dilatation as shown here

Pathophysiology

Whether a cervical rib, anomalous first rib, or fibrous band, such a structure lies "schematically" in the position of the normal first rib, i.e., forming the floor of the scalene triangle. However, it is "higher" than the normal first rib, and thus invariably narrows this space. The high cervical rib pushes the subclavian artery above it so the artery is resting on the rib and arterial pulsation is constantly beating against the rib. In time, the wall of the artery, which is in contact with the rib, becomes fibrotic from continuous trauma. The arterial wall thickens in that spot and when enough fibrosis accumulates inside the artery, stenosis occurs. Arterial flow is accelerated in the stenotic area and turbulence develops distal to the stenosis.

When there is enough turbulence to produce vibrations, post stenotic dilatation of the artery can occur, but only if the vibrations elicit a bruit and thrill. Arterial stenosis that fails to produce vibrations in the proper sound range is not associated with post stenotic dilatation. Experiments have demonstrated that the most effective vibrations are those of very low frequencies, 25–35 Hz [3, 4]. These vibrations weaken elastin fibers and may destroy links between collagen fibers, making the arterial walls more distensible and subject to dilatation under normal arterial pressure. Once dilatation begins aneurysm formation soon develops, and as the aneurysm enlarges, mural thrombus forms against the lateral walls. Stenosis that does not result in post-stenotic dilatation still produces turbulence that results in post-stenotic eddy currents and subsequent thrombus formation just distal to the stenosis (see algorithm, Fig. 77.3). These processes occur silently. Most patients are unaware of their abnormal rib and even more unaware of the thrombus forming in either their subclavian artery aneurysm or distal to subclavian stenosis. Once thrombus develops

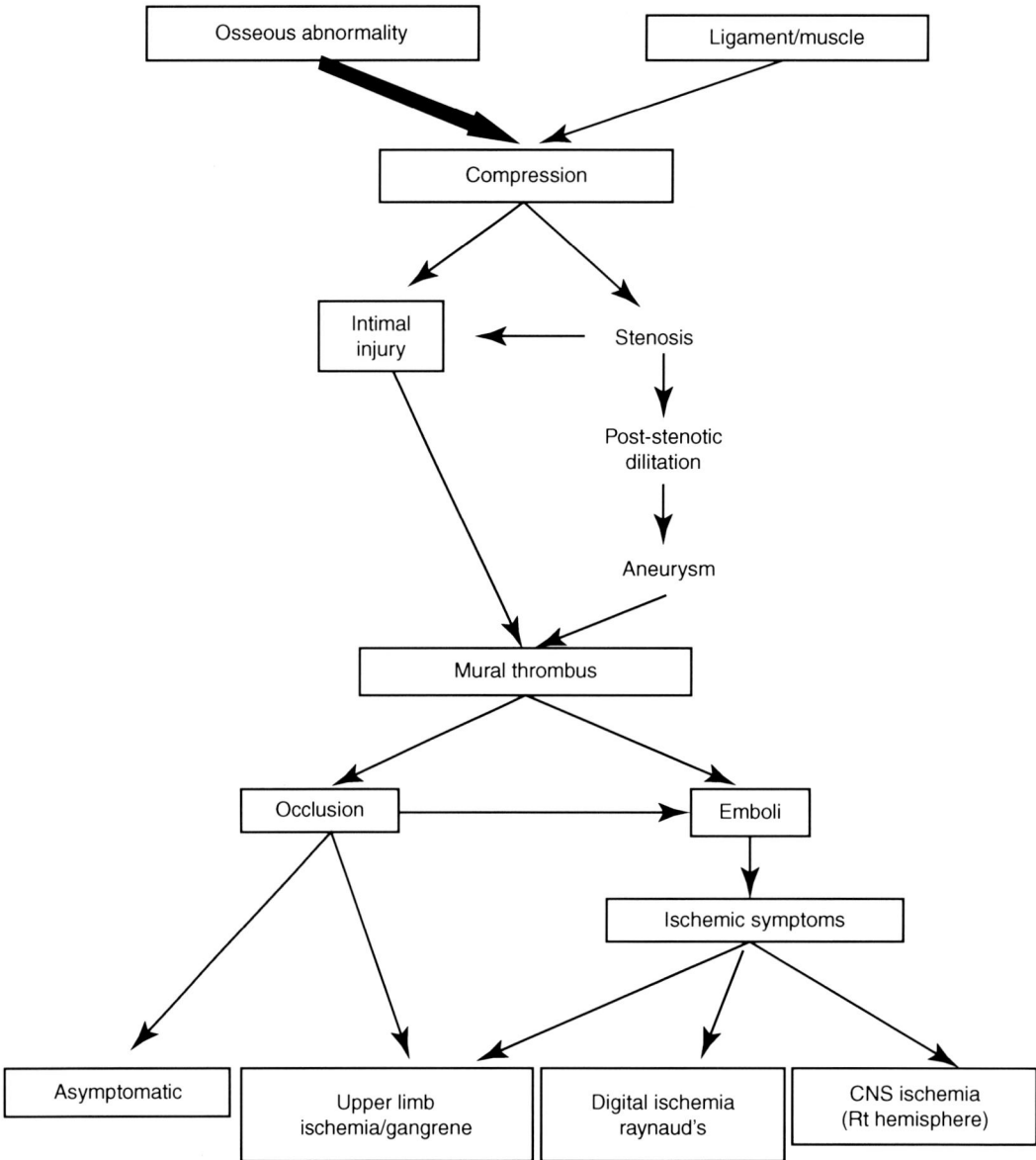

Fig. 77.3 Algorithm of pathophysiology of complications seen in aTOS (Reprinted from Sanders and Haug [5]. With permission from Wolter Kluwers Health)

it is just a matter of time before embolization occurs. An embolus small enough to lodge in digital arteries produces a white, numb, painful finger which is frequently the first symptom causing a patient to seek medical attention. In other patients the first symptom comes from a larger embolus occluding the brachial and/or radial and ulnar arteries resulting in limb-threatening ischemia.

An example of a patient with an embolus from a stenosis without aneurysm formation is shown in Fig. 77.4a. This image demonstrates an elevated subclavian artery with a filling defect representing the stenosis (note that the stenosis is slightly distal to the cervical rib). After resecting the cervical rib, the diseased arterial segment was resected and end-to-end anastomosis accomplished without difficulty. The postoperative film

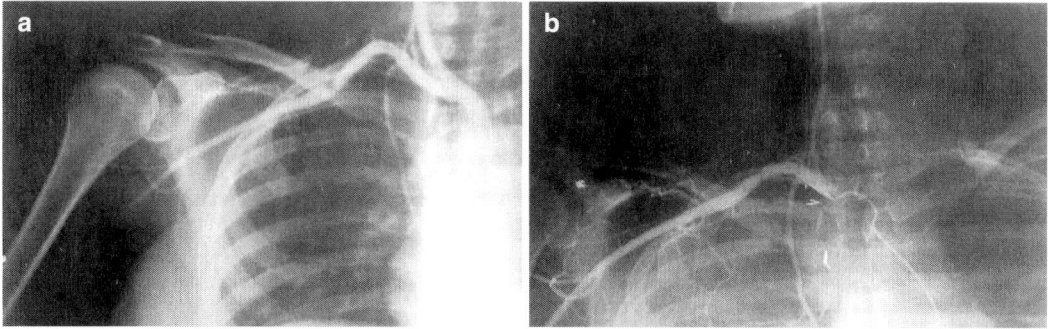

Fig. 77.4 Arteriography in a 32 year old woman with a right cervical rib and embolization to the right arm and hand. (**a**) Preoperative film demonstrating high lying subclavian artery elevated by a cervical rib plus stenosis of the artery where thrombus formed and embolized down the arm. The thrombus is seen behind the superimposed clavicle. (**b**) Postoperative arteriogram following resection and end-to-end anastomosis revealing a lower lying artery made possible by excising the abnormal rib. The descent of the artery permitted resection of 2 cm of artery and end-to-end anastomosis. In this patient there was no right first rib. The cervical rib was fused to the second rib (Reprinted from Sanders and Haug [6]. With permission from Wolter Kluwers Health

(Fig. 77.4b) reveals the subclavian artery lying lower because the rib is gone. Descent of the artery permits excision of 2–3 cm of artery and still allows an end-to-end anastomosis.

References

1. Kieffer E, Ruotolo C. Arterial complications of thoracic outlet compression. In: Rutherford RB, editor. Vascular surgery. 3rd ed. Philadelphia: WB Saunders Co.; 1989. p. 875–82.
2. Sanders RJ, Hammond SL, Rao NM. Thoracic outlet syndrome: a review. Neurologist. 2008;14:365–73.
3. Roach MR. Changes in arterial distensibility as a cause of poststenotic dilatation. Am J Cardiol. 1963; 12:802–15.
4. Roach MR, Melech E. The effect of sonic vibration on isolated human iliac arteries. Can J Physiol Pharmacol. 1971;49:288–91.
5. Sanders RJ, Haug CE. Thoracic outlet syndrome: a common sequela of neck injuries. Philadelphia: JB Lippincott; 1991. p. 213.
6. Sanders RJ, Haug CE. Thoracic outlet syndrome: a common sequela of neck injuries. Philadelphia: JB Lippincott; 1991. p. 215.

Clinical Presentation and Patient Evaluation in ATOS

Ali Azizzadeh and Robert W. Thompson

Abstract

Arterial thoracic outlet syndrome (TOS) is a rare condition most frequently observed in relatively young, active, and otherwise healthy individuals. It is typically caused by a bony anatomic abnormality, leading to subclavian artery compression, poststenotic dilatation with aneurysmal degeneration and/or ulceration, and mural thrombus formation with distal embolization to the arm and/or hand. The clinical presentation of arterial TOS occurs in four settings: (1) upper extremity claudication due to fixed or positional subclavian artery obstruction, resulting in exercise-induced arm symptoms of fatigue, muscle cramping, heaviness and pain; (2) acute or subacute upper extremity ischemia due to thromboembolism, resulting in pain, numbness and/or tingling, cold sensation, and a pale or mottled appearance in the hand and/or fingers. (This is often associated with sustained digital vasospasm, which may be complicated by fingertip ulceration or digital gangrene); (3) an asymptomatic pulsatile mass in the supraclavicular space, typically found in association with a cervical rib; and (4) the presence of symptoms of neurogenic TOS in a patient with a cervical rib, with an incidental finding of a subclavian artery aneurysm identified on physical examination or imaging studies. In this chapter, we review the clinical presentation of arterial TOS and use of history, physical examination, and imaging studies to establish a sound diagnosis of this potentially limb-threatening condition.

A. Azizzadeh, MD, FACS (✉)
Department of Cardiothoracic and Vascular Surgery,
University of Texas Medical School,
Memorial Hermann Heart and Vascular Institute,
6400 Fannin St., Suite 2850, Houston,
TX 77030, USA
e-mail: ali.azizzadeh@uth.tmc.edu

R.W. Thompson, MD
Department of Surgery, Section of Vascular Surgery,
Center for Thoracic Outlet Syndrome, Washington
University, Barnes-Jewish Hospital,
Campus Box 8109/Suite 5101 Queeny Tower 660 S
Euclid Ave, St. Louis, MO 63110, USA
e-mail: thompson@wudosis.wustl.edu

K.A. Illig et al. (eds.), *Thoracic Outlet Syndrome*,
DOI 10.1007/978-1-4471-4366-6_78, © Springer-Verlag London 2013

Introduction

Arterial thoracic outlet syndrome (TOS) is a rare condition most frequently observed in relatively young, active, and otherwise healthy individuals [1–4]. Arterial TOS is typically caused by a bony anatomic abnormality, leading to subclavian artery compression, poststenotic dilatation with aneurysmal degeneration and/or ulceration, and mural thrombus formation with distal embolization to the arm and/or hand. Arterial TOS is commonly caused by abnormal osseous structures, such as cervical ribs, anomalous first ribs, fibrocartilagenous bands and hypertrophic callus from healed clavicular fractures [2, 4, 5]. Cervical ribs displace the brachial plexus and subclavian artery forward where the artery is compressed between the abnormal rib, the anterior scalene muscle, and the first rib. While the association between a cervical rib and arterial symptoms was first reported by Sir Astley Cooper in 1818, Coote reported the first surgical procedure for arterial TOS in 1861 at St. Bartholomew's Hospital in London, where he removed an exostosis of the transverse process of the seventh cervical vertebrae to treat an ischemic hand [6]. The term "thoracic outlet syndrome" was coined by Peet and colleagues in 1956 [7].

Epidemiology

Examination of the published literature reveals that arterial TOS is the least frequent form of TOS. In a series of more than 5,000 patients published by Urshel and Kourlis, the incidence was 6 % [8]. Other large, single-institution series have reported an incidence of arterial TOS of 1–3 % [9–12]. The mean age at presentation is 37 years, with an equal proportion of men and women affected. Abnormal osseous structures are consistently present in this population. The relative frequency of anatomic abnormalities causing arterial TOS is listed in Table 78.1. Interestingly, a recent cadaveric study reported the incidence of cervical ribs to be <0.5 % in the general population, and showed that cervical ribs can be associated with histopathologic changes in the brachial plexus.

Table 78.1 Bony abnormalities associated with arterial TOS

Abnormality	Frequency (%)
Cervical rib	65
Anomalous first rib	20
Fibrocartilagenous band	8
Clavicular fracture	7
Elongated C7 transverse process	1

Data compiled from five large clinical series representing a total of 119 patients with arterial TOS

As a result, subtle neurological symptoms may also be present in this patient population [13].

Clinical Presentation

The clinical presentation of arterial TOS occurs in four settings: (1) upper extremity claudication due to fixed or positional subclavian artery obstruction, resulting in exercise-induced arm symptoms of fatigue, muscle cramping, heaviness and pain; (2) acute or subacute upper extremity ischemia due to thromboembolism, resulting in pain, numbness and/or tingling, cold sensation, and a pale or mottled appearance in the hand and/or fingers. (This is often associated with sustained digital vasospasm, which may be complicated by fingertip ulceration or digital gangrene); (3) an asymptomatic pulsatile mass in the supraclavicular space, typically found in association with a cervical rib; and (4) the presence of symptoms of neurogenic TOS in a patient with a cervical rib, with an incidental finding of a subclavian artery aneurysm identified on physical examination or imaging studies. Confusion can arise in patients presenting with symptoms that are primarily attributable to brachial plexus compression (neurogenic TOS), where there is positional ablation of the radial pulse on arm elevation, or in those with secondary hand/finger vasospasm due to sympathetic overactivity. However, neither of these situations are considered to represent arterial TOS.

Patients with arterial TOS are often young and healthy, and they frequently report vigorous use of the arm in occupational or recreational activities. Due to the chronic nature of the arterial injury, extensive collateralization has often developed.

As a result, the presenting symptoms may be limited to arm claudication with exercise, especially in overhead positions. The symptoms may be described as pain, cramping, heaviness, and heightened cold sensation. Unfortunately, patients often do not seek medical evaluation, or the serious nature of the condition is not appreciated, until embolization and ischemic complications have developed. These can include digital ulceration, gangrene, vasomotor symptoms (Raynaud's phenomenon), loss of palpable pulses and paresthesias. Acute ischemic symptoms secondary to subclavian artery thrombosis, as well as embolization to the brachial, radial and ulnar arteries, can occur. Rare instances of acute stroke, secondary to retrograde embolization of subclvian artery thrombus to the vertebral circulation, have also been reported [14–18].

Patient Evaluation

History

The diagnosis of arterial TOS starts with a detailed history and physical examination of the neurovascular and musculoskeletal structures of the neck, shoulder, arms and hands, and extends to additional diagnostic studies. The history should include the patient's occupational, athletic, and recreational physical activity, as well as any history of trauma.

A history of repetitive overhead activity at work (e.g., electricians, baseball players), carrying of heavy objects on the shoulder or in the hand (e.g., backpacks, brief cases), or any prolonged posture (e.g., sitting, typing) should be documented. The timing, location, distribution, character and intensity of pain, as well as any exacerbating and alleviating factors, should be noted. Aggravation of symptoms with the upper extremity in the elevated position is often reported. Paresthesias attributable to the lower brachial plexus (C8 and T1) may also be present in patients with arterial TOS.

Physical Examination

The physical examination begins with inspection of the hands for evidence of cyanosis, erythema, discoloration, ulceration, and gangrene, as well as thenar or hypothenar muscle atrophy (Fig. 78.1). Next, palpation of bilateral carotid, brachial, radial and ulnar pulses should be performed. A decrease or absence of the distal pulses is not uncommon if significant embolization has already occurred. A palpable, bony prominence in the supraclavicular fossa often represents a cervical rib, and a palpable pulsation in the same area may represent a subclavian artery aneurysm. Point tenderness over the scalene triangle may be present if

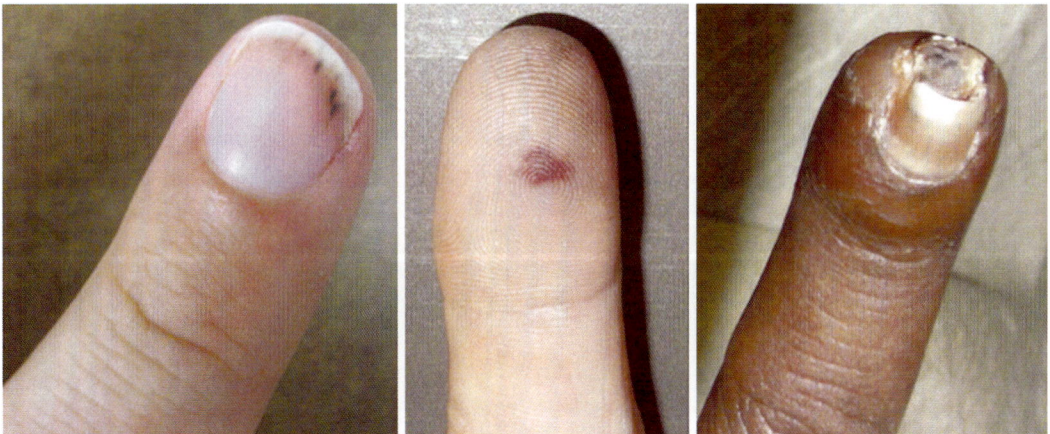

Fig. 78.1 Digital emboli in arterial TOS. Photographs illustrating three examples of patients that presented with digital emboli and were found to have arterial TOS

a neurogenic component of TOS is present. Auscultation over the supraclaviacular and infraclavicular spaces should be performed at rest and during arm abduction. Bruits may be most noticeable when the arm is moving from a resting position into full abduction and external rotation, but will disappear once the pulse is completely obliterated. A thorough neurological examination, including sensory, motor and reflex testing, is essential. Muscle weakness or atrophy should be noted. Blood pressure measurements should be obtained in bilateral upper extremities, with the pressure in the affected extremity expected to be approximately 30 mmHg lower than the unaffected extremity in the presence of a subclavian artery occlusion.

Provocative Testing

Although provocative tests have a relatively low sensitivity and specificity (approximately 72 and 53 %, respectively), the reproduction of symptoms during certain maneuvers may help support the diagnosis of arterial TOS [19, 20]. Furthermore, it is important to note that the false positive rate of more than one provocative maneuver in the asymptomatic patients is 56 % [21]. Regardless, the clinician who evaluates patients with arterial TOS should be aware that no single physical examination maneuver can unequivocally establish the presence or absence of the condition.

The Adson's test is considered positive if obliteration or diminution of the radial pulse is noted after "having the patient take a long breath, elevate his chin and turn it to the affected side" [22]. The Roos, or elevated arm stress test (EAST), is performed by having the patient abduct and externally rotate both arms in a 90° angle while rapidly flexing and extending the fingers. Reproduction of symptoms within 20 seconds is considered a positive test [23]. The Wright's test is positive when a decrease in the radial pulse or reproduction of symptoms is

noted with hyperabduction of the pectoralis minor (axillary interval) [24, 25]. The patient sits in a comfortable position with the head forward, while the arm is passively brought into abduction and external rotation to 90° without tilting the head or flexing the elbow more than 45°. Finally, the costoclavicular maneuver is performed with the patient in a sitting position. The examiner assists the patient in performing scapular retraction, depression, elevation, and protraction, each for 30 seconds. The patient is monitored for changes in the pulse or reproduction of symptoms [25, 26]. Patients with arterial TOS often have more than one positive provocative test, and in the presence of negative test results, other clinical diagnosis should be considered.

Imaging Studies

Once the diagnosis of arterial TOS is suspected based on history and physical examination, additional adjunctive studies are required for confirmation. Plain chest x-rays are performed to evaluate for a cervical rib or other bony abnormalities (Fig. 78.2). Duplex ultrasound can visualize a subclavian artery aneurysm, and segmental pressure testing with digital waveforms can be conducted at baseline and with provocative maneuvers. Reduced arterial pulse waveforms can be seen at rest, or during the performance of various positional maneuvers, secondary to embolization or arterial compression. Either computed tomography, magnetic resonance imaging or catheter-based angiography is performed to assess the location and extent of arterial pathology (Fig. 78.3). These tests need to be performed both at rest and with the arm in overhead position. Laboratory diagnostic studies are used to rule out other systemic conditions (e.g., hypercoagulable disorders, connective tissue disease, and vasculitis) that can mimic arterial TOS.

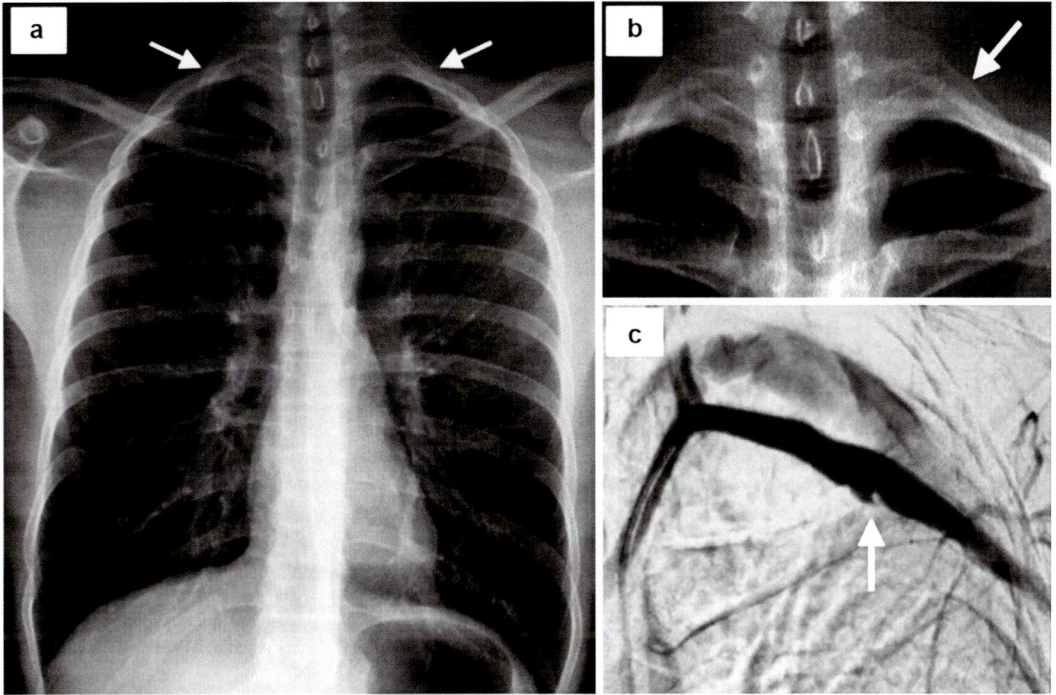

Fig. 78.2 Radiographic imaging in arterial TOS. Imaging studies in a young man who presented with left-sided digital emboli and ischemic hand symptoms. (**a**) Anterior-posterior chest x-ray demonstrating bilateral cervical ribs (*arrows*). (**b**) Magnified view of the chest x-ray, illustrating cervical rib on the symptomatic left side (*arrow*). (**c**) Catheter-based left subclavian arteriogram, demonstrating relatively mild poststenotic dilatation of the subclavian artery with a focal area of ulceration on the inferior aspect of the artery (*arrow*). This area of ulceration was associated with mural thrombus at the time of thoracic outlet decompression and subclavian aneurysm repair, confirming it as the source of distal emboli

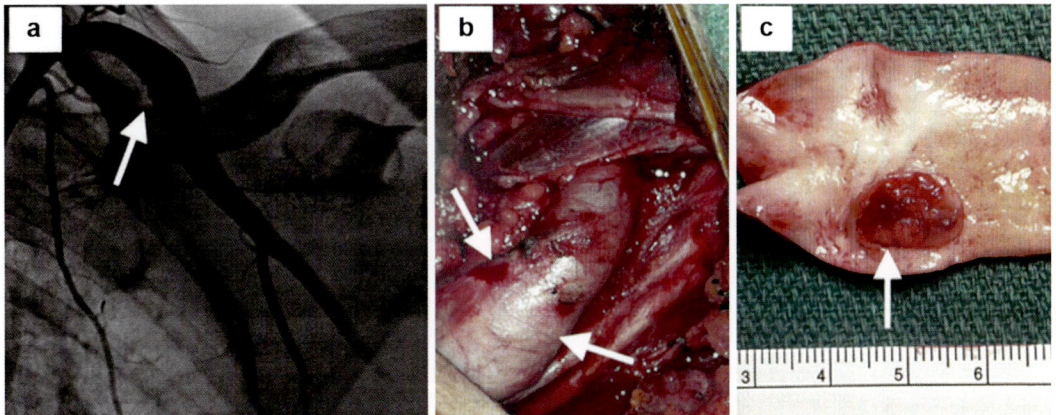

Fig. 78.3 Subclavian artery aneurysm. Photographs of a young man with left hand ischemia and a left-sided cervical rib. (**a**) Preoperative arteriogram demonstrating a subclavian artery aneurysm with minimal surface irregularity (*arrow*). (**b**) Operative exposure from the left side, demonstrating the site of arterial compression between the anterior scalene muscle, first rib, and cervical rib, and a moderate-sized subclavian artery aneurysm (*arrows*). (**c**) Opened surgical specimen of the excised subclavian artery aneurysm, demonstrating a focal area of mural thrombus within the site of ulceration (*arrow*), which served as the source of distal emboli

References

1. Sanders RJ, Haug C. Review of arterial thoracic outlet syndrome with a report of five new instances. Surg Gynecol Obstet. 1991;173:415–25.
2. Durham JR, Yao JS, Pearce WH, Nuber GM, McCarthy Jr W. Arterial injuries in the thoracic outlet syndrome. J Vasc Surg. 1995;21:57–69.
3. Thompson RW, Driskill MR. Neurovascular problems in the athlete's shoulder. Clin Sports Med. 2008;27:789–802.
4. Criado E, Berguer R, Greenfield L. The spectrum of arterial compression at the thoracic outlet. J Vasc Surg. 2010;52:406–11.
5. Casbas L, Chauffour X, Cau J, Bossavy JP, Midy D, Baste JC, Barret A. Post-traumatic thoracic outlet syndromes. Ann Vasc Surg. 2005;19:25–8.
6. Coote H. Exostosis of the left transverse process of the seventh cervical vertebra, surrounded by blood vessels and nerves; successful removal. Lancet. 1861;1:360–1.
7. Peet RM, Hendriksen JD, Anderson TP, Martin GM. Thoracic outlet syndrome: evaluation of a therapeutic exercise program. Proc Mayo Clin. 1956;31:281–7.
8. Urschel HC, Kourlis H. Thoracic outlet syndrome: a 50-year experience at Baylor University Medical Center. Proc Bayl Univ Med Ctr. 2007;20:125–35.
9. Sanders RJ, Hammond SL, Rao NM. Diagnosis of thoracic outlet syndrome. J Vasc Surg. 2007;46(3):601–4.
10. Cormier JM, Amrane M, Ward A, Laurian C, Gigou F. Arterial complications of the thoracic outlet syndrome: fifty-five operative cases. J Vasc Surg. 1989;9:778–87.
11. Nehler MR, Taylor LMJ, Moneta GL, Porter JM. Upper extremity ischemia from subclavian artery aneurysm caused by bony abnormalities of the thoracic outlet. Arch Surg. 1997;132:527–32.
12. Gelabert HA, Machleder HI. Diagnosis and management of arterial compression at the thoracic outlet. Ann Vasc Surg. 1997;11:359–66.
13. Tubbs RS, Louis RGJ, Wartmann CT, Lott R, Chua GD, Kelly D, Palmer CA, Shoja MM, Loukas M, Oakes WJ. Histopathological basis for neurogenic thoracic outlet syndrome. J Neurosurg Spine. 2008;8:347–51.
14. Symonds CP. Two cases of thrombosis of subclavian artery with contralateral hemiplegia of sudden onset, probably embolic. Brain. 1927;50:259–60.
15. Fields WS, Lemak NA, Ben-Menachem Y. Thoracic outlet syndrome: review and reference to stroke in a major league pitcher. AJR Am J Roentgenol. 1986;146:809–14.
16. Naz I, Ziad S. Cerebral embolism: distal subclavian disease as a rare etiology. J Pak Med Assoc. 2006;56:186–8.
17. Lee TS, Hines GL. Cerebral embolic stroke and arm ischemia in a teenager with arterial thoracic outlet syndrome: a case report. Vasc Endovascular Surg. 2007;41:254–7.
18. Hugl B, Oldenburg A, Hakaim AG, Persellin ST. Unusual etiology of upper extremity ischemia in a scleroderma patient: thoracic outlet syndrome with arterial embolization. J Vasc Surg. 2007;45:1259–61.
19. Nichols AW. Diagnosis and management of thoracic outlet syndrome. Curr Sports Med Rep. 2009;8(5):240–9.
20. Gillard J, Pérez-Cousin M, Hachulla E, Remy J, Hurtevent JF, Vinckier L, Thévenon A, Duquesnoy B. Diagnosing thoracic outlet syndrome: contribution of provocative tests, ultrasonography, electrophysiology, and helical computed tomography in 48 patients. Joint Bone Spine. 2001;68:416–24.
21. Nord KM, Kapoor P, Fisher J, Thomas G, Sundaram A, Scott K, Kothari MJ. False positive rate of thoracic outlet syndrome diagnostic maneuvers. Electromyogr Clin Neurophysiol. 2008;48:67–74.
22. Adson AW. Surgical treatment for symptoms produced by cervical ribs and the scalenus anticus muscle. Surg Gynecol Obstet. 1947;85:687–700.
23. Roos DB, Owens JC. Thoracic outlet syndrome. Arch Surg. 1966;93:71–4.
24. Wright IS. The neurovascular syndrome produced by hyperabduction of the arms: the immediate change produced in 150 normals and the effect on some persons of prolonged hyperabduction of the arms as in sleeping and in certain occupations. Am Heart J. 1945;29:1–19.
25. Watson LA, Pizzari T, Balster S. Thoracic outlet syndrome part 1: clinical manifestations, differentiation and treatment pathways. Man Ther. 2009;14(6):586–95.
26. Falconer MA, Weddell G. Costoclavicular compression of the subclavian artery and vein. Lancet. 1943;2:539–43.

Management of Digital Emboli, Vasospasm, and Ischemia in ATOS

79

Robert W. Thompson

Abstract

Unilateral digital ischemia is one of the most common presenting problems in patients with arterial TOS, leading to numbness, tingling, cold and painful sensations, cyanotic or pale discoloration, delayed capillary refill in the fingers, and non-healing fingertip ulceration. Diagnostic evaluation requires differentiation between proximal and distal arterial sources of thromboembolism, localized digital artery occlusion, and primary vasospasm. Digital emboli typically accompany arterial TOS as a result of mural thrombus formed within an area of aneurysmal degeneration in the subclavian (or axillary) arteries. While there are a variety of medical treatments to help reduce local symptoms of digital ischemia and vasospasm, definitive management depends on surgical control of the proximal source of thromboembolism. Additional interventions, such as thromboembolectomy and intra-arterial infusion of thrombolytic agents and/or vasodilators, are valuable adjuncts toward achieving optimal outcomes.

Clinical Presentation

Unilateral digital ischemia is one of the most common presenting problems in patients with arterial TOS [1, 2]. The principal symptoms include numbness, tingling, cold and painful sensations, cyanotic or pale discoloration, and delayed capillary refill in the fingers. Non-healing fingertip ulceration may be present, particularly in patients with longstanding symptoms (Fig. 79.1). On physical examination the brachial, radial and/or ulnar pulses may be absent or decreased in the presence of a proximal arterial occlusion, with diminished blood pressure in the affected arm. Digital ischemia may also exist with

R.W. Thompson, MD
Department of Surgery, Section of Vascular Surgery,
Center for Thoracic Outlet Syndrome, Washington
University, Barnes-Jewish Hospital,
Campus Box 8109/Suite 5101 Queeny Tower 660 S
Euclid Ave, St. Louis, MO 63110, USA
e-mail: thompson@wudosis.wustl.edu

K.A. Illig et al. (eds.), *Thoracic Outlet Syndrome*,
DOI 10.1007/978-1-4471-4366-6_79, © Springer-Verlag London 2013

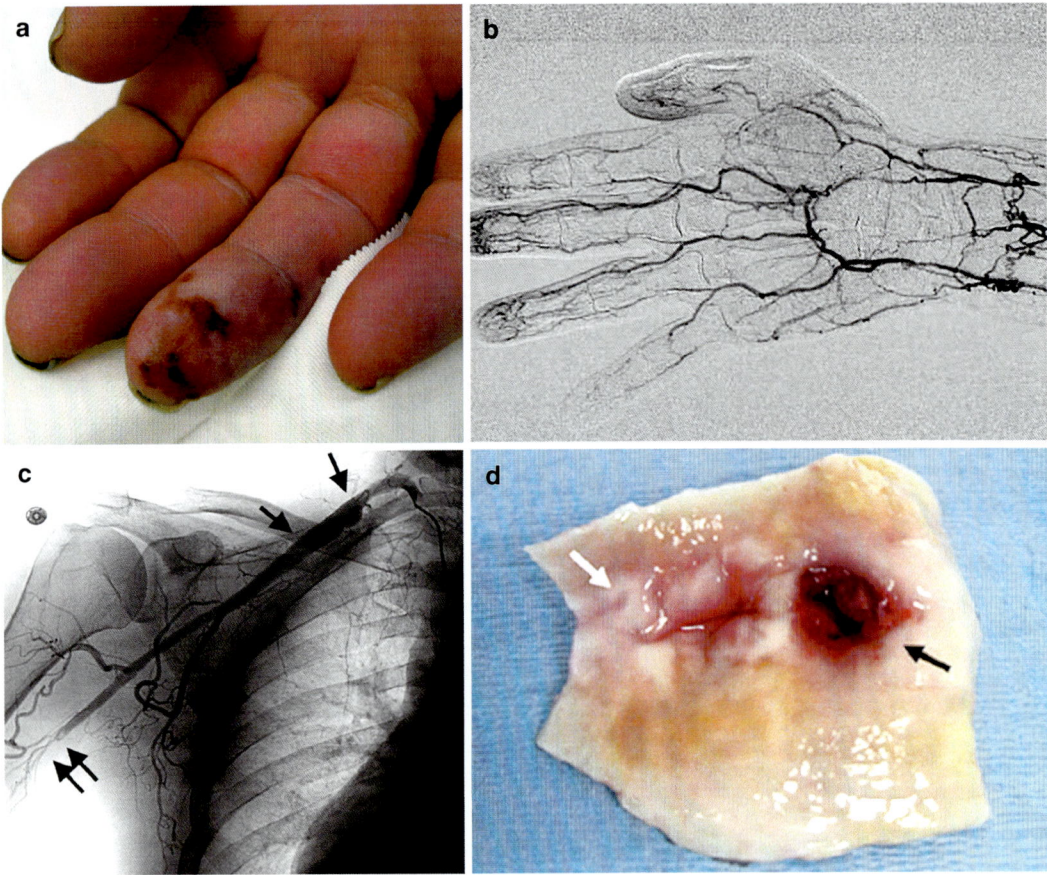

Fig. 79.1 Digital ulceration due to arterial emboli. Patient presenting with non-healing fingertip ulcerations in the *right hand* (**a**). Arteriography demonstrated digital artery occlusions due to emboli from a proximal source (**b**), and revealed a proximal brachial artery occlusion (**c**, *double arrows*) and a subclavian artery aneurysm (**c**, *arrows*). A right cervical rib was also present. Following thoracic outlet decompression with resection of the cervical and first ribs, the subclavian aneurysm was excised and the subclavian artery repaired with an interposition bypass graft. The surgical specimen demonstrated intimal thickening (**d**, *white arrow*) and a deep intimal ulcer filled with chronic thrombus as the source of distal emboli (**d**, *black arrow*)

normal radial and ulnar pulses if the site of arterial obstruction is solely within the vessels of the hand, which can occur with digital artery embolism from a more proximal site or with digital artery thrombosis secondary to local trauma. Digital ischemia usually coexists with and is exacerbated by local vasospasm and cold intolerance. In some circumstances, primary vasospasm can also result in digital ischemia in the absence of arterial thrombosis or embolism. The potential causes of digital ischemia are summarized in Table 79.1.

Diagnosis

The diagnostic evaluation of digital ischemia requires differentiation between proximal and distal arterial sources of thromboembolism, localized digital artery occlusion, and primary vasospasm [3]. Upper extremity embolism arising from the heart usually leads to occlusion of the axillary or brachial arteries by a relatively large thrombus, and can be effectively evaluated by echocardiography and Duplex ultrasound studies of the upper extremity. In most cases of distal embolism

Table 79.1 Differential diagnosis of digital ischemia

Thromboembolism from a cardiac source

  Arrhythmia, valvular disease, septal defect (paradoxical)

Thromboembolism from a proximal arterial source

  Aorta: endothelial erosion, ulceration, or penetrating ulcer

  Subclavian or axillary arteries: aneurysm, occlusion, stenosis or ulceration

Thromboembolism from a distal arterial source

  Brachial, radial or ulnar arteries: local trauma

  Palmar arteries: hypothenar hammer syndrome

Systemic diseases associated with vasculitis

  Scleroderma, rheumatoid arthritis, polyarteritis nodosa, takayasu's, beurger's disease

Local vascular diseases

  Hemangioma, arteriovenous malformation, glomus tumor, synovitis

Primary digital artery thrombosis

  Local repetitive trauma

Primary vasospasm

  Raynaud's disease, cold exposure, tobacco use, cocaine

in a young, otherwise healthy individual, an arterial source must be considered. Although vascular laboratory studies may increase suspicion of an arterial lesion, this is best evaluated by catheter-based (transfemoral) selective arteriography, with positional views of the neck and upper arm and high-resolution views of the hand (Fig. 79.2). This may also be accomplished in some settings with contrast-enhanced computed tomography (CT) or magnetic resonance imaging (MRI), but catheter-based arteriography remains the most accurate and definitive approach.

If a proximal arterial source of embolism cannot be identified, primary digital artery thrombosis and/or vasospasm is suspected. Digital artery thrombosis can be caused by localized repetitive trauma, such as that occasionally seen in baseball players secondary to pressure exerted on a specific site in the index or middle finger when gripping or throwing the ball. Another arterial lesion localized within the hand is the "hypothenar hammer" syndrome, where degeneration of the distal ulnar artery as it crosses the hamate bone is caused by chronic repetitive trauma to the base of the hand, resulting in thromboembolism to the digital arteries. Finally, primary digital artery spasm (in the

absence of embolism or thrombosis) may be the result of localized injury in combination with sustained cold exposure and/or use of tobacco, cocaine or other vasoconstrictive agents.

Digital emboli typically accompany arterial TOS as a result of aneurysmal degeneration in the subclavian or axillary arteries (Figs. 79.1, 79.2, and 79.3) [4–7]. Mural thrombus formed within an aneurysm in these locations is particularly prone to embolize to distal vessels, since the axillary and subclavian arteries are subject to a great deal of motion during the course of normal daily upper extremity activity, and because arterial TOS is usually associated with cervical ribs or other bony anomalies [8]. Embolic occlusion may occur in the distal brachial, radial or ulnar arteries, or may be confined to the small digital vessels.

Treatment

A variety of medical treatment options have been described for the initial treatment of digital ischemia and vasospasm (Table 79.2) [3]. While these measures may help reduce local symptoms, definitive management depends on identifying the underlying cause and surgical treatment for any proximal and/or distal arterial lesion. In many cases ongoing medical treatment for digital ischemia is also required despite satisfactory surgical control of the proximal source of thromboembolism, such as a subclavian artery aneurysm. This may include interventions such as thromboembolectomy and intra-arterial infusion of thrombolytic agents and/or vasodilators, either at the time of the principal operation or as secondary procedures performed during the follow-up period. Cervical sympathetic (stellate ganglion) blockade with local anesthetic is a useful adjunct in differentiating persistent digital vasospasm that may be responsive to vasodilator treatment. If sympathetic blockade provides effective but only short-duration relief of finger and hand symptoms, surgical approaches to cervical sympathectomy or digital artery sympathectomy can also be considered. While cervical sympathectomy can be readily performed in conjunction with primary thoracic outlet decompression procedures,

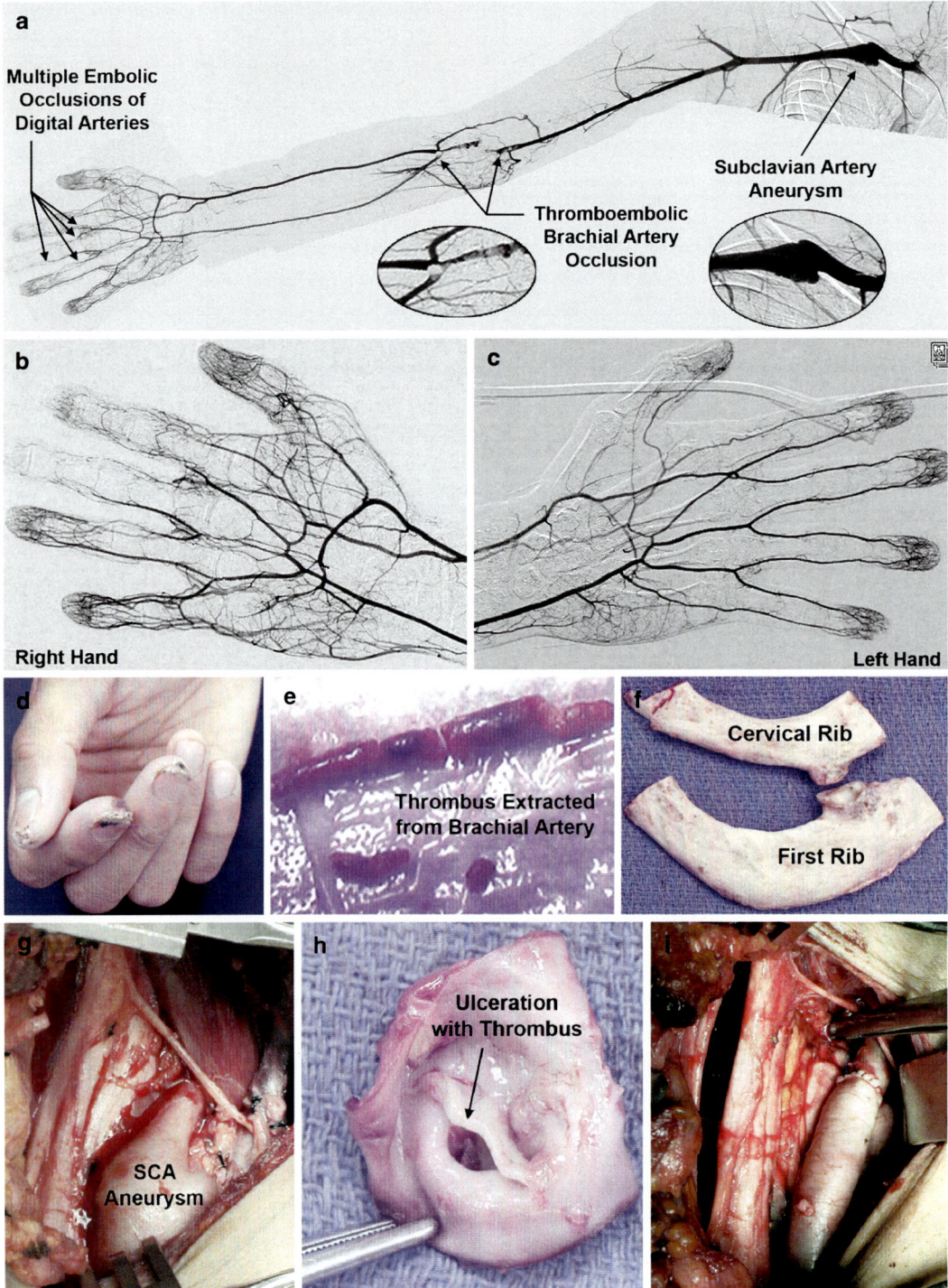

Fig. 79.2 Subclavian artery aneurysm causing digital ischemia. Patient presenting with right hand ischemia, with an upper extremity arteriogram demonstrating a subclavian artery aneurysm, thromboembolic occlusion of the distal brachial artery, and multiple embolic digital artery occlusions (**a**). Magnified arteriographic views of the affected right hand (**b**) and normal left hand (**c**) illustrate the differences in perfusion that led to ischemic fingertip lesions in the right hand (**d**). A brachial artery thromboembolectomy and patch angioplasty repair was initially performed (**e**), followed several days later by thoracic outlet decompression with resection of the cervical and first ribs (**f**). The subclavian artery aneurysm (**g**) was excised, with the specimen demonstrating intimal ulceration with thrombus (**h**), and an interposition arterial graft repair was performed (**i**)

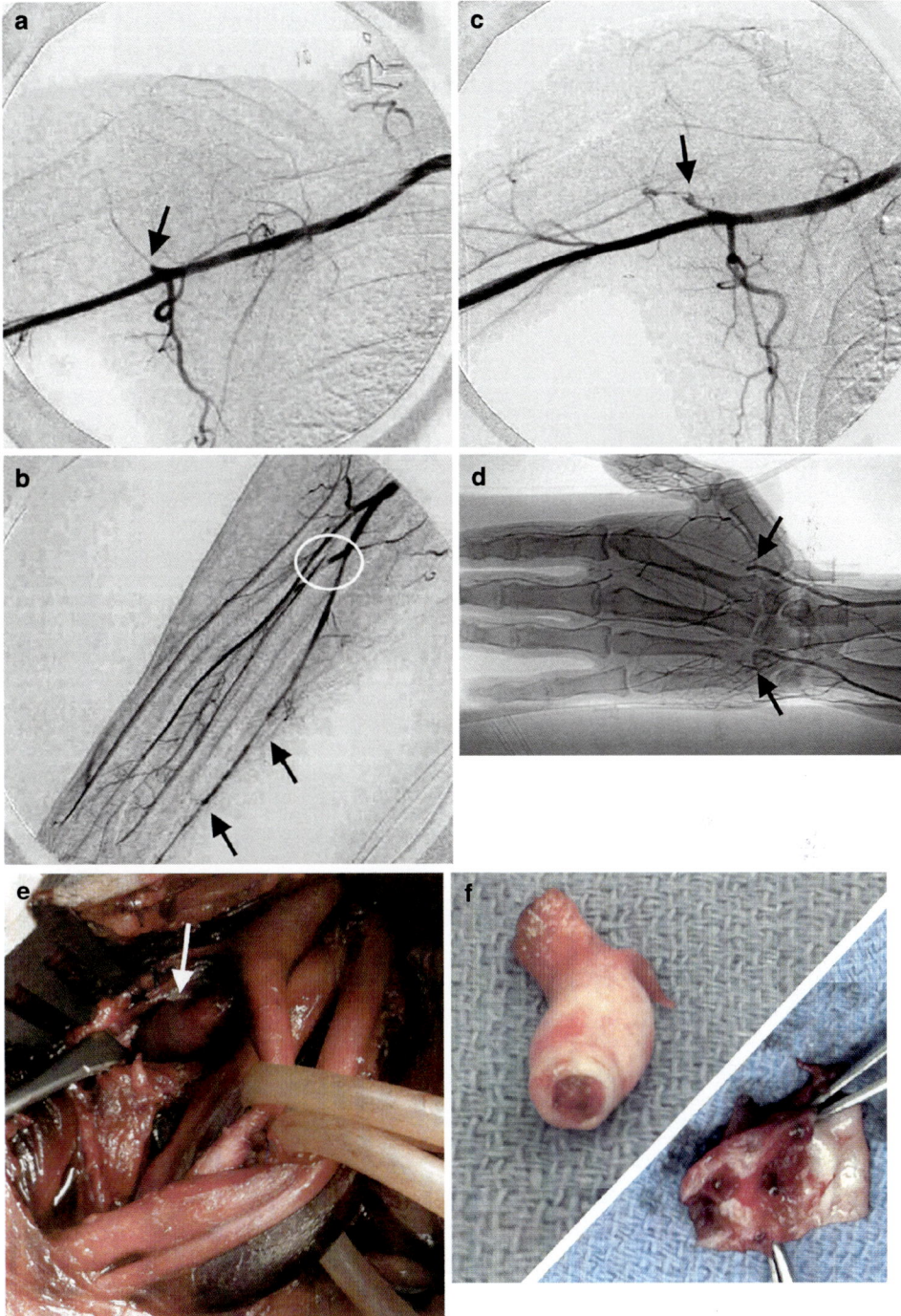

Fig. 79.3 Upper extremity thromboembolism caused by axillary artery branch vessel aneurysms. (**a–b**) An otherwise healthy overhead throwing athlete presented with digital ischemia. Arteriography demonstrated occlusion of a right posterior circumflex humeral artery aneurysm (**a**, *arrow*) and multiple emboli to the interosseus and ulnar arteries (**b**, *arrows*). (**c–f**) Professional baseball pitcher presenting with digital ischemia in the throwing hand. Arteriography demonstrated occlusion of a right posterior circumflex humeral artery aneurysm (**c**, *arrow*), with embolic occlusion of the radial and ulnar arteries in the hand (**d**, *arrows*). Operative exploration demonstrated a branch vessel aneurysm (**e**, *white arrow*), which was ligated and excised. The operative specimen revealed thrombus within the occluded aneurysmal lesion (**f**) (Adapted from Duwayri et al. [7]. With permission from Elsevier)

Table 79.2 Medical management of digital ischemia

Environmental measures
    Eliminate tobacco exposure; avoid cold exposure; limit arm activity

Anticoagulation
    Intravenous heparin (Dose adjusted to PTT > 2.5 normal)
        Subcutaneous heparin (e.g., lovenox 1 ug/kg sc BID)
        Warfarin (Dose adjusted to INR >2.0)

Antiplatelet agents
    Aspirin (325 mg po QD); clopidogrel (75 mg po BID)

Vasodilators
    Calcium channel blockers (e.g., nifedipine 10 mg po QID)
        ACE inhibitors (e.g., enalapril 5–10 mg po QD)
        Angiotensin receptor blockers (e.g., losartan 25–50 mg po QD)
        Nitrates (e.g., Topical nitropaste, sublingual TNG prn; isordil 5–10 mg po QD-BID)
        Phosphodiesterase-5 inhibitors (e.g., viagra 25 mg po QD)
        Pentoxiphylline (e.g., trental 400 mg po TID)

Interventions
    Intra-arterial thrombolytic infusions (e.g., TPA)
    Intra-arterial vasodilator infusions (e.g., papaverine, PGE)
        Cervical sympathetic (Stellate ganglion) blocks

Abbreviations: *ACE* angiotensin converting enzyme, *INR* international normalized ratio, *PGE* prostaglandin E, *PTT* partial thromboplastin time, *TNG* trinitroglycerine, *TPA* tissue plasminogen activator

it is particularly effective when performed as an independent operation using minimally invasive video-assisted thoracoscopic surgery (VATS) approaches [9]. The general outcomes of treatment for patients with digital ischemia and vasospasm are difficult to estimate, since they are largely dependent on the specific cause, extent, and duration of thrombosis, in addition to the specific forms of treatment used.

Intraoperative Administration of Thrombolytic and Vasodilator Agents

For patients with arterial TOS and pronounced digital ischemia that have undergone surgical treatment for the embolic source, intraoperative infusion of vasodilator agents, such as prostaglandin E (PGE) may be an effective means to improve arterial supply to the hand and digits. This approach may also be effective when performed as an independent procedure during follow-up. Initially introduced in our institution by Dr. Juan Parodi, we perform these procedures with intra-arterial access under general anesthesia, due to a substantial amount of pain that can accompany pharmacological vasodilatation in ischemic tissues.

Percutaneous access to the femoral artery is obtained with a small-caliber angiographic sheath and a guidewire is passed into the aorta under fluoroscopic guidance. An arch arteriogram is performed to guide selective placement of the catheter into the distal brachial artery, and high-resolution arteriographic images are obtained of the hand and digits. Intraoperative arterial infusion is performed with approximately 500 mL of saline containing PGE (1 μg/mL). Arterial pressure is closely monitored through the femoral artery sheath and the infusion rate is adjusted to maintain mean blood pressure above 60 mmHg. During PGE infusion there will be obvious vasodilatation in the skin of the forearm and hand, usually with a sharp demarcation just distal to the site of the infusion catheter. Vasodilator infusion is typically followed by intraarterial infusion of a thrombolytic agent, such as 2 mL saline containing 1 mg/mL tissue plasminogen activator (TPA). Following this, infusion of the vasodilator PGE and the thrombolytic agent TPA are alternated over a period of approximately 45 min, to achieve a total of 500 μg PGE and 4–6 mg TPA. Repeat arteriography is performed at the end of the procedure to demonstrate if there is improved perfusion of the hand and digital arteries, but occlusive lesions of the digital vessels are typically unchanged. Nonetheless, most patients exhibit a marked improvement, with the hand and fingers appeared warm, pink and well-perfused, with brisk capillary refill. Intra-arterial infusion of vasodilator and thrombolytic agents may be repeated several times over a period of 1–2 months, in an effort to obtain maximal and long-lasting improvement.

References

1. Criado E, Berguer R, Greenfield L. The spectrum of arterial compression at the thoracic outlet. J Vasc Surg. 2010;52:406–11.
2. Durham JR, Yao JS, Pearce WH, Nuber GM, McCarthy Jr W. Arterial injuries in the thoracic outlet syndrome. J Vasc Surg. 1995;21:57–69.
3. Herrick AL. Contemporary management of Raynaud's phenomenon and digital ischaemic complications. Curr Opin Rheumatol. 2011;23(6):555–61.
4. Nichols AW. Diagnosis and management of thoracic outlet syndrome. Curr Sports Med Rep. 2009;8(5): 240–9.
5. Thompson RW, Driskill MR. Neurovascular problems in the athlete's shoulder. Clin Sports Med. 2008;27: 789–802.
6. Thompson RW, Petrinec D, Toursarkissian B. Surgical treatment of thoracic outlet compression syndromes. II. Supraclavicular exploration and vascular reconstruction. Ann Vasc Surg. 1997;11(4):442–51.
7. Duwayri YM, Emery VB, Driskill MR, Earley JA, Wright RW, Paletta GAJ, Thompson RW. Axillary artery compression causing upper extremity thrombosis and embolism in the elite overhead throwing athlete: spectrum of pathology and outcomes of treatment. J Vasc Surg. 2011;53:1329–40.
8. Sanders RJ, Hammond SL. Management of cervical ribs and anomalous first ribs causing neurogenic thoracic outlet syndrome. J Vasc Surg. 2002;36(1):51–6.
9. Coveliers HM, Hoexum F, Nederhoed JH, Wisselink W, Rauwerda JA. Thoracic sympathectomy for digital ischemia: a summary of evidence. J Vasc Surg. 2011;54(1): 273–7.

ATOS in the Competitive Athlete

80

Gregory J. Pearl

Abstract

Arterial complications of thoracic outlet syndrome are secondary to repetitive compressive trauma to the subclavian artery. ATOS is typically associated with anomalous bony structures such as a cervical rib, anomalous first rib, or callous and angulation of the clavicle due to previous fracture. Fibrocartilaginous bands may also cause arterial compression. Arterial manifestations that develop secondary to post traumatic subclavian arterial pathology in the athlete are also most commonly seen in those competitive individuals possessing underlying bony abnormalities in the outlet. However, awareness and recognition of potential arterial abnormalities other than the subclavian artery is paramount in the thorough evaluation and appropriate treatment of arterial manifestations in the high performance athlete.

Introduction

Arterial complications of thoracic outlet syndrome are secondary to repetitive compressive trauma to the subclavian artery. ATOS is typically associated with anomalous bony structures such as a cervical rib, anomalous first rib, or callous and angulation of the clavicle due to previous fracture. Fibrocartilaginous bands may also cause arterial compression. Arterial manifestations that develop secondary to post traumatic subclavian arterial pathology in the athlete are also most commonly seen in those competitive individuals possessing underlying bony abnormalities in the outlet. However, awareness and recognition of potential arterial abnormalities other than the subclavian artery is paramount in the thorough evaluation and appropriate treatment of arterial manifestations in the high performance athlete.

Signs and Symptoms

Although arterial TOS is the least common type of thoracic outlet syndrome, the ischemic complications caused by the arterial thrombosis or thromboembolization pose the potentially most serious sequelae for the athlete. The most common manifestation of ATOS is hand or digital

G.J. Pearl, MD
Department of Vascular Surgery,
Baylor University Medical Center,
621 N. Hall Street, Suite 100, Dallas,
TX 75226, USA
e-mail: gregp@baylorhealth.edu

K.A. Illig et al. (eds.), *Thoracic Outlet Syndrome*,
DOI 10.1007/978-1-4471-4366-6_80, © Springer-Verlag London 2013

Fig. 80.1 Cross sectional
duplex image of subclavian
artery aneurysm with
endoluminal loosely attached
mural thrombus

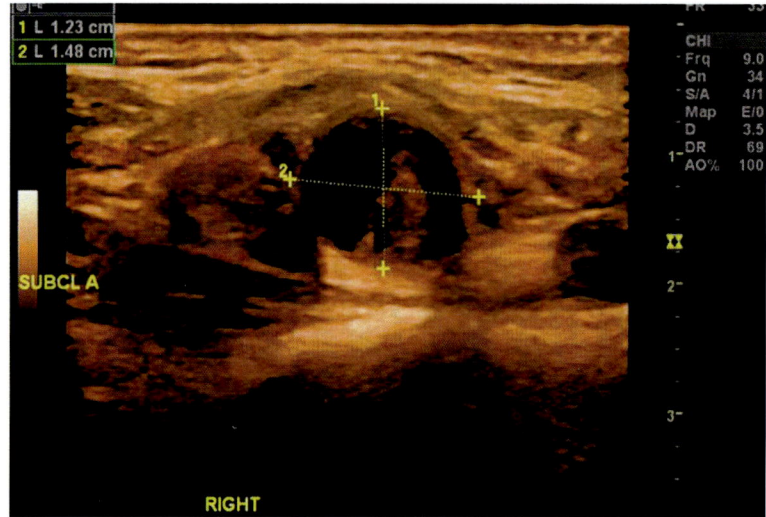

ischemia secondary to thromboembolization
from endoluminal damage or aneurysmal change
in the subclavian artery [1]. This presentation
may be quite obvious with ischemic skin changes
such as digital ulceration, or may be more subtle
such as the development of ipsilateral Raynaud's
syndrome or complaints of arm "claudication".
The high performance athlete, especially baseball
pitchers, may complain of coolness, color
changes, or digital or hand pain that is exacerbated with throwing, especially if playing in cool
weather. The development of painful and sensitive "calluses" on their throwing hand, which
actually represents ischemic digital ulceration, is
a common finding. One professional baseball
pitcher complained to the author that his fingertips
felt as though they had been "sanded with
sandpaper".

Clinical findings on exam may include a palpable pulsatile supraclavicular mass, palpable
cervical rib, and/or evidence of micro-embolization
to the hand and digits (manifest as tender skin
ulceration at the tips of the fingers or splinter
hemorrhages). Examination may reveal diminished or absent ipsilateral upper extremity pulses
in the resting position with thrombotic occlusion
of the axillary or subclavian artery, or pulses may
be readily palpable in the extremity in the setting
of micro-embolization. As in most TOS patients,
provocative maneuvers to demonstrate arterial
compression are non-specific and probably

superfluous, particularly if an arterial complication has already occurred. Duplex ultrasound
may be performed in the office and is useful in
interrogating the subclavian and axillary arteries
to evaluate for aneurysmal change, endoluminal
irregularities or thrombosis (Fig. 80.1). The brachial, radial, and ulnar arteries and palmar arch
may also be surveyed with duplex ultrasound for
thromboemboli or occlusion in the assessment of
the upper extremity runoff vessels [2] (Fig. 80.2).
Digital plethysmography is useful in demonstrating diminished digital perfusion seen with micro-
embolization. CT angiography may be performed
and is very accurate in demonstrating exact area
of arterial compression, arterial occlusion or
aneurysmal formation, but catheter based angiography may still be required to best define and
delineate the occlusive pattern in the hand
(Fig. 80.3). Arteriography may also be required
to identify an occult aneurysm of the posterior
circumflex humeral or subscapular arteries.

In contrast to the "non-athlete" presenting
with upper extremity ischemia, differential diagnosis of the source of these symptoms in the
competitive athlete includes several unusual entities and relates primarily to localization of the
arterial region responsible for the thrombo-em-
boli. (Table 80.1) As mentioned previously,
source lesions may be located in the subclavian
artery at the thoracic outlet, at the axillary artery
in the sub-pectoral space or at the level of the

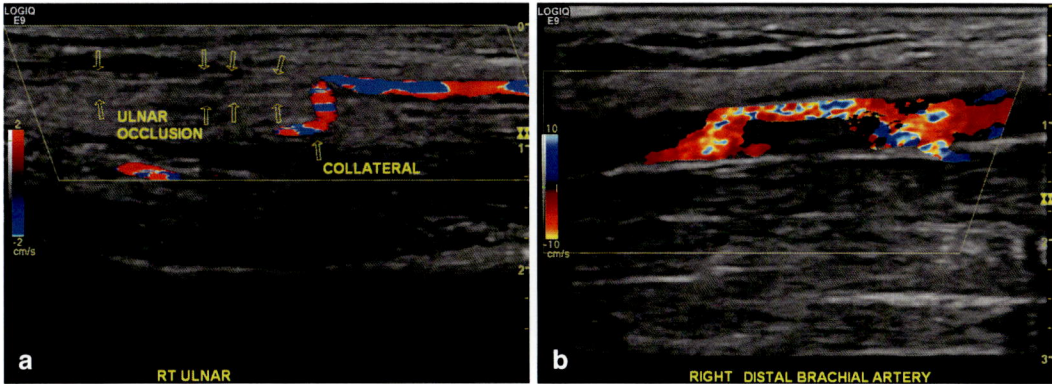

Fig. 80.2 (**a**) Long axis duplex image demonstrating complete occlusion of distal ulnar artery with collateralization. (**b**) Long axis duplex image of brachial artery with nonocclusive organized thrombus

humeral head, or in the posterior circumflex humeral artery aneurysm in the quadrilateral space. In baseball catchers, no proximal source lesion may be present and hand ischemia in this group may simply be secondary to occlusion from direct repetitive trauma to the palmar and digital branches in the hand itself.

Treatment

There is no role for conservative therapy in ATOS, especially in the competitive athlete whose goal is not only resolution of their symptoms, but, just as importantly, to get back to full athletic activities at a high level of performance (i.e., often return to work). The tenets of surgical treatment include relief of the arterial compression, correction of the source of thromboembolization, and restoration of digital perfusion. The requisite procedure will depend on the site of the arterial source of the lesion and associated compression, the severity of the attendant arterial damage, and the extent and location of the distal thromboembolization.

In the athlete with ATOS, decompression of the subclavian artery involves, at the very least, a thorough anterior and middle scalenectomy. In the presence of obvious bony abnormalities, all areas of demonstrable compression should be addressed. These would include resection of cervical or anomalous first ribs and/or division and excision of any fibrocartilaginous bands in

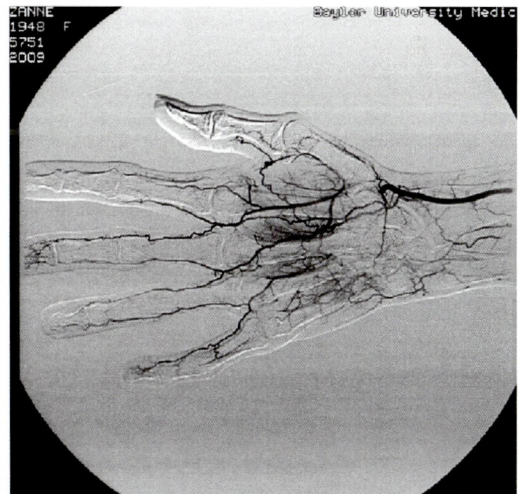

Fig. 80.3 Mag view of right hand from selective upper extremity arteriogram revealing radial and ulnar artery occlusions, occluded palmar arch, and multiple digital arterial occlusions

addition to scalenectomy. In the athlete with ATOS, our practice is to routinely perform first rib resection in the absence of obvious bony or fibrocartilaginous abnormalities, as we do not feel that scalenectomy alone offers adequate decompression of the outlet in these very active individuals. Leaving the first rib intact serves as a potential point for adhesions of the neurovascular structures and consequent persistence or recurrence of symptoms. Resection of the first rib also facilitates operative exposure for any necessary arterial reconstruction performed at the time of the decompression.

Our preference for decompression of the outlet is a supraclavicular or para-clavicular approach [3]. We feel that this approach offers the best exposure for thorough decompression as well as for concomitant arterial reconstruction. If a subclavian aneurysm is identified as the proximal source of thromboembolization to the extremity, aneurysm resection and reconstruction with interpositioning grafting should be performed. Lesser degrees of subclavian arterial injury with non-aneurysmal changes may be repaired with thrombo endarterectomy and patch angioplasty. Minimal arterial changes with no demonstrable residual thrombosis or evidence of intimal disruption may be treated conservatively in certain select cases with the expectation for remodeling and healing of the arterial changes following decompression. Distal revascularization may be accomplished with arterial thrombolysis

Table 80.1 Differential diagnosis of ATOS in athletes

Subclavian artery aneurysm
Subclavian artery endoluminal injury with thrombus
Axillary artery thrombosis
Axillary branch artery aneurysm
Posterior circumflex humeral artery
Anterior circumflex humeral artery
Subscapular artery
Traumatic palmar and digital artery occlusion

prior to the open decompression or with open thromboembolectomy performed concomitantly with the outlet decompression through an antecubital trans-brachial approach.

Repetitive compressive injury to arteries outside the thoracic outlet also occurs in the competitive athlete [4]. Awareness and recognition of these sites as potential sites of thromboemboli is paramount, particularly in the absence of apparent subclavian arterial pathology. The humeral head, pectoralis minor muscle, and other muscle groups around the shoulder are hytrophied in the throwing athlete. These overdeveloped structures cause compression, and, when combined with traction and rotational forces placed on the arteries around the shoulder with the repetitive motion of throwing, intimal injury with thrombosis or embolization or medial and adventitial disruption and consequent aneurysm formation can occur. Aneurysms of the posterior circumflex humeral artery and, less commonly, the anterior circumflex humeral artery and subscapular arteries leading to embolization and hand ischemia are well recognized. (Fig. 80.4) Thrombus develops within these aneurysms and is extruded and propelled into the axillary artery and embolizes into the distal circulation. Subluxation of the humeral head that occurs with forceful throwing motion may cause repetitive trauma and compression to the axillary artery leading to thrombosis, as described

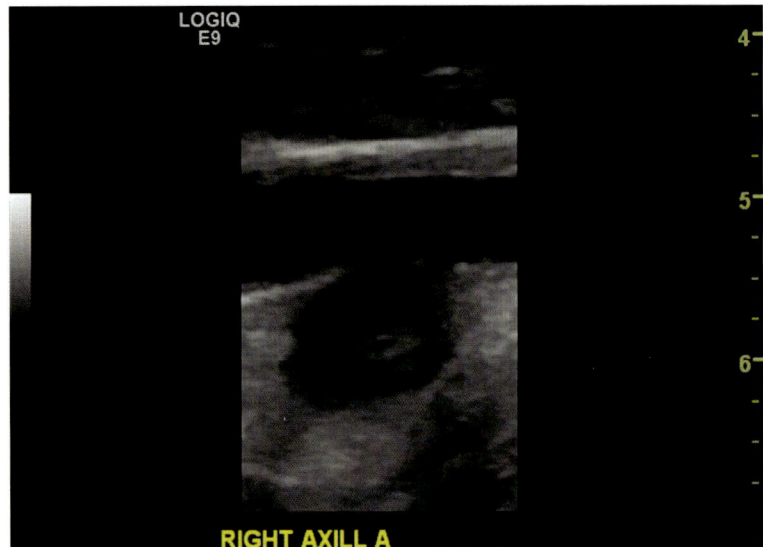

Fig. 80.4 Duplex image of posterior circumflex humeral artery aneurysm with mural thrombus in professional baseball pitcher who presented with subacute digital ischemia

by Rohrer and colleagues [5]. Treatment for these arterial injuries depends on location and extent of injuries and may include circumflex humeral aneurysm ligation or coiling or resection and interposition grafting of the axillary artery [6]. Decompression of the subpectoral space may be required with pectoralis minor tenotomy in certain select cases.

Summary

Diagnosis and treatment of ATOS in the competitive athlete poses specific circumstances not typically encountered in the general population. In addition to recognition of injury to the subclavian artery, recognition that other potential sites of arterial injury outside of the thoracic outlet may serve as a source of distal thromboembolization is necessary. Injury at these other arterial sites is exceedingly rare in the absence of strenuous repetitive activity with the arm, but is well recognized in the competitive athlete for this reason. The expectations of the high performance athlete typically far exceed those of the general TOS population. As a group, they expect not just correction and resolution of their ischemic symptoms but also anticipate a return to full athletic

activity at a high level in a relatively short period of time (and may depend on this activity for income). With proper diagnosis and treatment, including the help of experienced trainers or sports medicine specialists for supervision of the rehabilitation program, the expectations of this generally young, healthy, highly motivated group of individuals may be readily met.

References

1. Cormier JM, Amrane M, Ward A, et al. Arterial complications of the thoracic outlet: fifty-five operative cases. J Vasc Surg. 1989;9:778–87.
2. Ouriel K. Noninvasive diagnosis of upper extremity vascular disease. Semin Vasc Surg. 1998;11:54–9.
3. Thompson RW, Petrinec D, Toursarkissian B. Surgical treatment of thoracic outlet syndrome II, supraclavicular exploration and vascular reconstruction. Ann Vasc Surg. 1997;11:442–51.
4. Durham JR, Yao JS, Pearce WH, Nuber GM, McCarthy WJ. Arterial injuries in the thoracic outlet syndrome. J Vasc Surg. 1995;21:57–69.
5. Rohrer MF, Cardallo PA, Pappas AM, Phillips DA, Wheeler HB. Axillary artery compression and thrombosis in throwing athlete. J Vasc Surg. 1990;11:761–8.
6. Arko FR, Harris JE, Zarins CK, Olcott IV C. Vascular complications in high performance athletes. J Vasc Surg. 2001;33:935–42.

Congenital Abnormalities, Cervical Ribs, and Related Bony Abnormalities

81

Carlos A. Selmonosky and Poblete Raul Silva

Abstract

The presence of bony abnormalities in the thoracic outlet, most commonly abnormalities of the transverse process of the seventh cervical vertebra, cervical ribs, and abnormalities of the first thoracic ribs, are often responsible for vascular and neurological complications in patients with a diagnosis of thoracic outlet syndrome (TOS). The diagnosis of TOS should be considered if one or more of these bony abnormalities are found in a patient complaining of paresthesias and or pain anywhere in the upper extremities, neck and/or shoulder pain, or noncoronary chest pain. Early diagnosis can prevent vascular and neurological complications.

Introduction

Congenital bony abnormalities, while not common, are not infrequently seen on radiographic examination of asymptomatic persons, and are especially common in patients with arterial thoracic outlet syndrome (ATOS). These abnormalities are, in order of incidence (Table 81.1):

1. Anomalies of the transverse process of the seventh cervical vertebra,
2. Cervical ribs, and
3. Anomalies of the first rib.

C.A. Selmonosky, MD (✉)
Department of Medicine, Inova Fairfax Hospital,
3784 B Madison Lane, Falls Church, VA 22041, USA
e-mail: renee.sinkez@inova.org

P.R. Silva, MD
Equipo de Cirugia Vascular, Depto Cirugia,
Hospital Militar de Santiago,
Av. Larrain 9100, Santiago 6680481, Chile
e-mail: raulps@vtr.net

These should all be fairly easy to recognize with minimal practice in plain chest and cervical spine radiographs (Fig. 81.1) and the radiologist should report these anomalies with a full description, if present. While such abnormalities can certainly exist in patients without demonstrable problems, their presence in a patient complaining of paresthesias and/or pain in the upper extremity, pain in the neck or shoulder, or noncoronary chest pain should strongly suggest that TOS is the cause of these symptoms

Evaluation and Management

The physical examination in a patient with potential TOS should include inspection of the supraclavicular area for bony firmness, a pulsatile mass, and/or a bruit. Rarely, a supraclavicular fullness or mass is present (Fig. 81.2), which if fixed, bony, solid and sometimes tender may represent a cervical or abnormal rib. Such abnormalities are more common in females.

Table 81.1 Bony abnormalities in TOS

Congenital and acquired anomalies responsible for neurovascular compression at the thoracic outlet

Bones	Description
Abnormal transverse process of the seventh cervical vertebra	Elongated, enlarged, deformed
	Origin of a band attached to the first rib (Ross II)
Cervical rib	Complete, incomplete
	Fused with a pseudo-arthro-sis to the first rib
	Origin of a band inserting in the first rib (Ross I)
Abnormal first rib	Hypoplastic, abnormal shape and position
	Joint with first rib with a psudo-arthrosis
	Fracture, tumors (rare)
Clavicle	Abnormal shape and length, fractures, tumors

Other anatomical structures

Congenital or acquired abnormalities of the scalenus and subclavius muscles, brachial plexus, subclavian artery and vein, vertebral artery

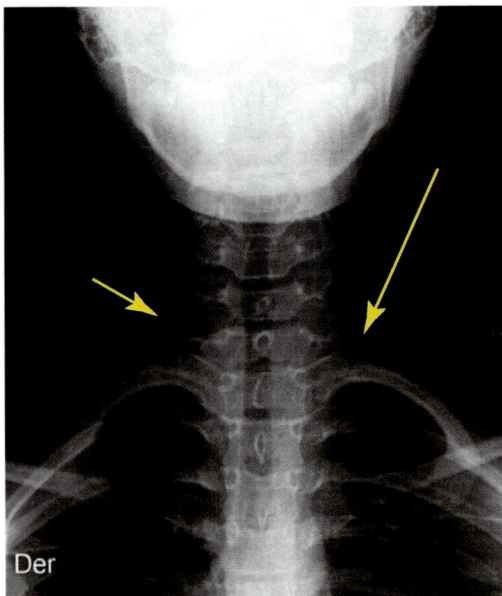

Fig. 81.1 Chest radiograph showing an abnormal transverse process of the seventh cervical vertebra on the right (*short arrow*) and short cervical rib with articulation with the spine on the left (*long arrow*)

Proper diagnosis requires radiological studies, including computerized tomographic (CT) examination if plain films are not diagnostic. Occasionally a fracture with excessive callus [1] or malunion of the clavicle [2] can compress the neurovascular bundle and present in a similar fashion.

The presence of such a bony abnormality is not in and of itself an indication for surgery [3], as most are asymptomatic. Reported prevalences vary according to the population studied, the methods used to perform the study, the definition of a "bony abnormality," and the degree to which such problems are looked for, factors that together account for the wide variability in reported rates. In patients undergoing thoracic outlet decompression, such findings are obviously common, and are most common in patients with arterial TOS (ATOS). Makhoul [4] found an incidence of 8.5 % of cervical and abnormal first ribs in 200 patients undergoing thoracic outlet decompression. Bilbey [5] found that a bony abnormality was present in 18 of 27 patients (81.5 %) with a diagnosis of TOS, while only two of 21 asymptomatic subjects (9.5 %) undergoing similar radiological examinations had a similar abnormality. Redembach [6] found bony abnormalities in 46 % of 250 cadaver dissections; and in 72 patients with surgically treated TOS the same authors found bony abnormalities in 83 % of their patients. By contrast, such bony abnormalities are only present in 0.5–2.94 % [7, 8] of the general population when radiographs performed for other reasons are examined. If these bony abnormalities are not present in patients with a clinical diagnosis of TOS, a CT of the cervical spine will frequently show abnormalities of the transverse process of the seventh cervical vertebra not seen in plain radiographs.

The embryologic basis for and interdependence of the various anomalies occurring in the thoracic outlet are discussed in Chaps. 2 and 13 and are further reviewed in Keating [9] and While [10]. Cervical ribs and abnormal C7 transverse processes have a familial inheritance pattern [11–13]. Interestingly, cervical ribs are associated with sacralization of the lumbar spine [14], and a high prevalence of cervical ribs has been found in children with cancer [15].

Fig. 81.2 Supraclavicular mass (*arrows*) in a patient with a bony abnormality

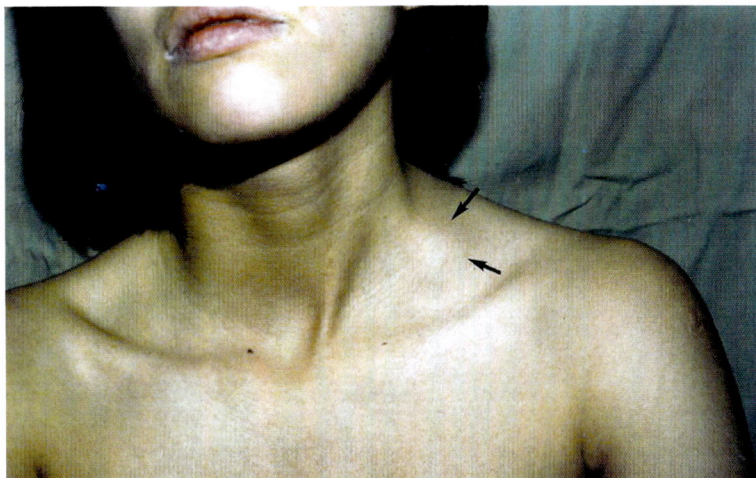

Anomalies of the Transverse Process of the Seventh Cervical Vertebra

Common anomalies of the C7 transverse process include elongation, enlargement, and deformity, the latter with a shape of a beaking tip pointing downward (Fig. 81.3, which also illustrates the difference between a prominent C7 transverse process(left side) and a true cervical rib (right side)). What exactly constitutes an abnormal C7 transverse process is not clear and has been the subject of several reports. Dominguez [16] studied 3,228 chest and spine radiographs in 6,456 thoracic outlet areas and found that the normal C7 transverse process measures 28 mm in females and 29.5 mm in males. Brantigan and Roos [17] define the C7 transverse process as abnormal if it extends beyond a line connecting the tips of C6 and T1. Hare [18] found wide variation in length and shape, with processes ranging from 5 mm short of to 8 mm beyond this line. In agreement with Gillatt [19], Hare stated that the shape appears to be a better guide to define an abnormal C7 transverse process, with an apophysomegaly and/or a sharp tip pointing downward being abnormal. Hare also found that pathologic C7 transverse processes were frequently present on the asymptomatic contralateral side.

The incidence of an abnormal C7 transverse process in radiologic studies in the general population is varied. Brewin [8] found an incidence of 2.2 % in a London population, Pioner [20], 1.84 % in a general population, and Palma [21], 4.98 % in an isolated Italian village where other

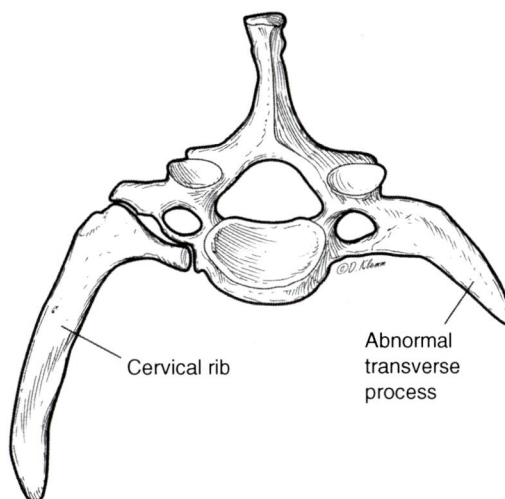

Fig. 81.3 Diagram of an abnormal transverse process (*patient's left side*) and cervical rib (*patient's right*). (Courtesy of Dave Klemm, Georgetown University School of Medicine.)

factors may have influence the incidence. By contrast, Redenbach [6] found 24 abnormal transverse processes in 500 thoracic outlet dissections in 250 cadaver specimens yielding an incidence of 9.1 %, although "abnormal" was simply defined as a C7 transverse process longer than that of T1.

Patients with TOS in general (and probably even more so with ATOS) are thought to have a higher incidence of bony abnormalities, cervical ribs being best studied. Bilbey [5] found that 66 % of patients with a diagnosis of TOS but no obvious bony abnormalities had an abnormally elongated C7 transverse process when evaluated by CT.

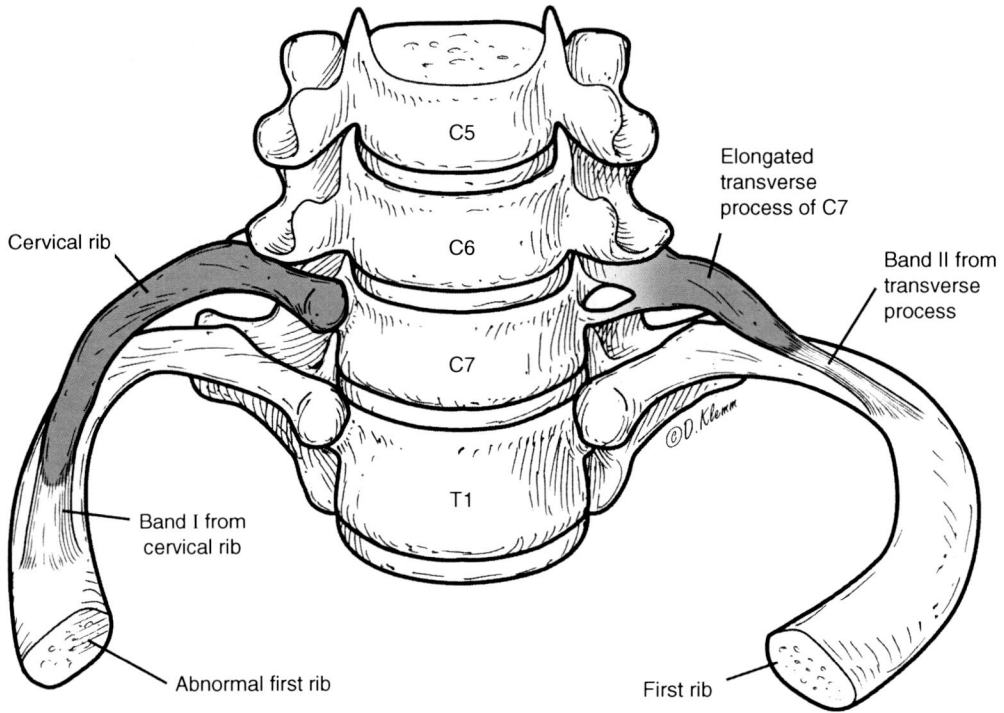

Fig. 81.4 Diagram of an abnormal seventh cervical vertebral process on the left with a Roos Type 2 band, and cervical rib on the right with a Roos Type 1 band. Note the abnormal right first rib with tight, "J-shaped" curve (Courtesy of Dave Klemm, Georgetown University School of Medicine.)

Table 81.2 Roos' classification of congenital fibromuscular bands at the thoracic outlet: roos's bands

Type	Origin	Insertion
1	Tip of incomplete cervical rib	First rib
2	Tip of abnormal transverse process of seventh cervical vertebra	First rib
3	Fibromuscular band neck of first rib	Behind scalene tubercle of the first rib
4	Large middle scalenus muscle transverse process 1–5 cervical vertebra	Anterior to the scalenus tubercle of the first rib
5	Scalenus minimum muscle transverse process 6–7 cervical vertebra	Posteriorly in the first rib
6	Scalenus minimum muscle transverse process 6–7 cervical vertebra	Sibson fascia covering the cupola
7	Long fibromuscular band from the lower part of the middle scalenus muscle	Anterior part of the first rib or sternum
8	Fibromuscular band arising from the anterior scalene muscle	Costal cartilage of the first rib and subclavian muscle
9	Sharp-edged fribro-muscular band	Along the posterior inner surface of the first rib
10	A double fibrous band forms over the cupola of the lung	Posterior limb to middle third of the first rib
	Posterior limb arises from the cervical rib or neck of the first rib	Anterior limb to the sternum or costal cartilage of the first rib

Based on data from Brantigan and Roos [17]

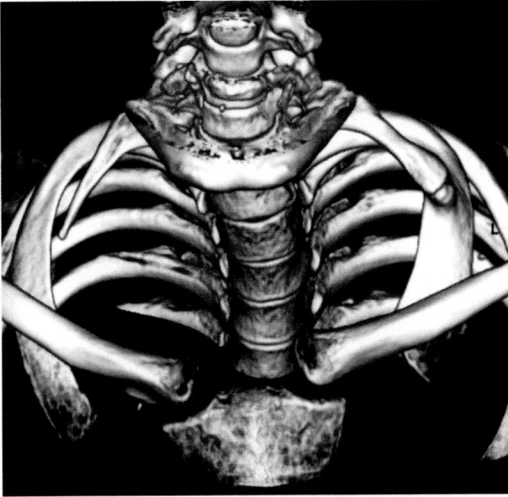

Fig. 81.5 CT reconstruction showing an incomplete cervical rib in the right and fusion of the left cervical rib with the first rib

As described in the next section, most cervical ribs are not calcified all the way to their insertion onto the first rib and the connecting fibrous band is the source of symptoms. Similarly, a fibrous band (classified by Roos [22] as a Type 2 band) arising from the tip of the C7 transverse process alone (i.e., without a cervical rib being present) and inserting into the first rib can be the cause of compression of the brachial plexus (Fig. 81.4). These fibromuscular bands insert in the bony structures and insert in the first rib and other anatomical components of the thoracic outlet (see Table 81.2 for a full description of Roos' classification).

Cervical Ribs

A cervical rib can be *complete*, defined as a bony insertion into the sternum or first rib, or *incomplete*, ending free in the soft tissues or being connected to the first rib by a fibrous band (Fig. 81.5). If bilateral, they are often of different lengths. Short ribs (less than 5 cm) usually have a fibrous band arising from their tips which attaching to the first rib, classified by Roos [22] as a Type 1 band.

As illustrated in Figs. 81.3 and 81.4 the term "cervical rib" should be only used when a true costovertebral joint is present at the body and the

transverse process of the seventh cervical vertebra. Abnormal transverse processes are fused with the body of the vertebra.

Some cervical ribs are fused with the first rib by means of a pseudoarthrosis (Fig. 81.5) that produces compression of the neurovascular bundle and, often, the subclavian artery [23].

A long cervical rib, more than 5 cm in length, is frequently associated with vascular TOS (although neurological compression commonly occurs) [3, 4, 24], while shorter cervical ribs are more commonly responsible for neurological symptoms. Cervical ribs are bilateral in 50–80 % of cases, and are associated with significant symptoms 10–20 % of the time when they are present [3, 7].

The incidence of cervical ribs in the general population varies because of the different geographic areas and methods used to arrive to the diagnosis. Using review of radiographic studies in general populations, Atasoy [7] found an incidence of 0.5–0.6 %, Brewin [8], 0.74 %, Thompson [25], 0.45–1.5 %, and Sanders [3], 1 %. In a special Anatolian population Gulekon [26] found an incidence of 3 %, again suggesting that other factors were present.

As discussed above, cervical ribs are more commonly seen in patients with ATOS. Sanders reported this to be 4.5 % in his experience [3].

Anomalies of the First Thoracic Ribs

A normal first rib originates from the first thoracic vertebra with two synovial joints, one to the body of the vertebra and another to the transverse process of the first thoracic vertebra. An abnormal first rib is hypoplastic, thinner, and may be completely articulated with the sternum or be incomplete with different lengths bilaterally. It is usually positioned slightly higher than a normal first rib and may have a more vertical "J" shape in contrast with the normal first rib which circumscribes a 180° angle (Figs. 81.4 and 81.6) [24, 27–29]. While an abnormal first rib can articulate with the sternum, more frequently it is fused with the second rib or the tip ends in the soft tissues. While sometimes subtle, such a rib should be diagnosed

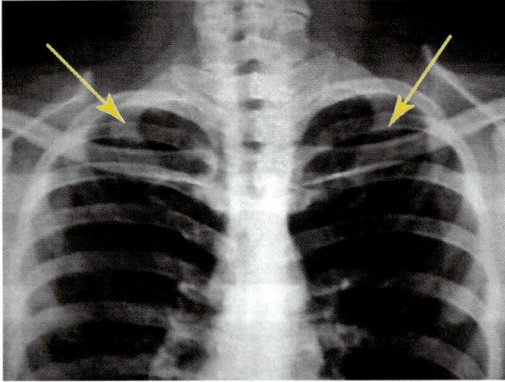

Fig. 81.6 Chest radiograph showing abnormal first ribs bilaterally (*arrows*)

with plain chest and cervical spine radiographs (Fig. 81.6). Sanders believes that the shape of the first rib on radiological studies of the chest usually predicts whether it will require surgical resection for NTOS and, although uncontrolled, his results are good using this algorithm [3]. The incidence of anomalies of the first thoracic rib range from 0.21 to 0.34 % [27, 30], and the incidence of bilaterally is similar to that of cervical ribs.

Vascular symptoms and complications of predominantly arterial TOS are common in patients with abnormalities of the first rib [3, 29–31]. Patients with symptoms suggesting ATOS as the predominant complaint were found by Cormier [24] to be associated with bony abnormalities in 70–100 % of cases, and Criado [31] found bony abnormalities in 66 % of patients operated on because of complications of predominantly arterial TOS.

Finally, abnormal first thoracic ribs are often fused with the second rib by a large exostosis or pseudoarthrosis that may compress the subclavian artery [29, 32]. Rib excision is indicated if vascular signs and symptoms are present; if not, close followup should be initiated because of the high probability of vascular complications in the future.

Fractures

Acquired isolated first rib fractures may also produce compression of the neurovascular bundle at the thoracic outlet. Nonunion [33] and/or an exuberant callus will compress the neurovascular structures, preferentially the subclavian artery

with subsequent severe subclavian artery complications. If any history of first rib (or, more commonly, clavicular) fracture is present in a patient with any form of TOS, this should be considered the cause of the problem until proved otherwise.

Summary

In summary, while the presence of a bony abnormality significantly increases the chances of ATOS being present, most patients with such an abnormality do not have symptoms. Although widely varying definitions make accurate assessment of prevalence very difficult, it is probably fair to say that major abnormalities are present in 1–2 % of the general population, 10–50 % of patients with TOS, and 66–100 % (perhaps) of patients with ATOS. By contrast, only 10–20 % of patients with such an abnormality will develop TOS.

References

1. England JO. AAEM case report 33: costoclavicular mass syndrome. American Association of Electrodiagnostic Medicine. Muscle Nerve. 1999;22(3):412–8.
2. Yoo MJ, Seo JB, Toong B, Kim PK, Lee JH. Surgical treatment of thoracic outlet syndrome secondary to clavicular malunion. Clin Orthod Surg. 2009;1(1):54–7.
3. Sanders RJ, Hammond SI. Management of cervical ribs and anomalous first ribs causing neurogenic thoracic outlet syndrome. J Vasc Surg. 2002;36(1):51–6.
4. Makhoul RG, Machleder HI. Developmental anomalies at the thoracic outlet. An analysis of 200 consecutive cases. J Vasc Surg. 1992;16:534–45.
5. Bilbey JG, Muller NL, Connell DG, Luoma AA, Nelems B. Thoracic outlet syndrome: evaluation with CT. Radiology. 1989;171(2):381–4.
6. Redembach DM, Nelems B. A comparative study of structures comprising the thoracic outlet in 250 human cadavers and 72 cases of thoracic outlet syndrome. Eur J Cardiothorac Surg. 1998;13:353–60.
7. Atasory E. Thoracic outlet syndrome anatomy. Hand Clin. 2004;2:7–14.
8. Brewin J, Hill M, Ellis H. The prevalence of cervical ribs in a London population. Clin Anat. 2009;22:331–6.
9. Keating DR, Amberg JR. A source of potential error in the roentgen diagnosis of cervical ribs. Radiology. 1954;62(5):688–94.
10. While JC, Popell MH, Adams R. Congenital malformations of the first thoracic rib: a cause of brachial

neuralgia which simulates the cervical rib syndrome. S Gyn-Obstet. 1945;81:643.

11. Boles JM, Missoum A, Mocquard Y, Goas HY, Bellet M. Familial anomaly of the seventh cervical vertebra. Radio-clinic comparison in a fourteen member family. J Radiol. 1982;63(4):273–7.

12. Shapera J. Autosomal dominant inheritance of cervical ribs. Clin Genet. 1987;31(6):386–8.

13. Weston WJ. Genetically determined cervical ribs – a family study. Br J Radiol. 1956;29:455–6.

14. Erken E, Ozer HT, Gulek B, Durgun B. The association between cervical rib and sacralization. Spine. 2002;27(15):1659–64.

15. Merks JH, Smets AM, Van Rijn RR, Kobes J, Caron HN, Maas M, Hennekam RC. Prevalence of rib anomalies in normal Caucasian children and childhood cancer patients. Eru J Med Genet. 2005;48(2):113–29. E-pub 2005 Feb 12.

16. Dominguez LE, Hernandez JL, Santa Cruz LMH. Radiological measurement of the transverse process of the seventh cervical vertebra. Acta Med GP. 2004;2(4):235–42.

17. Brantigan CO, Roos DB. Etiology of neurogenic thoracic outlet syndrome. Hand Clin. 2004;20: 17–22.

18. Hare WS, Rogers WJ. The scalenus medius band and the seventh cervical transverse process. Diagn Imaging. 1981;50(5):263–8.

19. Gilliatt RW, Le Quesn PM, Logue V, Sumner AJ. Wasting of the hand associated with a cervical rib or band. J Neurol Neurosurg Psychiatry. 1970;33: 615–24.

20. Pionnier I, Depraz H. Congenital abnormalities, statistical studies of 10000 radiographs. Radiol Clin. 1956;25:170–86.

21. Palma A, Cerini F. Variation of the transverse apophysis of the 7th cervical vertebra: anatomic radiological study of an isolated population. Arch Ital Anat Embriol. 1990;95(1):11–6.

22. Roos DB. Congenital anomalies associated with thoracic outlet syndrome. Am J Surg. 1976;132(6):771–8.

23. Edwards PR, Moody AP, Harris PL. First rib abnormalities in association with cervical ribs: a cause for postoperative failure in the thoracic outlet syndrome. Eur J Vasc Surg. 1992;6(6):677–81.

24. Cormier JM, Amrane M, Ward A. Arterial complications of the thoracic outlet syndrome. Fifty five operative cases. J Vasc Surg. 1989;9:787–9.

25. Thompson RW, Driskill M. Thoracic outlet syndrome: neurogenic. In: Cronenwett JL, Johnston KW, editors. Rutherford's vascular surgery. 7th ed. Philadelphia: Saunders/Elsevier; 2010. p. 1878–98.

26. Gulekon IN, Barut C, Turgut HB. The prevalence of cervical ribs in an Anatolian population. Gizi Med J. 1999;10:149–52.

27. Siderys H, Walker D, Pittman JN. Anomalous first rib as a cause of the thoracic outlet syndrome. JAMA. 1967;199(2):133–4.

28. Hasimoto H, Nikaido Y, Kurokawa S, Myamoto K, Sakeki T. Thoracic outlet syndrome due to first rib anomaly: a case report. No Shrinkel Geku. 1994; 22(11):1063–6.

29. Baumgartner F, Nelson RJ, Robertson JM. The rudimentary first rib. A cause of thoracic outlet syndrome with arterial compression. Arch Surg. 1989;124(9):1090–2.

30. Sanders RS, Haug CI. Thoracic outlet syndrome: a common sequela of neck injuries. Philadelphia: Lippincott Williams & Wilkins; 1991.

31. Criado E, Bergner R, Greenfield L. The spectrum of arterial compression at the thoracic outlet. J Vasc Surg. 2010;52(2):406–11.

32. DiFiore JW, Reid JR, Drummond-Webb J. Thoracic outlet syndrome in a child – transaxillary resection of anomalous first rib. J Pediat Surg. 2002;37(8): 1220–2.

33. Wiesler ER, Chloro GD, Xu NM, Li Z. A rare cause of thoracic outlet syndrome. Arch Orth Trauma Surg. 2008;128(1):33–5.

ATOS in the Pediatric Age Group

82

Linda M. Harris and Purandath Lall

Abstract

ATOS in children is frequently associated with anatomic abnormalities. It may present in a variety of ways, similar to those seen in adults, and should be considered in young patients presenting with either upper extremity or cerebral ischemic symptoms. Surgical intervention should be strongly considered in this young population due to the frequent presence of anatomic abnormalities and the excellent response typically seen in these patients.

Thoracic Outlet syndrome most commonly affects adults in the 30–50 year age range. Arterial TOS is the least common subtype in this population, occurring in less than 1 % of patients by some reports [1]. Many large series of TOS include children, but without further comment or analysis. In adults, NTOS is the most common variant. In children, however, vascular TOS – including both arterial and venous subtypes – appears to be much more common than in adults. Patients in a recent study of vascular TOS (22 arterial, seven venous, and one combined) were, on the average, 26.1 years of age, much younger than the typical NTOS series [2]. Arterial TOS

may present in a variety of ways, including ischemic symptoms from embolization (either prograde or retrograde), development of an aneurysm, or arterial impingement with upper extremity claudication type symptoms with use.

Blank and Connar published a series describing complications of TOS in 1974, and identified a 12 year old boy with occlusion of the subclavian artery at the level of an anomalous first rib [3]. In 2000, Okereke described subclavian dilatation in a 16 year old girl with upper extremity ischemic symptoms which resolved after resection of a cervical rib and fibrous band [4]. The first report of an arterial aneurysm secondary to TOS in a child was probably published by Reid in 2002 [5]. They found a dilated subclavian artery in a 6 year old boy, who presented with a pulsatile neck mass. He demonstrated pulse obliteration with abduction, and was found to have pseudarthrosis between the first and second ribs. He underwent transaxillary first rib resection, with division of the anterior scalene and resection of fibrous bands with 6 month postoperative

L.M. Harris, MD (✉)
Department of Surgery, Kaleida Health,
3 Gates Circle, Buffalo, NY 14209, USA
e-mail: lharris@kaledahealth.org

P. Lall, MD
Department of Surgery, VA WNY Health Care System,
3495 Bailey Avenue, Buffalo, NY 14215, USA
e-mail: purandath.lall@va.gov

K.A. Illig et al. (eds.), *Thoracic Outlet Syndrome*,
DOI 10.1007/978-1-4471-4366-6_82, © Springer-Verlag London 2013

MRA demonstrating improvement in the stenosis and a decrease in the poststenotic dilatation of the subclavian artery. A subsequent case report was published by Sen in 2007 who described an 8 year old boy with subclavian artery poststenotic dilitation and a cervical rib articulated to the first rib on the left, who responded well to surgery without further complications [6].

Despite its rarity, several larger series of ATOS in children do exist. Vercellio presented the first true series on pediatric TOS syndromes in 2003 [7]. In his review, 26 % of all patients operated at his institution during the time period were nonadult, ranging in age from 8 to 16 years old, with four boys and four girls (and in the subsequent 6 months three additional children presented with TOS who were not included in this series). He classified the lesions as venous in 75 % and neurogenic in 25 %, but found associated arterial symptoms in three patients (one venous and two neurogenic patients). All patients had symptomatic improvement at a follow-up of 18 months, with one developing recurrent venous thrombosis and symptoms. This was the first study to identify the higher prevalence of vascular TOS in children.

The second reported series, by L.G. Arthur, described outcomes in 25 children ranging in age from 12 to 18 [8]. Forty-four percent of these patients had VTOS and 8 % ATOS, yielding a 52 % rate of vascular TOS, and the authors concluded that vascular complications were more common in children than adults. Both cases of arterial TOS were seen in females, and were characterized by upper extremity claudication. Neither patient with arterial TOS developed embolization or aneurysm in this series.

Due to the paucity of good data on TOS in children, we reviewed our experience with 12 pediatric TOS patients, finding that 38 % of operated patients less than 20 years of age had ATOS, 38 % neurogenic, and 24 % venous [9]. Our youngest symptomatic patient was 8 years old. Most patients with ATOS were identified fairly rapidly, with a mean diagnostic time of 2.2 months after onset of symptoms, while mean time to diagnosis for VTOS was 7.6 months and NTOS 34 months. Delay in surgery greater than 6 months

from diagnosis correlated with increased time to resolution of symptoms irrespective of TOS type. Two patients required brachial embolectomy for upper extremity ischemia prior to their TOS surgery, and a third required repair of a subclavian aneurysm with bypass at the time of the rib resection. All patients with arterial TOS underwent evaluation for other sources of embolization and were found to be negative. Postoperative improvement or resolution of symptoms occurred in 100 % of the early onset patients. Rigberg and Gelabert, however, found no cases of ATOS in a series of 18 children (33 % had VTOS) [10].

Embolization with ischemia is clearly the worst outcome from arterial TOS. Several reports highlight the presence of this disorder in children. Edwards described a 20 year old cross country college athlete who presented with embolization to the brachial artery requiring cervical rib resection [11]. In our series two children required embolectomy of the affected arm [9], and one 19 year old male was described by Monica who developed upper extremity ischemia and was found to have occlusion of the brachial and radial arteries secondary to embolus from a stenotic subclavian artery. He had suffered several episodes of traumatic shoulder dislocation at the age of 12 [12]. Ozcakar described a patient with delayed limb growth due to intermittent compression of the subclavian artery in a 17 year old girl [13]. She was found to have a smaller and paler left hand and MRA confirmed subclavian compromise with hypertrophied left middle and posterior scalene muscles. She was, however, treated non-operatively with physical therapy and apparently improved without surgical intervention.

In addition to arm ischemia, ATOS can cause cerebral symptoms due to retrograde embolization of the vertebral on either side or right carotid (overall, cerebral ischemia is more commonly reported on the right side, likely due to the proximity of the common carotid origin to the affected subclavian artery). Gooneratne described a 21 year old male who presented with stroke after a history of right arm pain for 1 month [14]. He was found by MRI to have bilateral pontine infarcts, a right cervical rib with stenosis of the subclavian artery 1 cm distal to the right vertebral artery, poststenotic dilation of the subclavian artery with occlusion of the distal axillary artery, and basilar artery occlusion secondary to embolus. All other workup for embolic source and for hypercoagulable states was negative. Yamaguchi also described a case of acute basilar artery occlusion in a 22 year old with left subclavian artery occlusion due to ATOS [15]. The patient initially presented with unilateral Raynaud's syndrome, and was found to have compression on the artery from an "elevated" first rib. He presented with a cerebellar infarct, and underwent resection of the affected first rib. Prior published a small series of five patients, including a 21 year old woman with bilateral cervical ribs who developed multiple transient ischemic attacks which did not resolve until her cervical rib and associated fibrous band were resected [16]. Blank and Connar described an 18 year old woman with bilateral cervical ribs, upper extremity ischemia, and a brainstem infarct (who refused surgery) [3] and Matsen a 19 year old female who 6 months following an MVA was found to have an ischemic upper extremity with occlusion of the brachial artery and negative thrombophilia workup [17]. She subsequently developed headache, dizziness, right sided facial numbness, difficulty swallowing, and ataxia, dysarthria, and right eye ptosis, and MRI demonstrated a medullary stroke. She was found on angiography to have occlusion of the axillary and brachial arteries with aneurysmal degeneration of the subclavian artery and sluggish right vertebral flow with embolic occlusion. Lee described a teenage girl who developed a cerebral embolic stroke and arm ischemia from ATOS [18]. She had been diagnosed 3 months prior to the stroke with TOS, and then presented with simultaneous loss of pulses to the right extremity and left sided weakness of both the upper and lower extremities. Diagnostic studies included an MRI/A, which demonstrated occlusion of the R MCA with infarct, while DSA demonstrated occlusion of the right subclavian artery at the midclavicle with bilateral cervical ribs. Cardiac echocardiogram was negative, but she was found to be heterozygous for Factor V Leiden mutation. She underwent thrombectomy and resection of the cervical rib and bypass with GSV, as well as anticoagulation for the cerebral infarct, but was left with persistent left sided weakness at follow-up due to the stroke. Finally, Sharma described an 18 year old male who presented with a right basal ganglia infarct due to subclavian compression from a cervical rib with poststenotic arterial dilation and occlusion with abduction [19]. The patient had claudication symptoms in the upper extremity prior to the stroke, and apparently did well after subsequent cervical rib resection.

It is evident from the discussion above that most of what we know about ATOS in "children" is derived from individual case reports and very small series, almost certainly because of the rarity of this disorder. Like VTOS, however, it seems that younger patients have a higher incidence of ATOS in general. Two possible explanations exist. First is the possibility that NTOS is relatively rare before adulthood. This would not increase the prevalence of ATOS itself, but would lead to the perception (either in the literature or one's clinical practice) that vascular TOS in general is more common, as a greater number of young patients would exhibit such symptoms. Secondly, however, is related to etiology. ATOS tends to be associated with a defined anatomic abnormality (such as cervical or anomalous first ribs) and, as such, may be more likely to present before adulthood.

In summary, our knowledge of ATOS in children is incomplete, but available data suggest that it should be treated according to the same general principles used in adults. Children are frequently found to have anatomic abnormalities to account for their symptoms, such as cervical ribs or bands. Children with arterial TOS should strongly be considered for operative intervention to prevent ischemic complications from embolization, which can be devastating and lead to stroke as well as arm symptoms.

References

1. Sanders RJ, Hammond SL, Rao NM. Thoracic outlet syndrome a review. Neurologist. 2008;14(6):365–73.
2. Davidovic LB, Kostic DM, Jakovljevic NS, et al. Vascular thoracic outlet syndrome. World J Surg. 2003; 27:545–50.

3. Blank RH, Connar RG. Arterial complications associated with thoracic outlet compression syndrome. Ann Thorac Surg. 1974;17(4):315–24.
4. Okereke CD, Mavor A, Naim M. Arterial thoracic outlet compression syndrome: a differential diagnosis of painful right supraclavicular swelling? Hosp Med. 2000;61(9):672–3.
5. Reid JR, Morrison ST, DiFiore JW. Thoracic outlet syndrome with subclavian aneurysm in a very young child: the complementary value of MRA and 3D-CT in diagnosis. Pediatr Radiol. 2002;32:22–4.
6. Sen S, Discigli B, Boga M, et al. Thoracic outlet syndrome with right subclavian artery dilatation in a child – transaxillary resection of the pediatric cervical rib. Thorac Cardiovasc Surg. 2007;55:339–41.
7. Vercellio G, Baraldini V, Gatti C, et al. Thoracic outlet syndrome in paediatrics: clinical presentation, surgical treatment, and outcome in a series of eight children. J Pediatric Surg. 2003;38(1):58–61.
8. Arthur LG, Teich S, Hogan M, et al. Pediatric thoracic outlet syndrome: a disorder with serious vascular complications. J Pediatric Surg. 2008;43:1089–94.
9. Maru S, Dosluoglu H, Dryjski M, Cherr G, Curl GR, Harris L. Thoracic outlet syndrome in children and young adults. Eur J Vasc Endovasc Surg. 2009;38:560–4.
10. Rigberg DA, Gelabert H. The management of thoracic outlet syndrome in teenaged patients. Ann Vasc Surg. 2009;23:335–40.
11. Edwards NM, Casey R, Johnson R. Extensive arterial embolus in the arm of a college runner with thoracic outlet syndrome: a case report. Clin J Sport Med. 2009;19(4):331–2.
12. Monica JT, Kwolek CJ, Jupiter JB. Thoracic outlet syndrome with subclavian artery thrombosis undetectable by magnetic resonance angiography. J Bone Joint Surg Am. 2007;89:1589–93.
13. Ozcakar L, Malas FU, Erol O. A 17-year-old girl with a small left hand: thoracic outlet syndrome is on the agenda. Clin Pediatric. 2008;47(1):80–2.
14. Gooneratne IK, Gamage R, Gunarathne KS. Pearls & oy-sters: distal subclavian artery – a source of cerebral embolism. Neurology. 2009;73(July 14):e11–12.
15. Yamaguchi R, Kohga H, Kurosaki M, et al. Acute basilar artery occlusion in a patient with left subclavian artery occlusion due to first rib anomaly – a case report. Neurol Med Chir (Tokyo). 2008;48:355–8.
16. Prior AL, Wilson LA, Gosling RG, et al. Retrograde cerebral embolism. Lancet. 1979;2(8151):1044–7.
17. Matsen SL, Messina LM, Laberge JM, et al. SIR 2003 film panel case 7: arterial thoracic outlet syndrome presenting with upper extremity emboli and posterior circulation stroke. J Vasc Interv Radiol. 2003;14:807–12.
18. Lee TS, Hines GL. Cerebral embolic stroke and arm ischemia in a teenager with arterial thoracic outlet syndrome: a case report. Vasc Endovasc Surg. 2007;41(3):254–7.
19. Sharma S, Kumar S, Joseph L, et al. Cervical rib with stroke as the initial presentation. Neurol India. 2010;58(4):645–7.

Differential Diagnosis, Decision-Making, and Pathways of Care for ATOS

83

William H. Pearce

Abstract

The diagnosis of arterial thoracic outlet syndrome (ATOS) is made when the patient's *primary* symptoms are arterial in nature even though the patient may also have neurogenic or venous symptoms. The neurovascular bundle in the thoracic outlet is compressed when the arm and shoulder are placed in certain positions in many patients without symptoms. In some, however, repeated injury may occur and produce arterial wall injury leading to endothelial ulceration, clot formation, post-stenotic aneurysmal dilatation, digital embolization, forearm vessel occlusion, and/or proximal arterial occlusion. This process is often silent and progressive. Subclavian-axillary artery lesions may be produced by either abnormal bony structures or normal structures that become abnormal with certain arm positioning.

Introduction

The diagnosis of arterial thoracic outlet syndrome (ATOS) is made when the patient's *primary* symptoms are arterial in nature even though the patient may also have neurogenic or venous symptoms. The neurovascular bundle in the thoracic outlet is compressed when the arm and shoulder are placed in certain positions in many patients without symptoms. In some, however, repeated injury may occur and produce arterial wall injury leading to endothelial ulceration, clot formation, post-stenotic aneurysmal dilatation, digital embolization, forearm vessel occlusion, and/or proximal arterial occlusion. This process is often silent and progressive. Subclavian-axillary artery lesions may be produced by either abnormal bony structures or normal structures that become abnormal with certain arm positioning. This chapter will review the differential diagnosis, clinical decision making, and clinical pathways in patients who present with arterial lesions in the thoracic outlet.

Differential Diagnosis

The differential diagnosis of upper extremity ischemia is large. Table 83.1 describes the many lesions that may affect the upper extremity.

W.H. Pearce, MD
Department of Surgery, Division of Vascular Surgery,
Feinberg School of Medicine, Northwestern University,
676 North St. Clair Suite 650, Chicago, IL 60611, USA
e-mail: wpearce@nmh.org

K.A. Illig et al. (eds.), *Thoracic Outlet Syndrome*,
DOI 10.1007/978-1-4471-4366-6_83, © Springer-Verlag London 2013

Table 83.1 Differential diagnosis

Non atherosclerotic vascular disease
SLE, CREST, scleroderma
Buerger's aisease
Fibromuscular aysplagia (FMD)
Vasculitis
Giant cell
Takayasu
Uremic arteriopathy
Diabetes mellitus
Atherosclerosis
Stenosis/occlusion
Atheroembolism
Degenerative aneurysms
Hematologic process
Hypercoagulopathies
Cryofibrinogenemia
Leukofibrinogenemia
Trauma
Occupational
Orthogenic
Iatrogenic/penetrating
Arterial thoracic outlet
Cryptogenic

In general, the disease processes can be categorized based upon the arteries affected. Small digital vessel occlusions may be caused by emboli from a proximal source or by Berguer's disease, connective tissue disease, or uremic arteriopathy. When the disease process is located in the subclavian-axillary arteries the problem is most commonly Takayasu's arteritis, atherosclerosis, giant cell arteritis, or ATOS. Atherosclerosis is most commonly seen at the origin of the great vessel (proximal subclavian and/or innominate arteries). Both Takayasu's disease and giant cell arteritis also affect the subclavian and axillary arteries, but in these situations the disease processes tend to be more diffuse and can present with tubular stenosis, occlusion, and/or multiple vessel involvement.

Subclavian-axillary artery disease is readily demonstrated by standard contrast arteriography or CT or MR arteriography. The clinical presentation of patients with ATOS is similar to that of other patients with upper extremity ischemia. The majority of patients present with silent ischemia, splinter hemorrhages, digital ischemia,

and/or arm symptoms related to exercise induced muscle ischemia [1–4]. Patients with ATOS may have coexisting neurogenic symptoms, depending on the patient's particular anatomy, as the artery and nerves both run through the scalene triangle. By definition, however, the dominant symptoms are arterial in nature in patients with the diagnosis of ATOS. In other words, while many patients with NTOS have hypoperfusion inducible by stress maneuvers, *a patient with true arterial damage leading to local or distal symptoms* has ATOS.

The key to diagnosing ATOS is to exclude the other diseases that affect the subclavian-axillary arteries and to look for either abnormal bony structures or normal structures which are compressing the subclavian-axillary arteries or branches. Virtually every patient with ATOS has a bony abnormality or a defined, objective, acquired structural problem. These patients are generally healthy, very active, and present in their second to fourth decades. There appears to be no difference in the gender distribution in patients with bony ATOS in general, although there is a male predominance in high-performance throwing athletes in whom normal structures become pathologic [5–8].

Clinical Decision Making

The first step in the evaluation of patients with upper extremity ischemia is to determine whether or not another underlying disease process is present. After history and physical examination, most such problems can be ruled out rapidly by noting normal levels of inflammatory serum markers such as C-reactive peptide (CRP) levels or erythrocyte sedimentation rates and absence of atherosclerotic risk factors (most notably, young age). If no evidence of other problems exist, suspicion for ATOS is high and the structures that are producing the arterial lesion should be sought out and the degree of distal embolization assessed. It is stressed again that in virtually all cases either an abnormal bony structure is present, the patient has developed hypertrophied muscles, or the patient (often a throwing athlete) has put the arm

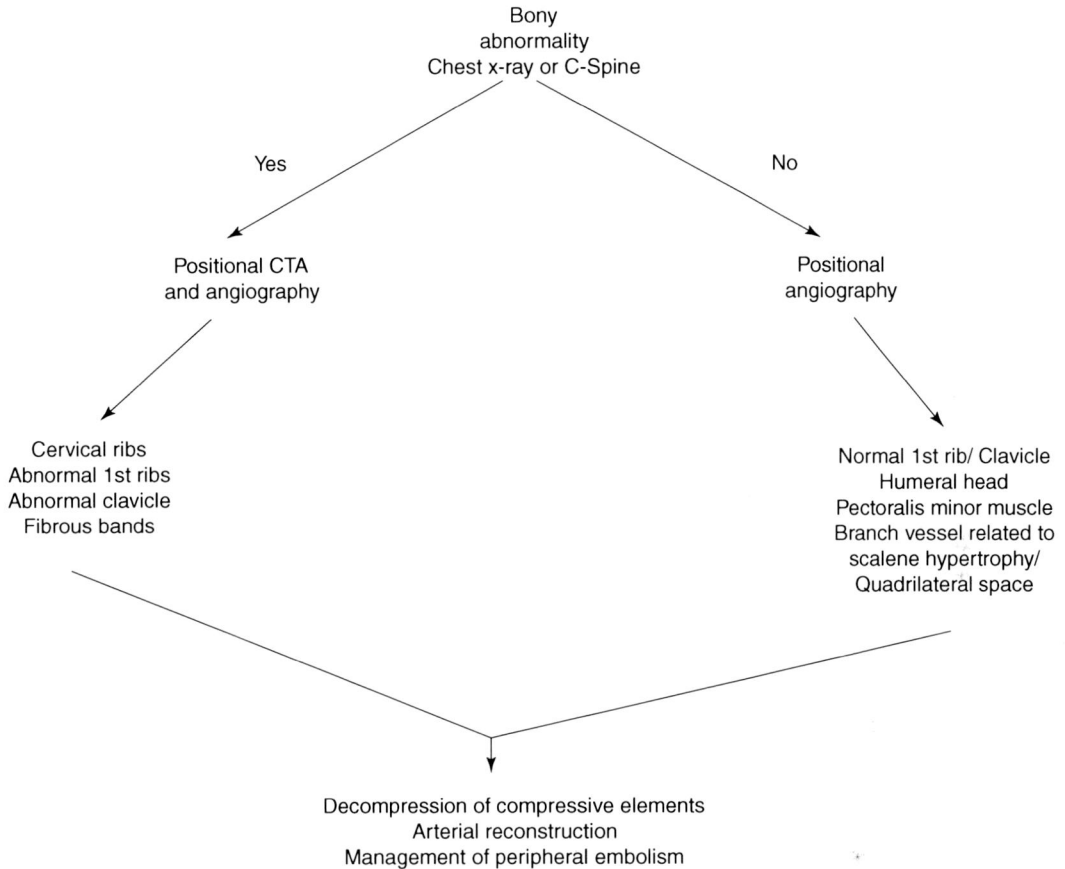

Fig. 83.1 Clinical decisions/clinical pathways

in such extreme positioning that normal structures have become the damaging element (Fig. 83.1). An arterial lesion acting as an embolic source may be located in a branch vessel or in the main axial artery itself. Emboli have been shown to have arisen from the thyrocervical trunk, the third portion of the subclavian artery at the costoclavicular space, the artery at the pectoralis minus muscle and the quadrilateral space, and at the third portion of the axillary artery at the humeral head [9–16].

Defined abnormal "bony" structures that commonly produce subclavian-axillary artery lesions include true cervical ribs, fibrous bands arising from cervical ribs (and abnormal C7 transverse processes and the first rib itself, at times), and clavicular fractures with malunion and callus formations. In high-performance athletes normal structures can become pathologic, including the

costoclavicular junction, anterior scalene muscle, quadrilateral space, and the humeral head.

To understand these relationships and the specific anatomy with enough detail to plan treatment, it is important to use imaging that defines the anatomy *at rest and with positioning*. Plain radiographs, CT and MR imaging, and, of course, contrast arteriography are all useful to determine the bony structures that are producing the impingement (see Chap. 54). CTA is particularly useful, since both the artery and bones are depicted in relationship to one another [17]. The shoulder joint changes remarkably as the arm is moved from the side to an elevated position, and all imaging should be performed with the arm by the side and in an abducted, externally rotated position. A disadvantage of CTA is the lack of clear definition of forearm and digital vessels and the inability to put the arm in full abduction and external rotation (as a pitcher would during the pitching motion). Standard contrast arteriography can provide detailed information regarding the forearm and digital vessels – correction of the problem at the thoracic outlet must be combined with treatment of whatever distal embolization has occurred.

In patients in whom there are normal bony structures, however, CTA is not particularly useful. In these patients the intent is to find branch vessel occlusions or aneurysms, external compression by normal structures such as the humeral head or the first rib, and to define the runoff vessels, and catheter-directed selective arteriography is the best test. Branch vessel occlusions are often subtle and require careful evaluation of muscular vessels. The thyrocervical trunk, the axillary artery beneath the humeral head, and the posterior circumflex artery should all be carefully examined [11–15]. As discussed above it is also invaluable have the patient assist the radiologist by putting the arm in the extreme positioning that occurs during pitching motions. These patients have highly flexible joints and are able to place their shoulders in positions that are uncommon in the normal patient population.

Clinical Pathways

Surgical treatment for ATOS must address three things: the patient's compressive elements, the underlying proximal arterial lesion, and the degree of peripheral embolization.

In most instances the compressive elements are addressed first. These may be cervical ribs, fibrous bands, clavicular fractures [18, 19], or hypertrophied muscles. At operation, it is extremely important to include the arm in the operative field to allow mobility of the shoulder joint for intraoperative evaluation of the bony thoracic outlet. The thoracic outlet can be assessed by placing a finger between the clavicle and first rib and placing the shoulder in different positions. Most patients with ATOS will have a cervical rib. These are best resected via a supraclavicular approach after the artery has been mobilized, and these patients will often have an elongated

subclavian artery (an infraclavicular incision is sometimes needed for full exposure) (see Chap. 85). Reconstruction of the artery is essential if any abnormality exists. In patients in whom the pathology is a clavicular fracture that has healed with a large callus formation, a decision needs to be made regarding whether resection of the clavicle is needed (see Chap. 64) or whether simply trimming the callus thus providing a large space for the arterial reconstruction to pass is adequate. It is absolutely essential to place the reconstructed artery in a space that is not to be harmed by residual calluses, fibrous bands, or bony structures; restenosis is likely to occur unless these structures are removed.

In patients in whom there is hypertrophy of normal muscular structures, the treatment has traditionally been to resect the muscle and to ligate the branch vessel that has become abnormal. Such patients can have hypertrophied scalene muscles with thyrocervical artery enlargement and thrombosis, pectoralis minor syndrome (compression of the axillary artery by this muscle), and/or quadrilateral space syndrome (compression of the axillary nerve and posterior humeral circumflex artery by the teres major and minor and triceps muscles and humerus). It is not possible to enlarge this latter space, but simply ligating the posterior circumflex artery is usually adequate (freeing the axillary nerve in this space has also been described [13, 20]).

One of the more problematic lesions of the distal portion of the axillary artery is compression and injury by the humeral head in high-performance, often throwing athletes (see Chap. 80). Humeral head compression produces an endovascular fibrosis not dissimilar to fibromuscular disease, and lesions in this space are difficult to treat because this fibrosis surrounds the neurovascular bundle and is associated with significant inflammation. Once the artery is freed a variety of techniques have been employed to treat this lesion. Some surgeons prefer bypass from the proximal subclavian to the distal axillary artery, while others recommend patch angioplasty. Series are small and there is no definitive information regarding the most appropriate treatment of these patients.

Conclusions

Arterial TOS is uncommon and treatment is challenging. An accurate and appropriate diagnosis is critical, as there are several disease processes that affect the subclavian-axillary vessels. Interestingly, the majority of these are associated with an underlying vasculitis, have high recurrence rates if not treated appropriately, and occur in similar demographic groups to those with ATOS. It is important to recognize that both abnormal and normal structures may produce arterial lesions in the thoracic outlet. While abnormal structures are readily identified with CTA, patients with no bony abnormalities often have normal structures that have become pathologic. In these instances arteriography is essential. Once the culprit lesion has been identified, the clinical decision must be made as to what structures need to be resected and the method in which arterial reconstruction should be performed. It must remembered that many of these patients are young and very active, and in many instances their livelihood depends upon supranormal functioning of the upper extremity.

References

1. Cormier JM, Amrane M, Ward A, et al. Arterial complications of the thoracic outlet syndrome: fifty-five operative cases. J Vasc Surg. 1989;89:778–87.
2. Scher LA, Veith FJ, Samson RH, et al. Vascular complications of thoracic outlet syndrome. J Vasc Surg. 1986;3:565–8.
3. Short DW. The subclavian artery in 16 patients with complete cervical ribs. J Cardiovasc Surg. 1975;16:135–41.
4. Eden KC. The vascular complications of cervical ribs and first thoracic rib abnormalities. Br J Surg. 1939;27:111–39.
5. Durham JR, Yao JS, Pearce WH, et al. Arterial injuries in the thoracic outlet syndrome. J Vasc Surg. 1995;21:57–69.
6. Rohrer JM, Cardullo PA, Pappas AM, et al. Axillary artery compression and thrombosis in throwing athletes. J Vasc Surg. 1990;11:761–9.
7. Schneider K, Kasparyan NG, Atlchek DW, et al. An aneurysm involving the axillary artery and its branch vessels in a major league baseball pitcher; a case report and review of the literature. Am J Sports Med. 1999;27:370–5.
8. Dugas JR, Weiland AQJ. Vascular pathology in the throwing athlete. Hand Clin. 2000;16:477–85.
9. Tullos NS, Irwin WD, Woods AW, et al. Unusual lesions of the pitching arm. Clin Orthop. 1972;88: 169–89.
10. Finkelstein JA, Johnston KW. Thrombosis of the axillary artery secondary to compression by the pectoralis minor muscle. Ann Vasc Surg. 1993;7:287–90.
11. McCarthy WJ, Yao JST, Schafer MF, et al. Upper extremity arterial injury in athletes. J Vasc Surg. 1989;9:317–27.
12. Reekers JA, den Hartog BM, Kuyper CF, et al. Traumatic aneurysm of the posterior circumflex humeral artery: a volleyball player's disease? J Vasc Interv Radiol. 1993;4:405–8.
13. Hoskins WT, Pollard HP, McDonald AJ. Quadrilateral space syndrome: a case study and review of the literature. Br J Sports Med. 2005;39:39.
14. Vlychou M, Spanomichos G, Chatziiannou A, et al. Embolization of a traumatic aneurysm of the posterior circumflex humeral artery in a volleyball player. Br J Sports Med. 2001;35:136–7.
15. Dijkstra PF, Westra D. Angiographic features of compression of the axillary artery by the musculus pectoralis minor and the head of the humerus in the thoracic outlet compression syndrome. Radiologia Clin. 1978;47:423–7.
16. Nijhuis HHAM, Müller-Wiefel HM. Occlusion of the brachial artery by thrombus dislodged from a traumatic aneurysm of the anterior humeral circumflex artery. J Vasc Surg. 1991;13:408–11.
17. Matsumura JS, Rilling WS, Pearce WH, et al. Helical computed tomography of the normal thoracic outlet. J Vasc Surg. 1997;26:727–35.
18. Fujita K, Matsuda K, Sakai Y, et al. Late thoracic outlet syndrome secondary to malunion of the fractured clavicle: a case report and review of the literature. J Trauma. 2001;50:332–5.
19. Mandal AKJ, Jordaan J, Missouris CG. Fractured clavicle and vascular complications. Emerg Med J. 2004;21:646–50.
20. McAdams TR, Dillingham MF. Surgical decompression of the quadrilateral space in overhead athlete. Am J Sports Med. 2008;36:528–32.

ATOS is an uncommon but clinically challenging entity. This condition typically involves formation of an aneurysm of the subclavian artery related to the presence of a cervical rib. An alternative form is also described with positional compression of the axillary artery against the head of the humurus. Excellent diagnostic procedures are available for ATOS, with arteriography being the gold standard. These patients may first present with arterial thromboembolic complications which require urgent intervention. In Chap. 52, vascular surgeons with extensive experience in ATOS provide a framework for both catheter-based and surgical management of this condition.

Dr. Illig provides a detailed review the role of endovascular intervention in patients presenting with distal emboli in the upper extremity or occlusion of the axillary-subclavian artery. The techniques of chemical and mechanical arterial thrombolysis are described, and the role of endovascular stenting is discussed. Like many experienced TOS surgeons, Dr. Illig cautions against the routine use of arterial stents in this location.

Drs. Singh and Fanciullo outline the surgical approaches to the axillosubclavian including the supraclavicular, infraclavicular and combined approaches. They also discuss the deltopectoral approach if more distal exposure into the upper arm is required.

ATOS may occur from lesions of the axillary artery created by compression against the head of the humerus. This is most commonly seen in overhead athletes such as baseball players. Drs. Azizzadeh and Thompson discuss their approach to the diagnosis of positional compression of the axillary artery, as well as their technique for resection and arterial reconstruction.

Surgical Techniques: Thrombolysis and Endovascular Intervention for ATOS

84

Karl A. Illig

Abstract

Patients with arterial thoracic outlet syndrome (TOS) most commonly present with distal emboli, either to the brachial, radial or ulnar arteries, or to the palm and digital vessels (most common). While endovascular intervention can be of benefit, digital emboli are often resistant to thrombolysis and brachial artery emboli can be easily removed surgically under local anesthetic, so the role of thrombolysis in arterial TOS is limited. However, if a large, proximal vessel is acutely occluded (most common in the setting of a subclavian artery aneurysm or in recurrent arterial TOS), preliminary thrombolysis can reestablish flow and define the anatomy prior to surgical repair, which must include bony decompression of the thoracic outlet. Almost no data exist regarding the use of endovascular stents or stent-grafts in this location. Indeed, such a treatment approach is generally discouraged, and if contemplated, must be accompanied by thoracic outlet decompression and unusually close followup.

Introduction

Arterial TOS is relatively rare, accounting for less than 1 % of cases of TOS in most large collected series [1]. This condition usually presents with either episodic or chronic upper extremity arterial obstruction leading to arm claudication from subclavian artery occlusion or to acute ischemia from aneurysmal degeneration and distal embolization; very rarely, severe limb-threatening ischemia may occur after acute subclavian artery thrombosis. Conventional endovascular techniques can be considered in any patient with arterial TOS but are especially helpful in patients with an acutely occluded vessel. The majority of this chapter will thereby deal with treatment for occlusion of the axillary-subclavian artery (either as a primary problem or in recurrent arterial TOS), although other roles for endovascular intervention will also be discussed.

Diagnosis

Most patients presenting with severe ischemia will have a recognizable diagnosis of arterial TOS, as evidenced by a young, otherwise, healthy

K.A. Illig, MD
Department of Surgery, Division of Vascular Surgery,
University of South Florida, 2 Tampa General Circle,
STC 7016, Tampa, FL 33606, USA
e-mail: killig@health.usf.edu

patient with a cervical rib, a pulsatile mass in the neck, and a history of arm claudication or fingertip emboli; severe ischemia is also frequent in patients with recurrent arterial TOS, suggested by a history of previous surgical treatment for a cervical rib, so the diagnosis should be quite straightforward. The diagnosis of acute axillary or subclavian artery thrombosis should also be readily apparent, as such patients usually present with relatively acute arm ischemia. However, this is not always the case, as there is a rich supply of collateral vasculature around the base of the neck, shoulder and axilla, and the patient may be surprisingly symptom-free. As a result, the patient may present with non-urgent symptoms. Physical examination is obviously critical. A patient with severe hand pain, diminished sensation and discolored fingers in the presence of a palpable brachial and/or radial pulse has probably had discrete emboli to the hand, while a patient with severe forearm and hand pain, often with paralysis, may have had more proximal (brachial artery) macroembolism. There is usually an easily palpable pulsatile mass immediately above the clavicle, corresponding to a dilated subclavian artery displaced anteriorly by a cervical rib, which is typically nontender.

Duplex ultrasound examination is also potentially useful in this situation. In addition to helping localize the site of embolization and confirming obstruction, it is important to determine if the artery is aneurysmal just beyond the rib. If so, replacement or bypass will likely be needed, and thrombolysis may be a less favorable option. Ultrasound studies may also help document the extent to which the distal circulation is compromised (e.g., brachial-brachial-index, digital waveforms). Based on a high clinical suspicion and initial Duplex studies, it often appropriate to initiate anticoagulation treatment with intravenous heparin, to help limit progression of distal thrombus while further studies are conducted. Following this, the most important step in diagnosis depends on more detailed vascular imaging, obtained by contrast enhanced CT-, MR- or catheter-based arteriography.

It is an axiom of endovascular intervention for vascular thrombosis that success is most likely if intervention is performed within 14 days or so after thrombosis. This is usually not a problem if the patient presents acutely, but if the patient has minimal symptoms they may present with a relatively well-organized thrombus resistant to dissolution. Because mural thrombus may form over a long period of time and progressive accumulation of emboli to the forearm arteries may not cause symptoms until blood flow to the hand is severely compromised (giving rise to a clinical impression of acute symptoms), the actual duration of thrombus or emboli is often difficult to determine prior to attempts at thrombolysis. This may be one reason for failures in the use of thrombolytic treatment in this setting.

Finally, causes of upper extremity ischemia other than arterial TOS must be considered and the angiographic appearance can help. Proximal subclavian artery stenosis in an elderly patient is almost certainly due to atherosclerosis, while a young patient with a recent febrile illness could have either Takayasu's (proximal lesion) or giant cell (upper arm) arteritis. The diagnosis of true arterial TOS would be most likely in a young, healthy, perhaps athletic patient with no other significant risk factors or symptoms to suggest atherosclerosis or inflammatory arteritis, who presents with acute occlusion of the subclavian artery where it passes over the first rib. The suspicion of arterial TOS is raised to near-certainty if a cervical rib is also seen on radiography, particularly when there is a corresponding history of intermittent claudication in the arm.

Technique

Whatever the etiology, thrombolysis can be considered if suspicion is high for acute thrombosis of the axillary-subclavian artery in the region of the first rib. Intervention is straightforward and follows the principles of any vascular intervention. Access is usually most convenient via the femoral artery route, although it helps to have the ipsilateral arm prepped into the sterile field. The patient is anticoagulated with intravenous heparin, and a guiding catheter or angiographic sheath is placed and positioned selectively into the affected subclavian artery. In the young, healthy patients typically affected by arterial TOS, the risk of vertebral or right carotid artery embolization from thrombus at the tip of the angiographic sheath is probably more theoretical than actual, but should always be kept in mind during prolonged procedures.

Essentially all endovascular interventions are performed over a guidewire, and thus a wire must initially be passed across the lesion as a fundamental requirement for any intervention. If the thrombus is relatively fresh, a hydrophilic wire will generally pass quite easily. A combination of angled catheters and wires, in various sizes and stiffnesses, are often needed. Retrograde access from the brachial artery in the arm can also be attempted, if angulation of the anatomy and/or length of access is felt to hinder success from the femoral artery. If a subclavian artery aneurysm is present making "reentry" into the normal vessel beyond the occlusive lesion more difficult, entry from both ends of the vessel and snaring the wire to pull it through the lesion can also be performed.

Once successful passage of the guidewire has been achieved, dissolution or removal of clot is the next goal. There are two choices: rapid pharmacomechanical thrombolysis and relatively "slow" conventional thrombolysis via an infusion catheter. Often both techniques are used. Pharmacomechanical thrombolysis, as the name implies, refers to several different techniques that combine instillation of a clot-dissolving drug and use of a mechanical technique for clot removal. The Trellis device (Bacchus, Santa Clara, CA) physically breaks up clot by means of a rotating sinusoidal wire within an isolated segment of the artery that is controlled by balloons at either end and laced with tissue plasminogen activator (t-PA; Genentech, San Francisco, CA). Unfortunately, this technique is best suited for long, nonbranching tubes, and the subclavian artery is poorly-suited anatomically for this device. Another option is the Arrow-Trerotola PTD device (Arrow International, Reading, PA), which is essentially a small catheter-based "egg-beater" designed to macerate clot. Although the resulting microemboli are easily absorbed by the

lungs when this approach is used for venous thrombus, this device is probably not well-suited for arterial thrombus.

A third possibility is use of the Angiojet (Possis Medical, Minneapolis, MN) technique, usually using the "Power-Pulse" setting. "Power-Pulse" is a technique (hardware and software being part of the commercial package) whereby a t-PA/saline solution (usually 10 mg in 240 mL) is forcibly injected into the clot itself through multiple sideholes in the infusion catheter, and then allowed to sit and "mature" within the thrombus for 20 or 30 min. Following this, conventional Angiojet pharmacomechanical thrombolysis is performed (the Angiojet removes thrombus by aspiration, using a high velocity fluid jet which creates suction).

The pharmacomechanical approach to thrombolysis is highly successful if there is acute thrombus present, and it can usually be completed in a single session. Although distal microembolization can occur, such emboli are laced with t-PA and usually respond to an additional period of conventional t-PA infusion. Finally, if residual thrombus is present, consideration can be given to leaving the catheter in place overnight, for conventional thrombolytic treatment according to established protocols.

Once the artery is opened, the underlying problem causing the thrombosis must be identified and corrected, which almost always means surgical resection of the cervical and first rib. In the relatively uncommon event that the artery is completely normal following thrombolysis, thoracic outlet decompression with rib resection may be all that is required. If the artery appears only mildly dilated but is otherwise relatively normal following rib resection, further arterial reconstruction is probably not necessary. Conversely, if the subclavian artery is dilated to aneurysmal proportions (twice the diameter of the adjacent normal artery), especially if distal embolization has occurred or if there is surface ulceration and/or mural thrombus, the vessel should be resected and replaced. Intraoperative arteriography can be useful at this stage of the operation if the subclavian artery appears relatively normal in diameter, as it can detect surface ulceration or stenosis that might otherwise be overlooked. Another technique that may have application in this setting is the use of intravascular ultrasound (IVUS). For example, passage of an IVUS catheter across the subclavian artery may provide more detailed information about the presence of mural thrombus, wall thickening or surface ulceration, in which case the subclavian artery is repaired.

Although endovascular stents have been placed in the subclavian artery, this should be approached with a great deal of caution as the long-term results of this approach are completely unknown. Indeed, arterial TOS occurs in young active patients and there is considerable motion in the subclavian artery, particularly with arm elevation, so stent placement in this setting can be expected to have a substantial failure rate. Consequently, very few reports of arterial stenting in the thoracic outlet have been published.

Other Scenarios

Many patients with arterial TOS will present with isolated distal microembolization, without thrombus in a proximal major vessel. Preoperative thrombolysis in this situation is unlikely to yield benefit, for two reasons. First, with distal emboli it is not possible to provide true catheter-directed intra-thrombus delivery of the thrombolytic agent, due to the small size, multiple sites, and distal location of the emboli. The best that can be accomplished in this regard is "whole-limb" infusion proximally, and it is unclear how much active ingredient can actually reach the site(s) of occlusion. The second major problem is likely even more important: in this situation, the occluding material is likely to be chronic mural thrombus from the proximal source rather than acute thrombus as seen in the setting of acute occlusion, especially if a subclavian or axillary artery aneurysm is present. Acute digital emboli that occur during proximal intervention (being made up of fresh, t-PA-laced clot) may respond well to continued limb perfusion with TPA, but chronic digital emboli that occur in an isolated manner most likely will not.

It is often tempting to consider placement of a covered endovascular stent (or "stent-graft") across any arterial lesion. As described above, the long-term results of such an approach in arterial TOS are not known, and we stress that the cervical and/or first rib(s) must still be surgically resected for optimal management. Stent-graft placement might be appropriate in a rare patient with a well-defined subclavian artery aneurysm, particularly if the lesion is judged to be too difficult to resect or if the patient is considered to be at particularly high risk for surgical treatment. It is notable in considering this approach that flexible covered stents usually require large sheath sizes, and a brachial artery or combined brachial/femoral approach, perhaps with through-and-through wire control to improve trackability, may be required. It is also important to consider anatomical constraints, such as the necessity of preserving the vertebral artery or the inability to satisfactorily isolate large branch vessels (e.g., the internal thoracic or thyrocervical trunk), which may preclude the utility of stent-grafts for lesions in this location.

Results

There are essentially no clinical series and only isolated case reports dealing specifically with thrombolysis and stenting of the axillary-subclavian artery for arterial TOS. Hood and colleagues described six patients who presented with arm claudication (three) or acute ischemia (three); all of the latter had hand emboli and none had an occluded axillary-subclavian artery [2]. Two of the patients with forearm emboli improved with preoperative thrombolysis. All patients underwent thoracic outlet decompression, and two required further arterial intervention (one having subclavian aneurysm resection and one having endarterectomy). While all 17 patients with "vascular TOS" in their series did relatively well, the results of the arterial and venous groups were not separately described.

Thus, few data exist regarding arterial stenting or stent-graft placement in arterial TOS, although stents placed in the subclavian vein for venous TOS are recognized to have an extremely high rate of failure [3]. A case report published more than a decade ago described deformation of a covered, self-expanding stent within 3 months of placement in the subclavian artery, but this was almost certainly located distal to the first rib [4]. Malliet and colleagues report three cases of arterial TOS, all with subclavian artery aneurysm formation, which were treated with endovascular stent-grafting followed by cervical and/or first rib resection (up to 2 months after intervention) [5]. Interestingly, although all three of these patients did well with patent devices 1–6 years later, two had developed early occlusion of the endoprosthesis requiring secondary thrombectomy procedures. It is also significant that the same two patients had exhibited recurrent symptoms during the interval between the initial endovascular treatment and thoracic outlet decompression. The largest series of patients with arterial TOS (n=55) was published in 1989; although 69 % of the patients presented with "embolic occlusion" there was no mention of endovascular intervention in this series [6].

References

1. Lee JT, Dua MM, Hernandez-Boussard TM, Illig KA. Surgery for TOS: a nationwide perspective. J Vasc Surg. 2011;53:100S–1S.
2. Hood DB, Kuehne J, Yellin AE, Weaver FA. Vascular complications of thoracic outlet syndrome. Am Surg. 1997;63:913–7.
3. Urschel HC, Patel AN. Paget-Schroetter syndrome therapy: failure of intravenous stents. Ann Thorac Surg. 2003;75:1693–6.
4. Sitsen ME, Ho GH, Blankensteijn JD. Deformation of self-expanding stent-grafts complicating endovascular peripheral aneurysm repair. J Endovasc Surg. 1999;6:288–92.
5. Malliet C, Fourneau I, Daenens K, Maleux G, Nevelsteen A. Endovascular stent-graft and first rib resection for thoracic outlet syndrome complicated by an aneurysm of the subclavian artery. Acta Chir Belg. 2005;105:194–7.
6. Cormier JM, Amrane M, Ward A, Laurian C, Gigou F. Arterial complications of the thoracic outlet syndrome: fifty-five operative cases. J Vasc Surg. 1989; 9:778–87.

Surgical Techniques: Approach to the Axillosubclavian Artery

85

Michael J. Singh and Dustin J. Fanciullo

Abstract

Exposure of the axillosubclavian artery can be challenging due to the surrounding bony structures, bulky pectoralis muscles, and adjacent nerves. A thorough understanding of the thoracic outlet anatomy facilitates surgical exposure of both the subclavian and axillary arteries. However, given the complex anatomy within a confined surgical field, even to an expert exposure of these vessels is certainly not without risk. This chapter will serve as a review of both the supraclavicular and infraclavicular approaches to the axillosubclavian artery.

Introduction

Exposure of the axillosubclavian artery can be challenging due to surrounding bony structures, bulky pectoralis muscles, and adjacent nerves. A thorough understanding of the thoracic outlet anatomy facilitates surgical exposure of both the subclavian and axillary arteries. However, given the complex anatomy within a confined surgical field, even to an expert exposure of these vessels is certainly not without risk. This chapter will serve as a review of both the supraclavicular and infraclavicular approaches to the axillosubclavian artery.

M.J. Singh, MD, FACS, RPVI (✉)
Department of Surgery,
University of Rochester Medical Center,
601 Elmwood Avenue, Box 652,
Rochester, NY 14642, USA
e-mail: singhmj@upmc.edu

D.J. Fanciullo, MD, RPVI
Private Practice, Vascular Surgery,
Rochester, NY, USA

An important point should be made regarding planning. Vessels in the groin, legs, arms, and even abdomen are surrounded only by soft tissue, and an experienced and talented vascular surgeon can approach such vessels very quickly if emergencies arise or a traumatic or surgical injury is present. The brachiocephalic vessels, importantly including the subclavian and axillary arteries, do not afford this luxury, and emergent proximal exposure frequently requires time consuming bony resection or division. For this reason we suggest an unusually reasoned, thoughtful planning process prior to exposure of these vessels.

Anatomy

The right subclavian artery and right common carotid artery both originate from the innominate artery. The left subclavian artery originates directly off the aortic arch distal to the left common carotid artery. Infrequently, aberrant right

Fig. 85.1 The extra-thoracic subclavian artery can be exposed through a supraclavicular incision. Transecting the anterior scalene muscle will expose the vessel. Three major branches originate from the subclavian artery and are: the internal mammary, vertebral and thyrocervical trunk

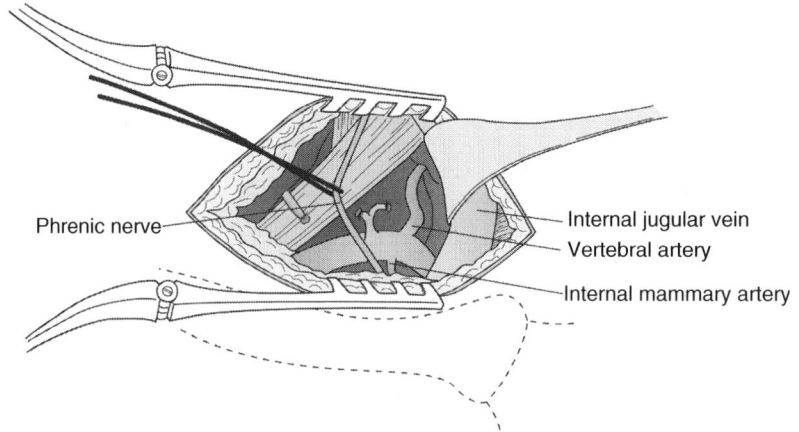

Phrenic nerve

Internal jugular vein
Vertebral artery
Internal mammary artery

subclavian artery anatomy is discovered. In these cases, the right subclavian artery originates from the descending thoracic aorta distal to the left subclavian artery. A supraclavicular incision provides excellent exposure of the extra-thoracic subclavian artery. Releasing the anterior scalene muscle provides direct visualization of the vessel. At this level three major branches off the subclavian artery are found – from medial to lateral they are the internal mammary artery, vertebral artery and thyrocervical trunk (Fig. 85.1) [1].

The subclavian artery transitions to the axilliary artery at the lateral edge of the first rib. The lateral boundary of the axillary artery is defined by the lateral edge of the terres major muscle; distal to this boundary the axillary artery becomes the brachial artery. The pectoralis minor muscle divides the axillary artery into three segments. The first segment is medial to the pectoralis minor, the second is deep to the muscle and the third segment is distal. The first axillary segment contains one branch, which is the supreme thoracic artery. The second segment has two branches, which are the thoracoacromial and lateral thoracic arteries. The third segment has three branches; from medial to lateral the subscapular, medial humeral circumflex and lateral humeral circumflex arteries. (Figs. 85.2 and 85.3)

Supraclavicular Approach

The supraclavicular approach is well suited for any operation requiring the exposure of the subclavian artery or brachial plexus. Further, this approach is unique in that it provides excellent exposure of all anatomic structures associated with the thoracic outlet (See also Chap. 29).

Under general anesthesia, the patient is placed in the supine position with the head turned away from the operative side. A transverse shoulder roll can be utilized to extend the neck and flatten the supraclavicular fossa. Care should be taken to avoid hyperextending the neck. The surgical field is then prepped to include the entire extremity, neck, shoulder and upper chest.

The sternal notch, clavicle, and sternocleidomastoid muscle are identified. A transverse incision is made 1 cm superior the clavicle starting just lateral to the sternal portion of the sternocleidomastoid muscle. (Fig. 85.4) This incision should be 8–10 cm in length and parallel the clavicle.

The incision is deepened by use of the superficial cervical aponeurosis, platysma muscle, and clavicular portion of the sternocleidomastoid muscle are all divided. The external jugular vein will be identifiable and should be ligated. Care should be taken when dividing the sternocleidomastoid muscle as the internal jugular vein lies just beneath it. Once identified, the internal jugular vein should be mobilized and retracted medially. If this exposure is to be performed on the patient's left side, careful dissection along the internal jugular vein is mandatory to avoid injury to the thoracic duct which travels posterior. The duct drains into the superior aspect of the confluence between the left internal jugular and subclavian veins. If injured, the duct should be identified and ligated to prevent the development of a lymphocutaneous fistula formation.

Fig. 85.2 Proximally the axillary artery is anatomically defined by the lateral margin of the first rib and distally by the lateral edge of the teres major muscle. The pectoralis minor muscle divides the axially artery into three segments

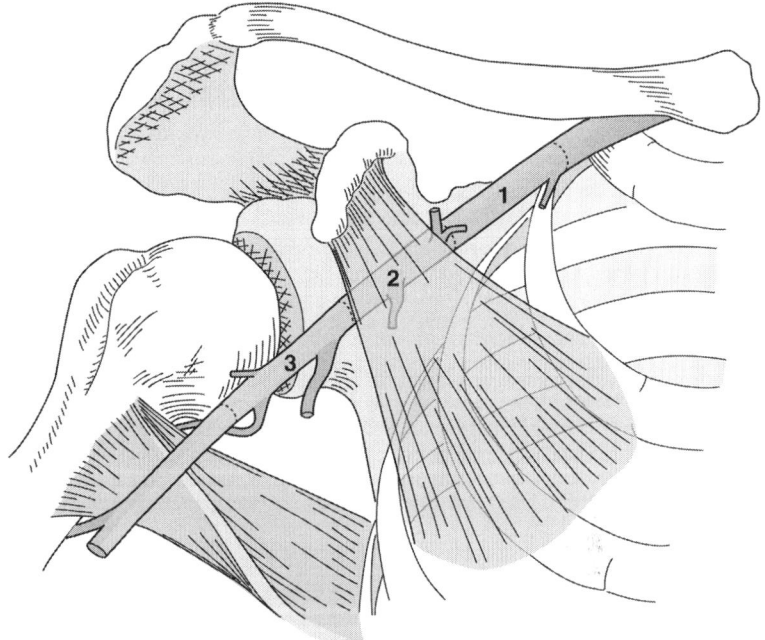

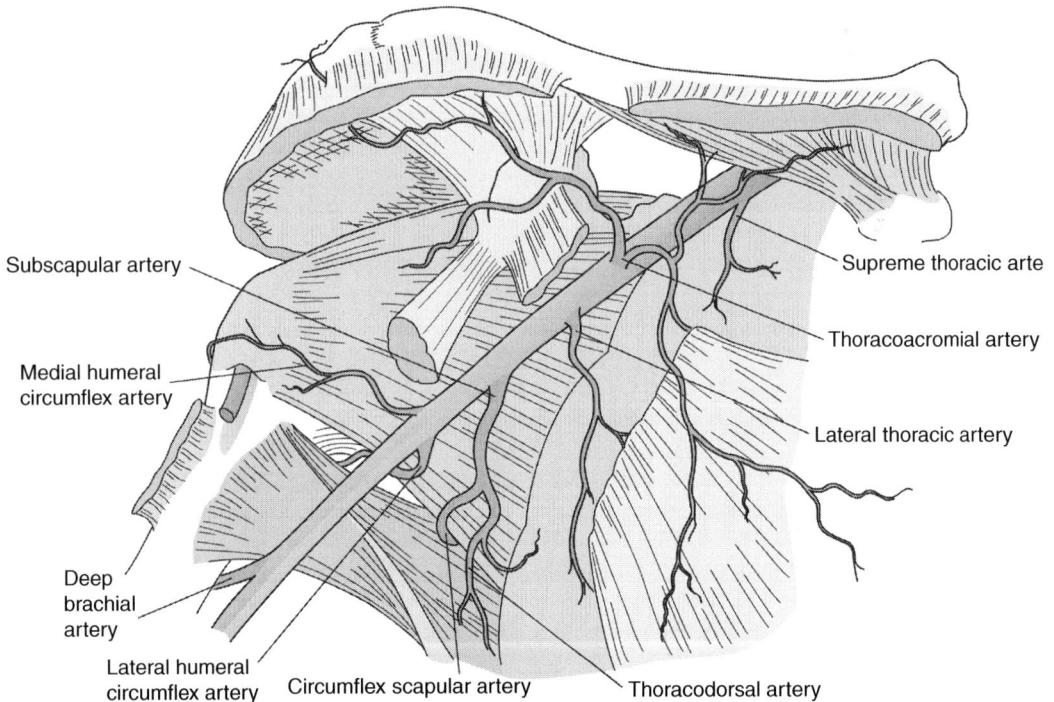

Fig. 85.3 Branches of the axillary artery are: supreme thoracic artery, thoracoacromial artery, lateral thoracic artery, subscapular artery, medial humeral circumflex artery and the lateral humeral circumflex artery

Just deep and medial to the internal jugular vein is the common carotid artery. The location of the vagus nerve is most often posterior and lateral to the common carotid artery. The scalene fat pad which lays deep to the platysma should be dissected along its medial border and reflected

Fig. 85.4 The patient is placed supine with neck slightly extended and rotated away from the surgical site. The transverse supraclavicular incision in placed 1 cm superior to the clavicle. The platysma and clavicular portion of the sternocleidomastoid muscle are transected

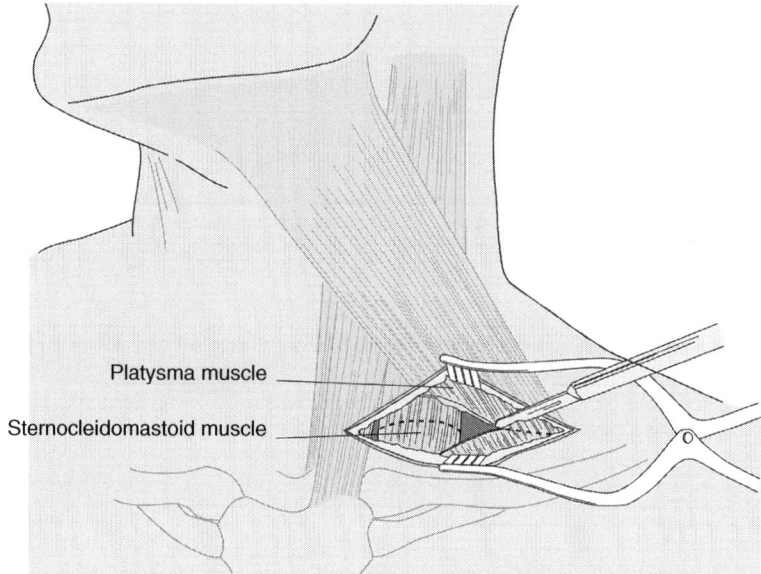

Platysma muscle

Sternocleidomastoid muscle

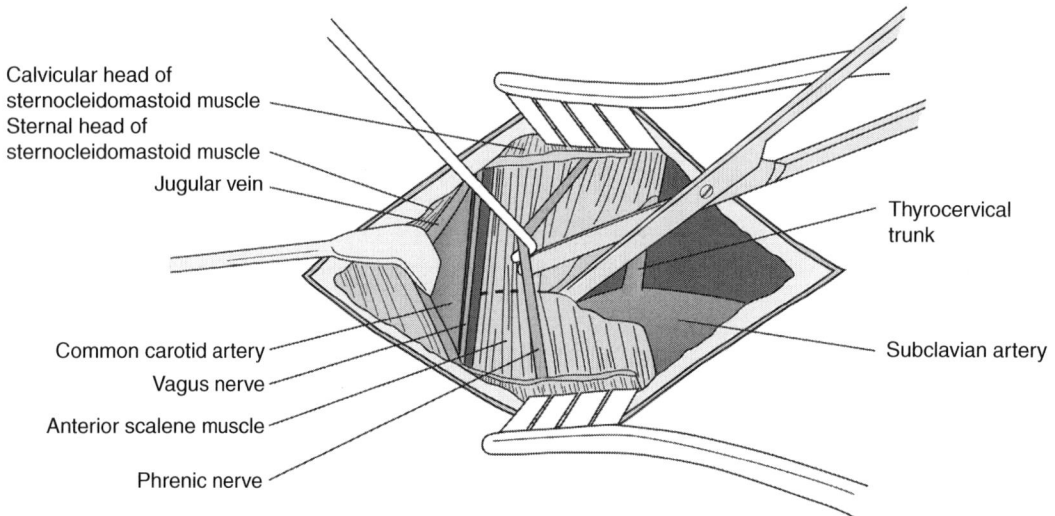

Calvicular head of sternocleidomastoid muscle

Sternal head of sternocleidomastoid muscle

Jugular vein

Thyrocervical trunk

Common carotid artery

Vagus nerve

Anterior scalene muscle

Phrenic nerve

Subclavian artery

Fig. 85.5 After mobilizing the scalene fat pad, the phrenic nerve coursing lateral to medial will be found lying on top of the anterior scalene muscle. The nerve should be gently mobilized and the anterior scalene muscle sharply released from its insertion on the first rib

laterally to provide exposure of the anterior scalene muscle. Prior to any scalene muscle dissection, it is of paramount importance to identify the phrenic nerve which lies superficial to the anterior scalene muscle and typically courses obliquely from lateral to medial (Fig. 85.5). Once identified, the nerve is mobilized and gently retracted medially with a vessel loop. Placing a right angle clamp behind the anterior scalene muscle facilitates the transection of its tendinous insertion on the first rib.

Once the anterior scalene muscle has been transected, 3–5 cm of the subclavian artery will easily be visualized. The C5 and C6 nerve roots will be found laterally. On the left side, the subclavian artery is slightly deeper and less accessible. After isolating the subclavian artery dissection of it branches vessels is helpful and includes the

Fig. 85.6 A horizontal infraclavicular incision will expose the pertoralis major muscle (PMA). Once fibers of the PM are separated, the clavopectoral fascia (CPF) and pectoralis minor muscle (PMI) are readily seen. The pectoralis minor is transected with cautery

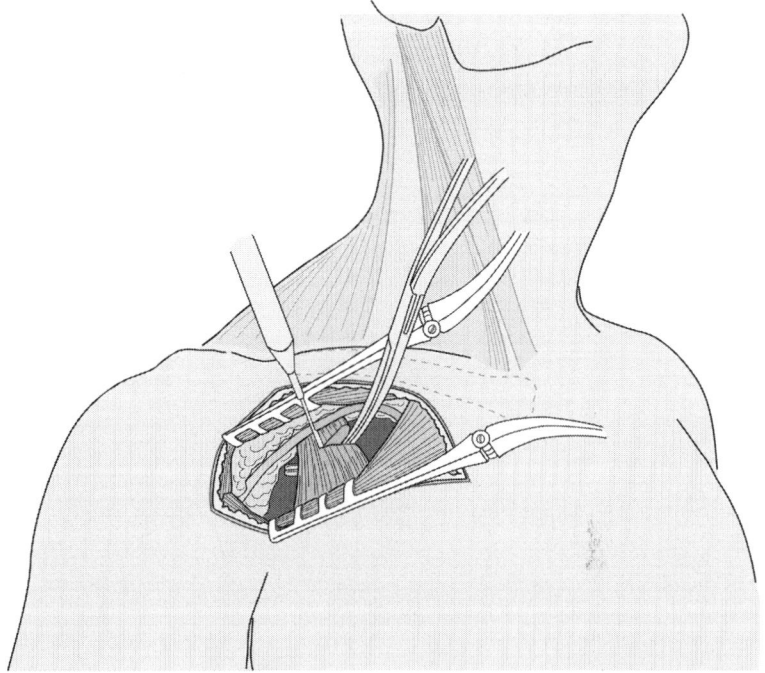

vertebral artery, internal mammary artery, and thyrocervical trunk (Fig. 85.1) [2–5].

Infraclavicular Approach

As described above, the axillary artery is comprised of three anatomic segments. All three are easily approached through an infraclavicular incision. The first segment, extending from the lateral border of the first rib to the medial border of the pectoralis minor, is the best location to serve as a donor artery in the construction of extra-anatomic bypasses as movement with arm extension is minimal.

In preparation for surgery, the patient should be placed supine on the operating room table. When exposure is being performed for ATOS, the entire upper extremity, supraclavicular area, and thorax should be prepped and draped in a sterile fashion. If the patient requires an extra anatomic bypass to the lower extremity, the ipsilateral arm should be abducted 45–60°.

A horizontal skin incision is made one fingerbreadth inferior to the clavicle. It should start approximately 1–2 cm below the medial

third of the clavicle and extend laterally to the deltopectoral grove for a distance of 8–10 cm. The incision is deepened with electrocautery through the subcutaneous tissue and pectoralis major fascia. A dissection plane is created between the pectoralis major muscle fibers. This blunt or sharp dissection separates the muscle fibers and exposes the superficial surface of the clavipectoral fascia. This fascial layer is incised to expose the underlying pectoralis minor muscle. The pectoralis minor is transected near the coracoid process. (Fig. 85.6) Crossing superficial to this muscle are the acromiothoracic artery and vein. If traced medially, these two vessels will guide the surgeon to the axillary artery and vein.

Using sharp dissection, the axillary sheath is opened. The first structure encountered within the axillary sheath is the axillary vein. To expose the artery, which lies deep and superior to the vein, gentle caudal retraction on the axillary vein should be applied. Once the vein is retracted, dissection continues along the axillary artery until enough length is achieved to perform an anastomosis. If the dissection is extended laterally, one must be careful to identify and preserve the branches of the brachial plexus [1, 2]. (Fig. 85.7)

Fig. 85.7 Distal exposure of the axillary artery and vein can be obtained by extending the infraclavicular incision laterally. Using sharp dissection, the axillary sheath is opened. The first structure encountered within the axillary sheath is the axillary vein. To expose the artery, which lies deep and superior to the vein, gentle caudal retraction on the axillary vein should be applied

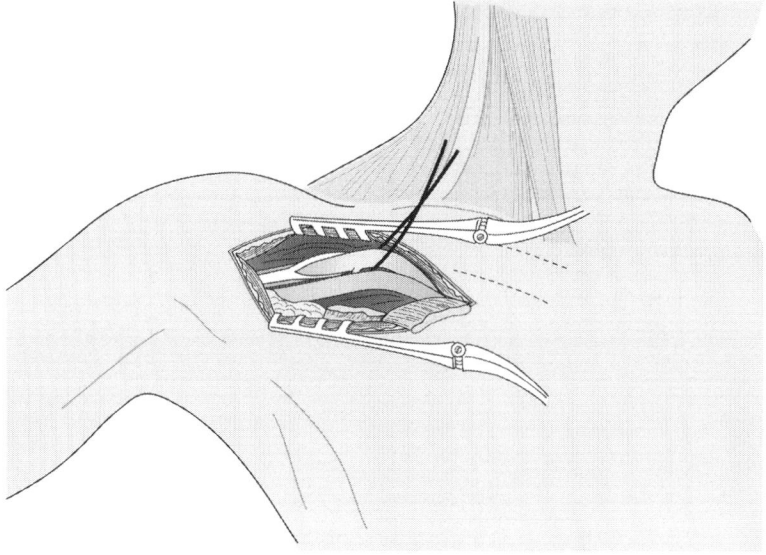

Fig. 85.8 A combined supraclavicular and infraclavicular approach may be necessary for large axillosubclavian artery aneurysms

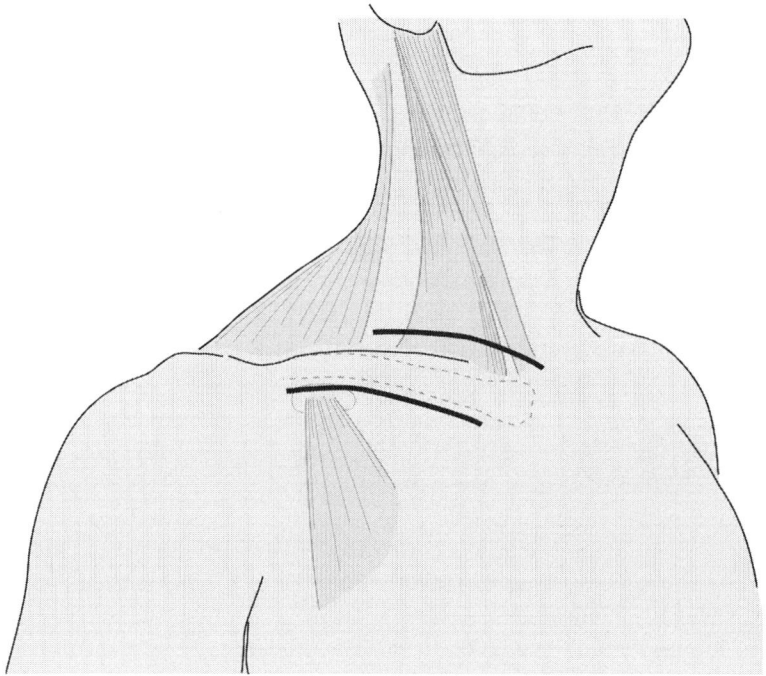

Deltopectoral Approach

If distal axillary artery exposure is necessary, extending the incision onto the upper arm may be necessary. The lateral portion of the incision should extend to the intersection of the anterior border of the deltoid muscle and the external border of the biceps muscle. The superficial location of the cephalic vein places it in harm's way and should be preserved if possible.

Combined Supraclavicular and Infraclavicular Approach

Occasionally a combined supraclavicular and infraclavicular approach is necessary for large axillosubclavian artery aneurysms or traumatic arterial injuries. In these situations excellent arterial exposure can be obtained using a combined approach which avoids the morbidity associated with resection of the clavicle (Fig. 85.8).

References

1. Hallett J, Mary H. In: Branchereau A, Berguer R, editors. Vascular surgical approaches. 1st ed. Armonk: Futura Publishing Company, Inc.; 1999. p. 43–54.
2. Thompson R, Driskill M. In: Cronenwett J, Johnston KW, editors. Rutherford's vascular surgery. 7th ed. Philadelphia: Saunders; 2010. p. 1878–98.
3. Zarins CK, Gewertz BL. Atlas of vascular surgery. 2nd ed. Philadelphia: Elsevier, Inc.; 2005. p. 40–9.
4. Saunders RJ, editor. Thoracic outlet syndrome: a common sequela of neck injuries. 1st ed. Philadelphia, PA: Lippincott; 1999.
5. Vogelin E, Haldemann L, Constantine M, Gerber A, et al. Long-term outcome analysis of the supraclavicular surgical release for the treatment of thoracic outlet syndrome. Neurosurgery. 2010;66:1085–92.

Surgical Techniques: Axillary Artery Reconstruction for ATOS

86

Ali Azizzadeh and Robert W. Thompson

Abstract

Extrinsic compression of the distal axillary artery or its immediate branches can cause unique vascular lesions that represent a variant of arterial TOS. These lesions are occasionally reported in overhead athletes, such as baseball pitchers and volleyball players, for whom positional compression of the artery opposite the head of the humerus has led to aneurysm formation, with thrombosis and/or embolism to the arteries of the arm or hand. The unique clinical setting of these lesions requires different considerations from those applicable to other forms of TOS or vascular disease. This chapter describes the spectrum of pathology and the outcomes of treatment for compressive axillary artery lesions, with particular emphasis on the methods of surgical treatment and the subsequent return to high-performance overhead athletic activity.

Introduction

The most typical form of arterial thoracic outlet syndrome (TOS) involves development of a subclavian artery aneurysm, caused by compression of the subclavian artery within the scalene trian-

A. Azizzadeh, MD, FACS (✉)
Department of Cardiothoracic and Vascular Surgery,
University of Texas Medical School,
Memorial Hermann Heart and Vascular Institute,
6400 Fannin St., Suite 2850, Houston, TX 77030, USA
e-mail: ali.azizzadeh@uth.tmc.edu

R.W. Thompson, MD
Department of Surgery, Section of Vascular Surgery,
Center for Thoracic Outlet Syndrome,
Washington University, Barnes-Jewish Hospital,
660 S Euclid Avenue, Campus Box 8109/Suite 5101
Queeny Tower, St. Louis, MO 63110, USA
e-mail: thompson@wudosis.wustl.edu

gle at the level of the first rib. This usually occurs in conjunction with a congenital cervical rib or first rib anomaly, with formation of mural thrombus and embolic occlusion of distal arteries in the arm and/or hand. Similar pathologic and clinical findings can develop from lesions in the distal axillary artery or its immediate branches, also caused by extrinsic compression, thereby representing a variant of arterial TOS (Fig. 86.1) [2]. Compressive lesions of the axillary artery have been occasionally reported in overhead athletes since the early 1970s, particularly in baseball pitchers and volleyball players [3–6]. The rare nature of these lesions and their unique clinical setting requires different considerations from those applicable to other forms of vascular disease. This chapter describes the spectrum of pathology and the outcomes of treatment for

K.A. Illig et al. (eds.), *Thoracic Outlet Syndrome*,
DOI 10.1007/978-1-4471-4366-6_86, © Springer-Verlag London 2013

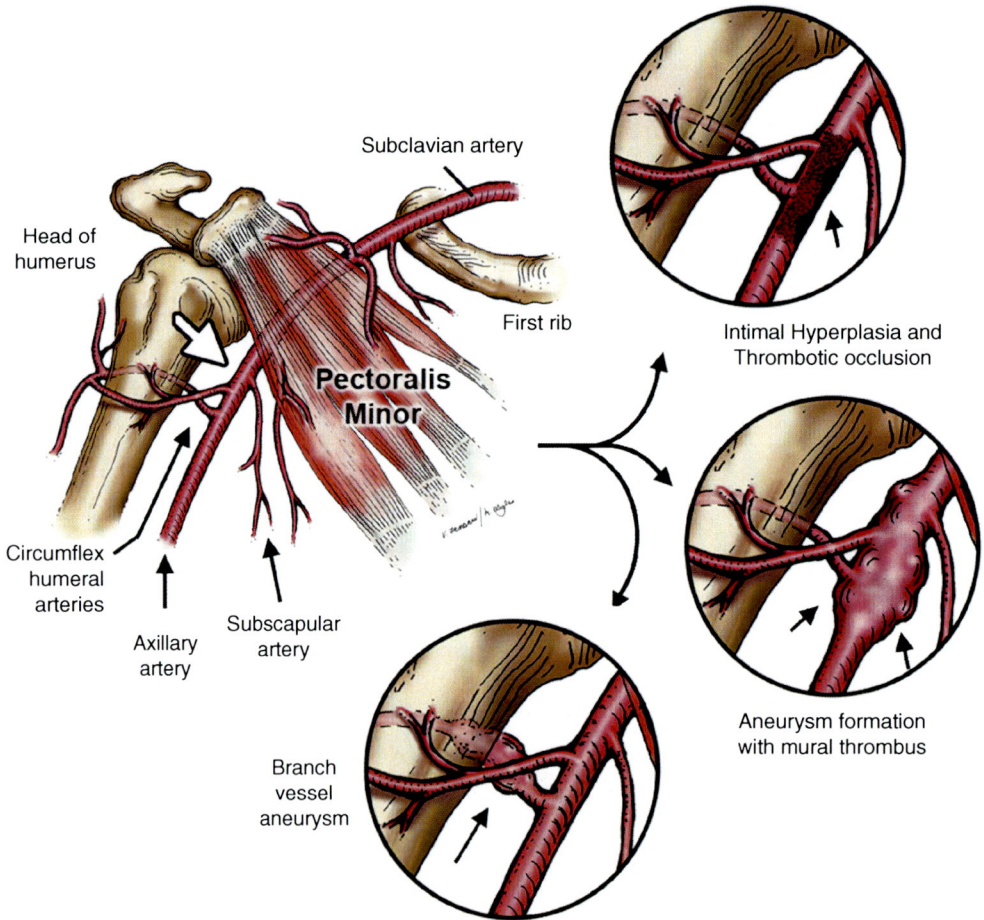

Fig. 86.1 Pathogenesis of axillary artery lesions. Compression of the third portion of the axillary artery by anterior displacement of the humeral head during the overhead throwing motion. The axillary artery is relatively fixed in position at this site by the overlying fascia, branch vessel origins, and the pectoralis minor muscle. Repetitive compression can lead to intimal hyperplasia with stenosis, or aneurysm formation, with or without thrombotic occlusion. Similar lesions may also arise in the adjacent axillary artery branches (subscapular and circumflex humeral arteries) (Adapted from Duwayri et al. [1]. With permission from Elsevier)

axillary artery lesions in the high-performance overhead throwing athlete, with particular emphasis on the methods of surgical treatment and the subsequent return to athletic activity.

Clinical Presentation, Diagnosis, and Initial Management

Presenting symptoms include early and pronounced arm fatigue, finger numbness, Raynaud's syndrome and cold hypersensitivity in the hand and/or fingers, rest pain in the hand, and localized fingertip discoloration, consistent with cutaneous digital embolism. Digital ulcerations, non-healing wounds, or palpable bony abnormalities are sometimes present. A clinical diagnosis of upper extremity arterial insufficiency is often initially suspected by the examining physician. Non-invasive vascular laboratory studies, including brachial-brachial indices and forearm/digital waveforms, often confirm the clinical impression of arterial insufficiency. Computed tomography (CT) or magnetic resonance (MR) arteriograms, as well as standard upper extremity arteriography, can be used for definitive diagnosis. Diagnostic findings include stenosis or occlusion of the distal axillary artery at rest or with arm

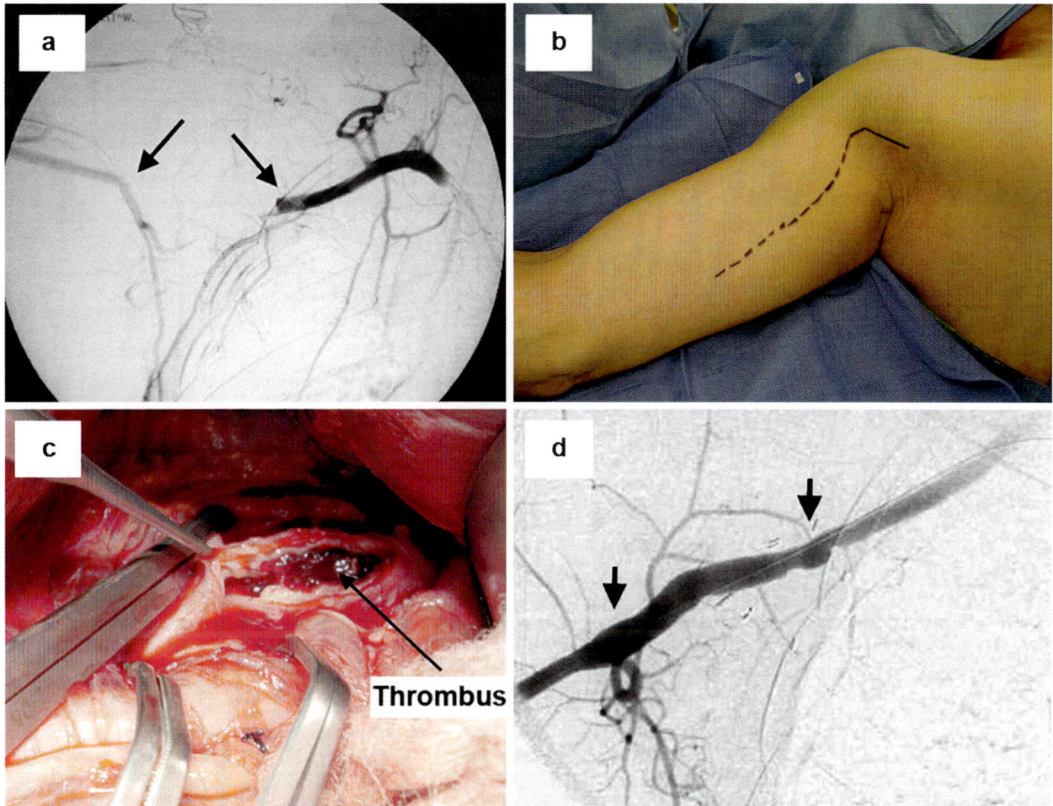

Fig. 86.2 Axillary artery thrombosis. (**a**) Initial arteriogram demonstrating occlusion of the right axillary artery in a 29 year-old baseball pitcher. (**b**) Surgical exploration through an upper arm incision, (**c**) revealing acute thrombosis of the distal axillary artery, superimposed on an area of intimal thickening caused by focal intimal hyperplasia. (**d**) The excised arterial segment was replaced by an interposition vein graft, illustrated on a completion arteriogram (Adapted from Duwayri et al. [1]. With permission from Elsevier)

elevation. Branch vessel occlusion may also be seen. Patients with axillary artery occlusions can undergo catheter directed intra-arterial thrombolysis. However, balloon angioplasty and stent placement is not recommended. Following the initial diagnostic studies and interventions, patients are maintained on therapeutic anticoagulation with subcutaneous low molecular weight heparin and/or warfarin prior to definitive treatment.

Surgical Treatment

Diagnostic upper extremity arteriography is performed with the affected arm at rest and in the overhead elevated position (Fig. 86.2a). Intravascular ultrasound (IVUS) may also be employed to assess pathological characteristics of the arterial wall, such as intimal thickening or aneurysmal dilatation. Surgical exploration is performed through an upper medial arm incision (Fig. 86.2b). The distal (third) portion of the axillary artery is exposed and circumferentially mobilized from its surrounding fascia, with gentle retraction of the axillary vein and brachial plexus nerves. The axillary artery branch vessels (subscapular and circumflex humeral arteries) are also mobilized and controlled. The location of the axillary artery lesion is identified by direct palpation and reference to the diagnostic arteriogram, with proximal and distal control obtained where the vessel appears normal (Fig. 86.2c). In our experience, the axillary artery pathology is usually confined to the third portion of the vessel or its branches (lateral to the pectoralis minor

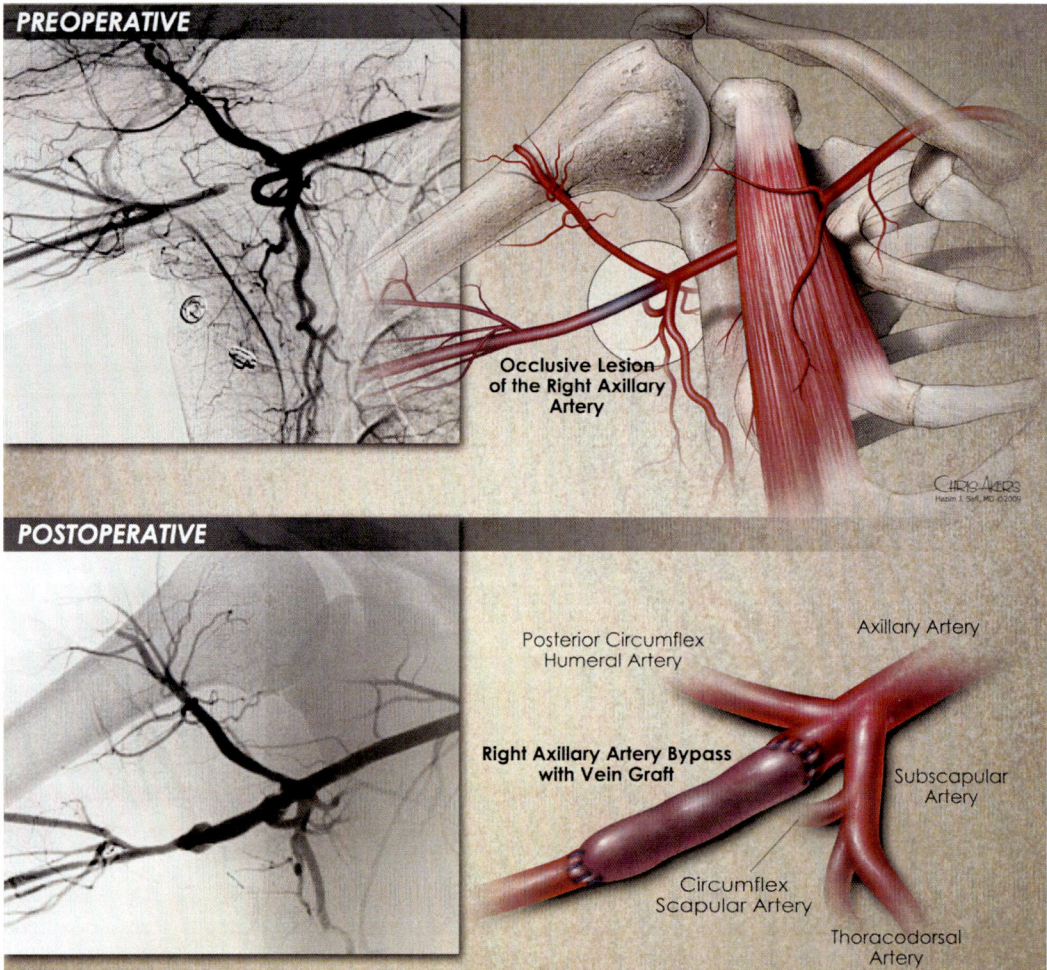

Fig. 86.3 Repair of axillary artery lesion. Preoperative arteriogram and illustration depicting occlusion of the distal right axillary artery. At surgical exploration, the affected segment of axillary artery was excised and replaced with a reversed saphenous vein graft bypass, with preservation of the subscapular, thoracodorsal, circumflex scapular, and posterior circumflex humeral artery branches, as depicted by the postoperative arteriogram (Courtesy of Chris Akers, Hazim J. Safi, MD © 2009)

muscle). In rare instances when the lesion extends more proximally, control of the artery can be obtained through a transverse infraclavicular incision. Division of the pectoralis minor muscle is not usually required for vascular exposure.

The affected segment of the axillary artery is excised and the artery is reconstructed with a reversed saphenous vein interposition bypass graft (Fig. 86.2d). These bypass grafts are placed with widely beveled, end-to-end anastomoses, after measuring the appropriate length of the graft while the arm is placed in overhead extension to avoid subsequent tension, torsion or compression by the humeral head during overhead positioning. In addition, the distal anastomoses are created to incorporate at least one of the axillary artery branch vessel origins (subscapular and/or circumflex humeral arteries) (Fig. 86.3). Occasionally, an axillary artery thrombectomy is required. Focal lesions may be treated with a saphenous vein patch rather than a bypass graft. In patients who have lesions confined to the axillary artery branch

Table 86.1 Classification and staging of axillary artery lesions

Lesion type	Arteriographic findings and surgical pathology		
Type I	Patent axillary artery with positional compression alone		
Type II	Fixed axillary artery stenosis or occlusion ± Positional compression		
Type III	Axillary artery aneurysm formation ± Positional compression		
Type IV	Axillary artery branch vessel aneurysm or occlusion (Circumflex humeral or subscapular arteries)		
Lesion stage	Distal arteriographic findings		
	Brachial artery	**Radial and ulnar arteries**	**Palmar arch**
	Across elbow	**Through forearm and wrist**	**Through hand**
Stage 0	Patent	Both patent	Patent
Stage 1	Occluded	Both patent	Patent
	Patent	One occluded	Patent
Stage 2	Occluded	One occluded	Patent
	Patent	Both occluded	Patent
Stage 3	Occluded	Both patent	Interrupted
	Patent	One or both occluded	Interrupted
Stage 4	Occluded	One or both occluded	Interrupted
"D" Modifier	Presence of digital artery emboli or occlusions		

Adapted from Duwayri et al. [1]. With permission from Elsevier

vessels, simple ligation and excision of the aneurysm, without axillary arteriotomy or direct reconstruction, is sufficient. A classification and staging system for axillary artery lesions, based on a combination of arteriographic findings and surgical pathology, is shown in Table 86.1. In our experience, fixed axillary artery stenosis or occlusion with or without positional compression (Type II) is the most commonly encountered abnormality. Angiographic evidence of thromboembolism distal to the elbow is also very common in this patient cohort.

Intraoperative completion arteriography following treatment of the axillary artery or branch vessel lesion is prudent. Selective injections with the arm at rest and in overhead elevation are obtained. The distal circulation is assessed from the brachial artery to the hand. If residual distal thromboembolism is encountered, brachial artery exploration and thrombectomy, along with intraarterial thrombolysis and vasodilator infusion into the distal vessels of the forearm, is performed. Upon completion of the operative procedure, a closed-suction drain is placed into the axillary space for 24–48 hours, and therapeutic anticoagulation

is resumed (intravenous heparin followed by conversion to warfarin) along with antiplatelet therapy (clopidogrel).

Postoperative Care

Postoperative anticoagulation and antiplatelet therapy is maintained for approximately six weeks. Physical therapy is also continued for six weeks, with an initial focus on restoration and maintenance of upper extremity range of motion while restricting vigorous overhead activity and upper-body weight lifting. This is allowed to progress to upper-body strengthening and throwing, beginning six weeks after surgery, with an emphasis on maintaining proper posture and shoulder mechanics during overhead motion. Planned secondary imaging studies (CT, MR or angiography) are performed four to six weeks after surgical treatment, to evaluate the axillary artery reconstruction and distal circulation prior to the return to more vigorous upper extremity exercise. Anticoagulation is discontinued six weeks after surgery, at which time patients are permitted more vigorous athletic rehabilitation, overseen by a team physician and trainer.

Discussion

The overhead throwing position involves 90–120° of shoulder abduction, excessive external arm rotation, and full wrist pronation [7]. During this maneuver, the third portion of the axillary artery is potentially subject to compression by the head of the humerus distal to the pectoralis minor muscle, where the artery is relatively fixed in position by its surrounding fascia and branch vessel origins (the subscapular and circumflex humeral arteries). Anterior translation of the glenohumeral joint and axillary artery compression with the arm in the throwing position has been demonstrated by ultrasound [8]. Cadaveric and angiographic studies have also documented that abduction and external rotation of the arm can cause compression of the axillary artery by the humeral head, acting as a fulcrum [9, 10]. Moreover, tethering of the third portion of the axillary artery can result in stretch injury to its branch vessel origins during the extremes of arm abduction and external rotation, particularly where the posterior circumflex humeral artery passes into the quadrilateral space [11, 12].

Repetitive positional compression of the distal axillary artery or its branches has been sporadically reported in baseball players and other competitive overhead athletes. A recent review of the literature revealed 46 cases, including 28 (61 %) with axillary artery pathology and 18 (39 %) with lesions of the axillary artery branch vessels, with the majority (70 %) occurring in baseball players (Table 86.2) [2]. It is evident that these lesions are typically caused by chronic vessel wall injury and frequently associated with intimal hyperplasia, stenosis, and thrombus formation, as well as distal embolization to smaller vessels. More abrupt and substantial axillary artery injury may result in acute thrombotic occlusion or dissection, and progressive medial degeneration can lead to aneurysm formation in the axillary artery or its branches. Even though small in size, the turbulent flow in these aneurysms readily produces mural thrombus that has a high propensity to embolize to the distal extremity, particularly during repetitive movement at the level of the shoulder joint.

This condition is probably under-recognized, in part because symptoms resembling arm claudication, digital numbness and circulatory changes are not uncommon in high-performance, overhead throwing athletes. In this setting, such symptoms are often initially attributed to fatigue and musculoskeletal etiologies. Collegiate and professional athletes are usually first evaluated by their team physicians, who need to have a high index of suspicion when these symptoms arise acutely or when they are associated with pulse deficits, pallor, or differences in temperature. The variety of presenting symptoms reinforces the need for team physicians to remain vigilant in evaluating unusual or persistent upper extremity complaints.

Noninvasive vascular laboratory testing may be used in diagnosis, as brachial-brachial indices may be abnormal with axillary artery occlusion and digital waveforms may be dampened in cases with distal thromboembolism. These studies can be deceptive, however, as normal results may be obtained in the resting position when there is only positional compression of the axillary artery. Plain films may reveal cervical ribs in cases of subclavian artery compression in the thoracic outlet, but are normal in cases of axillary artery compression. Angiography remains the most important and essential diagnostic study, whether performed by catheter-based techniques or contrast-enhanced MR or CT. Angiograms should be performed with the arm both at rest and in the overhead position (90–120° shoulder abduction, full external rotation), with good visualization of the axillary artery, its branches, and the more distal vessels.

Conclusion

Repetitive positional compression of the axillary artery is a rare but important problem in the elite overhead throwing athlete. It can cause a spectrum of pathology, including focal intimal hyperplasia, aneurysm formation, segmental dissection, and branch vessel aneurysms or occlusions. Prompt recognition of these lesions is crucial, given their propensity toward thrombosis and distal embolism. Positional arteriography is necessary for

Table 86.2 Axillary artery and branch vessel lesions in competitive athletes

Year	Author (ref)	No. of patients (sport)	Types of lesions	
1989	McCarthy [13]	4 Patients (3 BB, 1 SB)	3 A×A Positional compression	
			1 Branch artery occlusion	
1990	Nuber [4]	6 Patients (BB)	5 A×A Positional compression	
			1 Branch artery occlusion	
1990	Rohrer [9]	1 Patient (BB)	1 A×A Thrombosis	
1993	Reekers [14]	1 Patient (VB)	1 Branch artery aneurysm	
1995	Kee [15]	2 Patients (BB)	2 Branch artery aneurysms	
1998	Todd [16]	2 Patients (BB)	2 A×A Aneurysms	
1999	Schneider [5]	1 Patient (BB)	1 A×A Aneurysm	
2000	Caiati [17]	1 Patient (TN)	1 A×A Dissection	
2000	Ikezawa [18]	2 Patients (1 VB, 1 TN)	1 Branch artery aneurysm	
			1 Branch artery thrombosis	
2001	Arko [19]	5 Patients (NA)	1 A×A Aneurysm	
			4 Branch artery aneurysms	
2001	Ishitobi [20]	4 Patients (BB)	4 A×A Thrombosis	
2001	Vlychou [21]	1 Patient (VB)	1 Branch artery aneurysm	
2006	McIntosh [22]	2 Patients (VB)	2 Branch artery aneurysms	
2006	Simovitch [23]	1 Patient (BB)	1 A×A Positional compression	
2006	Takach [24]	1 Patient (BB)	1 A×A Positional compression	
2007	Baumgarten [25]	1 Patient (BB)	1 Branch artery aneurysm	
2008	Seinturier [26]	1 Patient (NA)	1 Branch artery aneurysm	
2009	Ligh [27]	1 Patient (BB)	1 A×A Positional compression	
2010	Duwayri [2]	9 Patients (BB)	5 A×A Thrombosis	
			2 Branch artery aneurysms	
			1 A×A Dissection/Compression	
			1 A×A Positional compression	
Totals		46 Patients	12 A×A Positional compression	26.1 %
		(32 BB, 70 %)	10 A×A Thrombosis	21.7 %
		(1 SB, 2 %)	4 A×A Aneurysms	8.7 %
		(5 VB, 11 %)	2 A×A Dissection/Compression	4.3 %
		(2 TN, 4 %)	3 Branch artery occlusions	6.5 %
			15 Branch artery aneurysms	32.6 %

Adapted from Duwayri et al. [1]. With permission from Elsevier
Abbreviations: *BB* baseball, *SB* softball, *TN* tennis, *VB* volleyball, *NA* not available

accurate diagnosis and thrombolysis may be useful as initial management when axillary artery thrombosis is present. However, balloon angioplasty and placement of axillary artery stents should be avoided. Anticoagulation should be instituted upon confirmation of the diagnosis, along with referral for surgical treatment as soon as feasible. Full functional recovery can be anticipated within several months following surgical treatment, consisting of mobilization and segmental reconstruction of the diseased axillary artery, or ligation and excision of branch artery aneurysms, as well as concomitant management of any distal thromboembolism.

References

1. Duwayri YM, Emery VB, Driskill MR. Positional compression of the axillary artery causing upper extremity thrombosis and embolism in the elite overhead throwing athlete. J Vasc Surg. 2011;53: 1329–40.

2. Duwayri YM, Emery VB, Driskill MR, Earley JA, Wright RW, Paletta GAJ, Thompson RW. Axillary artery compression causing upper extremity thrombosis and embolism in the elite overhead throwing athlete: spectrum of pathology and outcomes of treatment. J Vasc Surg. 2011;53:1329–40.

3. Tullos HS, Erwin WD, Woods GW, Wukasch DC, Cooley DA, King JW. Unusual lesions of the pitching arm. Clin Orthop Relat Res. 1972;88:169–82.

4. Nuber GW, McCarthy WJ, Yao JS, Schafer MF, Suker JR. Arterial abnormalities of the shoulder in athletes. Am J Sports Med. 1990;18:514–9.

5. Schneider K, Kasparyan NG, Altchek DW, Fantini GA, Weiland AJ. An aneurysm involving the axillary artery and its branch vessels in a major league baseball pitcher. A case report and review of the literature. Am J Sports Med. 1999;27(3):370–5.

6. Jackson MR. Upper extremity arterial injuries in athletes. Semin Vasc Surg. 2003;16:232–9.

7. Fleisig GS, Barrentine SW, Escamilla RF, Andrews JR. Biomechanics of overhand throwing with implications for injuries. Sports Med. 1996;21:421–37.

8. Stapleton CH, Herrington L, George K. Anterior translation at the glenohumeral joint: a cause of axillary artery compression? Am J Sports Med. 2008;36:539–44.

9. Rohrer MJ, Cardullo PA, Pappas AM, Phillips DA, Wheeler HB. Axillary artery compression and thrombosis in throwing athletes. J Vasc Surg. 1990;11(6):761–8, discussion 768–9.

10. Dijkstra PF, Westra D. Angiographic features of compression of the axillary artery by the musculus pectoralis minor and the head of the humerus in the thoracic outlet compression syndrome: case report. Radiol Clin (Basel). 1978;47:423–7.

11. Cahill BR, Palmer RE. Quadrilateral space syndrome. J Hand Surg Am. 1983;8:65–9.

12. Reeser JC. Diagnosis and management of vascular injuries in the shoulder girdle of the overhead athlete. Curr Sports Med Rep. 2007;6:322–7.

13. McCarthy WJ, Yao JST, Schafer MF, Nuber G, Flinn WR, Blackburn D, Suker JR. Upper extremity arterial injury in athletes. J Vasc Surg. 1989;9:317–27.

14. Reekers JA, den Hartog BM, Kuyper CF, Kromhout JG, Peeters FL. Traumatic aneurysm of the posterior circumflex humeral artery: a volleyball player's disease? J Vasc Interv Radiol. 1993;4:405–8.

15. Kee ST, Dake MD, Wolfe-Johnson B, Semba CP, Zarins CK, Olcott C. Ischemia of the throwing hand in major league baseball pitchers: embolic occlusion from aneurysms of axillary artery branches. J Vasc Interv Radiol. 1995;6(6):979–82.

16. Todd GJ, Benvenisty AI, Hershon S, Bigliani LU. Aneurysms of the mid axillary artery in major league baseball pitchers: a report of two cases. J Vasc Surg. 1998;28:702–7.

17. Caiati JM, Masters CM, Todd EJ, Benvenisty AI, Todd GJ. Symptomatic axillary artery dissection in a tennis player: case report. Am J Sports Med. 2000;28:411–2.

18. Ikezawa T, Iwatsuka Y, Asano M, Kimura A, Sasamoto A, Ono Y. Upper extremity ischemia in athletes: embolism from the injured posterior circumflex humeral artery. Int J Angiol. 2000;9:138–40.

19. Arko FR, Harris EJ, Zarins CK, Olcott C. Vascular complications in high-performance athletes. J Vasc Surg. 2001;33(5):935–42.

20. Ishitobi K, Moteki K, Nara S, Akiyama Y, Kodera K, Kaneda S. Extra-anatomic bypass graft for the management of axillary artery occlusion in pitchers. J Vasc Surg. 2001;33:797–801.

21. Vlychou M, Spanomichos G, Chatziioannou A, Georganas M, Zavras GM. Embolisation of a traumatic aneurysm of the posterior circumflex humeral artery in a volleyball player. Br J Sports Med. 2001;35:136–7.

22. McIntosh A, Hassan I, Cherry K, Dahm D. Posterior circumflex humeral artery aneurysm in 2 professional volleyball players. Am J Orthop (Belle Mead NJ). 2006;35:33–6.

23. Simovitch RW, Bal GK, Basamania CJ. Thoracic outlet syndrome in a competitive baseball player secondary to the anomalous insertion of an atrophic pectoralis minor muscle: a case report. Am J Sports Med. 2006;34:1016–9.

24. Takach TJ, Kane PN, Madjarov JM, Holleman JH, Nussbaum T, Robicsek F, Roush TS. Arteriopathy in the high-performance athlete. Tex Heart Inst J. 2006;33:482–6.

25. Baumgarten KM, Dines JS, Winchester PA, Altchek DW, Fantini GA, Weiland AJ, Allen A. Axillary artery aneurysm with distal embolization in a major league baseball pitcher. Am J Sports Med. 2007;35:650–3.

26. Seinturier C, Blaise S, Maufus M, Magne JL, Pasquier B, Carpentier PH. A rare cause of embolic ischemia of the hand: an isolated aneurism of a branch of the axillary artery. J Mal Vasc. 2008;33:225–8.

27. Ligh CA, Schulman BL, Safran MR. Case reports: unusual cause of shoulder pain in a collegiate baseball player. Clin Orthop Relat Res. 2009;467:2744–8.

Part XII

Arterial TOS: Outcomes and Future Directions

Outcomes After Treatment of ATOS

87

Gregory J. Pearl

Abstract

Although the least common form of the group, without recognition and timely treatment the ischemic complications of arterial thoracic outlet syndrome (ATOS) can lead to tissue loss and thus may cause the most severe and disabling sequelae of all. ATOS can present as a single ischemic event due to acute thrombotic occlusion of the subclavian or axillary artery or it may present more insidiously with extremity pain and fatigue or subtle signs and symptoms of digital ischemia. Effective and successful treatment of arterial TOS and its direct relative, positional axillary artery compression or its branches, requires a high level of suspicion and early recognition. As demonstrated in numerous series as well as our own, excellent outcomes are achieved with prompt correction of the compressive mechanism and appropriate adjunctive revascularization as needed. Failures arise with the delay in diagnosis and treatment due to the development of fixed occlusive lesions in the runoff arterial beds. Results are excellent in patients with subclavian arterial lesions at the first rib, but poorer in those with positional axillary artery compression due to non-first rib pathology.

Introduction

Although the least common form of thoracic outlet syndrome (TOS), without recognition and timely treatment the ischemic complications of arterial involvement (ATOS) can lead to pain and tissue loss and may cause the most severe and disabling sequelae of all. Fields' report of a stroke in a major league baseball pitcher with

ATOS serves as an extreme case in point of the devastation that may be caused by a single thromboembolic event in a high performing, otherwise healthy athletic individual [1]. As discussed in previous chapters, the clinical presentation of ATOS may be manifest as a single ischemic event due to acute thrombotic occlusion of the subclavian or axillary artery; or it may present more insidiously with extremity pain and fatigue or subtle signs and symptoms of digital ischemia. In either case, timely diagnosis and treatment is key to achieving a successful, durable result and offer the best chance for an excellent long term outcome in this generally young, active group of patients.

G.J. Pearl, MD
Department of Vascular Surgery,
Baylor University Medical Center,
621 N. Hall Street, Suite 100, Dallas, TX 75226, USA
e-mail: gregp@baylorhealth.edu

K.A. Illig et al. (eds.), *Thoracic Outlet Syndrome*,
DOI 10.1007/978-1-4471-4366-6_87, © Springer-Verlag London 2013

Cumulative Results

The results of treatment for ATOS are generally excellent. Cormier et al. [2] described the long term outcome of 55 procedures for subclavian arterial complications in TOS. Distal embolization had occurred in 35 (64 %) of the patients. Emboli in the arm were treated with transbrachial embolectomy but distal emboli in the hand and digits were not treated. Thirty-nine patients were available for long-term follow-up. There were no minor or major amputations and 90 % reported complete freedom from any symptoms. Four of the patients reported exertional related discomfort in the forearm that was non-disabling. Kieffer and Ruotolo [3] also reported excellent outcomes in 97 % of treated patients, noting only a single digit amputation and just one graft occlusion with mean follow-up of 43.7 months.

In a later report, Durham et al. [4] retrospectively reviewed the experience at Northwestern University with 34 patients treated for ischemic complications of arterial thoracic outlet syndrome. Twenty-two patients were found to have a subclavian artery injury and 12 lesions of the axillary artery or its branches. In the subclavian group, all patients underwent thoracic outlet decompression. Additionally, 15 patients required subclavian artery reconstruction with resection and interposition grafting or patch angioplasty. Seven patients underwent decompression alone and observation for a minimal arterial injury. Two of the subclavian arterial reconstructions required re-operation; one bypass for graft thrombosis on postoperative day 82 with successful thrombectomy, and a second required excision of a vein graft for aneurysmal degeneration and replacement with a new vein graft. Both of these revisions remained patent at the time of the report. Five patients required axillary artery reconstruction, four with vein patch angioplasty, one of which had concomitant axillary to interosseous artery bypass; and one patient underwent interposition grafting with greater saphenous vein. All five axillary reconstructions remain patent at the time of the report. All of the patients in the axillary artery group were either higher performance athletes or manual laborers. The five patients in

this group that did not undergo axillary artery reconstruction or decompression were treated with modification in their throwing motion or modification of their activities at work. There were no amputations in this group and all patients experienced improvement or relief of their symptoms.

Thompson and colleagues [5] have recently reported on their experience in the treatment of nine patients with lesions of the axillary artery or its immediate branches, which represented 19 % of the patients treated on their service with ATOS over the past decade. All patients were operated upon through an upper medial arm approach. Direct repair of the axillary artery with saphenous vein interposition grafting in five patients and thrombectomy with vein patch angioplasty in two were performed. Two patients were treated with ligation and excision of a circumflex humeral aneurysm. Two of the nine patients in the series required transbrachial thromboembolectomy with intra-arterial thrombolysis and vasodilator infusion into the distal vascular bed. All patients had an uncomplicated postoperative recovery and were subsequently maintained on anticoagulation for several weeks.

Two of the nine patients required secondary operative procedures, one at 2 years after experiencing recurrent ischemic symptoms in the digits that was found to have distal extension of chronic thrombus in the hand as well as stenosis of the proximal anastomosis of the saphenous vein interposition graft. This patient was treated with radial artery thrombectomy, vasodilator infusion and balloon angioplasty of the anastomotic stenosis. He required video assisted trans-thoracic sympathectomy 2 years later for persistent ischemic digital symptoms. The second patient experienced thrombosis of an extended saphenous vein bypass graft 1 month post-operatively due to proximal compression of the vein graft at the level of the first rib. He underwent supraclavicular first rib resection and subclavian to axillary bypass with externally supported PTFE. This new graft occluded at 1 year and was successfully treated with catheter directed thrombolysis. Eight of the nine patients returned to professional careers following treatment for at least some period of time and secondary patency rates of 100 % and assisted primary patency rate of 89 % were achieved.

The Baylor Experience

Our own experience in the treatment of ATOS at parallels that observed in the previous reports. Patency rates and outcomes in our series are excellent, with durable arterial reconstruction after 9 years and with rare exception, the patients return to full strenuous activities, competitive or otherwise.

Over a period of 10 years we have treated 31 patients with ATOS (unpublished series). At a mean follow-up of 37 months, we have observed no graft occlusions, graft failures or instances of recurrent upper extremity embolization in 23 patients in the subclavian artery group. All of these patients experienced complete relief of symptoms as well as resolution of all ischemic sequelae in the arm, hand or digits.

Eight patients comprised our axillary artery group, all of whom underwent axillary artery reconstruction. Two of these patients, both of whom are professional major league baseball players, experienced recurrent or persistent ischemic symptoms in their arm or hand, and important observations may be made in the examination of these two failures. Both players had presented with distal thromboemboli and digital ischemia secondary to posterior circumflex humeral artery aneurysms. Both players underwent saphenous vein interpositioning grafting of the axillary artery with exclusion of the posterior circumflex humeral aneurysm and preservation of the anterior circumflex humeral artery. Both underwent concomitant brachial artery exploration with transbrachial thromboembolectomy. Due to the chronicity of the thromboemboli, thrombus extraction was unsatisfactory. The brachial artery was closed with patch angioplasty and both patients were maintained on systemic anti-coagulation postoperatively.

One of the professional ballplayers was a pitcher and was unable to return to pitching at the major league level due to persistent exertional related symptoms in his forearm and hand. He went into coaching but continued to experience vasospastic problems in the hand and digits. Fifteen months following the axillary artery reconstruction, he was living and coaching in Alabama and underwent re-evaluation with upper extremity arteriography for persistent symptoms which revealed the saphenous interposition graft to be widely patent with no evidence of compression with provocative maneuvers. He demonstrated persistent distal occlusive lesions from the original thromboembolic event. He was placed on calcium channel blockade and has done well with his current level of activities and avoidance of cold exposure.

The second patient was a shortstop who continued to experience vasospastic symptoms in the affected hand. A radial artery to radial artery bypass graft with saphenous vein was performed in an attempt to alleviate these persistent ischemic symptoms; however the radial artery reconstruction occluded in the early postoperative period, most likely secondary to compromised run off in the hand. He recovered satisfactorily with dramatic improvement in his symptoms. He returned to professional baseball but sequently developed an acute thrombotic event of his brachial artery during spring training in Florida. He underwent emergent brachial artery exploration and thrombectomy. Arteriography confirmed that the saphenous vein interposition graft placed for the axillary artery reconstruction remained widely patent and again demonstrated no evidence of any compression with provocative maneuvers. Following the thrombotic event, he continued to experience profound exertional symptoms in the forearm and hand and returned to Dallas where we discovered his brachial artery had rethrombosed. Re-exploration was performed with thrombectomy and intraoperative arteriography which demonstrated extremely compromised runoff in the forearm. Extended patch angioplasty was performed on the brachial artery and carried down onto the proximal ulnar artery. Completion arteriogram revealed improvement of flow into the forearm vessels and hand. His upper extremity arterial reconstruction remains patent; however, he has elected not to return to his baseball career at the present time. Both of these cases illustrate the long term adverse sequelae of delay in diagnosis and treatment for the thromboembolic complications of arterial thoracic outlet syndrome, and illustrate the difficulties created by extensive chronic distal embolization with loss of outflow.

Cumulative Results

Review of several series as well as our own reveals that thoracic outlet decompression in conjunction with judicious, selective subclavian artery reconstruction as indicated yields excellent, primary patency rates in excess of 90 %, secondary patency rates as high as 100 %, as well as excellent durable functional recovery in nearly all patients.

Conversely, patients with positional axillary artery compression appear to represent a more diverse group in regard to treatment options and somewhat less predictable outcomes. The combination of the axillary artery patients from the Northwestern, Washington University, and Baylor series yields a total of 29 patients. This combined group is compromised of 13 saphenous vein interposition grafts, 7 vein patch angioplasties with or without concomitant thrombectomy, 2 posterior, circumflex humeral aneurysm ligation/excisions, and 5 patients in whom no reconstructive treatment was pursued and simple modification of their activities was recommended. Four of the 29 patients required secondary or tertiary operative procedures for graft thrombosis/stenosis or brachial and/or distal arterial thrombosis. This group required more adjunctive procedures such as distal arterial bypass, vasodilatation infusion, intraoperative thrombolysis or subsequent sympathectomy than the subclavian group. As expected the more complex multimodal therapy required to treat the thromboembolic sequelae in this group resulted in the failure of 10 of the 29 patients in this combined group to return to full, unrestricted symptom free activity.

Summary

Effective and successful treatment of arterial TOS and its direct relative, positional axillary artery compression or its branches, requires a high level of suspicion and early recognition. As demonstrated in numerous series as well as our own, excellent outcomes are achieved with prompt correction of the compressive mechanism and appropriate adjunctive revascularization as needed. Failures arise with the delay in diagnosis and treatment due to the development of fixed occlusive lesions in the runoff arterial beds. This may result in suboptimal functional recovery due to the persistence of exertional related ischemic symptoms, or lead to an increased risk of subsequent acute thrombotic ischemic events in the setting of a discontinuous runoff bed.

References

1. Fields WS, Lemak NA, Ben-Menachem Y. Thoracic outlet syndrome: review and reference to stroke in a major league pitcher. AJNR Am J Neuroradiol. 1986; 7:73–8.
2. Cormier JM, Amrane M, Ward A, Laurian C, Gigou F. Arterial complications of the thoracic outlet syndrome: fifty five operative cases. J Vasc Surg. 1989; 9:778–87.
3. Kieffer E, Ruotolo C. Arterial complications of thoracic outlet compression. In: Rutherford RB, editor. Vascular surgery. 3rd ed. Philadelphia: WB Saunders Co; 1989. p. 875–82.
4. Durham JR, Yao JST, Pearce WH, Nuber GM, McCarthy WJ. Arterial injuries in the thoracic outlet syndrome. J Vasc Surg. 1995;21:57–70.
5. Duwayri YM, Emery VB, Driskill MR, Earley JA, Wright RW, Paletta GA, Thompson RW. Positional compression of the axillary artery causing upper extremity thrombosis and embolism in the elite overhead throwing athlete. J Vasc Surg. 2011;5: 1329–40.

Assessment and Treatment of Recurrent/Residual ATOS

Stephen J. Annest and Richard J. Sanders

Abstract

Recurrent ATOS is uncommon and can be limb threatening. It can be due to several causes including failure to recognize arterial pathology when excising cervical or anomalous first ribs, failure to recognize an abnormal rib when repairing subclavian artery pathology, thrombosis of a subclavian artery or a previous arterial repair, or development of stenosis in a previously repaired subclavian artery. Patients may present with arm and hand claudication or acute upper limb ischemia caused by graft thrombosis or distal emboli. Depending on the etiology, treatment may include excision of an abnormal rib, thrombectomy or replacement of the subclavian artery or previous bypass graft, or distal embolectomy. In addition, the potential contribution of sympathetic nerves to the ischemic condition should be evaluated and addressed.

Introduction

Arterial thoracic outlet syndrome (TOS) is very uncommon. It represents approximately one percent of all patients with TOS, although in the pediatric population, the percentage of vascular TOS compared to neurogenic TOS is substantially higher [1]. Arterial TOS can be separated into two types- complicated and uncomplicated-based on whether or not injury to the subclavian artery has developed in the form of stenosis, aneurysm, distal embolization, or occlusion. The majority of cases of arterial TOS, those without arterial injury or distal embolization, can be effectively treated by thoracic outlet decompression without arterial repair, even if mild arterial dilation beyond the rib has occurred [2–4]. Future development of arterial symptoms is not seen is these patients, with rare exceptions [5, 6]. In contrast, those patients in whom arterial injury was part of the initial presentation are at risk for recurrence, including those in whom the artery was repaired. Recurrence can be limb threatening and result in functional impairment [6].

S.J. Annest, MD, FACS (✉)
Department of Vascular Surgery, Vascular Institute of the Rockies, Presbyterian St. Luke's Medical Center, 1601 East 19th Avenue, Suite 3950, Denver, CO 80218, USA
e-mail: annest@vascularinstitute.com

R.J. Sanders, MD
Department of Surgery, HealthONE Presbyterian-St. Lukes Hospital, 4545 E. 9th Ave #240, Denver, CO, 80220, USA
e-mail: rsanders@ecentral.com

K.A. Illig et al. (eds.), *Thoracic Outlet Syndrome*,
DOI 10.1007/978-1-4471-4366-6_88, © Springer-Verlag London 2013

Etiology

Recurrence of symptoms following previous surgical therapy for arterial TOS occurs in the following instances: (1) At the first operation, the abnormal, impinging rib was excised, but the pathology in the subclavian artery and/or distal embolic occlusion in the affected arm was not recognized or left untreated [7]. (2) At the first operation the artery was repaired but the underlying osseous defect was unrecognized or left untreated. This occurs most often where an abnormal first rib is the compressing structure. These ribs can be difficult to identify as being anomalous and are easily overlooked by surgeons as well as by radiologists [8]. (3) The initial arterial repair developed thrombosis or stenosis. This is seen with both vein and prosthetic grafts and has been reported following endovascular stent-graft placement into the abnormal subclavian artery [9]. (4) Arterial occlusion occurs upon halting anticoagulants or altering anti-platelet therapy following initial arterial reconstruction. This signals the likelihood of an intra-luminal lesion in the repaired artery. (5) Non-arterial neurogenic symptoms may develop due to scar formation, which entraps the brachial plexus nerves following surgical dissection in either the axilla or supraclavicular fossa. An unresected first rib may be a contributing factor, or the entrapping tissue may consist of scarred muscle and soft tissue fibrosis [7, 9]. (6) Rarely, arterial injury occurs not at the level of the subclavian artery but more distally, at the third portion of the axillary artery, with compression by the head of the humerus or from the overlying pectoralis minor muscle tendon. This may be unrecognized at the time of initial treatment or during follow-up for recurrent symptoms. These patients are frequently heavy laborers or high level athletes [4, 10, 11].

Pathology

Two types of pathology are seen in recurrent arterial TOS: The first is distal emboli to the upper extremity, or rarely, retrograde emboli into the cerebral circulation, emanating from thrombus in a patent but diseased subclavian artery [12–14].

The natural history of distal embolism is progressive limb ischemia and limb loss [15]. The second pathologic occurrence is subclavian artery or bypass graft thrombosis, usually occurring without showering emboli.

Symptoms

Patient complaints may be similar to those that the patient presented with prior to the initial operation. However, the onset may now be more acute and consist of coolness of the arm, cold intolerance, paresthesias, color changes, claudication, pain, and tenderness of a finger, hand, or palm, and progressive weakness of the arm. The cause is ischemia secondary to emboli lodging in the brachial artery and distal arterial branches. Alternatively, an acute proximal arterial thrombosis results in decreased blood flow and oxygenation of the arm. Depending on the severity and duration of ischemia, these patients may present with rest pain, fingertip ulceration, and tissue loss.

Physical Examination

Physical findings may include diminished or absent pulses at the antecubital fossa or wrist, a pale or cyanotic hand, a recognizable difference in skin temperature compared to the unaffected extremity, delayed capillary refill, a bruit or mass in the neck, a palpable supraclavicular rib, reduced blood pressure of the affected limb, hand weakness, digital ischemia, or early tissue necrosis.

Diagnostic Tests

Non-invasive tests of potential use include bilateral upper extremity segmental pressures and wave-forms, finger photoplethysmography, color-flow duplex scanning of the subclavian and distal extremity arteries of the affected side, and x-rays of neck and chest. Early arterial imaging is essential, being performed by either CT or MRI angiography or by trans-femoral arteriography, the latter being perhaps of most use in that views of the hand may be of higher quality. Imaging should include visualization from the origin of the subclavian artery to the hand vessels. If trans-femoral arteriography is selected, the treatment team also has access to initiate therapy immediately upon interpreting the diagnostic study.

Management

Urgent intervention to re-establish blood flow to the arm is to be considered in all cases of recurrent arterial TOS. Initial therapy often employs immediate catheter-directed thrombolysis prior to definitive operative repair [10]. The decision to use thrombolytics or not is based in part on surgical judgment as to whether the degree of ischemia will allow the added time necessary for this step in treatment. With the use of thrombolytic agents infused directly into the obstructed vessels, acute thrombosis and emboli may be substantially cleared, whereas chronic embolic occlusions often are not [16].

The optimal surgical approach will depend upon the specific pathology. In every case the subclavian artery will require treatment, because it is either occluded or acting as the source of distal emboli. If bony or soft tissue abnormalities are present, they must be removed as the presumed cause of ongoing subclavian arterial injury [15]. If distal emboli remain after thrombolysis, or if thrombolysis is deemed inadvisable, then surgical thromboembolectomy is required to restore arterial flow.

When distal arterial occlusion is chronic and extensive, with no response to catheter-directed thrombolysis, the use of systemic heparin has been advocated as initial treatment moving to surgical exploration if motor and sensory impairment persists for greater than 6 h [17]. Intra-arterial vasodilator infusion during arteriography, followed by 2–4 days of heparin and Dextran infusion, has also been used [18].

Treatment of the Subclavian Artery

If the subclavian artery was not previously replaced, it almost always requires repair or replacement. Open repair necessitates supraclavicular and often infraclavicular exposure to provide safe control of the vessel. If the artery is patent and on external examination appears to be normal, it should be opened and visually inspected. Any intra-luminal pathology is then corrected [17, 19].

The abnormal section of artery may be amenable to endarterectomy and patch repair, or it may require excision with primary repair using an end-to-end arterial anastomosis. In other circumstances, an arterial bypass graft may be necessary to restore arterial flow to the arm. Reversed saphenous vein or autologous external iliac artery have been the preferred graft materials, but prosthetic graft are also acceptable conduits in this setting [20]. Re-lining the artery by placement of an endoluminal stent-graft is also an alternative that may be considered.

Graft Thrombosis and Embolization

If a subclavian artery bypass graft has thrombosed, thrombolytic therapy should be considered prior to graft thrombectomy or replacement. Graft occlusion usually presents with limb ischemia but without imminent limb threat, as often no distal embolization has occurred to further compromise the distal arterial tree (this must of course be verified by arterial imaging). As initial therapy, either catheter-directed thrombolysis or pharmaco-mechanical thrombolysis via a transfemoral approach, with distal embolic protection, can be considered. Thrombolytic therapy does require advanced interventional skills and it may not be advisable when there is an imminent threat to the limb. However, when successful, thrombolysis and concurrent interventional treatment of the culprit arterial lesion may obviate the need for reoperative open surgery. In all other circumstances, open surgical repair of the stenotic or occluded graft is recommended (Fig. 88.1).

When embolization has occurred, the patent subclavian artery bypass graft is the most likely source of the emboli. The bypass graft can be managed by replacement, ligation and bypass, or by lining it with an endoprosthesis. In a reoperative setting, a subclavian-to-distal axillary artery bypass may be the safest choice, because of the

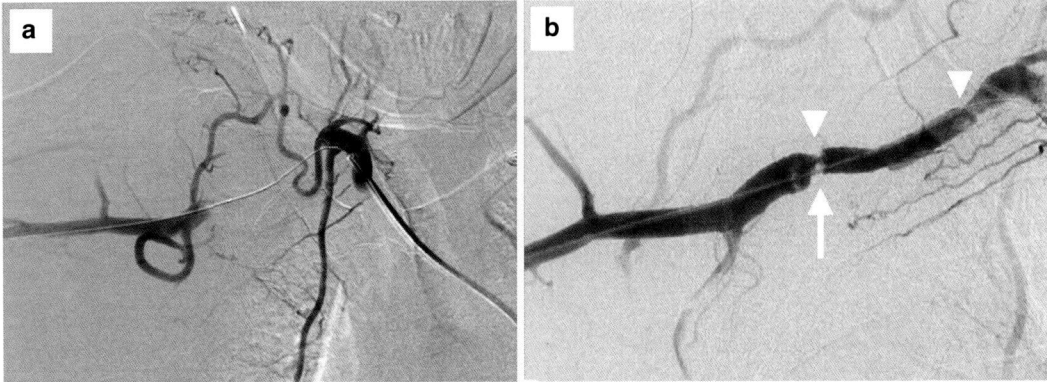

Fig. 88.1 Recurrent arterial TOS. A 44-year-old man underwent surgical treatment for a post-stenotic subclavian artery aneurysm caused by a cervical rib anomaly, with resection of the cervical and first ribs and an interposition prosthetic graft replacement of the subclavian artery. He was asymptomatic until 10 year later, when he developed an ankle fracture requiring use of crutches for several weeks and developed ischemic symptoms in the right upper extremity. (**a**) Right upper extremity arteriogram demonstrating thrombotic occlusion of the right subclavian artery bypass graft, with collaterals reconstituting the axillary artery and no distal thromboembolism. (**b**) Follow-up arteriogram after catheter-directed intra-arterial thrombolytic therapy, which reopened the subclavian artery bypass graft (*arrowheads*) and revealed an underlying high-grade stenosis at the distal anastomosis (*arrow*). This stenosis was successfully treated by prosthetic patch angioplasty [Courtesy of Robert W. Thompson, MD (Washington University, St. Louis)]

hazards of working in a scarred field in the proximal infraclavicular fossa, where the brachial plexus cords surround the axillary artery. If extensive scar makes dissection of the proximal subclavian artery hazardous, the common carotid artery, easily exposed at the level of the omohyoid muscle, may serve as a suitable inflow source. In this patient population, the carotid artery is usually a healthy vessel, and its suitability as an inflow source can be further assessed by use of carotid duplex scanning or by the arch arteriogram obtained when the upper extremity is evaluated.

Endovascular Stent-Grafts

In situations where a previously untreated subclavian artery aneurysm or stenosis is found, stent-graft insertion via the transfemoral or brachial artery approach offers the possibility of avoiding re-entry into a previously dissected surgical field. Long-term outcomes with prosthetic endovascular stent-grafts are variable, with reports of stent-graft occlusion at 1 year [12]. We have treated four such patients. Two patients re-occluded within the first 3 months, shortly after discontinuing warfarin, and they were successfully treated by thrombolysis and placement of additional stents at the margins of the previous stent-grafts. These repairs remain patent at the time of this writing. A third patient presented with an asymptomatic decrease in blood pressure in the operated left extremity, and was found to have an in-stent stenosis which was treated by balloon angioplasty (Figs. 88.2, 88.3, and 88.4). Another series with a similar experience was reported by Malliet et al. [21]. Based on these experiences, we now treat patients that have undergone stent-graft repair with warfarin for 6 months, before converting to long-term treatment with clopidogrel or aspirin. Importantly, we usually elect to correct the abnormal artery using direct open repair in this young healthy population. In addition, we monitor all subclavian artery interventions, both endovascular and open, with serial color flow duplex scans and upper extremity segmental pressures and waveforms in order to recognize graft narrowing prior to the development of thrombotic occlusion.

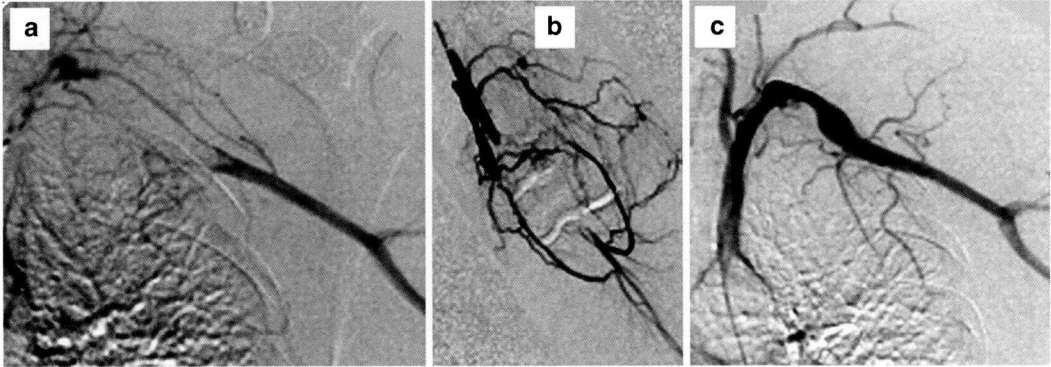

Fig. 88.2 Recurrent arterial TOS. Angiographic images depicting a patient with recurrent arterial TOS. (**a**) Left subclavian artery with occlusion before initial management with thrombolytic therapy. (**b**) Embolic occlusion of the left brachial artery, which was subsequently treated by thrombolysis. (**c**) Aneurysm of the left subclavian artery visualized after thrombolysis. This was treated with resection of the first and cervical ribs and a subclavian-to-axillary artery bypass using an 8 mm diameter PTFE graft

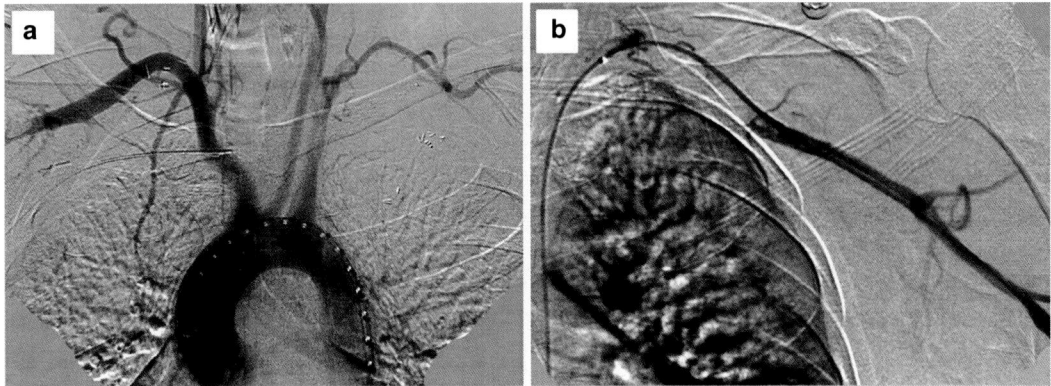

Fig. 88.3 Recurrent arterial TOS. Angiographic images of patient depicted in Fig. 88.2. (**a**) Nine months after the initial procedure, the left subclavian artery was noted to be occluded 2 days after the patient had undergone contralateral (*right*) transaxillary first rib and cervical rib resection. (**b**) Complete occlusion of the left subclavian artery bypass graft with distal emboli. Treatment included pharmaco-mechanical thrombolysis (Angiojet) followed by placement of a 7 mm diameter by 50 mm long Viabahn stent-graft inside the previous 8 mm PTFE graft, and brachial artery embolectomy performed through the brachial artery angiographic sheath

Retained Abnormal Ribs

Bony pathology, when present, usually represents an anomalous first rib or unresected cervical rib, and as the presumed cause of the recurrence, such lesions must be removed. Rib resection can be performed through the same supraclavicular incision that is used for the arterial repair. Alternatively, a transaxillary approach is a reasonable option, especially if the supraclavicular route was used at the first operation and endovascular correction of the subclavian artery is planned. The supraclavicular approach does not permit resection of the anterior portion of the first rib, but in arterial TOS this is unnecessary.

Distal Emboli

The subclavian artery should be treated first, before addressing distal embolic occlusions, so that if additional emboli are released during the course of the subclavian repair, they can be removed during the concurrently performed embolectomy. Most patients presenting with ischemic fingers and hands

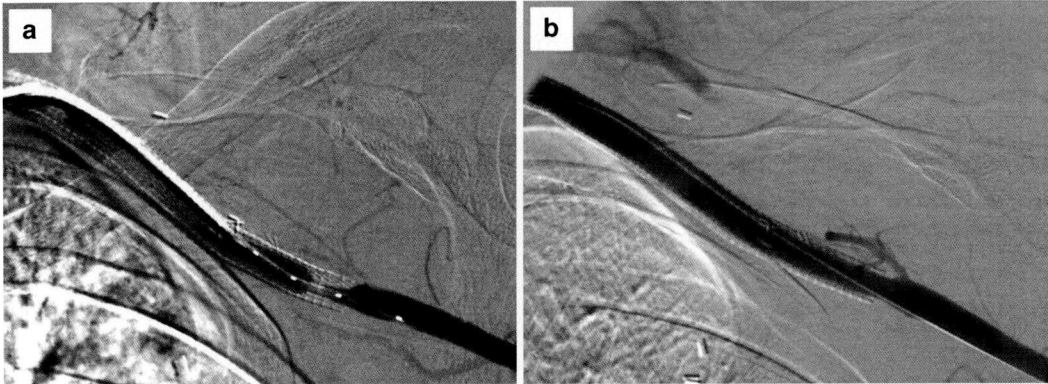

Fig. 88.4 Recurrent arterial TOS. Angiographic images of patient depicted in Fig. 88.2. (**a**) At follow-up 15 months after left subclavian artery stent-graft placement, the patient was noted to have 40 mmHg difference in blood pressure between arms and an abnormal Doppler signal in left arm. An arteriogram revealed a smooth in-stent restenosis of the distal aspect of the stent-graft. (**b**) The in-stent restenosis was treated with balloon angioplasty to 6 mm diameter (Angiosculpt) with resolution of the stenosis

will have emboli lodged in the brachial and/or forearm arteries. Open surgical thromboembolectomy via an antecubital incision provides an opportunity for thorough extraction of emboli causing occlusion of the arm and forearm vessels. After creating a brachial arteriotomy, balloon embolectomy catheters are passed distally into the radial and ulnar arteries, as well as retrograde into the brachial artery, until normal proximal pulsatile arterial flow is restored. For direct reconstruction, the radial and ulnar arteries may also be easily entered by extending the "S" shaped antecubital incision to the origins of these vessels beyond the brachial artery. Balloon embolectomy catheters may be carefully passed proximally into the axillary and subclavian arteries, taking great care to keep the balloon distal to the vertebral artery orifice.

Completion arteriography may reveal occlusion of the palmar arch and digital arteries. Attempts to perform embolectomy distal to the level of the wrist are associated with a high incidence of early re-occlusion. Intra-arterial infusion of thrombolytic drugs into the circulation of the hand may also be attempted, but to date this approach appears to have questionable benefit. Experience has shown that if the primary arteries proximal to the hand are reopened, distal ischemia will gradually resolve because of development of additional collateral arterial flow [17].

Sympathectomy

Sympathectomy has long been considered a potential adjunct in relieving distal ischemia [17, 22]. Other authoritative authors consider its use to be controversial [3]. Therefore, especially in the older surgical literature, it has been common practice to include dorsal sympathectomy to the operative procedure for any patient who initially presents with acute or chronic distal ischemia. Two alternatives exist: injection of the sympathetic chain with a long acting local anesthetic during rib resection, or neuromodulation by implantation of a dorsal column nerve stimulator [23]. The effects of spinal cord stimulation (SCS) on vascular tone in the peripheral circulation have been studied extensively in the laboratory and observed clinically. Research suggests that SCS reduces peripheral sympathetic vascular tone, augmenting blood flow to both skin and muscle in the limb. The effects of SCS are blunted by chemical and surgical sympathectomy [24–26].

References

1. Arthur LG, Teich S, Hogan M, Caniano DA, Smead W. Pediatric thoracic outlet syndrome: a disorder with serious vascular complications. J Pediatr Surg. 2004; 43:1089–94.

2. Sen S, Discigil B, Boga M, Ozkisacik E, Inci I. Thoracic outlet syndrome with right subclavian artery dilatation in a child: transaxillary resection of the pediatric cervical rib. Thorac Cardiovasc Surg. 2007;55:322–41.

3. Scher LA, Veith FJ, Haimovici H, Samson RH, Ascer E, Gupta SK, Sprayregen S. Staging of arterial complications of cervical rib: guidelines for surgical management. Surgery. 1984;95:644–8.

4. Durham JR, Yao JS, Pearce WH, Nuber GM, McCarthyIII WJ. Arterial injuries in thoracic outlet syndrome. J Vasc Surg. 1995;21:57–70.

5. Short DW. The subclavian artery in 16 patients with complete cervical ribs. J Cardiovasc Surg. 1975;16:135–41.

6. Craido E, Berguer R, Greenfield L. The spectrum of arterial compression at the thoracic outlet. J Vasc Surg. 2010;52:406–11.

7. Connell JL, Doyle JC, Gurry JF. The vascular complications of cervical rib. Aust NZ J Surg. 1980;50:125–30.

8. Coletta JM, Murray JD, Reeves TR, Velling TE, Brennan FJ, Hemp JR, Hall LD. Vascular thoracic outlet syndrome: successful outcomes with multimodal therapy. Cardiovasc Surg. 2001;9:11–5.

9. Sanders RJ, Haug C. Review of arterial thoracic outlet syndrome with a report of five new cases. Surg Gynecol Obstet. 1991;173:415–25.

10. Galabert HA, Machleder HI. Diagnosis and management of arterial compression at the thoracic outlet. Ann Vasc Surg. 1997;11:359–66.

11. Duwayri YM, Emery VB, Driskill MR, Earley JA, Wright RW, Paletta GA, Thompson RW. Axillary artery compression causing upper extremity thrombosis and embolism in the elite overhead throwing athlete: spectrum of pathology and outcomes of treatment. J Vasc Surg. 2011;53:1329–40.

12. Vierhout BP, Zeebregts CJ, van den Dungen JJAM, Reijnen MMPJ. Changing profiles of diagnostic and treatment options in subclavian artery aneurysms. Eur J Vasc Endovasc Surg. 2010;40:27–34.

13. Al-Hassan HK, Sattar MA, Eklof B. Embolic brain infarction: a rare complication of thoracic outlet syndrome. J Cardiovasc Surg. 1988;29:322–5.

14. Naz I, Sophie Z. Cerebral embolism: distal subclavian disease as a rare etiology. J Pak Med Assoc. 2006;56:186–8.

15. Davidovic LB, Kostic DM, Jakovljevic NS, Kuzmanovic IL, Simic TM. Vascular thoracic outlet syndrome. World J Surg. 2003;27:545–50.

16. Hood DB, Kuehne J. Vascular complications of thoracic outlet syndrome. Am Surg. 1997;63:913–7.

17. Cormier JM, Amrane M, Ward A, Laurian C, Gigou F. Arterial complications of the thoracic outlet syndrome: fifty-five operative cases. J Vasc Surg. 1989;9:778–87.

18. McCarthy WJ, Yao JST, Schafer MF, Nuber G, Flinn WR, Blackburn D, Suker JR. Upper extremity arterial injury in athletes. J Vasc Surg. 1989;9:317–27.

19. Heyden B, Vollmar J. Thoracic outlet-syndrome with vascular complications. J Cardiovasc Surg. 1979;20:531–6.

20. Wylie EJ, Stoney RJ, Ehrenfeld WK, Effeney DJ. Thoracic outlet syndromes. In: Wylie EJ, Stoney RJ, Ehrenfeld WK, Effeney DJ, editors. Manual of vascular surgery, Comprehensive manuals of surgical specialties, vol. II. New York: Springer; 1986. p. 249–71.

21. Malliet C, Fourneau I, Daenens K, Maleux G, Nevelsteen A. Endovascular stent-graft and first rib resection for thoracic outlet syndrome complicated by an aneurysm of the subclavian artery. Acta Chir Belg. 2005;105:194–7.

22. Banis JC, Rich N, Whelen RJ. Ischemia of the upper extremity due to non cardiac emboli. Am J Surg. 1977;134:131–9.

23. Naver H, Augustinnsson LE, Elam M. Vasodilating effect of spinal dorsal column stimulation is mediatiated by sympathetic nerves. Clin Auton Res. 1992;2:41–5.

24. Linderoth B, Gunasekera L, Meyerson BA. Effects of sympathectomy on skin and muscle microcirculation during dorsal column stimulation: animal studies. Neurosurgery. 1991;29:874–9.

25. Gaber JN, Lifson A. The use of spinal cord stimulation for severe limb threatening ischemia: a preliminary report. Ann Vasc Surg. 1987;1:578–82.

26. Sagher O, Huang MS. Mechanisms of spinal cord stimulation in ischemia. Neurosurg Focus. 2006;21(6):E2.

Directions in Clinical Research on ATOS

89

Ali Azizzadeh, Louis L. Nguyen, and Robert W. Thompson

Abstract

Arterial thoracic outlet syndrome (TOS) is the least frequent but likely most complex form of TOS. It most frequently occurs in relatively young, active, and otherwise healthy individuals. It is primarily caused by bony abnormalities, such as cervical ribs and anomalous first ribs. In this condition, longstanding subclavian artery compression leads to poststenotic dilatation and ulceration or aneurysmal degeneration, followed by occlusive thrombosis or mural thrombus formation with distal embolization to the arm and/or hand. Many clinical questions regarding diagnosis and optimal management of arterial TOS remain unanswered. The development of an international registry for patients with arterial TOS, along with standards for characterizing patients and reporting clinical outcomes, would provide useful data to help guide the optimal management of this rare and challenging clinical condition.

A. Azizzadeh, MD, FACS (✉)
Department of Cardiothoracic and Vascular Surgery,
University of Texas Medical School,
Memorial Hermann Heart and Vascular Institute,
6400 Fannin St., Suite 2850, Houston, TX 77030, USA
e-mail: ali.azizzadeh@uth.tmc.edu

L.L. Nguyen, MD, MBA, MPH
Department of Vascular and Endovascular Surgery,
Brigham and Women's Hospital,
75 Francis Street, Boston, MA 02115, USA
e-mail: llnguyen@partners.org

R.W. Thompson, MD
Department of Surgery, Section of Vascular Surgery,
Center for Thoracic Outlet Syndrome,
Washington University, Barnes-Jewish Hospital,
Campus Box 8109/Suite 5101 Queeny Tower,
660 S Euclid Avenue, St. Louis, MO 63110, USA
e-mail:thompson@wudosis.wustl.edu

Introduction

Arterial TOS is the most rare form of TOS and is most frequently observed in relatively young, active, and otherwise healthy individuals [1–4]. The condition is often caused by osseous structures, such as cervical ribs, anomalous first ribs, fibrocartilagenous bands and hypertrophic callus from healed first rib or clavicular fractures [2, 5, 6]. The pathophysiology is related to longstanding subclavian artery compression, poststenotic dilatation, and ulceration or aneurysmal degeneration, followed by occlusive thrombosis or mural thrombus formation with distal embolization to the arm and/or hand. Due to the rarity of this condition, there are no large prospective clinical trials involving patients with arterial

K.A. Illig et al. (eds.), *Thoracic Outlet Syndrome*,
DOI 10.1007/978-1-4471-4366-6_89, © Springer-Verlag London 2013

TOS. Therefore, the diagnosis and care of patients with arterial TOS is largely based on principles derived from caring for other types of TOS, as well as standard vascular surgical techniques in dealing with the complications of arterial TOS. In this chapter, we explore some of the clinical questions related to arterial TOS that need further study and organize these questions into the stage of care at which these issues arise.

Diagnosis and Imaging

Among patients who present with acute upper extremity ischemia, arterial TOS is only one of many possible causes. A high suspicion for the diagnosis should be considered, however, in young patients, especially those who participate in athletics or in occupations with repetitive arm motion. Initial imaging studies should include plain chest and cervical spine x-rays to evaluate for osseous abnormalities. Additional imaging obtained in the course of treatment for these patients should include visualization of the subclavian artery for the presence of an aneurysm. The choice of imaging modality may depend on the urgency of the presentation. Computerized tomography angiography (CTA) and magnetic resonance angiography (MRA) both provide excellent imaging of the aortic arch, subclavian artery and axillary artery, though anomalous bony structures are better viewed with CTA and soft tissue structures are better seen with MRA.

Traditional angiography provides detailed imaging of the proximal vessels and the distal extremity vessels that are otherwise difficult to image with conventional CTA and MRA. Visualization of the distal vasculature is particularly important in patients suspected of having thromboembolism. A recently published series reported that the incidence of arterial compression at the thoracic outlet may actually be underreported [4]. The authors recommend routine arterial imaging for patients evaluated with TOS who have a bony abnormality or an examination that shows an arterial abnormality.

Uncertainty exists for patients who present with incidentally discovered cervical ribs or elongation of the C7 transverse process (apophysomegaly). The estimated prevalence of cervical ribs and C7 apophysomegaly is approximately 0.75 % and 2.2 %, respectively [7]. In the absence of symptoms of arterial TOS, it is unclear what imaging or follow up is needed for patients who present with incidental cervical ribs and apophysomegaly. Since arterial TOS is usually asymptomatic until the clinical sequelae of aneurysmal degeneration, thrombus formation, and distal embolization occur, it is prudent to follow these patients with serial imaging. Future research, through observational studies, is needed to determine the time-course over which arterial abnormalities develop and the optimal type and frequency of surveillance imaging in this patient population.

Research Directions

- Who should be screened for or suspected of having ATOS?
- What is the most appropriate diagnostic test to screen for cervical ribs or other osseous abnormatilities?
- What is the appropriate follow up for patients with asymptomatic cervical ribs or C7 apophysomegaly?
- What is the most appropriate imaging modality to screen for subclavian artery aneurysms?
- Do all patients diagnosed with ATOS require angiography?
- What are the implications of arterial signs in a patient with neurogenic TOS?

Treatment

A selection of published case series of patients undergoing surgery for arterial TOS are listed in Table 89.1 [1, 2, 4, 5, 8–16]. This review of the literature revealed fewer than 450 cases of arterial TOS reported over three decades. This signifies the rarity of this pathology and the importance of relying on the clinical experience with other types of TOS for the best management of these patients. There appears to be a significant correlation between arterial TOS and the presence of osseus abnormalities, especially cervical

Table 89.1 Selected case series on treatment of arterial TOS

Author	Type of TOS, # of patients					F/U years	Treatment		Ex/Good results (%)
	A	V	N	C	R		TA	SC	
Dunwayri [8]	47	178	347	–	–	1.2	–	527	89
Sanders [21]	11	75	2,375	–	–	–	–	–	–
Degeorges [9]	38	27	15	96	–	7.5	107	69	84
Urschel and Razzuk [10]	240	264	2,210	–	1,221	–	2,714	–	–
Jamieson and Chinnick [11]	29	12	368	–	–	4	380	29	72
Hempel et al. [12]	18	47	705	–	–	>2	–	770	86
Lindgren et al. [13]	3	2	146	24	–	2	175	–	59
Wood et al. [15]	20	20	81	–	2	5.5	123	–	89
Kieffer et al. [16]	38	–	–	–	–	3.6	–	33	87

Type of TOS: *A* arterial, *V* venous, *N* neurogenic, *C* combined, *R* recurrent, *F/U* followup in years. Treatment: *TA* transaxillary, *SC* supraclavicular, *Ex/Good* percent of patients with excellent or good results

ribs and anomalous first ribs [4, 6]. Although the transaxillary approach has been utilized by many authors to effectively decompress the thoracic outlet for neurogenic and venous TOS, exposure and reconstruction of the subclavian artery is best achieved with the patient supine through supraclavicular or paraclavicular exposure [4, 17]. This allows for the greatest surgical access to the subclavian and axillary vessels, the brachial plexus, and the relevant musculoskeletal structures. Using a combination of transaxillary and supraclavicular approaches has also been reported [10].

Surgical decompression with removal of osseus abnormalities is recommended for patients with arterial TOS. In the presence of a cervical rib, removal of both the first and cervical rib is often recommended [4, 6, 10, 17], but it is still unclear whether removal of the cervical rib alone provides adequate decompression. Studies of cadavers with cervical ribs have revealed histological changes of fibrosis in the lower brachial plexus nerve trunks [18]. This evidence suggests that neurolysis of the brachial plexus and first rib resection may be beneficial in patients who undergo decompression for arterial TOS, since at least some proportion of symptoms in these patients may be attributable to concomitant neurogenic TOS. For patients with distal emboli and compromised circulation in the hand, concomitant dorsal (cervical) sympathectomy has also been advocated [10, 19].

For patients with minimal poststenotic dilation of the subclavian artery, relief of the proximal stenosis without arterial reconstruction is usually sufficient [10]. However, no long-term studies exist that have followed these dilated segments to see if they are prone to later aneurysmal dilation or thrombosis, and it is worth emphasis that surface ulceration and mural thrombus formation can occur even with minimal arterial dilatation. It appears well established that when authentic aneurysmal degeneration of the subclavian artery is present, excision of the affected segment with interposition grafting is required. However, the choice of the optimal conduit for this type of bypass is debatable, and use of both autogenous and prosthetic conduits has been reported. Long-term comparative studies regarding the patency rates of different conduits in patients with arterial TOS is lacking. Extrapolating the data from other anatomical beds, however, it would appear that autogenous conduits would be preferable. It is notable that there is often a size mismatch between the greater saphenous vein (GSV) and the subclavian artery, making reversed GSV a less than ideal choice. Spiral grafts of the GSV may correct the size mismatch, but are often cumbersome and time-consuming to construct. Use of the autogenous iliac artery has been described for subclavian artery repair [20], and other suitable options for bypass graft conduits include the superficial femoral vein or cryopreserved femoropopliteal artery. The use of prosthetic grafts, constructed from either Dacron or polytetrafluoroethylene (PTFE), has also been reported, and these widely used conduits have excellent outcomes in carotid-subclavian bypass procedures for atherosclerosis. At present, the choice of conduit for subclavian artery reconstruction in arterial TOS appears to be largely based on surgeon preference. The use and duration of postoperative anticoagulation is also widely variable among published studies, but for patients with extensive distal embolization who undergo thrombectomy and vascular reconstruction, a significant period of anticoagulation seems advisable.

Research Directions

- Does removal of a cervical rib or other osseous abnormality constitute adequate ATOS decompression? Do first ribs always need to be resected as well?
- What is the most appropriate conduit for subclavian artery aneurysm repair? Autogenous or prosthetic?
- What is the most suitable autogenous conduit for repair of the subclavian artery? Greater saphenous vein, femoral vein, external iliac artery, or cryopreserved femoral artery?
- If autogenous conduits are preferred, is a greater saphenous vein with a significant size mismatch appropriate?
- What is the proper management of distal upper extremity embolization? Open thrombectomy or thrombolysis prior to decompression?
- How soon after thrombolysis should the ATOS decompression procedure be performed? Same admission, or electively?

Outcomes and Follow-Up

The reported results of surgery for arterial TOS reveal excellent or good outcomes in the majority of patients. Following decompression and arterial reconstruction at the thoracic outlet, the status of the distal vasculature plays the most important role in the functional recovery of the patient. Extensive emboli that have led to chronic occlusion of the forearm and hand vessels are often irreversible. Revascularization of the distal

vasculature using thrombolysis or open thrombectomy following thoracic outlet decompression is recommended in this setting, especially in the presence of acute ischemia. Simultaneous dorsal (cervical) sympathectomy has also been recommended by some authors, as a means to optimize microvascular circulation and lower the risk for digital ulceration or tissue loss [10]. A relatively simple classification system has been used by most authors to assess functional outcomes, graded as follows: (1) excellent results characterized by no pain and an easy return to preoperative professional and leisure daily activities; (2) good results with intermittent pain that is well tolerated, and a possible return to preoperative professional and leisure daily activities; (3) fair results with intermittent or permanent pain that is poorly tolerated, as well as a difficult return to preoperative professional and leisure daily activities; and (4) poor results when symptoms are not improved or are aggravated. The reported follow-up regimen for patients undergoing decompression for arterial TOS is unfortunately widely variable. It nonetheless seems prudent that patients undergoing arterial reconstruction for arterial TOS should be followed on a regular basis with physical examination and noninvasive ultrasound assessment of upper extremity circulation, and perhaps intermittent imaging evaluation.

Research Directions

- What is the appropriate medical therapy (anticoagulation, clopidogrel, or aspirin) after ATOS decompression and subclavian artery aneurysm repair? How long should it be continued?
- What is the natural history of a subclavian artery poststenotic dilation after ATOS decompression?
- What is the follow-up regimen of patients after ATOS decompression? How often should they be seen? What diagnostic tests should be ordered?

Conclusion

Arterial TOS is the least frequent but likely most complex form of TOS. The diagnosis and management of these patients is based on the cumulative experience of physicians who have expertise in the care for patients with all forms of TOS. Many clinical questions regarding this condition remain unanswered, yet randomized clinical trials and even satisfactory observational studies are not feasible. The development of an international registry for patients with arterial TOS, along with more uniformly-applied standards for characterizing patients and reporting clinical outcomes, would be an immense step in collecting more useful data to help guide the optimal management of this challenging clinical condition.

References

1. Sanders RJ, Haug C. Review of arterial thoracic outlet syndrome with a report of five new instances. Surg Gynecol Obstet. 1991;173:415–25.
2. Durham JR, Yao JS, Pearce WH, Nuber GM, McCarthy Jr W. Arterial injuries in the thoracic outlet syndrome. J Vasc Surg. 1995;21:57–69.
3. Thompson RW, Driskill MR. Neurovascular problems in the athlete's shoulder. Clin Sports Med. 2008;27: 789–802.
4. Criado E, Berguer R, Greenfield L. The spectrum of arterial compression at the thoracic outlet. J Vasc Surg. 2010;52:406–11.
5. Casbas L, Chauffour X, Cau J, Bossavy JP, Midy D, Baste JC, Barret A. Post-traumatic thoracic outlet syndromes. Ann Vasc Surg. 2005;19:25–8.
6. Sanders RJ, Hammond SL. Management of cervical ribs and anomalous first ribs causing neurogenic thoracic outlet syndrome. J Vasc Surg. 2002;36(1): 51–6.
7. Brewin J, Hill M, Ellis H. The prevalence of cervical ribs in a London population. Clin Anat. 2009;22: 331–6.
8. Dunwayri YM, Emery VB, Driskill MR, Earley JA, Wright RW, Paletta GA Jr, Thompson RW. Positional compression of the axillary artery causing upper extremity thrombosis and embolism in the elite overhead throwing athlete. J Vasc Surg. 2011;53(5): 1329–40.
9. Degeorges R, Reynaud C, Becquemin JP. Thoracic outlet syndrome surgery: long-term functional results. Ann Vasc Surg. 2004;18(5):558–65.
10. Urschel Jr HC, Razzuk MA. Neurovascular compression in the thoracic outlet: changing management over 50 years. Ann Surg. 1998;228:609–17.
11. Jamieson WG, Chinnick B. Thoracic outlet syndrome: fact or fancy? A review of 409 consecutive patients who underwent operation. Can J Surg. 1996;39:321–6.
12. Hempel GK, Shutze WP, Anderson JF, Bukhari HI. 770 consecutive supraclavicular first rib resections for thoracic outlet syndrome. Ann Vasc Surg. 1996;10:456–63.
13. Lindgren SHS, Ribbe EB, Norgren LEH. Two year follow-up of patients operated on for thoracic outlet syndrome: effects on sick-leave incidence. Eur J Vasc Surg. 1989;3:411–5.
14. Thompson JF, Webster JH. First rib resection for vascular complications of thoracic outlet syndrome. Br J Surg. 1990;77:555–7.
15. Wood VE, Twito R, Verska JM. Thoracic outlet syndrome: the results of first rib resection in 100 patients. Orthop Clin North Am. 1988;19:131–46.
16. Kieffer E, Jue-Denis P, Benhamou M, Richard T, Palombo D, Natali J. Arterial complications in the thoracobrachial outlet syndrome: surgical treatment of 38 cases [Article in French]. Chirurgie. 1983;109:714–22.
17. Thompson RW, Petrinec D, Toursarkissian B. Surgical treatment of thoracic outlet compression syndromes. II. Supraclavicular exploration and vascular reconstruction. Ann Vasc Surg. 1997;11:442–51.
18. Tubbs RS, Louis RGJ, Wartmann CT, Lott R, Chua GD, Kelly D, Palmer CA, Shoja MM, Loukas M, Oakes WJ. Histopathological basis for neurogenic thoracic outlet syndrome. J Neurosurg Spine. 2008;8:347–51.
19. Thompson RW. Treatment of thoracic outlet syndromes and cervical sympathectomy. In: Lumley JSP, Siewert JR, Hoballah JJ, editors. Springer surgery atlas series: vascular surgery. London: Springer; 2004.
20. Wylie EJ, Stoney RJ, Ehrenfeld WK, Effeney DJ. Thoracic outlet syndromes. In: Wylie EJ, Stoney RJ, Ehrenfeld WK, Effeney DJ, editors. Comprehensive manuals of surgical specialties, manual of vascular surgery, vol. II. New York: Springer; 1986. p. 249–71.
21. Sanders RJ, Hammond SL, Rao NM. Diagnosis of thoracic outlet syndrome. J Vasc Surg. 2007;46:601–4.

Part XIII

Additional Topics Related to Thoracic Outlet Syndrome

TOS: The Perspective of the Patient

90

Karl A. Illig

Abstract

As all who care for patients with this problem can attest, thoracic outlet syndrome (TOS) is perhaps the best example of a diagnosis that is slow to be made. Symptoms can be obscure and at first mild, many primary care physicians are unfamiliar with the syndrome, and some even doubt its existence. As a result, the diagnosis is frequently delayed by months or even years, and patients are often told that "it's all in your head" in one way or another.

Although this is a textbook for practitioners, we felt that because of these factors hearing about the process directly from patients would be extremely helpful. Practitioners who care for these patients pride themselves on doing the right thing, but this is inevitably after the diagnosis is made. *What does the patient with TOS go through?*

As all who care for patients with this problem can attest, thoracic outlet syndrome (TOS) is perhaps the best example of a diagnosis that is slow to be made. Symptoms can be obscure and at first mild, many primary care physicians are unfamiliar with the syndrome, and some even doubt its existence. As a result, the diagnosis is frequently delayed by months or even years, and patients are often told that "it's all in your head" in one way or another.

Although this is a textbook for practitioners, we felt that because of these factors hearing about the process directly from patients would be extremely helpful. Practitioners who care for these patients pride themselves on doing the right thing, but this is inevitably after the diagnosis is made. *What does the patient with TOS go through?*

Vignette 1: A Motor Vehicle Accident and Physical Therapy

One moment can change your life forever. I was driving a sleek sports car—my first ever—and had stopped for a red traffic light at a city intersection. My mind relaxed, wandered briefly. Presto: the light turned green. My foot pressed the gas. My eyes locked on the road ahead.

K.A. Illig, MD
Department of Surgery, Division of Vascular Surgery,
University of South Florida,
2 Tampa General Circle, STC 7016,
Tampa 33606, FL, USA
e-mail: killig@health.usf.edu

K.A. Illig et al. (eds.), *Thoracic Outlet Syndrome*,
DOI 10.1007/978-1-4471-4366-6_90, © Springer-Verlag London 2013

I didn't see the car that whizzed toward the intersection. I didn't see as it came from the right, a streak of dark green appearing out of nowhere. In seconds, it slammed into the passenger side of my car, bound us together, twirled us around in sickening choreography and then flung us apart. Two thousand pounds of metal and I hadn't seen it—that is, until it was too late.

It took 72 h to realize something wasn't right. No bones were broken; no skin punctured. No, but suddenly the injury became so hellish, so hard to explain—it was here, it was there. Why was sitting so excruciating? Why did turning my head from side to side feel like someone was knifing me in the back and in the chest at the same time? Why did the left side of my face hurt—what the hell was all this *tugging*? People thought I was nuts: *Tugging?*

Over the next few months I understood: everything that used to be pleasurable was now the opposite. *Honey, don't touch my hair—it hurts. Dad—no, please, don't hug me; it hurts. Dinner and a movie—oh, absolutely not.* My idea of a good time involved being prone for 10 min without pain. Hello, thoracic outlet syndrome.

Over the next 5 years, until the syndrome began to abate, pain sought me out. It moved and morphed inside my body, it elongated time. It was crafty and powerful, something, I finally realized, much too complex to be harnessed by the single word *pain*. So I stretched my vocabulary. To name each instance of pain was one small step towards conquering it—or so I believed. I tossed out "hurt." In its place came replacements: seared, throbbed, ached, and burned, *shattering*. One pain was so fast and sharp it crackled through my arm: only the metaphor of an electrical shock would do.

Here's what I know now: Thoracic outlet syndrome is essentially a disorder of nerve compression. It creates a symphony of responses in the body—that's a polite way to say you never know when the pain is going to land or even where the pain's going to hit. It might center with singular precision or spray, like machine-guy fire, with wild abandon. Oh, what a tangled web. You've got nerves that run through your neck and chest, pass through the space above the collarbone, ride into your arm, reach below your shoulder bone, for example. Offshoots from these nerves turn

backwards to the spine, greedily including the neck and head in front, the shoulder blades in back, and downward, into chest and breast. And each nerve has the ability to cause exquisite pain.

Activities of daily life (ADL's), those benign tasks that include getting dressed, changing sheets, shampooing hair, washing dishes, vacuuming the carpet, shopping for groceries—these were my enemies. I hated ADL's; they had to be done and yet were my downfall, causing my symptoms to flare wildly. Driving was one of the worst triggers. Turning the steering wheel, swiveling my head during a routine parallel park, bouncing—ouch—over a pothole, each caused pain to rip through me.

I was eventually referred to a physical therapist who initiated the ENVEST protocol that taught me how to heal myself. Life moved forward, bit by bit. The ENVEST protocol was working. My daughter, three at the time of my accident, turned four, then five, then six. At some point, I decided not to look back. No, I'd never ice skate again, nor jog 4 miles, nor swim a mile three times a week. I'd never write a book, as I had done before. But I could take a walk with my kid. I could take on short writing assignments. I bought voice recognition software, to save my hands and arms and chest even, from the distal impacts of tapping the keyboard. I bought a standing workstation so I could work without sitting down. I committed to a mantra: forward motion. I asked for help with things large and small: "Hey—could you unscrew the lid from that jar for me?"

Fast forward to today. I wake up without pain. I go to sleep without pain. I drive (with a steering wheel redesigned especially for those with a disability) all over town. I walk almost 4 miles a day. I swim—slowly, yes, and not nearly as far as I used to—in a warm (92°) pool for the disabled. I do my own grocery shopping. I cook.

Vignette 2: Repetitive Data Entry and Physical Therapy

There is hope. I suffered with shooting pains in my arms for the past 7 years. Over the last year it crept up into my chest and right armpit and shoulder and I was diagnosed with Thoracic Outlet Syndrome

(TOS). I laid on the floor at work and cried every night at home. With physical therapy guidance I am 95 % better. I still have flare-ups and it is not smart for me to sit for periods of more than an hour. I now know what to do to help myself get better and I'm not in fear. My break through came New Year's Eve 2010 weekend – the extreme chronic *pain* transitioned into *discomfort* and *sensation.*

Here are some observations taken from my experience:

- It is important to stay within the boundaries of the exercises that were given to me. I am tempted to do more – to push – but that is not the way to healing. More is not better. Stay in the range where exercises *feel good.*
- Thinker Pose is KEY. This is what led to my breakthrough on New Year's Eve. I thought this was a silly exercise. Once I finally started doing it all the time, I was 50 % better in 1 week. I still do it when I get up from sitting, get up from the toilet, open doors, carry bags and get out of the car.
- Do breathing exercises slowly and pay gentle attention. I slow down until I feel the swampy feeling in my shoulder move and let go. I begin to feel the shoulder-joint area loosen. I breathe and rock the pelvis until I feel the swampiness loosen in my shoulder and it begins to creak and move.
- I'm always aware of dropping my breath into my lower belly when walking. This gets it out of my chest where tension can build.
- For me, doing two sets of breathing/walking/breathing per day worked. So that would be an hour's worth of physical therapy twice per day. One set before lunch and one before dinner. The trio of breathe/walk/breath allowed things to loosen up more with the second breathe session each time.
- Hot baths help relax everything.
- Stay warm, especially in chest area.
- Make the floor your friend. I lay flat on my back a lot.
- Download and relax to Scott Gauthier's *Welcome to Earth.* Guided relaxation. AMAZING.
- Thermacare heat packs (buy at drugstore) can be stuck to the chest and worn all day.
- Main thing that changed everything was doing the Thinker Pose with my strong arm and

using the weak arm to reach in the cupboard, slip on shoes, open a drawer, push a door, and pick up anything.
- Let people help you.
- Move slower. I don't do any sudden movements. I move throughout the house more gently. Jerky movements inflame my pain.
- Sleeping: When sleeping on my back I prop up my Right shoulder (injured shoulder) with a pillow so there is no gravity pulling down on it. When sleeping on my side, I sleep on my Left side. I pile two big pillows on top of each other and hug them so my right arm is draped over them, parallel to the bed, propped up high.
- Work: I changed my career so that I don't have to sit in front of a computer all day. I decided to leave to pursue a career in teaching high school.
- It is hard for me to get on the floor sometimes but once I'm there the exercises feel so good. At first they didn't feel like anything. Now I love them.
- Stand and sway or lay on the floor. Do as little sitting as possible.
- Do exactly what protocols say to do. It will work. I had to suspend my disbelief because all the exercises seemed like they couldn't possibly do anything.
- Do not assume that because you completed an exercise on 1 day, you can do it without pain on the next day.
- You must do the exercises mindfully and incrementally to determine if they are causing pain. Rushing through them can cause a setback.
- Working Too Hard to Progress: Just because you are not progressing to the next exercise, it does not mean the pain will stay longer. Much relief can be had from the simple breathing exercises, the thinker pose, and the adjustment to your daily living.
- Do not try to force yourself through each stage of the exercises hoping to get to the next one. If you feel pain, any pain, stop. It might be that you even need to skip or modify an exercise because you are not able to do it without pain. Work with the physical therapist closely to determine what works for you.

- Don't Say I Can't: I always say pain is a great motivator. Yes, the exercises take up quite a bit of time, especially in the beginning. As you begin to work them into your day you will learn to do them more efficiently.

Vignette #3: Venous TOS and Surgery

I could always click my clavicles as a child. The loud crunching sound made by my clavicles caused my parents significant distress. We sought the medical advice of pediatricians, pediatric orthopedists, and orthopedists. Each physician reassured us there was nothing wrong. I noticed as a teenager my arms, specifically by biceps and deltoids, were large for my small frame. During my freshman year of college, I threw a heavy tote-bag over by left arm and immediately experienced shooting, electric-like pain throughout my left arm. Eager to stay at school, I ignored the numbness, low-grade throbbing, and swelling in my arm for several days. When my parents visited me 4 days later my dad, a physician, commented on the large size and firmness of my left arm. An abnormal spider vein in my left arm led my father to suspect I had Paget-Schroetter syndrome, but my lack of other symptoms like hand swelling and arm discoloration made him uncertain of this diagnosis. Again, determined to remain at school I dismissed my father's concern.

Unconvinced by my reassurances, my father decided to ultrasound my left arm the following day. With his diagnosis of Paget-Schroetter syndrome confirmed by the ultrasound I went to the hospital where I had a venogram—yet another confirmation of the diagnosis. Subsequently, I underwent a balloon dilation of the occluded subclavian vein which failed. I then received 24 h of catheter directed thrombolysis followed by repeat balloon dilation; both of which failed. My physicians advised that I have a rib resection. Both the surgery and a postoperative balloon dilation attempt failed to open the occluded vein. At this point in time, I was discharged from the hospital. Over a 12 month span, the swelling slightly decreased in my left arm. Eighteen months later I have several prominent, non-bulging veins that can see by the naked eye. Based on my experience, I highly recommend patients with TOS make sure their physicians are well educated about this diagnosis.

Vignette #4: Bilateral VTOS and Secondary NTOS and Surgery

I was diagnosed with bilateral venous thoracic outlet syndrome. I underwent urgent surgery on my left side, and 3 months later I elected to have surgery on my right side. My postoperative experiences significantly differed.

After undergoing an urgent rib resection on my left side, which failed to open the occluded vein, I developed increasing electric-like pain in my arm and back over the next 6 months. Three months after my first emergent surgery I had an elective rib resection on my right side for VTOS. Immediately postoperatively I experienced high levels of pain which necessitated that I take prescription pain medication for 3 weeks. Within a day postoperatively, however, I began moving the arm and performing nerve glides. I performed these nerve glides three times a day for the first 6 months, and 18 months later I still perform these stretches twice a day. These simple exercises significantly increase arm and shoulder mobility and dramatically reduce nerve pain. When my pain from the right-sided elective surgery started to taper off 4 months after the operation, I suspected the intensifying pain on my left side was abnormal. I decided to seek a second opinion when I realized my decision to defer my spring semester of college was based on the continued postoperative pain from the earlier surgery (left) rather than the postoperative pain from the second surgery (right).

Based on my symptoms, which comprised of severe, electric-like shocks radiating throughout my arm and back, my second opinion physician suggested that the problem was secondary NTOS due to scar tissue formation and perhaps inadequate rib resection and that I have a reoperation. Eager to try any remedy that would provide me with enough relief to sleep at night and function during the day, I agreed. Postoperatively, the surgeon noted the rib and cartilage had grown back, and the vein still remained occluded. Immediately after surgery the severe electric-like pain in my arm and back significantly decreased. My pain levels from the surgery required that I remain on prescription pain medications for approximately 3 weeks. After the 3 week period, I took and still continue to take non-opiate prescription and non-prescription anti-inflammatory medications. A day after the surgery, however, I again started nerve glides twice a day, and I still a year later perform nerve glides twice daily. My pain levels were significantly reduced postoperatively to the extent that I could return full time to college. I experienced and still experience, 12 months after surgery, electric-like pain in my back and arm along with general muscle pain and inflammation. To help alleviate some of the nerve pain, I apply a lidoderm patch nightly to the symptomatic area. I also go for weekly massage appointments and apply heat to the symptomatic areas; both treatments seem to significantly reduce the muscle pain. I experienced and am still continuing to experience the most promising gains from acupuncture. I started treatment 8 months postoperatively. After three treatments the swelling in my left arm significantly reduced, and now both arms look nearly identical. Some 3 months after starting acupuncture, the nerve pain in my arm and back has significantly reduced. And, overall my mobility has dramatically increased. In my opinion, clinicians should encourage their patients to try nerve glides and acupuncture because I personally derived great benefits from both.

Vignette #5: Recurrent NTOS (in a Physician)

In 2005, I began experiencing pain and numbness in my left hand when operating. An EMG ruled out carpel tunnel syndrome, but a MRI revealed a small C6–C7 disk protrusion. The physicians thought this was the etiology of my pain and I was treated with multiple spinal steroid injections. As my symptoms progressed, it increasingly affected my clinical abilities. Unsure if my

diagnosis was correct, I went to a tertiary care center where I was diagnosed with bilateral NTOS. I underwent an unsuccessful first rib resection on my left side followed by an equally unsuccessful anterior scalenectomy.

By this time, my pain and numbness had progressed where I was no longer able to perform surgery or clinic work that required my arms to be elevated. I was forced to close my practice. Over the next 4 years, my symptoms and quality of life worsened. I contacted my previous surgeon at the Mayo Clinic and inquired about trying the surgery on my right side. The response was no, since the previous surgery had not worked on the left.

I then started researching other physicians that were doing work in TOS and sought a "third opinion." After an evaluation and review of the previous surgery, this surgeon agreed to perform surgery on my right side. He performed a right first rib resection, full anterior and middle scalenectomy, and pectoralis minor tenotomy. Within a couple of months, I could see a clear improvement. I returned 3 months later and repeated the surgery on the left side, and continued aggressive physical and occupational therapy over the next year. By Sept of 2011, I was able to return to my practice of obstetrics and gynecology with no restrictions. I am very grateful to this surgeon and his team for their willingness to try other procedures and for restoring my ability to practice medicine, and want to emphasize the critical importance of seeking care from a team that concentrates on this disorder and ensuring that when surgery is performed it is proper and complete.

Vignette #6: An NTOS Journey

The phone call from my physiatrist was abrupt – "The good news is that you don't have a blood clot; the bad news is that I'm pretty sure you have Neurogenic Thoracic Outlet Syndrome." My heart sank-- I knew it was a difficult diagnosis already, having spent 3 years, with three physicians, undergoing a myriad of exams and tests; and I also knew how difficult of a condition it was to treat. Already having been in physical therapy under his care, my physiatrist went on to tell me that he really didn't have any resources for me to consult and that most times when he made a surgical referral, the physician on the receiving end would run the other way to avoid a TOS patient. Continued PT was his recommended protocol; he didn't know of anyone in my metropolitan area that he'd trust with my case. How could that be– with all of the renowned area hospitals and two world-class medical schools, was there no one here who could help me?

So, I did what most people do– I went right to the internet. If you have seen a patient with TOS, you know we are a desperate, and consequently resourceful group. We spend hours on the internet, we pore over published papers, we dwell on websites and blogs with information and case studies, and we search for the best physician teams in the country. I visited the websites of every hospital organization in my state looking for a specialist, but to no avail. One specialist was identified and excitedly e-mailed, but was found to be comfortably retired with no one having taken over this portion of his practice. Through our e-mail engagement, however, he found me a referral, and when I began to do my research I felt like I had found the Holy Grail I had been seeking.

I can trace my symptoms back to 2006, starting with pain in my right wrist, forearm and elbow. My PCP suspected carpal tunnel syndrome, but all of the neurological tests were normal. Possibly tendonitis? A few rounds of steroids improved the situation temporarily. Then blow-drying my hair or holding a telephone caused my arm to ache and feel as heavy as a boulder. I have been a fitness fanatic my whole life, and had recently changed my workouts to include rowing and aggressive yoga practices with repeated plank poses, push-ups and hand stands. We surmised that the new symptoms had something to do with this new regimen, so I abandoned these forms of exercise. Over the next year or so, these new symptoms would not subside, and progressed to a constant dull pain on the right side of my neck and upper back. By this time, I had a cadre of professionals lined up to help deal with these distressing symptoms– I had a chiropractor, accu-

puncturist, massage therapist, and a Reiki practitioner. I was spending about $100 per week on all of these pain management techniques!

In 2009 I became desperate for a diagnosis and treatment. I was quite frightened when now my right hand would turn cold to the touch, and change to a mottled pink color when I would partake in various activities, especially using my computer every day. Arms at my side– pink and tingly right hand; arms extended at a keyboard– cold right hand; arms overhead– ache in right arm; and still the persistent pain in the neck. I couldn't even tell the temperature of my son's bath water with my hand. I began working with a physiatrist who suspected TOS after his first clinical exam. An MRI of my neck and C-spine showed no abnormalities, so he prescribed PT. Unfortunately, this resulted in no improvement and even a worsening of the symptoms. The physician found a new PT to work with who supposedly had experience with the condition– but that was no better. Then more MRIs and a dynamic arterial Doppler test led to the phone call mentioned above.

That's when my search for a knowledgeable physician led me to the right place in 2010. I assembled a binder that captured the 4 years of my journey– test results, PT reports, dictated physician office visit notes, and even my own symptom log. During our first visit, I knew I had found the right physician who had expertise in the condition, and the understanding of what I had endured to bring me to travel 600 miles to find him. He made the diagnosis of NTOS, and with information from a scalene muscle block, believed that both my anterior scalene and pectoralis minor muscles were involved. We agreed to try more PT with coordinated care through the TOS specialists at his center. After a year of minimal improvement, we again conferred and weighed the options of full decompression surgery vs. isolated pectoralis minor tenotomy (PMT). After discussing success rates and recovery times, I decided that PMT alone was the option I wanted to pursue as a next step, and in June, 2011, this was done. The surgery went as planned and I remain in physical therapy now 4 months later.

I wish I could report a full recovery from all of my NTOS symptoms. The pain in the right side of my neck has been significantly reduced and my hand no longer turns pink; however, the intolerable cold right hand and achy upper arm symptoms are still with me. Also, new symptoms are present now– numbness during the night that wakes me up from sleep and periodic paresthesias during the day. Most upsetting is that I now have symptoms on my left side, which were likely masked due to the magnitude of the right-sided problem– and I do have bilateral cervical ribs. I have no regrets in my decision to undergo the PMT as a first step, but am now at a crossroads: Do I accept these distressing symptoms that interfere with my daily life as my "new normal", or do I undergo a full decompression surgery and hope for a full recovery? As crazy as it sounds, I have found myself wishing my condition had presented as venous TOS– then there would have been a clear decision to operate further.

Thinking back over the past 5 years, I can give you countless examples of how my life has changed due to my NTOS. I think you have an idea of the time, money and resources I have invested into my treatment. I am an executive at a Fortune 500 company and I avoid business travel as best I can, because I know that pulling my briefcase or suitcase on wheels through an airport will cause a flare-up of symptoms. I use a heating pad or ice pack at least a few times each week before bed. Riding a bike with my 9-year old son is very painful, and I can no longer throw around a baseball with him or join him in bowling. I spend time wondering if this condition will degenerate even further and impact the use of my arms. I worry that I won't be able to hold a grandchild because my arms will ache, and I am concerned that my condition will continue to degenerate and that I will possibly suffer from permanent nerve damage.

Is my condition terminal? Absolutely not: I know there are many more consequential diagnoses I could have than NTOS. Unfortunately, the symptoms, the unpredictability of whether each day is going to be a "good day" or a "bad day", and the sheer pain and discomfort are with me every single day and serve as constant reminders of this chronic, difficult condition.

Nerve and Arterial Injury After First Rib Resection

91

William H. Pearce

Abstract

Surgery for Thoracic Outlet Syndrome (TOS) is associated with potential injuries. The thoracic inlet, where surgery for neurogenic, venous, and arterial TOS is performed, is a compact anatomic region containing the brachial plexus, phrenic nerve, long thoracic nerve, subclavian vein and artery, and pleura of the lung. The nature of injury is often related to the specific operation performed, and neurovascular injuries following thoracic outlet decompression are much more likely to result in disability than such an injury in the lower extremity. Paramount to preventing injuries to the neurovascular bundle of the upper extremity and associated structures is a thorough understanding of the region's anatomy along with knowledge of common and uncommon variants.

Introduction

Surgery for Thoracic Outlet Syndrome (TOS) is fraught with potential for injury to critical structures. The thoracic outlet, where surgery for neurogenic, venous, and arterial TOS is performed, is a compact anatomic region containing the brachial plexus, phrenic nerve, long thoracic nerve, subclavian vein and artery, and pleura of the lung. Pneumothoraces are the most common complication, and hardly avoidable as the pleura forms the posterior surface of the rib and is open during rib resection [1]. However, injury to any of the other structures may occur during thoracic outlet decompression and can often be associated with significant morbidity. The nature of injury is often related to the specific operation performed.

Neurovascular injuries following thoracic outlet decompression are much more likely to result in disability than such an injury in the lower extremity. Femoral nerve paralysis, for example, may simply prevent extension of the knee joint, and a peroneal nerve injury is well treated with bracing. If an upper extremity nerve injury does occur, however, particularly to the brachial plexus, substantial implications follow because the use of the hand is so important. Morbidity is also greater because exposure is more difficult – while access to proximal arteries in the lower extremities is easily accomplished using a

W.H. Pearce, MD
Department of Surgery, Division of Vascular Surgery,
Feinberg School of Medicine, Northwestern University,
676 North St. Clair, Suite 650, Chicago, IL 60611, USA
e-mail: wpearce@nmh.org

retroperitoneal approach, for example, upper extremity vascular access can require median sternotomy, a trap door incision, or even claviculectomy. Paramount to preventing injuries to the neurovascular bundle of the upper extremity and associated structures is a thorough understanding of the region's anatomy obtained through high quality imaging, along with knowledge of common and uncommon variants. This chapter will review the available literature and current recommendations for nerve and vascular injuries which occur during surgery for the TOS.

Nerve Injuries

Irrespective of the surgical approach – transaxillary, supraclavicular, or any combination thereof, the overall risk of nerve injuries is similar, ranging from 0 to 2 % for phrenic and long thoracic nerve injures but higher for brachial plexus and perhaps when scalenectomy is performed (Table 91.1) [2–5].

Interestingly, there is no clear evidence that neurovascular injuries are specific to the experience or training of the surgeon, and even experienced and well trained surgeons may have one or more of these complications. This is probably due in part to the anatomic variability common in this region. Roos described the fibrous bands and muscle abnormalities that may occur in the region as normal variants [6]. Perhaps the most concerning anatomic variability is in the brachial plexus

itself, nicely described by Tibbs and colleagues [7, 8]. The brachial plexus classically is made up of the C5 to T1 nerve roots. However, the brachial plexus may be "prefixed," meaning it has a large C4 and small T1 contribution, or "postfixed," meaning a small contribution from C5 and a large contribution from T2 – in other words, it may be either more proximal or more distal on the axial spinal column. In a patient with a postfixed brachial plexus (large contribution from T2), for example, excessive traction or inadvertent dissection may result in damage to this structure. The brachial plexus is also further affected by abnormalities within the cervical spine as well as by variable interdigitations of nerve fibers within the brachial plexus itself. In fact, the traditional dermatome distribution described in many anatomy texts is only a rough guide to the high degree of variabilities seen in the brachial plexus [8].

Nerve injuries can occur as the result of either traction or transection. Traction injuries may occur during transaxillary exposure as the result of excessive force placed on the arm, or during supraclavicular exposure as the result of nerve retraction. There is a higher preponderance of phrenic nerve injuries with a supraclavicular approach as one would expect. There appears to be a similar distribution in brachial plexus injuries between the two approaches, however (Table 91.1). The long thoracic nerve may be injured during either supraclavicular or transaxillary exposure. As encountered during supraclavicular exposure, the long thoracic nerve

Table 91.1 Complications associated with thoracic outlet surgery: a comparison of different procedures

Injury	Author	Operation transaxillary	Anterior/middle scalenectomy	Supraclavicular first rib resection
Plexus	Sanders	2.7 %		2.5 %
	Sharp	3.5 %		37.5 % (small series)
	Leffert	12		
	Chang (NIS)	0.6 %		
Phrenic	Sanders	0.9 %	6 %	2.2 %
	Axelrod			0.6 %
Long Thoracic	Sanders	0	0	0.4
Arterial	Sanders	0	0	0.4
Venous	Sanders	2	1.4	1.1 %
"Vascular"	Chang (NIS)	1.74 %		
Pneumothorax	Sanders	9 %	0.4 %	2.5 %

emerges from the middle scalene, where it is vulnerable during dissection of this muscle and exposure of the rib, and courses laterally. The nerve then passes along the thoracic wall and can be seen and injured during a dissection of the first rib in the transaxillary approach. In most instances, this results in winging of the scapula that is of little consequence, and if injury is due to traction, it often resolves with time. However, the lack of stability in the shoulder joint may produce abnormalities in other muscle groups and create new symptoms, and the winging itself may cause significant disability in a person whose vocation or avocation requires use of the arms over the level of the shoulders.

It should be noted that nerve injuries described in the literature are almost always self-reported by the operative surgeon and not by an unbiased observer. Cherington described five patients who underwent thoracic outlet surgery and were seen independently by the author [9]. All five had clear evidence of injury to the brachial plexus with the ulnar nerve being predominantly affected. In two other cases, the patients suffered significant postsurgical complex regional pain syndrome (CRPS), and one also experienced substantial hemorrhage during the operative procedure. While this is in no way an unbiased sample, it is probably safe to say that the literature probably provides an underestimate of the true incidence of nerve injuries. In a recent retrospective review of the Nationwide Inpatient Sample Database (sampling cases from 1993 to 2003) Chang found that of a total of 2,016 cases, 12 patients (0.6 %) suffered brachial plexus injuries and 35 (1.74 %) vascular injuries [10]. There was no difference between teaching and nonteaching hospitals for brachial plexus injury.

The management of nerve injuries is evolving [11–15]. Microsurgical techniques have evolved to the point where distal nerve transfers are more effective than reconstruction of a brachial plexus injury. Nerve regrowth is 1–1.5 mm/day, but unfortunately the motor endplates may degenerate before the nerve completely regrows (12–18 months). Furthermore, if too much time has elapsed from the injury to the time of referral the endplate may have degenerated. Direct nerve repair is thus only recommended if regrowth of the nerve is anticipated to occur before motor endplate degeneration. For laceration injuries, direct repair or grafting may be performed. For traction injuries, observation for at least 3 months is recommended since many such problems will resolve spontaneously [12, 15]. For all these reasons, while repair can be attempted at the initial surgery, it is better to observe the patient's recovery and then to perform a peripheral nerve transfer if a permanent problem is present. By the same token, it is critically important not to wait beyond the time in which the muscle so deteriorates that reintervention is of little effect.

EMGs should be performed at 3 and 5 months. If nerve recovery does not occur at 5 months, peripheral nerve transfer should be performed prior to atrophy of the neuromuscular junctions. Nerve grafts have been performed in proximal lesions, but again because of the long distance of nerve regeneration required they have been less successful than nerve transfers. In patients in whom the injury is delayed beyond 6 months in which there is no chance for nerve transfers to be effective tendon transfers may improve upper extremity function. The most important factor regarding upper extremity function is flexion at the elbow joint and some apposition of the digits.

Vascular Injuries

Vascular injuries during thoracic outlet surgery are rarely reported, both because of their rarity but also probably because they are simply fixed at that time. In addition, there is little long-term data on outcomes associated with these proximal injuries. Finally, many neurologic injuries probably occur as the "result" of a vascular injury as inadvertent clamping of nerves may occur during attempts to control excessive bleeding.

In Changs NIS analysis, vascular injuries occurred in 1.74 % of cases, and, in contrast to nerve injuries, occurred at a higher rate nonteaching (2.69 %) versus teaching (1.34 %) hospitals (p=0.03). The nature of each injury was obviously unknown [10]. Sanders found that venous injuries occur more commonly during transaxillary exposure (2 %) versus scalenectomy or supraclavicular first rib excision (0.4 and 1.1 % respectively) [3]. Most vascular injuries are associated with avulsion of side branches with traction, and are simply managed by clipping or suture repair. Such side branch arteries include the thyrocervical or costocervical artery branches of the subclavian artery, or the superior or lateral thoracic artery branches of the axillary artery, and even ligation carries with it no clinical consequence. Venous tributaries of the axillary and subclavian veins may similarly be injured and are best treated with packing and suture ligation. Because of the limited visibility during transaxillary rib exposure and the use of very large instruments such as a right angle rib cutter, "past-pointing" may occur beyond the rib leading to vessel injury. For this reason, many surgeons have opted to use Kerrison rongeurs or another mechanism to increase visibility (endoscopes) and take every action to protect the vascular structures. Venous vascular injuries which occur at the costoclavicular junction may be difficult to control depending upon the exposure. Transaxillary exposures are the most difficult and may require the patient's wound be packed and placed in the supine position for an anterior approach. The reader is cautioned that an infraclavicular approach does not usually allow exposure proximal enough to repair such an injury, and a supraclavicular approach is likely best.

Comment

The patient should be made aware of these potential complications prior to surgery for TOS. Because of the catastrophic nature of these injuries, the patient will certainly have disability, because of the critical function of the hand in daily living. It also appears that the upper extremity may be more prone to complex regional pain syndrome than the lower extremity (See Chap. 92) and this will also be severely debilitating. A clear understanding of the operative field and its potential abnormalities will help prevent some of these injuries. However, even in the most experienced hands these injuries occur, either due to mild traction on the nerves, postoperative bleeding, anatomic variability, or other as yet unknown factors.

References

1. Barbalat ES, Pearce WH. Thoracic outlet syndrome—Which way to go? In: Eskandari MK, Morasch MD, Pearce WH, Yao JST, editors. Vascular surgery: therapeutic strategies. Shelton: People's Medical Publishing House; 2010.
2. Axelrod DA, Proctor MC, Geisser ME, et al. Outcomes after surgery for thoracic outlet syndrome. J Vasc Surg. 2001;33:1220–5.
3. Sanders RJ, Pearce WH. The treatment of thoracic outlet syndrome: a comparison of different operations. J Vasc Surg. 1989;10:626–34.
4. Sharp WJ, Nowak LR, Zamani T. Long-term follow-up and patients' satisfaction after surgery or thoracic outlet syndrome. Ann Vasc Surg. 2001;15:32–6.
5. Leffert RD, Perlmutter GS. Thoracic outlet syndrome. Results of 282 transaxillary first rib resections. Clin Orthop. 1999;368:66–79.
6. Roos DB. Congenital anomalies associated with thoracic outlet syndrome. Anatomy, symptoms, diagnosis, and treatment. Am J Surg. 1976;132:771–8.
7. Loukas M, Tubbs RS, Stewart D. An abnormal variation of the brachial plexus with potential clinical significance. West Indian Med J. 2008;57:403–5.
8. Pellerin M, Kimball Z, Tubbs RS, et al. The prefixed and postfixed brachial plexus: a review with surgical implications. Surg Radiol Anat. 2010;32:251–60.
9. Cherington M, Happer I, Machanic B, et al. Surgery for thoracic outlet syndrome may be hazardous to your health. Muscle Nerve. 1986;9:632–4.
10. Chang DC, Lidor AO, Matsen LS. Reported in-hospital complications following rib resections for neurogenic thoracic outlet syndrome. Ann Vasc Surg. 2007;21:564–70.
11. Cardenas-Mejia A, O'Boyle CP, Chen K-T, et al. Evaluation of single-, double-, and Triple-nerve transfers for shoulder abduction in 90 patients with supraclavicular brachial plexus injury. Plast Reconstr Surg. 2008;122:1470–8.
12. Schessler MJ, McClellan WT. The role of nerve transfers for C5-C6 brachial plexus injury in adults. W V Med J. 2010;106:12–7.
13. Colbert SH, Mackinnon SE. Nerve transfers for brachial plexus reconstruction. Hand Clin. 2008;24:341–61.
14. Kozin SH. Nerve transfers in brachial plexus birth palsies: indications, techniques, and outcomes. Hand Clin. 2008;24:363–76.
15. Mackinnon SE, Colbert SH. Nerve transfers in the hand and upper extremity surgery. Tech Hand Up Extrem Surg. 2008;12:20–33.

Postoperative Complex Regional Pain Syndrome

Rahul Rastogi

Abstract

Complex regional pain syndrome (CRPS) is a complex, multifaceted, disabling and disproportionate spectrum of pain, vasomotor, sudomotor and trophic changes resulting from surgical or traumatic injury. There is some evidence that CRPS may play a primary role in thoracic outlet syndrome (TOS) patients, but because surgery is so often provided as a treatment for TOS there is an increased overall risk of development of CRPS in this patient group to start with. The pathophysiology of CRPS involves peripheral neurogenic inflammation and an intricate interaction of peripheral and central mechanisms involving the somatosensory, somatomotor and autonomic nervous systems. Due to lack of a specific diagnostic test, diagnosis remains clinical and laboratory tests supportive. Clinical diagnosis is made by the presence of sensory, vasomotor, sudomotor, and motor/trophic symptoms and signs as defined by the "Budapest criteria". Treatment is challenging and a comprehensive approach including education, prevention, rehabilitation, psychotherapy, pharmacotherapy, and interventional modality seems logical. Early diagnosis, treatment and preemptive measures in high-risk patients are critical.

Introduction

Complex regional pain syndrome (CRPS) is a complex, multifactorial, disproportionately debilitating condition associated with pain and sensorimotor and autonomic dysfunction that arises after traumatic or surgical injury [1].

Patients often present with localized peripheral inflammatory changes that variably progress to a systemic condition. TOS and CRPS co-exist; the relationship between the two is inconsistent and poorly described [2].

Since its first description in 1864 by Mitchell [3], multiple terms have been used to describe this condition: Sudeck's atrophy, algoneurodystrophy, reflex sympathetic dystrophy (RSD), reflex neurovascular dystrophy, causalgia, and sympathetic maintained pain, to name several. In 1994 the International Association for the study of Pain (IASP) accepted the term CRPS

R. Rastogi, MD
Department of Anesthesiology, Washington University School of Medicine, 660 S. Euclid, Box 8054, St. Louis, MO 63110, USA
e-mail: rastogir@anest.wustl.edu

to replace this older, sometimes confusing terminology. CRPS is further divided into two subgroups – CRPS 1 for symptoms without identifiable nerve injury (replacing RSD) and CRPS 2 where pain is associated with specific nerve injury (replacing causalgia). Although they differ according to the inciting event, both subgroups of CRPS have a similar clinical presentation [3].

Epidemiology of CRPS

The overall incidence and prevalence of CRPS after traumatic or surgical injury is extremely variable, ranging from 5 to 26 % [4, 5]. The majority of these patients' symptoms resolve spontaneously in the first few months [5], although a subset of patients experience persistent symptoms. It affects females more than males, with ratios in the range of 2:1–4:1 [4]. CRPS often initially involves a single extremity (usually upper [5]), but can later spread to other body parts. Interestingly, while spontaneous spread to a contralateral (53 %) or ipsilateral extremity (32 %) occurs, diagonal spread is almost always secondary to new trauma [6]. It affects all ages, but patients with spontaneous onset and familial predisposition tend to be younger in age with severe disease phenotype [7]. Overall recurrence rate of CRPS is 1.8 % per patient per year [8].

The post-surgical incidence of CRPS is not clearly known, but ranges from 2 to 14 % after various procedures [9–11]. By contrast, the recurrence rate of CRPS in patients who require repeat surgery at the same anatomic site can be as high as 70 % [5], but can be reduced by utilization of preemptive sympathetic blockade [12].

Clinical Features of CRPS

CRPS is a progressive painful disease with intensity disproportionate to the causative injury. It presents in one of three clinical stages:
- Stage 1, Sudomotor changes: color and temperature changes, increase sweating, restricted mobility (hours to weeks).
- Stage 2, Vasomotor changes: edema, stiffness, osteoporosis, diminishing regional hair and nail growth, tremors and weakness (weeks to months).
- Stage 3, Trophic changes: significant muscle atrophy, loss of mobility, osteoporosis, and regional deformity from muscle contractures. It is an irreversible stage (months to years [13]).

Although CRPS is a progressive disease, after 1 year most of the signs and symptoms are well developed and progression is only moderate despite increasing disease duration [5].

Pathophysiology of CRPS

The etiology and pathophysiology of CRPS are unclear. Several factors correlate with CRPS including trauma, sprain, surgical procedures, burns, and even venipuncture. More "passive" conditions such as stroke, tumors, multiple sclerosis, an infection involving nerves, seizures, spinal degenerative disease, herpetic zoster, barbiturate use, and anti-tuberculosis drugs also seem to be associated with CRPS. In approximately 10 % patients the cause of CRPS remains unknown [14].

Several mechanisms have been proposed for the development of CRPS, which can be broadly understood by assigning them to peripheral, or central/sympathetic categories.

Peripheral mechanisms are responsible for peripheral sensitization and tissue ischemic-reperfusion injury [15]. Peripheral injury resulting in neurogenic and peripheral tissue inflammation is a hallmark of CRPS, evidenced by presence of pro-inflammatory cytokines and neuro-specific neuropeptides in CRPS blister fluid analysis. There is also peripheral sympathetic overactivity through increased adrenoceptor hypersensitivity and sprouting of newer sympathetic connection in the dermis [4]. These peripheral changes cause stimulation and sensitization of nociceptors which results in ectopic firing activity, leading to so-called "peripheral sensitization".

Central/sympathetic mechanisms are felt to arise as the result of constant input from the periphery to the spinal cord which leads to release of neuropeptides at the dorsal horn. Sympathetic overdrive occurs as the result of sprouting of sympathetic nerve fibers. These make new neural connections in the dorsal horn resulting in "central sensitization" through involvement of Neurokinin-1 and N-methyl-D-aspartate (NMDA) receptors [16]. The continuous barrage of signals from the periphery and to the cortex results in alteration in sensory-discriminative (abnormal referred sensations, distorted body perception), affective-motivational (impaired learning, emotional changes, motor dysfunction from fear) and somatosensory cortical reorganization (decrease representation of affected limb) [3].

These mechanisms, operating in tandem, result in excessive peripheral vasoconstriction and produce a state of oxidative stress in the form of decreased tissue oxygenation, local acidosis, and release of free radicals. Oxidative stress in presence of an endothelial nitric oxide (vasodilator) and endlthelin-1 (vasoconstrictor) imbalance accelerates the cascade of micro-vascular ischemia- reperfusion injury cascade to produce progressive CRPS symptoms [4, 15].

Finally, genetic factors are associated with increased risk of CRPS, suggesting further mechanistic possibilities. Various studies show polymorphism of pro-inflammatory mediator genes in CRPS patients, including TNFα promoter genes, human leucocytes antigens (HLA), acetyl cholinesterase (ACE) I/D genes, and alpha 1a-adrenoceptors genes [4, 17].

Diagnosis

The diagnosis of CRPS is essentially clinical, and is based upon extensive history and physical examination. Various laboratory tests are largely supportive but not conclusive [14]. Currently used diagnostic criteria were proposed through a consensus symposium in 2005 at Budapest [18], described in Table 92.1 ("Budapest criteria"). Clinical examination includes a detailed patient history focusing on inciting events and nature of symptoms and a comprehensive physical examination focused on detailed neurological

Table 92.1 Diagnostic criteria for complex regional pain syndrome

1. Continuing pain, disproportionate to inciting injury	
2. There is no other diagnosis that explains the signs and symptoms	
3. Must have at least one SYMPTOM in three of the four categories	
Sensory	Hyperesthesia and/or allodynia
Vasomotor	Temperature asymmetry and/or skin color changes and/or skin color asymmetry
Sudomotor	Edema and/or sweating changes and/or sweating asymmetry
Motor/trophic	Decreased range of motion and/or motor dysfunction (weakness, tremor, dystonia) and/or trophic changes (hair, nail, skin)
4. Must have at least one SIGN at time of evaluation in two of the four categories	
Sensory	Hyperalgesia (to pinprick) and/or allodynia (to light touch and/or temperature sensation and/or deep somatic pressure and/or joint movement)
Vasomotor	Temperature asymmetry (>1 °C) and/or skin color changes and/or asymmetry
Sudomotor	Edema and/or sweating changes and/or sweating asymmetry
Motor/trophic	Decreased range of motion and/or motor dysfunction (weakness, tremor, dystonia) and/or trophic changes (hair, nail, skin)

examination. The criteria are self-evident; a positive finding in all four categories is required for diagnosis.

Laboratory tests are not conclusive for the diagnosis of CRPS, but are primarily used to rule out other disorders [4, 14]. Imaging can aid in the diagnosis as the presence of patchy demineralization of long bone epiphyses in plain radiographs may point towards late stages of CRPS. Intestinal edema and vascular hyper-permeability seen on magnetic resonance imaging (MRI) suggests acute disease, while muscle atrophy, fibrosis, and fatty infiltration suggest chronic CRPS [19]. Triple phase bone scans are helpful to recognize early phase CRPS (increased bone metabolism) if increased Technetium Tc99 uptake is seen, and late if decreased [20]. Nerve conduction studies [21] can occasionally help differentiate CRPS1 from CRPS2 in the early phase of the disease. Because temperature differences between affected and healthy extremities is common, objective testing can be helpful to identify subtle differences and produce objective findings [21]. Finally, autonomic function tests including infrared thermometry, quantitative sudomotor axon reflex testing, thermoregulatory sweat testing, and laser Doppler imaging have been utilized to study the abnormal autonomic function in affected limbs [21].

Management

Since the disease is a complex, multifaceted biopsychosocial disorder, effective management is understandably multimodal – pharmacological, interventional, rehabilitative, and psychological [3, 14]. The goals of therapy are to reduce pain and improve function without causing harm (Fig. 92.1).

Numerous pharmacologic agents have been tried in management of CRPS over the years [22],

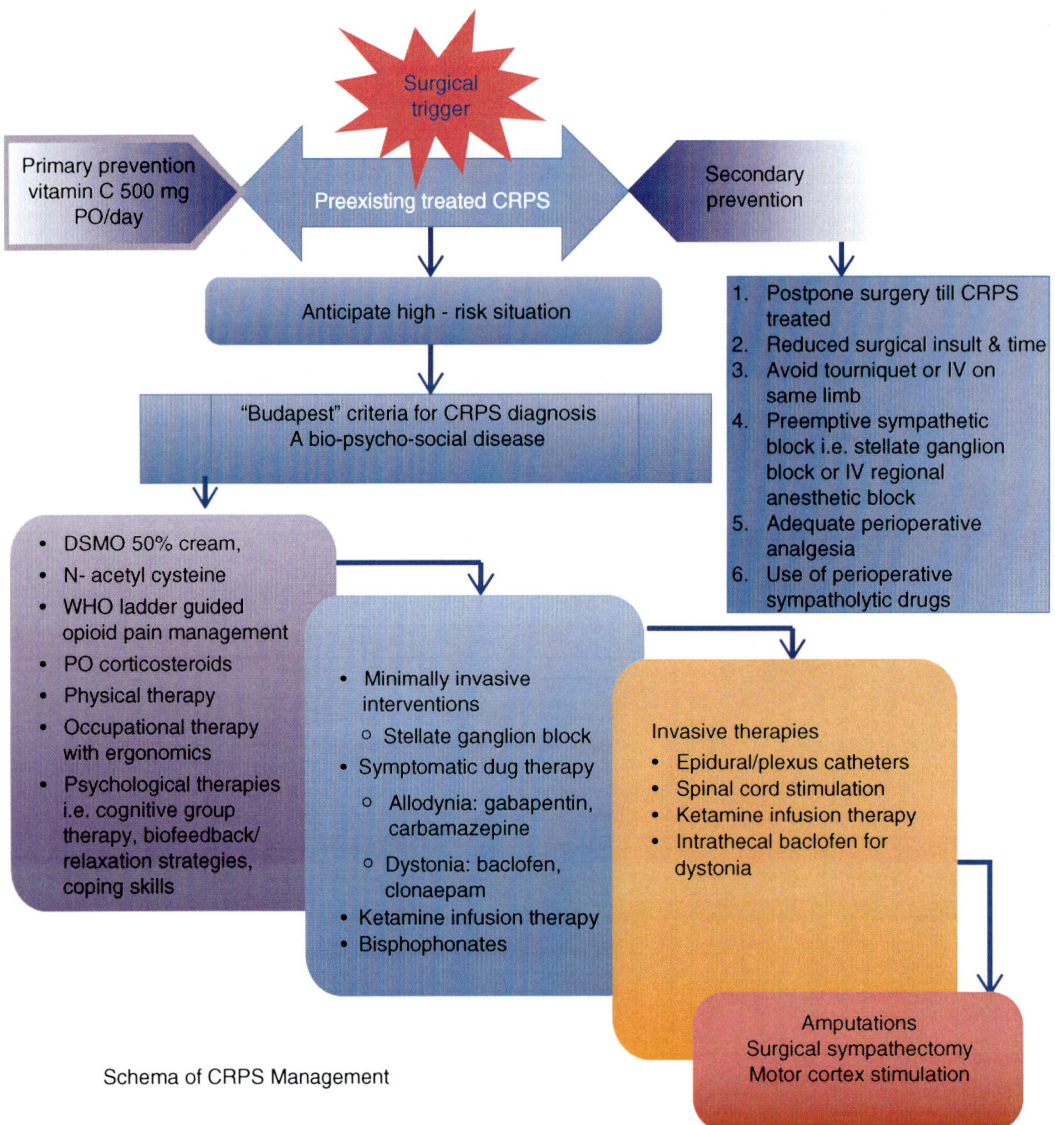

Fig. 92.1 Scheme for postoperative CRPS management

but no pharmacological agent alone or in combination has been able to provide consistent and long-lasting benefit in patients with CRPS. Bisphosphonates [22, 23] (intravenous alendronate, intravenous palmidronate, oral alendronate etc.), free radical scavengers [22, 24] (vitamin C, 50 % dimethylsulfoxide cream, N-acetylcysteine, mannitol etc.), and immune-modulating agents (steroids, tumor necrosis alpha antagonists etc.) have reportedly improved pain and other CRPS symptoms in several studies, while calcitonin, clonidine, anticonvulsants (gabapentin etc.) have had limited efficacy [22]. Ketamine, a potent NMDA-blocking agent, has demonstrated effectiveness in various studies [22, 25], although safety data for long-term and repetitive usage is unknown.

Interventional sympathetic blockade (stellate ganglion) is efficacious in recurrent CRPS when used prophylactically, although limited success is seen with therapeutic use [26]. Various agents (lidocaine, guanethidine, clonidine, Ketanserin- a serotonin receptor antagonist, lidocaine with steroid, lidocaine with bretylium etc.) administered via intravenous regional block have failed to demonstrate efficacy [22].

Neuromodulation by means of spinal cord stimulation has been shown to be efficacious for functional improvement and analgesia as compared to other surgical modalities [27, 28]. Targeted stimulation of damaged peripheral nerves shows benefit in patients with CRPS-2 [29]. Experience with transcutaneous electrical nerve stimulation (TENS) remains limited, while intrathecal drug delivery (Baclofen) improves dystonic symptoms but has not been shown to be of benefit in patients with other CRPS symptoms [22].

Surgical sympathectomy has been shown to help the subset of patients who had a significant decrease in pain after sympathetic block. Unfortunately 10 % of such patients fail to see any benefit at all, 28 % experience an increase in pain 1 year post-sympathectomy and 9–37 % develop new spreading CRPS [30, 31]. Additionally, there is a 24 % risk of post-sympathectomy neuralgia associated with sympathectomy irrespective of the surgical approach [31].

Cognitive behavioral therapy, graded physical therapy, mirror therapy, graded motor imagery, occupational therapy, and acupuncture have all been used within multimodal management protocols. While some improvement in pain and swelling can be seen, no differences in objective impairment, disability, and handicap assessment are usually found [14, 22].

Finally, as a last resort, amputation of the affected limb has been used as a management strategy, although results are limited [32].

Prevention

Because successful management of CRPS remains unpredictable at best, the best strategy should be to prevent or decrease the risk of CRPS. It has been suggested that once a diagnosis of CRPS is established it may remain in a dormant phase, but can recur suddenly [33]. Relapse rates for CRPS are as high as 13 % even with the utilization of interventions intended to reduce relapse [34].

The use of vitamin C in 500 mg daily oral doses has been shown to decrease the incidence of CRPS after traumatic injury and after operation [35]. The obvious question is in which patients to apply prevention strategies to; the answer remains obscure.

Secondary preventive measures are those that decrease the risk of CRPS relapse [34]. Such strategies include postponing surgical intervention until CRPS symptoms have resolved [34], minimizing the use of tourniquets or placement of intravenous lines on the same side of the CRPS-treated extremity, peri-operative vasodilators to increase blood flow, and mannitol as a free radical scavenger [36]. Most importantly, utilization of preemptive sympathetic blockade of the targeted extremity has been shown to reduce the relapse rate from 72 to 10 %, preemptive analgesia to as low as 1 % [37].

Summary

While CRPS is a multifaceted biopsychosocial painful disorder of perplexing pathophysiology, trauma and/or surgical injury remains the most common inciting event. All of these factors have relevance to TOS. To date, the diagnosis relies primarily on a careful history and physical examination with specific criteria delineated by the "Budapest criteria". Befitting the multifactorial etiology and complex presentation, the treatment approach is multipronged. Unfortunately, even with optimal management outcome remains unpredictable. In light of this, it cannot be overemphasized that there is a pressing need for early diagnosis and adequate management of symptoms to prevent progression to chronicity, which is much harder to treat.

References

1. Schwartzman RJ, Erwin KL, Alexander GM. The natural history of complex regional pain syndrome. Clin J Pain. 2009;25(4):273–80.
2. Kaymak B, Ozcakar L. Complex regional pain syndrome in thoracic outlet syndrome. Br J Sports Med. 2004;38(3):364.
3. Maihofner C, Seifert F, Markovic K. Complex regional pain syndromes: new pathophysiological concepts and therapies. Eur J Neurol. 2010;17(5):649–60.
4. de Mos M, de Bruijn AG, Huygen FJ, Dieleman JP, Stricker BH, Sturkenboom MC. The incidence of complex regional pain syndrome: a population-based study. Pain. 2007;129(1–2):12–20.
5. Sandroni P, Benrud-Larson LM, McClelland RL, Low PA. Complex regional pain syndrome type I: incidence and prevalence in Olmsted county, a population-based study. Pain. 2003;103(1–2):199–207.
6. van Rijn MA, Marinus J, Putter H, Bosselaar SR, Moseley GL, van Hilten JJ. Spreading of complex regional pain syndrome: not a random process. J Neural Transm. 2011;118(9):1301–9.
7. de Rooij AM, de Mos M, Sturkenboom MC, Marinus J, van den Maagdenberg AM, van Hilten JJ. Familial occurrence of complex regional pain syndrome. Eur J Pain. 2009;13(2):171–7.
8. Veldman PH, Goris RJ. Multiple reflex sympathetic dystrophy. Which patients are at risk for developing a recurrence of reflex sympathetic dystrophy in the same or another limb. Pain. 1996;64(3):463–6.
9. Prosser R, Conolly WB. Complications following surgical treatment for Dupuytren's contracture. J Hand Ther. 1996;9(4):344–8.
10. Cameron HU, Park YS, Krestow M. Reflex sympathetic dystrophy following total knee replacement. Contemp Orthop. 1994;29(4):279–81.
11. Shinya K, Lanzetta M, Conolly WB. Risk and complications in endoscopic carpal tunnel release. J Hand Surg [Br]. 1995;20(2):222–7.
12. Goldner JL. Causes and prevention of reflex sympathetic dystrophy. J Hand Surg [Am]. 1980;5(3):295–6.
13. Kumar S, Mackay C, O'Callaghan J, De'Ambrosis B. Complex regional pain syndrome after dermatological surgery. Australas J Dermatol. 2008;49(4):242–4.
14. Raja SN, Grabow TS. Complex regional pain syndrome I (reflex sympathetic dystrophy). Anesthesiology. 2002;96(5):1254–60.
15. Coderre TJ. Complex regional pain syndrome: what's in a name? J Pain. 2011;12(1):2–12.
16. Woolf CJ, Thompson SW. The induction and maintenance of central sensitization is dependent on N-methyl-D-aspartic acid receptor activation; implications for the treatment of post-injury pain hypersensitivity states. Pain. 1991;44(3):293–9.
17. Herlyn P, Muller-Hilke B, Wendt M, Hecker M, Mittlmeier T, Gradl G. Frequencies of polymorphisms in cytokines, neurotransmitters and adrenergic receptors in patients with complex regional pain syndrome type I after distal radial fracture. Clin J Pain. 2010;26(3):175–81.
18. Harden RN, Bruehl S, Stanton-Hicks M, Wilson PR. Proposed new diagnostic criteria for complex regional pain syndrome. Pain Med. 2007;8(4):326–31.
19. Nishida Y, Saito Y, Yokota T, Kanda T, Mizusawa H. Skeletal muscle MRI in complex regional pain syndrome. Intern Med. 2009;48(4):209–12.
20. Wuppenhorst N, Maier C, Frettloh J, Pennekamp W, Nicolas V. Sensitivity and specificity of 3-phase bone scintigraphy in the diagnosis of complex regional pain syndrome of the upper extremity. Clin J Pain. 2010;26(3):182–9.
21. Rommel O, Malin JP, Zenz M, Janig W. Quantitative sensory testing, neurophysiological and psychological examination in patients with complex regional pain syndrome and hemisensory deficits. Pain. 2001;93(3):279–93.
22. Tran DQH, Duong S, Bertini P, Finlayson RJ. Treatment of complex regional pain syndrome: a review of evidence. Can J Anaesth. 2010;57:149–66.
23. Yanow J, Pappagallo M, Pillai L. Complex regional pain syndrome (CRPS/RSD) and neuropathic pain: role of intravenous bisphosphonates as analgesics. Scientific World Journal. 2008;8:229–36.
24. Perez RS, Zuurmond WW, Bezemer PD, et al. The treatment of complex regional pain syndrome type I with free radical scavengers: a randomized controlled study. Pain. 2003;102(3):297–307.
25. Schwartzman RJ, Alexander GM, Grothusen JR, Paylor T, Reichenberger E, Perreault M. Outpatient intravenous ketamine for the treatment of complex regional pain syndrome: a double-blind placebo controlled study. Pain. 2009;147(1–3):107–15.
26. Ackerman WE, Zhang JM. Efficacy of stellate ganglion blockade for the management of type 1 complex regional pain syndrome. South Med J. 2006;99(10):1084–8.
27. Stanton-Hicks M. Complex regional pain syndrome: manifestations and the role of neurostimulation in its management. J Pain Symptom Manage. 2006;31(4 Suppl):S20–4.

28. Kemler MA, De Vet HC, Barendse GA, Van Den Wildenberg FA, Van Kleef M. The effect of spinal cord stimulation in patients with chronic reflex sympathetic dystrophy: two years' follow-up of the randomized controlled trial. Ann Neurol. 2004;55(1):13–8.

29. Hassenbusch SJ, Stanton-Hicks M, Schoppa D, Walsh JG, Covington EC. Long-term results of peripheral nerve stimulation for reflex sympathetic dystrophy. J Neurosurg. 1996;84(3):415–23.

30. Bandyk DF, Johnson BL, Kirkpatrick AF, Novotney ML, Back MR, Schmacht DC. Surgical sympathectomy for reflex sympathetic dystrophy syndromes. J Vasc Surg. 2002;35(2):269–77.

31. Hooshmand H, Hashmi M. Complex regional pain syndrome (CRPS) diagnosis and therapy. A review of 824 patients. Pain Digest. 1999;9:1–24.

32. Dielissen PW, Claassen AT, Veldman PH, Goris RJ. Amputation for reflex sympathetic dystrophy. J Bone Joint Surg Br. 1995;77(2):270–3.

33. Rocco AG. Comment on: abnormal contralateral pain responses from an intradermal injection of phenylephrine in a subset of patients with complex regional pain syndrome (CRPS). Pain. 2005;115(1–2):213–4. author reply 214.

34. Veldman PH, Goris RJ. Surgery on extremities with reflex sympathetic dystrophy. Unfallchirurg. 1995;98(1):45–8.

35. Cazeneuve JF, Leborgne JM, Kermad K, Hassan Y. Vitamin C and prevention of reflex sympathetic dystrophy following surgical management of distal radius fractures. Acta Orthop Belg. 2002;68(5):481–4.

36. Zyluk A, Puchalski P. Treatment of early complex regional pain syndrome type 1 by a combination of mannitol and dexamethasone. J Hand Surg Eur Vol. 2008;33(2):130–6.

37. Reuben SS. Preventing the development of complex regional pain syndrome after surgery. Anesthesiology. 2004;101(5):1215–24.

Anna Weiss and David C. Chang

Abstract

Quality of life (QOL) research provides a framework to judge outcomes, health status, and treatment effectiveness from the patient's point of view. It is important for surgical outcomes, particularly as medicine shifts emphasis from mortality to perceived health status and patient preference. QOL research can be useful in thoracic outlet syndrome (TOS), given the disease's weak objective findings. There is no tool specific for TOS, however generic or dimension-specific measures can apply. The Disability of the Arm, Shoulder and Hand survey (DASH), a dimension-specific measure, is used to evaluate symptoms and function of patients with upper extremity disability. General measures such as the Short Form 36 (SF-36) or SF-12 can also be used. TOS patients were administered the DASH and SF-12. At baseline, patients with TOS reported similar quality of life scores as patients with congestive heart failure, and DASH scores similar to patients with chronic rotator cuff injury. DASH scores post-operatively improved 0.85 points (P<.001) for neurogenic patients and 0.81 points (P<.001) for venous per month. The physical and mental component scores of the SF-12 also improved significantly over time (0.24 and 0.15 points per month respectively for neurogenic patients, and 0.40 and 0.55 points for venous patients). Therefore, in appropriately selected patients with TOS, surgical intervention can improve their quality of life.

A. Weiss, MD
Department of Surgery,
University of California, San Diego,
200 West Arbor Drive, #8402, San Diego,
CA 92103, USA
e-mail: a3weiss@ucsd.edu

D.C. Chang, PhD, MPH, MBA (✉)
Department of Surgery,
University of California, San Diego,
200 West Arbor Drive, #8401, San Diego,
CA 92103, USA
e-mail: dchang1@ucsd.edu

Introduction

Quality of life research provides a conceptual framework to judge patient outcomes, health status, and treatment effectiveness from the patient's point of view. Currently, most clinical research focuses on morbidity and mortality which are objective, provider-centered data, but those addressing healthcare delivery and quality improvement are beginning to focus more on

K.A. Illig et al. (eds.), *Thoracic Outlet Syndrome*,
DOI 10.1007/978-1-4471-4366-6_93, © Springer-Verlag London 2013

patient-centered data such as quality of life measures [1]. Quality of life measures have many potential uses to improve clinical practice, including the ability to facilitate communication, identify preferences, screen for and prioritize problems, and monitor changes or treatment responses [2]. Quality of life assessment also has extensive research applications: in descriptive research, it can characterize burden of disease and injury; in clinical research, it is used to test the efficacy of treatments. Quality of life research is increasingly important for analyzing surgical outcomes, particularly as modern medicine evolves and emphasis shifts from mortality to perceived health status, wellness, and patient preference.

Disease-Specific Quality of Life Measures

Quality of life measurements can be useful in thoracic outlet syndrome (TOS), especially given the disease's symptomatic diagnosis and relatively weak objective diagnostic criteria and variable symptoms. While venous TOS may be confirmed by ultrasound or venogram, no definitive diagnostic tests exist for neurogenic TOS. Since the diagnosis of TOS remains largely clinical, patients may often be seen by multiple physicians and labeled as either disabled or malingering. The same uncertainty exists in the evaluation of patient outcomes post-operatively, and to date, most evaluations have been based on unstructured subjective assessment. A structured, validated assessment of the quality of life and functional outcomes of TOS patients would be highly beneficial.

There are many types of quality of life measures. Generic measures exist, such as the Short-Form 36 (SF-36) which measure several general health domains. There are individualized measures, such as the Patient Generated Index, which allow patients to apply a weighted importance to each characteristic surveyed. There are dimension-specific measures, such as the Beck depression inventory, which measure one aspect of health. Finally, there are disease-specific measures,

which measure several health domains within one disease process [3].

There is no disease-specific quality of life measure for TOS, although several generic or dimension-specific measures can apply. The Disability of the Arm, Shoulder and Hand survey (DASH) was developed by the American Academy of Orthopaedics Surgeons as an outcomes tool to evaluate "upper extremity-related symptoms and measure functional status at the level of disability" [4, 5]. Concepts covered by the DASH include symptoms (pain, weakness, stiffness, tingling/numbness), physical function (daily activities, house/yard chores, errands, recreational activities, self-care, dressing, eating, sport/performing art), social function (family care, occupation, socializing with friends/family) and psychological function (self-image).

General measures such as the Short Form 36 (SF-36) can also be used for TOS patients. The popular SF-36 was developed from the Medical Outcomes Study in the early 1990s [6]. It provides scores for eight health domains, and reports these as physical and mental component summary scores (PCS and MCS). The SF-12 is a condensed version of the SF-36 (regression methods were used to select and score the "best" 12 items from the SF-36), has been shown to be highly predictive of full SF-36 scores [5], and thus is an especially useful tool to save time when patients have to answer more than one survey.

Theories of Quality of Life Research

Quality of life research by nature is based on patient survey. There are three fundamental principles of any survey research: acceptability, reliability, and validity.

Questions on a survey should be acceptable to the target population. This is assessed with focus groups to determine the appropriateness and ease of comprehension of the survey. In analysis, acceptability can be assessed with data completeness and score distributions. There should be less than 5 % missing data for the summary scores generated; more missing data suggesting that respondents have difficulty understanding the

Fig. 93.1 Demonstration of the concepts of reliability versus validity. Assume that the *gray circle* represents "truth," while the surrounding *white circle* represents "error:" the pattern of *checkmarks* (observations) shown in (**a**) would be both valid and reliable. Pattern (**b**) shows a situation where the observations are tightly clustered – reliable – but are in error, and the situation is thus not valid. The circumstance shown in pattern (**c**) represents validity – but the observations are scattered so not very reliable. Finally, pattern (**d**) is neither valid nor reliable

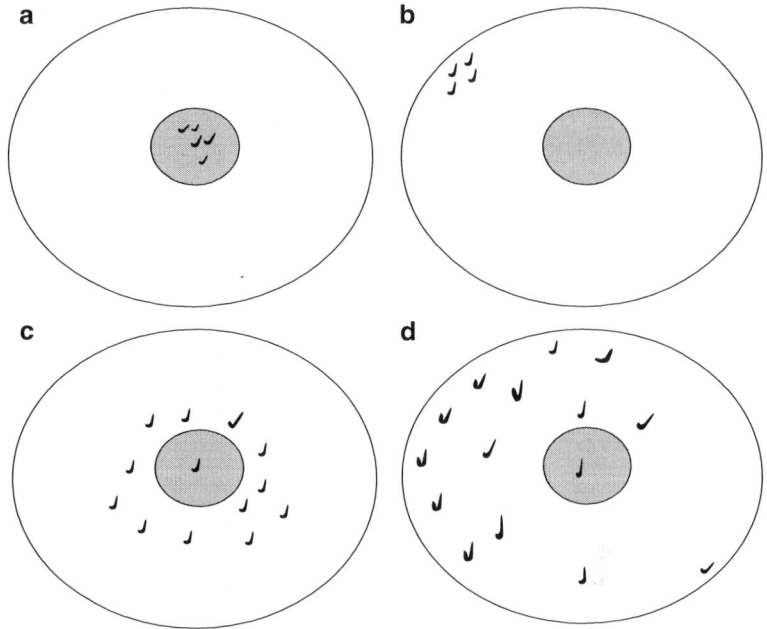

questions. There should be an even distribution of frequencies for each response category, with less than 10 % floor/ceiling effects—i.e., no more than 10 % of responses clustered at the low-end (floor) or high-end (ceiling) of the range of response categories. The presence of ceiling/floor effects would suggest that the questions may not be meaningful.

The concept of reliability is demonstrated by Fig. 93.1. Reliability is usually assessed with a test-retest reliability protocol, which involves administering the same survey on two different occasions, and then examining the correlation in scores between the two. The correlation should ideally be greater than 0.80. The time interval between tests should be short enough to ensure that no clinically meaningful change is likely to occur (e.g., both surveys should be pre-operative or both post-operative), but interval should be long enough to ensure that the subjects do not recall their answers to the first assessment. Problems with reliability may suggest that the questions have unclear or vague wording; a very clear question is unlikely to elicit a different response each time from a respondent.

Validity of a questionnaire is the concept that it should somehow represent the "truth", or some

gold standard. This is particularly difficult in quality of life research since there is no "gold standard" for quality measures. Validity is thus demonstrated indirectly, by showing that a questionnaire instrument "makes sense", and "behaves" as one would expect it to under different scenarios.

In turn, there are two major "validity" concepts: content and construct validity. Content validity means that a questionnaire "makes sense". It represents the concept that the content of the questionnaire is representative of the conceptual domain that it is intended to cover. This is usually assessed qualitatively during questionnaire development phase, or through focus groups.

Construct validity means that a questionnaire should "behave" as one would expect. There are two forms of construct validity: internal and external. Internal construct validity is the concept that questions meant to measure one concept should correlate with one another, while external construct validity is the correlation of concepts with those outside the current questionnaire. There are three methods to demonstrate external validity: Convergent, discriminant, and known-group differentiation validity. An instrument demonstrates convergent validity if it correlates well with another instrument that measures a similar construct. The degrees of correlations are expected to vary according to similarity of the concepts being measured by each instrument. For example, since DASH is dimension-specific and SF-36 is generic, correlations are in moderate range. Since DASH items are meant to capture physical issues, higher correlations are expected between DASH and the PCS of the SF-36, than the MCS. Discriminant validity is the opposite of convergent validity – a questionnaire demonstrates discriminant validity if it does *not* correlate with an instrument that measures a *different* concept. For example, the DASH, since it measures disability and not general health status, should not correlate with age and gender in healthy subjects. Finally, a questionnaire is said to have known-group differentiation validity if it can differentiate between patients that are known to be different. For example, DASH scores should increase (i.e., denoting more frequent symptoms) with increasing severity of TOS.

Quality of Life Data in Thoracic Outlet Syndrome

To date, there are limited data on quality of life and functional outcome of TOS patients, and much are based on unstructured subjective assessment. We thus decided to undertake a study to quantify the degree and characteristics of TOS patient disability using structured, validated patient-reported quality of life instruments, and to assess their long-term quality of life outcomes following transaxillary first-rib resection and scalenectomy for TOS [7].

Pre-operative patient demographics and post-operative clinical outcomes were abstracted from clinical records of patients treated by operation between February 2005 and March 2008 at the Johns Hopkins University TOS practice. The DASH and SF-12 were chosen to assess TOS patients' quality of life. Understandability and acceptability of the questionnaires were assessed by discussion with the first five patients.

These surveys were administered pre-operatively and then at 3, 6, 12, 18, and 24 months after surgery. Informed consent was obtained by the attending surgeon or the physician assistant in the clinic.

The PCS and MCS on the SF-12 scale were standardized and normalized to population data (mean 50, SD 10). Means were compared to population norms with one-sample t tests. Reliability of the survey package was assessed by test-retest reliability. Validity of the survey package was assessed by convergent validity via simple regression between SF scores and DASH. The rate of recovery was determined with population-averaged models using generalized estimating equations (GEE) method. Kaplan-Meier method was used to analyze time to return to work.

By June 2008, 70 of 105 eligible patients (66.7 %) completed the study protocol, returning 188 valid DASH surveys (124 neurogenic; 64 venous) and 243 SF-12 surveys (162 neurogenic; 81 venous).

Preoperative Status

There was no statistically significant difference in baseline survey scores, captured at the initial clinic visits, between the 70 patients who participated fully in this study, versus the other patients who did not participate further in this study (PCS 37.3 vs 37.9, MCS 44.1 vs 47.9, and DASH 41.9 vs 34.9, all P=ns).

Intervention

All patients had failed physical therapy prior to referral. Pre-operative treatments for the venous population included venography with clot lysis and anticoagulation if necessary. All patients underwent transaxillary first-rib resection and scalenectomy, followed by 2 months of post-operative physical therapy. All venous TOS patients also underwent venogram and dilatation 2 weeks following surgery, and anticoagulation if necessary.

Quality of Life Outcome

Separating baseline neurogenic and venous TOS patient data, it was found that neurogenic TOS patients had significantly worse PCS values than venous (33.8 vs. 43.6, P<.001). In contrast, there was no significant difference between their MCS scores (44.5 vs. 43.5, P=ns). The DASH scores were also significantly worse among neurogenic TOS patients than venous (50.2 vs 25.0, P<.001).

PCS scores for neurogenic patients improved 0.24 points (P<.001) and MCS scores improved 0.15 points per month on average (P=.01) (Fig. 93.2a). PCS scores for venous patients improved 0.40 points (P=.004) and MCS scores improved 0.55 points per month (P<.001) on average (Fig. 93.2b). DASH scores also improved 0.85 points (P<.001) for neurogenic patients and 0.81 points (P<.001) for venous patients per month on average. Additionally, the median time to normal quality of life for neurogenic patients was 23 months for physical and 12 months for mental function. For venous patients, the median time to normal quality of life was 11 and 8 months respectively. These quality of life recovery times were significantly longer than the time it took for the patients to return to full-time work or activity.

Return to Work

While 15/44 (34 %) of neurogenic patients and 2/26 (8 %) of venous patients were disabled or unemployed upon presentation, 22 (50 %)

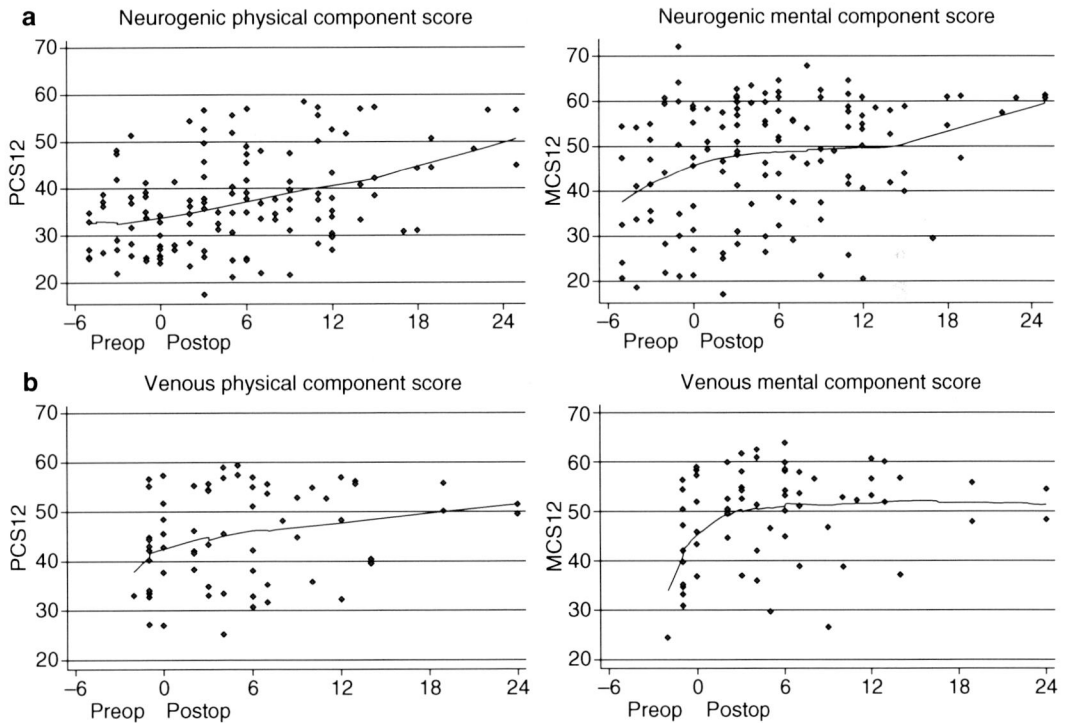

Fig. 93.2 Graphic representation of quality of life scores, including Physical Component Score (*PCS*) and Mental Component Score (*MCS*) for (**a**) neurogenic TOS patients, and (**b**) venous TOS patients. This graph was based on data from "Surgical intervention for thoracic outlet syndrome improves patient's quality of life" by Chang, Rotellini-Coltvet, Mukherjee and Freischlag. Preoperatively, neurogenic TOS patients had significantly worse Physical Component Score (PCS) values than venous (33.8 vs. 43.6, P<.001), and the DASH scores were also significantly worse among neurogenic patients (50.2 vs 25.0, P<.001). (**a**) Shows the PCS and MCS scores for neurogenic patients, you can see that the scores improved 0.24 and 0.15 points per month respectively. (**b**) shows the PCS and MCS scores for venous patients improved 0.40 and 0.55 points per month respectively (Based on data from Chang et al. [7])

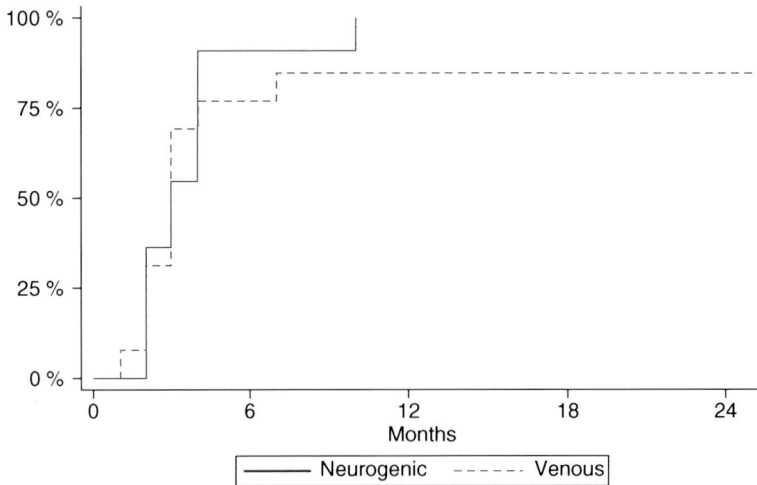

Fig. 93.3 The proportion of patients returning to full-time work or activity over time, this graph was based on results from "Surgical intervention for thoracic outlet syndrome improves patient's quality of life", Chang et al. While 34 % of neurogenic and 8 % of venous patients were disabled or unemployed pre-operatively, 50 % neurogenic and 77 % venous patients returned to full-time work or activity during the follow-up period. Half of patients returned by 4 months, and more than 75 % returned by 5 months. There was no statistically significant difference in the rate of return to work between neurogenic and venous patients (Based on data from Chang et al. [7])

neurogenic patients and 20 (77 %) venous patients eventually returned to full-time work or activity during the follow-up period. Additionally, there were two neurogenic patients and two venous patients who returned to part-time activity. The time course of returning to full-time work or activity is presented in Fig. 93.3. Half of the patients returned by 4 months, and more than 75 % returned by 5 months. There was no statistically significant difference in this rate of return to work between neurogenic and venous patients.

Discussion

While some risk factors predicting persistent post-operative disability in patients with TOS have been identified, measurement of long-term post-operative mental and physical functional outcomes has been lacking [8–12]. While there have been some attempts to assess such outcomes, these have focused on diffuse measures of patient satisfaction using unvalidated tools [13–16]. A recent report by Cordobes-Gual et al. presented functional data using the validated DASH instrument on 23

patients, but included only a single follow-up at approximately 4–6 months after surgery [17].

In contrast to these limited studies, the current study presents functional data on a larger group of patients (n = 70) followed over a longer period of time (up to 2 years) using objective, well-established quality of life instruments. Our findings suggest that despite the seemingly vague nature of their complaints, TOS patients suffer striking physical morbidity. The mean baseline PCS of 37.5 was approximately 1.3 standard deviations below the population norm, and was much worse than the mean scores reported by patients with chronic prostatitis (46.4), hypertension (46.5), or diabetes (44.8) and similar to that reported by patients with chronic heart failure (34.0) [18–20]. Similarly, the mean DASH score of 41.4 was similar to that reported by patients with chronic rotator cuff tears (43.7) [20]. The validity of TOS patients' physical complaints was further supported by their MCS being within one standard deviation of population norm.

Our data show that patients with venous and neurogenic TOS present with significant physical disability. Their quality of life profile in general is similar to patients with chronic heart failure, and, in relation to upper extremity function, similar to patients with chronic rotator cuff tears. Following first-rib resection, venous TOS patients typically improved both physical and mental quality of life in shorter periods of time than their neurogenic counterparts. Neurogenic and venous TOS patients returned to full-time work/activity within the same length of time postoperatively, although neurogenic patients required more secondary interventions. In both cohorts, patients returned to full-time work or activity before they returned to normal quality of life scores, suggesting patients are able to return to full-time work or activity while they are still recovering. Therefore, in appropriately selected patients with either neurogenic or venous TOS, surgical intervention can improve their quality of life over time.

Future Directions

Although quality of life instruments are structured and have undergone extensive validation testing, the verbal nature of these reports still presents a concern for some investigators, especially considering the diagnostic uncertainty in TOS patients.

A biomechanical validation of the quality of life reports would be valuable to confirm patient recovery following surgery as well as a possible tool to assist in making an objective diagnosis. One such tool would be an accelerometer, a device that measures changes in position over time. The most basic accelerometer is the pedometer, which measures the number of steps taken; an ankle version of the device, for example, has been used to measure ambulation among stroke patients [21]. Given the complexity of upper extremity function as compared to ambulation, the simple swinging motion of the arm is less important than the ability to raise the arm to a certain angle and hold it there. Therefore, an ideal accelerometer would measure three planes simultaneously, capturing abduction/adduction and flexion/extension of the arm, and would track the time data to determine

the total length of time that the arm is being used. This could then serve as an external validation of the quality of life data obtained in TOS patients. This could enhance the objectivity of outcomes measurement, and further advance the state of the clinical science in this field.

References

1. Neumayer L. How do (and why should) I use the National Surgical Quality Improvement Program? Am J Surg. 2009;198(suppl):S36–40.
2. Higginson IJ, Carr AJ. Measuring quality of life: using quality of life measures in the clinical setting. BMJ. 2001;322(7297):1297–300.
3. Garratt A, Schmidt L, Mackintosh A, Fitzpatrick R. Quality of life measurement: bibliographic study of patient assessed health outcomes measures. BMJ. 2002;324(7351):1417.
4. Hudak PL, Amadio PC, Bombardier C. Development of an upper extremity outcome measure: the DASH (disabilities of the arm, shoulder and hand) [corrected]. The Upper Extremity Collaborative Group (UECG). Am J Ind Med. 1996;29:602–8.
5. Kirkley A, Griffin S, Dainty K. Scoring systems for the functional assessment of the shoulder. Arthroscopy. 2003;19(10):1109–20.
6. Ware Jr J, Kosinski M, Keller SD. A 12-Item Short-Form Health Survey: construction of scales and preliminary tests of reliability and validity. Med Care. 1996;34(3):220–33.
7. Chang DC, Rotellini-Coltvet LA, Mukherjee D, De Leon R, Freischlag JA. Surgical intervention for thoracic outlet syndrome improves patient's quality of life. J Vasc Surg. 2009;49(3):630–5.
8. Gockel M, Lindholm H, Vastamäki M, Lindqvist A, Viljanen A. Cardiovascular functional disorder and distress among patients with thoracic outlet syndrome. J Hand Surg [Br]. 1995;20(1):29–33.
9. Yavuzer S, Atinkaya C, Tokat O. Clinical predictors of surgical outcome in patients with thoracic outlet syndrome operated on via transaxillary approach. Eur J Cardiothorac Surg. 2004;25(2):173–8.
10. Axelrod DA, Proctor MC, Geisser ME, Roth RS, Greenfield LJ. Outcomes after surgery for thoracic outlet syndrome. J Vasc Surg. 2001;33(6):1220–5.
11. Divi V, Proctor MC, Axelrod DA, Greenfield LJ. Thoracic outlet decompression for subclavian vein thrombosis: experience in 71 patients. Arch Surg. 2005;140(1):54–7.
12. Chang DC, Lidor AO, Matsen SL, Freischlag JA. Reported in-hospital complications following rib resections for neurogenic thoracic outlet syndrome. Ann Vasc Surg. 2007;21(5):564–70.
13. Sharp WJ, Nowak LR, Zamani T, Kresowik TF, Hoballah JJ, Ballinger BA, et al. Long-term follow-up

and patient satisfaction after surgery for thoracic outlet syndrome. Ann Vasc Surg. 2001;15(1):32–6.

14. Bhattacharya V, Hansrani M, Wyatt MG, Lambert D, Jones NA. Outcome following surgery for thoracic outlet syndrome. Eur J Vasc Endovasc Surg. 2003;26(2):170–5.

15. Degeorges R, Reynaud C, Becquemin JP. Thoracic outlet syndrome surgery: long-term functional results. Ann Vasc Surg. 2004;18(5):558–65.

16. Rochkind S, Shemesh M, Patish H, Graif M, Segev Y, Salame K, et al. Thoracic outlet syndrome: a multidisciplinary problem with a perspective for microsurgical management without rib resection. Acta Neurochir Suppl. 2007;100:145–7.

17. Cordobes-Gual J, Lozano-Vilardell P, Torreguitart-Mirada N, Lara-Hernandez R, Riera-Vazquez R, Julia-Montoya J. Prospective study of the functional recovery after surgery for thoracic outlet syndrome. Eur J Vasc Endovasc Surg. 2008;35(1):79–83.

18. McNaughton-Collins M, Pontari MA, O'Leary MP, Calhoun EA, Santanna J, Landis JR, et al. Quality of life is impaired in men with chronic prostatitis: the Chronic Prostatitis Collaborative Research Network. J Gen Intern Med. 2001;16(10):656–62.

19. Baker DW, Brown J, Chan KS, Dracup KA, Keeler EB. A telephone survey to measure communication, self-management, and health status for patients with heart failure: the Improving Chronic Illness Care Evaluation (ICICE). J Card Fail. 2005;11(1):36–42.

20. Tashjian RZ, Henn RF, Kang L, Green A. The effect of comorbidity on self-assessed function in patients with a chronic rotator cuff tear. J Bone Joint Surg Am. 2004;86A(2):355–62.

21. Busse ME, Pearson OR, Van Deursen R, Wiles CM. Quantified measurement of activity provides insight into motor function and recovery in neurological disease. J Neurol Neurosurg Psychiatry. 2004;75(6):884–8.

Medicolegal Issues in TOS

Kevin J. Adrian

Abstract

The care by a physician of a patient suffering from thoracic outlet syndrome can often require the physician to become involved in legal proceedings. Frequently patients who suffer from this condition will pursue claims in a workers' compensation, personal injury or medical malpractice case, and the physician may simply be asked to offer testimony regarding the care they provided the patient. The physician may also, of course, be named as a defendant should he or she's care be called into question in a medical malpractice case. Finally, a non-treating physician may be asked to review a medical malpractice matter either for the plaintiff or the defendants. For the physician witness, this chapter will address the need to be fully apprised of causation standards in various legal settings prior to offering such opinions, and further issues regarding patient confidentiality laws. For the physician as a possible defendant to a medical malpractice lawsuit, means to limit exposure to such suits is discussed, along with what the physician can expect from the litigation process and his or her responsibilities in that process. Finally, with regard to physicians as expert witnesses in thoracic outlet syndrome cases, the practical and ethical guidelines and qualifications for such expert work established by the American Association for Thoracic Surgery (AATS), the Society of Thoracic Surgeons (STS), and Society for Vascular Surgeons (SVS) is discussed.

The care by a physician of a patient suffering from thoracic outlet syndrome can often require the physician to become involved in legal proceedings. Frequently patients who suffer from this condition will pursue claims in a workers' compensation, personal injury or medical malpractice case, and the physician may simply be asked to offer testimony regarding the care they provided the patient. The physician may also, of course, be named as a defendant should he or she's care be called into question in a medical malpractice case. Finally, a non-treating physician may

K.J. Adrian, BS, JD
800 Market Street, Suite 1100,
St. Louis, MO 63101, USA
e-mail: kadrian@bjpc.com

K.A. Illig et al. (eds.), *Thoracic Outlet Syndrome*,
DOI 10.1007/978-1-4471-4366-6_94, © Springer-Verlag London 2013

be asked to review a medical malpractice matter either for the plaintiff or the defendants.

Physician as Witness

There exists in the medical community some debate as to whether repetitive activities can in fact cause thoracic outlet syndrome, and significant debate as to the exact repetitive activities and duration of such activities that will give rise to the syndrome. Frequently reported work activities thought to give rise to thoracic outlet syndrome are typing, working on an assembly line, and repetitive lifting. Patients with thoracic outlet syndrome which they attribute to work activities will often pursue a workers' compensation action.

Workers' compensation in general is a no fault system to compensate workers who experience disability as a result of their work activities. In other words, the employee need not prove negligence on the part of his employer. Instead, the employee must prove that the work activities caused a medical condition which requires medical treatment and/or has caused temporary or permanent disability.

One or both attorneys to a workers' compensation action may wish to depose the physician evaluating and treating the thoracic outlet syndrome patient. Unlike personal injury or medical malpractice cases, the request for deposition may come before surgery is actually performed. In many states, the employer will directly pay for medical care, and thus treatment must be pre-approved. Counsel for the employee or employer may request the physician's deposition to establish a causal relation between work and the need for surgery.

The threshold for causation may differ greatly from state to state. In some states the causal requirement may be very strict and require that the work activities were the prevailing or primary factor in causing the injury. Conversely, some states have very lax causation standards, requiring as little as a statement from a physician that the work activities might or could have caused the condition or aggravated a pre-existing

condition. If asked to provide a deposition, a physician treating such a workers' compensation patient should inquire of the attorney requesting causation testimony the standard for causation which the state utilizes.

Traumatic events, such as motor vehicle accidents, may also lead to thoracic outlet syndrome, and such accidents may give rise to personal injury lawsuits. Again, the treating physician whose deposition is taken will be asked to offer testimony on causation and perhaps also the need for future treatment needs. The causation standard from state to state may differ, and thus a physician providing such a deposition should request the attorneys define the state's causation standard prior to offering such testimony.

It should be noted that when the physician is merely to serve as a fact witness in a case (as opposed to when the physician's care is the subject matter of the lawsuit), the attorneys for both sides may wish to speak with the physician prior to the deposition. Different states have different laws regarding ex parte meetings with defense attorneys. Therefore, if a defense attorney contacts a physician to discuss a plaintiff's treatment, it is advisable for the physician to consult with his or her administrator or attorney to determine whether such meetings are permitted.

Physician as Defendant

To prove a claim for negligence against a physician, a plaintiff must prove negligence on the part of the physician and that said negligence caused damages to the plaintiff. Negligence is shown by producing evidence and testimony that the physician deviated from the standard of care. Although the legally accepted definition of standard of care will vary to some degree from state to state, the standard of care can generally be defined as that degree of skill and learning ordinarily used under the same or similar circumstances by members of the medical specialty in question.

From the perspective of medical malpractice liability, there are steps that can be taken to limit exposure. It goes without saying that the practice of good medicine and attention to detail are the most important aspect of avoiding lawsuits. However, having a realistic informed consent discussion with the patient about their prognosis can be almost as valuable. The informed consent discussion is the foundation of the physician-patient relationship, and thus it is important to make the patient a partner in the treatment decisions. The patient should receive a detailed explanation of the cause of the problem, and the indication for and goals of surgery. Non-surgical alternatives should be discussed, and if they are not feasible for the patient, an explanation as to why not.

It is imperative that the risks of the surgery be fully provided to the patient in order for the patient to do a proper risk-benefit evaluation. The patient must be advised that surgical decompression may not completely alleviate all symptoms. All surgeries inherently involve risk and these general risks must be discussed. However, it is important that known risks specific to decompression surgery, such as temporary or even permanent nerve injury, be addressed. The course and duration of recovery should be discussed, and complications during that recovery, such as stenosis of the surrounding vessels or graft, discussed.

At the end of this discussion, the patient should be allowed to express their concerns regarding potential complications or risks. The physician must honestly address these concerns. Patients are less likely to sue when they feel their physician is responsive to their concerns and questions. Problems, and often lawsuits arise when patients feel as if they are being ignored or pushed into surgery.

A favorite mantra of plaintiffs' counsels is that "if it's not documented, it was not done." Although this is not accurate in the day-to-day practice of medicine, the most often heard regret we hear from physicians we represent is that they failed to document all of their activities and discussions with the patient. Although the statute of limitations for bringing a lawsuit varies from state to state, it is not uncommon for a medical malpractice case to go to trial 5–10 years after the treatment was provided. In the absence of detailed documentation, it is virtually impossible for a

physician to recall every last detail of what transpired. Furthermore, if there is no documentation, jurors are more likely to believe plaintiff's version. Although detailed documentation can be excessively time consuming in the busy practice of medicine, the added burden such documentation imposes will allow you to present the complete facts at trial. It should also be noted that experts for all parties to the suit will rely heavily on the documented notes in forming their opinions of the care provided and the merits, or lack thereof, of the case.

In determining what needs to be documented, often the documentation of what transpires before the actual procedure is most vital. Specifically, the records must show the factors which justified a diagnosis and treatment plan, and why more conservative non-surgical alternatives were not viable options. Similarly, risks and complications discussed with the patient during the informed consent discussion should be documented. Even if a complication is a known risk of the surgery, juries are less likely to find for the physician if the patient testifies that they were not advised of the risk and there is no documentation to refute this testimony.

A physician who is named as a defendant in a lawsuit will experience a wide range of emotions, and rightfully so as a lawsuit publically calls into question a physician's skill and competency. The stress is amplified as the physician recognizes that his or her actions will not be truly judged by a jury of his or her peers, but instead by laypersons with little or no medical training. Causing further stress is the fact that the individual who will be arguing the case for the doctor, the attorney, is not a physician and thus cannot possibly have the same expertise as the physician regardless of how long they have practiced or how many similar cases they have handled.

The physician must recognize that to achieve a successful defense, lines of communication between the physician and attorney must remain open and active throughout the course of the case. It is the attorney's job to walk the physician through the litigation process and to respond to any questions or concerns the physician may have. In turn it is the physician's job to educate the attorney on the medicine. The physician must become an active participant in the planning and strategy for the defense. Confidence in one's theory of the case is essential for the physician to present at trial as a knowledgeable and effective witness. The physician should also be actively involved in the selection of experts as the physician knows best which physicians nationally are respected as authorities in their field of medicine.

Despite the physician's prior experience with depositions in prior cases, it is often useful to conduct a "mock" deposition before being deposed in a particular case. In a mock deposition, the attorney will have a colleague from his or her firm pretend to be the plaintiff's attorney and ask the questions they anticipate will be posed at the real deposition. A court reporter will transcribe the mock deposition, which the physician will then have an opportunity to review and discuss with their attorney before the real deposition. This allows the physician an opportunity to identify potential problem areas and to work with their attorney to formulate answers to anticipated questions which will fully and accurately express their thoughts. Thorough preparation by reviewing all pertinent materials is essential for both the mock and real deposition.

As medical and anatomical terminology can be difficult for the jury to absorb or even understand, visual exhibits can make the difference in getting the jury to understand the physician's decision-making process in deciding to perform thoracic outlet syndrome decompression, and what the surgery itself entails. From the beginning of the case, the physician should actively look for visual aides which can be provided to assist the attorney and for possible use at trial.

Although the defense attorney strives to view all cases as defensible when first received, there are of course some medical malpractice cases with merit. Although difficult, the physician must identify potential areas of concern for the case as early as possible and openly identify those to his or her counsel. With that information, the attorney can properly assess the physician of possible exposure in the case and formulate a settlement strategy, if appropriate.

Physician as Expert Witness

One of the most important and controversial figures in malpractice litigation is the physician expert witness. The need for expert witnesses has engendered the need for clear definitions of their qualifications. This is particularly true for specialized surgeries such as thoracic outlet syndrome decompression. The American Association for Thoracic Surgery (AATS) [1] and the Society of Thoracic Surgeons (STS) [2] have both adopted qualifications for expert witnesses and guidelines for the behavior of AATS members rendering expert opinions in the legal system.

Both groups' qualifications mandate that the physician expert must have a current, valid and unrestricted license to practice medicine, should be a diplomate of a specialty board recognized by the American Board of Medical Specialties and be qualified by experience or demonstrated competence in the subject matter of the case. Further, the physician expert witness must be familiar with the subject matter of the case and the relevant standards of care at the time of the alleged occurrence, and have been actively practicing thoracic surgery at the time the incident leading to the litigation occurred. The expert must also be able to demonstrate evidence of continuing medical education relevant to the specialty and subject of the matter. Finally, the physician expert should be prepared to document the percentage of professional time spent in serving as an expert witness, should be willing to disclose the amount of fees or compensation obtained for such activities and the total number of times he has served as an expert in medical liability actions for patients and physicians.

The AATS and STS guidelines for the behavior of physicians acting as expert witnesses indicate that the physician expert has an ethical obligation to be impartial in legal proceedings, to refrain from adopting positions as advocates or partisans, and to testify for both plaintiffs and defendants. The physician expert is obligated to review all the relevant medical information in the case and testify to its content fairly, honestly and in a balanced manner. Any inferences the physician expert is asked to make should also be made according to the same standards of fairness, honesty and balance. The physician expert should not fail to distinguish between actual negligence and an unfortunate medical outcome such as recognized complications occurring as a result of medical uncertainty. Furthermore, within a reasonable time of providing testimony, the physician expert should review the standards of practice prevailing at the time and under the circumstances of the alleged occurrence including the relevant medical literature. The physician expert should state the basis for his or her testimony or opinion, and whether it is based on personal experience, specific clinical references, evidence-based guidelines, or a generally accepted opinion in the specialty field. Compensation of the physician expert witness should be reasonable and commensurate with the time and effort given to preparing for deposition or court appearance. It is unethical for a physician expert witness to link compensation to the outcome of a case. The physician expert witness is ethically and legally obligated to tell the truth and not to mislead or deceive by act or omission. Expert opinions, including statements rendered prior to the initiation of litigation, transcripts of depositions, and courtroom testimony, are subject to independent peer reviews. Moreover, the physician expert witness should willingly provide transcripts and other documents pertaining to the expert testimony to independent peer review if requested by his or her professional organization.

The AATS addresses expert witness testimony in its code of ethics [3]. Specifically, it is stated that expert witness testimony is considered the practice of medicine and is subject to peer review. Members whose testimony is false, deceptive, misleading or without medical foundation, or otherwise violates the code of ethics may be subject to disciplinary action by the AATS. Similarly, STS provides a mechanism through which STS members can lodge complaints against fellow members who may have violated the Society's standards for expert witnesses [4].

The Society for Vascular Surgeons has also instituted guidelines for testimony by a vascular surgeon serving as an expert witness in litigation [5]. These guidelines address impartial testimony, subject matter knowledge, and compensation. With regard to impartial testimony, the guidelines mandate that the vascular surgeon expert witness shall be an impartial educator for the attorneys,

jurors and the court. The expert shall represent and testify as to the practice behavior of a prudent vascular surgeon providing different viewpoints to the extent they exist, and shall identify any personal opinions that vary significantly from generally accepted vascular surgical practice. The vascular surgeon expert shall recognize and correctly represent the full standard of care and shall with reasonable accuracy state whether a particular action was clearly within, clearly outside of, or close to the margins of the standard of care. Most importantly, the vascular surgeon expert witness shall not be evasive for purposes of favoring one litigant over another, and shall answer all properly framed questions pertaining to his opinions.

With regard to subject matter knowledge, the guidelines instruct that a vascular surgeon expert witness shall have sufficient knowledge of and experience in the specific subjects on which he or she will opine to warrant designation as an expert, and ideally should hold current hospital privileges to perform the procedures in question. An expert is required to review all pertinent medical records before rendering an opinion, and should be very familiar with prior and current concepts of standard vascular surgical practices, and ideally should be able to demonstrate evidence of continuing medical education relevant to the subject matter of the case.

As to compensation, the guidelines indicate that a vascular surgeon expert witness should be prepared to document the percentage of his or her professional time spent as an expert witness. Experts shall not accept a contingency fee for providing expert services. Finally, the guidelines indicate that charges for medical expert opinion services shall be reasonable and commensurate with the time and effort given to preparing and providing expert witness services.

Conclusion

Thoracic outlet syndrome may give rise to a number of legal issues. Surgeons who perform decompression surgery inevitably will need to be involved in such proceedings, whether as a fact witness, defendant or expert witness. Regardless of the capacity for which the physician's testimony is requested, it is essential that the physician fully acquaint himself with the patient's medical issues prior to offering testimony. When the physician is a defendant to a lawsuit or serving as an expert witness, the physician must work with the attorney to educate the attorney on the medical issues, while in turn the attorney educates the physician of the appropriate legal standards and defenses.

References

1. Statement on the physician acting as an expert witness. http://www.aats.org/Association/Policies/Statement_ on_the_physician_Acting_As_An_Expert_Witness. html. Accessed 5 May 2011.

2. Statement on the physician acting as an expert witness. http://www.sts.org/about-sts/policies/statement-physi-cian-acting-expert-witness. Accessed 5 May 2011.

3. Code of ethics. http://www.aats.org/Association/Policies/Code_of_Ethics.html. Accessed 5 May 2011.

4. Expert witness grievance procedure. http://www.sts.org/about-sts/ethics/expert-witness-grievance-process. Accessed 5 May 2011.

5. Guidelines for testimony by vascular surgeons serving as expert witness in litigation. http://www.vascularweb.org/about/policies/Pages/expert-witness-guidelines.aspx. Accessed 5 May 2011.

Disability and Workman's Compensation Issues in TOS

Gary M. Franklin

Abstract

Reported outcomes of treatment for all surgical procedures are far worse among workers compensation patients than among those with general health benefits. Population-based observational studies among injured workers in Washington State demonstrate that more disability and greater cost are associated with surgery for TOS. Factors associated with disability among injured workers likely contribute to these poor outcomes, including multiple diagnoses and prolonged disability prior to diagnosis and treatment of TOS. Higher quality trials of treatments for TOS are needed, along with a more objective case definition of neurogenic TOS and development of measures that would reflect clinically meaningful outcomes of treatment.

Introduction-Workers' Compensation 101

Injured workers present special challenges to both primary care and specialty practitioners. The key issue in workers compensation relates to the fact that 5 % of injured workers account for 80–85 % of the costs in the system [1–3]. The reason for this is that the vast majority of workers who end up on long term disability, removing

them essentially from work and everyday activities for the rest of their lives, start out with a non-catastrophic injury: a low back or neck sprain, carpal tunnel syndrome, or knee or shoulder sprain. A discussion of *how* an injured worker could end up in such a state from a non-catastrophic injury, often with severe loss of lifetime wages and loss of social and work structure, is beyond the scope of this chapter. Suffice it to say that the risk factors for development of long term disability are both intrinsic to the worker (e.g., low recovery expectation, high fear avoidance) and extrinsic to the worker (e.g., delays in administrative processing, early inappropriate opioid use, inability for an employer to accommodate return-to-work) [4, 5].

Efforts at secondary prevention, or disability prevention, to be effective, must be implemented

G.M. Franklin, MD, MPH
Departments of Environmental
and Occupational Health Sciences,
Neurology, and Health Services,
University of Washington,
130 Nickerson St, #212, Seattle, WA 98109, USA
e-mail: meddir@uw.edu

K.A. Illig et al. (eds.), *Thoracic Outlet Syndrome*,
DOI 10.1007/978-1-4471-4366-6_95, © Springer-Verlag London 2013

early, within 2–3 weeks of injury, including screening for risk of disability and application of occupational health best practices. Even modest efforts at early disability prevention can save the life of one in five of the workers likely to go on to long term disability [6]. On the contrary, a worker who has been on wage loss compensation for 3 months is already 50 % likely to still be totally disabled at 1 year. The longer disability goes on, the worse the outcome. The same principal applies to effectiveness of surgical interventions. Every procedure we have investigated has worse outcomes the longer the duration of disability prior to the application of the procedure [7].

The 3 month point on the disability curve is critical since it is at that point the worker has really already developed chronic pain. Increasing evidence suggests that the locus of the pain shifts from the originally injured part related to acute and subacute pain to a brain (central) locus involved in chronic pain [8]. If this is true, can a focused surgical intervention aimed at the originally injured part have a reasonable chance to substantially rid the patient of pain if it is conducted months after the establishment of chronic pain? For work-related carpal tunnel syndrome and its surgery, for example, the later the diagnosis and the longer the duration of disability prior to surgical intervention, the worse the outcome [9, 10].

These important issues associated with disability in workers compensation are likely highly contributory to the dozens of studies that have demonstrated that procedures conducted among injured workers receiving workers compensation benefits have far worse outcomes than similar procedures conducted among patients receiving general health benefits [11]. For example, in this meta-analysis, patients receiving shoulder acromioplasty, lumbar spine fusion, lumbar discectomy, or carpal tunnel decompression were more than four times as likely to have an unsatisfactory outcome if they received these procedures through workers compensation benefits compared to receipt through general health benefits. No similar comparative studies have been conducted for thoracic outlet syndrome (TOS) surgery. However, even patients with TOS treated conservatively

had worse outcomes if they were on workers compensation [12].

The other crucial element, also related to time loss duration, is accuracy of diagnosis at the time of workers' compensation claim initiation. Workers with carpal tunnel syndrome (CTS) diagnosed at the outset of their workers compensation claim have far superior results from median nerve decompression than workers whose CTS diagnosis is delayed by weeks to months following claim initiation [10]. Because of diagnostic inaccuracy, and the patient being seen by various specialists focusing on different parts of the upper extremity, the "syndrome of the spreading diagnosis" is prevalent. Patients diagnosed with TOS receiving conservative management report worse outcomes if they have undergone prior cubital or median nerve release [12]. This "multiple diagnosis problem" is extremely significant with relationship to the diagnosis of TOS in the Washington State workers compensation system; on average, TOS has been the TENTH diagnosis among our injured workers.

All of these factors, taken together with issues related to accuracy and reliability of diagnosis of neurogenic TOS, likely contribute to the poor outcomes, described in greater detail below, of TOS surgery among injured workers in Washington State.

Outcomes of TOS Surgery in Workers' Compensation Patients

A recent Cochrane review of studies of outcome of TOS found no randomized or quasi-randomized studies comparing surgery to any other nonsurgical comparator [13]. The authors concluded that "there is a need for an agreed definition for the diagnosis of TOS, especially the disputed form, agreed outcome measures and high quality randomized trials that compare the outcome of interventions with no treatment and with each other." In the absence of high quality randomized trials, observational studies can provide valid evidence of effectiveness on a population basis, and better information than randomized trials on costs and adverse events. In addition, such observational studies are more reflective of real world application of interventions than highly controlled randomized trials [14].

More than a decade ago, we reported the Washington State workers compensation experience with TOS in a population-based cohort of 158 cases who were diagnosed between 1986 and 1991 [15]. This reported experience included ALL such operations conducted among State Fund claimants during that time period. At this time, there is still no other reported observational study that is population-based. Two smaller observational studies have reported outcomes from University-based case series. Novak et al. reported patient self-reported outcomes among 42 cases who received physical therapy (PT) [12]. The PT was applied on average after 38 months of symptoms, and patients reported outcomes about 1 year following PT. Almost 60 % (25/42) reported some symptomatic improvement, and 38 % (16/42) reported full work and recreational activities. Cases with workers' compensation or concomitant distal entrapment neuropathy fared worse. Bosma et al [16] reported a case series of 46 TOS patients, 24 operated and 22 conservatively treated, compared to a matched group of healthy controls, on quality of life. All TOS patients reported low QOL, regardless of treatment type. These authors recommend that improved patient selection could lead to improved outcomes.

Table 95.1 summarizes the time loss and medical cost outcomes for the Washington workers' compensation TOS cohort [15]. After adjusting for important covariates, such as the time from injury to TOS diagnosis, and for the duration of time-loss prior to TOS diagnosis, the odds of being totally disabled 1 year after surgery were nearly three times greater for those receiving TOS surgery. Over half (53 %) of TOS surgery patients were still totally disabled 1 year after surgery, compared to 16 % of TOS patients who received only conservative treatment. Neither the type of surgery, the presence/absence of provocative tests, or surgical experience predicted better surgical outcome. In a structured telephone interview conducted an average of 4.5 years following TOS surgery, 72.5 % reported being "limited a

Table 95.1 Time loss and medical costs for cases with and without TOS surgery diagnosed 1987 – 1989

Time loss, costs	TOS surgery	No surgery
Unadjusted		
	N = 74	N = 95
Mean medical costs, $	25,614	14,063
Percent on time loss at 1 year	56.8	21.1
Percent on time loss at 2 years	40.5	12.6
Adjusted[a]		
Mean medical costs, $	22,576	15,652
Percent on time loss at 1 year	52.7	15.8
Percent on time loss at 2 years	37.2	7.8

Adapted from Franklin et al. [15]. With permission from Wolter Kluwers Health
[a]Adjusted for age, cervical spine diagnosis, number of years from injury to diagnosis, sex, time loss in 6 months before diagnosis, previous injury, and previous surgery. All p values were <0.01

Table 95.2 TOS update, 2003–2007

	No surgery	Surgery
First diagnosis (353.0) in 2003–2007		
N	906	50
Injury to first TOS diagnosis, year	1.5	2.6
Pct still open as of 10/31/2009	20 %	60 %
For time loss cases only (through 10/31/2009)		
N	662	50
Mean time loss pre diagnosis, days	374	435
Mean time loss post diagnosis, days	587	1,132
Mean medical costs to date, $$	44,697	64,560
Mean time loss, paid to date, $$	52,298	86,424

lot" in rigorous activities. Finally, 31.7 % had at least one acute complication of surgery, 19 % with a pleural tear, and 7 % with pneumothorax or atelectasis. Almost 18 %, as recorded in the medical record, had at least one new sensory complaint following surgery.

Table 95.2 summarizes the Washington workers compensation TOS experience from cases identified in 2003–2007. The mean time loss

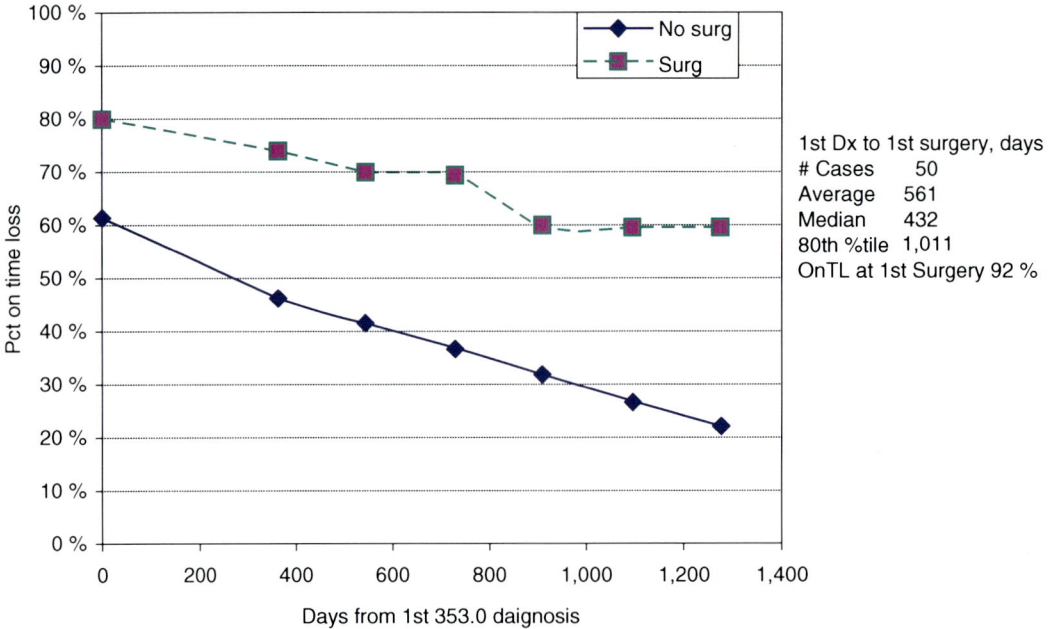

1st Dx to 1st surgery, days
Cases 50
Average 561
Median 432
80th %tile 1,011
OnTL at 1st Surgery 92 %

Fig. 95.1 Time to leaving time loss after diagnosis of thoracic outlet syndrome-Washington Workers Compensation, 2003–2007

Table 95.3 Total costs for 956 TOS cases first diagnosed in 2003–2007

	Cases	Time loss$$, ptd	Med aid$$, ptd	Total$$, ptd	Avg$$/case
No surgery	906	34,307,263	30,963,747	86,641,273	95,631
Surgery	50	4,321,193	3,228,003	10,580,286	211,606
Grand total	956	38,628,457	34,191,750	97,221,559	101,696

following TOS diagnosis in those receiving surgery was double that of those treated without surgery. Figure 95.1 shows the time to leaving time loss in cases who did and did not receive TOS surgery. Finally, Table 95.3 shows the total costs of all TOS cases. The total amount spent on all cases with a diagnosis of TOS was $97.2 million. The costs/case in those who received surgery ($211,606) were more than double the costs/case of the TOS cases treated conservatively ($95,631).

The Washington Workers Compensation TOS Surgery Guideline

Because of our reported experience with TOS and TOS surgery, our statutory Industrial Insurance Medical Advisory Committee recently developed a guideline [17, 18] that requires

objective evidence by electrodiagnostic studies of brachial plexus involvement before surgery for TOS can be approved. In addition, the results of scalene blocks are not considered a compelling reason to allow surgery in the absence of abnormal electrodiagnostic studies.

Conclusion

It is surprising that no high quality randomized trials are available on TOS comparing surgery to appropriate comparators. Observational studies suggest that conservative approaches such as targeted physical therapy can be effective. The experience of worse outcomes for most studied procedures in workers' compensation populations is probably related to confounding issues related to prolonged disability, inaccurate diagnosis of multiple upper extremity disorders, and risk factors for long term disability having nothing to do with medical care received. However, the WA population-based data, and smaller observational studies, also suggest that TOS surgery per se is associated with very poor outcomes in the injured worker population. More rigorous scientific study of potentially effective treatments for TOS, including surgery, will be critical to help inform future policy.

References

1. Cheadle A, Franklin G, Wolfhagen C, et al. Factors influencing the duration of work-related disability: a population-based study of Washington State workers' compensation. Am J Public Health. 1994;84: 190–6.
2. Hashemi L, Webster BS, Clancy EA, et al. Length of disability and cost of workers' compensation low back pain claims. J Occup Environ Med. 1997;39:937–45.
3. Hashemi L, Webster BS, Clancy EA, et al. Length of disability and cost of work-related musculoskeletal disorders of the upper extremity. J Occup Environ Med. 1998;40:261–9.
4. Turner JA, Franklin GM, Fulton-Kehoe D, et al. Early predictors of chronic work disability associated with carpal tunnel syndrome: a longitudinal workers' compensation cohort study. Am J Ind Med. 2007;50:489–500.
5. Turner JA, Franklin G, Fulton-Kehoe D, et al. ISSLS prize winner: early predictors of chronic work disability: a prospective, population-based study of workers with back injuries. Spine. 2008;33:2809–18.
6. Wickizer T, Franklin GM, Fulton-Kehoe D, et al. Centers on occupational health and education: final report on outcomes from the initial cohort of injured works, 2003–2005. http://www.lni.wa.gov/ClaimsIns/Providers/ProjResearchComm/OHS/default.asp. Accessed 5 July 2011.
7. Franklin GM, Wickizer TM, Fulton-Kehoe D, Turner JA. Policy-relevant research: when does it matter? NeuroRx. 2004;1:356–62.
8. Becerra L, Morris S, Bazes S, et al. Trigeminal neuropathic pain alters responses in CNS circuits to mechanical (brush) and thermal (cold and heat) stimuli. J Neurosci. 2006;26:10646–57.
9. Daniell WE, Fulton-Kehoe D, Chiou LA, Franklin GM. Work-related carpal tunnel syndrome in Washington State workers' compensation: temporal trends, clinical practices, and disability. Am J Ind Med. 2005;48:259–69.
10. Daniell WE, Fulton-Kehoe D, Franklin GM. Work-related carpal tunnel syndrome in Washington State workers' compensation: utilization of surgery and the duration of lost work. Am J Ind Med. 2009;52:931–42.
11. Harris I, Mulford J, Solomon M, et al. Association between compensation status and outcome after surgery: a meta-analysis. JAMA. 2005;293:1644–52.
12. Novak CB, Collins ED, Mackinnon SE. Outcome following conservative management of thoracic outlet syndrome. J Hand Surg [Am]. 1995;20:542–8.
13. Povlsen B, Belzberg A, Hansson T, Dorsi M. Treatment for thoracic outlet syndrome. Cochrane Database Syst Rev. 2010;(20):CD007218.
14. Dreyer NA, Tunis SR, Berger M, et al. Why observational studies should be among the tools used in comparative effectiveness research. Health Aff. 2010;29:1818–25.
15. Franklin GM, Fulton-Kehoe D, Bradley C, Smith-Weller T. Outcome of surgery for thoracic outlet syndrome in Washington State workers' compensation. Neurology. 2000;54:1252–7.
16. Bosma J, Engeland MI, Leijdekkers VJ, et al. The influence of choice of therapy on quality of life in patients with neurogenic thoracic outlet syndrome. Br J Neurosurg. 2010;24:532–6.
17. Washington State Department of Labor and Industries. Medical treatment guidelines. http://www.lni.wa.gov/ClaimsIns/Providers/TreatingPatients/TreatGuide/default.asp. Accessed 5 July 2011.
18. The National Guideline Clearinghouse. Work-related neurogenic thoracic outlet syndrome: diagnosis and treatment. http://www.guidelines.gov/content.aspx?id=24159. Accessed 5 July 2011.

Internet-Based Patient and Clinician Resources for TOS

96

Linda M. Harris and Purandath Lall

Abstract

Internet access and usage for medical conditions is common amongst patient and physicians and can be a resourceful tool for both groups in the management of patients with thoracic outlet syndrome. There are multiple educational, easily accessible websites that provide non-biased, up to date treatment options for TOS. Websites should be scrutinized for their content, potential for commercial and personal bias and "updated history" to avoid medical pitfalls.

Introduction

The terms "Internet" and "World Wide Web" are often used in everyday speech without much distinction. However, the Internet and the World Wide Web are not one and the same. The Internet is a global system of interconnected computer networks. In contrast, the Web is one of the services that run on the Internet. It is a collection of interconnected documents and other resources, linked by hyperlinks and URLs (Uniform Resource Locator). In short, the Web is an application running on the Internet [1].

L.M. Harris, MD(✉)
Department of Surgery, Kaleida Health,
3 Gates Circle, Buffalo, NY 14209, USA
e-mail: lharris@kaledahealth.org

P. Lall, MD
Department of Surgery, VA WNY Health Care System,
3495 Bailey Avenue, Buffalo, NY 14215, USA
e-mail: purandath.lall@va.gov

Background

Internet usage has become commonplace amongst both patients and physicians. Unfortunately, the quality of health information available on the internet is extremely variable, putting quality health care at risk if patients rely on inaccurate information. Surveys indicate anywhere between 40 and 80 % [2, 3] of patients utilize the internet to search medical information. The internet can clearly be a benefit to both physician and patient. Good information on the internet can augment doctor- patient information, but inaccurate information can lead to failure to comply with appropriate treatment, delay in treatment, or use of unproven or worthless therapy (e.g. chelation). Physicians can be proactive in facilitating effective use of the internet for medical diseases by recommending appropriate sites to assist patients in gathering additional information on their conditions and treatment. In an unpublished study by the authors, 91 % of patients would like to visit a website created by

K.A. Illig et al. (eds.), *Thoracic Outlet Syndrome*,
DOI 10.1007/978-1-4471-4366-6_96, © Springer-Verlag London 2013

their own physician, and 90 % would like for their physicians to have a list of recommended websites based on disease process (versus 17 % preferring to search for information without guidance). Furthermore, this interaction may increase discussion between the patient and the health care provider, hopefully decreasing the impact of erroneous information.

In a study of patient use of the internet, Diaz et al. [4] surveyed 1,000 primary care patients. Of the 512 who responded, 60 % felt that the information on the internet was the same as or better than information from their doctors. Alarmingly, 59 % did not discuss this information with their doctors. In this study, Diaz [4] reports that 58 % used the internet to determine medication or procedure side effects, while 41 % looked for alternative or complementary care and 41 % utilized the internet for a second opinion.

Semere et al. [5], investigated "Parent usage of the internet for medical information" to first determine parents' access to and use of the Internet for information relating to their child's health, second, to investigate parents methods of searching for such information, and, third, to evaluate the information found in relation to its readability, accuracy, and influence. They concluded many parents use the Internet for additional medical information, but they do not access this information frequently. The overwhelmingly positive impression of online health information suggests parents are unaware of the dangers of encountering misleading sources, an issue of special concern when considering the amount of influence this information carries.

Some general recommendations on patient internet use include:

- Not to use the internet as a substitute for the physician,
- Preferential use of government or medical society sponsored health sites,
- Attention to when the site was last updated,
- Looking for journal references,
- Wariness of sites associated with attempts to sell products/services, and
- Primary use of trusted medical sites (such as WebMD).

With this said, the internet can be useful by reinforcing information given by the physician, providing images to facilitate patient understanding, providing access to support groups (perhaps most important for uncommon diseases/therapies), providing printed material for the patient to share with family/friends, and providing information on where to find specialists for patients.

Resources for Patients

There are multiple available search engines and websites that provide information on TOS. The first site we would recommend for patients is the American TOS association site, atosa.org/thoracic-outlet-syndrome [6]. This site provides basic information on the types of TOS, symptoms, diagnoses, and possible therapies. The site also provides links to a research library, support groups, and a physician locator service, although this function is limited to physician members of the organization and is not an exhaustive or complete list of competent physicians who treat TOS. The Society for Vascular Surgery website also provides a physician locator service by state which can be useful for patients, http://www.vascularweb.org/vascularhealth/Pages/thoracic-outlet-syndrome.aspx [7].

The National Organization for Rare Diseases provides a brief report e-mailed to the patient at no cost. The report was copyrighted in 2009, and reviews the various types of TOS, symptoms, causes, related disorders, standard therapy and testing, as well as therapy: http://www.rarediseases.org/search/rdblist.html [8]. The site offers a link to Clinicaltrials.gov [9] which describes any current research studies on the subject, as well as the American Chronic pain Association.

An excellent referral website for patients is MedlinePlus, the National Institutes of Health's Web site for patients and their families and friends: http://www.nlm.nih.gov/medlineplus/thoracicoutletsyndrome.html [10] (Fig. 96.1). Produced by the National Library of Medicine, it

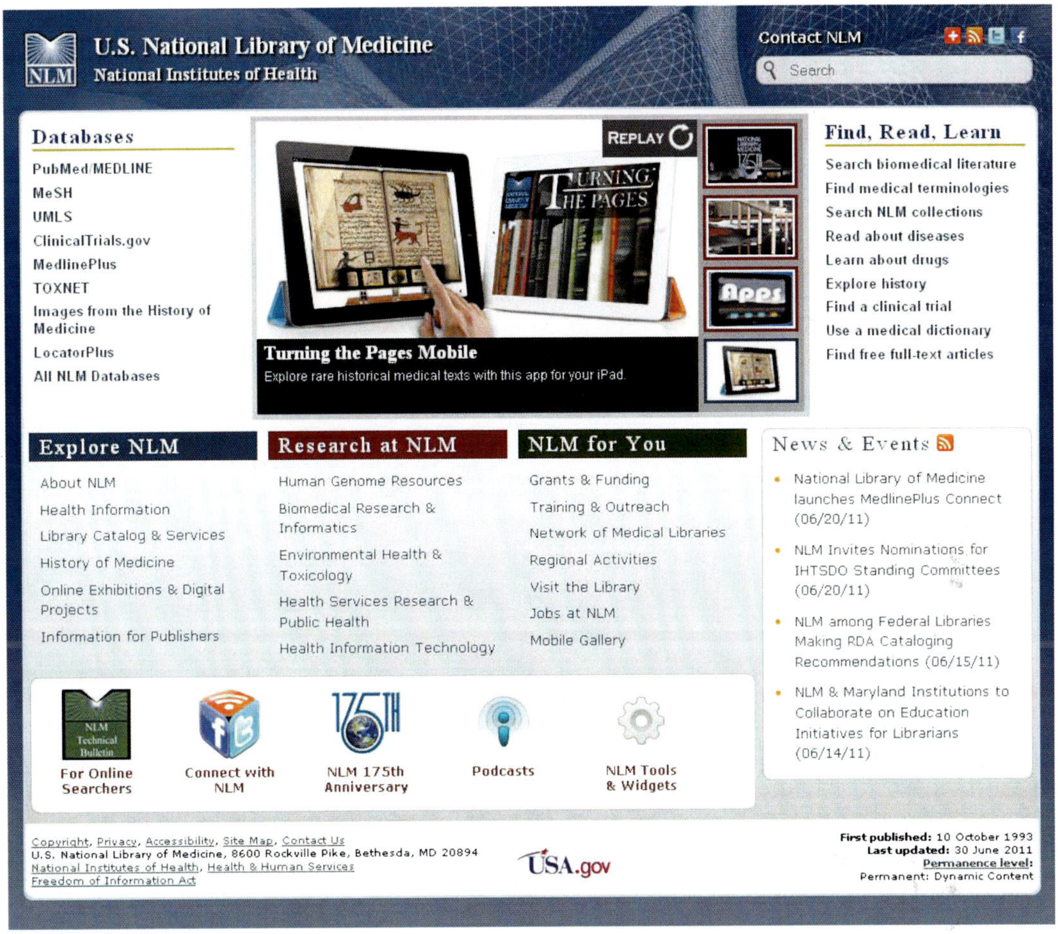

Fig. 96.1 NIH website providing basic information on TOS including symptoms, treatment, prognosis, and complications (Courtesy of the National Library of Medicine)

"provides information about diseases, conditions, and wellness issues in language you can understand". MedlinePlus offers reliable, up-to-date health information, anytime, anywhere, for free". This webpage is constructed with an easy to read layout including "the basics, research, and a reference to directories and organizations that treat TOS". There is an external link that redirects the user to the SVS webpage on TOS treatment and patient handouts in English and Spanish language.

The website http://www.ninds.nih.gov/disorders/thoracic/thoracic.htm [11] available through the National Institute of Neurological Disorders and Stroke (NINDS) is also a good starting page for both patients and physicians. There are multiple "clickable icons" on the webpage that will redirect the user to clinical trials, treatment options, prognosis, research, organizations and additional resources form MEDLINE plus. The webpage offers patient brochures in English and Spanish options and also has a "listen" option enabled by readspeaker.

A site with a good overview of TOS written at the patient level is http://www.mdguidelines.com/thoracic-outlet-syndrome [12]. Sites from respected national organizations with pages on TOS also include http://www.mayoclinic.com/health/thoracic-outlet-syndrome/DS00800 [13]. A site by Dr Saunders, http://www.tos-syndrome.

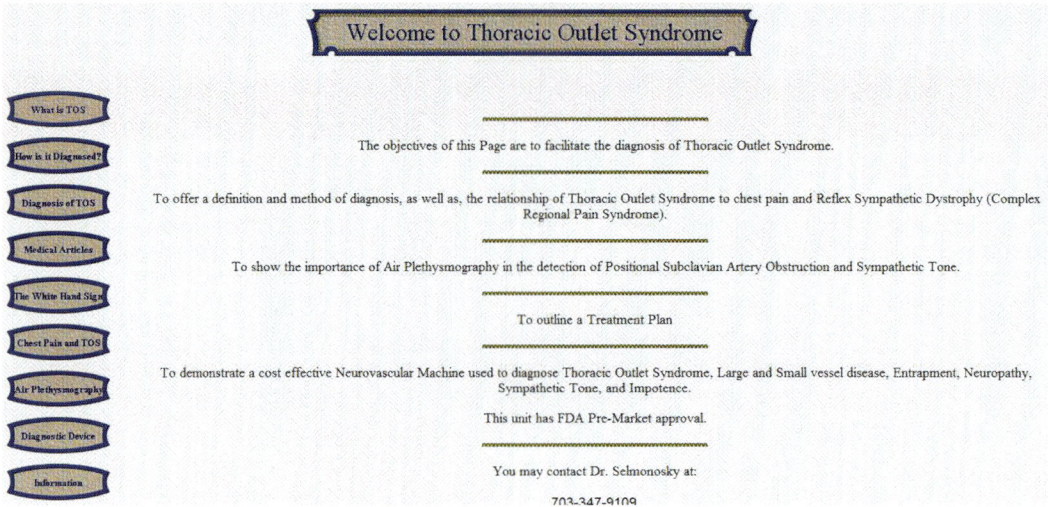

Fig. 96.2 Physician website provides multiple clickable icons to information on diagnosis, treatment, and reference articles (Courtesy of Dr. Carlos A. Selmonosky)

com [14] (Fig. 96.2), provides good information, although there is an effort to sell equipment for diagnosis on the site.

MedicineNet, Inc., owned and operated by WebMD and part of the WebMD Network. The website describes itself as "an online, healthcare media publishing company. It provides easy-to-read, in-depth, authoritative medical information for consumers via its robust, user-friendly, interactive website." The webpage http://www.medicinenet.com/thoracic_outlet_syndrome/article.htm [15] provides a good overview of TOS, including etiology, signs and symptoms and treatment in layman terms. There is also a "patient to patient" case report edited by a physician included on the webpage.

A growing source of information for patients is Wikipedia [16]. Wikipedia defines itself as "a multilingual, web-based, free-content encyclopedia project based on an openly editable model. Wikipedia's articles provide links to guide the user to related pages with additional information. Wikipedia is written collaboratively by largely anonymous Internet volunteers who write without

pay. Anyone with Internet access can write and make changes to Wikipedia articles (except in certain cases where editing is restricted to prevent disruption or vandalism). Users can contribute anonymously, under a pseudonym, or with their real identity, if they choose." While much of the information from this source may be accurate, it is not peer-reviewed and thus at some risk for misinformation. It currently does provide useful information for both patients and physicians including the definition, classification and treatment options. There is a paragraph on notable people who suffered with TOS including athletes and musicians. Most of the content however, is written in medical terminology and will probably be difficult reading for the patients. At the end of the webpage, multiple external links and references are provided to help the patient acquire more information if needed, including the SVS webpage.

Finally, Facebook, a popular networking and social media site, also provides several sites with general information, pictures of surgical incisions, and access to chat groups. One such site is http://www.facebook.com/home.php#!/group.php?gid=15231937182 [17]. Patients may also find others with TOS through internet support groups, such as searching Thoracic Outlet on http://www.dailystrength.org/ [18]. Once caution with support groups, is that the information provided from these groups is not medically verified. However, it may still be useful for patients with chronic conditions to be in contact with others with similar situations for emotional support. Youtube also provides SVS-sponsored presentations directed towards patients regarding TOS by Julie Frieschlag http://www.youtube.com/watch?v=yU0EyY5W8uU [19], Ben Chang, Greg Moneta and Karl Illig which briefly review various types of thoracic outlet syndrome.

Resources for Healthcare Professionals

For a significant portion of practicing physicians, the Internet has become a critical component of how they seek medical information. In a survey conducted by Hall and Partners [20] (commissioned by Google), 86 % of U.S. physicians use the Internet to gather health, medical or prescription drug information. Of physicians who use the Internet for health information, 92 % accessed it from an office setting, 88 % from home, and 59 % from a mobile device. Seventy-one percent said they start their research with a search engine, 92 % of those using Google. Fifty eight percent 58 % of physicians searched more than once per day – including 65 % of primary care physicians. Of physicians who start with a search engine, 57 % use terms related to conditions and 36 % use terms related to treatments and trials. While the most common action taken after an online search was to conduct further research (48 %), about a third of the surveyed physicians said they had made a change to a patient's medication as a result of a search, or had initiated new treatment.

For physicians, the internet can provide evidence-based studies, societal or consensus conference recommendations, and videos of procedures which the surgeons may be less comfortable with. A site by Dr Harold Urschel and a prior patient with TOS, www.thoracicoutletsyndromes.com/index.html [21] (Fig. 96.3), provides information at the physician level for diagnosis, surgical therapy, etiology, recurrence, as well as many images. http://www.youtube.com/watch?v=D_jBR0J_sSo [22] is a movie of a supraclavicular resection of a cervical rib by a neurosurgeon which may be useful for training programs or for physicians more comfortable with the transaxillary approach.

The internet can also provide videos that may be useful in the medical management of TOS patients. Videos may provide exercise and stretching programs that may be useful to educate local physical therapists unfamiliar with TOS, or to provide additional help for patient home therapy. However, videos on Youtube can be discontinued at any time. The following site provides images of clinical exam positions as well as therapeutic stretches for patients to perform, and may be useful for educating physical therapists, http://www.nismat.org/ptcor/thoracic_outlet [23].

Conclusions

The internet will continue to play an increasing role in medical care as more of the population is computer savvy. Young physicians rely more on the internet and electronic textbooks than on hardcopy texts and journals. Patients are also turning to electronic resources at a higher rate. It is imperative that physicians interact with patients and discuss information garnered from outside sources to decrease the risk of adverse outcomes due to inaccurate or biased websites. Used properly, the internet can assist the patient and surgeon by reinforcing useful information, and providing images, support systems, as well as information on new developments in the field.

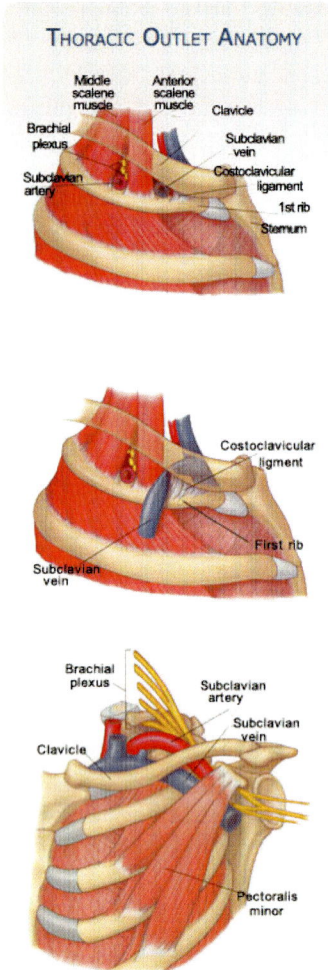

Thoracic Outlet Syndromes

Thoracic outlet syndrome (TOS) refers to compression of one or more of the neurovascular structures traversing the superior aperture of the chest. Previously, the name was designated according to the etiologies of compression, such as scalenus anticus muscle, costoclavicular ligament, hyperabduction, cervical rib, or first rib syndromes. Peet coined the term "thoracic outlet syndrome" in 1956 to designate compression of the neurovascular bundle at the thoracic outlet.

Nerve Compression

The symptoms of nerve compression most frequently observed are pain, paresthesias (numbness and tingling) and motor weakness. Pain and paresthesias are segmental in 75% of cases, 90% involving the ulnar nerve distribution. The onset of pain is usually insidious and commonly involves the neck, shoulder, arm, and hand. The pain and paresthesias may be precipitated by strenuous physical exercise or sustained physical effort with the arm in abduction and the neck in hyperextension.

Vein Compression

The axillary subclavian vein traverses the tunnel formed by the clavicle and subclavius muscle anteriorly, the scalenus anticus muscle laterally, the first rib posterior-inferiorly, and the costoclavicular ligament medially. In most patients with thrombosis of the axillary subclavian vein (Paget-Schroetter Syndrome), the costoclavicular ligament congenitally inserts further lateral than normal. Thus, when the scalenus anticus muscle hypertrophies the vein is occluded, rather than simply compressed.

Arterial Compression

Aneurysm (with emboli) or occlusion of the artery may occur. The diagnosis is suspected by the history, physical examination, and Doppler studies and is confirmed with arteriography. Therapy for arterial compression depends on its degree of involvement. Symptoms of arterial compression include coldness, weakness, easy fatigability of the arm and hand, and pain that is usually diffuse.

Sympathetic Compression

Compression of the sympathetic nerves in the thoracic outlet may occur alone or in combination with peripheral nerve and blood vessels. The sympathetics are intimately attached to the artery as well as adjacent to the bone. It may cause atypical chest pain (pseudoangina) which simulates cardiac pain, or excessive cold, sweaty upper extremities.

Home   Etiology   Diagnosis   Treatment   Recurrence   About Us   Contact

Fig. 96.3 Physician website that is easy to navigate, well illustrated, with multiple clickable icons regarding basic information, etiology, diagnosis, therapy, and recurrence for TOS (Courtesy of Harold C. Urschel, Jr., MD and Associates)

References

1. The key and critical objectives of "The W3C Technology Stack". World Wide Web Consortium. http://www.w3.org/Consortium/technology. Accessed 13 May 2011.

2. Baker L, Wagner T, Singer S, Bundorf M. Use of the internet and e-mail for health care information: results from a national survey. JAMA. 2003;289(18):2400–6.

3. Assessing the quality of information to support people in making decisions about their health and healthcare, Picker Institute, BMA-Picker Institute. http://www.pickereurope.org/page.php?id=48. Accessed 5 May 2011.

4. Diaz J, Griffith R, Ng JJ, Reinert S, Friedmann P, Moulton A. Patients' use of the internet for medical information. J Gen Intern Med. 2002;17(3):180–5.
5. Semere W, Karamanoukian HL, Levit M, et al. A pediatric surgery study: parent usage of the internet for medical information. J Pediatr Surg. 2003;38:560–4.
6. The key and critical objectives of the American TOS Association. http://atosa.org/main. Accessed 6 May 2011.
7. The key and critical objectives of the Society for Vascular Surgery website. http://www.vascularweb.org/vascularhealth/Pages/thoracic-outlet-syndrome.aspx. Accessed 6 May 2011.
8. The key and critical objectives of the National Organization for Rare Diseases. http://www.rarediseases.org/search/rdblist.html. Accessed 6 May 2011.
9. The key and critical objectives of the National Organization for Rare Diseases. http://clinicaltrials.gov/. Accessed 6 May 2011.
10. The key and critical objectives of MedlinePlus. http://www.nlm.nih.gov/medlineplus/thoracicoutletsyndrome.html. Accessed 6 May 2011.
11. The key and critical objectives of the National Institute of Neurological Disorders and Stroke. http://www.ninds.nih.gov/disorders/thoracic/thoracic.htm. Accessed 6 May 2011.
12. The key and critical objectives of the MD Guidelines site. http://www.mdguidelines.com/thoracic-outlet-syndrome. Accessed 6 May 2011.
13. The key and critical objectives of the Mayo Clinic. http://www.mayoclinic.com/health/thoracic-outlet-syndrome/DS00800. Accessed 6 May 2011.
14. The key and critical objectives of a site by Richard J. Sanders, MD. http://www.tos-syndrome.com. Accessed 6 May 2011.
15. The key and critical objectives of a site MedicineNet, Inc. http://www.medicinenet.com/thoracic_outlet_syndrome/article.htm. Accessed 6 May 2011.
16. The key and critical objectives of a site named Wikipedia. http://www.wikipedia.org/. Accessed 6 May 2011.
17. The key and critical objectives of Facebook. http://www.facebook.com/home.php#!/group.php?gid=15231937182. Accessed 6 May 2011.
18. The key and critical objectives of internet support groups. http://www.dailystrength.org/. Accessed 6 May 2011.
19. The key and critical objectives of Youtube. http://www.youtube.com/watch?v=yU0EyY5W8uU. Accessed 13 May 2011.
20. The key and critical objectives of Connecting with PhysiciansOnline. www.fdasm.com/docs/Connecting%20with%20Physicians%20Online%20Webinar%20Deck--%20final.pdf. Accessed 13 May 2011.
21. The key and critical objectives of the site by Harold C. Urschel Jr., MD www.thoracicoutletsyndromes.com/index.html. Accessed 6 May 2011.
22. The key and critical objectives of Youtube. http://www.youtube.com/watch?v=DjBROJsSo. Accessed 6 May 2011.
23. The key and critical objectives of the Nicholas Institute of Sports Medicine and Athletic Trauma. http://www.nismat.org/ptcor/thoracic_outlet. Accessed 6 May 2011.

Establishing a TOS-Focused Practice

97

Karl A. Illig, Robert W. Thompson,
Julie Ann Freischlag, Dean M. Donahue,
and Peter I. Edgelow

Abstract

Patients with thoracic outlet syndrome, especially neurologic, typically require many more resources than the typical vascular, thoracic, or neurologic patient. As such, a dedicated TOS clinic pays major dividends, in terms of time, resources, and patient and provider satisfaction. Such a clinic should include, at a minimum, a provider, physician extender, and physical or occupational therapist truly interested in the problem, along with logistical support for the documentation and paperwork required. If local resources permit, a neurodiagnostician with interest in modern, objective diagnostic and therapeutic block techniques is valuable, as are a psychologist or even a psychiatrist. Educational materials can be made available to patients ahead of time, streamlining the visit itself. Such a clinic does not need to be free-standing or full-time, but can exist "virtually" within a conventional clinic simply by designating a time when patients and providers can all assemble. Such a clinic vastly improves the care of patients with VTOS, and acts as a surprisingly effective marketing tool in most communities.

K.A. Illig, MD (✉)
Department of Surgery, Division of Vascular Surgery,
University of South Florida,
2 Tampa General Circle, STC 7016, Tampa,
FL 33606, USA
e-mail: killig@health.usf.edu

R.W. Thompson, MD
Department of Surgery, Section of Vascular Surgery,
Center for Thoracic Outlet Syndrome,
Washington University, Barnes-Jewish Hospital,
Campus Box 8109/Suite 5101
Queeny Tower, 660 S Euclid Ave, St. Louis,
MO 63110, USA
e-mail: thompson@wudosis.wustl.edu

J.A. Freischlag, MD
Department of Surgery,
Johns Hopkins Medical Institutions,
720 Rutland Avenue 759 Ross,
Baltimore, MD 21205, USA
e-mail: jfreisc1@jhmi.edu

D.M. Donahue, MD
Department of Thoracic Surgery,
Massachusetts General Hospital,
Blake 1570, 55 Fruit Street, Boston, MA 02114, USA
e-mail: donahue.dean@mgh.harvard.edu

P.I. Edgelow, DPT
Graduate Program in Physical Therapy, UCSF/SFSU,
2429 Balmoral St., Union City, CA 94587, USA
e-mail: peteriedgelow@aol.com

K.A. Illig et al. (eds.), *Thoracic Outlet Syndrome*,
DOI 10.1007/978-1-4471-4366-6_97, © Springer-Verlag London 2013

Introduction

Imagine this scenario: You are halfway through a busy clinic, pretty much on time although the waiting room is three-quarters full and you see rooms with charts on the door, a couple of new patients with carotid disease and a routine post-bypass followup visit. A patient awaits with a medium-sized thoracoabdominal aneurysm who will need some time. You enter the room of the next patient, however, and notice two things: she is young, and she has a foot-high stack of old charts and pain diaries on the chair next to her (Fig. 97.1). The chief complaint says "thoracic outlet syndrome symptoms for 4 years/causalgia," and she has driven three hours to get to your office. Two things go through your head: "Every single person in my office is going to be mad," and "there goes my day."

Patients with suspected TOS, perhaps more so than any other entity a surgeon sees, are best treated in a formal, disease-dedicated clinic. These patients require more time to evaluate, require more time for education, decision-making, and implementation of plans, have more associated diagnoses, and carry with them almost inevitably more paperwork (both to read and to fill out). A smoothly running clinic can be brought to a grinding halt by anything more than a very straightforward TOS case, and apart from the physician's personal unhappiness at a late day, this event produces ripples of unhappiness for everyone involved in the day's work. A TOS clinic does one very major thing: it *concentrates resources*. First and foremost, such concentration allows the best possible care for the TOS patient, and second, elimination of these patients from the "regular" clinic allows that clinic to run much more smoothly and those patients (and staff, referring physicians, and doctor) to be infinitely happier.

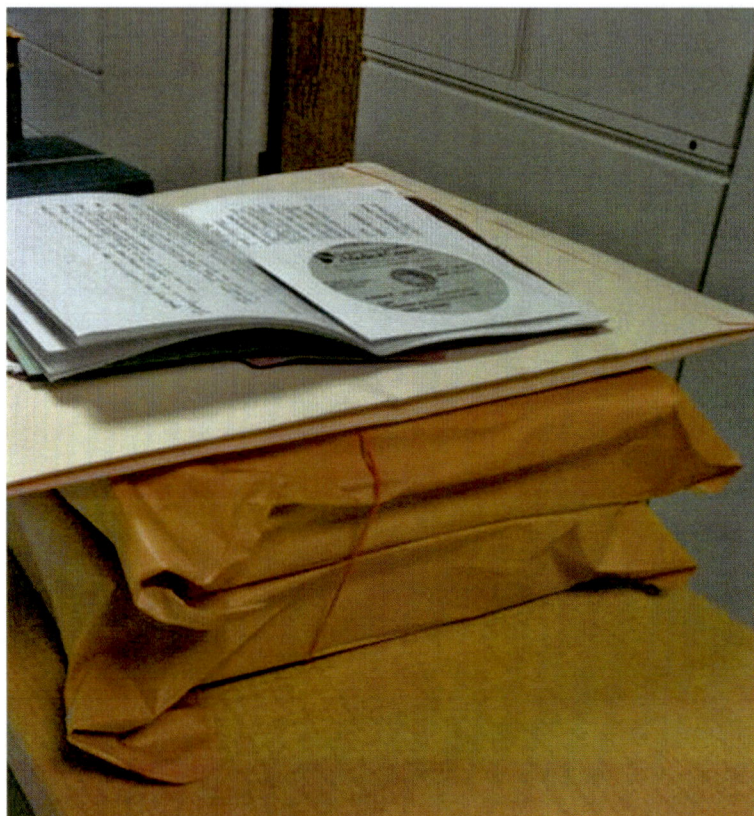

Fig. 97.1 "Typical TOS patient" chart

Concentration of Resources

As discussed above, these patients have unique needs that may be best met (and uniquely so) by concentration of resources. Such resources include educational materials and methods, personnel, evaluation from multiple perspectives simultaneously, facilities for managing paperwork, time for chart review and lengthy dictation, and, perhaps most importantly, a mindset allowing plenty of time for a thorough, focused evaluation without worrying about other patients backing up in exam rooms.

Education is unusually critical for this entity. TOS is a diagnosis that is poorly understood by patients and referring practitioners alike. In addition, a thorough understanding of this entity can be therapeutic, and even agreeing upon a diagnosis can be amazingly helpful to these often beleaguered patients (in one large specialty practice, more than 50 % of patients do not receive the correct diagnosis for a mean of 2 years [1]). As such, patients with TOS require more education than most. Everyone dealing with TOS quickly evolves a "spiel," and while annoyingly repetitive, going over this ten times in a day once every couple of weeks is probably preferable to doing it once every clinic day. Even more useful are prerecorded video programs outlining the basic facts and anticipated protocols surrounding this diagnosis, which can be set up in the waiting room or used as a previsit orientation program before personalized evaluation. Finally, if dedicated space is available, written materials (wall or brochures) can be set up as permanent tools (educational materials can, of course, be sent to affected patients in advance, but this is not a specific advantage of a dedicated clinic).

Concentration of personnel is perhaps the most significant benefit of a TOS clinic. As described in multiple chapters above, this may be the most "multidisciplinary" diagnosis that a surgeon or neurologist will face. At a minimum, it is suggested that the physician work with a dedicated midlevel provider (nurse practitioner or physicians' assistant) who is interested in this diagnosis and patients who have it and a physical or occupational therapist. One of the most important benefits of this is the ability to *evaluate the patients from multiple perspectives simultaneously*. Rather than sequentially see each "team" and repeat their story over and over, one long, thorough visit by at least the "medical" and "physical therapy" personnel together allows the most complete data gathering and highest patient satisfaction. Each "team" can gather needed data by questioning, but each will also find opportunities to interject, ask additional questions, seek to modify answers, and consult together in real time. In the editors' experience, something is learned by both patients and providers and care improved in virtually every encounter of this type.

This is only the minimum, and should be practical in virtually every environment. Even more advanced protocols are feasible. For example, with increasingly accurate predictive value of neurointerventional maneuvers (see Chap. 20), an argument can be made for near-universal application in patients with NTOS. Even if not practical in one physical setting, the block team can set aside their own concentrated clinic day and save time for same-day referrals (particularly helpful as many patients will travel considerable distances to such a clinic). It has also been increasingly recognized (see Chap. 8) that a large percentage of patients have problems in addition to this diagnosis, such as depression, opioid dependence, or chronic regional pain syndrome, that significantly alter treatment strategies and responses to same. For this reason, a psychologist, psychiatrist, pain physician, neurologist, or other appropriate professional should, at a minimum, be available for consultation on a same-day basis; if the clinic is busy enough, on-site presence can probably be justified (and some clinics are run by non-surgeons as described below).

Paperwork needs are unusually important when treating patients with TOS, as all interested practitioners can attest. The patient almost always brings things to the encounter for the physician to help with, most commonly disability forms. Work excuses, work limitation evaluation, legal questions, and prescription requests are also commonly seen. Concentration of thought regarding these and the assistance of an interested midlevel provider convert an onerous chore into something much easier to perform (and perform correctly the first time). Equally important, however, is the paperwork the practitioner brings to the table. First are documents needed for the individual clinical encounter, including patient self-description of the chief complaint as well as past history information. Again, this can be mailed ahead of time, but as a TOS-specific form is often very different from a conventional vascular, thoracic, neurosurgical, or neurologic "generic encounter" form, concentrating these all on 1 day helps the practitioner correctly evaluate them. Finally, of increasing importance are ancillary data collection forms, directed at function, the psychological effects of the condition, and, importantly, data collection for evaluation of outcomes (see Appendix).

Adequate time for thorough evaluation of past records and thorough, detailed dictation is, we feel, another critical benefit of a TOS clinic, especially when combined with concentration of personnel as described above. A full-day TOS clinic might have new patients scheduled at 30, 45, or even 60 min intervals. The patient can be exposed to taped educational materials ahead of time, and the midlevel provider, physical therapist, neurologist, and psychologist can all spend individual time with the patient, as needed (assuming an initial combined visit as described above). All of these periods allow the responsible practitioner intervals for chart review, planning of therapy, and dictation, the latter being particularly important. Having a limited number of patients rationally scheduled on a dedicated day (without adding on emergent patients as is often needed during a normal clinic day) allows a thorough, methodical approach to each patient in turn.

Finally, a dedicated day often allows streamlined testing, including plain chest and cervical spine radiographs, perhaps nerve conduction testing in patients with NTOS, and noninvasive lab testing in patients with vascular TOS. Again, if these resources are not available in the clinic itself, concentrating TOS patients on certain days creates the opportunity to set up such services on a same day, walk-in basis.

Other Benefits

Several other benefits are created by the establishment of a TOS clinic. First and foremost, the patients and referring practitioners are immediately apparent that this is an entity that is "real" and is judged important by the TOS practitioner. Every single practitioner who treats this disease hears some variant of "no one believes me" or "no one knows anything about TOS" on nearly a daily basis, and in our experience just walking through the door of a focused clinic makes such patients extremely happy. In addition to treating patients with compassion, the very concept that someone is taking them seriously and "it's not all in my head" is, we feel, highly therapeutic. Second is the marketing benefit. Establishing such a clinic allows better communication with referring physicians, making them more aware that this diagnosis exists and giving them a place to send such patients. Again, the patients benefit, but in virtually every case that such a clinic is established, business is quickly brisk. Finally, concentration of resources makes the logistics of record-keeping much easier, for both assessment of individual outcomes and academic investigation.

Practical Considerations

A brief outline of a successful TOS clinic is as follows.

- Physical plant and resources:
  - Usually section of conventional clinic set aside for TOS patients only on appropriate days. In almost all cases there is not enough business for a separate office, but even if clinic is weekly or monthly, appropriate signage (waiting area) and dedicated examination rooms are highly desirable. A separate entrance from the waiting room to the clinic area, again so marked, is valuable for psychological (and logistical) reasons.
  - Educational materials and forms available in the waiting area
  - Strongly consider preparing video educational materials. While these can be

available in the waiting area, they are probably most effective if presented to each patient in an examining room prior to being seen by a practitioner. Separate films should be created for neurogenic, venous, and arterial TOS.

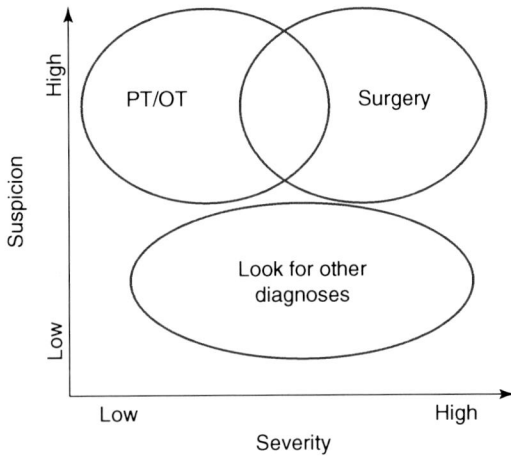

Fig. 97.2 Algorithm to guide discussion of options. This is posted on the walls of the examining room (or written on a whiteboard)

– Educational materials, including models and/or posters, on display in the exam room
– Simple treatment algorithms (fully worked out or whiteboard-based (Fig. 97.2)) on display in the examination rooms to guide discussion.
– Pre-printed prescription pads on hand – commonly used medications, testing, physical and occupational therapy referral forms, and so on.
– Pre-existing contact and referral information available when a common non-TOS diagnosis is made – shoulder, neck or carpal tunnel problems, for example.
– Strongly consider syndrome-specific flowchart (Fig. 97.3) outlining plans, timelines, and decision points, to be evaluated at each visit with the patient.
• Personnel present for each clinic, at a minimum:
– TOS physician.
– Nurse practitioner or physicians' assistant *who is truly interested in this condition.*

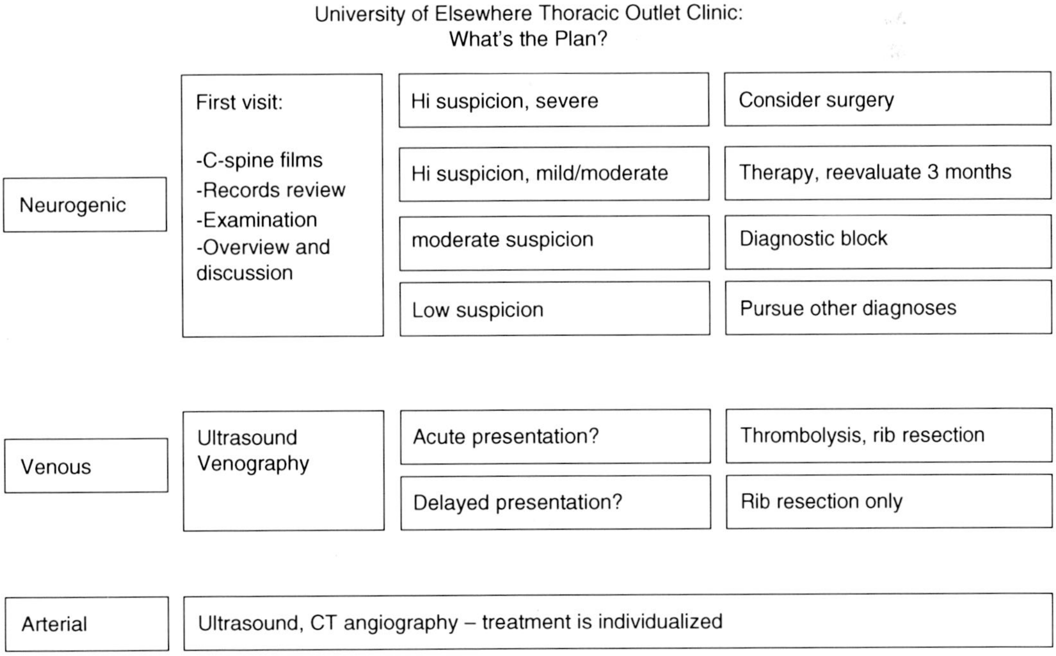

Fig. 97.3 An example of a general algorithm to give to the patient to guide treatment (this may vary from location to location and practitioner to practitioner)

This person (or persons) should be available for all clinics, and should be expected to handle paperwork, phone calls (patients and other providers), test results, and logistics regarding these patients on non-TOS clinic days.

- Physical or occupational therapist *who is truly interested in this condition*. Again, this person should be present on all clinic days; even though actual treatment facilities will usually not be co-located, their presence is critical for evaluating problems, determining who is most appropriate for treatment, and dealing with subsequent logistics. Many patients will be from out of town, and we have found a direct therapist-to-therapist discussion with whoever will be treating such a patient very useful.
- Personnel highly useful if volume allows, or at a minimum "on call" for same-day walk-in consultation:
  - Neurologist or other pain physician interested in treating patients with chronic pain conditions,
  - Psychologist or other appropriate practitioner interested in treating patients with depression or associated psychological conditions (including substance abuse/dependence),
  - Neurologist or neurointerventionalist interested in and skilled at diagnostic block techniques. This practitioner must be familiar with up-to-date, objective, blinded treatment protocols (see Chap. 20).
  - A facility adept at performance and interpretation of nerve conduction studies,
- Testing resources co-located or nearby with same-day availability:
  - Noninvasive vascular lab for vascular TOS,
  - Radiographic facilities for plain films, and
  - Depending on level of interest and skill, pre-established cross-sectional imaging protocols set up in advance for CT or MR venography and imaging of the neurogenic thoracic outlet.

- Prior to visit:
  - Invest time in creating TOS-specific self-reporting forms, as above (See appendix), perhaps dedicated to the specific form of TOS.
  - Attempt to determine if the patient's symptoms are neurogenic, venous, or arterial, and provide such education and information forms as appropriate, and
  - Provide the patient with written educational materials, as appropriate, self-reported history forms, and initial/baseline functional and emotional status instruments (such as SF-36, DASH, and CBSQ forms) to be filled out ahead of time.
- At first visit (Fig. 97.3):
  - Cervical spine and chest radiographs ordered prior to being seen with films immediately available electronically (or hard copy) at the time of arrival.
  - If vascular TOS, perform noninvasive testing prior to practitioners' visit.
  - After check in, 15 min for video/other "generic" education; practitioner(s) can review old records and results of spine radiographs and noninvasive testing during this time.
  - Basic initial generic history review and exam by midlevel provider, if needed.
  - Thorough TOS-focused history and physical examination by physician, midlevel provider, and physical or occupational therapist *together*.
  - Detailed, specific discussion, again together, of the problem at hand, unique situation, diagnosis, degree of certainty, and plan
    - If testing or further imaging is needed (or patient to be enrolled in a clinical or research protocol), set up at this time and make followup appointment,
    - If physical therapy is needed, therapist spends time with patient to make plans,
    - If referral to pain physician, psychologist, or other field needed, set up at this time.
    - If operation is recommended, set up at this time.

- At each follow up visit:
  - Repeat functional and psychological testing (minimum SF-36, DASH, and CBSQ) as above. This will allow longitudinal analysis of outcomes, but is also strongly recommended as needed global data collection for outcomes research purposes.
  - Individual encounters will vary depending on the treatment provided and results thereof.

Summary

Patients with thoracic outlet syndrome, especially neurologic, typically require many more resources than the typical vascular, thoracic, or neurologic patient. As such, a dedicated TOS clinic pays major dividends, in terms of time, resources, and patient and provider satisfaction. Such a clinic should include, at a minimum, a provider, physician extender, and physical or occupational therapist truly interested in the problem, along with logistical support for the documentation and paperwork required. If local resources permit, a neurodiagnostician with interest in modern, objective diagnostic and therapeutic block techniques is valuable, as are a psychologist or even a psychiatrist. Educational materials can be made available to patients ahead of time, streamlining the visit itself. Such a clinic does not need to be freestanding or full-time, but can exist "virtually" within a conventional clinic simply by designating a time when patients and providers can all assemble. Such a clinic vastly improves the care of patients with VTOS, and acts as a surprisingly effective marketing tool in most communities.

Reference

1. Lee JT, Dua MM, Chandra V, Hernandez-Boussard TM, Illig KA. RR18. Surgery for thoracic outlet syndrome: a nationwide perspective. J Vasc Surg. 2011; 53(6):100S–101S.

Appendix

Suggested Forms to Gather Information from Patients with TOS

Three forms seem to be most useful for patients with thoracic outlet syndrome, and we urge all who treat this disorder to use them for data collection:

DASH (Disabilities of the Shoulder and Hand): Copyrighted by The Institute for Work & Health 2006. All rights reserved.

Obtain at: http://www.dash.iwh.on.ca/ (September 24, 2012)

SF-36 (Short Form - 36): Copyrighted by The Medical Outcomes Trust/QualityMetric Incorporated 2002. All rights reserved.

Obtain at: http://www.sf-36.org/ (September 24, 2012)

CBSQ (Cervical Brachial Symptom Questionnaire): Courtesy of Pain Physician, American Society of Interventional Pain Physicians? Printed on pages to follow.

K.A. Illig et al. (eds.), *Thoracic Outlet Syndrome*,
DOI 10.1007/978-1-4471-4366-6, © Springer-Verlag London 2013

Cervical Brachial Symptom Questionnaire ("CBSQ")

NAME_____   DATE_____

READ INSTRUCTIONS FIRST. This form is important for measuring the outcome of treatment.
Based on your experiences in the PAST WEEK, answer the following questions regarding how often
symptoms would be likely to increase if you were to engage in certain activities.
Circle the number corresponding to how likely it would be for symptoms to increase during an activity
so much that you would have to stop or modify the activity.
DO NOT LEAVE ANY BLANKS.
If a CONSTANT ongoing symptom would not be more noticeable during the activity, mark the answer "0."
If a symptom would increase during half of the instances of the activity, mark the answer "5."
Only mark "10" if your symptoms would increase during EVERY instance of the activity.

1.   Pain going down the arm increases with neck movement, as in turning, flexing or extending the neck.

    0   1   2   3   4   5   6   7   8   9   10
It would NEVER happen this past week   This past week, it would happen ALWAYS

2.   Pain in the arm or shoulder increases instantly with brief shoulder movement as in throwing something or
       in reaching behind the body.

    0   1   2   3   4   5   6   7   8   9   10
It would NEVER happen this past week   This past week, it would happen ALWAYS

3.   Hand or arm aches or fatigues with arm exercise, particularly with overhead or outstretched positioning.

    0   1   2   3   4   5   6   7   8   9   10
It would NEVER happen this past week   This past week, it would happen ALWAYS

4.   Hand or arm swells after arm exercise, including after any activities that require repetitive arm
       movements.

    0   1   2   3   4   5   6   7   8   9   10
It would NEVER happen this past week   This past week, it would happen ALWAYS

5.   Sensations of tingling or numbness in the hand or arm increase when reaching overhead or outwards.
       Examples include brushing hair or blow-drying hair, reaching for an overhead shelf, or working with arms
       overhead as in painting a ceiling or screwing in light bulbs.

    0   1   2   3   4   5   6   7   8   9   10
It would NEVER happen this past week   This past week, it would happen ALWAYS

6.   Sensations of tingling or numbness increase in the hand or arm when awakening from sleep.

    0   1   2   3   4   5   6   7   8   9   10
It would NEVER happen this past week   This past week, it would happen ALWAYS

7.   Sensations of tingling or numbness increase in the hand or arm with repetitive finger movements as in writing, typing, sewing, playing musical instruments or assembling objects.

0	1	2	3	4	5	6	7	8	9	1 0

It would NEVER happen this past week   This past week, it would happen ALWAYS

8.   Sensations of tingling or numbness increase with prolonged or forceful grasping as in holding a steering wheel to drive, using tools, handling office instruments or controlling industrial equipment.

0	1	2	3	4	5	6	7	8	9	10

It would NEVER happen this past week   This past week, it would happen ALWAYS

9.   Sensations of tingling or numbness increase while bending elbow or leaning on elbow, for example, while holding telephone receiver or leaning on a desk.

0	1	2	3	4	5	6	7	8	9	10

It would NEVER happen this past week   This past week, it would happen ALWAYS

10.   Hand is clumsy or weak while trying to hold onto objects or while attempting to open jars, use keys to open a lock, pull zippers or button clothing.

0	1	2	3	4	5	6	7	8	9	10

It would NEVER happen this past week   This past week, it would happen ALWAYS

11.   Pain is caused by experiences that ordinarily are not painful. Examples include a light touch to the hand, arm, or neck, such as a light draft, the rub and tug of clothing, or the touch of something moderately hot or cold.

0	1	2	3	4	5	6	7	8	9	10

It would NEVER happen this past week   This past week, it would happen ALWAYS

12.   Disabling pain that can last into the next day is caused by activities that ordinarily produce only mild discomfort. Examples include a light exercise session, a physical therapy treatment or a physical examination.

0	1	2	3	4	5	6	7	8	9	10

It would NEVER happen this past week   This past week, it would happen ALWAYS

13.   Symptoms have occurred with the above activities in the past without recurrence in the past week.

        yes   no   (circle your answer)   If the answer is "yes", please list by number and explain on back.

14.   Hand becomes blue, red, swollen, sweaty or hot.   Yes   No   (circle answer)   If "yes" explain on back.

Cervical brachial symptom questionnaire

Name ————————————————

Mark where you feel pain with horizontal
or vertical lines. Mark sensory changes
with diagonal lines. If different pains or specific
items in the questionnaire, then indicate
by the question number.
Use next page if necessary.

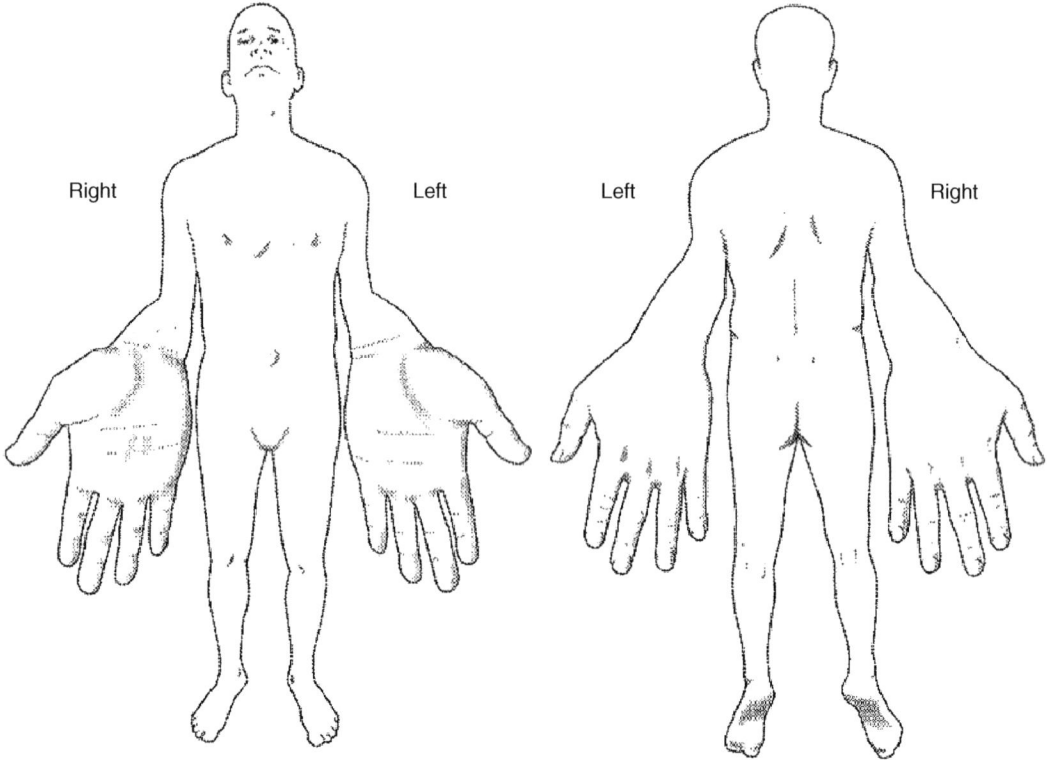

Right   Left   Left   Right

≡≡≡ or |||||| Mark pain

\\\\\ or ///// Mark numbness or sensory disturbance including tingling

Index

K.A. Illig et al. (eds.), *Thoracic Outlet Syndrome*,
DOI 10.1007/978-1-4471-4366-6, © Springer-Verlag London 2013

Printed by Publishers' Graphics LLC
ICISO140211.15.17.1